Clinical Surgery

Clinical Surgery

4th Edition

M. Asif Chaudry BA(Hon) MA BM BCh(Oxford) MD FRCS

Consultant Robotic Oesophageal & Gastric Cancer Surgeon
The Royal Marsden NHS Foundation Trust
London, UK

Shahnawaz Rasheed B Clin Sci (Hons) MBBS DIC PhD FRCS

Consultant Colorectal Surgeon
The Royal Marsden NHS Foundation Trust
Gastrointestinal Unit
London, UK
Medical Director, Humanity First International, Surrey, UK
Executive Director, Inspiral Health, London, UK

James Kinross FRCS PhD

Senior Lecturer in Surgery and Consultant Surgeon
Department of Surgery and Cancer
Imperial College London, St Mary's Hospital
London, UK

Associate Editor
Stella Nikolaou

Research Associate
The Royal Marsden NHS Foundation Trust
Gastrointestinal Unit
London, UK

For additional online content visit Elsevier eBooks+

ELSEVIER   London New York Oxford Philadelphia St Louis Sydney 2023

First edition 2001
Second edition 2005
Third edition 2012
Fourth edition 2023

Notices

Practitioners and researchers must always rely on their own experience and knowledge in evaluating and using any information, methods, compounds or experiments described herein. Because of rapid advances in the medical sciences, in particular, independent verification of diagnoses and drug dosages should be made. To the fullest extent of the law, no responsibility is assumed by Elsevier, authors, editors or contributors for any injury and/or damage to persons or property as a matter of products liability, negligence or otherwise, or from any use or operation of any methods, products, instructions, or ideas contained in the material herein.

ISBN: 978-0-7020-7050-1
IE ISBN 978-0-7020-7051-8

Content Strategist: Alexandra Mortimer
Content Development Specialist: Rebecca Gruliow
Project Manager: Julie Taylor
Design: Patrick Ferguson
Illustration Manager: Muthukumaran Thangaraj
Illustrator: MPS North America, LLC/TNQ
Marketing Manager: Deborah Watkins

Printed in the UK

Last digit is the print number: 9   8   7   6   5   4   3   2   1

 Working together to grow libraries in developing countries

www.elsevier.com • www.bookaid.org

Clinical Surgery

4th Edition

M. Asif Chaudry BA(Hon) MA BM BCh(Oxford) MD FRCS

Consultant Robotic Oesophageal & Gastric Cancer Surgeon
The Royal Marsden NHS Foundation Trust
London, UK

Shahnawaz Rasheed B Clin Sci (Hons) MBBS DIC PhD FRCS

Consultant Colorectal Surgeon
The Royal Marsden NHS Foundation Trust
Gastrointestinal Unit
London, UK
Medical Director, Humanity First International, Surrey, UK
Executive Director, Inspiral Health, London, UK

James Kinross FRCS PhD

Senior Lecturer in Surgery and Consultant Surgeon
Department of Surgery and Cancer
Imperial College London, St Mary's Hospital
London, UK

Associate Editor
Stella Nikolaou

Research Associate
The Royal Marsden NHS Foundation Trust
Gastrointestinal Unit
London, UK

For additional online content visit Elsevier eBooks+

ELSEVIER   London New York Oxford Philadelphia St Louis Sydney 2023

First edition 2001
Second edition 2005
Third edition 2012
Fourth edition 2023

ISBN: 978-0-7020-7050-1
IE ISBN 978-0-7020-7051-8

Content Strategist: Alexandra Mortimer
Content Development Specialist: Rebecca Gruliow
Project Manager: Julie Taylor
Design: Patrick Ferguson
Illustration Manager: Muthukumaran Thangaraj
Illustrator: MPS North America, LLC/TNQ
Marketing Manager: Deborah Watkins

Printed in the UK

Last digit is the print number: 9   8   7   6   5   4   3   2   1

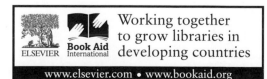

Contents

Foreword

We are delighted to write a foreword for the 4th edition of Clinical Surgery. The practise of surgery has changed enormously over the past decade with life changing innovations. These innovations include surgical robotics, laparoscopic technologies, three-dimensional printing, and artificial intelligence which have already revolutionized the world of surgery. Surgeons now require a different set of knowledge and skills, and their role will change even more with innovations from further collaboration with multidisciplinary experts. New diagnostic methodologies, with advances in genomics, immunotherapy, and radiotherapy, will improve the diagnostic error and help with specific targeted drug and surgical therapies. These will change the role that surgery plays in many areas. For example, it will require earlier intervention, be more accurate, less invasive with faster recovery times, and hopefully with less risk of harm; all for the benefit of our patients. The focus will be on the prevention of diseases, improving quality of life, and maintaining good health, rather than on the illness itself. All important factors in the context of an increasingly elderly population, along with a changing relationship between the doctor and the patient.

Medical schools have altered their curricula to incorporate these changes in the practise of medicine. These newer technologies have been included, with support from a strong evidence base. Over recent years more attention has been given to ethics and communication to be in line with the General Medical Council's duty of candour, emphasizing the importance of honesty in communication with patients and their families when things go wrong.

This edition has therefore undergone a major transformation to address these new issues. We are therefore pleased to see chapters on surgical ethics, leadership and management of a surgical team, assessment and management, and health promotion.

The book is still divided into three sections with new and useful chapters covering a wealth of information. The first section has been totally reordered and includes sections on basic mechanisms, for example, on cell growth and differentiation, infection, inflammation, innovation, along with more practical chapters on procedures and assessment. The second section discusses common surgical conditions and includes chapters on skin disorders, plastic surgery, and trauma. The last section includes evidence-based medicine, ethics, and we were pleased to see a chapter on global surgery. With the current rapid mobility of populations across the world due to faster travel, turmoil due to war and migration, all doctors will be faced with a multitude of different diseases from around the globe.

This new edition will be widely read and is an excellent companion to our own *Kumar and Clark's Clinical Medicine* textbook. We hope that these books will help you in both your undergraduate and postgraduate careers. We, as doctors and healthcare professionals, are privileged to treat our patients and improve healthcare for us all.

Parveen J. Kumar
Michael L. Clark

List of Contributors

The editor(s) would like to acknowledge and offer grateful thanks for the input of all previous editions' contributors, without whom this new edition would not have been possible.

Mudussar Ahmad, MBBS MRCS FRCS Tr & Orth.
Consultant Trauma and Orthopaedic Surgeon, Barking, Havering & Redbridge University Hospitals NHS Trust, London, UK
Trauma and orthopaedic surgery

Dimitri Amiras, MBBS BSc FRCR
Consultant Musculoskeletal Radiologist, Imperial College Healthcare NHS Trust, London, UK
An introduction to radiology and diagnostic imaging
Interventional radiology

George Asimakopoulos, PhD FRCS(CT)
Consultant Cardiovascular and Thoracic Surgeon, Department of Cardiac Surgery, Royal Brompton and Harefield Trust, London, UK
Common surgical conditions of pulmonary disease

Alan Askari, MB ChB MSc DIC PhD FRCS
East of England Deanery, Cambridge, UK
Evidence based medicine

Thanos Athanasiou, MD PhD MBA FECTS FRCS
Department of Cardiothoracic Surgery, Imperial College Healthcare, Hammersmith Hospital, London, UK
Evidence based medicine

Tipu Aziz, MD DMedSci FRCS FMedSci FFPMRCA
Professor of Neurosurgery, University of Oxford, Oxford, UK
Common neurosurgical conditions

Silvia Bagué, MD
Consultant Histopathologist, Sarcoma Unit, The Royal Marsden NHS Foundation Trust, London, UK
Sarcoma

Emily Barrow, BSc (Hons) MBChB (Hons) PhD
Department of Surgery and Cancer, Imperial College London, St Mary's Hospital, London, UK
Surgical technology and innovation

Nebil Behar, MBChB MSc(Surg Sci) FRCS(Gen Surg)
Consultant Emergency Surgeon, Chelsea and Westminster Hospital NHS Trust, London, UK
Emergency general surgery

Ondina Bernstein, BMBS BMedSci MRCS FRCR EBIR
Consultant Vascular and Interventional Radiologist, Imperial College Healthcare NHS Trust
London, UK
An introduction to radiology and diagnostic imaging
Interventional radiology

Ricky Harminder Bhogal, PhD FRCS
Consultant Hepato-Pancreatico-Biliary Surgeon, The Royal Marsden NHS Foundation Trust
Honorary Faculty, Institute for Cancer Research, London, UK
Common upper gastrointestinal surgical conditions and their management
Surgical pathology of the liver, pancreas and biliary tract

Catherine J. Bradshaw, MBChB MSc FRCS (Paed)
Consultant Paediatric Surgeon, Bristol Royal Hospital for Children, University of Bristol and Weston NHS Foundation Trust, Bristol, UK
Principles of paediatric surgery

Tim W. R. Briggs, MD (Res) MCh (Orth) FRCS
Consultant Orthopaedic Surgeon – Royal National Orthopaedic Hospital, Stanmore, UK
Trauma and orthopaedic surgery

Elaine Burns, MBCHB FRCS PhD
Consultant Colorectal Surgeon and Honorary Senior Lecturer, St Mark's Hospital - The National Bowel Hospital, Middlesex, Harrow, UK
Leadership and the surgical team and management

M. Asif Chaudry, BA(Hon) MA BM BCh(Oxford) MD FRCS
Consultant Robotic Oesophageal & Gastric Cancer Surgeon, The Royal Marsden NHS Foundation Trust, London, UK
Common upper gastrointestinal surgical conditions and their management

Aswin Chari, MA BMBCh MRCS
Neurosurgical Registrar, Department of Neurosurgery, Great Ormond Street Hospital, London, UK
Common neurosurgical conditions

Peter Clarke, BSc(Hons) MBChB FRCS(ORL)
Consultant Head and Neck Surgeon, Imperial College Healthcare NHS Trust, London, UK
Common surgical conditions of head and neck

Joseph F. Cosgrove, MB BS FRCA FFICM
Consultant in Anaesthesia and Intensive Care Medicine, Newcastle upon Tyne Hospitals, UK
Surgical ethics

Rebecca Cui, BMed MS
Department of General Surgery, Royal Prince Alfred Hospital, Sydney, Australia
Leadership and the surgical team and management

Lord Ara Darzi, OM KBE PC FRS MD FRCS FMedSci FREng
Department of Surgery and Cancer, Imperial College London, St Mary's Hospital, London, UK
Surgical technology and innovation

Annalisa Dolcet, MD
Institute of Liver Studies, King's College Hospital, London, UK
Organ transplantation

George Garas, BSc (Hons) MBBS (Dist) PhD DIC FRCS (ORL-HNS) FEBORL-HNS (Gold medal)
Consultant ENT/Thyroid/Head & Neck Surgeon (Surgical Oncology), Head & Neck Unit, Queen Elizabeth Hospital Birmingham, University Hospitals Birmingham NHS Foundation Trust, Birmingham, UK;
Honorary Clinical Senior Lecturer, Department of Surgery and Cancer, Imperial College London, St Mary's Hospital, London, UK
Surgical technology and innovation

Amy Godden, MD MRCS MBBS BSc
Registrar in General Surgery, Royal Marsden Hospital, London, UK
Common breast surgical conditions

Robert Goldin, MD MEd FRCPath
Professor of Pathology, Department of Metabolism, Digestion and Reproduction, Faculty of Medicine, Imperial College London, London, UK
Disorders of growth, differentiation and morphogenesis

Mevan Gooneratne, MBBS MA (Dist) BSc PGCME
Consultant Anaesthetist, The Royal London Hospital, Barts Health, London, UK
Consultant lead for Pre-assessment and Vascular Anaesthesia
Perioperative management and postoperative complications

Nigel Heaton, MB BS FRCS
Professor of Transplant Surgery, Consultant Adult and Paediatric Liver Transplantation and HPB Surgery, King's College Hospital NHS Foundation Trust, London, UK
Organ transplantation

Thom C. C. Hendriks, MD PhD
Surgeon in training, Radboudumc, Nijmegen, The Netherlands
Global surgery

Johnathan G. Hubbard, MBBS MD FRCS(Gen) FEBS
Consultant Endocrine Surgeon, Guy's & St Thomas' Hospitals and King's College Hospital, London, UK
Common endocrine surgical conditions

Samer Jallad, MBBS MRCS MSc PhD FRCS (Urol)
Consultant Urology Surgeon, Frimley Health NHS Foundation Trust, Frimley, UK
Common urological conditions

Simon Jordan, MB BCh MD FRCS
Consultant Thoracic Surgeon, Royal Brompton and Harefield Trust, London, UK
Common surgical conditions of pulmonary disease

Meera Joshi, MBBS AICSM BSc.(Hons) PhD FRCS
Honorary Research Fellow, Faculty of Medicine, Department of Surgery and Cancer, Imperial College London, St Mary's Hospital, London, UK
Small-bowel disease and intestinal obstruction

Rajiv Kaila, MBBCh MRCS MSc MFSEM(UK) FEBOT
Fellow Trauma and Orthopaedic Surgeon, Joint Reconstruction Unit, The Royal National Orthopaedic Hospital NHS Trust, Stanmore, London, UK
Trauma and orthopaedic surgery

Ramanathan (Nathan) Kasivisvanathan, BMedSci(Hons) BMBS (Hons) FRCA MSc
Head of Anaesthesia and Perioperative Medicine, The Royal Marsden NHS Foundation Trust, London, UK
Perioperative management and postoperative complications

Aamir Z. Khan, FRCS Eng (Gen)
Consultant Surgeon, The Royal Marsden NHS Foundation Trust, London, UK
Surgical pathology of the liver, pancreas and biliary tract

Aadil A. Khan, MPH PhD FRCS (Plast.)
Consultant Plastic Surgeon, The Royal Marsden NHS Foundation Trust, London, UK
Principles of plastic surgery

James Kinross, FRCS PhD
Senior Lecturer in Surgery and Consultant Surgeon, Department of Surgery and Cancer, Imperial College London, St Mary's Hospital, London, UK
Pharmacology in surgical practice
Cancer/Principles of surgical oncology

Louis John Koizia, MBBS BSc MRCP
Consultant Physician and Geriatrician, Imperial College Healthcare NHS Trust, London, UK
The older surgical patient

Tristan R. A. Lane, MBBS BSc PhD FRCS(Vasc)
Consultant Vascular Surgeon, Cambridge Vascular Unit, Addenbrookes Hospital, Cambridge University Hospitals NHS Trust, Cambridge, UK, Honorary Senior Clinical Lecturer, Section of Vascular Surgery, Department of Surgery and Cancer, Imperial College London, London, UK
Common vascular surgical conditions

Graham Lawton, BSc DMCC MD FRCS (Plast.)
Head of Speciality Plastic Surgery Imperial Healthcare NHS Trust, Honorary Clinical Senior Lecturer Imperial College London, London, UK
Inflammation, wound healing and surgical immunology

Daniel R. Leff, PhD FRCS
Reader in Surgery and Honorary Consultant Oncoplastic Breast Surgeon, Department of Surgery and Cancer, Imperial College London, St Mary's Hospital, London, UK
Common breast surgical conditions

Azeem Majeed, MD FRCP FRCGP FFPH
Professor of Primary Care and Public Health, Imperial College London, Charing Cross Hospital, London, UK
Health Promotion and Disease Prevention

George Malietzis, MBBS MSc PhD DIC FRCS colorectal
Honorary Clinical Lecturer, Department of Surgery and Cancer, Imperial College London, St Mary's Hospital, London, UK
Evidence based medicine

Erik Mayer, BSc (Hons) MBBS (Hons) MRCS PhD FRCS (Urol) FFCI
Clinical Reader, Department of Surgery & Cancer, Imperial College London, St Mary's Hospital, London, UK, Consultant Surgeon, The Royal Marsden NHS Foundation Trust & Imperial College Healthcare NHS Trust, London, UK
Common urological conditions

Andrew McLeod, MB BS FRCA
Consultant Anaesthetist, The Royal Marsden NHS Foundation Trust, London, UK
Surgical ethics

Mary Miller, MSc Dip Learning & Teaching FRCP
Consultant in Palliative Medicine, Sobell House, Honorary Senior Clinical Lecturer in Palliative Medicine, University of Oxford, Oxford, UK
Director OxCERPC (Oxford Centre for education and research in palliative care)
The dying surgical patient

Hemel N. Modi, MRCS MEd PhD
Specialty Registrar in Hepatobiliary & Pancreatic Surgery, Addenbrookes Hospital, Cambridge University Hospitals NHS Trust, Cambridge, UK
Honorary Research Fellow, Department of Surgery and Cancer, Imperial College London, St Mary's Hospital, London, UK
Surgical technology and innovation

Rebecca Morrison, BSc (Hons), MBChB
Department of Pathology, Imperial College London, St Mary's Hospital, London, UK
Disorders of growth, differentiation and morphogenesis

Jamie Murphy, BChir PhD FRCS FASCRS
Senior Lecturer and Consultant in Colorectal Surgery, Department of Surgery and Cancer, Imperial College London, St Mary's Hospital, London, UK
Common anal conditions

Stella Nikolaou
Research Associate, Royal Marsden Hospital, Gastrointestinal Unit, London, UK
Common colorectal surgical conditions
Global surgery

David Nott, OBE FRCS
Professor of Practice (Surgery), St Mary's Hospital, London, UK
Royal Marsden NHS Foundation Trust, London, UK
Trauma surgery/principles of trauma care

Ching Ling Pang, MA (Oxon) BMBCh FRCA
Consultant Anaesthetist, Royal London Hospital, London, UK
Perioperative management and postoperative complications

Nikhil Pawa, MD LLM MSc FRCS
Consultant Colorectal and General Surgeon, Chelsea and Westminster Hospital NHS Foundation Trust, London, UK
Small-bowel disease and intestinal obstruction

George Peck, MBBS BSc FRCP
Consultant Physician and Geriatrician, Department of Trauma and Orthopaedics, Imperial College Healthcare NHS Trust
Honorary Clinical Senior Lecturer, Division of Surgery, Imperial College London, London, UK
The older surgical patient

Erlick Pereira, MA(Camb) DM(Oxf) FRCS(Neuro.Surg) SFHEA
Reader in Neurosurgery and Consultant Neurosurgeon, St George's, University of London, London, UK
Common neurosurgical conditions

Roshani V. Patel, MRCS MEd MBBS BSc
Clinical Research Fellow, Department of Surgery and Cancer, Imperial College London, UK; St Mark's Hospital, Harrow, UK
The principles of assessment and management of the surgical patient

Kieran Power, MB BCh BAO BMed Sci, MSc Surg Sci, MSc Aesthetic Surg, FRCS Plast
Consultant Plastic Surgeon and Head of Department, The Royal Marsden NHS Foundation Trust, London, UK
Principles of plastic surgery

Sanjay Purkayastha, MD FRCS
Consultant in General, Upper GI & Bariatric Surgery, St Mary's Hospital, London, Associate Professor, Surgery and Cancer, Imperial College, London, UK
Bariatric and metabolic surgery

Mahim I. Qureshi, MA (Oxon), MBBS (AICSM), MRCS, PhD
Academic Clinical Lecturer in Vascular Surgery, University of Bristol, North Bristol NHS Trust, Bristol, UK
Practical procedures

Shahnawaz Rasheed B, Clin Sci (Hons) MBBS DIC PhD FRCS
Consultant Surgeon, Royal Marsden Hospital, Gastrointestinal Unit, London, UK; Medical Director, Humanity First International; Surrey, UK, Executive Director, Inspiral Health, London, UK
Common colorectal surgical conditions
Global surgery

Celia Riga, BSc MBBS MD FRCS
Head of School, London Surgery HEE, Consultant Vascular Surgeon & Clinical Senior Lecturer, Imperial College London, London, UK
Common vascular surgical conditions

Phoebe Roche, MB BCh BAO, DoHNS, MCh, MD, FRCS (ORL-HNS)
Consultant Otolaryngologist, Head & Neck Surgeon, Bart's Health, NHS Trust, London, UK
Honorary Clinical Lecturer, Department of Targeted Intervention, Head and Neck Academic Centre, UCL, London, UK
Common surgical conditions of head and neck

Magda Sbai, MBBS BSc (Hons) MRCP
Consultant Geriatrician, POPS Team, Consultant Lead for POPS GI and Gynae Surgery, Department of Ageing & Health, Guy's and St Thomas' Hospital, London, UK
The older surgical patient

Armine Sefton, MD FRCP FRCPath
Consultant Microbiologist, The Princess Alexandra Hospital NHS Trust and Emerita Professor, Barts and the London School of Medicine and Dentistry, London, UK
Surgical infection

Shaun Selvadurai, MBBS BSc (Hons) MRCS DOHNS
Core Surgical Trainee, Imperial College Healthcare NHS Trust, St Mary's Hospital, London, UK
Inflammation, wound healing and surgical immunology

David Shipway, MA (Oxon) BM BCh MRCP(UK) FRCP (London)
Consultant Physician and Perioperative Geriatrician, Departmental Lead, Geriatric Medicine, Southmead Hospital, North Bristol NHS Trust, Bristol, UK, Honorary Senior Clinical Lecturer, University of Bristol
The older surgical patient

Constantinos Simillis, BSc MBBS AICSM PGC MA MD FRCS FEBS
Consultant Colorectal and General Surgeon, Cambridge Colorectal Unit, Addenbrooke's Hospital, Cambridge University Hospitals NHS Foundation Trust, Cambridge, UK
Small-bowel disease and intestinal obstruction

Neil Smart, MBBS (Hons) PhD FRCSEd FEBS-AWS (Hon)
Consultant Colorectal Surgeon, Royal Devon & Exeter Hospital & Associate Professor, University of Exeter Medical School, Exeter, UK
Hernia

Myles Smith, MB BCh BAO PhD FRCSI FRCS
Consultant General Surgeon and Surgical Oncologist, Sarcoma and Melanoma Unit, The Royal Marsden NHS Foundation Trust, London, UK
Skin disorders
Sarcoma

Maria Souvatzi, MD, MSc, FRCS
Consultant Colorectal Surgeon, Imperial College NHS Healthcare Trust, London, UK
Common anal conditions

Alan Thompson, BSc (Hons) MBBS (Hons) MS FRCS (Urol)
Consultant Urological Surgeon, The Royal Marsden NHS Foundation Trust, London, UK
Common urological conditions

Alexander von Roon, PhD FRCS

Consultant Colorectal Surgeon, University College London Hospitals NHS Foundation Trust, London, UK

The principles of assessment and management of the surgical patient

Bee Wee, CBE MB BCh FRCP FRCGP SFFMLM Hon DSc PhD

Consultant in Palliative Medicine, Oxford University Hospitals NHS Foundation Trust, Associate Professor and Official Fellow, Harris Manchester College, University of Oxford, Oxford, UK

The dying surgical patient

Michelle Wilkinson, FRCS PhD

General Surgery SpR, Sarcoma and Melanoma Unit, The Royal Marsden NHS Foundation Trust, London, UK

Skin disorders

Peter Willson, BSc MBBS FRCS(gen)

Consultant Surgeon, Keyhole Clinics Ltd, The New Victoria Hospital, Kingston-upon-Thames, Surrey, UK

Practical procedures

Alec A. Winder, BM FRACS

Fellow General Surgery and Surgical Oncology, Sarcoma and Melanoma Unit, The Royal Marsden NHS Foundation Trust, London, UK

Sarcoma

Derek KT. Yeung, MRCS BMBS BMedSci

General Surgery Registrar and Clinical Research Fellow, Department of Surgery & Cancer, Imperial College London, London, UK

Bariatric and metabolic surgery

Abbreviations

A&E	accident and emergency	CQC	Care Quality Commission
AAA	abdominal aortic aneurysm	CSF	cerebrospinal fluid
ABGs	arterial blood gases	CSSD	central sterile supply department
ABPI	ankle:brachial pressure index	CT	computed tomography
ACE	angiotensin-converting enzyme	CVA	cerebrovascular accident
ACL	anterior cruciate ligament	CVP	central venous pressure
ACTH	adrenocorticotrophic hormone	DCIS	ductal carcinoma in situ
ADH	antidiuretic hormone	DGH	district general hospital
AEE	activity energy expenditure	DIC	disseminated intravascular coagulation
AFP	alpha-fetoprotein		
AION	anterior ischaemic optic neuropathy	DIT	dietary-induced thermogenesis
APC	antigen-presenting cell	DMSA	dimercaptosuccinic acid
APPT	accelerated partial thromboplastin time	DSA	digital subtraction angiography
		DTPA	diethylene-triamine-penta-acetic acid
APUD	amine precursor uptake and decarboxylation	DTSI	deep-to-superficial incompetence
ARDS	adult respiratory distress syndrome	DVT	deep-vein thrombosis
ARMD	age-related macular degeneration	ECF	extracellular fluid
ATLS	advanced trauma life support	ECG	electrocardiogram
ATP	adenosine triphosphate	ECMO	extracorporeal membrane oxygenation
AV	(1) atrioventricular; (2) arteriovenous		
AVM	arteriovenous malformation	EEG	electroencephalogram
BMR	basal metabolic rate	EGF	epidermal growth factor
BMT	best medical therapy	ELISA	enzyme-linked immunosorbent assay
BP	blood pressure		
BPH	benign prostatic hyperplasia	EMG	electromyography
BST	basic surgical training	ENT	ear, nose and throat
CA 19-9	carbohydrate antigen 19-9	ER	oestrogen receptor
CABG	coronary artery bypass grafting	ERCP	endoscopic retrograde cholangiopancreatography
CAD	coronary artery disease	ESR	erythrocyte sedimentation rate
CCD	charge couple device	FDPs	fibrin degradation products
CCK	cholecystokinin	FEV^1	forced expiratory volume in the first second
CCST	Certificate of Completion of Specialist Training		
		FFA	free fatty acids
CDC	Centers for Disease Control	FNA	fine-needle aspiration
CEA	(1) carcinoembryonic antigen; (2) carotid endarterectomy	FNAC	fine-needle aspiration cytology
		FNH	focal nodular hyperplasia
CLI	critical limb ischaemia	FSH	follicle-stimulating hormone
CNS	central nervous system	FVC	forced vital capacity
COPD	chronic obstructive pulmonary disease	GA	general anaesthetic
		GCS	Glasgow Coma Score
CPAP	continuous positive airways pressure	G-CSF	granulocyte colony-stimulating factor
CPB	cardiopulmonary bypass		
CPP	cerebral perfusion pressure	GFR	glomerular filtration rate

GI	gastrointestinal
GMC	General Medical Council
GnRH	gonadotrophin-releasing hormone
GORD	gastro-oesophageal reflux disease
GTN	glyceryl trinitrate
HAART	highly active antiretroviral therapy
hATI	human anti-tetanus immunoglobulin
hCG	human chorionic gonadotrophin
HDU	high-dependency unit
HRT	hormone replacement therapy
HST	higher surgical training
i.m.	intramuscular
i.v.	intravenous
IABP	intra-aortic balloon pump
ICF	intracellular fluid
ICP	intracranial pressure
ICU	intensive care unit
IFN	interferon
IL	interleukin
INR	international normalized ratio
IVN	intravenous nutrition
IVU	intravenous urogram
JVP	jugular venous pressure
L	litre
LA	local anaesthetic
LAD	left anterior descending coronary artery
LATS	long-acting thyroid stimulators
LCA	left coronary artery
LCIS	lobular carcinoma in situ
LDH	lactate dehydrogenase
LH	luteinizing hormone
LHRH	luteinizing hormone-releasing hormone
LMA	laryngeal mask airway
LMWH	low-molecular-weight heparin
LVEDP	left ventricular end-diastolic pressure
MAG3	technetium-99m mercaptoacetyltriglycine
MAP	mean arterial pressure
MCV	mean corpuscular volume
MG	myasthenia gravis
MHC	major histocompatibility complex
MODS	multiple organ dysfunction syndrome
MOSF	multiple organ system failure
MRCP	magnetic resonance cholangiopancreatography
MRI	magnetic resonance imaging
MRSA	methicillin-resistant *Staphylococcus aureus*
MS	multiple sclerosis
MSU	midstream urine
NHS	National Health Service
NICE	National Institute for Clinical Excellence
NSAID	non-steroidal anti-inflammatory drug
NSCLC	non-small-cell lung cancer
NTN	National Training Number
NVE	native valve endocarditis
NYHA	New York Heart Association
OA	osteoarthritis
OPSI	overwhelming postsplenectomy infection
PABA	p-aminobenzoic acid
PACS	picture archive and communication system
PAD	peripheral arterial disease
PCA	patient-controlled analgesia
PCL	posterior cruciate ligament
PCR	polymerase chain reaction
PCT	Primary Care Trust
PE	pulmonary embolism
PEEP	positive end-expiratory pressure
PEG	percutaneous endoscopic gastrostomy
PET	positron emission tomography
PGA	persistent generalized lymphadenopathy
PiCCO	pulse-induced contour cardiac output
PNO	pneumothorax
PONV	postoperative nausea and vomiting
PPV	positive-pressure ventilation
PR	progesterone receptor
PSP	peak systolic pressure
PTA	percutaneous transluminal angioplasty
PTC	percutaneous transhepatic cholangiography
PTCA	percutaneous transluminal coronary angioplasty
PTH	parathyroid hormone
PUJ	pelviureteric junction
PUO	pyrexia of unknown origin
PVD	posterior vitreous detachment
PVE	prosthetic valve endocarditis
RA	rheumatoid arthritis
RAPD	relative afferent pupillary defect
RAS	renal artery stenosis
RCA	right coronary artery
REE	resting energy expenditure

RP	Raynaud's phenomenon	TIBC	total iron-binding capacity
RSI	repetitive strain injury	TNF	tumour necrosis factor
RTI	respiratory tract infection	TNM	tumour–node–metastasis
RVF	rectovaginal fistula	TPN	total parenteral nutrition
SA	sinoatrial	TRH	thyrotrophin-releasing hormone
SAC	Specialist Advisory Committee	TRUS	transrectal ultrasound
SCC	small-cell carcinoma	TSH	thyroid-stimulating hormone
SCFAs	short-chain fatty acids	TSSU	theatre sterile supply unit
SCID	severe combined immune deficiency	TUR	transurethral resection
SIRS	systemic inflammatory response syndrome	U&E	urea and electrolytes
		UGI	upper-gastrointestinal
SPECT	single-photon emission computed tomography	UICC	Union for International Cancer Control
		UTI	urinary tract infection
SpR	Specialist Registrar	VATS	video-assisted thoracic surgery
TBW	total body water	VIP	vasointestinal peptide
TEE	total energy expenditure	VMA	vanillylmandelic acid
THI	tissue harmonic imaging	VVF	vesicovaginal fistula
TIA	transient ischaemic attack	WBC	white blood cell

SECTION 1

General Issues

1

Inflammation, Wound Healing and Surgical Immunology

Wounds

Damage to the human integument is more commonly referred to as a wound.

Wounds may be described in many ways, based on the time of causation, anatomical location, the underlying aetiology or by the dominant tissue types in the wound bed. Each description serves a purpose in classifying the type of wound and attempting to advise the clinician as to the appropriate management.

A wound can be defined as a breakdown in the continuity of the epithelial layer of skin with or without loss of underlying connective tissue. This can occur following an injury to the skin, underlying tissue or organs as a result of surgery, physical trauma (incision, blow, chemical, temperature, shear force) or disease, such as leg ulcers or malignancy.

Anatomy and Physiology of the Skin

The skin is the largest organ of the body and has many functions:
- Protection
- Sensation
- Thermoregulation
- Vitamin D synthesis
- Aesthetics and communication

There are three functional layers to the skin: epidermis, dermis and hypodermis.

Epidermis – Largely consists of stratified epithelium; the epidermis undergoes a constant cell cycle. New keratinocytes migrate from the basal layer to the outer layer, flatten, and then shed off in a 28–35-day cycle. This renewal of cells is essential to wound healing.

The epidermis consists of five layers (Box 1.1).

Dermis – Main role is to support and provide nutrition to the epidermis; primarily consisting of irregular connective tissue (collagen, elastic fibres and extrafibrillar matrix) which create structural stability. Within this structure many important cell types are found, including: fibroblast, inflammatory cells, blood and lymph vessels, nerve endings, mechanoreceptors and thermoreceptors. Additionally, apocrine glands, sebaceous glands and hair follicles are found in this layer. Dermal thickness varies throughout the body from less than 0.5 mm thick in the eyelids to almost 1 cm thick on the back.

Hypodermis – Anchors skin and offers support to dermis. Primarily consists of adipose tissue, connective tissue and blood vessels.[1]

- **Stratum Corneum:** Tough, waterproof outer layer, providing protection, and assisting with homeostasis of skin pH and temperature.
- **Stratum Lucidum:** Present in areas subjected to more frequent pressure exposure.
- **Stratum Granulosum:** Layer of keratinocytes where cells lose their nuclei and progressively flatten and die. Helps reduce water loss from epidermis.
- **Stratum Spinosum:** Layer of polyhedral keratinocytes, important in synthesizing cytokeratin, which form desmosomes that allow strong connections between cells.
- **Stratum Basale:** Basement membrane. One cell thick, providing a definitive border between dermis and epidermis.

Wound Healing

Wound healing is a complex and dynamic process that varies depending on the location and type of wound that is formed. Fundamentally all wounds heal similarly, following four phases: haemostasis, inflammation, proliferation (reparative) and remodelling (consolidative).

Haemostasis

Haemostasis[2–5] is a process that causes bleeding to stop and therefore keeps blood within damaged blood vessels. The haemostatic system limits blood loss by highly regulated interactions between components of the vessel wall, platelets and soluble plasma proteins (referred to as coagulation factors). Initially, the coagulation process was portrayed by two groups in Seattle and Oxford as a 'cascade' or 'waterfall' of pro-enzyme reactions, each converted by a series of proteolytic reactions into an active enzyme resulting in the production of thrombin and, ultimately, the formation of an insoluble fibrin clot. Two limbs were described depending on whether the processes were independent of extravascular factors (intrinsic) or relied upon exposure of the blood to substances outside the circulation (extrinsic) (Fig. 1.1).

This simple format aided understanding and simplified the processes by removing the extensive list of synonyms prevalent in the literature and by providing defined sequences of reactions. Each coagulation factor was given a Roman numeral according to the order in which it was discovered. Fibrinogen was discovered first and so became factor I, followed by prothrombin (PT/factor II) and tissue factor (TF/factor III). It was not portrayed as a comprehensive explanation and the activation of factor V was included without any supportive evidence.

The cascade theory gained widespread acceptance and some authors emphasized the intrinsic pathway to the detriment of the extrinsic. The model was modified over the years as some coagulation factors were found to be cofactors with no enzymatic activity (tissue factor, factor V and factor VIII.) The extrinsic pathway also gained further acceptance, most probably as it explained the utility of the prothrombin time in clinical scenarios. It was not until the isolation of bovine TF in 1981 that investigators were able to identify a unique glycoprotein responsible for 'the thromboplastic' effect, as this had previously been thought to be a generalized activity of tissues outside the circulation.

The problem with the cascade theory was that, whilst it supported the laboratory evidence of the various interactions, it was unable to explain the mechanisms of haemostasis in clinical scenarios and could not be utilized to predict which patients with various known deficiencies would go on to have problematic bleeding. Why, for instance, in the absence of FVIII and FIX (haemophilia A and B), did not the extrinsic system take over and secure haemostasis independently of the failed intrinsic limb? The interactions that make up the cascade theory were thought to take place solely within the plasma. Recent models emphasize the importance of cellular elements with the intrinsic and extrinsic systems operating in parallel on different cell surfaces. This 'cell-based model of haemostasis' divides the process into three (overlapping) phases that occur on differing cell surfaces and not solely within the plasma.

These phases are initiation, amplification and propagation. Following blood vessel injury, the vessels immediately contract to slow the flow of blood to the injured area. This is followed by localization of platelets to the site of vessel injury. The platelets adhere to collagen and von Willebrand factor (vWF) exposed within the blood vessel lining after injury to the endothelium. The interaction with vWF enables the platelets to bind both to other plasma proteins and to other platelets, leading to the formation of a loosely associated platelet plug.

Coagulation is then initiated by formation of a complex between thromboplastin tissue factor (TF), exposed as a result of vessel wall injury, and circulating FVII or activated FVII (FVIIa). Platelet plug formation and the initiation phase of coagulation are simultaneous processes. Approximately 1% of the total FVII is normally present in the activated form in the circulation. Upon binding to TF, FVII is activated to FVIIa.

FVII is a vitamin-K-dependent glycoprotein comprised of 406 amino acids. Cleavage of a single peptide bond converts the single chain inactive FVII into the double chain active FVIIa. The binding of calcium to the activated glycoprotein changes the configuration of the FVIIa, facilitating the binding of TF and phospholipid.

TF is a membrane-bound glycoprotein expressed on cells in the sub-endothelium and is not normally exposed to circulating blood. Once exposed to the blood, TF serves as a high affinity receptor for FVII/FVIIa.

FVIIa bound to TF initiates the coagulation cascade by activating FX. FXa then combines with FVa to form a *prothrombinase complex* which causes a small volume of thrombin to be produced on the TF bearing cell. This is

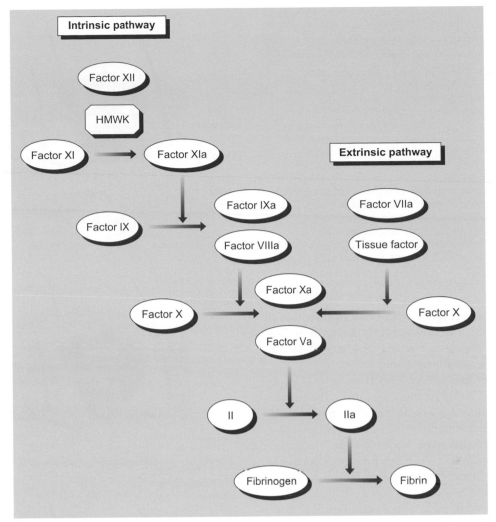

• **Fig. 1.1** Illustration of the 'Cascade' or 'Waterfall' Theories of Coagulation. HMWK, High Molecular Weight Kininogen

not enough thrombin to form a clot but does lead to the next step, which occurs on the phospholipid platform provided by the platelets. On the platelet, due to a positive feedback mechanism involving FVIII, FIX and FXI, a much larger amount of thrombin is formed, termed the 'thrombin burst', which leads to production of a competent clot. This is the basis of the 'cell-based model' which is summarized underneath.

1. Local vasoconstriction – Damage to a vessel causes vasoconstriction, both directly and indirectly, via platelets which are recruited to site of tissue damage and release vasoconstrictor mediators.
2. Formation of platelet plug – Platelets, derived from megakaryocytes, are recruited to sites of endothelial damage. Glycoprotein receptor-Ibα (GP1bα) on the platelet surface interact with von Willebrand factor (vWF), only expressed at sites of endothelial disruption and vascular injury. This causes 'rolling' of platelets and further interactions between platelet receptors (GPVI/Integrinα2β1) and the exposed subendothelial collagen. Upon adhesion, a cascade of intraplatelet events occur, causing a

reduction in intracellular cyclic adenosine and guanine monophosphates (cAMP and cGMP), and a subsequent increase in intracellular Ca2+. This stimulates the release of cytosolic, granule bound mediators, such as ADP, 5HT3 and TXA2 which act in an autocrine and paracrine manner to further activate the platelet and promote aggregation. This forms an unstable, primary plug which requires further consolidation.[3,4]
3. Activation of clotting cascade – This involves interaction between multiple plasma proteins ultimately resulting in the conversion of fibrinogen to fibrin. Fibrin is deposited at sites of tissue injury, creating a meshwork which stabilizes the platelet plug and seals damaged vasculature.

Tissue factor exposed on subendothelial tissue binds factor VII, which is auto-activated to form a TF-VII complex. This converts factor X to its active form (Xa). TF-VII complex also activates factor IX (IXa), which itself generates more factor Xa with assistance of activated factor VIII (VIIIa). Factor VIIIa accelerates the rate factor IXa activates factor X by more than one thousand-fold. Factor Xa, and its co-factor Va, creates a complex which

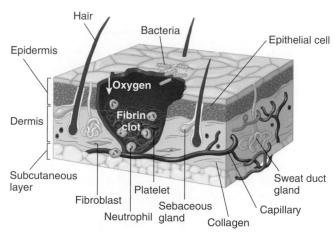

A: Haemostasis

catalyses the conversion of prothrombin to thrombin in sufficient quantity. Thrombin quickly activates fibrinogen to fibrin on the platelet surface, resulting in the formation of a stable haemostatic plug.[3,4]

Further activation of factor X by TF-VII complex is inhibited by the tissue factor pathway inhibitor. The amount of factor Xa produced is insufficient to sustain coagulation and becomes reliant on activation via the factor IXa/VIIIa pathway. At this stage, however, sufficient thrombin has been produced to catalyse further activation of factor VIII and factor V, therefore promoting a positive feedback cycle.

1 Fibrinolysis This takes place over a period of 7–12 days, where the fibrin in the wound is dissolved as the site of injury is healed and vascular integrity is restored.

Inflammation[1,2,5]

Inflammation describes an innate response to tissue damage. Characterized by redness (rubor), swelling (tumor), heat (calor) and pain (dolor), inflammation prepares the tissue for repair. Inflammation during wound healing is a similar response to what is seen in acute inflammation of any cause (Box 1.2).

Surrounding haemostasis, a number of inflammatory markers are released resulting in arteriole vasodilation and venule constriction, increased tissue permeability, intercellular oedema, cellular proliferations and migration of leucocytes into the damaged area. This results in an increase in blood flow to the wound site, aiding recovery but also resulting in the redness and heat associated with acute inflammation.

Fig. 1.2 illustrates the classic stages of wound repair. As chemokine and inflammatory mediators concentration increases, phagocytes, predominantly polymorphonuclear neutrophils (PMNs), leave the capillaries and enter the site of tissue damage. Here they engulf and destroy pathogens and debris, presenting pathogen as non-self-matter,

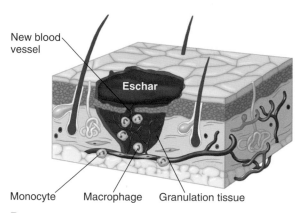

B: Proliferative

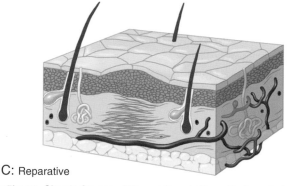

C: Reparative

• **Fig. 1.2** Classic Stages of Wound Repair (From Gurtner et al. Nature https://doi.org/10.1038/nature07039)

recruiting further phagocytes and also members of the adaptive immune system such as T-helper cells, releasing additional proinflammatory cytokines and activating macrophages. Bacteria within the wound site are killed through the release of free radicals.

After 48–72 hours macrophages replace the PMNs as the predominant cell type, and digest apoptotic PMNs. They arrive largely as monocytes before maturing to macrophages. They phagocytose tissue debris and bacteria, releasing proteolytic enzymes to break down damaged tissue. Additionally, macrophages release chemokines and growth factors important in the proliferative phase of wound healing.

Proliferative (Reparative) Phase[1,2,5]

The proliferative phase overlaps with the inflammatory phase, with the focus now on building new tissue to fill the wound space. Approximately 3 days after initial injury, inflammation begins to subside and fibroblasts begin to enter the wounds. Fibroblasts are attracted to the wound by growth factors (PDGf, TGF-β) and fibronectin, initially adhering to the fibronectin. Fibroblasts synthesize and secrete strands of collagen which later becomes the basis of the new extracellular matrix. Additionally, they secrete other growth factors including vascular endothelial growth factor (VEGF), keratinocyte growth factor (KGF) and epidermal growth factor (EGF) (promoting proliferation and migration of keratinocytes).

Angiogenesis occurs in the damaged areas forming capillary loops. Endothelial cells migrate towards tissue damage, attracted by fibronectin, cytokines released by platelets and macrophages, and by tissue hypoxia (and increased levels of lactic acid). The process additionally requires clot lysis, stimulated by plasminogen and break down of earlier ECM by collagenases and metalloproteinases.

Collagen, fibronectin, glycoproteins, glycosaminoglycans and hyaluronic acid are deposited to form provisional ECM. Initially, the collagen formed is in a disordered manner; however, stress applied to the wound causes realignment of the fibres in the direction of the stress forces.

The collection of inflammatory cells, new capillaries, fibroblasts and provisional ECM together are referred to as granulation tissues. Granulation tissue is fragile and readily bleeds. It continues to grow and begins to contract through the effects of specialized myofibroblast (differentiated fibroblasts under growth factor influence). Contraction of myofibroblasts with realignment of collagen fibres is essential to the restoration of the tensile strength of the tissue. This process of contraction occurs over a 5–15-day period; however, it may take longer. The myofibroblasts migrate to the edge of the wound, attaching themselves to the wound edge and ECM and contract, contributing to wound contracture. Simultaneously, fibroblasts are laying collagen down within the wound.

Additionally, in large open surface wounds, epithelial cells (largely basal keratinocytes) from wound edges migrate across granulation tissues, attracted by growth factors secreted by fibroblasts, in addition to the lack of contact inhibition caused by the epithelial disruption and nitric oxide produced by PMNs. They detach from their basal membrane and neighbouring cells through dissolution of desmosomes and releasing of integrins from the cell's intermediate filaments. At the same time, new keratinocytes are produced at the wound edge, stimulated by growth factors. The migrating keratinocytes secrete further growth factors and lay down proteins to form a new basement membrane until they meet in the middle, at which point contact inhibition prevents further proliferation.

This process continues until the entire wound is re-epithelialized. Nerve endings begin to redevelop and tissue starts to rearrange itself, achieving 70–80% of its original tensile strength by 3 months. However, at this stage the tissue remains fragile and prone to interruption or failure which can result in the formation of non-healing areas.

Maturation (Consolidative Phase)[1,2,5,6]

During the maturation phase, the newly formed collagen within the wound undergoes constant remodelling. Disordered type III collagen is degraded via the action of collagenases and matrix metalloproteinases, with collagen synthesis occurring simultaneously producing well-organized, stronger and cross-linked type I collagen. This destructive process is carefully balanced with tissue inhibitors of metalloproteinases. Where the balance between degradation and synthesis is disrupted, rather than maturation and quiescence of cellular activity occurring over 12 months, collagen may be produced excessively resulting in red, hypertrophic scar tissue; if extending beyond the margins of the initial wound, this is known as a keloid.

Additionally, as remodelling occurs, the vascularity of the wound decreases, causing scar tissue to become paler as granulation vessels undergo apoptosis.

Recovery of Tensile Strength

During initial preparative phases, the wound's opposed edges consists only of adherent fibrin, resulting in a tensile strength of zero. As collagen accumulates during the reparative phase, the tensile strength increases rapidly to ~50% of its pre-injury strength at 3 months. After 6–12 months when a strong cross-linked scar of type 1 collagen has been formed, it reaches the maximum tensile strength it will achieve of ~80% of its pre-injury strength.[5,6]

Factors Involved in Wound Healing[1,7]

Wound healing is a sum of interrelated events whose common aim is restoration of injured tissues.[7] We have spoken of the complex interplay of this dynamic system, including the multiple components involved (epidermal cells, extracellular matrix, proteolytic enzymes, etc.), in addition to the environment and homeostatic and systemic signals required (cytokines, chemokines and growth factors, etc.). The normal response as described (haemostasis, inflammation, proliferation and remodelling) can be impaired by a number of factors.

Aetiology of the Wound

The degree of damage, and therefore the ability of a wound to heal, is directly related to the causation of the wound, and the energy transferred to the tissue. For example, a precise surgical incision made with minimal damage to surrounding tissue will heal efficiently. In contrast, a large blunt trauma, resulting in an open fracture, would create a significant amount of force to surrounding tissues, a greater area of damage and therefore a more prolonged healing process. Wounds that heal promptly within less than 10 days may suffer from some pigmentation changes but are very likely to form good scars; wounds that heal within 21 days again predominately have good scar characteristics; however, wounds that heal after 21 days have a very high chance of generating poor scars.

Local Factors

- *Desiccation* – moist environment aids wound healing
- *Tissue maceration* (e.g. urinary/faecal incontinence) – promote infection and delay healing
- *Foreign bodies/infection*
- *Ischaemia/smoking/toxins*
- *Local cancer* (e.g. basal cell, squamous cell cancer, malignant melanoma)
- *Venous insufficiency* – results in venous stasis/pooling of blood containing waste products and high CO_2 content, impairing healing and promoting ulcer formation
- *Pressure* – pressure may impede blood flow to the wound and surrounding tissues, thereby creating a hypoxic environment delaying healing
- *Trauma* – wounds may heal slowly, or fail to heal at all, in an environment in which they are repeatedly traumatized or deprived of local blood supply
- *Radiation*

Systemic Factors[1]

- Chronic disease (e.g. diabetes mellitus, renal disease)
- Nutritional deficiencies (e.g. deficiency of protein or vitamins)
- Congenital healing disorders (e.g. Ehlers–Danlos syndrome, Marfan's syndrome)
- Alcoholism
- Iatrogenic steroid use
- Chemotherapeutic agents (e.g. methotrexate)
- Radiotherapy
- Advanced aged
- Distant cancer
- Uraemia

Mature scar formation, while not synonymous with normal skin, successfully achieves the goal of restoring tissue integrity; this 'normal wound healing', however, lies on a spectrum. Fibroproliferative disorders resulting in hypertrophic scar and keloid formation represent 'over healing', whereas patients with chronic wounds and atrophic scar represent under healing.[1]

Acute Wounds

An acute wound may be defined as those that present without undue delay. The iatrogenic surgical incision is the

• BOX 1.3   Acute Wounds Are Often Grouped According to Mechanism

- *Incised wounds.* Usually caused by a clean sharp-edged object such as surgical knife, or piece of glass, without significant contamination.
- *Lacerated wounds.* Usually a result of blunt trauma causing tearing of tissue due application of force beyond limits of tissue elasticity.
- *Burn wounds.* Injury caused by heat, radiation, electricity, friction or chemicals. Classically but not exclusively confined to the skin.
- *Blast wounds.* Caused by interaction of the body with the peak over pressure blast wave and blast energized fragments.

ultimate acute wound but any break in the integrity of the skin as previously described that attends in the immediate post-insult period is an acute wound. Box 1.3 summarizes types of acute wounds. However, acute wounds can be further broken down into **simple** or **complex** dependent on the involvement of deeper structures.

Chronic Wounds

Chronic wounds can be described as non-healing wounds which persist over 6 weeks,[1] although any wound presenting after undue delay may in practice be labelled as chronic. Non-healing, chronic wounds cause significant morbidity to patients, both psychologically and physically. Chronic wounds often result in impaired physical mobility, pain and emotional stress, in addition to causing familial and social isolation. Furthermore, chronic wounds represent a significant socio-economic burden on the healthcare system: outpatient wound management, absence from work, loss of employment, requirement for assistance with activities of daily living, transportation for medical appointments and expense of self-care and medication.[7]

Pathophysiology of Chronic Wounds

For wounds to heal successfully, complex interactions between multiple processes are required as outlined above. If any component is disrupted, non-healing wounds can result. A number of factors have been shown to be instrumental to the formation of chronic wounds.

Matrix Metalloproteinases (MMPs)[7–10]

Proteolysis of extracellular components is an important step during normal wound healing, encouraging cell migration and angiogenesis. Exacerbated proteolytic processes can cause uncontrolled tissue degradation, which may result in development of a non-healing chronic wound. ECM is produced in similar amounts by fibroblasts found in chronic wounds when compared to normal fibroblasts. In contrast, chronic wound fluid contains a significantly higher proportion of MMPs compared to acute wound fluid, resulting in suppression of cell proliferation and angiogenesis, in addition to increasing degradation of ECM, impairing adequate tissue repair.

MMPs are a family of zinc-dependent endopeptidases capable of degrading virtually all extracellular components and basement membrane proteins at neutral pH.[8–10] Additionally, MMPs function in the regulation of enzymes, growth factors, cytokines and chemokines. Thus MMPs are essential to ECM composition and cell proliferation. Fibroblasts cultured in stress-free type I collagen lattice demonstrate an increased expression of MMP2 and MMP14 compared to those cultured under mechanically stressed type I collagen lattice, suggesting that, under tension, a 'fibrotic' phenotype is favoured.[11] This is utilized in clinical practice, whereby wound edges are approximated under tension, favouring ECM accumulation and wound healing.[8,11]

MMP expression is controlled by inflammatory cytokines such as interleukin (IL)-1β, IL-6, and tumour necrosis factor (TNF)-α, which promote their expression,[7,12] and by tissue inhibitor of metalloproteinases (TIMPs) and plasma inhibitors (α2-macroglobulin, α1-protease inhibitor),[13] which control their activity. TIMPs are glycoproteins produced by fibroblasts which bind with high affinity to active MMPs forming irreversible complexes. Fibroblasts in chronic wounds have been shown to have increased levels of TIMP-1 and TIMP-2, thereby reducing the level of MMP-1 and MMP-2, limiting their capacity for ECM remodelling. TIMPS can also participate in cell apoptosis and cell proliferation. Thus, the final tissue repair outcome is a result of a fine balance between TIMPS and MMPs.

Three MMPs in particular have been found to be important in the underlying mechanism that perpetuates non-healing wound conditions: MMP-1, MMP-2 and MMP-9.

MMP-1 expression is important in wound re-epithelization.[8,14] It is produced by basal keratinocytes, in normal and chronic wounds, after contact with type 1 collagen. Its expression is promoted by a number of growth factors including transforming growth factor (TGF)-α, TGF-β1, epidermal growth factor (EGF), and hepatocyte growth factor[15,16] and its production is arrested when the wound is closed, in conjunction with reducing levels of cytokines such as IL-1α.[17]

MMP-2 expression is important in angiogenesis and matrix remodelling. MMP-2 cleaves multiple sites of type I and III collagen, in addition to fibronectin, elastin and laminin, type IV collagen and anchoring fibrils of hemidesmosomes. Higher concentrations are seen more frequently in elderly people, and contribute to chronic wound development due to excessive degradation of ECM.

MMP-9 is vital to tissue repair due to its important function of degradation of type IV collagen. This promotes basal keratinocyte detachment and endothelial cell invasion during the early stages of wound healing.[18] MMP-9 also degrades type VII collagen located in anchoring fibrils of the dermal-epidermal attachment,[18] in addition to dissolving ECM proteins such as gelatine, collagen (type I, V, VII, and XIV), vitronectin, aggrecan, elastin and entactin.[19] Therefore higher concentrations in chronic wounds may contribute to the underlying mechanism which perpetuates non-healing wounds.

Serine Proteinases[7]

Neutrophils are one of the first cell lineages to arrive at a wound site. Their role is to remove damaged tissues, bacteria and foreign material through phagocytosis and subsequent degradation. Neutrophils produce the majority of serine proteases found in non-healing chronic wounds, and are essential to the wound healing process. It has been shown that the fragments caused by over expression of serine proteases at wound sites can exert a chemotactic effect over other neutrophils, resulting in a cycle perpetuating a non-healing state.[5,20]

Integrins[7]

Integrins are heterodimeric receptors that allow communication between extracellular membrane components and intracellular cytoskeleton. This connection is essential in stimulating intracellular pathways which maintain high concentrations of growth factors, important for cell proliferation, differentiation, migration[21] and, therefore, tissue repair. One example is αvβ6, an epithelial cell receptor, whose expression is induced in migrating keratinocytes at wound edges during the first weeks of tissue repair until re-epithelialization is complete.[22,23] αvβ6 favours adhesion and migration of epithelial cells and production of constituents required in early wound matrix formation. After 14 days, levels decrease, except within keratinocytes found in chronic wounds, where αvβ6 integrin maintain a strong up-regulation.[23]

Chemokines[7]

Chemokines are small proteins which act on cell surface receptors, inducing chemotaxis over several cell populations. For example, the CXC subset mainly recruits neutrophils and lymphocytes, whereas the CC subset recruits monocytes and lymphocytes. As such, they play a key role in tissue remodelling and angiogenesis with various chemokines additionally inducing the expression of MMPs in leukocytes.

Replicative Cell Senescence[7]

Replicative cell senescence describes the irreversible incapacity of diploid cells to enter or complete the S phase of the cell cycle, thereby ceasing to replicate further. Characteristically, cells appear larger, with a number of local findings being described, including increased production of cytokines, chemokines (e.g. CCL2, IL-15), oxygen free radicals, MMPs and TIMPs.

Replicative cell senescence of fibroblasts has been a mechanism hypothesized to be involved in non-healing ulcers. Compromised fibroblasts are larger than non-senescent fibroblasts, with a slower growth rate. In vitro stimulation of senescence fibroblasts has shown a deficient ability to express genes during late G1 phase and S phase, suggesting senesced fibroblasts perpetuate resistance to apoptosis, resulting in a persistent immune/inflammatory response and impairment in wound healing.[24,25] Other studies have demonstrated that fibroblasts in chronic wounds exhibit a distinct phenotype compared to senesced fibroblasts.[26]

Growth Factors[7]

Growth factor dysregulation is thought to play a key role in the phenotype of non-healing ulcers. A combination of increased amount of growth factor, superimposed bacterial infection, hypoxia and ageing promotes a prolonged inflammatory response, often seen in chronic wounds. A number of growth factors have been shown to play a significant role:

HIF-1-VEGF/SDF-1: Hypoxia is a key feature of chronic wounds. Hypoxia-Inducible Factor (HIF-1) is a canonical transcription factor, which contains an α sub-unit that is degraded in the presence of oxygen and iron (Fe^{2+}) through prolyl hydroxylases (PHDs).[27–29] Hypoxia prevents this degradation, allowing it to promote expression of a number of proteins including VEGF and stromal-derived factor-1 (SDF-1). VEGF encourages angiogenesis, with SDF-1 enhancing recruitment of progenitor cells to damaged tissue. Wounds treated with SDF-1 have demonstrated beneficial effects through recruiting bone marrow progenitor cells, promoting healing. Modulation of HIF-1 expression through use of iron chelating agents, which both inhibit PHDs and deplete iron, have shown to reduce oxidative stress,[30] enhance neovascularization and promote wound healing in diabetic wounds.[31,32]

FGF-2: A potent cytokine for stimulation of neovascularization. Its effects are typically mediated via interactions with tyrosine kinase receptors, activating signalling pathways which regulate endothelial cell proliferation and migration. FGF-2 has been shown to be upregulated in the setting of ischaemia. Low levels of FGF-2 have been seen in the setting of diabetes and non-healing wounds.[33]

PDGF: Produced by a variety of cells, including platelets, fibroblasts and endothelial cells, PDGF binds to PDGF receptors on endothelial cells, exerting angiogenic effects, influencing endothelial cell proliferation and migration. PDGF produced by platelets is additionally important in chemotactically recruiting inflammatory cells, such as neutrophils, fibroblasts and monocytes.[34] PDGF-based therapies have been shown in animal models of diabetes to increase fibroblast proliferation and vascular density with accelerated wound closure.[34] Recombinant human PDGF has successfully been used in treatment of diabetic foot ulcers.

TGF-β: Multi-factorial protein with three main isoforms, TGF-β1, TGF-β2 and TGF-β3, which bind to their respective receptor (T-βR1, 2 and 3). T-βR3 has been shown to be related to angiogenesis, whilst T-βR1/2 receptor has been implicated in scarring and fibrosis.[35,36] Dysregulation of TGF-β1 has been implicated in keloid scar formation.[37]

Common Chronic Wounds

Four main groups of chronic wounds are discussed in more detail, vascular (venous or arterial), diabetic and pressure ulcers. Although occurring in a variety of settings, they all share the presence of altered blood flow, varying degrees of hypoxia and the propensity for microbial colonization and subsequent infection.

Venous Ulcer[7]

Venous ulceration accounts for 80% of non-healing ulcers and occurs due to circulatory insufficiency and venous hypertension, most commonly above the medial malleolus or 'Gaiter area'. Typical features of chronic venous ulcers include: oedema, cellulitis, epidermal eczema, haemosiderin deposits resulting in cutaneous hyperpigmentation and fibrous dermal tissue, surrounding varicose veins.[1,7] Venous ulcers are usually superficial, with irregular, shallow borders and are typically painless containing granulation tissue and cloudy exudate. Histologically, subcutaneous septal fibrosis and fat cysts are seen with dermal accumulation of collagen bundles, degradation of elastic fibres, with an increased level of inflammatory markers and loss of normal tissue architecture through the effacement of dermal papillary structures.[38] They exhibit fibrotic cuffs encasing dermal capillary vessels, which constitute a predominant factor in the pathogenesis of non-healing venous ulcers due to the limitation of oxygenation and nutrients between blood and dermal tissue, in addition to the entrapment of inflammatory cells, cytokines and enzymes, resulting in endothelial damage.[38,39]

Arterial Ulcers[1]

Arterial ulcers occur as a result of peripheral arterial disease or arterial insufficiency, where there is a reduction in blood supply, particularly to the periphery of limbs. This can range from mild arterial insufficiency resulting in intermittent claudication, to critical limb ischaemia resulting in tissue death and necrosis. Peripheral arterial disease accounts for approximately 10% of leg ulcers in the UK; however, they can occur as a mixed picture with concomitant venous disease.

Arterial insufficiency occurs for a number of reasons. These include atherosclerosis and deposition of cholesterol plaques within arteries, destruction of the microvascular circuit from diseases such as diabetes and hypertension or from smoking. Similarly, age-related hardening of arteries, with reduction in elasticity and vasoconstriction, can also cause arterial insufficiency. Peripheral arterial disease often manifests in microvascular circulations and at end or arterial trees first; therefore, extremities and underlying tissue are at greatest risk of tissue death. This can lead to destruction of skin integrity and result in non-healing ulcers.

Typically, arterial ulcers have a deep, punched out appearance with steep edges. Surrounding skin may be thin, shiny and hairless, feet may be pale, cool or discoloured and there may be prolonged capillary refill.

Diabetic Ulcers[1,7]

Non-healing wounds represent one of the significant long-term morbidities associated with diabetic patients. Most diabetic ulcers occur at pressure points on the foot as a result of a triad of peripheral neuropathy, joint deformity and local trauma.[40] These ulcers are usually superficial and painless and exhibit necrotic bases with irregular margins, often surrounded by other signs of diabetic disease, including thin dry skin, hair loss and surrounding paraesthesia. Local ischaemia occurs as a result of both macrovascular and microvascular disease. Macrovascular disease is related to a high burden of atherosclerosis in larger vessels, particularly below the knee, seen in diabetic patients, resulting in claudication, muscle atrophy, poor pulses and delays in capillary refill time. Microvascular disease is largely due to thickening of basement membrane, compounded by glycosylated haemoglobin, impairing nutritional and oxygen exchange.[41,42]

Key to the non-healing nature of diabetic ulcers is the impaired immune response and poor chemotactic recruitment of inflammatory cells to the site of injury. This results in inadequate activation of the initial wound healing process and increases the risk of bacterial infection. Once an adequate inflammatory response has occurred, they switch to a distinctive and prolonged cellular infiltration with a high concentration of macrophages and B cells, with low concentration of CD4 T cells,[43] resulting in a sustained expression of chemokines and stimulators for MMP production. Cutaneous ulcers from diabetic individuals show increased concentration of several MMPs compared to traumatic wounds in non-diabetic patients. Prolonged exposure to hyperglycaemia, generating glycation of proteins, has also been shown to disturb cellular response and affect wound healing.[43]

Pressure Ulcers

Pressure ulcers represent another type of delayed wound healing (Box 1.4). Pressure ulcers occur in patients where mobility is impaired for a prolonged period of time, such as elderly patients or patients in the intensive care unit. They occur as a result of prolonged compression, friction or sheer force on areas of body, usually on bony prominences, impairing the perforating arteries ability to perfuse tissue, inducing tissue necrosis. It is important to consider that the skin is relatively resistant to ischaemia and therefore the surgeon should be alert to the presence of deeper tissue involvement beyond the obvious area of skin necrosis.

Pressure ulcers exhibit elevated expression of MMP-2 and MMP-9, with significantly higher concentrations of activated MMP1 and MMP-8 and lower concentrations of TIMP-1 compared to normal healing wounds.

> **• BOX 1.4 Pressure Ulcers Are Commonly Described by Clinical Stage**
>
> Stage I: Intact skin with non-blanchable area of redness of a localized area.
> Stage II: Partial thickness loss of dermis, resulting in shallow open ulcer with red, pink wound bed without slough
> Stage III: Full thickness tissue loss. Subcutaneous fat may be visible; however, bone, tendon and muscle are not exposed. Slough may be present.
> Stage IV: Full thickness with exposed tendons or muscle. Sough or eschar may be present on parts.

Granulation tissue from ulcers contain high levels of proteinases including uPA, neutrophil elastase and cathepsin G, without equivalent anti-proteinase molecules, resulting in a proteolytic environment, impairing the tissue repair process.[44–46]

Acute Wound Management

Incised

Incised wounds are associated with surgical instruments or sharp agents such as knives and glass. Typically, there is no lost tissue and minimal additional adjacent cellular injury. Following haemostasis these can be closed, i.e. primary closure. All but the most superficial wounds must be explored prior to closure for two main reasons:

1. For effective irrigation, evacuation of haematoma and removal of foreign bodies, both of which may become a nidus for infection.
2. To document and repair, if required, damage to underlying structures such as nerves, tendons, blood vessels, fractures and viscera.

Lacerated Wounds

Typically, wounds resulting in tearing of tissue following blunt trauma or sheering forces applied to the skin. A combination of mechanical lavage and surgical excision must be used to debride all devitalized tissues, visible contamination and foreign bodies. The extent of this debridement will be determined by the degree of energy transfer through the wound and the volume of necrotic material.

Tissue viability may be difficult to judge at the index debridement. Tissue may be contused as a result of injury, degloving injuries (where deep fascia is sheered from overlying skin) which can cause loss of cutaneous blood supply and progressive skin necrosis, or 'fickle fat' that appears initially normal but undergoes late necrosis. In these circumstances, the wound is best left open, and re-inspected at intervals, so-called 'second look' surgery prior to delayed primary closure.

The classic examples of evolving wounds that benefit from further inspection are those due to blast or ballistic injury where delayed primary closure is the mainstay of treatment.

Historically, wounds left beyond 6 hours were felt to have a significant inoculum of bacteria and therefore were at much greater risk of infection. Whilst the early administration of appropriate antibiotics in the context of open cutaneous wounds has been shown to minimize infective sequelae, the protracted use of antibiotics only seems to select out resistant strains of microorganisms. Most modern guidance recommends broad spectrum antibiotic use for a maximum of 72 hours. Antibiotics should then be stopped and, if concerns remain, then wound should be sampled to facilitate targeted antibiotic therapy.

When confronted with a wound presenting in a delayed fashion, utilize the principles outlined in the management of lacerated and evolving wounds. Gain surgical control of the wound by removal of foreign and devitalized material. Plan accordingly once the wound is clean and healthy.

Infected Wounds

Infected wounds should be managed with meticulous debridement and removal of all foreign and necrotic material. Tissue specimens should be sent urgently to facilitate targeted antibiotic therapy and wound swabs should be used only when representative tissue specimens are not practicable or to do so would cause undue delay.

If the patient's condition precludes targeted antibiotics, then broad spectrum therapy should be commenced as soon as possible as per local policies. Debridement should be expedited and urgent Gram stain requested. The role of surgery is in diagnosis of the causative pathogen, source control and in delivering a clean healthy wound suitable for delayed primary closure or reconstruction.

However, surgical incisions and access sites may well be the infected wound. Surgical site infections (SSIs) are 'infections of the incision or organ space that occur after surgery' and they represent a significant global health problem. Prevention is better than cure: almost 50% of SSIs could be avoided by implementing known evidence-based solutions, such as adequate glycaemic control, maintaining normothermia and avoidance of hypoxia.

Arrest of Bleeding (Surgical Haemostasis)

To achieve successful closure of wound, a dry wound with minimal oozing is essential. Failure to achieve adequate control of bleeding causes problems as blood:
- acts as a space-occupying lesion preventing wound edge contact, therefore requiring a larger gap to be bridged and more fibrous scar tissue.
- may result in a haematoma, an accumulation of clot which is lysed causing further cytokine-mediated inflammation, synthesis of reactive oxygen and activation of complement.
- may lead to infection as haematoma provides an ideal environment for bacterial proliferation.

A number of methods are employed to stop bleeding in clinical practice.

Compression

Compression of a focus of bleeding, for example through packing a bleeding cavity, or directly applying pressure to a bleeding vessel, helps prevent blood loss while providing time for, and aiding, normal haemostasis to be achieved. 5 minutes of compression allows contraction of small vessels, platelet aggregation and coagulation, and therefore arrest of bleed. However, these processes must be normal for effective haemostasis to be achieved.

Ligation

The damaged vessel is picked up using haemostat (surgical clip) and tied off with a ligature utilizing either absorbable or non-absorbable material. Absorbable sutures have the advantage that once haemostasis is achieved and a thrombus is formed behind the ligature, the suture material dissolves, reducing foreign material present in the wound bed. The disadvantage is that if the suture dissolves too quickly before adequate haemostasis is achieved, particularly in the presence of sepsis, this may result in secondary haemorrhage. Large vessels are more often ligated with non-absorbable sutures for this reason.

Thermal Coagulation/Diathermy (see Ch. 14)

First introduced in the early twentieth century, thermal coagulation is used to facilitate haemostasis and/or the cutting of tissue. This is achieved through using a diathermy, which converts normal electrical current into high frequency alternating current (HFAC). This HFAC produces heat which coagulates blood vessels and cuts through tissue.

There are two types: monopolar and bipolar diathermy.
- Monopolar: HFAC emitted from diathermy via an active electrode is conducted through the patient's body to a large-area contact plate and thence to earth.
- Bipolar: HFAC from diathermy between two points of instrument (bipolar forceps), creates an independent completed electric circuit.

Small vessels can be precisely dealt with using either technique. When used for cutting through soft tissue, a continuous wave form is produced, creating an arc between the electrode and the tissue, vaporizing water in cells and disrupting tissue continuity.

Clipping and Stapling

Blood vessels and other small tubes (e.g. cystic ducts), can be occluded by metal or synthetic clips, delivered using special forceps. Larger vessels may be transected using vascular stapling instruments and, in the context of microsurgery, small metal clips secure haemostasis avoiding the detrimental heat generated as a consequence of electrocautery and preserving blood flow within the adjacent vascular pedicle.

TABLE 1.1   Summary of Long-Acting Haemostatic Agents.

Agent	Mode of Action	Uses	Risks
Bone wax	Tamponade	Bone surface	Infection, delayed bone union
Gelatine foams	Activates extrinsic coagulation system	Small vessel bleeding	Avoid closed spaces as pressure effects may cause nerve damage
Oxidized cellulose	Activates extrinsic coagulation system	Raw bleeding surfaces	Low pH may increase inflammation and interfere with thrombin-based agents
Microfibrillar collagen	Platelet adherence and activation	Bleeding surfaces	Not effective if thrombocytopenic
Thrombin (± gelatine matrix)	Converts fibrinogen to fibrin, activates coagulation	Raw bleeding areas	Allergic reaction especially to bovine products
Fibrin sealants	Thrombin and fibrinogen mixed at site of bleeding to form fibrin clots	Raw bleeding surfaces and tissue sealant, e.g. dura	
Polyethylene glycol hydrogels	Cross-linking polymers in wound	Sealing vascular anastomoses and adhesion prevention	Swells up to four times volume over 24 hours
Glutaraldehyde cross-linked albumin	Cross links albumin to cell proteins in wound to form protein scaffold for haemostasis	Seals vascular suture lines in arterial surgery	Allergy, constriction of nerves or other tissues
Fibrin dressings	Freeze-dried thrombin and fibrinogen on gauze dressing	Large raw surfaces	
Chitin/chitosan dressings	Vasoconstriction, mobilization of red cells, platelets and clotting factors	Emergency control of wound bleeding	Allergy (shellfish product)
	Absorbs water and concentrates red cells, platelets and clotting factors	Emergency control of wound bleeding	Foreign body reaction to product

Adapted from Achneck et al. A comprehensive review of hemostatic agents: efficacy and recommendations for use. Annals of Surgery 2010;251:217–228.

Ultrasonic Instruments

High frequency ultrasonic instruments produce cutting and coagulation of tissue at lower temperatures than diathermy.

Topical Haemostatic Products[6]

A host of topical haemostatic products are available to aid surgical haemostasis (Table 1.1).

When to Stop Anticoagulation

Prior to certain elective surgeries, anticoagulation should be withheld in order to minimize haemorrhagic complications. Warfarin should be stopped 5 days prior to major elective surgery as it has a half-life of approximately 36 hours and, once it is itself ineffective, vitamin K-dependent clotting factors require synthesis before clotting returns to normal. Direct oral anticoagulants (DOACs) need to be withheld prior to surgery based upon their half-life and the renal function of the patient. A summary of half-life and bleeding risks for DOACs can be seen in Table 1.2.

The advice regarding anti-platelet therapies is less clear but continuing low-dose aspirin anti-platelet therapy results in a 1.5 times higher incidence of postoperative bleeding complications. However, the risk of postoperative thrombosis needs to be judged against the risk of adverse bleeding. For most invasive non-cardiac procedures, aspirin therapy can be continued but, if the risk of bleeding is deemed high, aspirin should be omitted from 3 days prior until 7 days after surgery. NICE is expected to publish its guidance on pre-operative anticoagulation in 2020 and updates can be found here: https://www.nice.org.uk/guidance/indevelopment/gid-ng10072

Wound Closure

Whilst it is useful to consider all the options available to you when confronted with a wound, it is potentially more

TABLE 1.2 Half-Lives of Commonly Used DOACs.

Renal function (CrCl, mL/min)	Estimated half-life (h)	Low bleeding risk (h)	High bleeding risk(h)
Dabigatran			
≥80	13	24	48
≥50 to <80	15	24–48	48–72
≥30 to <50	18	48–72	96
Rivaroxaban			
≥30	9	24	48
<30		48	72
Apixaban			
≥30	8	24	48
<30		48	72
Edoxaban			
≥30	10–14	24	48
<30		48	72

CrCl, Creatinine clearance; DOAC, direct oral anticoagulant.
From Keeling et al. Peri-operative management of anticoagulation and antiplatelet therapy. Br J Haematol 2016;175(4):602–613.

helpful to perform this mental exercise before creating the wound in the first instance. Have a plan and also a fall-back position, even if that position is dressings and on-going review. Certain traumatic wounds by their very nature have no easy options, whilst elective surgical incisions will immediately demand to be closed primarily.

The Reconstructive Ladder

Historically, the reconstructive ladder (Fig. 1.3) offers a simple framework to guide the clinician. The lowest rung on the ladder is the simplest, increasing in complexity as one ascends. Unlike a ladder, it is possible to jump rungs or start on at the level that serves the patient best.

Primary Wound Closure

The method used to close wounds should be the simplest and safest available. To ensure the most acceptable scar is achieved, haemostasis must be precise as the breakdown products of retained haematoma contain free radicals that are cytotoxic. In addition, haematoma represents an excellent growth medium for bacteria with the concomitant risk of sepsis. In primarily closed wounds, there should be minimal tissue tension and suture material should be as narrow as possible while maintaining adequate extrinsic strength. Wounds heal between sutures and not at the suture. It is also

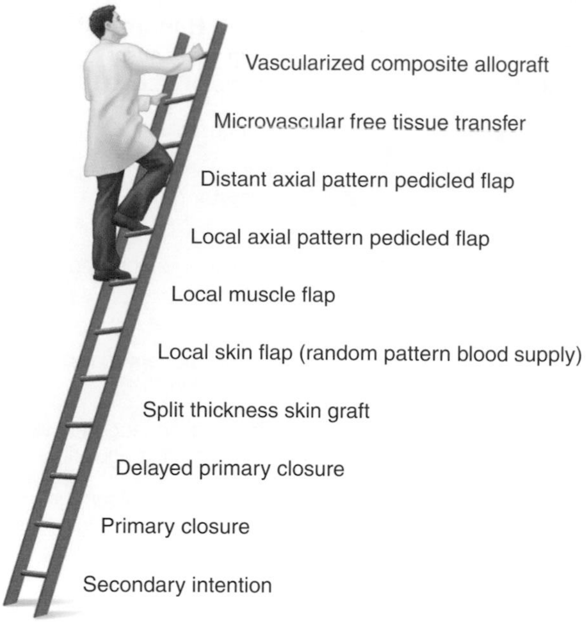

Vascularized composite allograft
Microvascular free tissue transfer
Distant axial pattern pedicled flap
Local axial pattern pedicled flap
Local muscle flap
Local skin flap (random pattern blood supply)
Split thickness skin graft
Delayed primary closure
Primary closure
Secondary intention

• **Fig. 1.3** The Reconstructive Ladder

better to have a longer scar more sympathetically positioned than a short scar in an obtrusive or less than ideal location.

Circular wounds are converted to an ellipse, whose long axis lies parallel to or within the skin crease for the most acceptable scar. The wound is closed in such a manner so as the edges are closely opposed and slightly everted. Holding the skin with any surgical instrument causes additional local trauma but the use of fine-toothed surgical forceps and skin hooks minimizes these insults. Tissue tension is avoided by ensuring tissue approximates easily and can be assisted with a buried subcutaneous suture or adhesive tape to redistribute tension. The quality of the final scar is a result of a combination of operative technique and individual biological healing characteristics. Certain anatomical locations are also high risk for unsightly scars, with the 'cloak' distribution of anterior chest and deltoid region particularly unrewarding.

Needles

Straight needles are held in the hand, similar to ordinary sewing. The thread is usually swaged inside a hollow blunt end, with the point of the needles containing a triangular cutting edge to aid penetrating collagenous tissue. Curved needles are usually designed to be held with a needle holder, being either a cutting edge, reverse cutting edge or round-bodied. Curved cutting needles are often large, and used for closing wounds where penetration of tough fascial layers may be needed. These are the most common cause of needlestick injuries to surgeons and assistants. As a result, more surgeons are using heavy blunt-tipped needles to avoid this risk.

Round-bodied needles are often smaller and used for precise work on viscera (e.g. intestines), nerve and blood vessels. Microsurgical sutures, such as those used in vascular surgery, are usually of this type. Reverse cutting needles have

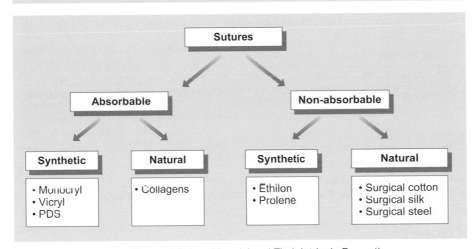

Suture type	Absorbable	Non-absorbable	Monofilament	Multifilament
Vicryl	✓			✓
PDS	✓		✓	
Monocryl	✓		✓	
Nylon		✓	✓	
Prolene		✓	✓	
Silk	✓			✓

Sutures

Absorbable
- **Synthetic**
  - Monocryl
  - Vicryl
  - PDS
- **Natural**
  - Collagens

Non-absorbable
- **Synthetic**
  - Ethilon
  - Prolene
- **Natural**
  - Surgical cotton
  - Surgical silk
  - Surgical steel

• **Fig. 1.4** Types of Suture Material and Their Intrinsic Properties

a cutting surface on the convex edge, and are used for tough tissue such as skin and subcuticular sutures.

Curved needles vary in their curvature and are described as the proportion of a completed circle: 1/4, 3/8, 1/2 and 5/8 are most commonly used, depending on access to the area requiring suturing.

Suture

Sutures are used for ligation of blood vessels and closing of wounds. They may be synthetic or natural, absorbable or non-absorbable, monofilament or braided. Absorbable materials are broken down by proteolysis (catgut) or hydrolysis (new synthetic absorbable sutures such as polyglycolic acid). Absorbable sutures have the advantage that they do not persist as foreign material, and therefore, if wounds become infected, bacteria cannot colonize suture permanently. Catgut (denatured collagen from treated sheep intestinal submucosa) was the original absorbable suture (a summary is provided in Fig. 1.4). Its main disadvantage was that its rates of dissolution meant it was not suitable for any form of distraction, as it would not last long enough for intrinsic tensile strength to recover. This would be further accelerated if the wound was infected. Synthetic absorbable sutures can have their rate of dissolution manipulated, and therefore can be used in a variety of circumstances.

Non-absorbable sutures are preferred in some cases, due to the fact that reassurance tensile strength will be maintained until wound healing reaches an adequate stage. They are not affected by hydrolysis or proteolysis and maintain tensile strength for a prolonged period time, almost permanently.

Their permanence does promote a variable inflammatory response, worse in natural products such as silk, and less so with synthetic materials such as polyamide (nylon), and polypropylene (Prolene). Natural materials are only available in braded form, creating a further nidus for bacteria to colonize between the individual strands. When infection occurs in these wounds, they usually only resolve with removal of the suture. A similar issue is seen in synthetic non-absorbable sutures; however, these are usually monofilaments which slide easily throughout tissue and are less favourable to bacterial colonization.

SUTURE SIZE AND DIAMETER

Non-absorbable and synthetic absorbable sutures USP size	Diameter limits (mm)	Metric size
10-0	0.020–0.029	0.2
9-0	0.030–0.039	0.3
8-0	0.040–0.049	0.4
6-0	0.070–0.099	0.7
5-0	0.100–0.149	1
4-0	0.150–0.199	1.5
3-0	0.200–0.249	2
2-0	0.300–0.339	3
1-0 or 0	0.350–0.399	3.5
1	0.400–0.499	4
2	0.500–0.599	5
3, 4	0.600–0.699	6

• **Fig. 1.5** Suture Size and Diameter

Suture Gauge

Originally, the suture diameter was based on gauge 1, at the time the finest available. As time has progressed, finer suture materials have become available, with the introduction of gauge 0, 00 and further down to 10-0 used in microsurgery. Modern metric gauge is 10 × diameter of a suture material in mm (Fig. 1.5).[24,25]

Other Methods of Closure[6]

Staples

Similar in design to the familiar office stapler, surgical staples have been adapted to introduce a row or circle of staples. Titanium is preferred for internal staples as it produces less tissue reaction and is non-magnetic; therefore, it is compatible with MRI scanning. Stainless steel is commonly used in skin staples where cost and the ability for subsequent removal favours them. Staples are used in a number of circumstances:

- Skin: shortening time taken for wound closure
- GI tract: when anastomosing sections of bowel of different diameters, such as sub-total colectomies, and for speed in damage-control operations leaving the bowel in discontinuity
- Lung: resection can be done, where staggered staple lines are delivered preventing an air leak, and in trauma situations, where non-anatomical lung resection can be performed readily by the non-expert
- Minimal access surgery: suturing can be technically difficult and time-consuming

Tapes

Used in skin closure, useful in minor wounds and where cosmetic outcome is important (e.g. face), as skin puncture marks from sutures are avoided. Once the wound is healed they can be peeled away.

• BOX 1.5 Properties of the Ideal Wound Dressing

Provide physical protection
Provide protection from contamination
Be non-irritant
Help debride the wound
Promote epithelialization
Promote granulation
Be cheap and readily available
Provide absorption of discharge from the wound surface
Eliminate infection and therefore accelerate healing

Adhesives

Glues, particularly cyano-acrylate preparations (Histoacryl), are used sometimes in closure of minor skin wounds. They are particularly useful in children as injection of local anaesthetic can be avoided. They work through polymerization when they come into contact with tissue moisture, resulting in a firm adhesive bond forming. Their disadvantage is poorly opposed tissue cannot be realigned. When utilized in combination with other wound closure strategies, adhesives can help to reduce surgical site infections.

Closure of the Abdominal Wall

Laparotomy results in significant tension over the incision. A mass closure technique is used, whereby heavy sutures are inserted across all deep layers of subcutaneous tissues and fascia, distributing tension over a large suture–tissue interface. Continuous sutures obey Jenkins rule, whereby the suture length is approximately four times the length of the wound.

Sutures should be placed approximately 1 cm apart and 1 cm into tissue on each side of wound. Non-absorbable sutures with gauge 0 or 1 are usually used.

If it is not possible to close the abdominal wall due to distension, oedema of viscera or in damage-control scenarios, the surgical team may choose to leave the abdominal cavity open at the index procedure (laparostomy.)

The open abdomen may be packed with gauze dressings, closed with a plastic sheet sewn to wound edges or topical negative pressure wound therapy utilized. Laparostomy wounds may be addressed by delayed primary closure, component separation (where aspects of the abdominal wall are dissected free form one another) or alternatively the wound may be left open and allowed to heal by secondary intention with subsequent skin grafting of the granulating wound bed.

Dressings[1,6]

Wounds which are open or have been closed are commonly covered with some form of dressing. Dressings have multiple purposes but the ideal dressing is outlined in Box 1.5.

Types of Dressing

The different types of wound dressings available are summarized in Table 1.3, and are discussed further below.

TABLE 1.3 **A Summary of the Different Types of Wound Dressings.**

Generic Dressing Type	Common brands	Indications	Contraindications	Type of Wound
Hydrocolloids • **Hydrating**	Granuflex Duoderm Hydrocol Comfeel	Dry or low exudating wounds	Heavily exudating (wet) wounds Any risk of gas gangrene	Pressure ulcers, leg ulcers, surgical wounds Dehisced wounds Traumatic wounds Ruptures blisters
Foams (adhesive or non-adhesive) • **Absorbent**	Biatin Lyofoam Allevyn	Moist, moderate or heavily exudating wounds (moist, not wet)	None	All wound types
Film • **Neither absorbent or hydrating**	Hydrofilm C-View Tegaderm Opsite	On fragile, vulnerable skin with no exudate, or on low exudating wounds if an alginate of hydrofibre is applied to wound first	None	Superficial wounds of all types and on vulnerable skin or scar tissue
Alginates • **Absorbent**	Sorbsan Kaltostat	All wounds with any levels of moisture. Can be moistened to 20% if wound dry	None	All wound types. Not suitable for completely dry wounds. Used to fill deeper wounds to skin level, before further dressing applied
Hydrofibre • **Absorbent**	Aquacel (plain)	All wounds with any levels of moisture. Can be moistened to 20% if wound dry	None	All wound types. Not suitable for completely dry wounds. Similar use to alginates
Hydrogel/hydrogel sheet • **Hydrating**	Actiform cool (sheet) Intrasite (gel and sheet) Nu-gel Aquagel	For dry or very low exudating wounds	Heavily exudating (wet) wounds Infected wounds Any risk of gas gangrene	All wound types
Non-Adherent • **Not absorbent or hydrating**	Silicone or knitted fabrics Mepitel Urgotulle	To prevent dressings adhering to a wound	None	All wound types. Often used to prevent primary dressing from adhering to skin, or used with vacuum-assisted closure devices
Other Dressing Types	Absorbent pad, e.g. kerramax, eclipse Surgipads, Gamgee, gauze, dressing pads	Except highly absorbent pads, minimal use of this dressing in modern wound care	Not for open wounds	Only wet wound types. Rarely used as frequently adheres to wound making removal painful
Antimicrobials	Silver/silver impregnated Honey/honey impregnated Iodine/iodine impregnated	Infected wounds	None	All infected wounds

Antimicrobial Dressings[1]

Honey/Honey Impregnated

Medical grade honey has anti-inflammatory and antimicrobial properties. Honey promotes an hyperosmotic environment that promotes autolytic debridement (removal of debris from wound bed), and kills and reduces bacteria levels. It is cost effective and effective against a number of bacteria especially pseudomonas species.

The disadvantage of honey is its osmotic properties may result in a wet wound which promotes bacterial growth. Similarly, not all bacteria are killed by honey; in fact, some thrive on the sugar, resulting in rapid bacterial growth. Therefore, when used, close monitoring is required to ensure dressing is changed before becoming saturated. Similarly, dressings must be used cautiously in patients with diabetes.

Iodine and Iodine Impregnated Dressings

Commonly chosen as first-line antimicrobial due to its low cost. There are two main types:

1. Cadexomer iodine is placed in ointments and pastes. Free iodine is released when exposed to wound exudate, acting as an antiseptic on the wound surface. Additionally, it can absorb exudate and aid de-sloughing of wound debris. Common examples include Iodoflex and Iodosorb. Disadvantages are that there are increasing degrees of bacterial resistance encountered, in addition to the risk of systemic absorption when applied to large wounds. It is contraindicated in pregnant patients, breastfeeding patients, patients with thyroid conditions or patients taking lithium.
2. Povidone iodine is used when impregnated on knitted viscose dressing incorporated in a hydrophilic polyethylene glycol base, which facilitates prolonged release of iodine onto the wound bed. A common example is Inadine dressing. Disadvantages are they are rapidly deactivated by wound exudate and therefore maintaining a sustained antimicrobial effect is difficult. When employed they should be changed regularly.

Silver Impregnated Dressing

Silver has a broad spectrum of antimicrobial activity secondary to damage of cell walls and inhibition of cell division. Currently it has no known bacterial resistance. The only contraindication to silver dressings are allergies and dressings containing silver sulphadiazine, which contain silver salts that may be absorbed causing blood disorders and skin discolouration.

There are four main groups of silver dressings:

1. Dressings that release nanocrystalline silver into the wound (Acticoat)
2. Dressings that absorb bacteria and exudate (Aquacel Ag)
3. Dressings that both release silver and absorb exudate (Contreet Foam)
4. Dressings that release a silver compound (Flamazine and Urgotul)

There is some weak evidence to suggest that silver dressings may impair keratinocyte migration and therefore wound healing but the main disadvantage of silver dressings relates to their high cost.

Topical Negative Pressure Wound Therapy (TNPWT)

This increasingly common dressing purports to confer benefit by applying a negative pressure at the wound bed. The science behind this is ill-defined but it prevents wound edge separation and pulls the edges together via a process of macrodeformation as tissue adapts to an applied force. Microdeformation applies at a cellular level with reduction in oedema, increased angiogenesis, favourable perfusion and formation of granulation tissue.

Negative pressure is applied to the wound bed from a pump via an open pore sponge or a gauze-based dressing. The airtight seal required is constructed by placing an impermeable film across this dressing and the adjacent skin. The negative pressure can be exerted in a continuous or intermittent fashion and the negative pressure can vary with most common commercial systems allowing the clinician to select from -50 mmHg to -125 mmHg.

TNPWT has improved the care of a number of differing types of wounds especially dehisced median sternotomy wounds, open abdomens, debrided pressure sores and large irregular traumatic wounds. Contra-indications to TNPWT application include malignancy, active bleeding, exposed dura/bowel and undebrided/necrotic tissue.

Summary

An understanding of the physiology of wound healing allied with a thorough knowledge of the patient's pathophysiology and disease processes allows the operating surgeon to select the optimum wound closure technique from their armamentarium. Whilst some dressings are convenient and comfortable, no dressing has been shown to confer significant advantage.

References

1. Peate I, Glencross W. *Wound Care at a Glance: At a Glance Series.* Oxford: Wiley Blackwell; 1979.
2. Gurtner GC, Werner S, Barrandon Y, Longaker MT. Wound repair and regeneration. *Nature.* 2008;453(7193):314–321. Available from https://doi.org/10.1038/nature07039.
3. Patrono C, Andreotti F, Arnesen H, et al. Antiplatelet agents for the treatment and prevention of atherothrombosis. *Eur Heart J.* 2011;32(23):2922–2932.
4. Eikelboom JW, Hirsh J, Spencer FA, Baglin TP, Weitz JI. Antiplatelet drugs: antithrombotic therapy and prevention of thrombosis, ninth ed. American College of Chest Physicians Evidence-Based Clinical Practice Guidelines. *Chest.* 2012;141(suppl 2):e89S–e119S.
5. Longaker MT, Gurtner GC, et al. Wound healing: an update. *Regen Med.* 2014;9(6):817–830. Available from https://doi.org/10.2217/RME14.54.

6. Thompson JN. Wound healing and management. In: Henry MM, Thompson JN, eds. *Clinical Surgery*. 3rd ed. Elsevier, London: 2012 [chapter 8].

7. Tredget EE, Gharary A, Scott PG, Medina A. Pathophysiology of chronic nonhealing wounds. *J Burn Care Rehabil*. 2005;26(4):306–319. Available from https://doi.org/10.1097/01.BCR.0000169887.04973.3A.

8. Harding KG, Morris HI, Patel GK. Science, medicine and the future: healing chronic wounds. *BMJ*. 2002;324:160–163.

9. Trengove NJ, Staecy MC, MacAuley S, et al. Analysis of the acute and chronic wound environment: the role of proteases and their inhibitors. *Wound Repair Regen*. 1999;7:442–452.

10. Lobemann R, Ambrosch A, Schultz G, Waldmann K, Schiweek S, Lehnert H. Expression of matrix-metalloproteinases and their inhibitors in the wounds of diabetics and non-diabetic patients. *Diabetologia*. 2002;45:1011–1016.

11. Tomasek JJ, Halliday N, Updike DL, et al. Gelatinase A activation is regulated by the organization of the polymerized actin cytoskeleton. *J Biol Chem*. 1997;272:7482–7487.

12. Dasu MR, Barrow RE, Spices M, Herndon DN. Matrix metalloproteinase expression in cytokine stimulated human dermal fibroblasts. *Burns*. 2003;29:527–531.

13. Wysoki AB, Kusakabe AO, Chang S, Tuan TL. Temporal expression of urokinase plasminogen activator, plasminogen activator inhibitor and gelatinase-B in chronic wound fluid switches from a chronic to acute wound profile with progression to healing. *Wound Repair Regen*. 1999;7:154–165.

14. Parks W. Matrix metalloproteinases in repair. *Wound Repair Regen*. 1999;7:423–432.

15. Pilcher BK, Gaither-Ganim J, Parks WC, Welgus HG. Cell type-specific inhibition of keratinocyte collagenase-1 expression by basic fibroblast growth factor and keratinocyte growth factor. A common receptor pathway. *J Biol Chem*. 1997;272:18147–18154.

16. Sudbeck BD, Pilcher BK, Welgus HG, Parks WC. Induction and repression of collagenase-1 by keratinocytes is controlled by distinct components of different extracellular matrix compartments. *J Biol Chem*. 1997;272:22103–22110.

17. Barone EJ, Yager DR, Pozez AL, et al. Interleukin-1 alpha and collagenase activity are elevated in chronic wounds. *Plast Reconstr Surg*. 1998;102(4):1023–1027.

18. Han YP, Tuan TL, Hughes M, Wu H, Garner WL. Transforming growth factor-beta and tumour necrosis factor-alpha-mediated induction and proteolytic activation of MMP-9 in human skin. *J Biol Chem*. 2001;276(25):22341–22350.

19. Hartlapp I, Abe R, Saeed RW, et al. Fibrocytes induce an angiogenic phenotype in cultured endothelial cells and promote angiogenesis in vivo. *FASEB J*. 2001;15:2215–2224.

20. Rao CN, Ladin DA, Liu YY, Chilukuri K, Hou ZZ, Woodley DT. Alpha 1-antitrypsin is degraded and non-functional in chronic wounds but intact and functional in acute wounds: the inhibitor protects fibronectin from degradation by chronic wound fluid enzymes. *J Invest Dermatol*. 1995;105:572–578.

21. Powell DW, Mifflin RC, Valentich JD, Crowe SE, Saada JI, West AB. Myofibroblasts. I. Paracrine cells important in health and disease. *Am J Physiol*. 1999;277:C1–C9.

22. Breuss JM, Gallo J, DeLisser HM, et al. Expression of the beta 6 integrin subunit in development neoplasia and tissue repair suggests a role in epithelial remodeling. *J Cell Sci*. 1995;108:2241–2251.

23. Häkkinen L, Koivisto L, Gardner H, et al. Increased expression of beta 6- integrin in skin leads to spontaneous development of chronic wounds. *Am J Pathol*. 2004;164:229–242.

24. Pang JG, Chen KY. Global changes of gene expression at late G1/S boundary may occur in human IMR-90 diploid fibroblasts during senescence. *J Cell Physiol*. 1994;160:531–538.

25. Shelton DN, Chang E, Whittier PS, Choi D, Funk WD. Microarray analysis of replicative senescence. *Curr Biol*. 1999;9:939–945.

26. Stephens P, Cook H, Hilton J, et al. An analysis of replicative senescence in dermal fibroblasts derived from chronic leg wounds predicts that telomerase therapy would fail to reverse their disease-specific cellular and proteolytic phenotype. *Exp Cell Res*. 2003;283:22–35.

27. Callaghan MJ, Chang EI, Seiser N, et al. Pulsed electromagnetic fields accelerate normal and diabetic wound healing by increasing endogenous FGF-2 release. *Plast Reconstr Surg*. 2008;121(1):130–141.

28. Robson MC, Phillips LG, Lawrence WT, et al. The safety and effect of topically applied recombinant basic fibroblast growth factor on the healing of chronic pressure sores. *Ann Surg*. 1992;216(4):401–406; discussion 406–408.

29. Ohura T, Nakajo T, Moriguchi T, et al. Clinical efficacy of basic fibroblast growth factor on pressure ulcers: case-control pairing study using a new evaluation method. *Wound Repair Regen*. 2011;19(5):542–552.

30. Bergeron RJ, Wiegand J, McManis JS, Bussenius J, Smith RE, Weimar WR. Methoxylation of desazadesferrithiocin analogues: enhanced iron clearing efficiency. *J Med Chem*. 2003;46(8):1470–1477.

31. Botusan IR, Sunkari VG, Savu O, et al. Stabilisation of HIF-1 alpha is critical to improve wound healing in diabetic mice. *Proc Natl Acad Sci*. 2008;105(49):19426–19431.

32. Sundin BM, Hussein MA, Glasofer S, et al. The role of allopurinol and deferoxamine in preventing pressure ulcers in pigs. *Plast Reconstr Surg*. 2000;105(4):1408–1421.

33. Cross MJ, Claesson-Welsh L. FGF and VEGF function in angiogenesis: signalling pathways, biological responses and therapeutic inhibition. *Trends Pharmacol Sci*. 2001;22(4):201–207.

34. Heldin CH, Westermark B. Mechanism of action and in vivo role of platelet-derived growth factor. *Physiol Rev*. 1999;79(4):1283–1316.

35. Simo R, Carrasco E, Garcia-Ramirez M, Hernandez C. Angiogenic and antiangiogenic factors in proliferative diabetic retinopathy. *Curr Diabetes Rev*. 2006;2(1):71–98.

36. Penn JW, Grobbelaar AO, Rolfe KJ. The role of the TGF-β family in wound healing, burns and scarring: a review. *Int J Burns Trauma*. 2012;2(1):18–28.

37. Le M, Naridze R, Morrison J, et al. Transforming growth factor Beta 3 is required for excisional wound repair in vivo. *PLoS ONE*. 2012;7(10):e48040.

38. Herouy Y, Aizpurua J, Stetter C, et al. The role of the urokinase-type plasminogen activator (uPA) and its receptor (CD87) in lipodermatosclerosis. *J Cutan Pathol*. 2001;28:291–297.

39. Cowin AJ, Hatzirodos N, Holding CA, et al. Effect of healing on the expression of transforming growth factor beta(s) and their receptors in chronic venous leg ulcers. *J Invest Dermatol*. 2001;117:1282–1289.

40. Boulton AJ. The diabetic foot; a global view. *Diabetes Metab Res Rev*. 2000;16(suppl 1):S2–S5.

41. Goova MT, Li J, Kislinger T, et al. Blockade of receptor for advanced glycation end-products restores effective wound healing in diabetic mice. *Am J Pathol.* 2001;159:513–525.

42. Jeffcoate WJ, Price P, Harding KG. Wound healing and treatments for people with diabetic foot ulcers. *Diabetes Metab Res Rev.* 2004;20(suppl 1):S78–S89.

43. Loots MA, Lamme EN, Zeegelaar J, Mekkes JR, Bos JD, Middlekoop E. Differences in cellular infiltrate and extracellular matrix chronic diabetic and venous ulcers versus acute wounds. *J Invest Dermatol.* 1998;111:850–857.

44. Wysocki AB, Kusakabe AO, Chang S, Tuan TL. Temporal expression of urokinase plasminogen activator, plasminogen activator inhibitor and gelatinase-B in chronic wound fluid switches from a chronic to acute wound profile with progression to healing. *Wound Repair Regen.* 1997;7:154–165.

45. Rogers A, Burnett S, Moore J, Shakespeare P, Chen J. Involvement of proteolytic enzymes—plasminogen activators and matrix metalloproteinases—in the pathophysiology of pressure ulcers. *Wound Repair Regen.* 1995;3:273–283.

46. Yager DR, Nwomeh BC. The proteolytic environment of chronic wounds. *Wound Repair Regen.* 1997;7:433–441.

47. Knight B. *Forensic Pathology.* 2nd ed. London: CRC press; 1996.

2

Pharmacology in Surgical Practice

CHAPTER OUTLINE

Safe Prescribing

Medication safety can be improved by utilizing the five R's: right drug, right route, right time, right dose and right patient (Box 2.1). Medication errors are barriers that prevent the right patient from receiving the right drug in the right dose at the right time through the right route of administration at any stage during medication use, with or without the occurrence of adverse drug events. The most common prescribing errors are incorrect drug, incorrect dose, allergies, and drug–drug interactions.

Adverse drug events (ADEs) are common in surgery and these errors may occur at all stages of the surgical patient pathway. Preventable ADEs (pADEs) are defined as medication-related harm caused by a medication error; the incidence of ADEs during admission ranges from 1.7 to 51.8 ADEs per 100 admissions. In fact, medication errors account for 15% of all surgical adverse events.[1] This is in part exacerbated by the fact that surgical patients are often taking multiple medications and they typically receive anaesthesia and analgesics during the surgical intervention and during the postoperative period. Surgical patients are also often subjected to medication changes due to the intervention, due to the presence of co-morbidities, and/or due to the multiple in-hospital transfers during the surgical pathway.[2]

It is therefore important to tailor prescriptions for individual patients, identifying allergies, pregnancy, lactation, age, co-morbidities, breastfeeding, size and patient weight. The surgeon must be familiar with the medications they prescribe and needs to know the medications in their specialty that are associated with high risk of adverse events. A summary of the GMC good prescribing practice can be found in Box 2.2, and more information can be found here: https://www.gmc-uk.org/-/media/documents/Prescribing_guidance.pdf_59055247.pdf

The first national audit of all cases of life-threatening anaphylaxis in NHS hospitals between 2015 and 2016 demonstrated 48% of the 266 cases reviewed were found to have been caused by antibiotics administered to prevent surgical site infections. Thirty-three percent were caused by neuromuscular blocking agents. Other triggers included the antiseptic chlorhexidine (9%) and Patent Blue V dye (4.5%) used to identify lymph vessels during breast surgery. These were preventable, and assessment of the risk of allergic reaction is an essential component of good prescribing practice and the WHO checklist. Adherence to guidelines for investigating anaphylaxis also remains low. Only 16% of patients were seen in an allergy clinic within the ideal 6-week wait time, and the 18-week target for appointments was breached in nearly a quarter of cases.[3] On discharge, communication with the primary care team is critical for ensuring that all changes to prescriptions made during the surgical journey are safely handed over. This is achieved through the discharge summary and by clearly explaining these changes to the patient.

Right Drug
Right Route
Right Time
Right Dose
Right Patient

• BOX 2.2 **Good Prescribing Practice**

You must keep up to date with, and follow, the law, our guidance and other regulations relevant to your work.

You must recognise and work within the limits of your competence.

- In providing clinical care you must:
  - prescribe a medicine or treatment, including repeat prescriptions, only when you have adequate knowledge of the patient's health, and are satisfied that the medicine or treatment serves the patient's needs
  - provide effective treatments based on the best available evidence
  - check that the care or treatment you provide for each patient is compatible with any other treatments the patient is receiving, including where possible self-prescribed over-the-counter medications.

You must make good use of the resources available to you.

Documents you make to formally record your work, including clinical records, must be clear, accurate and legible. You should make records at the same time as the events you are recording or as soon as possible afterwards.

Clinical records should include:

- relevant clinical findings
- the decisions made and actions agreed, and who is making the decisions and agreeing the actions
- the information given to patients
- any drugs prescribed or other investigation or treatment
- who is making the record and when.

From GMC, 2021. Good practice in prescribing and managing medicines and devices. General Medical Council, www.gmc-uk.org/ethical-guidance/ethical-guidance-for-doctors/good-practice-in-prescribing-and-managing-medicines-and-devices.

A Basic Introduction to Pharmacology

Drug Metabolism

Drug metabolism is the biochemical transformation of pharmaceuticals in the body, required to create hydrophilic chemicals which can be more easily excreted by the kidneys and in bile. The liver is the most significant site of drug metabolism, where a series of enzymatic reactions change the physical structure and therefore chemical properties of molecules. This detoxification can be considered in four phases, outlined in Box 2.3.

The significance of this is that surgery may fundamentally disrupt each of these phases (for example, by keeping patients nil by mouth and preventing adequate uptake, through surgical disruption of the GI tract or modification of liver function).

Pharmacokinetics

Rather than the effect a substance has on the body, pharmacokinetics examines the effect the body has on the substance.

• BOX 2.3 **The Phases of Drug Metabolism**

- Phase 0 – uptake of drugs into cells
- Phase I – modification. Addition of reactive or polar groups using oxidation, reduction and hydrolysis, allowing phase II to be conducted. This step may activate a prodrug, inactivate an active agent or not change the action of a molecule and is commonly performed by the cytochrome P450 system of enzymes. If a molecule is rendered sufficiently hydrophilic, then excretion is possible after this phase
- Phase II – conjugation. Products of phase I can be conjugated to hydrophilic molecules to increase their water solubility and therefore potential for excretion. Such processes include glucuronidation (by UDP-glucuronosyltransferases), sulphation (by sulphotransferases) and acetylation (by N-acetyltransferases)
- Phase III – export of metabolites from cells using energy-dependent transporters

Following administration, it describes how agents are absorbed, distributed around the body, undergo metabolism and are eventually excreted. This process is complex, with differing chemical properties of pharmaceuticals, routes of administration, access to body compartments and interactions with host tissues.

Important principles in pharmacokinetics:

- Absorption:
  - Absorption rate – the rate with which administered medications reach the blood stream
  - Bioavailability – the proportion of a medication that enters the systemic circulation unchanged after administration (intravenous drugs have a bioavailability of 100%). After absorption, oral medications enter the hepatic portal system and often undergo first-pass metabolism in the liver, decreasing the bioavailability
- Distribution:
  - Unbound fraction – the proportion of a medication which is unbound to serum glycoproteins and is therefore considered active
  - Volume of distribution – the volume necessary to contain the entirety of an administered medication based on the plasma concentration
- Elimination:
  - Elimination rate – combined rate of excretion and metabolic elimination
  - Half-life – the time required for elimination of 50% of the absorbed quantity of a medication
  - Clearance – the difference between arterial and venous plasma concentrations are used to determine the volume of plasma that is completely cleared per unit time

Again, these factors should be considered when making perioperative prescribing decisions during surgical procedures. This is because surgery can cause fundamental changes in haemodynamics, physiological shifts, baseline metabolism and protein catabolism and anabolism. Moreover, it influences gastric emptying, which prevents the delivery of orally administered drugs to their major site of absorption, the small bowel. Distribution is also influenced by changes in blood volume, a dynamic circulation and changes in the extracellular fluid compartment, circulating plasma protein levels that bind drugs (e.g. albumin and alpha 1-acid glycoprotein). In addition, the renal elimination of drugs is affected in patients postoperatively, although the effects of biliary clearance are more challenging to define. Given the large and often rapid changes in pharmacokinetics in the perioperative period, the surgeon must remain vigilant to changes in drug efficacy and toxicity. The absorption of those drugs with known bioavailability is also of great importance in patients undergoing bypass surgery. It is important to consider the effect of obesity on pharmacokinetics independent of the bypass procedure, because it leads to a dramatic drop in body mass over a relatively short period of time. This may be associated with reversals in the influence of obesity on drug disposition to characteristics more in line with leaner patients. However, very little detail is known on this topic and more data is required before we can offer personalized therapeutic strategies.

Considerations for Medications After Surgery

Despite surgical procedures most commonly focusing on a single body system, it is a significant and underestimated stress to the body. Surgery results in a combination of tissue damage, variations in perfusion and oxygenation, organ support, electrolyte imbalance, handling of the gastrointestinal tract and hypothermia, which can all trigger a systemic metabolic response mediated by the release of cytokines and adrenal hormones. This has the potential to impact drug metabolism long past the surgical date, influencing factors such as drug absorption, metabolism and excretion.

Impact on Drug Absorption

It is common for medications to be administered via the oral route postoperatively, with gastrointestinal absorption having the potential to vary widely compared to the immediate intravenous route. Paresis of the stomach, small bowel and colon leads to delayed transit of medications, with poor blood supply decreasing passive absorption by lowering the concentration gradient across the mucosa. Patients may have mechanical reasons why medications are unable to successfully reach the section of the gastrointestinal tract where they are absorbed, such as following resection, formation of a stoma or ongoing mechanical obstruction. An example is cyanocobalamin (vitamin B_{12}), where resection of the terminal ileum or a proximal stoma can result in negligible oral absorption. A shortened gastrointestinal tract from significant resection or proximal-distal internal bypass (whether surgical or as a consequence of fistulating disease) can decrease the total absorptive surface area. Furthermore, a decreased transit time in cases of diarrhoea may give an insufficient opportunity for prodrugs to be activated by colonic microbes resulting in these drugs being lost in the faeces without absorption (sulphasalazine is a notable example).

Impact on Drug Excretion

Patients have many risk factors for developing renal dysfunction in the postoperative period, the route by which the majority of drugs and their active metabolites are cleared. Reduced renal blood flow can be caused by poor oral intake, insufficient intravenous fluid replacement, sepsis, haemorrhage and excessive gastrointestinal and third space fluid losses. Antidiuretic hormone is released at times of systemic stress and acts to reduce urine output, whilst some medications are directly nephrotoxic. Post-renal failure can be mediated by urinary tract obstruction from urinary retention.

Insufficient renal clearance risks the accumulation of active agents with either an excessive medicinal effect or toxic side effects. The active morphine metabolite morphine-6-glucuronide is renally excreted and will accumulate in renal failure, resulting in side effects such as respiratory depression. Aminoglycosides such as gentamicin are not metabolized and instead excreted into the urine unchanged. Renal dysfunction risks their accumulation, with direct nephrotoxicity demonstrated at increased plasma concentrations, contributing to a progressive accumulation. In the majority of clinical scenarios, medications which pose such risks can still be used, with either dose adjustment or monitoring sufficient.

Impact on Drug Metabolism

The liver is the primary source of drug metabolism and, therefore, any insult which modulates enzyme function will impact the efficacy of drug metabolism. Hepatocyte hypoxia can be caused by reductions in blood flow, anaemia or systemic hypoxia, which has been demonstrated to reduce the functions of enzymes through a lack of oxygen to use as a substrate and reduction in oxygen-dependent cofactors such as ATP. This appears to affect phase I oxidases greater than phase II conjugases, with evidence of variable impact on CYP subtypes. Expression of some CYP enzymes is reduced by pro-inflammatory cytokines released during surgery (such as IL-1, IL-6 and TNF-β) and CYP enzymes are known to be regulated by glucocorticoids.

Drug metabolism can also be influenced by factors which directly affect their serum concentration. The stress response of surgery reduces plasma albumin, which is responsible for binding to many acidic and neutral drugs such as digoxin and phenytoin. A1-acidoglycoprotein binds basic drugs such as lidocaine and is increased after surgery. Furthermore, acid-base disturbance (a common postoperative issue) will vary the percentage of a drug that is unbound and active in the plasma, producing an unpredictable clinical effect.

Commonly Used Drugs in Surgical Practice

Clearly all patients must be assessed from a holistic perspective and the management of co-morbidities must be closely managed in the perioperative phase. This is particularly the case in the diabetic patient, or those with a strong cardiovascular or respiratory history. However, these issues are individually addressed in Chapters 7, 8, 9 and 10. Only those drugs specific to surgical intervention will be discussed here.

TABLE 2.1	Examples of Commonly Used Analgesic Regimens in the Early Postoperative Period for a Healthy, 70-Kg Male.	
Grade of Surgery	**Example**	**Regular Analgesia**
Minor	Lipoma removal	Paracetamol 1 g PO QDS +/– Codeine 30 mg PO QDS
Moderate	Arthroscopy	Co-dydramol 1 g/20 mg PO QDS Diclofenac 50 mg PO TDS
	Hernia repair	Co-dydramol 1 g/20 mg PO QDS +/– Ibuprofen 400 mg PO TDS
Major	Laparotomy	Paracetamol 1 g i.v. QDS Diclofenac 50 mg PO TDS Morphine PCA (1 mg bolus, 5-minute lockout)
	Hip replacement	Paracetamol 1 g PO QDS Diclofenac 50 mg PO TDS Oxycodone SR 10 mg PO BD

BD, Twice daily (bis die); *co-dydramol*, combined paracetamol and codeine; *i.v.*, intravenously; *PO*, per oral; *PRN*, as required (pro re nata); *QDS*, four times daily (quarter die sumendum); *SR*, sustained release; *TDS*, three times daily (ter die sumendum).

Analgesia

Pain is the unpleasant experience when a noxious substance, tissue damage or anticipated tissue damage is encountered, which causes withdrawal, metabolic and conscious responses. Conversely, analgesia is the absence of pain after experiencing a stimulus which would be expected to be painful. This can be achieved in a variety of ways but the most common, and focus of this section, is analgesic medications.

It is necessary to consider the biology and anatomy of pain formation in order to most effectively use analgesic agents. A normal reaction to tissue damage (whether surgical or non-surgical) is the release of pain-mediating mediators such as bradykinin, histamine and prostaglandins, which act synergistically to stimulate afferent nociceptive fibres. Once in the dorsal horn of the spinal cord, these fibres release substance P (increasing the rate of nociceptor firing) and synapse with secondary neurons, to transmit the signal to the thalamus and eventually somatosensory cortex. Medications can therefore be focused at different points on this pathway in order to modulate or eliminate the sensation of pain.

Why Treat Surgical Pain?

It is self-evident that the psychological consequences of pain are detrimental to a patient's wellbeing and this provides the most apparent rationale for instigating therapy. However, there are further reasons to provide analgesia. Pain after abdominal or thoracic surgery can result in a patient being bedbound for the immediate postoperative days, with an inhibition of deep breathing or coughing to avoid the pain. Poor expansion of the lung bases will cause atelectasis which may develop into a pneumonia, providing a mortality risk and extension of hospital stay. Following routine hip or knee joint replacement, early mobilization is paramount for quality rehabilitation and can only be achieved with effective analgesia. Furthermore, the physiological responses to pain are tachycardia and vasoconstriction, which can stress vulnerable myocardium. Pain in the postoperative period significantly increases the risk of morbidity and it should therefore be treated

as a surgical emergency that requires immediate treatment. It is morally and ethically unjustifiable to leave a patient in pain.

Which Analgesic to Choose?

The analgesic choice, dose and route of administration varies widely across clinical practice and needs to be focussed to the specific clinical scenario, asking questions such as:

1. Which agents have the mechanism of action to most optimally address the cause of pain?
2. What is the preferred duration of action?
3. Do the risks of side effects of certain routes of administration outweigh the benefits?
4. What anatomical pattern of analgesia is required?

There are guiding principles which should be applied to help direct answers to the above questions, based upon the WHO's analgesia ladder originally proposed in 1986 for management of cancer pain. Analgesics should be given orally if possible, at regular intervals, should be tailored to the patient's interpretation of pain intensity with regular review, prescribed with the patient's involvement in the decision-making process and there should be personalized dosing (in consideration of factors such as tolerance, body weight and co-morbidities).

A combination of analgesic agents is often required for the management of pain caused by surgery or surgical pathologies (Table 2.1). Medications can often work synergistically and therefore this approach can avoid higher doses of analgesics with a greater burden of side-effects.

Common Analgesics

Paracetamol

The mechanism of action of paracetamol is poorly understood, but it is a highly effective analgesic and is staple in almost all regimens. Side effects are rare and it is most commonly administered intravenously or orally.

Non-Steroidal Anti-Inflammatory Drugs (NSAIDs)

NSAIDs inhibit the cyclooxygenase enzymes (subtypes 1 and/or 2) which acts to decrease the production of eicosanoids such as prostaglandins (nociceptive mediators). Common examples used for surgical pain are ibuprofen, diclofenac and parecoxib, with routes of administration that include oral, intravenous, intramuscular and rectal. A significant side effect of NSAIDs is gastric ulceration and potential bleeding, as the gastro-protective effects of prostaglandins are lost (including stimulation of mucus and bicarbonate secretion). Furthermore, NSAIDs can cause pre-renal dysfunction (vasoconstriction of afferent arteriole through prostaglandin deficiency leading to acute tubular necrosis) and drug-induced interstitial nephritis.

Opioids

Most balanced anaesthetic techniques use opioids for analgesia. Opioid analgesics mimic endogenous opioid compounds which act at opioid receptors. There are three types of receptor:

- OP1 or δ (delta)
- OP2 or κ (kappa)
- OP3 or μ (mu)

Opioid analgesics mimic endogenous opioid compounds which act to centrally suppress nociceptive stimulus transmission. The most relevant receptor is the μ subtype, with agonists acting to block afferent neurons releasing substance P in the dorsal horn and by stimulating descending inhibitory neurons from the midbrain. Drugs such as morphine and diamorphine have medium-term effects which last 2–4 hours. Shorter-acting opioid derivatives, such as fentanyl and alfentanil, are used intraoperatively for shorter procedures. Opioids can be administered by a number of different routes (see the section on postoperative analgesia).

Opioids are excellent analgesics for surgical patients with a wide variety on the available routes of administration. However, they suffer from notable side effects:

- Respiratory depression is mediated via the brainstem and this can cause resistance to hypercapnia with reduced drive to breathe. This can be life-threatening and lead to respiratory arrest, with naloxone (antagonist to opioid receptors) used as the antidote.
- Gastrointestinal side effects include nausea and vomiting from stimulation of the chemoreceptor trigger zone (co-administration with anti-emetics is advised) and constipation.
- Itching and urticaria caused by histamine can be stimulated by some opioids.
- Tolerance and addiction are features of longer-term use of opioid analgesics.

Morphine – A potent and commonly used analgesic, which can be used in immediate and long-acting preparations. It is metabolized by the liver to active metabolites which are excreted by the kidneys, raising the possibility of accumulation in renal dysfunction.

Diamorphine – This is the diacetyl ester of morphine, with greater analgesic and euphoric properties due to greater lipid solubility; resulting in a smaller required dose.

Fentanyl – This is a synthetic opioid with analgesic effects in the region of 100 times greater than morphine. It is very lipid soluble, such that it crosses the blood brain barrier rapidly for a fast effect (1–2 minutes) and short duration of action (in the region of 30 minutes). It has advantages over morphine in that it is less likely to cause itching and has greater cardiovascular stability. Fentanyl is most commonly used for surgical patients intra- and immediate postoperatively, with some ward-based use in the form of intravenous patient-controlled analgesia (PCA) or orally as a lollipop.

Tramadol – This is an opioid analgesic which also has action as a serotonin-noradrenaline (norepinephrine) reuptake inhibitor. It is most commonly administered orally, intramuscularly or intravenously; with metabolism in the liver and excretion via the kidneys. It is less likely to cause constipation than morphine.

Codeine – This opioid has relatively weak affinity for the μ-receptor but is a prodrug of morphine through conversion in the liver. Five to ten percent of patients are slow metabolizers due to a lack of appropriate enzyme, resulting in little analgesic effect. Codeine is used orally for mild to moderate pain, with 4–6-hour duration of action.

Oxycodone – This is a semi-synthetic opioid which can be used in both immediate and sustained-release preparations for moderate to severe pain.

Patient-Controlled Analgesia

The morphine is housed in the reservoir of a pump system and connected to an intravenous cannula; the patient controls the delivery of the drug by pressing a button which causes the device to deliver a predetermined dose (Fig. 2.1).

There follows a period (lock-out time) when a further press is ineffective, which protects against over administration. Use of such a device allows the patient to determine analgesic dose according to perceived pain. The device also gives the patient confidence that analgesia is readily available when necessary. Opioids can also be administered as part of an epidural regimen, usually in combination with a local anaesthetic. However, it is important to note that more-involved pain management techniques such as this need more-intensive nursing and are probably unsuitable for most general surgical wards.

Drugs Used in General Anaesthesia

Intravenous Induction Agents

Ideally the agent used should have a rapid onset of effect, with rapid production of unconsciousness. It should have few side effects on the cardiovascular and respiratory systems and be quickly metabolized to aid speedy recovery.

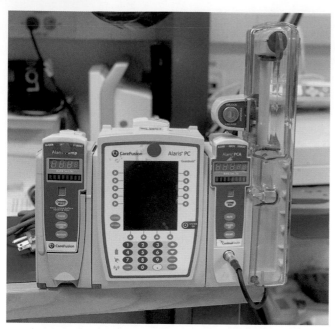

• **Fig. 2.1** A PCA Infusion Pump (From Kan K, Levine WC. *Anesthesia Equipment*, 3e, Elsevier, 2021, pp 351–367, Fig. 16.16)

Thiopental (Thiopentone)

Introduced into clinical practice in 1932, this drug is a sulphur analogue of pentobarbitone (a barbiturate). It produces unconsciousness in less than one brain–arm circulation time (about 30 seconds). It is then redistributed to the fat and muscle compartments, so its effects wear off relatively quickly. Unfortunately, it needs to be used very carefully because too large a dose can cause a severe fall in blood pressure, especially in those who have other factors which can contribute, e.g. hypovolaemia and impaired vasomotor tone. In common with all anaesthetic induction agents, it causes marked respiratory depression. Although painless on intravenous injection, extravasation into the tissues or accidental intra-arterial injection can cause pain and distal ischaemia.

Propofol

This simple molecule (2,6-di-isopropylphenol) has become extremely popular. It has a fast onset of action and is metabolized very rapidly by the liver and other organs. This means that the agent has very few hangover effects and results in a very bright, clear-headed recovery – it is ideal for day-care surgery. Its rapid metabolism also allows use as a continuous infusion, either for a short anaesthetic or as sedation on the intensive care unit. In common with thiopental (thiopentone), it can cause marked falls in blood pressure and markedly depresses respiration. Unfortunately, it is sometimes painful on intravenous injection, and to prevent this, many anaesthetists add a small dose of local anaesthetic (lidocaine (lignocaine)) to the solution.

Ketamine

This phencyclidine derivative is somewhat different from the other agents. It can be used as a sedative or to induce anaesthesia. Interestingly, systolic blood pressure is usually raised by ketamine, and respiration is not depressed except by very large doses. It is also a good analgesic. Unfortunately, it is associated with a high incidence of postoperative hallucinations. It may be used as the sole anaesthetic agent in those with shock and thus has a role in military surgery.

Inhalational Maintenance Agents

Once anaesthesia has been induced, it must be maintained, usually by inhalational agents. These are mainly ether derivatives (methyl-ethyl ethers) and hydrocarbons. They are mostly liquids at room temperature and are administered through special vaporizers on the anaesthetic machine, which are calibrated to allow specified concentrations of the vapour to be added to the oxygen and other gases in use for ventilation.

Sevoflurane, Desflurane, Isoflurane and Enflurane

These modern ether derivatives are all useful agents because they have a rapid onset and offset of action. Sevoflurane is pleasant to inhale and is often used to induce anaesthesia by the inhalational route in children who are intolerant of needles. Desflurane is less pleasant but, because it has a very rapid offset of action, is quite frequently used in day-case surgery, where rapid recovery is desirable. Isoflurane is an older agent in common use which has a relatively quick offset of action and has low levels of cardiovascular side effects. Enflurane is similar to isoflurane.

Nitrous Oxide

The gas is supplied in blue cylinders which can be connected to the anaesthetic machine. It is an analgesic gas (colloquially known as laughing gas). Special meters on the anaesthetic machine allow it to be mixed in known proportions with oxygen. Because of its analgesic properties, it is widely used in childbirth.

Neuromuscular Blocking Agents

Muscle relaxant drugs are often used as part of a balanced anaesthetic to allow intubation of the trachea and controlled respiration by intermittent positive pressure ventilation. This is usually necessary for prolonged or major surgery, particularly in the abdomen or thorax. It is also necessary in some emergency situations. Muscle relaxants may also be used to facilitate assisted ventilation for long periods of time in the intensive care unit. There are two main types of agent:
- Depolarizing – These first stimulate contraction by their action at the neuromuscular junction and then produce paralysis. The only clinically important depolarizing muscle relaxant is suxamethonium chloride.
- Non-depolarizing – By contrast, these do not cause any muscle activity before relaxation. These are

competitive blockers (see below) at the acetylcholine receptors on the neuromuscular junction. Drugs such as atracurium, vecuronium and pancuronium are examples.

The effects of these drugs can be reversed by the administration of acetylcholinesterase inhibitors, such as neostigmine, which increase the concentration of acetylcholine in the neuromuscular junction by preventing its breakdown. The increased concentrations of acetylcholine then compete with neuromuscular blocking drugs (hence the term competitive blockers) for receptors at the neuromuscular junction, and muscle power returns.

Suxamethonium
Suxamethonium is a depolarizing neuromuscular blocking agent which provides very rapid muscle relaxation (within 30 seconds). It is therefore very useful in emergency work where rapid control of the airway is essential to avoid aspiration of stomach contents. Its effects usually wear off in 2–3 minutes. It is metabolized by plasma cholinesterase (also known as pseudocholinesterase). It does have side effects, as follows:
- postoperative muscle pain
- bradycardia
- release (e.g. in the severely burned) of potassium from muscle cells into the bloodstream, which may cause cardiac arrest
- suxamethonium apnoea – approximately 1 in 3000 of the population have an inherited defect in cholinesterase which causes the muscle-paralysing effects to be prolonged, and anaesthesia and respiratory support must be maintained until the effects wear off
- acute anaphylactic shock (rare)
- malignant hyperpyrexia – a rare condition in which temperature control fails and death may follow

Vecuronium, Atracurium, Rocuronium and Pancuronium
These are longer acting, competitive muscle relaxants. They take longer than suxamethonium to relax the muscles (approximately 1–3 minutes) but their effects last longer (sometimes between half an hour and 1 hour). Vecuronium is a useful muscle relaxant with very few side effects. It is metabolized in the liver and excreted via the kidneys. Atracurium is also commonly used but can, as a side effect, release histamine; however, it has the advantage that it is degraded spontaneously in the bloodstream by a process called Hoffman degradation, which is dependent on the temperature and the pH of the plasma and is independent of liver and renal function. It can therefore be used in patients with renal or hepatic failure. Rocuronium is chemically similar to Vecuronium but has a quicker onset time of approx. 60 seconds. It has therefore been used in place of suxamethonium. Pancuronium is a much longer-acting muscle relaxant often used during prolonged procedures.

Other miscellaneous drugs
Benzodiazepines
These drugs are used for premedication (e.g. temazepam) and for short-acting intravenous sedation during procedures carried out under regional anaesthesia (e.g. midazolam).

Anti-emetics
Different classes of anti-emetics are used to prevent and treat postoperative nausea and vomiting. Metoclopramide and domperidone act at dopamine receptors in the midbrain. Anticholinergic agents (e.g. hyoscine) affect the so-called vomiting centre, also in the midbrain. Antihistamines (e.g. cyclizine) are effective but can cause sedation. 5HT 3 (homopentameric or serotonin) antagonists (e.g. ondansetron) are extremely effective, as are steroids (e.g. dexamethasone).

Local Anaesthesia
Local infiltrative anaesthesia is commonly used for a wide variety of day surgery procedures such as skin biopsy, excision, wound closure, tissue rearrangement, skin grafting, cauterization, non-ablative laser and ablative laser resurfacing. When performing procedures under general anaesthesia, it is good practice to combine this with local anaesthesia wherever possible to improve pain control postoperatively. Moreover, infiltrative, topical and local nerve block anaesthesia can also be combined if performing larger or more complex procedures without sedation or general anaesthetic.

Lidocaine, bupivacaine, levobupivacaine, prilocaine and ropivacaine are amides. They remain stable in solution and are metabolized by the liver. They cause a reversible conduction block in nerves by blocking the sodium channels in the nerve membrane. This disrupts the nerve action potential and inhibits propagation of the action potential along the axon. These agents also cause vasodilation, which increases their tissue absorption. When the skin is infiltrated, the action is almost immediate, owing to the small unmyelinated nerve fibres being rapidly penetrated by the local anaesthetic. These are the most commonly applied type of local anaesthesia, although esters such as cocaine, procaine, amethocaine and chloroprocaine are also used. They are becoming less popular because of the higher risk of allergy.

Allergy to lidocaine is rare, with a genuine immunological reaction representing only 1% of all adverse reactions to these medications. Toxicity is also rare, but the signs and symptoms tend to follow a progression of central nervous system (CNS) excitement. CNS toxic signs and symptoms occur at a lower serum level and are an early warning there may be a problem. The patient may complain of circumoral numbness, facial tingling, pressured or slurred speech, metallic taste, auditory changes and hallucinations, which may also be accompanied by hypertension and tachycardia. Ultimately, CNS depression may develop. Because amides also block sodium channels in myocardial cells, systemic dosing of local anaesthetics has a negative ionotropic effect and it may cause pacemaker suppression leading to bradycardia and sinus arrest. Of note, bupivacaine can initiate a refractory ventricular fibrillation which is difficult to defibrillate. In the event that there is a concern of toxicity, stop the administration of any further agents, administer oxygen, call for help and resuscitate. In the event of a cardiac arrest do not give lidocaine. If the patient does not respond rapidly to standard procedures, 20% lipid emulsion such as *Intralipid* should be given intravenously at an initial bolus dose of 1.5 mL/kg over 1 minute, followed by an infusion of 15 mL/kg per hour. After 5 minutes, if cardiovascular stability has not been restored or circulation deteriorates, give a maximum of two further bolus doses of 1.5 mL/kg over 1 minute, 5 minutes apart, and increase the infusion rate to 30 mL/kg per hour. Continue infusion until cardiovascular stability and adequate circulation are restored or maximum cumulative dose of 12 mL/kg is given.

Dose Calculations

Prior to administration, all injectable medicines must be drawn directly from their original ampoule or container into a syringe and should **never** be decanted into gallipots or open containers. Great care must be taken to avoid accidental intravascular injection; local anaesthetic injections should be given slowly in order to detect inadvertent intravascular administration. Calculating the correct dose of anaesthesia is a common challenge. A worked example for a 70-kg person can be found in Box 2.4. Each anaesthetic agent has its own dosing regimen and these are summarized in Table 2.2.

Each amide anaesthesia has its own distinct properties which can be leveraged depending on the operative requirement.

Lidocaine: It is effectively absorbed from mucous membranes and is a useful surface anaesthetic in concentrations up to 10%. Except for surface anaesthesia and dental anaesthesia, solutions should not usually exceed 1% in strength.

Prilocaine: This drug is closely related to lidocaine and is very similar in its clinical action. Its advantage is that it is more rapidly metabolized and hence less toxic. It can cause methaemoglobinaemia when used in high dosage (>600 mg). Methaemoglobinaemia causes a blue skin discolouration and results in false pulse oximeter readings.

Bupivicaine: It is commercially available in 0.25% and 0.5% solutions (with and without epinephrine (adrenaline)). It has a slow onset of action, taking up to 30 minutes for full effect. It is often used in lumbar epidural blockade and is particularly suitable for continuous epidural analgesia in labour, or for postoperative pain relief. It is the principal drug used for spinal anaesthesia. Bupivacaine is particularly cardiotoxic and should never be used in Bier's blocks. Bupivacaine binds tightly to tissues and thus has a long duration of action (up to 24 hours in some cases).

Levobupivicaine: Levobupivacaine contains the S enantiomer only of bupivacaine and it has a greater vasoconstrictive action and less motor block. It is also less cardiotoxic. It is typically used when rapid onset peripheral blockade or prolonged postoperative action is required.

Ropiviacaine: Ropivacaine is an aminoamide local anaesthetic and it is less toxic than bupivacaine.

Combinations of local anaesthesia may also be administered together to provide a combination of fast and long acting anaesthetic control.

Other Agents Commonly Added to Local Anaesthetic Agents

Epinephrine (adrenaline) (Box 2.5): It is not advisable to give this with a local anaesthetic injection in digits or appendages because of the risk of ischaemic necrosis. However, this agent is often added to local anaesthetics to cause vasoconstriction. This reduces the local anaesthetic absorption and thus prolongs the block duration and reduces toxicity.

Clonidine is an alpha-2 adrenoreceptor agonist. It prolongs and intensifies blocks when added to local anaesthetics. Adding clonidine 75–100 micrograms can extend the duration of peripheral blocks by 50–100% and for a Bier's block (IVRA) clonidine 150 micrograms can be added to the local anaesthetic solution. It reduces tourniquet pain and causes no adverse effects when the tourniquet is released. Clonidine is regularly used when prolonged postoperative analgesia is required.

Injection pain is associated with a low pH and cold solution. Thus, **sodium bicarbonate** raises the pH of the solution, which leads to a rise in the fraction of unionized local anaesthetic, enabling it to more readily penetrate the nerve membranes. This increases the speed of action and prolongs the duration and intensity of the block. The recommended dose is 1 mL of 8.4% sodium bicarbonate per 10 mL of local anaesthetic. There are also data to support the use of a slow infiltration rate, vibrating the skin, use of a warm (40°C) solution and cold air skin cooling to decrease the pain of local anaesthetic injection in adults. These can also be applied.

TABLE 2.2	Summary Dosing Data and Duration of Onset for Commonly Used Local Anaesthetic Agents.			
	Onset (min)	Duration (min)	Max Dose (mg/kg)	Max Mg (70-kg Person)
Lignocaine (1% or 2%) (Xylocaine)	2	15–60	3 mg/kg	220 mg (11 mL 2%) (22 mL 1%)
Lignocaine with adrenaline (epinephrine) (1% or 2%)	2	120–360	7 mg/kg	500 mg (25 mL 2%) (50 mL 1%)
Bupivicaine (0.25%) (Marcain)	5	120–240	2.5 mg/kg	175 mg (50 mL)
Bupivicaine with adrenaline (epinephrine)	5	180–420	3 mg/kg	225 mg
Prilocaine (0.5% or 1%) (Citanest)	2	30–90	7 mg/kg	500 mg (<70 kg) (50 mL 1%)
Ropivacaine (0.25%) (Naropin)	5	120–360	3 mg/kg	225 mg
Mepivacaine (1%) (Polocaine)	3–5	45–90	4 mg/kg	280 mg (28 mL 1%)
Mepivacaine (1%) with adrenaline (epinephrine)	4	120–300	7 mg/kg	400 mg

---

• BOX 2.5 The Administration of Epinephrine (Adrenaline) in Local Anaesthesia

Epinephrine is commercially available in two ampoule sizes:
- A 1 mL ampoule containing 1 mg (i.e. 1:1000)
- A 10 mL ampoule containing 1 mg (i.e. 1:10,000)
  Thus, a 1:10,000 solution of epinephrine contains 0.1 mg of epinephrine (or 100 micrograms) per mL
OR a 1:100,000 solution contains 10 micrograms per mL
OR a 1:200,000 solution contains 5 micrograms per mL
OR a 1:400,000 solution contains 2.5 micrograms per mL

• BOX 2.6 Summary of Risks and Advantages of Regional Anaesthesia

Advantages	Disadvantages/Risks
Avoids GA	Slower (may take 15 to 30 minutes)
Safe	Patient discomfort (on insertion or with numbness)
Patient preference for consciousness	Requires a skilled anaesthetist
Less postoperative nausea	Failure rate (up to 10%)
Faster discharge	Risk of nerve damage (<1 in 1000)
Cost effective	Potential for wrong site

Regional Anaesthesia

Regional nerve blocks are used for anaesthesia and/or analgesia during or after surgery, and also in the management of chronic pain (Box 2.6). Anaesthesia can be administered continuously via a catheter or as a single shot and is typically provided in surgery in one of the following routes:

Epidural analgesia or anaesthesia: The healthcare provider may inject medicine outside the spinal cord.

Spinal anaesthesia or analgesia: The healthcare provider may inject medicine in the fluid surrounding the spinal cord.

Peripheral nerve blockade: The healthcare provider may inject medicine around a target nerve causing pain.

Peripheral nerve blockade is a useful adjunct to general anaesthesia. It is delivered with a needle in close proximity to the target nerve. Anatomical landmarks, the detection of a 'click' when fascia is breached, and nerve stimulation can all be used to guide the needle-tip insertion. Increasingly, this is performed under ultrasound, e.g. an ultrasound-guided transversus abdominis plane block (Fig. 2.2). A peripheral nerve stimulator can also be used if the nerve carries motor fibres: a small electrical current is produced which elicits muscle twitching if the needle to be used for the block is close to the nerve. Ultrasound is now being used to introduce local anaesthetic close enough to the nerve without damaging it or the surrounding structures.

Bier's Block

Also known as intravenous regional anaesthesia, this has been classically used for reduction of Colles' fractures and is the exception to the rule that local anaesthetic should never be injected directly into the circulation. Systemic toxicity is prevented by the use only of prilocaine (the least toxic local anaesthetic) and by separating the intravenous local anaesthetic in

- **Fig. 2.2** A Transversus Abdominis Plane Block (From Keller, D.S., Transversus abdominis plane blocks: pilot of feasibility and the learning curve, *J Surg Res* 2016; 204:1:101-108, Elsevier)

the limb from the general circulation by a tourniquet until the agent is bound in the tissues – about 20 minutes. Deaths have resulted as a consequence of tourniquet failure.

Recently the risk of wrong site regional anaesthesia has been highlighted. On this basis, the Royal College of Anaesthetists have issued a checklist for interventional procedures under local anaesthesia or sedation (Fig. 2.3).

Epidural and Spinal Anaesthesia

In relation to nerve action, the introduction of local anaesthetic into the epidural or subarachnoid (spinal) spaces is similar to regional blockade, although the timescale and intensity differ. Both techniques involve the insertion of a needle into the midline between the spinous processes of adjacent vertebrae (Fig. 2.4). This form of anaesthesia is especially useful for surgery below the waist; blocks can be made as high as the mid-thoracic region, but associated abdominal and intercostal muscle weakness can interfere with the ability to breathe or cough. The epidural space is the more superficial of the two and is classically identified by the loss of resistance to injection of air or saline. Because an epidural injection does not puncture the dura, and therefore is well clear of the spinal cord, it can be done at any level in the vertebral column. In addition, wider-bore needles can be used, which allow the passage of a catheter into the epidural space and either 'top-ups' or continuous infusions. The local anaesthetic introduced into the epidural space has to diffuse through the epidural fat towards the nerve roots as they emerge from the dura; as a result, the block can take up to 20 minutes to become effective and may miss some nerve roots, leaving unblocked segments. It is generally less dense than a spinal anaesthetic. Larger doses of anaesthetic agent are also needed than for a spinal because the anaesthetic is injected further from its eventual site of action. With spinal anaesthesia, the dura is deliberately punctured to enter the subarachnoid space. The resulting persistent breach in the membrane can lead

to leak of CSF (cerebrospinal fluid) and be a cause of debilitating 'spinal' headache. To minimize this complication, very fine needles are used. Spinal anaesthetics are usually 'single shot' and last up to two hours. The spinal cord ends at the level of the body of L1; at or above this level, the cord is tethered and is at risk of being skewered by a needle; below this, there is the freely floating cauda equina and a needle tends to push the nerves away. In consequence, spinal anaesthetics are administered below the level of L1. The anaesthetic introduced is close to the nerves, and very small volumes can produce satisfactory blocks with very rapid onset. The agent introduced into the subarachnoid space can be 'floated' in the CSF towards the desired level of block above the level of insertion by appropriate positioning of the patient.

Complications

Epidural and spinal anaesthesia carry the same hazards as all other nerve blocks, but local complications in the central nervous system can be catastrophic, as follows:
- Infection in the vertebral column can result in meningitis or cord compression secondary to abscess formation.
- Haematoma can also lead to cord compression. This is a surgical emergency and requires urgent assessment and treatment.
- Epidural cannulae can shift over time or be misplaced from the beginning, so that inadvertent epidural venous cannulation can lead to rapid onset of local anaesthetic toxicity, and an unrecognized spinal tap can lead to an epidural dose being injected spinally, with dangerously high levels of block.
- Epidural and spinal anaesthetics block not only motor and sensory nerves but also vasomotor control; vasodilatation and a fall in the blood pressure may result.

Such anaesthetic blockade should never be performed without the same preparation and monitoring as for a general anaesthetic.

Antibiotics

Microbiology and antibiotic use are extensive and complex areas, with unique considerations to be had in the surgical setting. This section aims to explore and contextualize these topics within surgery rather than to replace dedicated microbiology or pharmacology sources of reference.

General Principles of Antibiotic Usage

There are a set of principles which underpin the use of antibiotics throughout healthcare, which are equally applicable in the surgical setting:
1. Antibiotic use and agent choices should be guided by the stewardship program of microbiology physicians at each healthcare institution. These guidelines factor in several issues including local resistance patterns, medication

Faculty of Pain Medicine Safety Checklist for:
Interventional Pain Procedures under local anaesthesia or sedation (adapted from the WHO surgical safety checklist).

Place addressograph label here

SIGN INTO THEATRE To be read out loud

☐ Initial team brief undertaken and staff members have introduced themselves.

Are the anaesthetic machine and monitors checked and emergency drugs drawn up or available?
☐ Yes   ☐ Not applicable

Is all the equipment available including image intensifier/radiographer when applicable?
☐ Yes   ☐ Not applicable

☐ Are all IRMER requirements met?
☐ Patient identity confirmed by local protocol?
☐ Site, procedure and consent confirmed?
   Is the procedure site marked?
☐ Yes   ☐ Not applicable

Does the patient require sedation?
☐ No   ☐ Yes, team notified and patient confirmed to be starved

Is the patient fasted by local protocol?
☐ Yes   ☐ No

Any special monitoring, equipment or positioning requirements?
☐ No   ☐ Yes

Does the patient have a known allergy?
☐ No   ☐ Yes

SIGN INTO THEATRE continued. To be read out loud

Females only: is the patient pregnant?
☐ No   ☐ Yes

Is the patient on anticoagulants (e.g. warfarin, apixaban, dabigatran or rivaroxaban), antiplatelets or at risk of bleeding for any other reason?
☐ No   ☐ Yes, confirm patient management in place: (e.g. anticoagulants stopped, necessary anticoagulation screen undertaken and recorded)

Does the patient have infection (systemic/locally at injection site)?
☐ No   ☐ Yes, proceed only in exceptional circumstances and record clinical reasoning.

Does the patient have diabetes?
☐ No   ☐ Yes, management in place

Does the patient have an ICD/Pacemaker/Implanted Pain device?
☐ No   ☐ Yes, state any special precautions required

Are there any other patient specific concerns?
☐ No   ☐ Yes

Is antibiotic prophylaxis required and been given?
☐ N/A   ☐ Yes

Signatures

A _____

B _____

FACULTY OF **PAIN MEDICINE** of the Royal College of Anaesthetists

continued overleaf...

TIME OUT (To be read out loud before start of pain procedure)

Physician, theatre nurse and registered practitioner verbally confirm:

Patient details, procedure and side?
☐ Yes   ☐ No

Required monitoring in place and sedation given (if necessary)?
☐ Yes   ☐ No

Any anticipated variations (e.g. diathermy pads required) or critical events?
☐ Yes   ☐ No

STOP BEFORE YOU BLOCK

Is everybody happy that the injections is about to be made to the correct side?
☐ Yes

(Compare consent form and theatre list and, if appropriate, involve patient).

Signatures

A _____

B _____

FACULTY OF **PAIN MEDICINE** of the Royal College of Anaesthetists

SIGN OUT (To be read out loud)

Before any member of the team leaves the operating room

Have all the needles, other sharps and diathermy pads been disposed of safely?
☐ Yes   ☐ No

Have any equipment problems been identified that need to be addressed?
☐ Yes   ☐ No

Are any variations to the standard recovery and discharge protocol planned for this patient?
☐ Yes   ☐ No

Is a plan for VTE required made (e.g. patients on anticoagulation)?
☐ Yes   ☐ Not applicable

Have any serial numbers of implanted devices been recorded and plans made for future care?
☐ Yes   ☐ Not applicable

Imaging:- Are appropriate images retained either electronic or hard copy retained?
☐ Yes

Has the procedure been documented?
☐ Yes

Signatures

A _____

B _____

This document is periodically updated based on user feedback and to ensure it meets the highest standards. To comment please contact fpm@rcoa.ac.uk

• **Fig. 2.3** Safety checklist for interventional pain procedures under local anaesthetic or sedation, Faculty of Pain Medicine of the Royal College of Anaesthetists, London. https://fpm.ac.uk/sites/fpm/files/documents/2019-08/Safety%20checklist%20for%20interventional%20pain%20procedures.pdf.

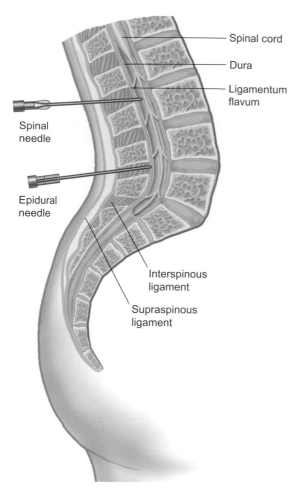

Spinal cord

Dura

Ligamentum flavum

Spinal needle

Epidural needle

Interspinous ligament

Supraspinous ligament

• **Fig. 2.4** The Anatomy of Spinal and Epidural Anaesthesia

availability, pharmacokinetics, pharmacodynamics and cost. These are designed to balance the benefits and risks associated with antibiotics, avoiding improper use such as starting antibiotics without clear evidence of infection and unnecessary prolonged administration.

2. Empirical antibiotic regimens are often used at the time of initial diagnosis while awaiting definitive pathogen identification from culture of swabs, body fluid or blood. Once sensitivities of these organisms have been defined, targeted narrow spectrum antibiotics should be administered.

3. Intravenous antibiotics should be switched to suitable oral alternatives when possible. This would often require there to be clinical resolution of sepsis, improvement in leucocytosis, toleration of oral fluids and the availability of a suitable oral alternative.

4. There are benefits to prescribing antibiotics in combination, such as a synergistic activity against target organisms. Furthermore, combinations ensure the bacteria are sensitive to at least one of the agents (given unknown resistance patterns), which increases the clinical response to infection and decrease the risk of resistance formation.

5. Regular clinical review of patients on antibiotics is crucial to track their progress and identify any deterioration early. This will allow interventions to improve the patient's outcome including change of antibiotic regimen

or use of surgical source control. Decisions regarding the use of antibiotics should involve regular discussions with local microbiology physicians.

6. Antibiotic choices should consider patient factors including existing medications, organ dysfunction, pregnancy status and variations in genetics.

Typical Pathogens Based on Body Site

There are a variety of factors which allow the physician to speculate about the pathogen or group of pathogens that are likely to be responsible for a given infection in a surgical patient, largely based on the body site affected (Fig. 2.5). These include adaptations to increase the virulence of certain pathogens, proximity to areas of certain bacterial populations, available routes of spread (including the surgical incision) and favourable tissue conditions for the pathogen. For this reason, empirical antibiotic regimens are different based on the body site being treated.

Antibiotic Types

Antibiotics are most commonly categorized by a mixture of their structure and their mechanism of action. Table 2.3 lists those that are commonly used in surgical patients, with it worth noting that those within the same classes often have similar pathogen coverage, clinical uses and side effects. The application of these to specific clinical scenarios will be explored later in this section.

Antibiotic Use in Prophylactic and Emergent Settings

Antibiotics can be administered to surgical patients preoperatively to prevent infections (prophylaxis) or to improve the outcomes from established infections (therapeutic).

The aim of prophylactic antibiotics given at the time of anaesthetic induction is to reduce the risk of surgical site infection with minimal impact on the patient's normal flora or the development of unwanted side effects. Patients can be stratified into three groups based on their risk and consequences of infection, with different antibiotic prophylaxis regimens recommended for each (Table 2.4).

Emergent use of antibiotics for the treatment of established infections is commonplace and is often used alongside surgical intervention to resolve the infection. In the case of a patient suffering with sepsis, these should be started within 1 hour to complement the other supportive measures to improve the patient's outcome (such as the use of intravenous fluid resuscitation). Surgical intervention is often indicated, such as when an infectious source requires definitive control and conservative measures would carry a higher morbidity and mortality risk than with the procedure. An example of this is faecal peritonitis from a perforated colonic diverticulum, where surgical source control (colonic resection and washout) is vital to avoid overwhelming sepsis and clinical deterioration. The duration of antibiotic therapy in this emergent setting

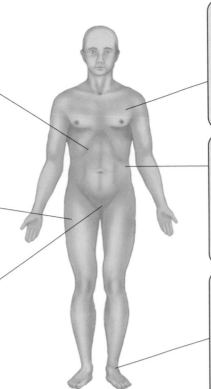

Hepatobiliary

Conditions: ascending cholangitis, cholecystitis, hepatic abcess.

Most likely to ascend from the GI tract
- **Gram –** (~90% e.g. *E. coli, Klesiella, Enterobacter*)
- **Gram+** (~10% e.g. *Enterococci*)

Joint and Prosthesis

Conditions: Septic arthritis, prosthetic infection.

Most likely to enter via the skin if an incision or trauma:
- **Gram +** (~90% e.g. *Stapylococci, Streptococci*)
- **Gram –** (~10% e.g. *Neisseria, gonorrhoeae, Pseudomonas aeruginosa*)

Urinary Tract

Conditions: catheter associated UTI, prostatitis, pyelonephritis.

Most likely to be gastrointestinal pathogens that ascend the urethra or associated with a catheter biofilm:
- **Gram –** (~90% e.g. *E. coli, Klebsiella, Enterobacter, proteus*)
- **Gram +** (~10% e.g. *Staphylococcus saprophyticus*)

Respiratory Tract

Conditions: hospital-acquired pneumonia, aspiration pneumonia

Pathogens differ in prevalence from community-acquired pneumonia:
- **Gram –** (e.g. *Haemophilus influenzae, Pseudomonas aeruginosa*)
- **Gram +** (e.g. MRSA, *Streptococcus pneumoniae*)

Peritonitis from Colorectal Source

Conditions: diverticulitis, appendicitis, colonic perforation

Pathogens most likely colonisers of the lower GI tract and infections are commonly polymicrobial:
- **Gram –** (e.g. *E. coli, Klebsiella, Enterobacter, Bacteroiides fragilis*)
- **Gram +** (<10% e.g. *Enterococci*)

Peritonitis from Colorectal Source

Conditions: infected leg ulcers, cellulitis

Pathogens are most likely from the skin and often initially as colonisers, creating polymicrobial infections:
- **Gram –** (e.g. *Pseudomonas aeruginosa, Klebsiella*)
- **Gram +** (e.g. *Staphylococci, Streptococci*)

• **Fig. 2.5** Common Infections Requiring Treatment in the Pre- and Postoperative Surgical Patient

TABLE 2.3 Best Practice for Prescribing an Antimicrobial for Perioperative Prophylaxis

Risk	Operative Features	Example Procedures	Prophylaxis Recommended	Example Regimen	If penicillin allergy
Low	Short duration (<2 hours) No use of prosthesis Surgery on clean tissue	• Open hernia repair without mesh • Simple hand surgery • Sinus surgery without a graft	None	-	
Medium	Clean-contaminated surgery Prolonged surgical time	• Colorectal resection • Cholecystectomy	IV antibiotics at induction only	Amoxicillin 1 g IV + gentamicin 3 mg/kg IV	Teicoplanin 400 mg IV + gentamicin 3 mg/kg IV
	Graft or prosthesis implantation	• Open aortic aneurysm repair • Total hip replacement • Aortic valve repair	IV antibiotics at induction and for 24 hours postoperatively	Ceftriaxone 2 g IV	Teicoplanin 400 mg IV gentamicin 5 mg/kg IV
High	Contaminated surgery Extensive dissection	• Colonic resection with significant spillage • Extensive peritoneal stripping with ascites	IV antibiotics at induction and for up to 5 days postoperatively	Amoxicillin 1 g IV + gentamicin 3 mg/kg IV + metronidazole 500 mg IV	Teicoplanin 400 mg gentamicin 3 mg/kg metronidazole 500 mg IV

Choice of antibiotics should be made according to data on pharmacology, microbiology and local guidelines which may vary. Be sure to check for allergies and be aware of the side effects of these medications, and adjust the dose where necessary for renal function (e.g. gentamicin). Single doses are indicated for the majority of procedures. The reason for antibiotic administration beyond one dose should be documented and comply with criteria such as significant intraoperative blood loss - >1.5 litre (re-dose following fluid replacement), prolonged procedures (>6 hours) or primary arthroplasty, where 24 hours prophylaxis is acceptable.

TABLE 2.4	Stratification of Patients by Procedure is Used to Guide Antibiotic Prophylaxis.			
Risk	Operative Features	Example Procedures	Prophylaxis Recommended	Example Regimen[b]
Low	Short duration (<2 hours) No use of prosthesis Surgery on clean tissue	• Open hernia repair without mesh • Simple hand surgery • Sinus surgery without a graft	None	–
Medium	Clean-contaminated surgery[a] Prolonged surgical time Graft or prosthesis implantation	• Colorectal resection • Cholecystectomy	i.v. antibiotics at induction only	1.5 g cefuroxime i.v. & 500 mg metronidazole i.v.
		• Open aortic aneurysm repair • Total hip replacement • Aortic valve repair	i.v. antibiotics at induction and for 24 hours postoperatively	1.5 g cefuroxime i.v. & 1.5 g vancomycin i.v.
High	Contaminated surgery[c] Extensive dissection	• Colonic resection with significant spillage • Extensive peritoneal stripping with ascites	i.v. antibiotics at induction and for up to 5 days postoperatively	1.5 g cefuroxime i.v. & 500 mg metronidazole i.v.

[a]Clean-contaminated surgery is defined as a procedure where the respiratory, alimentary or genitourinary tracts are entered but there is not significant contamination.
[b]These are typical antibiotic prophylaxis examples, with regimens often specific to individual healthcare providers. If a patient is MRSA positive on preoperative swabs, an additional dose of i.v. vancomycin would usually be recommended.
[c]Contaminated surgery is defined as a procedure where there is active infection (generally without purulence) or gross spillage of bowel contents. In this category, the antibiotics used for prophylaxis could also be considered part of a treatment regimen.

is tailored to the underlying diagnosis, clinical response of the patient, presence of bacteraemia and the timing of surgical control of the septic focus. Mild cholecystitis can often be managed with 5 days of oral antibiotics, whereas over 10 days of intravenous antibiotics can be needed for bacteraemia secondary to a slowly resolving pelvic abscess. Examples of regimens used in the emergent setting can be seen in Table 2.5.

Cautions

Antibiotic use is not without its risks and several factors always need to be considered when using them clinically:

• **Hypersensitivity and allergy:** This can present as anaphylaxis (type I, IgE mediated) or as a delayed response (types II–IV), with cross-reactivity between different antibiotic classes noted (particularly penicillins and cephalosporins). Antibiotics are the main cause of life-threatening allergic reactions during surgery. Teicoplanin causes 38% of antibiotic-induced anaphylaxis, despite accounting for only 12% of antibiotic use. Teicoplanin is regularly used for patients who report allergy to penicillin, but was associated with the highest incidence of life-threatening anaphylaxis (16.4 episodes per 100 000 administrations compared with 4.0 per 100 000 administrations for antibiotics overall). As 90% of patients who report penicillin allergy are not in fact allergic, better identification of true allergy is needed to reduce risk.[4]

• **Side effects:** These range from commonly reported nausea and gastrointestinal upset to potentially clinically significant side effects such as cholestasis with co-amoxiclav or tendon rupture with ciprofloxacin.

• **Development of resistant strains:** Bacteria are at risk of developing resistance to antibiotics when they are subjected to sub-lethal tissue concentrations. Furthermore, innately resistant bacteria (through mutation or incorporation of foreign genetic material) increase in prevalence from selective pressures as their susceptible peers perish from antibiotic use. This increases the risk of future infections being by a resistant organism which will not be susceptible to empirical therapies.

• **Increased risk of other infections:** Use of cephalosporins, penicillins, clindamycin and ciprofloxacin are associated with the development of *Clostridium difficile* colitis, which can cause life-threatening toxic megacolon. Furthermore, antibiotic use increases the risk of developing a fungal infection.

• **Medication interaction:** Medication interactions are increasingly common with the rise in polypharmacy. Antibiotics can inhibit or induce the cytochrome P450 complex which is a common enzyme for the metabolism of medications. An example is with ciprofloxacin, which inhibits CYP1A2 and its administration can increase the serum concentration of medications such as theophylline by up to 100%.

• **Long-term changes to host flora:** Systemic use of antibiotics has been demonstrated to change the composition of host microbial populations, which from long-term epidemiological studies appears to be correlated with the incidence of conditions such as asthma and colorectal adenomas.

Anticoagulants

Surgical patients are commonly in the unfortunate position that they present several risk factors for venous

TABLE 2.5 Sample Antibiotic Regimens for a Variety of Emergency Conditions in Surgical Patients.

Diagnosis	Initial Therapeutic. Regimen	Duration[a]	Rationale and Notes
Septic arthritis	2 g i.v. flucloxacillin 4h	At least 4 weeks but may be over 6 weeks in complicated cases	Flucloxacillin has excellent Gram+ cover, relevant for the likely pathogens of *Staphylococcus aureus* and *Streptococcal* species. Vancomycin may be substituted if MRSA suspected or ceftriaxone if gonococcal or Gram– suspicion
Moderate to severe intra-abdominal sepsis (including diverticulitis, appendicitis, colonic perforation, ascending cholangitis)	1.5 g i.v. cefuroxime TDS 500 mg i.v. metronidazole TDS +/– i.v. gentamicin OD	2–10 days depending on diagnosis	Cefuroxime has a good coverage of Gram– (and some Gram+), with the metronidazole covering anaerobes such as *Bacteroides*. Gentamicin gives additional Gram– cover and can be considered when there is significant evidence of sepsis. The duration of treatment largely depends on the timing of source control and resolution of clinical sepsis
Peritonsillar abscess	1.2 g i.v. benzylpenicillin QDS 500 mg i.v. metronidazole TDS	7 days	Penicillin covers the high likelihood of a streptococcal infection with metronidazole covering for anaerobes such as *Fusobacterium* and *Bacteroides*. Caution should be taken as there are increasing levels of penicillin resistance
C. difficile colitis	125 mg PO vancomycin QDS +/– 500 mg i.v. metronidazole	14 days	Vancomycin is not absorbed orally and therefore can act locally in the colonic lumen. When the colitis is severe, metronidazole can be added. Resistance to these agents is low
Acute prostatitis	500 mg PO ciprofloxacin BD	At least 2 weeks	Gram– such as *Escherichia coli* (>80% of prostatitis) and *Enterobacter* are the most common pathogens and are highly susceptible to ciprofloxacin. It has a high bioavailability and penetrates well into tissues, promoting oral administration
Necrotizing fasciitis	2 g i.v. ceftriaxone OD 1.2 g i.v. clindamycin i.v. i.v. amikacin OD	At least 2 weeks but often over 4 weeks	Broad-spectrum antibiotics are chosen to cover a wide range of pathogens in this potentially polymicrobial infection. Clindamycin gives additional anaerobic cover and decreases toxin production. After initial cultures, the antibiotics can be rationalised, and treatment duration is subject to repeated clinical review

[a]The duration of antibiotics is subject to ongoing clinical review and represents the total course length, where there is commonly a step-down to oral agents well in advance of course completion. OD = Once per day; TDS = three times per day; QDS = four times per day; i.v. = intravenous.

thromboembolism (VTE) – including increased age, general anaesthetic, co-morbidities, immobility, dehydration and presence of malignancy. A surgical patient developing either a deep venous thrombosis or pulmonary embolism has significant morbidity and mortality consequences. This is considered largely avoidable if appropriate measures for primary prevention are initiated early, of which administration of anticoagulants is a mainstay both as an inpatient and, in some cases, following discharge. Anticoagulation also has a role in a therapeutic setting, where treatment is required for established thrombotic disease of either the arterial or venous system.

Who Should Receive Pharmacological Prophylaxis for VTE?

On admission, every surgical patient should have their personalized risk for development of VTE both assessed and documented, with the understanding that this assessment may need to be updated later if clinical factors change. Although specific regimens differ between institutions, the principles for VTE prevention are universal. The lowest risk surgical patients are those with no established risk factors for VTE, which tends to include younger healthy patients, having relatively minor procedures in an ambulatory setting. In this cohort, conservative measures of VTE

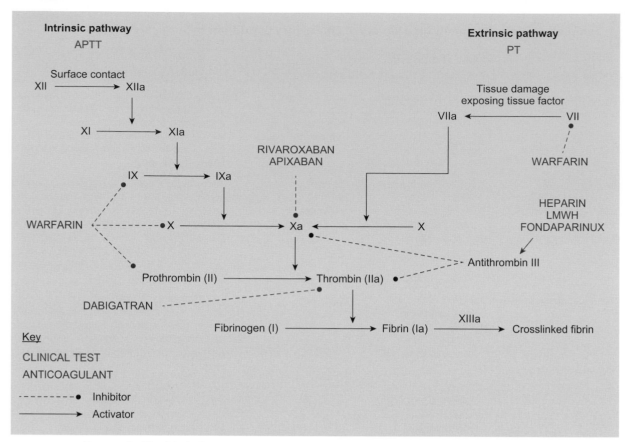

• **Fig. 2.6** A Simplified Coagulation Cascade, Noting the Site of Action for the Common Anticoagulants APTT, Activated partial thromboplastin time; LMWH, low molecular weight heparin; PT, prothrombin time.

prophylaxis are likely to suffice (including early mobilization and compression stockings). However, as soon as a patient's risk is clinically deemed to be moderate or high, it is likely that the benefits of pharmacological prophylaxis outweigh the risks.

A variety of anticoagulants can be used in the prophylactic setting, which is explored later in this section. They are commonly prescribed at doses significantly below that for therapeutic intention and therefore surgical re-intervention can be performed if necessary, without a reversal medication. Contraindications for anticoagulation include patients having active bleeding or at high risk of major bleeding (thrombocytopaenia, recent neurosurgery, recent gastrointestinal bleed, underlying coagulopathy or recent epidural anaesthesia).

There are cohorts of patients where prophylactic anticoagulation may be beneficial following discharge from hospital, often for a period of 2–4 weeks. These include patients having undergone colorectal resection for cancer or inflammatory bowel disease, following a large joint replacement or with significant joint immobility such as a cast for Achilles tendon rupture. Detailed guidance has been released by NICE on this topic, and this can be reviewed here: https://www.nice.org.uk/guidance/ng89.

The Coagulation Cascade and Common Anticoagulants

The coagulation cascade uses clotting factors created in the liver (with the exception of factor VIII) to convert soluble components into an insoluble fibrin mesh (Fig. 2.6). This can be triggered either by tissue damage (extrinsic pathway) or contact with exposed collagen (intrinsic pathway), with both ending in a common pathway by activating factor X. Anticoagulant medications can interact and influence this pathway in a variety of ways.

Unfractionated heparin (UFH) – Heparin potentiates the action of antithrombin III in its inhibition of thrombin and factor Xa. As a result of its short half-life (90 minutes), it is commonly administered intravenously twice daily for prophylaxis or as a continuous infusion for therapeutic dosing. For appropriate therapeutic UFH dosing, the activated partial thromboplastin time (APTT) is monitored and a ratio to a normal clotting time is given, with a target range of 2–2.5 most commonly applied. The anti-Xa level is also a measure of UFH dosing, which can be used in cases of suspected heparin resistance. The short half-life of UFH is such that surgical intervention can be performed shortly after the continuous infusion has ceased; however, in cases of overdose of significant bleeding, protamine sulphate can be given as an antidote. UFH has advantages over other types of anticoagulation as it is safer in renal failure and does not cross the placenta. A significant complication of UFH infusion is heparin-induced thrombocytopaenia, which has an incidence of approximately 2%.

Low molecular weight heparin (LWMH) – These are a subgroup of unfractionated heparins which have undergone depolymerization to decrease the chain length, changing the pharmacological profile and therefore how they are applied clinically. The mechanism of action is similar to UFH; however, LMWH have higher affinity for inhibiting factor Xa rather than thrombin. The half-life of LMWH is significantly longer, such that one or twice daily subcutaneous dosing is sufficient for either therapeutic or prophylactic use, which can often be self-administered by patients. Examples of LMWHs are enoxaparin, dalteparin and tinzaparin, all of which benefit from the lack of need for clinical monitoring and a lower risk of heparin induced thrombocytopaenia than UFH. Dose adjustment or switching to UFH may be required in renal failure due to reduced clearance.

Fondaparinux – This has a similar pentasaccharide structure to heparin and therefore acts in a similar way by binding to (and potentiating) antithrombin III; however, the lack of additional chain means this is not considered a heparin. It does not appear to cause thrombocytopaenia.

Warfarin – This is a derivative of coumarin which blocks the enzyme vitamin K epoxide reductase and abolishes the levels of active vitamin K, required for the production of the clotting factors II, VII, IX, X (in addition to proteins C and S). Warfarin is administered orally on a once daily regimen; however, the required dose varies significantly between patients. A usual starting dose is 5 mg and the international normalized ratio (INR) is then monitored to guide future dosing (aiming for an INR of 2–3 for the majority of indications). Warfarin is used for long-term anticoagulation rather than inpatient prophylaxis due to the duration required to achieve the anticoagulative effect and the relative difficulties in reversal. The effects of warfarin can be reversed by ceasing the medication (taking several days), the administration of vitamin K (approximately 8–12 hours), replenishment of factors with fresh frozen plasma (approximately 1 hour) or near-immediate reversal with prothrombin complex concentrates, depending on the clinical urgency. This medication is teratogenic and warfarin can interact with several foods and medications to cause a fluctuating INR.

Non-vitamin K antagonist oral anticoagulants (NOACs) – Since 2010 a variety of novel oral anticoagulants have been licensed, including dabigatran, apixaban and rivaroxaban. They act by either inhibiting factor Xa (noted by an 'xa' in the medication name) or thrombin. They are given orally with once daily dosing and do not require monitoring. An example of a NOAC being used in UK surgical practice is following total hip or knee replacement, where administration of dabigatran is recommended for 28 or 10 days, respectively.

Pharmacological Principles for Treatment of Malignancy

Anti-cancer drugs are administered to surgical patients to improve their outcome from neoplastic disease. This is commonly with curative intent, where they are used to complement operative resection in the goal of ensuring disease remission and extending disease-free survival. When used in the palliative setting, anti-cancer drugs aim to reduce the risk of disease progression, prolong overall survival and help alleviate symptoms.

There are a variety of medication types used in the treatment of malignancy:

- **Chemotherapeutics** – cytotoxic medications which target cells with a high proliferation rate, a hallmark of cancers. A variety of approaches are utilized to interrupt cell division, with medications commonly used to disrupt the synthesis of DNA and RNA. Categories of chemotherapeutics include anti-metabolites (structural imitators of natural compounds used in DNA synthesis), alkylating agents (addition of an alkyl group to guanine within DNA prevents correct double helix folding), inhibitors of mitosis (interaction with tubulin disrupts the metaphase) and topoisomerase inhibitors (interfering with topoisomerases in the control of the shape of DNA)
- **Small molecule therapy** – inhibitors of enzymes which are overexpressed or mutated in tumours, such as the receptor tyrosine kinases. An example is trastuzumab (Herceptin), a monoclonal antibody which causes down-regulation of the human epidermal growth factor receptor 2 in breast cancers
- **Hormonal therapy** – hormone blockers can be used to inhibit tumours where proliferation is hormonally driven. An example is degarelix, an antagonist of luteinizing hormone releasing hormone used in prostate cancer
- **Immunotherapies** – immune modulators to enhance the activity of the patient's immune system against cancer cells. An example is pembrolizumab, a monoclonal antibody to inhibit the programmed cell death protein 1 on lymphocytes, acting to promote detection of tumour cells by the immune system

The biological susceptibility of different tumour types demonstrates significant inter- and intra-tumour heterogeneity. This requires tailoring of chemotherapeutic regimens to both the primary cancer type in addition to any metabolic or genetic subtypes. This can often require combination therapy in addition to other modes of anti-cancer approaches such as radiotherapy. Combination therapy benefits from being able to maximize tumour cell death whilst avoiding unacceptable toxicity to the patient.

Timing of Administration

When used in conjunction with surgical intervention, the administration timing of pharmaceuticals is a significant consideration when striving for optimal efficacy. There are three general time periods: pre-, intra- and postoperative, with the following examples in colorectal cancer:

- **Neoadjuvant** – administration of agents in advance of surgical intervention, with the aim of achieving down-staging of the tumour or for the promotion of organ preservation. Long course neoadjuvant chemo-radio-therapy for locally advanced rectal cancer decreases local recurrence by up to 50%
- **Intra-operative** – chemotherapeutics given during operative resection. A novel approach over the past 15 years has seen patients with peritoneal carcinomatosis from advanced colorectal cancer undergo cytoreductive surgery (to remove all macroscopic metastatic disease), followed by delivery of hyperthermic intraperitoneal chemotherapy (HIPEC). Initial data using this technique demonstrated an improved overall survival from 12.5 to 22 months compared to systemic chemotherapy alone, with some new studies suggesting that these benefits are in fact mediated by the cytoreductive surgery component rather than the addition of HIPEC.[5] This remains contentious and new data are awaited
- **Adjuvant** – medications are given in the postoperative period. The presence of lymph node micrometastasis in a colonic surgical specimen increases the risk of future recurrent disease. When adjuvant chemotherapy is given in patients with nodal but not metastatic disease (stage III), the recurrence and mortality rates fall by up to 40%

The duration for which anti-cancer medications should be administered varies based on the cancer type, agent being used, toxicity profile and clinical response (Box 2.7). Therapeutic regimens are often initiated, and then patient review may prompt continuation of therapy, change of agents or ceasing of therapy. The strategy for chemotherapy is considered in more detail in Chapter 4.

Summary

Surgical patients are often co-morbid and they will be exposed to a large number of drugs during their inpatient stay. However, these can be very safely managed providing that the surgeon is aware of the fundamentals of basic pharmacology and safe prescribing. This requires the adoption of best local practices and checklists and a meticulous attention to detail.

• BOX 2.7 Examples of Chemotherapeutic Regimens in Cancers

Primary Organ	Example Regimen
Breast	12 weeks i.v. doxorubicin and cyclophosphamide followed by 8 weeks i.v. paclitaxel
Endometrial	18 weeks of i.v. carboplatin and i.v. docetaxel
Colorectal	12 weeks of i.v. oxaliplatin and PO capecitabine
Lung (non-small cell subtype)	12 weeks of i.v. cisplatin and i.v. vinblastine

References

1. de Vries EN, Ramrattan MA, Smorenburg SM, Gouma DJ, Boermeester MA. The incidence and nature of in-hospital adverse events: a systematic review. *Qual Saf Health Care.* 2008;17(3):216–223. https://doi.org/10.1136/qshc.2007.023622.
2. de Boer M, Boeker EB, Ramrattan MA, et al. Adverse drug events in surgical patients: an observational multicentre study. *Int J Clin Pharm.* 2013;35(5):744–752. https://doi.org/10.1007/s11096-013-9797-5.
3. Cook T, et al. *2018. Report and findings of the Royal College of Anaesthetists' 6th National Audit Project: perioperative anaphylaxis*; 2018.
4. Savic LC, Garcez T, Hopkins PM, Harper NJ, Savic S. Teicoplanin allergy - an emerging problem in the anaesthetic allergy clinic. *Br J Anaesth.* 2015;115(4):595–600. https://doi.org/10.1093/bja/aev307.
5. Smith ME, Nathan H. Cytoreductive Surgery and Hyperthermic Intraperitoneal Chemotherapy: Safety Is Only Half of the Story. *JAMA Netw Open.* 2019;2(1):e186839. https://doi.org/10.1001/jamanetworkopen.2018.6839.

3

Disorders of Growth, Differentiation and Morphogenesis

CHAPTER OUTLINE

Introduction

Growth, differentiation and morphogenesis are terms used to describe the numerous complex, highly regulated physiological processes that are fundamental to normal development and maintenance of health throughout life. Errors in growth, differentiation and morphogenesis during embryological development lead to congenital anomalies which, despite their nomenclature, may present to the surgeon in childhood or adulthood. For example, a child with Meckel's diverticulum usually presents before the age of 2 years with intestinal obstruction and intussusception, whereas an adult with a congenitally bicuspid aortic valve usually presents at 50–60 years of age with aortic stenosis. In addition, disorders of growth, differentiation and morphogenesis are seen in many organ systems as a result of disease. For example, patients with Grave's disease develop an enlarged thyroid gland due to abnormal growth of thyroid follicular epithelial cells, whilst patients with gastro-oesophageal reflux disease may develop Barrett's oesophagus, whereby oesophageal epithelial cells fail to show normal differentiation. Finally, all human cancers develop by manipulating the regulatory mechanisms that oversee growth, differentiation and morphogenesis and our improved understanding of these processes has paved the way for new therapeutic options.

An understanding of normal growth, differentiation and morphogenesis is essential in order to understand the related disorders that are commonly encountered in surgical practice. We will explore these processes and the regulatory mechanisms that oversee them before discussing associated disorders.

Growth

At a cellular level, growth is affected by cell size, number or both cell size and number. At a sub-cellular level, cell size is largely determined by the amount of intracellular protein, which depends on the balance between protein synthesis and protein degradation within a cell. For example, a muscle cell may increase in size due to increased myofibril synthesis. Conversely, cells may become smaller, by a process which includes autophagocytosis, when they receive inadequate nutrition and this is associated with protein catabolism. Cell number increases by cell division, which occurs in the last step of the cell cycle. Cell number decreases following cell death, which may be secondary to apoptosis (programmed cell death), necrosis (pathological cell death) or necroptosis (a form of programmed cell death which appears similar to necrosis). There are several other mechanisms of cell death including pyroptosis, autophagic cell death and ferroptosis, which we will discuss in further detail later on in this section.

At the tissue and organ level, growth is also affected by the amount of intercellular material (i.e. between individual cells) that is present. Intercellular material is synthesized by cells found within the connective tissue stroma, for example fibroblasts are stromal cells which secrete collagen and other extracellular matrix proteins. The terms used to describe these types of growth are shown in Table 3.1.

The Cell Cycle

The cell cycle is a tightly regulated sequence of events that lead to cell division, increasing the number of cells and resulting in growth (Fig. 3.1). There are four phases: gap 1 (G_1), synthesis (S), gap 2 (G_2) and mitosis (M). The cells which are not actively cycling are said to be quiescent and in G_0 phase. DNA synthesis occurs during S phase and cell division occurs at the end of M phase. G_1 and G_2 phases represent important regulatory times which are largely controlled by proteins called cyclins, cyclin-dependent kinases (CDKs) and CDK inhibitors (see Fig. 3.1).

Cyclins are so-named because they 'cycle' between high and low levels during the cell cycle. When a cyclin is present at increased levels, a corresponding CDK is activated and phosphorylates proteins within the cell that trigger progression onto the next phase of the cell cycle. On the other hand, CDK inhibitors can halt cell cycle progression by inhibiting

the action of CDKs. An important example of this is the Cyclin D1, CDK4, p16 and retinoblastoma (Rb) pathway: Cyclin D1 concentration is increased during G1 phase and forms a complex with CDK4 called the Cyclin D1-CDK4 complex. This Cyclin D1-CDK4 complex phosphorylates Rb and the cell progresses onto S phase of the cell cycle. p16 is a CDK inhibitor that functions by binding to CDK4 and preventing the formation of the Cyclin D1-CDK4 complex. This pathway is mutated in some human cancers (Clinical Correlation Box 3.1).

CLINICAL CORRELATION BOX 3.1

p16 is encoded by the CDKN2A tumour suppressor gene, which is sporadically inactivated in many cancers, e.g. up to 95% of pancreatic cancers. Inactivation of the CDKN2A gene leads to loss of the normal inhibitory function of p16 in G1 phase. There is no inhibition of the Cyclin D1-CDK4 complex, and Rb protein is hyperphosphorylated. As such, cells with this mutation divide uncontrollably. Pancreatic carcinoma is associated with a very poor prognosis and it is through understanding of its molecular mechanisms that new preventative strategies and treatments may emerge.

Germline mutations in CDKN2A are found in families with familial atypical multiple-mole melanoma syndrome. Of interest, these families are also at increased risk of pancreatic carcinoma.

Different cell types spend different amounts of time completing the cell cycle: the rapidly dividing cells of early embryogenesis spend around 30 minutes completing the cycle, while keratinocytes of the skin turn over around once every 50 days, and some cells may take months or years to complete the cell cycle. On the other hand, cells may permanently leave the cell cycle and lose the ability to divide: these cells are said to be terminally differentiated and cells within this category include neurones and cardiac myocytes. G1 phase shows the most variation in time between cell types, whilst S phase, G2 phase and M phase remain relatively constant in duration.

TABLE 3.1	Types of Growth
Multiplicative growth (Hyperplasia)	Growth due to an increase in cell number
Auxetic growth (Hypertrophy)	Growth due to an increase in cell size
Accretionary growth	Growth due to an increase in the amount of intercellular tissue, for example osteoid secretion by osteoblasts during bone growth

Adapted from Cross S. Underwood's Pathology: a Clinical Approach, sixth ed. Churchill Livingstone, Edinburgh; 2013.

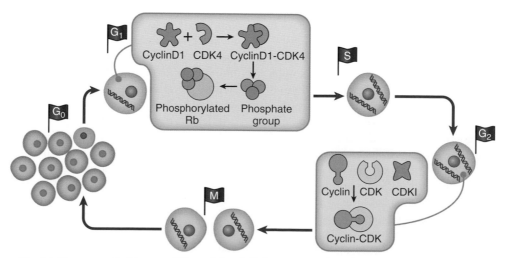

• **Fig. 3.1** Diagrammatic Representation of the Cell Cycle Including Expansion of G1, S, G2 and M Phases and Inclusion of Cyclin D1/CDK4/RB Regulatory Mechanism (Courtesy of L. Morrison.)

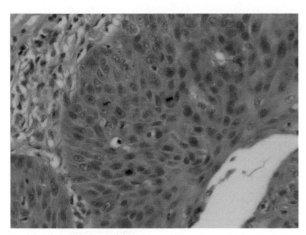

• **Fig. 3.2** This Histological Image of Dysplastic Epithelium Shows Numerous Mitotic Figures.

Cells in M phase can be seen relatively easily under the microscope because nuclear chromatin condenses (i.e. changes from heterochromatin to euchromatin) during mitosis and this can be visualized. The presence of a high number of mitoses or abnormal looking mitoses is used by the pathologist as evidence that the cell cycle is turning over at increased levels or occurring within mutated cells, and is one of the microscopic signs of cancer (Fig. 3.2).

Apoptosis

Apoptosis is a genetically programmed series of molecular events that culminates in the death and removal of unwanted or damaged cells from the body. Apoptosis can be thought of as complementary to mitosis in normal cell turnover and tissue homeostasis. As such, failure of apoptosis, which can be due to an increase or decrease in apoptotic activity, leads to a wide range of diseases. In the developing embryo, groups of cells must apoptose at set times and when this goes awry, it results in congenital malformations, for example, syndactyly (the failure of separation of the fingers). Congenital malformations will be discussed further in a later section of this chapter. Cancer cells often have mutations in genes that inhibit the apoptotic pathway, which allows them to survive and grow despite harbouring genetic mutations. Pathological apoptosis is the term used to describe apoptosis that occurs secondary to an underlying disease process which may be inflammatory or malignant. For example, apoptotic cells are seen in non-alcoholic fatty liver disease where they are known as acidophil bodies.

An apoptotic cell can be easily recognized under the microscope. In the initial stages of apoptosis, the cell is shrunken (and more acidophilic on Haematoxylin and Eosin staining) compared to its normal counterpart, and the nucleus is described as pyknotic (shrunken and more dense due to chromatin condensation) and starts to fragment. The cell then begins to entirely break down by releasing small cytoplasmic blebs from the cell membrane. These blebs detach from the cell and are seen as apoptotic bodies within the intercellular space. The apoptotic bodies are phagocytosed by macrophages with little to no associated inflammatory reaction (Clinical Correlation Box 3.2).

CLINICAL CORRELATION BOX 3.2

Physiological and Pathological Apoptosis

Hypertrophic and keloid scars are important causes of post-surgical functional and aesthetic impairment and represent defective wound healing. Under normal circumstances, a scar forms in wounds which are unable to completely regenerate, e.g. due to complete loss of regenerative cells by severe damage. This occurs through stages of inflammation, angiogenesis and the deposition and remodelling of extracellular matrix. Extracellular matrix is deposited and remodelled by fibroblasts which then undergo apoptosis, leaving behind collagen and fibrotic tissue. In hypertrophic and keloid scars, excessive amounts of collagen are deposited compared to that seen in a simple scar. This is, at least in part, due to failure of fibroblasts (which are the major source of collagen) to undergo normal apoptosis.

There are two pathways of apoptosis: the intrinsic and extrinsic pathways. The intrinsic pathway is a solely intracellular process and can be triggered by many factors that indicate to the cell that it is damaged or no longer required, e.g. detection of DNA damage, presence of misfolded protein or lack of growth factor stimulation (Clinical Correlation Box 3.3). The extrinsic pathway involves the action of an extracellular ligand and a 'death receptor'. This pathway is used by T-cells in the thymus as part of normal T-cell maturation. Both pathways culminate in the activation of cytosolic enzymes called caspases. Activated caspases, including caspase 3 and caspase 8, can directly degrade cellular organelles and activate other degradative enzymes, e.g. DNAses. Common techniques for identifying apoptotic cells include a technique which identifies the damage to the DNA (Terminal deoxynucleotidyl transferase dUTP Nick End Labeling (**TUNEL**)) or by the immunohistochemical demonstration of caspase 3 activation. The different regulatory proteins involved in the intrinsic and extrinsic apoptotic pathways are illustrated in Fig. 3.3.

CLINICAL CORRELATION BOX 3.3

The protein p53, also known as 'the guardian of the genome', is active during G_1 phase of the cell cycle and can trigger apoptosis in a cell that has accumulated DNA damage. This prevents a mutated cell from dividing – an important regulatory mechanism because division of mutated cells could lead to cancer. Sporadic mutations in TP53, the gene encoding p53, is the most commonly encountered mutation found in human cancer. Mutated p53 protein can be detected by immunohistochemistry and is used by pathologists in the diagnosis and prognostication of different cancers.

Germline mutations in TP53 are seen in families with Li Fraumeni syndrome. These families are at high risk of developing sarcomas, breast cancer, leukaemia and adrenal gland cancers.

- Growth factor signaling
- Misfolded protein
- DNA damage

✳ Cytochrome C

━ Mitochondrial membrane

━ Cytoplasm

⩗ APAF-1

○ Activated caspases

APOPTOSOME

A

Fas | Fas L

▲ Caspase-8

○ Activated caspases

B

• **Fig. 3.3** Intrinsic and Extrinsic Apoptotic Pathways (A) The intrinsic pathway of apoptosis can be triggered by a lack of growth factor stimulation, misfolding of protein or damage to DNA during the cell cycle. This results in leakage of cytochrome C across the mitochondrial membrane into the cytoplasm, where it binds to *APAF-1* (apoptosis-activating factor-1) and forms the apoptosome, resulting in caspase activation and apoptosis. (B) The extrinsic pathway is triggered by binding of FasL (a death ligand) to Fas (a death receptor), resulting in direct activation of caspase-8 and a subsequent cascade of caspase activation. (Courtesy of L. Morrison.)

Necrosis

Cell loss and altered growth may also occur by necrosis. In contrast to apoptosis, necrosis is always pathological and is a sign of underlying disease. Cell loss by necrosis is characterized by the loss of integrity of the cell membrane with leakage of intracellular protein into the surrounding tissue. This results in activation of the inflammatory response which is usually severe and may produce bystander damage to the adjacent normal tissue. Necrotic cells appear morphologically different to apoptotic cells (Fig. 3.4).

There are various patterns of necrosis that are seen depending on the initiating insult:

- Coagulative necrosis – This is seen as a consequence of ischaemia in all organ systems excluding the central nervous system. The cell nucleus disintegrates and the intracellular organelles break down, but 'ghost' outlines of anucleate cells are seen within preserved tissue architecture.

- Liquefactive necrosis – This is seen as a consequence of bacterial infection and abscess formation and as a result of ischaemic necrosis in the central nervous system. Liquefaction represents the complete disintegration of cells so that no remnant of the cell or tissue is left. This is seen in acute bacterial infection because the intense acute inflammatory reaction causes complete dissolution of the cells. It is also seen in central nervous system tissue because neural cells contain large amounts of lipid which rapidly dissolves.

- Fat necrosis – This is seen in the pancreas, breast and in adipose tissue as a result of activation of lipases. Lipases cleave triglycerides into fatty acids and glycerol. The fatty acids combine with calcium ions to form solid deposits of calcium that are often seen in this type of necrosis.

- Caseous necrosis – This is almost always seen in the context of mycobacterial infection (especially tuberculosis) and is so-named because of the gross 'cheese-like' appearance of the affected tissue. Microscopically, the necrotic material is granular.

- Fibrinoid necrosis – This is seen in vasculitis: fibrin and proteins leak out of necrotic vessel walls and accumulate

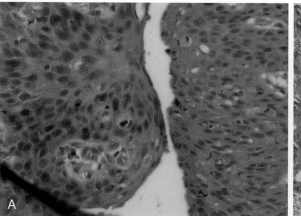
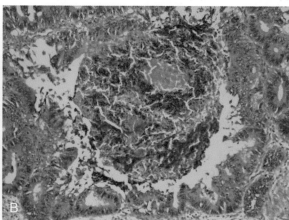

• **Fig. 3.4** Apoptotic Cell Versus Necrotic Tissue (Histological Image) (A) The apoptotic cell appears shrunken and its nucleus is pyknotic. There is no surrounding inflammation. (B) Necrotic tissue comprises cellular debris and inflammation.

around the outside of the dead blood vessel, seen as pink amorphous material.

- Gangrenous necrosis – This is the clinical term given to the appearance of tissue that has become necrotic as a result of interruption to its blood supply, e.g. gangrenous necrosis of the lower limb following acute or chronic limb ischaemia.

Necroptosis

Necroptosis is the term used to describe a type of cell death that shares features of both apoptosis and necrosis. Morphologically, cells undergoing necroptosis look similar to necrotic cells – the cells are swollen and the plasma membrane degrades with leakage of intracellular protein into the surrounding tissue and an inflammatory response. However, necroptosis also shares an important feature of apoptosis in that it is a regulated process that utilizes a genetically programmed intracellular signalling pathway. Receptor-interacting serine/threonine protein kinase 1 and 3 (RIPK1/RIPK3) are important triggers of necroptosis and can be activated by a variety of stimuli. Caspases, which are integral to apoptosis, are not active in necroptosis; in fact, experimental models have shown that caspases can inhibit necroptosis.

Necroptosis is seen in a variety of tissues and organs under physiological and pathological circumstances. Physiological necroptosis occurs in chondrocytes of the bone plate during longitudinal growth of long bones. Common examples of pathological necroptosis include cytomegalovirus infection, reperfusion injury and neurogenerative diseases such as Parkinson's disease.

Pyroptosis, Autophagic Cell Death and Ferroptosis

Pyroptosis, autophagic cell death and ferroptosis represent non-apoptotic forms of programmed cell death that are of emerging importance in a number of different disease states. Pyroptosis, also known as caspase 1-dependent programmed cell death, is seen in conditions associated with marked inflammation including bacterial infection, myocardial infarction and many different cancers. The main mediator is caspase 1 which, as well as activating important inflammatory mediators such as IL-1β and IL-18, causes cell death by disrupting membrane permeability with resultant leakage of intracellular contents into the interstitial space. The resultant histological appearance is similar to necrotic cell death with cellular debris and inflammatory cell infiltrate. Autophagic cell death is characterized by the accumulation of numerous autophagosomes – intracellular vesicles containing partly degraded cellular organelles. The accumulation of autophagosomes can be seen under the microscope as cytoplasmic vacuolations. Ferroptosis is a type of programmed cell death which requires intracellular iron stores and defective lipid peroxidation. It is important in neurodegenerative diseases including Huntingdon's disease.

Control of Growth

There are various factors that can influence growth including hormonal stimulation, biochemical changes, physical/mechanical demand, and changes in blood supply or innervation. These factors act by inducing different cellular signalling pathways, resulting in the switching on or off of certain genes.

Growth factors are biochemical molecules that can increase cell growth. Examples include epidermal growth factor, hepatocyte growth factor, platelet-derived growth factor and insulin-like growth factor. Despite its nomenclature, a single growth factor may show widespread growth-promoting effects on epithelial, mesenchymal and lymphoid cells.

There are many genes that can influence the cell cycle. Gene mutations in cancer tend to fall under the following categories:

- Proto-oncogenes: These genes encode proteins whose normal function is to promote cell growth. When mutated, the genes are instead known as 'oncogenes'. Examples include the *ras* oncogene in thyroid follicular carcinoma, leading to increased activity of a tyrosine kinase receptor.
- Tumour suppressor genes: These genes encode proteins whose normal function is to inhibit cell growth. Mutations in tumour suppressor genes cause loss-of-function of the protein product, e.g. loss of function of p53, leading to survival and proliferation of mutated cells.

More recently genes encoding micro-RNA (miRNA) have also been found to play a role in carcinogenesis. miRNAs are short segments of RNA that act by inhibiting the translation of mRNA into protein. Mutations in many different miRNA genes can lead to production of proteins that alter the cell cycle. These are discussed further later.

Disorders of Growth

Hyperplasia

Hyperplasia is defined as an increase in the size of an organ due to an increase in the number of its constituent cells, i.e. due to multiplicative growth of cells. Cells which show multiplicative growth must be capable of dividing, thus hyperplasia does not occur in organs composed of terminally differentiated cells. The increase in cell number translates to an increase in total cell mass, thus the tissue/organ appears physically enlarged to the naked eye and is increased in weight.

Hyperplasia is seen under normal physiological circumstances. There is hyperplasia of the endometrium during the menstrual cycle with rising levels of oestrogen and progesterone: the endometrium measures around 2 mm at menstruation and can increase up to 11 mm with each menstrual cycle. Furthermore, there is hyperplasia of the breast during puberty, pregnancy and lactation, again in response to changing hormonal levels. Hyperplasia can also be an adaptive response to damage or injury. The liver is one of the best studied examples of an organ that can adjust its

TABLE 3.2 **Pathological Hyperplasia: Examples.**

Organ	Cellular Changes	Clinical Features
Thyroid	Multiplicative growth of thyroid follicular epithelial cells, e.g. due to iodine deficiency	Multinodular goitre, neck lump, dyspnoea, dysphagia
Breast	Multiplicative growth of ductal epithelial cells	Usual-type epithelial hyperplasia, calcifications on mammography
Prostate	Multiplicative growth of glandular and stromal epithelial cells due to continued stimulation by androgens with increasing age	Benign prostatic hyperplasia and lower urinary tract symptoms
Endometrium	Multiplicative growth of endometrial glandular cells due to imbalance in oestrogen/progesterone levels	Endometrial hyperplasia and post-menopausal bleeding
Adrenal gland	Multiplicative growth of adrenal cortical cells due to increased levels of adrenocorticotropic hormone	Cushing's disease

TABLE 3.3 **Pathological Hypertrophy: Examples.**

Organ	Cellular Changes	Clinical Features
Heart – left ventricular hypertrophy	Auxetic growth of cardiac myocytes	Cardiac failure, arrhythmia, sudden death
Lung – hypertrophy of bronchial wall smooth muscle	Auxetic growth of bronchial smooth muscle cells	Asthma
Lung – hypertrophy of arterial wall smooth muscle	Auxetic growth of vascular smooth muscle cells within pulmonary artery and its branches	Pulmonary hypertension

growth in response to injury: following partial hepatectomy or paracetamol-induced necrosis, hepatocytes are able to proliferate and can regenerate the surrounding liver. This is regulated by growth factors such as hepatocyte growth factor and transforming growth factor-alpha, which cause hepatocytes to enter and progress through the cell cycle. Pathological hyperplasia is seen secondary to an underlying disease. Examples of pathological hyperplasia are shown in Table 3.2.

Hypertrophy

Hypertrophy is defined as an increase in the size of an organ due to an increase in the size of its constituent cells, i.e. due to auxetic growth of cells. There is increased synthesis of intracellular proteins, which accumulate in the cytoplasm and physically increase the size of the cell. This is usually associated with an increase in the functional capacity of the cell. Cells which show auxetic growth tend to be permanent cells that are not capable of dividing, or do so only very rarely, and most examples of hypertrophy are found in skeletal muscle, cardiac muscle or smooth muscle.

As with hyperplasia, hypertrophy can be physiological. The increase in muscle mass seen in athletes with weight training is due to an increase in the size of myocytes; there is no increase in the number of myocytes as these cells are

terminally differentiated and cannot divide. Moreover, the smooth muscle cells of the uterus increase in size, as well as in number, in pregnancy and the increase in cell size contributes to the physiological enlargement of the uterus. Examples of pathological hypertrophy, which occurs secondary to an underlying disease process, are detailed in Table 3.3.

Atrophy

Atrophy is defined as a decrease in the size of an organ due to a decrease in the size and/or number of its constituent cells. The cells decrease in size by degrading intracellular organelles and by reducing synthesis of intracellular proteins. The term autophagy is used to describe this 'self-eating' process by which a cell get rids of intra-cellular components. This involves the fusion of damaged organelles with lysosomes and, ultimately, the accumulation of the brown pigment lipofuscin, which is also known as 'wear and tear' pigment. Through these mechanisms atrophic cells are less metabolically active and thus have less demanding energy requirements than comparative cells of usual size. Cell number diminishes largely by apoptosis, which was discussed earlier in this chapter.

As with hyperplasia and hypertrophy, atrophy can occur under normal physiological circumstances. Examples of physiological atrophy include changes in the breast and

TABLE 3.4   Atrophy: Examples.

Type of Atrophy	Mechanism	Examples
Disuse atrophy	Decreased workload	Skeletal muscle atrophy following immobilization as a result of fracture
Denervation atrophy	Damage to nerves supplying a tissue or organ	Skeletal muscle atrophy following spinal cord injury Wasting of leg muscles in Charcot Marie Tooth disease
Lack of blood supply	Occlusion of blood vessels leading to ischaemia	Cerebral atrophy in elderly people with atherosclerosis of cerebral vessels
Pressure atrophy	Compression of a tissue or organ	Cerebral atrophy in tissue surrounding a primary brain tumour Atrophy in skin in immobile patients (bed sores)
Nutritional deficiency	Supply of nutrients fails to meet metabolic demands of the tissue	Cachexia in cancer patients
Hormone deficiency	Tissue hormone receptors lack stimulation	Addison's syndrome: lack of adrenocorticotropic hormone (ACTH) produced by anterior pituitary leads to atrophy of the adrenal gland

endometrium with the low levels of progesterone at the end of each menstrual cycle and following the menopause. In both cases, the trigger for this is the normal, physiological drop in a hormone.

Pathological atrophy has several causes; all result in the continued and progressive decreased supply or stimulation of an organ:

- disuse atrophy
- denervation atrophy
- lack of blood supply
- 'pressure' atrophy
- nutritional deficiency
- hormone deficiency

See Table 3.4 for examples of the different types of atrophy.

Differentiation

The 3.2 billion base pairs that make up the human genome are present in an identical sequence inside almost every cell type, yet there are vast functional and morphological differences in cells between and within organ systems. How is it that a neuron and a cardiac myocyte can harbour an identical genetic sequence yet appear so different and have such different roles? These changes are due to the process of differentiation, whereby genes are turned 'on' or 'off' within a cell, resulting in specific protein expression patterns. We will discuss the genetic basis of cellular differentiation and regulation of gene expression.

Genetic Mechanisms of Cellular Differentiation

Different genes are expressed in different tissues: the gene encoding the thyrotropin receptor is expressed in thyroid epithelial cells but is not expressed in, for example, gastric foveolar cells, which express the gene encoding the H^+/K^+ ATPase proton pump. This difference in gene expression between tissues is known as tissue-specific gene expression.

Moreover, genes may be expressed at different levels within a cell depending on the cell's external environment: the cells of the kidney and liver respond to hypoxia by increasing expression of the gene encoding erythropoietin. This is known as inducible gene expression. Other genes, known as 'housekeeping genes', are expressed at a constant rate in most cell types, e.g. the gene encoding ubiquitin. These phenomena are controlled by transcription and translation, which themselves can be influenced by chromatin structure and epigenetic mechanisms.

Transcription is the process in which a gene, encoded within a segment of DNA, is converted into RNA via the action of RNA polymerase. Transcription allows many copies of the gene to be made if the protein product is required in large amounts by the cell. Transcription is regulated by segments of DNA within (*cis*-regulatory elements) and at a distance from (*trans*-regulatory elements) the target gene, as well as proteins that bind to DNA (transcription factors). The segment of DNA which is transcribed is present on only one of the DNA strands, called the coding strand, and the RNA contains an identical sequence of base pairs, except thymine is replaced by uracil. DNA is transcribed from the 5' end to the 3' end.

Translation is the process in which mRNA is converted into protein. This usually occurs on the ribosome where tRNA, containing an anticodon and an amino acid molecule, binds to its corresponding codon which is present on the molecule of mRNA. Translation follows the genetic code whereby each codon is composed of three nucleotides and the complementary anticodon is linked to a particular amino acid. Translation is triggered by the universal 'start codon' (AUG) and is terminated by one of three 'stop codons' (UAG, UGA, UAA).

Gene expression is also controlled by a different type of RNA called microRNA. MicroRNA is encoded in the genome and is transcribed but is never translated into protein. Instead, it is involved in posttranscriptional silencing of gene expression by binding to segments of mRNA and directly inhibiting it or triggering its degradation.

Epigenetics and Cellular Differentiation

Epigenetics, that is inheritable changes in gene expression without any change in the underlying DNA sequence, plays a large part in normal growth and development and also in disease. Within the nucleus of the cell, the DNA molecule is wrapped around histones and this structure is called chromatin. In inactive cells, the chromatin can be seen under the light microscope as unevenly dispersed and dense heterochromatin, whereas the chromatin appears as the evenly dispersed and fine euchromatin in transcriptionally active cells. Only the genes that are found within the part of DNA that is 'unwrapped' from the histone can be transcribed and translated into protein. Modifications to histones such as methylation, acetylation and phosphorylation can all affect gene expression. Moreover, methylation of DNA itself can affect DNA-histone interactions and also gene expression. These modifications can be maintained within cell division and in this way can be passed on to different generations.

Stem Cells

Stem cells are undifferentiated cells that are able to give rise to all cell types during development and replace differentiated cell populations throughout childhood and adulthood, as well as having the capacity to 'self-renew' and thus give rise to more stem cells. They are defined by this self-renewal ability and by their unique ability to undergo 'asymmetric division', whereby each division of a stem cell gives rise to one differentiated cell and one 'replacement' stem cell.

Stem cells are classified according to the type(s) of the cell that they give rise to (i.e. the differentiation potential of the stem cell) or according to their origin. Table 3.5 outlines the classification of stem cells.

Embryonic stem cells are potentially useful because, as pluripotent stem cells that are capable of forming any cell type, they could in theory replace damaged tissue in conditions such as diabetes, heart disease and irreversible neurological diseases, e.g. Alzheimer's disease. There are, of course, complex ethical and moral issues surrounding the use of embryonic stem cells.

Stem cells are found in many different organ systems. In the small intestine, stem cells reside in the base of the intestinal crypts and give rise to absorptive epithelial cells and goblet cells that take part in normal digestion of foodstuffs. These cells have a relatively quick turnover time due to the harsh physical environment of the gut. In the hippocampus of the central nervous system, there is a small population of stem cells that give rise to hippocampal neurons that are thought to play a role in learning and memory throughout life.

Cancer Stem Cells

It is now known that many tumours harbour a tiny population of cancer stem cells within them. These cells are stem cells

Research Box

In 2012, part of the Nobel prize was awarded to Shinya Yamonaka and John B. Gurdon for the discovery of induced pluripotent stem cells (iPS). Their research involved the transformation of mature mouse-derived skin cells into stem cells capable of forming many types of differentiated tissues (i.e. pluripotent stem cells) by inducing the expression of four genes – OCT3/4, Sox2, Klf4 and c-myc. These 'induced pluripotent stem cells' are now being used all over the world in many different areas of research including drug discovery and development, and as potential treatments for neurodegenerative disease and macular degeneration.

TABLE 3.5   Classification of Stem Cells.

Classification Based on The Differentiation Potential of the Stem Cell	
Totipotent	Able to give rise to a complete organism including embryonic and extraembryonic tissues, e.g. fertilized egg
Pluripotent	Able to give rise to any cell type (endoderm, mesoderm or ectoderm)
Multipotent	Able to give rise to closely related families of cells
Oligopotent	Able to give rise to a small number of closely related cell types
Unipotent	Able to give rise to only one cell type
Classification Based on the Origin of the Stem Cell	
Embryonic	Stem cells derived from the inner cells of the blastocyst (forms around day 4 post-fertilization). These cells are pluripotent
Fetal	Stem cells derived from fetal tissue, e.g. blood or bone marrow
Perinatal	Stem cells derived from amniotic fluid, placenta or umbilical cord
Adult (tissue)	Stem cells that reside within the organ/ tissues of an adult
Induced pluripotent (iPS)	Stem cells derived from in-vitro genetic manipulation of differentiated human cells

in that they 'self-renew', and they are able to give rise to the population of tumour cells. This has important implications for cancer therapies and could explain mechanisms of tumour recurrence. Cancer stem cells have been reported in leukaemia, breast cancer, colorectal cancer and brain cancer, to name a few.

Control of Differentiation

The differentiation state of a cell is maintained and controlled by the local environment of the cell. A change in this local environment, for example a change in pH, change

TABLE 3.6	Pathological Metaplasia: Examples.	
Organ	**Cellular Changes**	**Clinical Features**
Lung	Squamous metaplasia	Seen in smokers, may progress to dysplasia and malignancy
Oesophagus	Columnar metaplasia	Barrett's oesophagus and increased risk of oesophageal adenocarcinoma
Stomach	Intestinal metaplasia	Occurs in the setting of *H. pylori* and confers an increased risk of gastric adenocarcinoma
Meckel's diverticulum	Gastric metaplasia Pancreatic metaplasia	Perforation and peritonitis of Meckel's diverticulum
Bladder	Squamous metaplasia	Occurs in the setting of recurrent UTI or schistosomiasis infection
Thyroid	Oncocytic (Hürthle cell) metaplasia	Occurs secondary to Hashimoto's disease

in hormones, etc., can lead to a change in the differentiation state of a cell. This may be physiological, for example due to a normal change in hormonal levels at puberty, but can also be pathological and in some cases can be a pre-cancerous change. Note that a differentiated cell cannot itself change its phenotype; instead, it is the underlying tissue stem cells that change and give rise to cells of a different differentiation.

Disorders of Differentiation

Metaplasia

Metaplasia is defined as the transformation of one fully differentiated cell type into another fully differentiated cell type. Metaplasia can be seen in epithelial cells (squamous metaplasia, columnar metaplasia) and in mesenchymal cells (lipomatous metaplasia, osseous metaplasia). The type of differentiation that is seen is given as a prefix to indicate the type of metaplasia that has occurred. An important feature of metaplasia is that it is reversible when the initiating stimulus is removed. For example, the squamous metaplasia seen in the lungs of smokers is reversible (over a number of years) if the smoking is stopped. This reversibility differentiates metaplasia from transdifferentiation.

Metaplasia can be physiological, for example as occurs in the cervix at puberty. With increasing oestrogen and progesterone levels at puberty, the cervix increases in mass and the columnar epithelial cells of the endocervix are seen on the part of the cervix that protrudes into the vagina as a 'cervical ectropion'. These epithelial cells are exposed to the acidic environment of the vagina and undergo squamous metaplasia – transformation from columnar to squamous epithelium. This occurs in an area known as the 'transformation zone' and it is this region that is the focus of the cervical screening programme as pre-cancerous change is most often found within these cells.

Table 3.6 discusses the types of metaplasia that can be seen in different pathological conditions.

Dysplasia

Dysplasia is defined as 'disordered cell growth' and is seen in two contexts. The first occurs following abnormal development of an organ with resultant congenital anomalies. Examples of this type of dysplasia include developmental dysplasia of the hip, whereby the femoral head and acetabulum show abnormal configuration; and renal dysplasia, in which part of or all of the kidney fails to develop leading to urinary obstruction and recurrent urinary tract infection. The second context in which the term dysplasia is used is as a pre-cancerous condition, generally affecting epithelia, in which epithelial cells show disordered growth and differentiation. We will focus on this type of dysplasia in this section.

Dysplasia is recognized by pathologists when examining tissue under the microscope. Compared to the normal epithelium, dysplastic cells show nuclear enlargement, hyperchromasia and increased mitotic figures. Whereas normal epithelial cells maintain a normal architecture, the dysplastic cells are haphazardly arranged and show no evidence of maturation. Dysplasia can occur with no known precursor but it is often seen in the setting of chronic inflammation or irritation, viral infection or following metaplasia (Fig. 3.5).

The morphological changes seen in dysplastic cells are due to underlying genetic mutations and epigenetic changes. For example, DNA methylation at the promoter region of tumour suppressor genes, and mutations in *TP53* gene. In fact, studies have shown that molecular changes can be detected before any morphological changes are seen under the microscope. It is thought that further research into the molecular mechanisms of dysplasia may help in identifying which patients will go on to develop an invasive cancer.

Dysplasia is often further classified as low-grade dysplasia and high-grade dysplasia depending on the severity and extent of the dysplastic change. When dysplasia involves the entire thickness of the epithelium, it is known as carcinoma in situ (CIS) or in situ neoplasia. By definition, the dysplastic cells do not breach the underlying basement membrane;

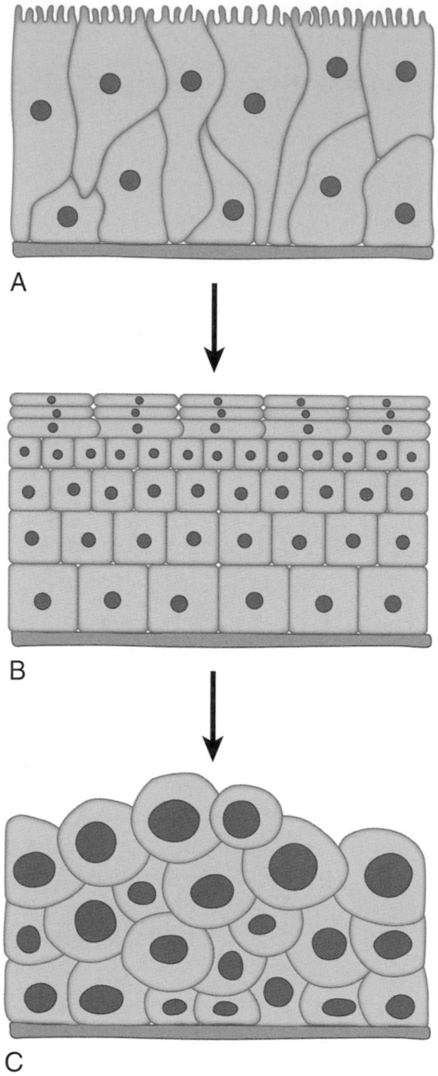

• **Fig. 3.5** Squamous Metaplasia and Dysplasia in the Lung (A) Normal respiratory-type epithelium is pseudostratified ciliated columnar epithelium and is found in the respiratory tract and bronchi. (B) In chronic smokers, there is squamous metaplasia of normal respiratory-type epithelium into stratified squamous epithelium due to chronic irritation and inflammation from irritants found in cigarette smoke. This is an adaptive change as squamous epithelium is able to withstand better the stresses associated with chronic irritation. The epithelium is organized with a single layer of basal cells lined up against the basement membrane and maturing layers of cells up to the surface. (C) Squamous metaplasia may undergo transformation into dysplasia. The dysplastic epithelium shows haphazardly arranged cells with nuclear enlargement, hyperchromasia and increased mitotic figures. Note that the dysplastic cells rest on an intact basement membrane. Invasion through it would signify the development of an invasive cancer. (Courtesy of L. Morrison.)

cells which have breached the basement membrane are classified as invasive cancer cells. There is a risk that dysplasia will progress to invasive cancer and the risk of progression is usually linked to the degree of dysplasia seen: high-grade dysplasia or CIS is at highest risk of progression to invasive cancer. Whilst both degrees of dysplasia may be reversible, low-grade dysplasia is more likely to reverse than high-grade

dysplasia. Table 3.7 discusses the different types of dysplasia seen in different organ systems.

Neoplasia

Neoplasia was defined by British oncologist R.A. Willis as 'an abnormal mass of tissue, the growth of which exceeds and is uncoordinated with that of the normal tissues and persists in the same excessive manner after cessation of the stimuli which evoked the change'. Neoplasia involves dysregulation of both growth and differentiation as neoplastic cells are able to divide in an unregulated fashion and behave differently from the normal cells of the tissue of origin. In malignant tumours, the cells often secrete proteins that allow them to degrade the basement membrane and invade through the intercellular tissue into blood vessels (vascular invasion), lymphatics (lymphatic invasion) or nerves (perineural/intraneural invasion). The molecular mutations that commonly result in neoplasia have been mentioned previously in this chapter.

Morphogenesis

Morphogenesis is the development of structure and form within organs and tissues. Morphogenesis is an extremely complex process that involves growth and differentiation, as well as regulated movement of groups of cells. Morphology, the study of structure, is one of the key methods used by pathologists in the diagnosis of disease.

Morphogenesis begins just after fertilization when the zygote, containing maternal and paternal chromosomes, undergoes multiple, rapid cell divisions in a process known as cleavage and forms the blastocyst in which there are two distinct groups of cells: the inner cell mass and the outer cell mass. These groups of cells go on to form different structures: the outer cell mass forms part of the placenta and the inner cell mass forms the embryo and extraembryonic membranes. How is it that the cells within the blastocyst are able to form these two distinct groups that are located in such an organized and predictable way? Research has shown that two transcription factors, Oct4 and nanog, are switched off in the outer cell mass but are switched on in the inner cell mass. This is thought to play at least part of a role in the difference we see within these two groups of cells.

Furthermore, at around week 3 of embryogenesis the cells form three distinct layers called endoderm, mesoderm and ectoderm in a process known as gastrulation. The formation of these three layers is essential in providing an organizational structure on which organogenesis is based: for example, the central nervous system is derived from the ectoderm, the heart and kidneys are derived from mesoderm and the gut is derived from endoderm. Moreover, the developing embryo shows clearly defined body axes – the craniocaudal, medial-lateral and dorsal-ventral axes. These axes are important in ensuring that cells migrate to and divide in the correct areas.

Morphogenesis is clearly an extremely complex process and involves a vast array of molecular and cellular processes,

TABLE 3.7	Dysplasia: Examples.	
Organ	**Dysplasia**	**Causative Agents**
Cervix	Carcinoma-in-situ (CIN): CIN-1, CIN-2 and CIN-3 of squamous epithelium	HPV virus: HPV 6 and 11 subtypes associated with CIN-1; HPV 16 and 18 subtypes associated with CIN-2 and CIN-3
Breast	Ductal carcinoma in-situ and lobular carcinoma in-situ	Risk factors identical to those for breast cancer – increased oestrogen exposure (early menarche, late menopause) and family history
Lung	Squamous dysplasia (low-grade and high-grade) and squamous carcinoma in-situ Atypical adenomatous hyperplasia and adenocarcinoma in-situ within lung parenchyma	Cigarette smoking Cigarette smoking
Skin	Bowen's disease (squamous carcinoma in-situ) Dysplastic naevus (mild, moderate, severe) Melanoma in-situ (superficial spreading, lentigo maligna and acral lentiginous)	UV exposure, immunosuppression UV exposure UV exposure, multiple dysplastic naevi
Oesophagus	Low-grade or high grade dysplasia of intestinal-type metaplasia in Barrett's oesophagus	Gastro-oesophageal reflux disease

CIN, Cervical intraepithelial neoplasia; HPV, human papillomavirus.

many of which are yet to be elucidated. We do, however, know that morphogenesis utilizes many of the growth and differentiation processes that we have discussed earlier in this chapter, including multiplicative and auxetic cell growth, and apoptosis. The process of cell migration is also very important in morphogenesis as this allows cells to move into their correct position and thus ensures that organs and tissues are sited correctly and appropriately. Cells are able to move via manipulation of the cell cytoskeleton, composed largely of actin and myosin filaments. Cell migration is stimulated by secretion of chemicals and creation of a chemical gradient that controls cell movement by chemotaxis.

Disorders of Growth, Differentiation and Morphogenesis During Embryogenesis

Disorders of growth, differentiation and morphogenesis during embryogenesis lead to congenital malformations. These are structural abnormalities that are present at birth but, as noted at the beginning of this chapter, may not present until later on in life. Congenital malformations have many different causes including genetic mutation, intrauterine infection, maternal alcohol consumption and maternal diabetes. In many cases, the cause is unknown. We will define the different terms used to describe congenital malformations and present a few examples in each category.

Agenesis

Agenesis is defined as the absence of a structure or organ due to a failure in its development, i.e. the structure or organ has

not developed at all during embryogenesis. There may be partial or complete agenesis of an organ. Agenesis can affect any organ, although one of the most commonly discussed examples of agenesis is in the kidney, where it is known as renal agenesis. Bilateral renal agenesis, affecting both kidneys, is incompatible with life. Unilateral renal agenesis affects up to 1 in 3000 live births. Affected patients may survive with only one kidney; however, this kidney often shows hypertrophic change as a compensatory effect and patients may go on to develop chronic kidney disease. In this example, the patient has a disorder of morphogenesis (unilateral renal agenesis) which has led to a disorder of growth (hypertrophy).

Atresia

Atresia is a congenital malformation that can affect any structure or organ that has a lumen, for example the oesophagus, trachea, biliary tree, pulmonary artery and small and large intestines. It is defined as the failure of luminal formation during embryogenesis, i.e. the normally tubular structure is instead completely solid. This is caused by a failure of physiological apoptosis. The consequences of atresia are usually severe and life-threatening because the normal passage of material, for example food and drink through the oesophageal lumen, is completely inhibited. As such, surgical correction is usually required shortly after birth. An example of atresia occurs in the biliary tree, where it is known as biliary atresia. Biliary atresia presents shortly after birth with jaundice, pale stools and dark urine, i.e. conjugated hyperbilirubinaemia. If detected at an early stage, biliary atresia may be treated surgically by anastomosing a loop of bowel to the liver hilum in order to allow bile drainage (hepato-portoenterostomy). In severe cases or in cases detected at a later stage, liver transplantation may be the only treatment option.

Hypoplasia

Hypoplasia is defined as the incomplete development of a structure or organ, i.e. the organ has at least partly developed but has failed to reach its normal size. Infants may be born with pulmonary hypoplasia whereby the lungs have failed to reach normal size and capacity. Pulmonary hypoplasia is often caused by pressure-effect from another structure or organ, for example a large diaphragmatic hernia. The lungs show a reduced number of bronchi and alveoli as well as a reduction in the number of pulmonary arterial branches. As a result, there is compensatory hypertrophy of existing arterial branches and this may lead to pulmonary hypertension.

Dysgenesis

Dysgenesis is defined as abnormal development of a structure or organ during embryogenesis, i.e. the structure or organ has developed, but appears abnormal. Dysgenesis may affect the male or female reproductive tracts, where it is known as gonadal dysgenesis. Gonadal dysgenesis is commonly seen in disorders affecting the sex chromosomes including Turner's syndrome and Klinefelter syndrome. Affected patients show 'streak gonads' whereby the normal gonadal tissue is replaced by fibrous tissue. The result is hypogonadism. In the testes, gonadal dysgenesis is a known risk factor for the development of testicular cancer.

Heterotopia

Heterotopia is a congenital malformation in which normal appearing tissue is found in an abnormal location. Another term for the same thing is a choristoma. This is often due to a failure in cell migration during embryological development. Examples include gastric heterotopia, in which small nodules of gastric mucosa are seen in the small and large intestine. These nodules of gastric mucosa can produce hydrochloric acid and this can result in ulcer formation and gastrointestinal bleeding. Another example of heterotopia is adrenal heterotopia, in which small nodules of adrenal tissue can be found anywhere in the body, including the abdominal wall, kidney and lung. Such lesions are usually asymptomatic but may be incidentally picked up on imaging, where they may mimic cancerous growths.

Hamartomas

These are localized malformations of the tissue normally found in a particular organ. An example is a pulmonary hamartoma which is composed of a nodular mass comprising an admixture of cartilage, smooth muscle and respiratory epithelium.

Further Reading

Allis CD, Jenuwein T. The molecular hallmarks of epigenetic control. *Nat Rev Genet*. 2016;17:487–500.

Angeli JPF, Shah R, Pratt DA, Conrad M. Ferroptosis inhibition: mechanisms and opportunities. *Trends Pharmacol Sci*. 2017;38:489–498.

Anversa P, Kajstura J. Ventricular myocytes are not terminally differentiated in the adult mammalian heart. *Circ Res*. 1998;83:1–14.

Battle E, Clevers H. Cancer stem cells revisited. *Nat Med*. 2017;23:1124–1134.

Bialik S, Kimchi A. Lethal weapons: DAP-kinase, autophagy and cell death: DAP-kinase regulates autophagy. *Curr Cell Bio*. 2010;22:199–205.

Columbano A, Shinozuka H. Liver regeneration versus direct hyperplasia. *FASEB J*. 1996;10:1118–1128.

Cooper G. *The Cell: A Molecular Approach*. 6th ed. Sunderland: Mass Sinauer Associates; 2013.

Cross S. *Underwood's Pathology: A Clinical Approach*. 6th ed. Edinburgh: Churchill Livingstone; 2013.

Giampietri C, Starace D, Petrungaro S, Filippini A, Ziparo E. Necroptosis: molecular signalling and translational implications. *Int l Cell Bio*. 2014. Article ID 490275.

Ilic D, Polak JM. Stem cells in regenerative medicine: introduction. *Br Med Bull*. 2011;98:117–126.

Kelley Bentley J, Hershenson MB. Airway smooth muscle growth in asthma. *Proc Am Thorac Soc*. 2008;5:89–96.

Kumar V, Abbas AK, Aster JC, eds. *Robbins and Cotran Pathologic Basis of Disease*. 9th ed. Philadelphia: Elsevier Saunders; 2015.

Naish J, Revest P, Syndercombe Court D. In: *Medical Sciences*. Edinburgh: Saunders Elsevier; 2009.

Raftery AT, Delbridge MS, Douglas HE. *Basic Science for the MRCS: A Revision Guide for Trainees*. 3rd ed. Elsevier Health Sciences; 2017.

Schoenwolf GC, Larsen WJ. *Larsen's Human Embryology*. 4th ed. Philadelphia: Churchill Livingstone; 2009.

Stolze I, Berchner-Pfannschmidt U, Freitag P, et al. Hypoxia inducible erythropoietin gene expression in human neuroblas tomacells. *Blood*. 2002;100:2623–2628.

Vande Walle L, Lamkanfi M. Pyroptosis. *Curr Biol*. 2016;26:568–572.

Voltaggio L, Cimino-Mathews A, Bishop JA, et al. Current concepts in the diagnosis and pathobiology of intraepithelial neoplasia: a review by organ system. *CA Cancer J Clin*. 2016;66:408–436.

Weinlich R, Oberst A, Beere HM, Green DR. Necroptosis in development, inflammation and disease. *Nat Rev Mol Cell Biol*. 2017;18:127–136.

Young B, Stewart W, O'Dowd G. *Wheater's Basic Pathology: A Text, Atlas and Review of Histopathology*. 5th ed. Edinburgh: Churchill Livingstone; 2011.

4

Cancer: Principles of Surgical Oncology

Introduction

Cancer is now the second leading cause of death in the United States with an estimated 1.735 million new cancer diagnoses predicted to be made in 2018 and over 600 000 cancer associated deaths.[1] Worldwide, in 2012 14.1 million new cancer diagnoses were made, with this estimated to rise to 23.6 million by 2030. Although currently lung, breast, prostate and colorectal cancers are the four most common cancer diagnoses (Fig. 4.1), incidence rates are changing in several of the more uncommon cancer types due to several influencing factors such as ageing population, lifestyle influences (smoking, obesity, alcohol intake, etc.), with pancreas and liver cancers projected to become the second and third most common cancers by 2030.[2] In addition, due to numerous factors, there is an increased lifetime risk of almost 40% of developing cancer.

The Presentation of Cancer

The different primary tumours may present with organ specific symptoms, which may allow earlier suspicion and diagnosis of certain tumours, such as a breast lump in breast cancer, or per-rectal bleeding in colorectal cancers. Other symptoms may be generic such as vague abdominal or back pain, weight loss, nausea or vomiting or abdominal distension. Many of these constitutional symptoms are associated more commonly with more advanced disease, and given their vague nature mimicking other medical conditions, diagnosis may be delayed in some cancers, such as

pancreatic cancer. For example, 25% of all colorectal cancers present acutely to the emergency room.

The difference in the stage of disease at presentation will largely influence the overall prognosis for different tumour types collectively. Therefore, prognosis for breast cancer is generally better than for pancreatic cancer due to more specific and early signs often being present, and with the establishment of screening programmes for the more common tumour types such as breast and colorectal cancers. In pancreatic cancer, only 20–25% of patients will have early stage disease suitable for surgery upfront, compared to 50%+ in early breast cancer at the time of initial diagnosis, reflected in the 5-year survival rate for pancreatic cancer being only 5%, whereas in breast cancer, stage III breast cancer has a 5-year survival rate of over 70% and stage IV has a 5-year survival rate of 20–25%.

Carcinogenesis and Growth

Controlled cellular proliferation occurs during embryogenesis, hypertrophy, healing, regeneration, repair and during the metabolic response to trauma and sepsis. In many instances, cellular replication occurs because growth factors bind to specific receptors on the cell surface and induce intracellular signals which activate the nucleus and cause cell division. Within the nucleus, nucleoproteins ensure accurate DNA replication, DNA repair and DNA transcription to messenger RNA. However, these biochemical processes are susceptible to damage and malfunction by mutations, deletions or amplifications of the genes which code for many of the

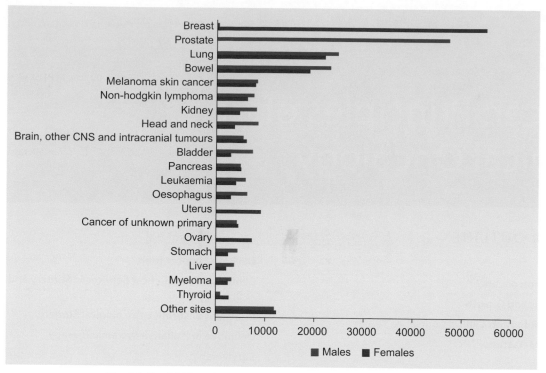

• **Fig. 4.1** Top 20 Most Common Cancers as Published by CRUK 2019[21]

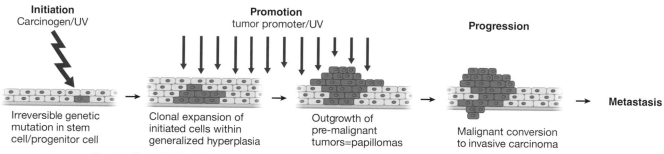

• **Fig. 4.2** The Initiation, Promotion and Progression of Cancer in the Example of Melanoma Metastasis requires the angiogenesis and escape from the primary organ of origin.

normal regulatory factors or their receptors. Mutations can occur either spontaneously or as a result of the interaction of aetiological factors with the DNA of the host (Fig. 4.2) setting the cells on a pathway towards cancer. Malignancy is the consequence of escape from the normal controlling factors for cellular replication.

At some point in the multi-step process of carcinogenesis, the transforming cell undergoes a number of genetic changes which result either in the unchecked expression of proto oncogenes or in abrogation of the function of tumour suppressor genes. These are constituents of the human genome which are associated with normal cellular proliferation and differentiation. They become implicated in carcinogenesis when their encoded proteins are overproduced, mutated or otherwise modified so that their function is abnormally expressed, rather than regulated. Unlike normal tissues where, in general, a cell divides only in order to replace one which has been lost, tumour cells fail to respond to the signals which regulate normal replication. The belief that all

tumours contain cells proliferating more rapidly than those in normal tissues is false. Most tumours enlarge because either the proportion of cells in the proliferative phase of the cell cycle (growth fraction) is greater than normal, or there is decreased cell loss from apoptosis (physiological cell death). It has been estimated that up to 50% of tumour cells are lost as a consequence of hypoxia, exfoliation, metastasis and destruction by host defences. Despite these losses, tumour cells adapt to the physiological selection pressures of their surroundings to achieve continuous advantage over the host. A further development of this adaptive nature is progression by which tumours become more aggressive with time and contain fewer cells which resemble their parent tissue, so producing cells with metastatic potential. A fundamental concept is that change to malignant behaviour on the part of cells does not result in a single disease process. The implications of cancer heterogeneity and evolution are significant as there may be heterogeneity between patients, cancers and within cancer types (Fig. 4.3).

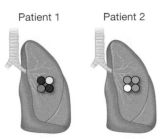
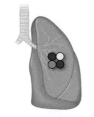
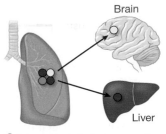

A Interpatient tumor heterogeneity   B Intratumor heterogeneity   C Intermetastatic heterogeneity   D Intrametastatic heterogeneity

• **Fig. 4.3** Types of Tumour Heterogeneity

CMS1 MSI immune	CMS2 canonical	CMS3 metabolic	CMS4 mesenchymal
14%	37%	13%	23%
MSI, CIMP high, hypermutation	SCNA high	Mixed MSI status, SCNA low, CIMP low	SCNA high
BRAF mutations		KRAS mutations	
Immune infiltration and activation	WNT and MYC activation	Metabolic deregulation	Stromal infiltration, TGF-β activation, angiogenesis
Worse survival after relapse			Worse relapse-free and overall survival

• **Fig. 4.4** Summary of Consensus Molecular Subtypes of Colorectal Cancer[4]

Advances in next-generation sequencing and bioinformatics have led to an unprecedented view of the cancer genome and its evolution. These have demonstrated the complex and heterogeneous clonal landscape of tumours of different origins and the potential impact of intratumor heterogeneity on treatment response and resistance, cancer progression and the risk of disease relapse (see Fig. 4.3). They have also provided novel frameworks for the objective phenotyping of tumour types based on biology rather than histological features. For example, an international consortium dedicated to large-scale data sharing and analytics across expert groups demonstrated marked interconnectivity between six independent classification systems for colorectal cancer coalescing into four consensus molecular subtypes (CMSs) with distinguishing features (Fig. 4.4).[3] Approaches such as this have been demonstrated in other cancers (e.g. breast)[4] where many more molecular subtypes of cancers are being discovered that vastly outnumber the classic histological descriptions. These approaches permit an objective, molecular descriptor of cancer to be made for trials, and are now being translated into routine clinical practice where they serve as tools for the stratification of therapy.

A deeper analysis of cancer biology has reinforced the importance of the tumour immune environment (e.g. CMS1 type 1 colorectal cancer). Tumour immune surveillance and immunoediting are fundamental drivers of the cancer phenotype; tumour immunoediting occurs in three main phases: elimination, equilibrium and escape. Elimination describes the initial damage and damage to tumour cells by the innate immune system, followed by presentation of the tumour antigens in the cellular debris to dendritic cells, which in turn present them to T-cells, leading to the production of tumour-specific CD4[1] and CD8[1] T-cells. These will be programmed to kill any remaining tumour cells. The equilibrium phase describes a state where tumour cells survive the initial elimination attempt but are not able to progress, and they are thus maintained in a state of equilibrium with the immune cells. Finally, in the escape phase, cancer cells grow and metastasize due to loss of control by the immune system. Escape occurs because cancer cells either express fewer antigens, lose their MHC class I expression or are able to protect themselves from T-cell attack by expressing immune checkpoint molecules on their surfaces. Immune checkpoint molecules are upregulated by cytokines produced by activated T-cells and are part of a normal negative feedback loop that prevents excessive tissue damage from inflammation. These checkpoints are mostly represented by T-cell receptor binding to ligands on cells in the surrounding microenvironment, forming immunological synapses which then regulate the functions of the T-cell, which become specialized, or 'polarized', to perform different activities. The precision healthcare revolution is now able to leverage these data to transform how oncologists phenotype cancer, and in turn guide and stratify therapy.

Influence of Biology on Clinical Course

In general, a tumour is of sufficient size to be clinically palpable when it contains 10^9 or more cells; however, at clinical presentation most tumours have many more cells than this. Even the smallest radiologically detectable breast carcinoma contains 10^7–10^8 cells. Patients usually die when the total has reached 10^{12}. This natural history is shown diagrammatically in Fig. 4.2.

Invasion and Metastasis

Carcinoma in situ is a collection of malignant cells confined by their normal basement membrane. This is the earliest stage at which a tumour may be histologically identified and implies that the tissue has changed under carcinogenic influences. The cells are both functionally and structurally altered – a state of dysplasia. This process may be multifocal, which implies that the remaining apparently normal cells are at increased risk of malignant transformation (e.g. the normal mucosa surrounding a colonic carcinoma). The advance of malignant disease is by:

- local tissue invasion through and beyond the basement membrane
- distant spread of cells (metastasis) to form autonomous tumour deposits

Invasion occurs when tumour cells start to secrete enzymes capable of digesting intercellular matrix. Many of these enzymes are now being characterized and their physiological or pharmacological inhibitors identified. Prominent among these enzymes are the matrix metalloproteinases. Through continued growth, suitably equipped cells can encroach upon and destroy adjacent organs (e.g. duodenal and bile duct obstruction from a pancreatic carcinoma). Tissue resistance to invasion is variable: arteries and tendons are rarely destroyed, but lymphatics and veins are commonly breached. Tumour cells have metastatic capacity when they are able to:

- invade adjacent tissues (especially veins and lymphatics)
- survive in unfamiliar tissue environments – bloodstream, peritoneal cavity
- sustain their own proliferation to form a focus of tumour cells

Although only about 1 in 10^6 tumour cells may have metastatic potential, many thousands of cells are shed from a tumour each day. Palpation or surgical manipulation of a tumour is known to increase shedding. Tumour metastases may themselves undergo further malignant progression and bear little pathological resemblance to the primary tumour.

Routes of Metastasis

Metastasis occurs through four possible routes (Fig. 4.5). Invasion of the lymphatics or veins allows the transport of viable invasive tumour cells to distant sites. The pattern of spread can be predicted for most tumours (e.g. breast and large bowel) and may be used to plan surgical removal of the primary tumour and possible sites of distant spread. Lymphatics usually accompany the arterial supply to an organ and so, in many instances, surgical removal of an organ which contains a tumour involves dissection of the arterial supply and removal of these vessels and their associated lymphatic tissue (e.g. radical gastrectomy, colectomy). Similarly, the venous drainage of an organ is an important determinant of venous metastatic spread. The identification of both intramural and extramural vascular invasion is an important prognostic indicator in rectal cancer. This can be identified by MRI. As surgical manipulation of any malignant tumour causes shedding of tumour cells into lymphatics and veins, some surgical procedures have been designed to reduce this by initially dividing the blood supply, especially the veins (e.g. ligation of the inferior mesenteric vessels before mobilizing a left-sided colonic tumour using a 'no-touch' technique).

Distribution of Metastases

The organ distribution of metastases varies with the type of tumour and is related to complex interactions between the migrating tumour cell and the capillary endothelium of the organ. Metastatic deposits may become sites from which tumour cells gain access to further vessels – metastases from metastases. In this way, tumours spread from the primary to predictable local metastatic sites, and then on to other less predictable places. Some tumours have a predilection for particular metastatic sites. Gastrointestinal malignancy tends initially to metastasize to the liver via the portal venous circulation; renal and breast carcinoma to the lungs. Bony metastases are relatively common in all terminal disease but there are five tumours that commonly metastasize to bone:

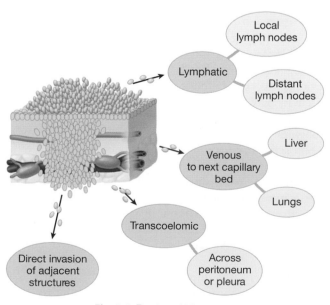

• **Fig. 4.5** Routes of Metastases

- breast
- prostate
- lung
- kidney
- thyroid

Occult Micrometastases

Microscopic tumour deposits, present at the time of original diagnosis and treatment but which escape detection, may emerge as metastases or recurrent disease some time later. They are of considerable importance in surgical oncology. Although they are often called recurrence, they are in fact the continued growth of residual tumour. Modern oncological management aims to include adequate treatment to deal with such micrometastases. This involves systemic therapy additional to local surgical measures – adjuvant therapy, if given after the operation, or neoadjuvant therapy if given prior to surgical extirpation.

Cancer Staging

Several eponymous staging systems are still in routine use (e.g. Dukes stage for colorectal cancer); however, these have largely been surpassed by the TNM staging system (American Joint Commission on Cancer (AJCC)). This has been devised for cancers to allow an assessment of tumour (T), nodal metastases (N) and distal metastases (M). The goal of having a site-specific staging system is to estimate prognosis, facilitate treatment planning, including the sequence of treatments, and allow comparisons of treatment for different stages. Generally, a combination of different 'T', 'N', and 'M' allows the cancer to be grouped into stages. Stages I–IV usually depict a tumour in the following state: stage 1 – early and superficial cancer, stage 2 – locally advanced, stage 3 – regionally advanced with lymph node metastases and stage 4 – distant metastatic disease. Note that the AJCC system is regularly updated, and an example of the staging for breast cancer can be seen online at the AJCC cancer staging site (https://www.facs.org/quality-programs/cancer-programs/american-joint-committee-on-cancer/cancer-staging-systems/). Although imaging is used to stage cancers preoperatively, cancer cannot be said to have been definitively diagnosed until histological confirmation has been achieved. The goals of a biopsy should be to provide a diagnosis that can be used to stratify therapy without excessive morbidity to the patient. Needle biopsy is not always adequate to aid treatment and, occasionally, the surgeon may be called upon to perform incisional or excisional biopsies. Lymphoma is a common tumour that may require a larger tissue sample to make the diagnosis.

Cancer Biomarkers

A biomarker is a defined characteristic that is measured as an indicator of normal biological processes, pathologic processes or responses to an exposure or intervention, including therapeutic interventions. Biomarkers can be considered individually or collectively as a composite biomarker.[5] Typically, cancer biomarkers are hormones, or functional subgroups of proteins such as enzymes, glycoproteins, oncofetal antigens and receptors. Furthermore, other changes in tumours, such as genetic mutations, amplifications or translocations, and changes in microarray-generated profiles (genetic signatures), are also types of cancer biomarkers (tumour markers) that are routinely applied in clinical practice. These are therefore generally applied across the following range of clinical scenarios:

1. Risk stratification of those patients at risk of disease. For example, the Integrative Analysis of Lung Cancer Etiology and Risk (INTEGRAL) Consortium for Early Detection of Lung Cancer or the Breast and Ovarian Analysis of Disease Incidence and Carrier Estimation Algorithm (BOADICEA) risk model to incorporate the effects of polygenic risk scores (PRS) and other risk factors (RFs).
2. Early detection – for large scale screening prior to disease becoming established, e.g. faecal immunochemistry testing for colorectal cancer.
3. Diagnostics – presence of cancer. These markers are expected to have high specificity and sensitivity; for example, the presence of Bence–Jones protein in urine remains one of the strongest diagnostic indicators of multiple myeloma.
4. Prognostic – clinical outcome, e.g. survival. For example, in testicular teratoma, human chorionic gonadotropin and alfa-fetoprotein levels can discriminate two groups with different survival rates.
5. Monitoring (serial or longitudinal biomarkers to detect a change in the extent of a disease). For example, the 21-gene recurrence score which is predictive of breast cancer recurrence and overall survival in node-negative, tamoxifen-treated breast cancer.
6. Therapeutic stratification – predictive biomarkers that determine whether an outcome is likely to be beneficial for a patient. For example, *HER2*, which predicts response to trastuzumab in breast cancer, or *KRAS*-activating mutations, which predict resistance to epidermal growth factor receptor (EGFR) inhibitors such as cetuximab in colorectal cancer.
7. Safety, e.g. toxicity.

Typical biomarkers in routine clinical use can be seen in Table 4.1.

Advances in omics technologies are increasing biomarker complexity, and increasingly multiple genomic, proteomic or metabolic features are used as a 'bar code' for a specific disease. For example, the use of genomic assays in human breast cancer has been endorsed by the National Institute for Clinical Excellence (NICE) and the American Society of Clinical Oncology (ASCO), and sophisticated scoring systems include the use of genetic signatures to refine the risk of recurrence, several of which are used clinically, such as Oncotype Dx in early breast cancer.[6] EndoPredict (EP) is a similar 15-point score based on an eight-gene panel which assigns patients to high- and low-risk groups. The reliability of the score is increased by incorporating clinical parameters (tumour size

TABLE 4.1 Common Biomarkers in Routine Clinical Use.

Cancer Biomarker Names	Alternative Names	Cancer Type	Clinical Use Based on ASCO and/or NACB Recommendations
HER2	ErtB2, NEU, CD340	Breast cancer	Select patients for trastuzumab therapy
PSA	Prostate-specific antigen, Kallikrein 3, KLK3	Prostate cancer	Screening (with DRE) Diagnosis (with DRE)
Alfa-fetoprotein	AFP, α-fetoprotein	Germ-cell cancer hepatoma cancer	Diagnosis Differential diagnosis or NSGCT Staging Detecting recurrence Monitoring therapy
Human chorionic gonadotropin- β	β-hCG	Testicular cancer	Diagnosis Staging Detecting recurrence Monitoring therapy
Calcitonin	Thyrocalcitonin	Medullary thyroid cancer	Diagnosis Monitoring therapy
CA125	Mucin 16, MUC16	Ovarian cancer	Prognosis Detecting recurrence Monitoring therapy
CA 15-3	Carcinoma antigen 15-3	Breast cancer	Monitoring therapy
CA 19-9	Cancer antigen 19-9, sialylated Lewis (a) antigen	Pancreatic cancer	Monitoring therapy
Carcinoembryonic antigen	CEA	Colon cancer	Monitoring therapy Prognosis Detecting recurrence Screening for hepatic metastases
ER	Oestrogen receptor	Breast cancer	Select patients for endocrine therapy
PgR	PR, NR3C3	Breast cancer	Select patients for endocrine therapy
Lactate dehydrogenase	LDH, LD	Germ cell cancer	Diagnosis Prognosis Detecting recurrence Monitoring therapy
Thyroglobulin	Tg	Thyroid cancer	Monitoring

ASCO, American Society of Clinical Oncology; DRE, digital rectal examination; NACB, National Academy of Clinical Biochemistry; NSGCT, non-seminomatous germ cell tumours.

and nodal status) in a score that has been named EndoPredict Clinical (EpClin).[7] EP and EpClin have better prognostic performance than routine surveillance, partly because of the addition of genomic data with nodal status and tumour size. The absence of an intermediate risk group in EP makes decision-making more straightforward.

Biomarkers must have high sensitivity, specificity and diagnostic accuracy, but in practice a large suite of biomarkers are applied for clinical decision making at specific points along the patient treatment journey. In practice, clinicians rely on several composition measures to make precise clinical decisions. These are illustrated by examining colorectal cancer as an exemplar condition (Table 4.2). Here it can be seen that treatment requires the use of circulating, tissue and imaging biomarkers.

The field of circulating tumour DNA (ctDNA) and its application in identifying patients with minimal residual disease (MRD) after surgery is rapidly developing in tandem with sequencing technologies to identify ctDNA.[8] Across multiple tumour types, detectable ctDNA postoperatively portends a poor prognosis and may identify the patients most likely to benefit from systemic treatment or intensified

TABLE 4.2 Current and Emerging Examples of Biomarkers for Guiding Prognosis or Therapy Selection in the Treatment of Colorectal Cancer.

Biomarker	Use	Details
Circulating		
Carcinoembryonic antigen (CEA)	Serum biomarker used clinically in surveillance for disease recurrence	A glycoprotein involved in cell adhesion. It has poor specificity as a diagnostic or screening biomarker but it is used to detect early recurrence
Circulating free tumour mRNA	Plasma biomarker for surveillance of disease recurrence	Detection of free cancer cell mRNA in the plasma of colorectal cancer patients is independent predictor of postoperative recurrence (https://www.esmoopen.com/article/S2059-7029(20)32699-5/pdf) Currently this approach requires mutation profiling of each patient's primary tumour prior to detection, and therefore is costly and time-consuming
DYPD mutations	Serum-based marker of increased risk of 5-FU toxicity	Dihydropyrimidine dehydrogenase (DPD) is a hepatic enzyme involved in the catabolism of uracil and thymine and is the initial rate-limiting enzyme in the metabolism of 5-FU in the liver; therefore deficiency is associated with increased toxicity secondary to impaired metabolism. Currently predictive adequacy is not accurate enough for screening all patients prior to therapy
Tissue		
MisMatch Repair (MMR) genes – MLH1, MSH2, MSH6 or PSM2	Tissue-based molecular biomarkers of Lynch syndrome	Lynch syndrome is an autosomal dominant condition with variable penetrance which leads to a lifetime risk of CRC of 80% if not screened and treated
High levels of microsatellite instability (MSI-H)	Tissue-based prognostic biomarker	Associated with improved prognosis even though MSI tends to be associated with poorly differentiated tumours (https://www.ncbi.nlm.nih.gov/pmc/articles/PMC7493692/)
Loss of heterozygosity of chromosome 18 (18qLOH)	Tissue-based prognostic biomarker	Chromosome 18 contains several important genes involved in carcinogenesis and 18qLOH is associated with chromosomal instability. It is also an independent poor prognostic indicator in patients with stage II disease
KRAS and BRAF	Tissue molecular markers of predicted response to anti-EGFR chemotherapy	KRAS encodes a g-protein, and BRAF encodes a protein kinase. Both are part of the ras/raf/mitogen-activated protein kinase intracellular pathway. The KRAS mutation predicts a complete lack of response to anti-EGFR therapy. BRAF mutation also has a predictive role in the response to therapy with anti-EGFR in cancers in patients with wild-type KRAS
Ki 67	Tissue-based predictive marker of the benefit of adjuvant chemotherapy in stage III colon cancer	Ki-67 is a monoclonal antibody that recognizes an antigen present in the nuclei of cells in all phases of the cell cycle except G_0. A marker of tumour proliferation – high expression is associated with an increased disease-free survival after adjuvant chemotherapy in stage III colon cancer
p53	Tissue-based potential prognostic marker of 5-year survival and predictor of response to adjuvant chemotherapy	p53 is a key regulator of cell growth control and plays a central role in the induction of genes that are important in cell cycle arrest and apoptosis following DNA damage. There is no general conclusion on the prognostic or predictive role of p53 in colorectal cancer yet but p53 mutation has been associated with significantly worse 5-year survival
p21	Tissue-based potential predictive marker of response to chemotherapy	p21, a cell cycle inhibitor, is transcriptionally regulated by p53 and mediates p53 dependent growth arrest. Additionally, p21 acts as an effector of multiple tumour suppressor pathways independent of the p53 tumour suppressor pathway. Some evidence that high expression is associated with poor response to chemotherapy in rectal cancer

Continued

TABLE 4.2	Current and Emerging Examples of Biomarkers for Guiding Prognosis or Therapy Selection in the Treatment of Colorectal Cancer—cont'd		
Biomarker	**Use**	**Details**
CDX2	Reduced expression of the protein associated with more advanced tumour stage, vessel invasion, and metastasis	Homeobox protein responsible for the maintenance of the intestinal phenotype. Five percent of patients do not express CDX2. CDX2 loss is an adverse prognostic factor and linked to molecular features of the serrated pathway
Imaging		
Extramural venous invasion (EMVI)	MRI and tissue-based prognostic marker and predictive marker of response to neoadjuvant therapy	Evidence of tumour cells in the vasculature outside the muscularis propria. Prognostic indicator associated with decreased disease-free survival. Evidence of EMVI regression on MRI is also a predictive marker of response to neoadjuvant therapy

CDX2, Caudal-type homeobox 2; *DYPD*, dihydropyrimidine dehydrogenase; *EGFR*, epidermal growth factor receptor; *FU*, flurouracil; *MRI*, magnetic resonance imaging

---

• **BOX 4.1**　**Examples of Decision Support Tools Commonly Deployed in Clinical Oncology for Prognostication, Risk and Treatment Stratification**

Multiple cancer types	MD Anderson	https://www.mdanderson.org/for-physicians/clinical-tools-resources/clinical-calculators.html
Multiple cancer types	Memorial Sloane Kettering	https://www.mskcc.org/nomograms
Multiple cancer types	Qcancer	https://www.qcancer.org/
Multiple cancer types	Oncoassist	https://oncoassist.com/adjuvant-tools/
Breast	Predict	https://breast.predict.nhs.uk/
Breast	CTS5 (online model for clinicians to predict late distant metastasis for women with ER-positive breast cancer who are recurrence-free 5 years after endocrine therapy)	https://www.cts5-calculator.com/
Colorectal risk assessment	NIH	https://ccrisktool.cancer.gov/
Prostate	Predict (compares outcomes from conservative management (or monitoring) with radical treatment (surgery or radiotherapy))	https://prostate.predict.nhs.uk/
Prostate	Prostate cancer risk prediction	http://www.prostatecancer-riskcalculator.com/

---

approaches. Conversely, patients without detectable ctDNA may be cured by surgery alone and may require either no postoperative treatment or de-escalated treatment. A number of ctDNA guided adjuvant trials in different disease are now underway to define the utility of ctDNA in this setting.

Decision Support Tools

In order to help both the clinician to explain and the patient to understand the complex data from the multitude of clinical trials, calculated risk scores have been devised for several tumour types, including early stage breast cancer and colorectal cancer. Decision support tools are numerous and can be found for all tumour types, stages and treatment (Box 4.1). They require caution in their interpretation as not all have been externally validated; however, our ability to understand the complexity of cancer-related data is advancing rapidly, driven by advances in data mining, predictive analytics, machine learning and artificial intelligence. A detailed analysis of these methodologies and analytical strategies are beyond this chapter. Needless to say, decision support tools are likely to become an increasingly important tool for both the surgeon and the patient.

Centralization of Cancer Services in Surgery and Cancer Strategy

In general, a higher volume of surgery is associated with lower postoperative mortality and morbidity (Box 4.2). Multiple studies have also demonstrated that there is unacceptable variation in the quality of, and outcomes from, specialist cancer services.

For this reason, best practice and NICE guidelines recommend minimum patient volumes for specialist cancer centres and minimum numbers of surgical procedures that should be carried out each year. The application of national cancer targets permits national benchmarking and performance to be measured. Within the UK, all patients must be seen within 2 weeks if referred by their GP to a specialist with a suspected cancer. From the time a decision is made to treat the patient, a time frame of 31 days is allowed before the first treatment must be given and no more than 62 days should pass between the point of referral and first treatment. Hospitals that allow patients

---

• **BOX 4.2** **Reasons for Centralization of Cancer Services**

Fragmentation of services
Insufficient planning of services
Workforce pressures
Unequal access to clinical trials and new treatments
Insufficient specialization to make the most of medical advances
Variation in oncological outcomes

---

to 'breach' from this pathway are liable to incur financial penalties (Fig. 4.6).

However, there have also been national strategies designed to improve outcomes from cancer treatment. The most recent of these was the NHS England National Cancer Strategy, *Achieving World-Class Cancer Outcomes*, produced by the Independent Cancer Taskforce. The taskforce looked at how cancer services are currently provided and set out a vision for what cancer patients should expect from the health service.[9] This included the establishment of 16 Cancer Alliances across the country to lead implementation of the strategy locally. With the three Alliances that form the Cancer Vanguard leading the pilot the plan was for these vanguards to roll out effective and efficient ways to plan, pay and direct the delivery of cancer services. At the core of this vision were the following:

- A radical upgrade in prevention and public health
- Drive a national ambition to achieve earlier diagnosis
- Establish patient experience as being on a par with clinical effectiveness and safety
- Transform our approach to support people living with and beyond cancer
- Make the necessary investments required to deliver a modern high-quality service, including
- Overhaul processes for commissioning, accountability and provision

The Role of the Oncological Surgeon

The role of the modern oncological surgeon is complex and it has evolved from a generalist role to a sub-specialism, driven by the pursuit of improved oncological outcomes.

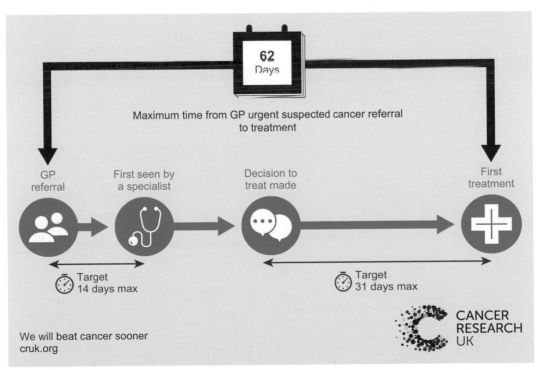

• **Fig. 4.6** Treatment Pathways and Patient Treatment Targets Employed in the NHS for Quality Assurance

The roles are outlined in Box 4.3. Surgery is predominantly in the curative setting, with palliative surgery limited to improvement of quality of life due to the physical effects of the cancer or prior treatments, such as adhesions causing bowel obstruction. Ablative techniques such as radiofrequency ablation have also been established in the treatment paradigms of cancers affecting liver and lung and they have transformed outcomes. The modern oncological surgeon has a portfolio of skills and will commonly be employed in delivering these modalities.

Patient Performance Scores

Patient performance is a critical factor in cancer care, as it is used to stratify therapy and prognosis. The Eastern Cooperative Oncology Group (ECOG) Scale of Performance Status is one such measurement. It describes a patient's level of functioning

---

• BOX 4.3   The Role of the Surgical Oncologist

1. To be an essential component of the multidisciplinary team that manages cancer patients
2. Diagnostics and staging, e.g. diagnostic laparoscopy
3. Therapeutic resection
4. Prophylactic surgery (e.g. BRCA 1- and 2-positive women requiring mastectomy)
5. Minimally invasive therapy and interventional radiology, e.g. ablation of metastatic disease
6. Palliative surgery procedures (e.g. debulking, bypass)

---

in terms of their ability to care for themselves, daily activity of living (ADL), and physical ability. These ADLs include basic activities such as getting dressed, eating and bathing, as well as more complex activities such as cleaning the house and working a regular job. A second commonly employed strategy is the Karnofsky performance status (Fig. 4.7).

Typically, performance status is used to assess both suitability for surgery and chemotherapy, and it is used in a longitudinal manner during therapy to assess treatment deconditioning.

The Multidisciplinary Team (MDT)

Alongside surgery, numerous modalities of treatments have been developed over the decades, most notably conventional chemotherapy, radiotherapy and, more recently, stereotactic radiosurgery, targeted agents and immunotherapy. Cancer treatment has therefore become more complex, and with it the decision-making process. The MDT was a critical innovation in the treatment of cancer and it has revolutionized how therapeutic decisions are made for cancer patients. However, there are both advantages and disadvantages to the MDT which are described in Box 4.4.

The typical team members are provided in Fig. 4.8. However, most importantly, the MDT should contain a member to advocate for the patient and to ensure that their wishes are expressed. The goal of the MDT is to ensure a consistent and high quality of oncological decision making and to consider all clinically appropriate treatment options

ECOG performance status	KARNOFSKY performance status
0–Fully active, able to carry on all pre-disease performance without restriction	100–Normal, no complaints; no evidence of disease 90–Able to carry on normal activity; minor signs or symptoms of disease
1–Restricted in physically strenuous activity but ambulatory and able to carry out work of a light or sedentary nature, e.g., light housework, office work	80–Normal activity with effort, some signs or symptoms of disease 70–Cares for self but unable to carry on normal activity or to do active work
2–Ambulatory and capable of all selfcare but unable to carry out any work activities; up and about more than 50% of waking hours	60–Requires occasional assistance but is able to care for most of personal needs 50–Requires considerable assistance and frequent medical care
3–Capable of only limited selfcare; confined to bed or chair more than 50% of waking hours	40–Disabled; requires special care and assistance 30–Severely disabled; hospitalization is indicated although death not imminent
4–Completely disabled; cannot carry on any selfcare; totally confined to bed or chair	20–Very ill; hospitalization and active supportive care necessary 10–Moribund
5–Dead	0–Dead

• **Fig. 4.7** Comparison of the ECOG and Karnofsky Performance Scores

even they cannot be provided locally. Standard treatment protocols for patients should be used whenever possible and patient suitability for trials should always be considered. Formal protocols are needed to manage referral of patient cases between MDTs and care plans should be communicated to other health professionals in the treatment pathway within a locally agreed timeframe.

Many MDTs occur within cancer networks either using a hub or spoke models (e.g. for anal cancer or specialist input). The regional care pathway provides a solid basis for uniform care, working according to evidence-based guidelines and further cooperation. There is good evidence that the MDT improves outcomes from surgery and it is now a critical for delivering high quality surgical care.

• BOX 4.4 Advantages and Disadvantages of the MDT

Advantage

- Structure and process of decision making
- Improved communication, coordination and decision making between healthcare professionals
- Evidence-based care
- Stratified care – tumour biology
- Holistic treatment – co-morbidities and social circumstances

Disadvantage

- May increase length of time to treatment
- MDT discussion not always advocated by national guidelines
- Not applied uniformly internationally
- Patient not present – consent and confidentiality
- Resource requirements, e.g. video links
- Time consuming
- Decisions may be biased towards riskier treatments
- Treatment decisions differ, especially in older patients and those with single organ metastases
- Grey legal area

Principles of Curative Oncological Surgery

The basic principles of surgery still follow those described by Halstead (Box 4.5). However, the modern cancer surgeon should adopt a personalized approach to surgery. This means performing the right operation on the right patient at the right time based on the right evidence. You should have a detailed appraisal of the preoperative imaging, pathological biopsy and patient anaesthetic assessment. The operative strategy should then be tailored according to the patient, the tumour type and stage.

• BOX 4.5 The Main Objectives of Oncological Surgery

1. Patient selection: Fitness for surgery and surgical approach
2. Surgery of the primary margin.
   a. Clear microscopic (R0) margin. As opposed to a microscopic positive margin (R1) or macroscopic margin (R2) which significantly worsens the prognosis of the patient
   b. 'No touch technique'
   c. Ensure maximum quality of life for the patient by removing only essential tissue where the evidence base supports it (e.g. wide local excision for breast cancer)
3. Surgery of the lymphatics a. Require removal of the draining lymph nodes for the purpose of staging and/or to achieve local control. Levels of prophylactic lymph nodes dissection vary according to tumour type and may increase surgical morbidity. Surgery in some tumours has become more conservative with the advent of sentinel node biopsy when lymph node metastases are not evident preoperatively
4. Surgery for metastatic disease.
   a. Surgery is increasingly performed on complex disease
   b. Both locally advanced and recurrent and systemic metastatic disease may be operated on (e.g. liver metastases) and these can be performed as synchronous or separate resections

---

Professional group	Discipline
Doctors	Surgeons Radiologists Histo-cytopathologists Oncologists (clinical and medical) Haematologists Palliative care specialists Other doctors (e.g. physicians, GP)
Nurses	Clinical nurse specialists Other nurses (e.g. nurse consultants, matrons, ward nurses etc)
Allied health professionals	Allied health professionals
MDT coordinators	MDT coordinators
Other (admin/clerical and managerial)	Other (admin/clerical and managerial)

• **Fig. 4.8** The Essential Components of the MDT

Adjuvant Treatment

The treatment of most solid tumours is multimodal, and as a result, the surgeon will often have to tailor therapy according to the requirements for treatment adjuncts. The term 'adjuvant therapy' was first used by Paul Carbone and his team at the National Cancer Institute in 1963. These therapies supplement primary surgery, aiming to reduce the risk of disease recurrence. The rationale for adjuvant therapy was originally discussed by a group of 23 surgeons who met in early 1957 to form the Surgical Adjuvant Chemotherapy Breast Project, later named the National Surgical Adjuvant Breast and Bowel Project (NSABP). They based their discussions on observations during the 1950s where patients who received systemic agents shortly after their 'curative' operations had better overall outcomes. The group devised the first trial consisting of the use of thiotepa (TSPA), an alkylating agent, for patients who had undergone radical mastectomy for early breast cancer. The first patient was enrolled and randomized on 4th April 1958, with accrual of 826 patients completed by October 1961. This study, called NSABP B-01, demonstrated the first evidence of systemic chemotherapy altering the natural history for a select premenopausal group with four or more positive lymph nodes. From this study, a multitude of different studies were developed in several different tumour types, including colorectal cancer, as well as using different treatment modalities, including systemic chemotherapy agents in combination, hormone therapy and radiotherapy. In recent years, immunotherapy has been shown to be beneficial adjuvant therapy, particularly in malignant melanoma.

The aim of adjuvant therapy is to reduce the risk of recurrent cancer through the early treatment of micrometastatic (minimal residual) disease, taking into account the short- and long-term toxicities of the therapies used. Although the NSABP B-01 study showed a positive survival effect of thiotepa, many surgeons were subsequently reluctant to use it due to significant toxicities. During these early years of the evolving fields of medical and clinical oncology, it was the rapid development of trial methodologies as much as the types and intensities of the adjuvant treatments which influenced heavily the resultant outcomes seen. This resulted in many adjuvant trials which either resulted in disappointing outcomes or adversely poorer outcomes. Several of the early trials were very complex designs, with many different questions being attempted to be answered in the same trial. Despite many of the negative trial outcomes, these studies are important in the field of oncology as they demonstrated it was possible to effectively run cooperative studies over a wide geographical area.

The early 1970s yielded a rapid increase in the number of adjuvant studies on the back of President Nixon's 1971 speech declaring a 'war on cancer' (https://dtp.cancer.gov/timeline/flash/milestones/M4_Nixon.htm). In February 1976, Gianni Bonadonna and colleagues published the seminal adjuvant breast cancer trial demonstrating a significant benefit in the use of combination chemotherapy in early breast cancer.[10] The relative benefit of adjuvant chemotherapy in a number of tumour types investigated since 1958 has been estimated to be between 30% and 50%.

In colorectal cancer, the use of adjuvant chemotherapy has become more refined over the decades; firstly, in the use of combination chemotherapy for higher risk disease, and more recently, in reducing the length of adjuvant treatment from 12 months, down to 6 months, and more recently, through the Innovation + Design Enabling Access (IDEA) collaboration initiative, to 3 months in select cases.[11] The dawn of the new millennium lead to the era of personalized medicine, where biomarkers are being developed to act as predictive and prognostic guides in determining adjuvant treatment. Worldwide, different chemotherapy agents have shown varying efficacies in different geographical populations, highlighting the possibility of a genetic influence on outcomes. Likewise, as we better understand the biology of inherited malignancies, such as Lynch syndrome, the efficacy of adjuvant therapy can be further refined. The toxicities associated with chemotherapy regimens include death due to a number of possible complications (although the frequency is generally under 5%), and some regimens carry a significant risk of morbid toxicities, such as neutropenic sepsis at a frequency of up to 30% in combination regimens. Other considerations include the effect of chemotherapy on fertility, particularly for younger patients, and survivorship issues such as long-term toxicities (for instance a one in five chance of peripheral sensory neuropathy with oxaliplatin), and risk of second malignancies due to the treatments used.

Hormone treatments have been long established in the treatment of advanced breast cancer, and have also been shown in several global large-population long-term follow-up studies to provide a significant benefit in risk reduction of recurrence. Several different options are available, depending on the menopausal status of the patient and side-effect profiles of the hormonal drugs. Recent data have suggested that longer hormone treatments in breast cancer, up to 10 years or more, confer additional clinically meaningful benefits, especially in such a common cancer type.

With the introduction of targeted agents into the treatment paradigms for advanced cancers, many trials have been conducted in most tumour types to see if a similar benefit can be obtained from their use as adjuvant therapies. Tumour types which have predominantly relied on targeted agents to treat advanced cancer, such as renal cell carcinoma, have shown inconsistent results for adjuvant targeted therapy between trials, whereby they do not have a role in the adjuvant setting outside clinical trials. A significant recent positive adjuvant trial in malignant melanoma has reported on prolonged relapse-free survival and overall survival in BRAF-mutated melanoma with the combination use of the targeted agents dabrafenib (BRAF inhibitor) and trametinib (MEK inhibitor).[12] Cancer immunotherapy is a rapidly expanding field that applies several strategies to augment tumour immunity. The shift is to focus on the biological phenotype of the tumour rather than its site of origin. A summary of these approaches can be found in Table 4.3.

TABLE 4.3	A Summary of Immunological Adjuvant Strategies.	
Drug Type	**Drug Exemplars**	**Disease Types**
Check point inhibitors	CTLA-4 (e.g. Ipilimumab), PD-1 (e.g. Nivolumab), PDL-1 (Atezolizumab)	Metastatic melanoma, urothelial carcinoma, non-small cell lung cancer
Adoptive cell transfer (CAR T-cell therapy) (currently experimental)	axicabtagene ciloleucel and tisagenlecleucel	B-cell lymphoma
Monoclonal antibodies	HER2 (e.g. ado-trastuzumab emtansine), CD52 (e.g. alemtuzumab), VEGF (e.g. bevacizumab), EGFR (e.g. cetuximab)	Metastatic breast cancer, B-cell chronic lymphoma, metastatic colorectal cancer, non-small cell lung cancer
Interleukins	Aldesleukin (IL2)	Melanoma, renal carcinoma
Interferons	Roferon-A [2a], Intron A [2b], Alferon [2a]	
Oncolytic virus therapy	Talimogene laherparepvec (Imlygic), or T-VEC (modified HSV)	Melanoma
Vaccine	Sipuleucel-T (a dendritic cell vaccine)	Metastatic prostate cancer

Monoclonal antibodies have been investigated in the adjuvant setting. Initial antibodies were murine analogues, and these typically have the suffix -omab. These have largely been replaced by chimeric (suffix -ximab) or humanized forms (suffix -zumab) which have an improved half life and efficiency. Human monoclonal antibodies (-umab) are produced using transgenic mice. The most notable established antibody is trastuzumab (anti-HER2 monoclonal antibody) in HER2 positive early breast cancer.[13] The use of monoclonal antibodies has been established in several other tumour types in advanced cancer, such as trastuzumab in gastric/oesophageal cancers, cetuximab/panitumumab in colorectal cancers and head and neck tumours, and bevacizumab in colorectal cancers and ovarian cancers. However, the use of these agents in adjuvant trials in several different tumour types have been disappointing, with no improvement in overall survival. Furthermore, in colorectal cancer, the use of monoclonal antibodies has resulted in outcomes which may be detrimental, highlighting the caution that the efficacy of treatments in advanced disease does not translate directly to efficacy in the adjuvant setting.

Immunotherapy has recently established itself as the mainstay of treatment for metastatic melanoma. Prior attempts to reduce the risk of recurrence in patients who undergo curative surgery had been limited by the lack of effective systemic agents, with chemotherapy being of very modest benefit in the advanced disease setting. However, immune modulation using interferon alpha (IFNα) was shown in both individual trials and in a subsequent meta-analysis to provide an improvement in overall survival; this came at the expense of significant, potentially life-threatening toxicity, meaning the clinical utility was limited depending on the patient, and required careful informed consent.

Following on from the success of checkpoint inhibitor (CPI) immunotherapies, such as ipilimumab, nivolumab and pembrolizumab in metastatic melanoma, adjuvant trials have recently reported an improved relapse-free survival and overall survival, both as single agent therapies and combination ipilimumab plus nivolumab, with the combination showing further benefit compared to monotherapy.[14] Currently, several other tumour types are being investigated for the role of immunotherapy in adjuvant treatment, especially where CPIs have demonstrated activity in the advanced settings.

A rapidly emerging immunotherapy approach is called adoptive cell transfer (ACT). This involves the isolation and in vitro expansion of tumour-specific T-cells, followed by infusion back into the patient. There are many forms of ACT, including those using techniques such as culturing tumour-infiltrating lymphocytes obtained directly from the tumour; isolating and expanding one particular T-cell or clone; or using T-cells that have been engineered in vitro to potently recognize and attack tumours. The most clinically advanced form of ACT is known as chimeric antigen receptor (CAR) T-cell therapies (CAR-T). Two products have been approved by both the US Food and Drug Administration (FDA) and the European Medicines Agency for use in this setting, namely axicabtagene ciloleucel[15] and tisagenlecleucel. However, despite early promise these therapies are currently in the early phase of their assessment and it is unclear if they will have a role in solid cancers. Moreover, they are not without side effects and they can cause severe cytokine-release syndrome (CRS) and neurotoxicity.

Oncolytic viruses are an emerging class of cancer therapeutics; viruses are genetically modified to lack virulence against normal cells but are able to invade and lyse cancer cells which have sacrificed many of their normal anti-viral cellular defences in order to amplify their growth potential. Lytic destruction triggers an immune response by the further release of tumour antigens. 'T-VEC' is a herpes simplex-1 virus (HSV-1) modified to express GM-CSF which further stimulates proliferation of immune cells, and it has been licensed for the treatment of melanoma. T-VEC is injected directly into areas of melanoma that a surgeon cannot remove.[16] Therapeutic vaccines are also rarely used (as opposed to prophylactic viruses, such as the human papillomavirus [HPV] vaccine). For example, Sipuleucel-T is licensed for the treatment of asymptomatic or minimally symptomatic castration-resistant prostate cancer (CRPC).[17]

Radiotherapy has also been used as adjuvant therapy in several specific clinical situations for specific tumour types. The use of routine adjuvant radiotherapy in early breast cancer has been controversial, but has been used to reduce the risk of local recurrence where surgical margins may remain positive when further surgery is not possible. In this situation, radiotherapy follows the completion of adjuvant systemic chemotherapy, to ensure any micrometastatic disease is targeted at the earliest opportunity. A similar approach may be used in individual cases for other solid tumours, including deep-seated tumours such as pancreatic cancers. Additionally, some patients who present with radiologically resectable localized deep-seated tumours, such as oesophageal/gastric cancers, may not be suitable surgical candidates due to co-morbidities. These patients can then undergo radical (definitive) radiotherapy to provide a 'sterile' field, usually after the patient has undergone previous chemotherapy to control disease and target potential micrometastatic disease initially. These patients may also receive concomitant chemotherapy with the radiotherapy which will act as a radiosensitizer.

Neoadjuvant Therapy

Neoadjuvant treatments are now used in several different tumours, in order to facilitate curative surgery. The initial rationale for neoadjuvant therapies was to achieve a response to convert patients with borderline resectable disease to subsequently undergo curative surgery. Neoadjuvant chemotherapy also has the potential to treat micrometastatic disease very early in the patient's treatment pathway with the potential to reduce future systemic relapse. In addition, the use of neoadjuvant therapies allows the oncologist to characterize the tumour's sensitivity to the treatments in vivo, which is something that is not possible solely with adjuvant therapy. Where patients may not respond, or progress, on the initial therapy, a change of treatment strategy may be required to try and convert patients to curative surgery. Knowledge of in vivo sensitivity may also influence choice of postoperative systemic chemotherapy, if appropriate, and increasingly total neoadjuvant strategies are being investigated in several tumour types.

More recently, the use of neoadjuvant therapy has allowed the ability to obtain further molecular information about the effect of therapies on the tumour cells, by being able to compare the original diagnostic biopsy samples with the subsequent surgical excision specimen. It has also afforded the opportunity to undertake 'window-of-opportunity' studies, comparing the early effects of novel treatment on prognosis and determining predictive biomarkers with the use of additional biopsies, either solid or liquid, early in the course of the neoadjuvant treatment, thus providing a deeper biological understanding, and a unique opportunity to correlate clinical with biological and/or radiological markers in vivo.

Furthermore, recent studies have shown that early breast cancer patients who undergo a complete pathological response (pCR) with no viable tumour cells present in the complete surgical excision specimen, will have a better overall prognosis with a greater relapse-free survival and overall survival. Similar analyses have been undertaken on other tumour types where neoadjuvant therapies are used, such as in rectal cancers, and gastroesophageal cancers.

The main risk associated with the use of neoadjuvant treatment, apart from the immediate toxicities, would be that patients who might have upfront resectable disease radiologically, could potentially progress if their tumour is resistant, turning a potentially curable tumour into either a locally advanced non-resectable tumour or development of metastatic disease. However, this might also identify patients with unfavourable biology destined to develop systemic disease and where potentially morbid surgery should be avoided. This will, however, depend on the tumour type and discussion with the patient. Secondly, some patients may experience significant toxicities from neoadjuvant treatment, which decondition them or exclude them from subsequent surgery.

Neoadjuvant monoclonal antibodies are currently used in HER2-positive early breast cancer, with recent approval by the FDA in the United States for pertuzumab to be used in combination with trastuzumab as dual HER2 blockade and docetaxel chemotherapy, with a significant increase in pCR rates. Regulatory bodies worldwide are now starting to recognize the importance of pCR rates in neoadjuvant therapies, and, based on this as a surrogate for overall survival, are granting accelerated approval pending mature data. This was the case for pertuzumab, which was granted accelerated approval in 2014, and subsequently achieved FDA full approval status in the neoadjuvant setting in 2018.

Currently, there are several ongoing phase III multicentre trials in various tumour types investigating the use of neoadjuvant immunotherapy, but at present, it remains unproven. It is expected that if early data suggest pCR rates show an improvement, they may also attain accelerated approval status by the FDA in the near future. Again, the window-of-opportunity studies provide immense opportunity to understand the impact of immune checkpoint inhibitors and predictive biomarkers through analysis on immune monitoring pipelines across multiple tumour types.

Radiotherapy has an established role in the neoadjuvant protocol for rectal tumours, where tumours which have threatened surgical margins radiologically at time of diagnosis, as identified by MRI, can potentially be downsized to maximize the chance of an R0 resection. Radiotherapy with concomitant chemotherapy (long-course chemoradiation) allows the most effective tumour shrinkage opportunity, with responses assessed by MRI pelvis. The development of improved protocols and imaging technologies for radiological assessment of response to treatment has lead towards the goal of achieving better surgical outcomes for these anatomically complex tumours.[18]

Definitive or Palliative Systemic Therapy

The earliest known descriptions of cancer are found in the ancient Egyptian papyrus scrolls dating from the period 1600 BCE in the Ebers papyrus and the Edwin Smith papyrus. Throughout recorded history, there have been many attempts to treat tumours with medicinal plant and herb extracts, including topical applications to treat tumours. The earliest most comprehensive list of such treatments was compiled by the Greek physician Dioscorides in the first century CE, which was used extensively for at least 1400 years. The idea of 'poisoning' tumours was established by the Arabic physician Ibn Sina in the 11th century CE, by the use of arsenic preparations, which were used in various forms for the next 600 years, with, however, significant toxicity. The use of systemic potassium arsenite by Lissauer in 1865 to treat chronic myelogenous leukaemia is considered by many to be the first recorded effective use of drugs to treat malignant disease. In the late 19th century, the famous surgeon, William Coley, developed a mixture of bacterial toxins (known as Coley's toxin) to regress several tumours. This concept is still employed successfully in modern oncology with the use of BCG in superficial bladder cancers and laid the foundations for cancer immunotherapy.

With the dawn of the 20th century, and the rise in financial opportunities to market different medicinal serums, there were many concoctions advertised as miracle cures to the desperate, despite a lack of any scientific or medical evidence. The term chemotherapy, however, was first used by the famous German chemist, Paul Ehrlich, in the early 1900s for drug treatment of infectious diseases. Subsequent anticancer drug development started in earnest at the end of the Second World War with the development of nitrogen mustards, initially by pioneers such as Dr Gustav Lindskog (for use in patients with lymphosarcoma) and Drs Wilkinson and Fletcher in the UK (for patients with Hodgkin's lymphomas). Further chemotherapeutic drugs, such as anti-folates, were established by Sidney Farber in acute leukaemias in children, giving rise to the class of drugs subsequently termed antimetabolites. Since the late 1940s, many different classes of compounds have been discovered, either through isolation from natural preparations or synthetically derived, which have formed the backbone of medical oncology, and continue to play an important role in the treatment of advanced cancer.

Through the establishment of clinical trials, these chemotherapy agents have been extensively tested in different tumour types, and in various combinations, to determine synergistic regimens. These have led to a vast number of different regimens used for different tumours, and at different stages of their advanced disease. The use of different targets in subsequent lines of treatment provided the strategy to further develop effective approaches, but incremental gains in many tumours have only been modest, with the patient's ability to undergo cytotoxic chemotherapy impaired generally by a worse clinical status in those considered for latter lines of therapy. Therefore, as a general principle, patients who receive cytotoxic chemotherapy often receive the most effective, but also often the most toxic, regimens earlier in their treatment paradigm as they are often more clinically robust than when latter lines of therapy are considered.

The use of these palliative therapies is to help control disease and symptoms, without substantial toxicities to risk affecting the quality of life of these patients and limiting the potential risk of death associated directly with the treatments administered. This overarching principle of palliative treatment often limits the length of duration of treatment and the number of lines of treatment, as by the nature of palliative treatments, these are for advanced disease with the aim for improved quality of life alongside prolongation of survival. The oncologist must therefore carefully consider and select the most appropriate treatment for the individual patient using the available clinical trial evidence, but also taking individual patient characteristics and beliefs into account.

Systemic cytotoxic chemotherapy has been in widespread clinical use for decades in almost all cancer types. They often have significant side effects, often aiding to the 'cancer phenotype' which can lead to negative perceptions towards patients. With more refined regimens and better supportive care measures, some of these toxicities are manageable, but others patients will endure throughout treatment, such as alopecia. Many conventional cytotoxic chemotherapy agents will have generic side effects, due to the nature of the treatments, by targeting more rapidly diving cells preferentially but not distinguishing malignant from non-malignant cells. Most commonly, the bone marrow can be affected, especially with cumulative doses of chemotherapy on established treatment giving rise to anaemia, leukopaenia, neutropaenia and thrombocytopaenia. Patients who undergo chemotherapy can also commonly experience fatigue, which may be a combination of tumour-related fatigue due to the hypermetabolic state of the disease, but also due to various hormone imbalances and cytokine release as a result of the cytotoxic drugs. With any cytotoxic drug treatment, patients must be carefully counselled about the risk of death associated with treatment, which can occur for various reasons (including neutropenic sepsis) and is generally under 5%. The cycle lengths of treatment regimens are often dictated by the time of onset of myelosuppression and length of time to bone marrow recovery, varying from daily dosing of oral agents up to monthly or longer for certain intravenous combinations.

Survivorship

The proportion of people predicted to survive a diagnosis of cancer is increasing by ~3% per year.[19] Indeed, cancer is now considered a chronic condition with an associated co-morbidity that demands long-term follow-up. The goal of cancer survivorship is to maintain a good quality of life, which typically means independence, normal physical and physiological function and a return to work. This has driven many of the advances in minimally invasive surgery which have aimed to reduce the functional and cosmetic impact of surgical treatment on the patient. However, there is variation of the definition of survivorship depending on whether it is thought to begin (1) at the time of diagnosis; (2) after the end of treatment; or (3) after a specified time has elapsed where the individual remains disease free (disease-free survival or DFS).[20]

Because survivorship varies between disease type, therapeutic intervention and geography, many guidelines have now been provided to help inform clinical practice (Box 4.6). For example, the National Comprehensive Cancer Network (NCCN) guidelines are evidence- and consensus-based for the treatment of patients with breast cancer.

However, survivorship generally follows the following principles:

1. **Management of the late effects of treatment and its associated symptoms:** For example, chemotherapy-induced nausea and vomiting, pain and peripheral neuropathy, bone loss with the possibility of subsequent osteoporosis, mucosal, dental and soft tissue problems of the head and neck, skin toxicity, lymphoedema, cardiovascular problems, fatigue, sleep disorders, cognitive function, depression and anxiety, fear of recurrence, eye problems, hormonal insufficiencies, infertility, amenorrhea, menopause, sexual dysfunction including impotence and lack of libido, urological problems, gastrointestinal problems and lung problems.

2. **Promoting positive health behaviours:** Physical activity, nutrition and weight management, stress management, reducing alcohol consumption, smoking cessation, avoidance of excessive exposure to UV radiation, avoiding worsening side-effects through the use of recreational drugs and encouraging the uptake of vaccinations.

3. **Rehabilitation:** Cancer and its treatment produce a multi-dimensional impact on patients' lives, affecting the physical, sensorial, cognitive, psychological, family, social and spiritual functional level. Rehabilitation should acknowledge this and typically this means employing a multidisciplinary team to support the symptoms of a chronic disease. Care should be provided in an outpatient setting and be provided by an expert.

4. **Physical and functional fitness:** The treatment of chronic fatigue and the prevention of deconditioning.

5. **Psychosocial care:** Between 30% and 50% of cancer survivors may experience psychological distress significant enough to warrant professional intervention sometime during the survivorship period. Psychological support should be offered to all patients.

6. **Prevention and detection of cancer recurrence:** Through surveillance, biomarker screening and patient education.

7. **Palliative care:** Palliative care requires a complete book to fully describe its importance. But its goals are to control physical, medical and functional symptoms, psychological and emotional problems, social, existential and spiritual needs. It is a personalized approach which employs a spectrum of treatments and "event assistance decision-making" around end-of-life issues. It is typically provided late in the patient's care pathway, but when it becomes apparent that cure is not possible, it should be bought forward as early as possible. This improves patient choice and quality of life, and provides the patient with time to make the most appropriate choices for them.

Patient support and advice is provided through charities such as the Macmillan charity.

• BOX **4.6** **National Guidelines on Cancer Survivorship**

ASCO	https://www.asco.org/news-initiatives/current-initiatives/cancer-care-initiatives/prevention-survivorship/survivorship
ACS	https://www.cancer.org/health-care-professionals/american-cancer-society-survivorship-guidelines.html
ESMO	https://www.esmo.org/Patients/Patient-Guides/Patient-Guide-on-Survivorship
NCCN	https://www.nccn.org/store/login/login.aspx?ReturnURL=https://www.nccn.org/professionals/physician_gls/pdf/survivorship.pdf

ACS, American Cancer Society; ASCO, American Society of Clinical Oncology; ESMO, European Society for Medical Oncology; NCCN, National Comprehensive Cancer Network.

Summary

Survival from cancer therapy has improved by 50% over the last 50 years, and rates will continue to climb through the adoption of precision based medical and surgical therapies. As the complexity of treatment increases, multidisciplinary care will remain at the core of precision cancer care, with the surgeon continuing to play a critical role.

References

1. Siegel RL, Miller KD, Jemal A. Cancer statistics, 2018. *CA Cancer J Clin.* 2018;68(1):7–30.
2. Rahib L, Smith BD, Aizenberg R, Rosenzweig AB, Fleshman JM, Matrisian LM. Projecting cancer incidence and deaths to 2030: the unexpected burden of thyroid, liver, and pancreas cancers in the United States. *Cancer Res.* 2014;74(11):2913–2921.
3. Guinney J, Dienstmann R, Wang X, et al. The consensus molecular subtypes of colorectal cancer. *Nat Med.* 2015;21(11):1350–1356.

4. Banerji S, Cibulskis K, Rangel-Escareno C, et al. Sequence analysis of mutations and translocations across breast cancer subtypes. *Nature*. 2012;486(7403):405–409.

5. Robb MA, McInnes PM, Califf RM. Biomarkers and surrogate endpoints: developing common terminology and definitions. *J Am Med Assoc*. 2016;315(11):1107–1108.

6. Olsson-Brown A, Piskilidis P, O'Hagan J, et al. The impact of the 21-gene recurrence score (Oncotype DX) on concordance of adjuvant therapy decision making as measured by the Liverpool Systemic Therapy Adjuvant Decision Tool. *Breast*. 2019;44:94–100.

7. Dubsky P, Filipits M, Jakesz R, et al. EndoPredict improves the prognostic classification derived from common clinical guidelines in ER-positive, HER2-negative early breast cancer. *Ann Oncol*. 2013;24(3):640–647.

8. Reinert T, Henriksen TV, Christensen E, et al. Analysis of plasma cell-free DNA by ultradeep sequencing in patients with stages I to III colorectal cancer. *JAMA Oncol*. 2019;5(8):1124–1131.

9. NHS. *Achieving World-Class Cancer Outcomes: A Strategy for England 2015–2020*; 2016.

10. Bonadonna G, Brusamolino E, Valagussa P, Veronesi U. Adjuvant study with combination chemotherapy in operable breast cancer. *Proc Am Assoc Cancer Res Am Soc Clin Oncol* 1975;16: 254.

11. Bregni G, Rebuzzi SE, Sobrero A. The optimal duration of adjuvant therapy for stage III colon cancer: the European perspective. *Curr Treat Options Oncol*. 2019;20(1).8.

12. Schadendorf D, Hauschild A, Santinami M, et al. Patient-reported outcomes in patients with resected, high-risk melanoma with BRAF(V600E) or BRAF(V600K) mutations treated with adjuvant dabrafenib plus trametinib (COMBI-AD): a randomised, placebo-controlled, phase 3 trial. *Lancet Oncol*. 2019;20(5):701–710.

13. Saad ED, Squifflet P, Burzykowski T, et al. Disease-free survival as a surrogate for overall survival in patients with HER2-positive, early breast cancer in trials of adjuvant trastuzumab for up to 1 year: a systematic review and meta-analysis. *Lancet Oncol*. 2019;20(3):361–370.

14. Menshawy A, Eltonob AA, Barkat SA, et al. Nivolumab monotherapy or in combination with ipilimumab for metastatic melanoma: systematic review and meta-analysis of randomized-controlled trials. *Melanoma Res*. 2018;28(5):371–379.

15. Neelapu SS, Locke FL, Bartlett NL, et al. Axicabtagene ciloleucel CAR T-cell therapy in refractory large B-cell lymphoma. *N Engl J Med*. 2017;377(26):2531–2544.

16. Masoud SJ, Hu JB, Beasley GM, Stewart 4th JH, Mosca PJ. Efficacy of talimogene laherparepvec (T-VEC) therapy in patients with in-transit melanoma metastasis decreases with increasing lesion size. *Ann Surg Oncol*. 2019;26(13):4633–4641.

17. Gulley JL, Mulders P, Albers P, et al. Perspectives on sipuleucel-T: its role in the prostate cancer treatment paradigm. *OncoImmunology*. 2016;5(4):e1107698.

18. Glynne-Jones R, Wyrwicz L, Tiret E, et al. Rectal cancer: ESMO Clinical Practice Guidelines for diagnosis, treatment and follow-up. *Ann Oncol*. 2017;28(suppl 4):iv22–iv40.

19. Guzzinati S, Virdone S, De Angelis R, et al. Characteristics of people living in Italy after a cancer diagnosis in 2010 and projections to 2020. *BMC Canc*. 2018;18(1):169.

20. Mullan F. Seasons of survival: reflections of a physician with cancer. *N Engl J Med*. 1985;313(4):270–273.

21. The 20 Most Common Cancers, UK, 2015. 2015. https://www.cancerresearchuk.org/health-professional/cancerstatistics/incidence/common-cancers-compared#heading-Zero.

5

Surgical Infection

This chapter begins with an introduction to infection and continues with a discussion about some infections that are common or important in surgical practice. It is not an exhaustive account. Surgical infections include both those that are established and present to surgeons and those that result from surgical interventions (iatrogenic).

INFECTION IN GENERAL

Importance of Infection

History

One hundred years ago, surgeons had few methods for the elimination of contamination from potential causes of infection. Infected wounds were treated by radical operations. Then Joseph Lister (1827–1912) discovered that meticulous technique and a spray of carbolic acid into and around the wounds of compound leg fractures reduced the incidence of infection, e.g. the use of antisepsis (destruction of infective organisms by physicochemical means) was followed by the development of asepsis (absence of infective organisms) in surgical procedures. The discovery by Paul Ehrlich (1854–1915) of chemical agents which could kill organisms dramatically changed the management of infection. In 1929, Sir Alexander Fleming discovered that a mould *(Penicillium)* inhibited bacterial growth and later won the Nobel Prize for this.

Incidence

The incidence of postoperative infection has fallen because of advances in sterilization techniques, antibiotic prophylaxis and surgical awareness. The risk is related to the type of surgery performed and the physiological status of the patient. In general surgery, operations have been classified into four risk groups (Table 5.1).

Morbidity and mortality

Postoperative infections cause increased morbidity, significant mortality, a prolonged stay in hospital and possible litigation.

Biology of Infection

Infection is defined as the proliferation of organisms in tissues and their invasion into places such as the blood. Colonization of parts of the body – e.g. the gastrointestinal tract and upper respiratory passages – is normal; 'normal flora' are important for health as they produce essential metabolites and prevent infection from more pathogenic organisms.

There is also frequent exposure of the body to contamination by other potentially invasive organisms, but infection remains comparatively rare. Its development depends on complex interactions between the organism, local factors and host defences (Fig. 5.1).

Organisms

Load

Experimental studies have shown that a certain quantity of organisms is required before infection results. Any wound is inevitably contaminated from the surrounding environment. The basis of simple first aid in traumatic wounds is the application of agents that selectively kill the organisms (antiseptics), decrease the load and, hence, reduce the chance of infection.

Pathogenesis and Virulence

Organisms capable of causing infection (pathogens) have varying virulence. Factors responsible include:
- direct growth, damaging surrounding structures by pressure and/or ischaemic effects, e.g. abscess formation
- production of bacterial toxins which cause a variety of effects, e.g. bacterial spread (streptokinase), cell damage (haemolysins), activation of cytokine cascades (Gram-negative endotoxin)
- synergy and interaction, e.g. combined promotion of infection by beta-haemolytic streptococci and anaerobic bacteria to produce rapidly spreading cutaneous gangrene (necrotizing fasciitis) where hyaluronidase from the streptococci cleave the fascial planes, allowing the infection to spread rapidly
- replication rate

Local Host Factors

The local environment has an impact on the chance of contamination resulting in an infection. Factors include:
- Ischaemia, which reduces the effectiveness of phagocytes and also aids the growth of anaerobic bacteria.
- Uncontrolled diabetes, which is associated with soft-tissue infections – the mechanism is multifactorial: local hyperglycaemia, microvascular disease and peripheral neuropathy.
- Haematomas, which provide an ideal environment for bacterial growth.

Host Defences

Mechanical, Physical and Chemical Barriers

Invasion is discouraged wherever a natural interface occurs between the tissues and surrounding environment.
- Skin is a mechanical barrier against organisms.
- Cilia in the respiratory tract keep contaminated secretions in constant movement towards the exterior.
- The acidic pH in the stomach destroys many organisms.
- Peristaltic movement discourages local organism growth.
- A competent ileocecal valve prevents reflux from large to small bowel.
- Flushing action of secretions such as tears and urine.
- Normal endogenous (commensal) flora on the skin and the GI tract provide a physical barrier by preventing the

TABLE 5.1	Classification of Risk of Wound Infection		
Type	**Definition**	**Example**	**Infection Risk (%)**
Clean	No breach of GI tract	Hernia, varicose veins	2
Clean–contaminated	Prepared GI tract opened	Elective colectomy	6
Contaminated	Unprepared bowel opened	Emergency colectomy	15
Dirty	Pus at operation site; perforated bowel	Perforated appendicitis	40

GI, Gastrointestinal.

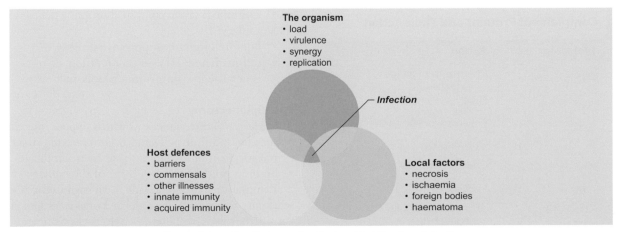

• **Fig. 5.1** Interaction Between the Factors That Produce Infection

adherence of foreign organisms, and some also secrete mucus to produce a chemical barrier.

Concomitant Illnesses
The general state of health of the patient can affect resistance to infection. The disorders thought to influence the incidence and course of infection through their effects on host defences are given in Box 5.1.

Natural Immunity

Phagocytic Cells: the Macrophage and the Neutrophil
Organisms that overcome the mechanical barriers of the skin, respiratory or GI tract are first attacked by these cells, which ingest and then kill them.

The Complement System
The complement system is a cascade of active proteins that attract phagocytic cells, increase vascular permeability and directly lyse pathogens (Table 5.2). Activation is either by the classical (antibody-mediated) or alternative (endotoxin-mediated) pathways.

Acquired Immunity

There are two types of acquired immunity: antibody-mediated and cell-mediated.

Antibody-Mediated Immunity
Organisms evading the first lines of defence encounter lymphocytes. B-lymphocytes secrete antibodies which are classically divided into five classes: IgM, IgG, IgA, IgD and IgE. Stimulation of antibody production is usually T-cell–dependent but some polysaccharides can stimulate B-cells directly. Antibodies protect the host by binding to the foreign antigen or act with complement proteins to opsonize, lyse and kill invading organisms. The classical pathway for complement activation involves the binding of C1-qrs, a calcium-dependent complex found in normal plasma, to IgG or IgM, which leads to the activation of C3, leading to an increase in vascular permeability, attraction of neutrophils and lysis foreign cells.

Cell-Mediated Immunity
Two different processes are involved:
- CD8 T-lymphocytes kill cells which contain replicating invaders, usually viruses.
- CD4 T-lymphocytes help macrophages to kill phagocytosed organisms.

Cytokines

Cytokines are small peptides, released by white blood cells, which act like hormones for the immune system. They allow communication between the different cell populations and control the response to infection (Table 5.3).

Immune Deficiency Syndromes

Defects in the innate or adaptive immune systems illustrate the importance of both in protection from infection:

Innate
- Primary:
  - complement disorders
  - phagocytic cell deficiencies: chronic granulomatous disease.
- Secondary:
  - burns
  - trauma (including surgical procedures)
  - presence of foreign bodies
  - corticosteroids.

Adaptive
- Primary:
  - B-cell deficiencies: Bruton-type agammaglobulinaemia
  - T-cell deficiencies: DiGeorge syndrome
  - combined: severe combined immune deficiency.
- Secondary:
  - humoral: immunosuppressive drugs
  - cell-mediated: HIV infection/AIDS
  - generalized: malnutrition, neoplasia.

Post-Splenectomy
The spleen has three functions which oppose infection:
- specific immunity – T- and B-lymphocyte production
- phagocytosis of foreign antigens by macrophages
- opsonin production

Removal of the spleen leads to an increased risk of overwhelming infection by encapsulated organisms like pneumococci. If the spleen is to be removed electively, vaccination against pneumococci, meningococci and *Haemophilus influenzae B*

• BOX 5.1   Factors Predisposing to Infection

- Malnutrition
- Malignancy
- Immunodeficiency
- Extremes of age
- Obesity
- Diabetes

TABLE 5.2   Complement Proteins and Their Action.

Active Molecule	Action
C3a	Chemoattractant for neutrophils Liberates histamine
C3b	Enhances phagocytosis
C5a	Opsonization
C8	Causes cells to leak
C9	Lyses antigens
C5–9	Chemoattractant for neutrophils

TABLE 5.3	Cytokines and Their Actions in Relation to Infection.	
Factor	**Source**	**Actions**
IL-1	Macrophages	Pro-inflammatory
IL-4	T-cells	T- and B-cell proliferation Macrophage activation
IL-6	T-cells	B-cell differentiation
IL-9	T-cells	Mast cell growth
IL-10	T- and B-cells macrophages	Cytokine inhibition
IFN-α	Multiple	Antiviral
IFN-γ	T- and NK cells	Antiviral
		Macrophage activation
		MHC induction
TNF-α	Monocytes	Cytotoxicity
		Cachexia, fever
TNF-β	T-cells	Inhibits T- and NK-cell activation
	Macrophages	
G-CSF	Macrophages	Granulocyte growth

G-CSF, granulocyte colony-stimulating factor; IFN, interferon; IL, interleukin; MHC, major histocompatibility complex; NK, natural killer; TNF, tumour necrosis factor.

should be done at least 2 weeks before the operation. After the operation, all patients should be on long-term prophylactic penicillin, or erythromycin/clarithromycin if penicillin allergic.

Infection Control and Prevention

Measures are required to protect the patient, other patients and healthcare personnel from infections which may be encountered during surgical management. Risks arise both from the environment and from the patient's endogenous flora.

Disinfectants

Disinfectants are substances that can kill most pathogenic organisms but not bacterial spores or slow viruses. Their main use is for cleaning instruments (e.g. endoscopes) and surfaces which cannot be sterilized by other means. Examples include:
- aldehydes, e.g. glutaraldehyde
- ethyl alcohol 60–90%
- chlorine-releasing agents, e.g. sodium hypochlorite (bleach)
- clear phenolics, e.g. Clearsol.

Antiseptics

These are disinfectants that can be used on living tissue.
Common examples include:
- aqueous or alcoholic 0.5% chlorhexidine
- aqueous or alcoholic 10% povidone-iodine.

Sterilization

This process involves the complete destruction of all organisms, including spores. A number of methods are available.

Protection for the Patient

The risk of infection of the surgical site (wound, anastomosis, peritoneal and other cavities) may be reduced in a number of ways.

Factors associated with increased risk of infection are:
- operation of more than 2 hours' duration
- abdominal procedures
- contamination, either endogenous or exogenous
- co-morbidities

When one or more of these is present, additional preventative measures should be considered, including the use of prophylactic antibiotics, although these are not a substitute for good surgical aseptic techniques. An assessment of the risk is made, based on the patient's medical state and the type of surgery to be done.

Aseptic Surgical Technique

Handwashing reduces the number of organisms found on the hands. Gloves should be put on with minimal contact between their external surface and the hand. Likewise, surgical gowns are put on so that the outside surface is never touched. Hair cover and masks are also worn.

Preparation of the Skin and Bowel

Skin

Antiseptics are used for the preparation of the skin before operation. Adherent plastic film placed onto the patient's exposed skin prior to incision may further reduce the chance of contamination from skin organisms.

Gastrointestinal Tract

This is discussed in Chapter 20.

Antibiotic Prophylaxis

Identification of Patients at Risk

Patients who are at high risk of infection, or in whom the risk may be low but infection would have serious consequences, should be given prophylactic antibiotics. There are operative and patient-related factors to consider:

- operative:
  - high risk of an infection – contaminated or dirty surgery (e.g. colectomy, trauma surgery)
  - placement of foreign materials, e.g. heart valve, arterial graft, joint replacement.
- patient:
  - immunosuppression
  - high-risk patients, e.g. previous foreign body implants, heart valve disease, peripheral vascular disease, obesity.

Choice of Antibiotic

This is determined by the likely infecting organisms. Most NHS trusts/units have agreed protocols tailored for type of operations and local resistance data. The chosen antibiotic should be:

- effective for the likely organisms, e.g. in gastrointestinal surgery, it must provide cover against Gram-negative bacteria and anaerobes
- cost-effective
- unlikely to promote resistance

Cephalosporins or glycopeptides are widely used for orthopaedic surgery. For gastrointestinal tract surgery, either a cephalosporin in combination with metronidazole or co-amoixiclav is commonly given (Table 5.4).

Dose and timing

The highest tissue concentration of antibiotic is required at the moment of tissue contamination. Usually one dose of chemoprophylaxis at the time of induction is sufficient unless the operation is long, there has been excessive blood loss or there are significant co-morbidities: in these cases, up to two further doses at appropriate intervals to complete 24 hours of prophylaxis may be required.

Route of administration

Intravenous

Adequate serum concentrations are guaranteed.

Oral

Sometimes used for patients undergoing certain minor procedures.

Rectal

Metronidazole suppositories are used by some gastrointestinal surgeons.

Topical

This route is used for specific circumstances, e.g. gentamicin-impregnated cement for orthopaedic prostheses.

Protection for Others

Other Patients

Continuous accurate monitoring of infections in the hospital environment can give early warning of potential problems and so allow early measures to be taken, such as temporary cessation of operations, isolation of patients and change in antibiotic regimens.

On the ward, patients who are highly infectious or colonized with resistant organisms should be isolated in side rooms. Clear instructions for staff and visitors about barrier nursing and use of gloves, aprons and use of appropriate masks must be given.

The increase in hospital-acquired infection has led to a greater emphasis on hand hygiene and aseptic technique. Before and after inspecting a wound (or touching a patient), all healthcare staff should clean their hands. If there is significant risk of infection, disposable gloves and aprons should be worn.

Patients who are admitted for elective joint surgery should not be placed next to someone with an infected wound; indeed, good practice would separate all elective clean surgery patients from those who might be infected. Many hospitals now screen all elective admissions for MRSA colonization. During the Covid 19 pandemic, UK hospitals have been screening all hospital admissions, both emergency and elective ones, for Covid.

In outpatient clinics, similar hygienic measures apply: paper covers to the examination couches; hand cleaning between patients; washing, disinfecting or sterilizing examination instruments such as endoscopes; and increasing use of disposables.

Healthcare Personnel

HIV drew attention to the protection of healthcare personnel from blood-borne viruses, although hepatitis B has caused far more infections in these personnel. HIV seroconversion following occupational injury is rare. Recently much attention has been drawn to the protection of healthcare personnel from respiratory viruses, particularly Covid 19 but also influenza, by the use of appropriate personal protective equipment (PPE).

Vaccination

All staff at risk should be vaccinated against hepatitis B and have a recent serological test to show adequate antibody levels. Currently, there are no effective vaccines against hepatitis C or HIV. Staff should also be encouraged to be vaccinatined against influenza and more recently against Covid 19.

TABLE 5.4 Common Antibiotics and Their Uses.

Antibiotic	Common Uses	Notes
Benzylpenicillin	Streptococcal infections	Most staphylococci are resistant due to beta-lactamase production.
Flucloxacillin	Treatment of wound infections and cellulitis	Active against staphylococci. Some activity against streptococci
Amoxicillin	Active against both Gram-positive and some Gram-negative organisms	Inactivated by beta-lactamases produced by many coliforms
Co-amoxiclav	Broad spectrum: active against Gram-positive and Gram-negative bacteria (but not *Pseudomonas* spp.) and anaerobes soft-tissue infections, pneumonia, UTI and for antibiotic prophylaxis of gastro-intestinal surgery and treatment of intra-abdominal infections	Combination of amoxicillin and clavulanic acid; latter acts to prevent action of beta-lactamases,
Piperacillin-tazobactam	Gram-positive and Gram-negative bacteria including *Pseudomonas* spp. and anaerobes	Reserved for severe infections, often used in combination with gentamicin or another aminoglycoside
Cefuroxime/cefotaxime	Broad spectrum: prophylaxis for bowel and biliary operations; treatment of GI conditions – cholecystitis, appendix mass, diverticulitis	Used in GI surgery often in combination with metronidazole; 5–10% of penicillin-allergic patients are also allergic to cephalosporins
Ceftazidime	Gram-negative infections including *Pseudomonas* spp.	Some improvement in activity against Gram-negative organisms compared with cefuroxime but poorer activity against staphylococci and streptococci
Meropenem	Broad spectrum: active against both Gram positive and most Gram-negative bacteria and anaerobes often reserved for use in ICU or on advice of consultant microbiologist	Carbapenem active against extended specrum beta-lactamase producing organisms (ESBL)-producing coliforms
Tetracycline	Pelvic inflammatory disease; other sexually transmitted diseases	Bacteriostatic rather than bactericidal; however, active against *Chlamydia*
Gentamicin/tobramycin/amikacin	Severe sepsis (in combination with a beta lactam +/– metronidazole); Prophylaxis during urinary tract instrumentation	Aminoglycoside active against Gram-negative organisms and *Pseudomonas*. Nephrotoxic – serum levels must be regularly checked
Erythromycin/clarithromycin	Soft-tissue and chest infections	Active against streptococci and for treatment of atypical pneumonia. Useful in those allergic to penicillin. Used in combination therapy for *Helicobacter pylori* infections
Vancomycin	Gram-positive infections in penicillin allergic patients and for MRSA. No activity against Gram-negative bacteria	Normally given i.v. by slow infusion over 100 minutes and levels need monitoring. Used orally to treat *C. difficile* infection
Teicoplanin	Similar uses to vancomycin. No activity against Gram-negative bacteria	Can be given by a slow i.v. injection and once daily
Trimethoprim	Urinary tract infections	Significant resistance now occurs
Nitrofurantoin	Urinary tract infections	First-line agent in many Trusts for lower urinary tract infections
Co-trimoxazole	*Pneumocystis* pneumonia	Relatively high incidence of skin rashes
Metronidazole	Anaerobic bacterial infections including dental abscesses; Gas gangrene; Amoebic infections	Metronidazole is not normally needed if amoxicillin-clavulanic acid, piperacillin- tazobactam or meropenem are used as these all have good anaerobic cover
Ciprofloxacin	Gram-negative infections including urinary tract infections and GI infections including *Salmonella*, *Shigella*, *Campylobacter*	Quinolones are the only group of oral antimicrobials active against *Pseudomonas* spp. Poor activity against Gram-positive bacteria. Implicated as a relatively common cause of infections due to *Clostridium difficile*.

ESBL, Extended spectrum beta-lactamase; GI, gastrointestinal; ICU, intensive care unit; MRSA, methicillin-resistant *Staphylococcus aureus*; UTI, urinary tract infection.

In order to monitor the incidence of occupationally acquired infection, sharp injuries must be reported and a serum sample obtained at the time, with another 3 months later. Post-exposure prophylaxis against HIV after injury from a high-risk patient is routinely offered.

DIAGNOSIS AND MANAGEMENT OF INFECTION

Prompt identification of the source and initiation of correct treatment are crucial to minimize infection related morbidity and mortality. Empirical antibiotic treatment as per local guidelines before the causative organism is identified may be required in patients with severe infections.

Features of Infection

History

The timing of a postoperative infection gives clues as to its cause. Wound infections do not usually become clinically manifest in the first 48 hours, and chest infections are a more likely cause of early sepsis. A leaking gastrointestinal anastomosis often presents with low-grade fever after 4 or 5 days. Deep-seated prosthetic infection may not be apparent for weeks or months. Direct questions for cough, dysuria or abdominal pain may focus further enquiry and investigation.

Physical Findings

An assessment, with measurement of pulse, blood pressure and temperature, gives an indication of severity. Full examination is essential in a surgical patient with pyrexia of unknown origin (PUO). Non-infective causes of PUO (deep vein thrombosis, haematoma, malignancy) should also be considered. Likely causes of infection include:
- chest
- surgical site (wounds, anastomoses) or areas adjacent to it (e.g. sub-phrenic spaces, pelvis)
- urinary tract, often secondary to catheterization
- intravenous lines

Investigation of Infection

Blood Sampling

- *Full blood count.* A raised white blood cell count suggests the presence of infection. However, severe infections can suppress the bone marrow and cause leucopoenia/anaemia/thrombocytopenia.
- *Blood culture.* It is important to take blood cultures and other samples as indicated before antibiotics are started because interpretation of results afterwards may become difficult. *Other* samples as indicated may include urine, sputum, wound swabs, pus, tissue.

- *Serological examination* to detect antibodies can identify specific infections in their recovery phase.

Microbiological Analysis

Appropriate samples should be sent for microbiological analysis. Specimens may include:
- swabs from contaminated or infected wounds
- drainage fluid
- urine
- stool for *Clostridium difficile* toxin testing
- tissue biopsies
  Methods of analysis include:
- direct microscopy
- Gram-staining of tissues and fluids can guide urgent treatment before a formal culture and sensitivity report is available; culture and sensitivity currently takes 24–48 hours
  In severe infections, empiric treatment should be started according to likely pathogens and likely sensitivities and then modified if required following test results.

Newer Microbiological Techniques

- *Enzyme-linked immunosorbent assay (ELISA)* is used to detect antibodies to an organism and is used to identify HIV and other viruses.
- *The polymerase chain reaction (PCR)* is increasingly used to identify a range of infections including TB, HIV and *Helicobacter pylori.*

Imaging

Localization of the source of infection is often a challenge. Ultrasound is often used as the first-line of imaging, but other techniques such as CT scanning or MRIs are frequently needed. Radionuclide imaging with labelled leucocytes is another technique used for localizing infection or inflammation.

General Measures

Basic treatment of infected wounds is summarized in Box 5.2. Other general measures include:
- resuscitation
- analgesia for pain
- anti-emetics
- analgesics
- cooling fans for high fever

Specific Measures

Antibiotics

The decision as to which antibiotics and when to start them is not always easy. Some fevers do not require antibiotics (e.g. postoperative pyrexia caused by DVT), and certain infections (e.g. abscesses) respond poorly to antibiotic therapy and require surgical intervention.

• BOX 5.2 Management of Infected Wounds

- Remove clips or stitches to open part of wound
- Surgically debride necrotic areas
- Take wound swab (although most wound infections do not need antibiotics)
- Mark area of cellulitis surrounding wound to assess efficacy of treatment
- Dress wound to keep it open, clean and comfortable
  - soaked gauze (saline, betadine or proflavine)
  - specialized dressings
  - avoid occlusive dressings which encourage anaerobic infection
- For complex or large wounds consider:
  - stoma wound bag
  - vacuum dressing
  - rarely the use of sterile larvae (maggots)

Drainage

A local collection of pus contains organisms that are relatively inaccessible to systemic antibiotics, acts as a toxic focus and may exert pressure effects on surrounding structures. Collections need draining either by:

- *Needle aspiration.* For abscesses that can be reached with a needle (sometimes under imaging control), aspiration and antibiotic therapy may be all that is required. The technique is particularly useful for areas where a scar is undesirable, such as on the face or breast.
- *Guided drainage.* Under image control, a tube drain can be inserted and left until the cavity has collapsed.
- *Open surgical drainage.* This is the most certain method.

Systemic Effects and Syndromes

Bacteraemia

The word 'bacteraemia' means simply bacteria in the blood. Blood is normally sterile but any minor trauma to a colonized area can cause a transient bacteraemia.

Septicaemia

In cases of septicaemia, bacteria are not just present in the blood but are multiplying. Clinical manifestations may include fever, tachycardia, hypotension, oliguria, Acute Respiratory Distress Syndrome (ARDS) and multiple organ failure. Blood cultures are often but not always positive. Causes of negative blood cultures include:

- low bacterial concentrations at the time of sampling
- prior administration of systemic antibiotics

Endotoxaemia

In some instances of severe sepsis, often with shock, organisms are not found, but circulating Gram-negative endotoxins can be demonstrated. Translocation of Gram-negative material from the gut and subsequent cytokine activation (notably tumour necrosis factor, TNF) has been proposed as the cause of this apparently sterile septic state.

Clinical features

Confusion, fever, hypotension and worsening malaise are warning signs. There may be symptoms related to a specific focus.

Investigation

Blood culture should be taken but may not always be positive. Raised white cell count is usual unless there is systemic suppression of white cell production by drugs, underlying illness or overwhelming sepsis.

Management

Emergency management of the septic patient is summarized in Emergency Box 5.1. Empirical antibiotic therapy should be started immediately after cultures have been taken. Any focus discovered should be eliminated as soon as possible, usually by drainage.

Systemic Inflammatory Response Syndrome

Nomenclature

Systemic inflammatory response syndrome (SIRS) is the name given to a physiological state of septic collapse. It is often, but not always, due to infection (Fig. 5.2). It embraces the terms 'sepsis', 'septic shock' and 'toxic shock'.

Pathophysiology

The central mechanism appears to be activation of macrophages and release of TNF. Oxygen supply to the tissues is reduced, and the situation is aggravated by cell injury which leads to deficient uptake of oxygen. The result is general tissue hypoxia and a build-up of lactic acid. Cytokine activation also occurs; TNF can produce this clinical pattern experimentally. The clinical picture is characterized by fever, hypotension, respiratory failure, oliguria and multiple organ failure, with hepatic and bone marrow suppression occurring as late events.

Generalized Fungal Infections

Causes are as follows:

- a severely compromised immune system, as in leukaemia, lymphoma or HIV infection or post chemotherapy
- prolonged administration of multiple antibiotics
  The commonest infection is with *Candida* spp.

Bacterial translocation

Some clinicians believe that ischaemic damage to the gut in the critically ill allows translocation of bacteria and toxins. Once bacteria have crossed the bowel wall, they may translocate to the respiratory system, which becomes colonized with enteric organisms.

Emergency Management of the Septic Patient

- Resuscitate, if necessary, with oxygen and i.v. fluids
- Identify likely cause – history, examination, case notes, temperature chart
- Take samples – blood cultures, swabs, urine
- Treat symptoms – lower fever with paracetamol or fans; analgesia
- Treat infection – best-guess antibiotics i.v.
- Identify cause – arrange imaging: chest X-ray, ultrasound, CT scan, MRI
- Plan definitive treatment
  - Transfer to high-dependency area if in septic shock
  - Antibiotics according to microbiology sensitivities
  - Ultrasound- or CT-guided drainage
  - Surgical drainage

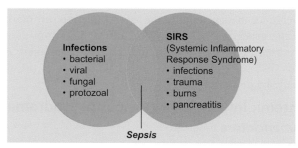

•**Fig. 5.2** Relationship Between Infection and Systemic Inflammatory Response Syndrome (SIRS)

Prevention

Selective Decontamination

To reduce endogenous bacterial load, selective decontamination of the digestive tract with topical, oral and intravenous antibiotics has been used but has not been widely adopted.

Immunomodulation

Immunoglobulins raised against the cell walls of Gram-negative organisms (antiendotoxins) have been protective in animal studies but have not improved mortality significantly in humans.

IMPORTANT INFECTIONS IN SURGICAL PATIENTS

Infections can arise as a result of surgical interventions or present as established infections that require surgical management.

The infections considered here are particularly common or important to surgical practice.

Some common antibiotics and their uses are given in Tables 5.4 and 5.5. When to use antibiotics and which ones to choose is not always clear. Most Trusts will have policies for the treatment of common infections. Many UK Trusts use Microguide.

Empirical treatment as per your hospital guidelines is often needed for sick patients, but may obscure the bacteriological diagnosis.

The selection of an antibiotic rests on:
- severity of infection
- site of infection
- likely organisms and sensitivities
- patient factors – age, sex, co-morbidities, being immunocompromised, allergies, pregnancy, renal function, etc.
- hospital policy

More expensive antibiotics often have a broader spectrum of activity but the broader spectrum an antimicrobial is, the more likely it is to disrupt normal flora, and encourage super-infection with more resistant bacteria and *Candida* spp. Hence broad-spectrum antimicrobials such as piperacillin-tazobactam and carbapenems are normally kept in reserve for severe infections or as second-line treatment and often require the approval of the consultant microbiologist.

Samples such as blood cultures should be taken before treatment is begun. Other factors to take into account are:
- dose
- route of administration
- frequency of administration
- duration (5–7 days' treatment is usually sufficient for most common bacterial infections)
- potential side effects
- toxicity – renal, ototoxicity, liver
- cost

Acquired Infections

Some infections arise as a consequence of an intervention or because of hospital admission. Common sources are listed in Box 5.3.

Clinical Features of Infection

Most wound infections can be identified by simple inspection for erythema and by palpation. A deeper infection may present insidiously, again with pyrexia, a rise in the white blood count or organ dysfunction such as prolonged postoperative ileus. Some deep infections are hard to detect and require special imaging techniques.

Management

Prevention

As described above, strict measures to reduce hospital-acquired infections must be observed. In particular the surgeon should:
- use meticulous technique to inflict minimal damage to tissues and to avoid a haematoma
- use prophylactic antibiotics where indicated
- maintain hand hygiene at all times
- ensure that peripheral and central intravenous cannulas are changed routinely
- avoid prolonged antibiotic treatment whenever possible
- comply with hospital infection control policies
- screen elective cases for infection and MRSA colonization prior to admission

Treatment

Antibiotics treat cellulitis surrounding a wound but cannot penetrate into an abscess. There is no substitute

TABLE 5.5 Examples of Typical Antibiotic Choices for Particular Clinical Infections.

Infection	First Choice	Alternatives
Chest infection	Benzylpenicillin + erythromycin	Co-amoxiclav (Augmentin) + erythromycin
Wound infection (cellulitis)	IV benzylpenicillin + flucloxacillin	Co-amoxiclav
Wound infection (abscess)	Aspiration + antibiotic	Flucloxacillin
Intra-abdominal infection (endogenous organisms likely)	Cefuroxime + metronidazole	Co-amoxiclav +/- gentamicin
		Cefotaxime
		Gentamicin
Cholecystitis-cholangitis	Amoxicillin-clavulanic acid or cefuroxime + metronidazole	Piperacillin-tazobactam (Tazocin)
Urinary tract infection	Trimethoprim	Nitrofurantoin, gentamicin
		Co-amoxiclav
Pelvic inflammatory disease	Tetracyclines + cefuroxime + metronidazole	
Severe sepsis	Amoxicillin + gentamicin + metronidazole or amoxicillin-clavulanic acid + gentamicin	Piperacillin-tazobactam, meropenem/imipenem
Methicillin-resistant *Staphylococcus aureus*	Intravenous vancomycin	Teicoplanin
Pseudomembranous colitis (*C. difficile*)	Oral vancomycin	Fidoxamycin
Gas gangrene	Penicillin + metronidazole or, piperacillin-tazobactam	Metronidazole

• BOX 5.3 Sources of Hospital-Acquired Infections

- The operative site – the wound, any anastomosis, the cavity in which the operation was done
- In relation to a prosthesis – joint, cardiac, other vascular or mesh used to repair a hernia
- Respiratory or gastrointestinal tract from translocation
- Urinary tract
- Infection from intravenous lines
- Cross infection, particularly methicillin-resistant *Staphylococcus aureus*
- *Clostridium difficile* from a person's faecal flora or occasionally from cross infection

for drainage in presence of pus. The common form of continued spread is peritonitis. If the infection has not localized, the only effective treatment is to re-explore and remove products of infection by lavage and control the cause of the infection, e.g. a leakage from an anastomotic suture-line.

Infection of a prosthesis is very serious. Although high-dose systemic antibiotics may work, the most effective treatment is to remove the prosthesis and not replace it until the infection has been controlled. However, some prostheses (e.g. heart valves and peripheral vascular grafts) cannot be removed without being immediately replaced.

Respiratory Tract

Definition

Infection of the respiratory tract includes a range of conditions: bronchitis, pneumonia, lung abscess and empyema. An element of alveolar under-expansion (atelectasis) after operation is common and can cause fever.

Organisms

The commonest organisms are *Streptococcus pneumoniae* and *Haemophilus influenzae* in patients recently admitted to hospital. Gram-negative organisms may cause postoperative chest infections especially if the patient has been in hospital for more than 4–5 days.

Clinical features

Symptoms

- fever
- cough
- breathlessness
- confusion from hypoxia

Physical findings

- cyanosis
- green/purulent sputum
- consolidation on chest examination

Investigation

- chest X-ray
- culture of sputum or bronchial washings
- arterial blood gas tensions

Management

Prophylaxis

- Do not perform elective surgery in the presence of uncontrolled respiratory infection.
- Postoperatively, provide adequate analgesia, physiotherapy and early mobilization.

Treatment

- Initial administration of oxygen with the aim of restoring normal blood gas tensions.
- Antibiotic administration; most hospitals have a policy for treating chest infections.

Urinary Tract

Definition

Urinary tract infection (UTI) encompasses a range of clinical conditions which include cystitis, pyelonephritis and perinephric abscess.

Organisms

Escherichia coli is the most common organism. Other Gram-negative bacteria include *Klebsiella* spp., *Pseudomonas* spp. and *Proteus mirabilis* or sometimes Gram-positive bacteria like *Enterococcus* spp. and coagulase-negative staphylococci.

Diagnosis

The urine of those with an indwelling catheter frequently contains organisms. Unless the patient is systemically unwell, this does not require treatment. The urine will not become sterile until the catheter is removed.

Clinical Features

Symptoms

Smelly urine, dysuria and, if a catheter is not in place, increased frequency are all symptoms of a UTI.

Physical Findings

In cystitis, these are unusual. In pyelonephritis, tenderness in the renal angles and fever may be found.

Investigation

Midstream or catheter drainage specimens should be taken before treatment is started, but best-guess antibiotic therapy can be started before culture results are available.

Management

Common first-line antibiotics include nitrofurantoin, trimethoprim, co-amoxiclav or gentamicin.

Clostridium difficile (pseudomembranous colitis)

Aetiology

Disturbance of normal colonic flora by antibiotics leads to colonization/overgrowth with *C. difficile*, an anaerobic spore-forming organism which produces an enterotoxin. Risk factors include:
- prolonged admission
- older age
- malignant disease
- broad-spectrum antibiotic use
- protein pump inhibitor use

Clinical Features

Symptoms

The patient develops profuse mucous diarrhoea usually after broad-spectrum antibiotics and may have an elevated WBC count and C-reactive protein (CRP) level.

Physical Findings

Fever and non-specific features of toxicity are common. The abdomen may be distended and tender. Sigmoidoscopy if performed reveals diffuse inflammation and, sometimes, the typical yellow membranous plaques.

Investigation

Diagnosis is made by the detection of *C. difficile* toxin in the stool.

Management

Stopping the antibiotics may be all that is needed in mild attacks. Oral metronidazole used to be the first line treatment but now oral vancomycin is the treatment of choice. Oral vancomycin is not systemically absorbed so levels are not required. Fidoxamycin can be considered for severe cases/relapses. Colectomy may be needed for:

- failure to respond to medical treatment
- toxic dilatation
- perforation

Faecal transplants are occasionally performed in patients with severe disease unresponsive to antimicrobial in an attempt to avoid colectomy.

Methicillin-Resistant *Staphylococcus aureus* (MRSA)

Methicillin is an antibiotic used to test sensitivity to flucloxacillin in the laboratory. MRSA are no more virulent than flucloxacillin-sensitive *S. aureus*, but are more difficult to treat. MRSA is particularly prevalent amongst elderly long-stay hospital or nursing home in-patients.

Clinical features

A patient may be colonized but have no signs of infection. Clinical manifestations are those of other *S. aureus* staphylococcal infection, with wounds and prostheses being particularly affected.

Investigation

Swabs should be taken from the wound, throat, nose, perineum and axilla and may be used for pre-admission screening. A rapid PCR-based test is also now available and may be particularly useful for testing emergency admissions.

Management

Most hospitals have a policy to deal with occurrences of MRSA, which consists of:
- isolation
- barrier nursing, including skin antiseptics
- topical mupirocin – an antibiotic agent related to vancomycin for local use only
- regular samples from the patient to ascertain if eradication has been achieved
- intravenous vancomycin or teicoplanin to treat serious infections

Eradication of MRSA is possible by these methods, but lack of compliance with the treatment or ineffective barrier nursing methods leads to failure in over 50% of cases. Colonization of the throat is particularly difficult to eradicate. The problem is an important issue in orthopaedic, vascular and cardiothoracic surgical patients. Standard antibiotics used for prophylaxis do not deal with MRSA.

The incidence of MRSA-related deaths in the UK has been reduced by the prevention strategies described above, but has not been eliminated.

Pyrexia of Unknown Origin

The cause of fever in the postoperative recovery period is not always apparent. However, infection is a common cause. Sources include:
- intravenous line
- abscess/collection
- urinary tract infection
- cholecystitis/pancreatitis in those convalescing from other disorders, particularly severe trauma
- pneumonia
- viral infections
  Other less common causes include:
- unresected tumour
- factitious
- collagen diseases

Established Infections in the Surgical Patient

Cellulitis and Wound Infections

Presents as reddening of the area, often with increased heat and swelling. It can affect any part of the body. Secondary cellulitis from intravenous lines or infected sutures is common. Two uncommon types worthy of mention are:
- Erysipelas – intradermal infection with streptococci. The organism produces streptokinase and spreads rapidly.
- Ludwig's angina – submandibular cellulitis, secondary to dental infection.

Organisms

Causative organisms are pyogenic streptococci (Group A, B, C and G), *S. aureus* and, occasionally, Gram-negative rods.

Clinical Features

Pain and fever are common, often with tenderness in the regional lymph nodes. Signs include a hot, tender, erythematous swelling with ill-defined margins and tender enlarged lymph nodes.

Management

Treatment with appropriate antibiotics – penicillin/amoxicillin for streptococci, flucloxacillin for staphylococci.

Established Abscesses

Definition

An abscess is a collection of liquefied leucocytes, dead tissue (slough) and organisms.

Organisms

The commonest pathogen is *S. aureus*. Depending on the site of the infection, other organisms are also common, such as gut bacteria (e.g. *E. coli*, enterococci and anaerobes in perianal and intra-abdominal collections).

Clinical Features

Symptoms
Abscesses close to the surface of the body cause pain from tension within the cavity. Deep-seated collections cause illness, fever and local pressure symptoms.

Clinical Findings
A tense, painful, red, hot and occasionally fluctuant swelling in a febrile patient is diagnostic. If there is doubt about whether pus is present, needle aspiration confirms the diagnosis and can sometimes be definitive treatment (e.g. breast abscess).

Investigation
Ultrasound and CT are useful to delineate deep-seated or multi-loculated collections. A raised WBC is common.

Management

Treatment is drainage, with the technique used being determined by the site and size of the abscess. Antibiotics are relatively ineffective in an established abscess but can partially control the symptoms surrounding cellulitis.

Gangrene

Definition

Gangrene is the presence of dead tissue. Two types occur:
- non-infected or dry (often colonized by bacteria and usually caused by ischaemia of a limb)
- infected (organisms are proliferating) or wet.
  Infected gangrene can be subdivided into clostridial and non-clostridial

Clostridial Gangrene (Gas Gangrene)

Organisms

Although other clostridia species or anaerobes can be involved, the predominant one is *Clostridium perfringens,* an anaerobic spore forming Gram-positive rods, present in the gut and soil. Modern surgical techniques and antibiotics have made this disease uncommon. Organisms multiply in dead muscle so removal of this is an effective method of both prophylaxis and management.

Clinical Features

Symptoms and Physical Findings. Severe pain and systemic illness lead to septic shock and death if untreated. Findings include a characteristic musty odour, blackening of overlying skin and watery brown discharge from a wound or sinus. Digital palpation may suggest presence of gas in the subcutaneous tissues. Prompt diagnosis and management is necessary.

Investigation. Imaging can demonstrate the presence of gas in the tissues. Gram-staining of wound discharge or tissue removed at operation shows the characteristic large Gram-positive rods.

Management (Box 5.4). Treatment is required before the bacteriological cultures are complete and includes:
- resuscitation
- high-dose beta-lactam (unless penicillin allergic), usually with metronidazole
- urgent surgical debridement of all necrotic tissue back to bleeding and viable structures; urgent amputation may be needed
- occasionally oxygen therapy in hyperbaric chamber is used

• BOX 5.4   Prophylaxis of gangrene and tetanus

The text deals with the management of established gas gangrene and tetanus. However, real advances have come from the recognition that good practice can prevent nearly all infections. For gas gangrene and non-clostridial gangrene, early adequate excision of dead and damaged tissue, avoidance of primary suture of high-risk wounds and systemic prophylactic antibiotics have made the conditions vanishingly rare. For tetanus, immunisation programmes are in place.

Non-Clostridial Gangrene

The two main types are:
- synergistic bacterial gangrene (Meleney's gangrene) – a mixed infection with a microaerophilic streptococci and *Staphylococcus aureus*, which spreads relatively slowly and affects chiefly the skin necrotizing fasciitis (Fournier's gangrene) – infection by streptococci and anaerobes, which spreads quickly and causes necrosis of fat and fascia with overlying secondary necrosis of skin.

Organisms

Pyogenic streptococci release toxins such as streptokinase and hyaluronidase which aid the spread of infection through the tissue planes.

Clinical Features

Symptoms and Physical Findings. In Fournier's (Fig. 5.3), there is rapid development of severe toxaemia. Black discoloration and breakdown of the skin, but without the crepitus of gas gangrene, occurs. Fournier's often affects the perineum.

Management
- Wide surgical debridement
- High dose, broad-spectrum beta-lactam such as piperacillin-tazobactam or meropenem plus or minus clindamycin or metronidazole.

Tetanus

Tetanus is a state of muscle spasm caused by an exotoxin produced by *Clostridium tetani*. Wounds contaminated with soil or faeces are the main predetermining cause.

Clinical features

The condition has an incubation period which varies from days to months. A better prognosis is associated with a longer incubation period. Tetanus should not occur if people have been immunized.

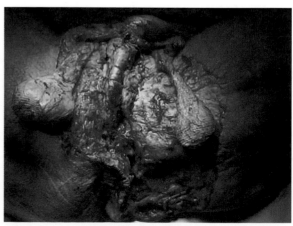

• Fig. 5.3 Wide Surgical Debridement of Scrotum and Perineum Needed to Cure Fournier's Gangrene

Investigation

Drumstick spores can be found in wound tissue and samples should be sent to the laboratory but treatment should commence on clinical diagnosis.

Management

- wide wound debridement
- tetanus immunoglobulin
- high-dose beta-lactam and metronidazole and seek expert advice

Candida Infection

Candida spp. are fungi which can cause opportunistic infections in sick patients, especially those on broad-spectrum antibiotics. Invasive fungal infections may be life threatening.

Pathological Features

The commonest sites are:
- oral and oesophageal
- perianal
- vaginal
- generalized in those with immunosuppression, blood disorders, long-term antibiotic treatment

Clinical Features

Findings include white plaques/discharge.

In generalized *Candida* infection, there are features of toxaemia and a lack of response to antibiotics.

Investigation

- microscopic evaluation of swabs or scrapings
- blood culture

Management

Local infection

Topical nystatin cream, mouthwash or pessaries suffice, although oral fluconazole is often used.

Generalized infection

Normally treated with intravenous agents, such as amphotericin, i.v. fluconazole or an echinocandin. Prophylactic systemic fluconazole (or other anti-fungal) is sometimes used in high-risk ICU patients.

HIV

Surgical presentation is the result of complications. Risk of cross-infection to healthcare personnel is minimal provided relevant precautions are taken. Modern highly active anti-retroviral treatment (HAART) has greatly improved the prognosis for HIV-infected patients, but they remain at increased risk of developing various malignancies including lymphoma, anal and oesophago-gastric cancer. Surgical involvement with these patients covers a wide range of conditions including:
- anal disease – warts, perianal abscess, carcinoma, and herpetic ulceration
- complications of drug injecting – abscesses at sites of injection, septic venous thrombosis, false arterial aneurysms
- lymph node biopsy for the diagnosis of associated disorders

Further Reading

Badia J, Casey A, Petrosillo N, Hudson P, Mitchell S, Crosby C. Impact of surgical site infection on healthcare costs and patient outcomes: a systematic review in six European countries. *J. Hospital Infect.* 2017;96:1–15.

Mazuski JE. *Surgical Infections, an Issue of Surgical Clinics.* Edinburgh: Saunders; 2009.

NICE guideline [NG125]. *Surgical site infections: prevention and treatment;* 2020. Last updated: 19 August 2020.

Taylor E, Williams J. *Infection in Surgical Practice.* London: Hodder Arnold; 2003.

UK Health Security Agency (UKHSA). *Surgical Site Infection (SSI): Guidance, Data and ANALYSIS;* Last updated: August 2021.

Velmahos GC, Vassiliu P, Demetriades D, et al. Wound management after colon injury: open or closed? A prospective randomized trial. *Am. Surg.* 2002;68(9):795–801.

6

Health Promotion and Disease Prevention

CHAPTER OUTLINE

Introduction

Over the last 100 years, societies across the world have seen a transition in the main causes of morbidity and mortality. For most of human history, infections and their complications have been responsible for the great majority of illness and death. However, as societies have become more affluent – resulting in changes such as better living conditions, improved housing and enhanced educational opportunities – and through the development of antibiotics and the implementation of immunization programmes, we have seen a dramatic decline in deaths from infections. In this period, there has been a concomitant rise in deaths from non-communicable diseases such as cardiovascular disease, cancer, diabetes, kidney disease and dementia; a change sometimes described as the 'epidemiological transition'.[1]

Many of these long-terms diseases that are now common in developed countries are closely linked to behavioural risk factors such as smoking, alcohol, poor diets, being overweight or obese or being physically inactive.[2] Making lifestyle changes such as stopping smoking, eating a healthier diet, increasing physical activity, losing weight and reducing alcohol consumption will all improve people's health and quality of life. These lifestyle changes will also result in improved outcomes for people undergoing surgical procedures, in addition to reducing the need for surgery (through a reduction in the frequency of problems that require surgical intervention).

The Ottawa Charter for Health Promotion defines health promotion as 'the process of enabling people to increase control over, and to improve, their health'.[3] Surgeons are not expected to be experts in health promotion. However, even very brief interventions from health professionals – such as offering some simple lifestyle suggestions – can result in beneficial changes to people's health. During their clinical practice – whether this is in outpatient, emergency department or inpatient settings – surgeons will see many patients with lifestyle-related conditions. This will include, for example, patients being considered for interventions such as joint replacement surgery, bariatric procedures and vascular surgery. In many cases, these patients will have potentially modifiable risk factors such as obesity or smoking. Each clinical contact should therefore be taken as an opportunity to raise awareness among patients of these adverse health behaviours and the benefits that can accrue through even modest positive changes in lifestyle.

Surgeons and their teams can also make positive contributions to people's health by encouraging them to take part in relevant screening and immunization programmes. This would include, for example, screening for conditions such as breast, colorectal and cervical cancer; and screening for aortic aneurysms. Immunization programmes would include those for children (such as measles, mumps and rubella), younger adults (such as meningitis immunization) and older adults (such as influenza, shingles and pneumococcal immunization). This advice is particularly important for people from marginalized communities, poorer people and people from minority groups, as they often have a lower uptake of preventive interventions.

KEY MODIFIABLE RISK FACTORS FOR LONG-TERM CONDITIONS

Smoking

Despite the decline in smoking rates in recent decades in the UK, smoking remains an important risk factor for a range of diseases including lung cancer, chronic lung disease and cardiovascular diseases such as coronary heart disease and peripheral vascular disease. In 2015, smoking-related diseases were estimated to have cost the National Health Service (NHS) in England around £2.6 billion (Table 6.1).[4] In addition to the costs to the NHS, there will also be substantial costs from smoking-related diseases to individuals, their families and carers and employers.

As well as the general health risks from smoking, smokers are also more likely to suffer from surgical complications. The adverse outcomes from smoking for surgical patients include higher risks, for example, of:

- Lung and heart complications
- Thrombo-embolic disease
- Postoperative infection
- Impaired wound healing
- Longer hospital stays
- Admission to an intensive care unit
- Emergency re-admission

Giving up smoking before surgery therefore improves outcomes for patients by reducing the risk of these complications and also saves money for health systems.[5] For example, a study of smokers who underwent coronary artery bypass graft surgery found that stopping smoking after undergoing surgery lowered the risk of death and repeat coronary procedures compared with patients who continued to smoke.[6]

Even very brief interventions by health professionals can lead to some people either giving up smoking entirely or cutting back on the number of cigarettes smoked. Surgeons should ensure that they ask about smoking status when they take a history and offer some encouragement for patients to give up smoking. The point in the care pathway when the patient and surgeon agree that surgery should take place will be a particularly important time to raise the importance of stopping smoking; for example, by emphasizing the improved outcomes following surgery if patients give up smoking.

To support the identification and referral of smokers to cessation services, the National Centre for Smoking Cessation and Training (NCSCT) has developed a method known as 'Very Brief Advice' (VBA; Box 6.1).[7]

Surgeons should be aware of the main risks from smoking and the benefits of smoking cessation. They should also be aware of how to signpost patients to other professionals or smoking cessation services for further advice and support. The pre-admission clinics that many hospitals now provide offer a good opportunity to raise the issue of smoking with patients and advise them of local smoking prevention services. For example, many hospitals will employ smoking cessation advisers who can spend more time counselling patients. Most parts of the UK will also have community-based smoking services that will accept self-referrals from patients. For hospital inpatients, advice on smoking should also be part of the discharge process when patients finally leave hospital following their inpatient stay.

Action on Smoking and Health (ASH), with support from the Royal College of Surgeons and other Royal Colleges, has produced a useful summary of what smokers should expect from the NHS before surgery (Box 6.2).[5]

Obesity

The prevalence of obesity is increasing globally and is predicted to increase still further in the next few decades. The Global Burden of Disease (GBD) Collaboration estimated

---

TABLE 6.1   Cost of Smoking to the NHS in England: 2015

NHS Event	Estimated Smoking-Related Burden
General practitioner visits	£794.0 million
Practice nurse visits	£111.7 million
Prescriptions	£144.8 million
Outpatient visits	£696.6 million
Hospital admissions	£851.6 million
Total	£2.6 billion

• BOX 6.1   Very Brief Advice

VBA has three components: Ask, Advise and Act.
1. Ask and record smoking status
2. Advise that the best way to give up smoking is through a combination of support from a smoking cessation service and medication.
3. Provide information and refer to a smoking cessation service. If the smoker is not ready to give up smoking, emphasis the risks of continuing to smoke.

• BOX 6.2   ASH Summary on Pre-Operative Smoking Support for Patients

- To be informed of the risks of smoking before surgery by all relevant health professionals
- To be referred to specialist stop smoking support where this is available
- To be given the opportunity to have behavioural support to help them quit
- To be provided with medication to support a quit attempt or temporary abstinence before surgery.

that in 2015 that around 108 million children and 604 million adults were obese worldwide. The overall prevalence of obesity was 5.0% among children and 12.0% among adults with large variations between countries and regions.[8] In the UK, around 27% of the population are currently obese (defined as body mass index of 30 or above), a prevalence of obesity that is amongst the highest in Europe.

Obesity is becoming linked to an increasing number of chronic diseases, including type 2 diabetes, cardiovascular disease, chronic kidney disease, liver disease, many types of cancer and arthritis and other musculoskeletal problems. Obesity and overweight currently contribute to around 4 million deaths globally, the majority of which are currently from cardiovascular disease. In the future, an increasing proportion of obesity-associated deaths will come from cancer.

In recent years, policy-makers both globally and in the UK have implemented numerous interventions to reduce rates of obesity. These include, for example, restrictions on advertisements of unhealthy foods; using taxes to increase the costs of high-calorie foods (such as a 'sugar tax' on high-calorie drinks); and the provision of weight management and reduction programmes. These interventions have thus far generally had limited or no effect on rates of obesity in societies, with the prevalence of obesity continuing to rise in the UK and elsewhere.

An intervention for obesity that has been shown to be effective is bariatric surgery, which will be covered elsewhere in this textbook. One key limitation of this intervention is that the capacity of health systems to offer bariatric surgery to patients who may potentially benefit it is generally very limited, with the number of people who may benefit from surgery far exceeding the availability of services.[9]

Physical Activity

Physical inactivity is one of the leading causes of preventable death from non-communicable disease worldwide. Despite the clear benefits of exercise on health, the number of people meeting recommended guidelines for physical activity remain low. The World Health Assembly has therefore identified tackling physical inactivity as one of its priority objectives in the fight against non-communicable diseases.

In England, only around 18% of adults are aware of national physical activity guidelines.[10] Knowledge of physical activity guidelines is also often poor among health professionals. National guidelines recommend at least 150 minutes of moderate aerobic activity for adults every week, supplemented by strength exercises at least 2 days every week (Box 6.3). Children and young people aged 5 to 18 years are recommended to engage in moderate to vigorous intensity physical activity for at least 60 minutes every day. On 3 days a week, this should also include exercises for strengthening muscles and bones such as hopping, skipping and jumping.

A regular exercise programme, in line with national guidance, can have substantial benefits on health through

---

• BOX 6.3　National Guidelines for Physical Activity for Adults Aged 19 to 64

At least 150 minutes of moderate aerobic activity such as cycling or brisk walking every week; and strength exercises on 2 or more days a week that work all the major muscles (legs, hips, back, abdomen, chest, shoulders and arms)
　Or:
　75 minutes of vigorous aerobic activity such as running or a game of singles tennis every week and strength exercises on 2 or more days a week that work all the major muscles (legs, hips, back, abdomen, chest, shoulders and arms)
　Or:
　a mix of moderate and vigorous aerobic activity every week – for example, two 30-minute runs plus 30 minutes of brisk walking equates to 150 minutes of moderate aerobic activity and strength exercises on 2 or more days a week that work all the major muscles (legs, hips, back, abdomen, chest, shoulders and arms)

---

reducing the risk of conditions such as type 2 diabetes, cardiovascular disease, cancer and musculoskeletal problems, as well as having positive effects on people's mental health. In addition, there are also substantial benefits to patients postoperatively with, for example, better survival rates.

Alcohol

Excessive alcohol consumption is an important cause of morbidity and premature mortality. Around 1.4% of all deaths registered in England and Wales are from excessive alcohol consumption and, in recent years, the number of alcohol-related deaths has been increasing. Most deaths from alcohol are from liver disease, which accounts for around 70% of all alcohol-related deaths. Alcohol is also frequently a cause of death from accidents and violence.

As well as the associated mortality, excessive alcohol consumption also contributes to morbidity from a wide range of physical and mental health problems. For example, in England, there are over 300 000 alcohol-related hospital admissions each year. As well as an increased risk of liver disease, excessive alcohol consumption also contributes to an increased risk of cancer (including mouth, bowel, gastric and liver cancer), heart disease, pancreatitis, mental health problems such as depression and suicide, and accidents and injuries. Alcohol also does not affect the drinker alone. There are also important adverse effects from alcohol on families, employers and society.

Surgeons should be aware of the major risks associated with excessive alcohol consumption and be able to advise patients on safe drinking levels and where they can obtain additional support. The four Chief Medical Officers in the UK published guidance on safe drinking levels in 2016 (Box 6.4). A routine medical history would include questions on alcohol consumption. People at high-risk from alcohol can be identified through tools such the CAGE Questionnaire and the AUDIT-C tool (Table 6.2). Patients who are identified as being at risk can then be offered brief advice on alcohol use and sign-posted to a specialist service for more intensive advice.

Diet and Nutrition

A healthy, balanced diet with a suitable calorie content is essential for good health. How much an individual needs to eat depends on factors such as how active they are. The average daily energy requirement for a man is about 10.5 MJ (2,500 kcal) and 8.4 MJ (2000 kcal) for a woman. Ideally, at least one-third of dietary intake should come from fruit and vegetables, with at least five portions of fruit and vegetables daily. A portion is defined as 80 g or one of the following:

- a slice of a large fruit such as a melon
- a whole piece of fruit such as an apple or banana
- two pieces of small fruit such as satsumas
- three tablespoons of cooked vegetables
- a bowl of mixed salad

BOX 6.4   UK Guidelines for Safe Drinking

- You are safest not to regularly drink more than 14 units per week, to keep health risks from drinking alcohol to a low level.
- If you do drink as much as 14 units per week, it is best to spread this evenly over 3 days or more. If you have one or two heavy drinking sessions, you increase your risks of death from long-term illnesses and from accidents and injuries.
- The risk of developing a range of illnesses (including, for example, cancers of the mouth, throat and breast) increases with any amount you drink regularly.
- If you wish to cut down the amount you are drinking, a good way to help achieve this is to have several drink-free days each week.
- If you are pregnant or planning a pregnancy, the safest approach is not to drink alcohol at all, to keep risks to your baby to a minimum.

The other key element of dietary intake is carbohydrates such as potatoes, bread, rice or pasta carbohydrates, choosing wholegrain versions where possible. In general, patients should be encouraged to reduce their intake of saturated fats, sugar and salt.

Illicit Drugs

Illicit drug use is an important cause of ill-health and death, particularly among younger adults. There were 2383 drug misuse deaths registered in England in 2016, an increase of 3.6% on 2015 and the highest figure on record. In addition to mortality, drug misuse and dependency can lead to a range of harms for the user including poor physical and mental health, unemployment, homelessness, family breakdown and a higher rate of criminal activity. Drug misuse also affects families and wider society, with an estimated cost to UK society of around £11 billion per year, in addition to its adverse effects on health, such as an increased risk of severe mental illness from cannabis and an increased risk of heart disease from drugs such as cocaine.

Risk factors for drug misuse include a family history of addiction, low income and socio-economic deprivation, homelessness, unemployment and poor mental health. Many of these problems cannot be addressed directly by health professionals but need to be tackled through wider societal initiatives. Although surgeons will not be expected to have a detailed knowledge of programmes to reduce the ill-health and mortality from drug misuse, as with other risk factors, this can be raised during a consultation and patients sign-posted to appropriate local services.

Mental Health

Mental illness is very common and the importance of its detection and management is continually reinforced to health professionals. Furthermore, mental health problems

---

TABLE 6.2   Alcohol Use Disorders Identification Test Consumption (AUDIT C) Tool

Questions	Scoring System					Your Score
	0	1	2	3	4	
How often do you have a drink containing alcohol?	Never	Monthly or less	2–4 times per month	2–3 times per week	4 or more times per week	
How many units of alcohol do you drink on a typical day when you are drinking?	0–2	3–4	5–6	7–9	10 or more	
How often have you had 6 or more units if female, or 8 or more if male, on a single occasion in the last year?	Never	Less than monthly	Monthly	Weekly	Daily or almost daily	

A total of 5 or more is a positive screen; 0 to 4 indicates low risk; 5 to 7 indicates increasing risk; 8 to 10 indicates higher risk; and 11 to 12 indicates possible alcohol dependence.

and physical health problems often co-exist, and as the UK population ages, we will see an increase in the number of people with co-existing physical health problems and mental health problems, such as depression and dementia. Mental health problems also contribute to the development of unhealthy lifestyles and long-term illness. The NHS has therefore placed increased emphasis on recognizing mental health as equally important as physical health. Patients with concurrent physical and mental health problems are often poorly managed because of the fragmentation of services between different healthcare providers. In many parts of the UK, the NHS is moving towards models of care whereby people with mental health problems can self-refer without the need for a formal referral from a health professional. This includes, for example, the Improving Access to Psychological Therapies (IAPT) programme in England whereby people with mental health problems, such as mild to moderate depression or anxiety, can refer themselves for therapy.

Another important issue in mental health globally is the increase in the number of people with dementia, a consequence of the rise in the number of older people in societies. People with dementia can be particularly challenging to manage in hospital settings. The move from their usual place of residence to an unfamiliar setting can lead to an increase in behavioural problems in these patients. Prolonged inpatient stays can also result in people with dementia becoming less independent and relying even more on their carers, and making it more difficult to discharge them once their treatment has been completed. It is therefore essential that the hospital environment encourages people with dementia to remain as independent as they can and that all hospital staff also encourage this independence.[11,12] These objectives can be reinforced by ensuring that clinicians have an understanding of dementia and a positive attitude to patients with dementia; can identify and assess cognitive impairment; and use an appropriate person-centred care plan which involves the families and carers of the patient.

STANDARDS FOR HEALTH PROMOTION IN HOSPITALS

It will be difficult for any health professional – including surgeons – to give effective health promotion messages to patients without adequate support from their employing institution. To facilitate this, the World Health Organization (WHO) has produced recommendations for health promotion in hospitals (Box 6.5). Through the dissemination and implementation of this guidance, the WHO hopes that hospitals can integrate health promotion into their routine activities; for example, by becoming a 'smoke-free zone'.

Funding for hospital services is gradually beginning to reflect these objectives; for example, by the awarding of incentive payments to hospitals to implement effective

---

BOX 6.5   Standards Advocated by WHO for Health Promotion

1. Hospitals have a written policy for health promotion. This policy must be implemented as part of the overall organization quality system and be aimed at improving health outcomes; and must be aimed at patients, relatives and staff.
2. The organizations' obligation is to ensure the assessment of the patients' needs for health promotion, disease prevention and rehabilitation.
3. The organization must provide the patient with information on significant factors concerning their disease or health condition and health promotion interventions should be established in all patients' pathways.
4. The management team accepts the responsibility to establish conditions for the development of the hospital as a healthy workplace.
5. There must be continuity and cooperation, with a planned approach to collaboration with other health service sectors and institutions.

---

health promotion policies. With the gradual move to more integrated health services in the NHS, the incentives and requirements for effective health promotion policies in hospitals will increase in future years.

Summary

Knowledge of the main determinants of health and the principles of health promotion is one of the core competencies of the postgraduate surgical syllabus in the UK. It is also a part of good medical practice and ensuring that surgeons – like other doctors and health professionals – practise in a holistic, patient-centred manner that addresses patients' wider health issues as well as the problem that requires immediate attention. Implementation of this knowledge and expertise in routine surgical practice will help improve the health of patients, as well as improving surgical outcomes and the burden of preventable ill-health in UK society.

References

1. Murray CJ, Barber RM, Foreman KJ, et al. Global, regional, and national disability-adjusted life years (DALYs) for 306 diseases and injuries and healthy life expectancy (HALE) for 188 countries, 1990–2013: quantifying the epidemiological transition. *Lancet.* 2015;386(10009):2145–2191.
2. Ezzati M, Riboli E. Behavioral and dietary risk factors for noncommunicable diseases. *N Eng J Med.* 2013;369(10):954–964.
3. World Health Organization. *Health Promotion: Ottawa Charter.* Ottawa: First International Conference on Health Promotion, 21 November 1986; 1995.
4. Public Health England. *Cost of Smoking to the NHS in England;* 2015. https://www.gov.uk/government/publications/cost-of-smoking-to-the-nhs-in-england-2015/cost-of-smoking-to-the-nhs-in-england-2015.

5. Action on Smoking & UK Royal Colleges. *Joint Briefing: Smoking and Surgery*. https://ash.org.uk/information-and-resources/briefings/briefing-smoking-and-surgery/.

6. Van Domburg RT, Meeter K, van Berkel DFM, et al. Smoking cessation reduces mortality after coronary artery bypass surgery: a 20-year follow-up study. *J Am Coll Cardiol*. 2000;36(3):878–883.

7. National Centre for Smoking Cessation and Training (NCSCT). *Very Brief Advice Training Module*. http://www.ncsct.co.uk/publication_very-brief-advice.php.

8. GBD 2015 Obesity Collaborators. Health effects of overweight and obesity in 195 countries over 25 years. *N Eng J Med*. 2017;377(1):13–27.

9. Ahmad A, Laverty AA, Aasheim E, Majeed A, Millett C, Saxena S. Eligibility for bariatric surgery among adults in England: analysis of a national cross-sectional survey. *JRSM Open*. 2014;5(1): 2042533313512479.

10. Knox ECL, Esliger DW, Biddle SJH, Sherar LB. Lack of knowledge of physical activity guidelines: can physical activity promotion campaigns do better? *BMJ Open*. 2013;3:e003633.

11. Waller S, Masterson A. Designing dementia-friendly hospital environments. *Future Hospital J*. 2015;2(1):63–68.

12. Dementia Action Alliance. *Dementia-Friendly Hospital Charter*; 2018. https://www.dementiaaction.org.uk/dementiafriendlyhospitalscharter.

7

The Principles of Assessment and Management of the Surgical Patient

Physiological Basis of Surgical Care

Water and Electrolyte Metabolism

Surgeons require an understanding of water and electrolyte metabolism. This is because illness and surgery cause shifts in normal fluid and electrolyte distribution and must be judiciously managed. This task is complicated by physiological differences between age groups, genders and body weights which must be appreciated to avoid erroneous fluid prescriptions (Table 7.1).

Body water distribution is summarized in Box 7.1, but it can also be compartmentalized into the following (Fig. 7.1):

- Intracellular fluid (ICF): The majority of body fluid is located inside the cells of the body (25 L)
- Extracellular fluid (ECF): The remainder of body fluid is located outside of the cells (17 L). This ECF is located in three spaces:
  - Intravascular (3 L)
  - Interstitial (14 L)
  - Third space (1 L)

Total Body Water (TBW)

- A 70-kg man has approximately 42 L (60% of TBW)
- In women, approximately 50% of body composition is water as they have more fat (fat has lower water content than muscle)
- TBW in infants is >60% of total body weight as they have very little fat
- The elderly have <50% TBW as their muscle mass, which has high water content, reduces with age
- Obese people have even less TBW compared to lean individuals, regardless of gender

Regulation of Fluid

There are a variety of homeostatic mechanism which regulate body fluid. Organs involved in these mechanisms include: kidneys, heart, lungs, adrenal glands, pituitary glands and parathyroid glands. The gastrointestinal tract also contributes significantly to fluid balance.

Dehydration

In dehydration, the circulating volume of water in the ECF reduces, thus causing an increase in the concentration of solute. The ECF osmolality is thus increased. Without homeostatic regulation, the concentration between the inside and outside of the cells would be different and water from the inside of the cell would move outside (to the area of high concentration) and this would cause cells to shrink and not function appropriately. However, homeostatic mechanisms exist to prevent this and to maintain tissue perfusion for cell metabolism.

Two important mechanisms that regulate fluid volume and thus blood pressure are the following (Fig. 7.2):

Renin–Angiotensin–Aldosterone System (RAAS)

- Juxtaglomerular cells at the afferent arteriole act as baroreceptors to detect reduction in blood pressure. The juxtaglomerular cells then release renin into the afferent arteriole.
- Renin then travels in the circulating blood to reach the liver where it cleaves angiotensinogen to angiotensin I.
- In the lung, angiotensin converting enzyme (ACE) coverts angiotensin I to angiotensin II.
- Angiotensin II:
  1. Acts as a general vasoconstrictor
  2. Acts on the adrenal gland to release aldosterone
     - Aldosterone acts on cells in the distal convoluting tubule (DCT) of the nephron to increase Na^+

reabsorption and thus water (water follows Na⁺). It also causes K⁺ secretion.

3. Acts on the hypothalamus which stimulates release of anti-diuretic hormone (ADH) from the posterior pituitary gland

Anti-Diuretic Hormone

- As blood perfuses the brain, the hypothalamus is able to detect any increases in osmolality (which reflects dehydration).

TABLE 7.1	Total Body Water as a Percentage of Body Weight for Age and Gender.[26]		
Age		Female	Male
Infant		>60%	>60%
Puberty to 39 years		52%	60%
40 to 60 years		47%	55%
>65 years		<50%	<50%

Adapted from Metheny, 2012

TABLE 7.2	Summary of Differences Between Plasma and Intracellular Electrolyte Concentrations.[26]	
Electrolyte	Plasma (mEq/L)	Intracellular (mEq/L)
Sodium Na⁺	142	10
Potassium K⁺	5	150
Magnesium Mg⁺⁺	2	40
Calcium Ca⁺⁺	5	–

Adapted from Metheny, 2012

• BOX 7.1 Typical Fluid Distribution in an Adult[2]

Electrolyte composition differs significantly between ICF and ECF compartments. The majority of sodium is located in the ECF compartment and most of the potassium is located in the ICF (Table 7.2). The most abundant electrolytes in the ICF are K⁺, Mg²⁺, Ph⁻ and negatively charged proteins. The most abundant electrolytes in the ECF are Na⁺, Ca²⁺, HCO₃⁻, and Cl⁻. Although the composition of the electrolytes differs between the two spaces, in homeostasis the concentration (or sum of cations and anions) match. The ECF water compartment fluctuates daily through input (oral fluid/food and metabolic water) and output (sensible losses: urine/faeces and insensible losses: skin/respiration) In clinical practice, plasma/serum concentrations (i.e. blood taken from venous/arterial sampling of the intravascular space) of electrolytes are used to reflect and give information on the ECF.

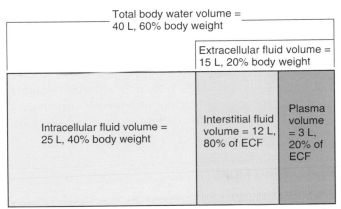

• **Fig. 7.1** Relationship of Sequestration of Intravenous Fluid and Body Water Compartments[23]

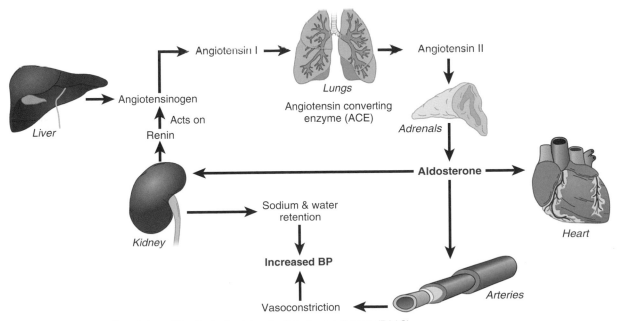

• **Fig. 7.2** Regulation of the Renin-Angiotensin-Aldosterone System (RAAS)

- The hypothalamus sends signals to the pituitary gland to release ADH into the blood.
- ADH reaches the kidneys (from circulating blood) and is filtered into the nephron. At the collecting ducts, ADH inserts a protein into aquaporin channels which allow water to be reabsorbed (i.e. the body is able to retain water).

Normal Gastrointestinal Physiology

Some further basic physiology of the gastrointestinal tract is required to be able to understand management of fluid/electrolyte imbalances that occur following gastrointestinal surgery. On average, 2 kg of food and drink is consumed daily: 500 mL of saliva is produced, 1–2 L of gastric juice and 1.5 L of pancreatico-biliary secretions. About 6 L of chyme (food, drink and secretions leaving the stomach) pass the duodenojejunal (DJ) flexure. Digestion in the upper jejunum adds further secretions until a predominant process of absorption occurs from the mid-jejunum. About 1 to 2 L of intestinal content reach the colon. The right colon functions mainly to absorb water and sodium and the left colon acts as a storage and propulsive organ.[1] The colon actively absorbs sodium and chloride against a concentration gradient (water follows) and thus there is very little sodium or chloride in normal stool. Surgery or complications of surgery disrupt normal digestion and absorption and lead to fluid and electrolyte disturbances.

Prescribing Fluid

Surgical incisions and resultant trauma cause a 'stress' response which results in increased levels of aldosterone, cortisol, ADH and catecholamines resulting in sodium and water retention in the peri-operative period. Practically this influences clinical practice as significantly less volumes of fluid prescription are required than may be realized. Careful assessment of fluid balance by clinical examination and review of fluid charts are required to avoid overzealous hydration of the patient (Table 7.3). Too little fluid and there is inadequate perfusion of vital organs as well as reduced flow to mesenteric vessels potentially compromising the operation site. Too much fluid and the patient may develop pulmonary oedema, gut dysfunction, ileus and potentially cause an oedematous anastomosis.

How to Calculate Daily Fluid Requirements for a Patient

Maintenance

The basic formula for calculating maintenance fluids in adults is as follows:
- 25–35 mL/kg per 24 h
- This is approximately 1500 to 2500 mL water per 24 h

TABLE 7.3	How to Calculate Fluid Needs After Surgery Based on a 70-kg Adult.[2]	
	Daily	
Basic Requirement	25 mL/kg	
Insensible losses	500 mL	
Potential ileus	500 mL (first day of surgery only)	
Gastrointestinal loss Nasogastric tube aspirate Vomit Stoma Fistulae Diarrhoea	Ascertain from fluid balance chart e.g. volume >750 mL/24 h	
Other losses		
Total		

Basic replacement of electrolytes is as follows:
- Na^+ 1 mmol/kg per day (50–100 mmol/24 h)
- K^+ 0.5–1 mmol/kg per day (40–80 mmol/24 h)

Replacement

On top of basic requirements, further fluid is required to replace third spacing, ileus, vomiting, high stoma outputs, fistula outputs, diarrhoea, nasogastric (NG) outputs and blood loss. Excess water is also lost with pyrexia and further fluid should be used to account for this. Fluid replacement should be calculated according to patient weight and calculations are made easier when a day is thought of as 25 hours.[2]

In addition to this, electrolytes that are being lost within certain fluids need to be included in fluid prescriptions (Table 7.4). It is important not to wait for serum levels of K^+ to fall if it is obvious that it is being lost, e.g. through vomiting.

Fluid prescription

Determining which fluids should be prescribed requires an understanding of the tonicity of the fluid and thus how quickly it is sequestered into the interstitial space or into the cells (Fig. 7.3). The different constituents of electrolytes in commonly prescribed fluids is outlined in Table 7.5. Note how one bag of 'normal' saline contains 154 mmol/L of sodium, thus far exceeding daily requirements.

Intravenous fluids can be classified as crystalloids or colloids.

Crystalloids

Definition: A solution of water containing ions (Na^+ and Cl^-) and/or small sugars (glucose). Crystalloids can be isotonic, hypertonic or hypotonic.

Isotonic: 0.9% Sodium Chloride
- Contains 154 mmol/L of Na^+ and Cl^-

TABLE 7.4   Compositions of Some Body Fluids.[23]

Body Secretion	Na+ mmol/L	K+ mmol/L	Cl– mmol/L	HCO3 mmol/L	Volume L/24 h
Gastric juice	20–60	14	140	0–15	2–3
Pancreatic juice	125–138	8	56	85	0.7–2.5
Bile	145	5	105	30	0.6
Jejunal juice	140	5	135	8	–
Ileal juice	140	5	125	30	–
Ileostomy adapted	50	4	25	–	0.5
Colostomy	60	15	40	–	0.1–0.2
Diarrhoea	30–140	30–70	–	20–80	Variable
Normal stool	20–40	30	–		0.1–0.25

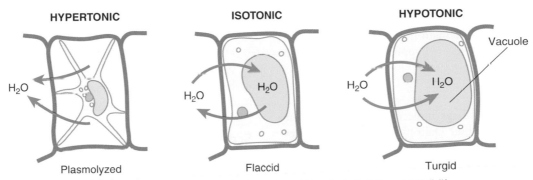

• **Fig. 7.3** Influence of Hypertonic, Isotonic and Hypotonic Solutions on Cells[24]

TABLE 7.5   Typical Properties of Commonly Used Intravenous Fluids.[23]

Type of Fluid	Sodium mmol/L	Potassium mmol/L	Chloride mmol/L	Glucose g/dL	Osmolarity mOsm/L	Plasma volume expansion duration (hours)[a]
Plasma	136–145	3.5–5.0	98–105	–	280–300	
5% Dextrose	0	0	0	5	278	
4% Dextrose/ 0.18% Saline	30	0	30	4	283	
0.9% 'normal' saline	154	0	154		308	0.2
0.45% 'half normal' saline	77	0	77		154	
Ringer's lactate	130	4	109		273	0.2
Hartmann's solution	131	5	111		275	0.2
Plasma Lyte 148	140	5	98		296	
Gelatine 4%	145	0	145		290	1–2

[a]Note how 1L of normal saline, Hartmann's solution, Plasma Lyte and Gelofusine all exceed daily requirement of sodium.

- Isotonic to plasma
- Freely crosses endothelial membrane
- Higher than the recommended daily allowance of Na^+
- Can be used for fluid resuscitation (but three times the amount of blood lost is required to replace the plasma volume)

Hypertonic: Balanced Crystalloids

- These are isotonic solutions containing Na^+, Cl^-, K^+, Ca^{2+}, lactate and bicarbonate
- Their function is to maintain ECF composition when large volumes of i.v. fluid are required in a short time
- They can be used for volume resuscitation
- Examples are Hartmann's solution, Plasma Lyte, Ringer's lactate

Hypotonic: 5% Dextrose

- This is water with 5% of sugar (glucose)
- The glucose is very quickly metabolized to leave water
- The remaining water is very quickly sequestered into the interstitial space and then into cells
- Poor plasma volume expansion (only 100 mL from 1000 mL of 5% dextrose will remain in the circulation)
- 5% Dextrose can cause severe hyponatraemia if given too quickly

Colloids

Definition: A solution of large molecules with a molecular weight of more than 10 000 Daltons. The large molecules cause an oncotic pressure which retains intravascular fluid. The most commonly used colloids are the gelatins. They act as plasma expanders.

Why Does Infusion for Normal Saline Cause Hyperchloraemic Metabolic Acidosis?

- When NaCl is added to water, the ions dissociate
- Water surrounds the charged ions
- Thus the following formula occurs: $NaCl + H_2O = HCl + NaOH$
- HCl is a strong acid and NaOH is a strong base
- The normal plasma concentration of Na is 140 and Cl is 100
- Therefore when 154 Na and 154 Cl in 1 L of water are infused into the blood, the chloride concentration increases a lot more that the Na, thereby producing more HCl and causing metabolic acidosis.

Resuscitation Fluids

Assessment of a patients' volume status should be made based on peripheral perfusion, pulse rate, blood pressure, JVP/CVP and urine output. If a patient is hypovolaemic, the cause of fluid loss should be considered. Management of haemorrhage is discussed separately below. Balanced crystalloids (Hartmann's solution or Ringer's lactate) or colloids (Gelofusine) can be used as appropriate. Fluid boluses of 200 mL should be administered immediately and once the fluid has finished, the patients' volume status should be reassessed.

There are three types of responses to fluid resuscitation in haemorrhage:

- Rapid response: vital signs return to normal, estimated blood loss is between 10% and 20%
- Transient response: there is a transient improvement in vital signs, but a recurrence of hypotension and tachycardia occurs. Blood loss may be between 20% and 40% and may be ongoing
- No response: vital signs remain abnormal, blood loss is estimated to be severe (>40%) and patient will need a blood transfusion

Features of Preoperative Assessment

The preoperative assessment allows:
- Proactive identification of co-existing medical illnesses
- Optimization of known medical conditions
- Identification of patients with high risk of complications
- Organization of postoperative care
- Examples of postoperative planning:
  - Day case vs in-patient
  - Ward vs HDU or intensive care unit (ICU)
- Planning safe discharge
  See Table 7.6 for a list of commonly requested investigations to assess fitness for surgery.

Scoring Systems

Scoring systems serve to stratify patients in terms of risk and allow for appropriate peri-operative planning. Two such scoring systems are the ASA and P-POSSUM.

ASA

See Table 7.7.

P-POSSUM (Portsmouth-Physiological and Operative Severity Score for the enUmeration of Mortality and Morbidity)

Risk predication of morbidity and mortality can be calculated with a variety of tools. For general surgery, P-POSSUM is one such tool. It is based on 12 physiological and 6 operative parameters and can provide a predictive risk of mortality and morbidity. This serves as a tool for decision making, including consent process, clinical governance and also for postoperative planning (HDU/ITU). There are criticisms that P POSSUM over predicts mortality in low-risk groups and at the extremes of age; this has led to speciality-specific elective POSSUM Scores for colorectal, vascular and upper GI surgery.

Special Considerations
The Frail Older Patient

About 8% of the UK population is now aged over 75 years and account for approximately 23% of surgical procedures.

TABLE 7.6   A Table of Commonly Requested Investigations to Assess Fitness for Surgery.[27]

System	Investigation	Possible Findings	Optimization Strategy
Respiratory	Chest radiograph	• Consolidation • Pleural effusion • Bronchiectasis • Cavitating lung lesion • Suspicious mass	Further imaging, e.g. CT Referral to respiratory physician Treatment for effusions or infections
	Lung function tests, e.g. spirometry and diffusion capacity for CO (DLCO)	Restrictive or obstructive pattern Impaired parenchymal function	Referral respiratory physician Discussions around optimal anaesthetic choice
Cardiovascular	Cardio Pulmonary Exercise Test (CPEX)	Impaired anaerobic threshold Poor oxygen uptake	Lifestyle and exercise recommendations Medical therapy, e.g. cardiovascular and respiratory
	Echo	Valvular disease Abnormal cardiac chamber structure and function Pulmonary hypertension	Refer to cardiologist or cardiac surgeon if required Respiratory physician if underlying disease
	ECG	• Arrhythmia • Evidence of previous MI	24-hour ECG monitoring Medical optimization
Renal	Serum Renal Function		
General	FBC	Anaemia	Iron studies Invasive investigation, e.g. gastroscopy Preoperative intravenous iron infusion
	Clotting	Coagulopathy	If caused by medicines, advice might need to be sought regarding bridging therapy
	Blood Glucose HbA1c		Patient may require review of diabetic medications to allow better control of diabetes preoperatively
	Group and Screen (G&S)		Hospital guidelines should be checked as to which operations require G&S and cross match.

CT, Computed tomography; CO (DLCO), diffusing capacity of the lungs for carbon monoxide; FBC, full blood count; MI, myocardial infarction.

It is estimated that by 2025 10% of the population will be aged over 75 years.[3] Special considerations include an age-related decline in physiological reserve which is compounded by illness, cognitive decline, frailty and polypharmacy. Frail patients are generally at higher risk from both elective and emergency surgery. Maintaining dignity of this vulnerable group is important.

Cardiorespiratory System

Ageing causes changes in the autonomic nervous system causing a reduced cardiac response to stress. This results in:

- Desensitization of β receptors; thus, the patient behaves as if they are 'β blocked'
- A reduced response to fluid losses due to inability to effectively increase cardiac output
- Baroreceptor dysfunction and reduced responsiveness to angiotensin II result in ineffective response to hypovolaemia

This may be further complicated in patients who have myocardial ischaemia and cardiac polypharmacy. There is age-related decline in lung and chest wall compliance and oxygen diffusion capacity.[3]

Renal System

Renal function declines with age and is affected further with co-morbidities such as hypertension and diabetes. Nephrotoxic drugs such as NSAIDS and ACE inhibitors can also cause renal impairment.[3]

Central Nervous System

Elderly patients may have impaired cerebral and cerebrovascular function and this can often contribute to postoperative delirium, thus affecting postoperative recovery and discharge. Peri-operative pain in the elderly is often underappreciated and ward doctors should try and use opioid-sparing analgesia in the elderly as per guidelines. Surgery or critical care must not be rationed on the basis of age; assessment of patient physiology and function are stronger predicators of outcome. Opportunities to optimize an elderly patient's pathophysiology include resuscitation before emergency surgery and pharmacological manipulation of chronic co-morbidities. Close collaboration and involvement of geriatrician/cardiologists/respiratory physicians is critical.[3]

TABLE 7.7	American Society of Anaesthesiologists Physical Status Classification for Assessing Fitness for Surgery for Adults (Separate Descriptions Exist for Paediatric and Obstetric Patients).	
ASA Physical Status Classification	**Description**	**Adult Examples**
1	A normal healthy patient	Healthy Non smoking No or minimal alcohol
2	Mild systemic disease	Smoker Social alcohol drinker Normal pregnancy Obesity (BMI 30 to 40) Well-controlled diabetes Well-controlled hypertension Mild lung disease
3	Severe systemic disease	Poorly controlled diabetes/hypertension COPD Morbid obesity (BMI >40) Alcohol dependence Implanted pacemaker History of >3 months of MI, CVA, TIA, or CAD/stents
4	Severe systemic disease which is a constant threat to life	Recent (<3 months) MI, CVA, TIA CAD/stents Ongoing cardiac ischemia Poor ejection fraction, sepsis, DIC
5	Moribund patient who is not expected to survive with or without the operation	Ruptured AAA Major trauma Intra-cranial haemorrhage with mass effect
6	A brainstem dead patient whose organs are being removed for donor purposes	

NOTE: The suffix E is used for emergency cases.

AAA, Abdominal aortic aneurysm; BMI, body mass index; CAD, coronary artery disease; CVA, cerebrovascular accident; DIC, disseminated intravascular coagulation; MI, myocardial infarction; TIA, transient ischaemic attack.

From ASA, 2020.

Obesity

In the UK, over a quarter of adults are now obese (BMI >30).[4] In the USA, over a third of the population are obese. The trend is set to continue to increase.[5] Obese patients have a number of associated cardiac, respiratory, metabolic and endocrine problems that are important for the surgeon to consider. Patients who are 'apple' shaped (typically male with central fat distribution) tend to carry more intra-abdominal fat and are more likely to have the associated metabolic syndrome, which is insulin resistance, hypertension and hypercholesterolaemia.[6] Patients who are 'pear' shaped (typically female) carry more external, peripheral fat and do not tend to have the associated metabolic syndrome. Obesity and associated hypertension causes significant strain on the heart. This can lead to heart strain, heart failure, ischaemic heart disease and arrhythmias, particularly atrial fibrillation. Patients with sleep apnoea can develop pulmonary hypertension. All obese patients should have an electrocardiogram (ECG).

Sleep disordered breathing describes both obstructive sleep apnoea (OSA) and obesity hypoventilation syndrome (OHS). Formal diagnosis is performed with a sleep study. Postoperative cardio-respiratory events and ICU admissions are more common.[7] It is important for patients established on CPAP to continue this postoperatively. Elective admission to critical care should also be considered. The STOP-BANG questionnaire can screen for sleep disordered breathing and a score of five or more indicates a high chance of the condition.[8] In addition, a venous bicarbonate of >27 mmol can indicate an underlying respiratory problem.

Diabetes is more prevalent in the obese population. It is thought to lead to insulin resistance.[9] Glycaemic control is important in the peri-operative period. Obese patients are hypercoagulable and prothrombotic. A venous thromboembolism (VTE) assessment should be performed on admission to hospital and pharmacological prophylaxis prescribed according to local guidance. The use of thromboembolic device (TED) stockings might not be practically possible, therefore mechanical devices (e.g. Flotron Therapy) might be more appropriate. Additionally, mobilization should be encouraged where possible.

Diabetes

Diabetes affects 6–7% of the UK population. As obesity levels rise, the prevalence of diabetes is expected to rise significantly. The peri-operative mortality of patients with diabetes is higher than the non-diabetic population. Patients with diabetes are likely to have associated cardiovascular disease including hypertension, ischaemic heart disease, stroke and renal impairment. Diabetic patients should be prioritized on the operating list to minimize the period of starvation, use of variable rate intravenous insulin infusions (VRII) and need for inpatient stay.

Diabetes and Preoperative Care

The term 'sliding scale' (intravenous insulin) is now termed 'variable rate intravenous insulin infusion' (VRIII). Patients with a short period of starvation (one meal missed maximum) can be managed with modification of their diabetic medications. This often means taking medicines as normal the day prior to surgery and either omission, adjustment of dose or taking as normal on the day of surgery. This should be addressed in preoperative assessment.[10] A VRIII is used for patients who miss more than one meal, type 1 diabetics who have not received any insulin, those with poor control or those undergoing emergency surgery. Patients whose diabetes is managed with lifestyle or once daily metformin do not require intervention.[10] Intraoperative glucose needs to be closely monitored and maintained between 6 and 10 mmol/L where possible.[10]

Diabetes and Postoperative Care

It is important to ensure that blood glucose levels are maintained postoperatively. Up to 12 mmol/L is acceptable. Operative stress can cause postoperative hyperglycaemia and poor control makes the patient more susceptible to infection. These risks can be minimized by good pain control, meticulous fluid and electrolyte replacement, pressure area surveillance and the return to normal eating, drinking and diabetic regimen as soon as possible.

Steroid Dependent Patients

Steroid usage can be either be short- or long-term. Complications can arise from adrenal suppression or the disease process itself. Surgery initiates a 'stress response' and the release of cortisol. This is impaired in steroid users and can lead to an Addisonian crisis. It is important to ascertain the steroid dose and the duration. Recent courses of steroids are important as well. Equivalent doses of steroids are: Prednisolone 10 mg = dexamethasone 1.6 mg = hydrocortisone 40 mg = methylprednisolone 8 mg daily. In general, doses of 5 mg/day of prednisolone or equivalent do not require cover; 10 mg/day or more prednisolone requires replacement. This applies to current usage or a course taken within the past 3 months. The replacement and dosage recommendations are then based on whether the surgery is minor,

moderate or major.[11] It is important to remember to continue intravenous-equivalent doses if the patient is unable to tolerate oral medicines.

The Multidisciplinary Team (MDT) Meeting

MDT meetings are often held for surgical specialities such as vascular, bariatric and oncological surgery. They often include an anaesthetist and other allied healthcare professionals. They aim to discuss and plan investigations and interventions in order to optimize patients for surgery.

Prehabilitation

Prehabilitation is a period of preoperative training with structured and sustained exercises in the run up to major surgery. It allows for an improvement in cardiovascular, respiratory and muscular health and is thought to lead to a lower rate of postoperative complications. It allows for patients to become active participants in their care.[12] Further clinical trials are underway.

Psychological Preparation

Undergoing surgery is a significant life event. Any surgery can cause the patient to experience fear and anxiety. Patients having major surgery (cardiac/vascular/transplant) or cancer surgery are likely to also experience significant psychological stress. Patients are unlikely to absorb information in one consultation and therefore it is important that patients are encouraged to attend appointments with a family member or friend and have further opportunities to discuss any concerns or anxieties with a specialist nurse, surgeon or allied healthcare professional.

The technicalities of the surgery should be explained to the patient in clear lay language and visual diagrams are strongly encouraged. Macmillan nurses and specialist nurse practitioners are a vital support for patients. Having a direct contact number means patients can access the team for further queries that arise either before or after surgery. Information leaflets, videos and patient support groups also provide useful resources for patients undergoing surgery.

The Postoperative Period

The assessment and management of postoperative patients is challenging and is complicated by physiological responses to large surgical incisions, trauma of surgery, postoperative analgesia and epidurals which make the assessment of abdominal pain difficult. It is recommended that surgeons examine postoperative patients at least twice a day in the postoperative period as changes in symptoms and pain are critical.

Careful history, examination, assessment of observation charts and laboratory investigations enable one to tease out what is a normal postoperative course and what features represent a postoperative complication.

Date and time	26th January 2018
Patient details	Miss Jemima Puddleduck DOB 5th July 1930 Hospital number 1234567
Elective/emergency	Emergency
Surgeon	Miss A. Jones
Assistant	Dr Y. Wong
Anaesthetist	Dr R. Singh
Operation	Laparotomy and division of band adhesion
Incision	Midline
Diagnosis	Small bowel obstruction secondary to congenital band adhesion
Findings	Band adhesion causing obstruction at mid ileum. Proximal small bowel distended Affected small bowel appeared viable Liver, colon, rectum, stomach and gallbladder all normal. Normal ovaries and uterus.
Procedure	Consent ✓ WHO Checklist ✓ Position: supine with arms wrapped Prepped and draped ✓ Midline incision Exploratory laparotomy performed. Small bowel delivered and examined from DJ flexure to TI. Band adhesion found at mid-ileum. Band divided. Wash with warm saline 1 L
Details of prosthetics used	Not applicable
Closure	Mass closure with loop PDS 0 Clips to skin Opsite dressing
Post operative plan	Epidural for 72 hours and wean NG on free drainage and 2 hourly aspiration Sips water for comfort only. Expect ileus Monitor one hourly urine output and fluid balance Encourage sitting out and mobilisation Chest physiotherapy and incentive spirometer No postoperative antibiotics 5000 units s/c dalteparin in 6 hours TEDS stockings
Signature	Miss A Jones Bleep number 1234

• **Fig. 7.4** Example Operation Note

This section will describe the following:
- Recommendation of what to include in the postoperative note and postoperative instructions
- Enhanced Recovery After Surgery (ERAS)
- The surgical ward round
- Postoperative complications
  - Recognition, management and prevention

Operative Note and Postoperative Instructions

A clear operative note for every operation/procedure is mandatory (ideally this should be typed) (Fig. 7.4). These notes travel with the patient to recovery and subsequently to the ward and clear instructions should be made so that nurses and doctors can understand postoperative plans and care.

Assessment of nutritional and fluid status

Electrolyte Disturbance	Causes
Hyponatraemia	Salt depletion with excessive water intake (diarrhoea and water drinking)
	Sequestration (burns/pancreatitis/ peritonitis/ascites)
	Severe cardiac failure
	Endocrine disturbances (adrenal insufficiency or hypothyroidism)
	Excessive water drinkers
	Drugs (morphine/clofibrate/barbiturates/ tricyclics/ antineoplastic agents
	Syndrome of inappropriate ADH secretion (SIADH) – pulmonary disease/neoplasia/cerebral disease
Hypernatraemia	Gastrointestinal losses (diarrhoea/fistula and vomiting)
	Renal losses (osmotic diuresis/ diabetes insipidus)
	Skin losses (sweating and burns)
	Iatrogenic causes (infusion of hypertonic saline)
Hypokalaemia	Gastrointestinal losses (vomiting/ diarrhoea/laxative abuse/fistula losses)
	Renal losses (diuretics/ hyperaldosteronism/renal tubular necrosis)
	Poor dietary intake
Hyperkalaemia	Pseudohyperkalaemia (haemolysis/ increases WBC or platelets)
	Renal failure
	Drugs (potassium sparing diuretics/ACE inhibitors)
	Adrenal insufficiency
	Tissue necrosis and rhabdomyolysis

Adapted from Nightingale, 2001, Chapter 17

Postoperative Instructions

A clear postoperative plan and instructions are vital for nursing staff and ward doctors to follow. With increasing shift work patterns, it is often the case that numerous team members look after patients in the postoperative period; thus, clear plans for effective handovers are vital. Postoperative instructions should include:

- Postoperative antibiotics (if required)
- Anticoagulation plan (prophylactic VTE) or, if heparin is required, time and plan for checking APTT ratio
- Monitoring of drains
- Nutrition plans
- Physiotherapy plans
- Stoma care
- Checking of full blood count (FBC)/electrolytes
- Analgesia
- NG – how often to aspirate

- How often to do observations (including target MAP and urine output)

Many specialities now use an 'enhanced recovery after surgery' protocol for operations. For colorectal surgery, this is often used for elective colorectal resections after cancer surgery. It is widely applied, often in the format of a booklet.

Enhanced Recovery After Surgery

In 2000, Henrik Kehlet published data reducing postoperative inpatient stays after elective open colorectal surgery to 2–3 days from an average of 6 to 12 days using a fast track multimodal rehabilitation programme focusing on optimal analgesia, stress reduction by use of regional anaesthesia, early enteral nutrition and early mobilization. The goals were to enhance recovery and reduce the complication rates using evidence-based practice.[13] The evidence base is now being expanded to provide ERAS protocols for many other surgical specialties including upper GI surgery, pancreatic resections, cystectomy, bariatric and liver surgeries.

ERAS is important because it reduces the risk of complications from surgery. Other benefits are reduced inpatient stay and improvement of patient experience. Furthermore, adherence to ERAS protocols is associated with reduced complications following colorectal surgery[14] and improved 5-year cancer specific survival.[15]

Preoperative Elements (for Elective Colorectal Resection)

- Information and counselling
  - Explaining to the patient what will happen during their hospital stay and explaining daily goals (breathing exercises, mobilization, nutrition) helps with adherence to ERAS
  - Empowering the patient – the patient should feel in control and take active part in their recovery
- No pre-med advised
- Avoidance of mechanical bowel preparation
  - Mechanical bowel preparation can result in dehydration and significant fluid and electrolyte shifts
  - Most centres avoid bowel preparation for right-sided colonic resections
  - There is controversy for bowel preparation in left-sided and rectal resections
  - There are some emerging data that show that preoperative bowel decontamination with oral antibiotics may reduce postoperative complications
- Preoperative fasting
  - Fasted of clear fluids for 2 hours
  - No solids for 6 hours
  - Clear carbohydrate-rich drink of 800 mL before midnight and 400 mL 2–3 hours before surgery

Intraoperative Elements

- Minimally invasive surgery
  - Laparoscopy: smaller wounds result in faster recovery

- Avoid routine use of NG tube
- Prevent intraoperative hypothermia
- Analgesia: avoid opiates; consider the use of spinal analgesia over an epidural, if appropriate; use of regular paracetamol, breakthrough NSAIDS after removal of epidural
- Avoid drains (limits mobility postoperatively)
- Avoid fluid imbalances; this is achieved by:
  - Avoidance of mechanical bowel preparation where possible
  - Minimizing preoperative starvation to 6 hours for solids and 2 hours for clear fluids
  - Intraoperative goal-directed fluid therapy with oesophageal Doppler
  - Restrictive fluid regimen intraoperatively
  - Avoiding sodium overload

Postoperative factors

- Analgesia: as above
- Pain and nausea control are crucial: excellent pain and nausea control are central to successful ERAS (see Ch 2).
- Early mobilization
  - 2 hours on day of surgery
  - 6 hours daily until day of discharge
- Nutrition
  - Oral nutritional supplements (400 mL/24 h until normal levels of food intake achieved)
  - Early oral food intake
- Discharge planning

Stoma Care

Stoma care begins before surgery. Patients should meet specialist stoma nurses to learn about stomas and psychologically prepare themselves for after the surgery. Patients should receive information to allay fears and anxieties. The stoma site should be marked preoperatively to take into account the position of the belt line, avoidance of bony prominences and visibility of stoma to allow patient to self-care. After discharge, patients need ongoing stoma care support.

Early Stoma Complications

- Ischaemia
  - Can occur due to tension or excessive ligation of mesentery
  - May initially appear purple and then progress to necrosis
  - Bedside assessment includes using a blood test tube and pen touch to assess proximal mucosa or puncture mucosa to assess for presence of bleeding
- Mucocutaneous separation (due to infection or inadequate approximation)
- High output stoma (see later)
- Skin corrosion
  - Stoma bags for ileostomy need to carefully cover the skin to avoid damage from corrosive properties of ileostomy effluent

Late Stoma Complications

- Prolapse
- Stenosis
- Retractions
- Fistula
- Parastomal hernia
  - Incidence can be as high as 50%
  - Risk factors include obesity, chronic cough, poor nutrition and wound sepsis

Surgical Drains

Surgical drains are commonly used. It is the surgeons' responsibility to indicate the reason for use, location of the drain, and clearly mark the drain. It is the surgeons' responsibility to instruct when the drain should be removed.

Surgical drains are used to:
- Remove existing collections of pus, fluid, or blood
- Prevent the build-up of collections (e.g. bile after bile duct surgery)
- Warn of potential life-threatening complications (e.g. bleeding post thyroidectomy or bleeding after a vascular anastomosis)

Risks of drains include:
- False reassurance: drains can become occluded and may not drain blood/bile, which is in fact accumulating inside the given cavity. If a drain is assessed in isolation, this can be falsely reassuring.
- Introduction of infection
- Injury to other organs/structures (if CT-guided or ultrasound (US)-guided drainage is used)

There are various types of surgical drains, including:
- Open passive drains
  - Corrugated drain: sheet drain which drain fluid through a gutter action
  - Penrose tube drain
  - Seton
- Closed passive drains
  - Robinson's drain
  - Chest drain (tube thoracostomy)
  - Nasogastric tube
- Closed active drains
  - Vacuum suction drain e.g. Redivac

Surgical Ward Round

The surgical ward round serves to monitor postoperative progress, engage patient in their postoperative recovery and to detect, treat and prevent postoperative complications. Poor quality ward rounds are associated with increase in preventable postoperative complications such as pneumonia or surgical site infection.[16] Assessing the postoperative abdomen is challenging and requires experience.

The ward round must have a structure. It should include the following elements.

History

- Pain assessment
- Nausea assessment
- Systems enquiry
  - Gastrointestinal tract:
    - Assessment of nausea, vomiting, bowel function and oral intake
  - Cardiorespiratory:
    - Assessment for dyspnoea and compliance with breathing exercises
    - If patient is not compliant, an enquiry into what is the limitation, e.g. pain
- Mobilization: ask if patients have been able to sit out of bed or walk
- Address ideas, concerns and expectations from patient

Examination

- Observe: look at the patient to assess their progress. For instance, is the patient sitting out in a chair reading or are they having difficulty getting out of bed?
- Assess the pulse: a tachycardia could imply infection, sepsis, hypovolaemia, PE, pain or an electrolyte disturbance causing arrhythmia.
- Auscultate the lungs: is there evidence of collapsed lungs or postoperative chest infection?
- Examine the abdomen
  - Inspection
    - Distention: may suggest ileus
  - Review the wound only when deemed necessary or when the dressing can be promptly changed (wound infection rates are higher if dressings are removed or changed too early)
    - The wound can generally be left undisturbed for 48 hours
  - Gentle palpation of the abdomen
    - Where is the pain?
    - Is it new?
    - Is in keeping with the postoperative course?
  - Assess drain output: What is in the drain?
    - Frank blood
    - Serous fluid
    - Haemoserous fluid
- Bile
  - Auscultate: Are there bowel sounds?

Review of Charts

- Observation chart
  - Look for trends in the pulse, blood pressure, temperature, saturations and respiratory rate
  - Patients on ß-blockers may not demonstrate tachycardia
- Fluid balance chart
  - input (oral/i.v.)
  - output (NG/urine/drains/vomit/stoma)
- Drug Chart
  - Check that venous thromboembolism prophylaxis is prescribed

- Review need for antibiotics
- Review analgesia and anti-emetics
- Prescribe intravenous fluids if required
- Laboratory tests
  - Review haemoglobin, inflammatory markers, renal function and electrolytes

Make a Plan for the Patient

Make plans for:
- Pain control
- Removal of catheters/drains/lines
- Nutrition
  - Oral nutrition: this should be started as soon as possible. Most patients having elective colorectal surgery can start oral nutrition within 24 hours.
  - NG feed: reserved for malnourished patients
  - Parenteral nutrition: for patients who are unable to eat or receive enteral feeds for >5 days.
- Mobilization
- Routine investigations: e.g. electrolytes
- Investigations and further management should be planned if patients are not progressing as expected or there is concern over postoperative complications (see later). Senior team members should be alerted and should review the patient.

Communication

Plans that have been made for the patient can only be executed if properly communicated to relevant team members and explanation for the daily goals given to the patients so that they can have as much control in their recovery as possible. Team members include:
- Nurses
- Physiotherapist
- Dietician
- Occupational Therapist
- Seniors

Postoperative Complications

All operations have a risk of complications. Complications can be:
1. Specific (these are the consequences of a particular surgical procedure)
2. General (occur after any operation, irrespective of its site, i.e. general anaesthetic itself) (Table 7.8)
   This classification can be further divided into:
1. Immediate
2. Early (within 30 days)
3. Late (after 30 days)
   All complications, no matter how minor, should be discussed at a regular clinical governance meeting. Severity of the complication are commonly graded using the Clavien-Dindo classification from grades I to IV. It has been found that the occurrence of any complication within 30 days of surgery affects long-term survival more than the patients pre-morbid state or intraoperative factors.[17]

TABLE 7.8	Example of Complications Related to Anterior Resection for Rectal Cancer.		
	Immediate	**Early**	**Late**
General	Trauma to mouth/teeth during GA	DVT/PE UTI CVP line sepsis Wound infection Pneumonia	DVT/PE
Specific	Injury to ureter/bowel/blood vessels/pelvic nerves/spleen	Anastomotic leak Collection Ileus	Incisional hernia Tumour recurrence LARS (low anterior resection syndrome)

CVP, Central venous pressure; DVT, deep vein thrombosis; GA, general anaesthetic; PE, pulmonary embolism, UTI, urinary tract infection.

Respiratory Complications

Three common respiratory postoperative complications are:
1. Atelectasis
2. Pneumonia
   a. Infective
   b. Chemical (aspiration pneumonia)
3. Pulmonary embolism

Respiratory Physiology

Respiratory Failure
- This is a clinical diagnosis based on an arterial blood gas
- A PaO_2 <8 kPa implies respiratory failure
- In type 1 respiratory failure:
  - $PaCO_2$ <6.5 kPa
  - It is due to a ventilation/perfusion mismatch
- In type 2 respiratory failure:
  - $PaCO_2$ >6.5 kPa
  - There is hypoventilation and the CO_2 cannot be blown off
  - Hypoxic drive

Atelectasis

Atelectasis is defined as the complete or partial collapse of a lung or lobe of a lung and develops when the alveoli become deflated. It most commonly occurs after major abdominal surgery (laparotomy) or thoracotomy.

Reduced chest expansion due to pain and splinting causes retention of secretions and alveolar collapse.

At risk patients include:
- Those with pre-existing chronic lung disease
- Obese patients
- Elderly patients
- Smokers
- Laparotomy/thoracotomy
Preventative strategies include:
1. Chest physiotherapy
   - Mobilization
   - Breathing exercises
   - Encouraging regular coughing to clear secretions
   - Incentive spirometry
   - Bubble positive expiratory pressure
2. Adequate analgesia to allow for breathing exercises

Pneumonia

Atelectasis can be superseded by bacterial infection causing pneumonia. Pneumonia is defined as the inflammation of the substance of the lungs. It is characterized by shortness of breath, dyspnoea, cough, productive sputum and fever. Chest radiograph may show consolidation.

Treatment is with oxygen, antibiotics and chest physiotherapy. If severe, with respiratory failure, patients may require non-invasive or invasive respiratory support.

Aspiration Pneumonia

Aspiration pneumonia is a serious and potentially fatal respiratory complication. It is caused by the acute aspiration of gastric contents into the lungs. Gastric content is highly corrosive owing to its acidity. Most common sites of aspiration pneumonia are the apical and posterior aspects of the right lower lobe due to bronchial anatomy.

High-risk patients include those who have/are:
- GI mechanical obstruction
- Postoperative ileus
- Pregnancy
Prevention:
- Immediate insertion of an NG tube after clinical suspicion of ileus or mechanical obstruction is life saving
- Nurse patients upright
- After immediate aspiration of gastric contents via NG tube, it should be left on free drainage with regular aspiration

Pulmonary Embolism (PE)

A pulmonary embolus occurs when a blood vessel supplying the lung becomes occluded with a clot. The clot is likely to have travelled from large veins in the pelvis, abdomen or legs via the heart. It is a medical emergency and both the surgeon and physician should be involved in the patient's care. CTPA (computerized tomography pulmonary angiogram) is gold standard for diagnosis.

Bedside Management of PE
1. High-flow oxygen through a non rebreather mask
2. I.V. fluid
3. Anti-coagulation with treatment dose LMWH

4. In the peri-operative period with a high risk of bleeding, an unfractionated heparin infusion with monitoring of APTT and close observations and Hb may be more suitable.

If there is evidence of circulatory collapse, inotropes may be required, thrombolysis/embolectomy may need to be considered in cases of massive PE.

VTE Prophylaxis

- Anticoagulation with LMWH
- Early mobilization
- TEDS stockings
- Mechanical VTE (can restrict mobilization)
- Inferior vena cava filter

Cardiovascular Complications

Important postoperative cardiovascular complications are:
1. Haemorrhage
2. Myocardial infarction

Pulmonary embolism (discussed earlier)

Haemorrhage

Haemorrhage can be classified as follows:
- Primary: occurs during the operation
- Reactionary: occurs immediately after the operation once BP and heart rate are normalized
- Secondary: occurs several days after the operation

Young patients, or a patient with a good physiological reserve, may not manifest signs of bleeding until they have lost a large volume of blood due to their ability to compensate (Table 7.9).

Types of response following initial fluid resuscitation (discussed above):
- Rapid response
- Transient/temporary response
- No response

Drains may not reliably indicate active bleeding.

Management

1. Oxygen
2. I.V. access × two large bore cannulae
3. FBC (to check Hb), clotting, cross match, venous blood gas (VBG) (for instant Hb check)
4. Major haemorrhage call (in the UK, the majority of trusts will have a major haemorrhage protocol to alert team members – anaesthetist, haematologist, surgeon and theatre staff)
5. Transfuse patient
   a. Type specific if available
   b. O-negative if type specific unavailable and patient unstable
6. Reverse any abnormal clotting with products. Thromboelastography (TEG) may guide the administration of blood products, especially in major bleeding or when unfractionated heparin has been administered recently, e.g. vascular or cardiac surgery
7. 1 g Tranexamic acid
8. Imaging (if patient is stable – it may be appropriate to arrange CT angiography to identify place of bleeding)
9. **Definitive management** to control source of bleeding:
   a. Interventional radiology (IR) embolization
   b. Return to theatre: trauma principles should apply. Patient is intubated after the surgeon has prepped and draped the patient.

Trauma triad of death referring to hypothermia, coagulopathy and acidosis will also apply and efforts to minimize this with correction of clotting, use of warmed products and mechanical warmed blanket should be made.

Gastrointestinal Complications

Important gastrointestinal complications following surgery include:
1. Ileus
2. High output stoma

TABLE 7.9 **Estimated Blood Loss (for a 70-kg Male) Based on Patient's Initial Presentation.**[28]

	Class I	Class II	Class III	Class IV
Blood loss (mL)	<750	750–1500	1500–2000	>2000
Blood loss (% blood volume) (like a tennis match)	<15%	15–30%	30–40%	>40%
Pulse	<100	100–120	120–140	>140
Systolic BP	Normal	Normal	Decreased	Decreased
Pulse pressure (mmHg)	Normal or increased	Decreased	Decreased	Decreased
Respiratory rate	14–20	20–30	30–40	>35
Urine output (mL/h)	>30	20–30	5–15	Negligible
CNS	Slightly anxious	Mildly anxious	Anxious – confused	Confused – lethargic
Initial fluid management	Crystalloid	Crystalloid	Crystalloid and blood	Crystalloid and blood

American College of Surgeons, 2012. ATLS Student Course Manual: Advanced Trauma Life Support, ninth ed. American College of Surgeons, Chicago.

3. Enterocutaneous fistula
4. Anastomotic leak
5. Collection

Ileus

Postoperative ileus is described as 'the transient cessation of coordinated bowel motility after surgical intervention which (Table 7.10) prevents effective transit of intestinal contents or tolerance of oral fluids'.[18] Ileus causes an accumulation of the gastrointestinal secretions, resulting in abdominal distention and vomiting. It is common after gastrointestinal surgery but also occurs after other types of surgery (vascular, gynaecological, urological and orthopaedic). A prolonged ileus is where symptoms have not resolved after 3 and 5 days for laparoscopic and open surgery, respectively.

Preventative measures can be taken to avoid development of ileus. Many elements from the ERAS protocol act to prevent ileus. This includes minimally invasive surgery, use of thoracic epidural/spinal analgesia to block sympathetic outflow and avoid opiate use. NG tubes are not used routinely but are used where ileus is likely (after emergency surgery for peritonitis). Avoiding fluid overload and electrolyte disturbances also prevents ileus. Once ileus is diagnosed principles of management includes insertion of NG tube (to avoid aspiration pneumonia), accurate fluid charts for inputs and outputs, restoration of normal physiology (by correction of electrolytes and fluid balance), exclusion of secondary causes (such as intra-abdominal sepsis, bowel inflammation or mechanical obstruction) and input of nutrition team if ileus becomes prolonged and patients likely to require TPN.

High Output Stoma

Initial normal output for a new ileostomy is 1.2 L/day and this gradually decreases over 2 to 3 months as there is adaptation of the ileostomy. A high output stoma is defined as >1.5 L of output per 24 hours and is clinically significant as it results in water, sodium and magnesium depletion and subsequent malnutrition. Although 100 cm of small bowel is required for survival, surgery leaving <200 cm is likely to cause a high output stoma. Other causes include proximal intermittent obstruction, medications, sepsis, ongoing inflammatory bowel disease.[19] Normal output for an adapted stoma is considered to be 700–800 mL/day.

Investigations

Investigation includes assessment of stoma, review of drug chart (increasing loperamide if necessary), ileoscopy and biopsies (to check for ongoing inflammatory disease) and cross-sectional imaging.

Initial Management

Initial treatment focuses on:
• reducing fluid and electrolyte losses
• hydrating patient (using i.v. fluid if necessary and aiming for urinary sodium >20 mmol/L)
• correcting underlying causes if possible
• strict fluid balance with daily weights and electrolytes:
  • oral fluid intake should be restricted to <1 L/24 h of hypotonic fluid
  • recommendation of 1 L/24 h of oral isotonic solution (e.g. St Mark's solution)
  • pharmacological treatments include loperamide 8 to 16 mg daily
  • if stoma output settles after 48 to 72 hours, oral fluid intake can be increased

Ongoing High Output Stoma

If there is ongoing high output stoma, the following measures can be considered:
• Fluid restriction should be continued with establishment of oral rehydration solutions (1 L St Mark's solution/24 h)
• Increase loperamide

TABLE 7.10	Causes of Postoperative Ileus.				
Action	**Process**	**Cause**	**Symptoms & Signs**	**Preventative Measures**	
Trauma of surgery	Activation of mast cells, monocytes and macrophages leading to release of histamine, TNF-a, protanoids and interleukins	Postoperative Ileus	• Nausea • Vomiting • Distention • Absolute constipation	Minimally invasive surgery	
Handling of bowel and anastomosis	Sympathetic stimulation Interference with electrochemical coupling		• Tachycardia • Hypotension • Abdominal pain • Reduced bowel sounds	Minimally invasive surgery	
Fluid overload	Intestinal oedema and stretch → reduced contraction of smooth muscle			Fluid restrict Goal directed therapy, e.g. with oesophageal Doppler (LiDCO)	
Opioid analgesia	Activation of opioid receptors; decreased intestinal motility			Avoid opiates	

Adapted from Bragg, et al., 2006.

- Reduction of secretions with high dose antacids
- Treatment of hypomagnesaemia
- Close monitoring of fluid and electrolyte balance
- Consideration of codeine phosphate 30 mg TDS, maximum dose of loperamide is 100 mg
- Octreotide can be trialled to further reduce secretions
- Nutrition team may need to consider long term TPN

How Does Oral Rehydration Solution Work?

When patients have a high output stoma, sometimes they erroneously drink hypotonic fluids (water, coffee, tea, carbonated drinks and juice) to try and rehydrate themselves. Having a high output stoma leads to increased sodium and water loss. The mucosal lining of the jejunum allows movement of sodium and water. However, if the luminal concentration of sodium is hypotonic (<90 mmol/L), then sodium will leave the plasma to rebalance the gradient; water will follow the sodium and, in a patient with high stoma output or diarrhoea, the patient will become dehydrated. St Mark's solution is a home-made electrolyte mix recipe of 20 g glucose, 2.5 g sodium bicarbonate and 3.5 g sodium chloride (salt) in 1 L of water. As it is a hypertonic solution, sodium and water are reabsorbed from the intestinal lumen into the blood.

Enterocutaneous Fistula

An enterocutaneous fistula is an abnormal communication between the gastrointestinal tract and the skin. It is most commonly due to postoperative complications (unrecognized injury of the bowel during the operation or partial disruption of the anastomosis). Other causes include distal obstruction, inflammatory bowel disease, previous irradiation, intestinal ischemia. Clinically, the patient is septic, and can initially present with what appears to be a discharging infected wound. Once opened, this is quickly followed by gastrointestinal content. A high output fistula is defined as an output of >500 mL/24 h. The higher the output, the more proximal the communication with the GI tract.

If the fistula is very high in the GI tract, significant water and electrolyte disturbances can occur; management includes strict fluid balance, daily weights, initially daily biochemistry and electrolytes, use of oral rehydration therapy, fluid restriction of hypotonic solutions, use of high dose antacids, and involvement of the nutrition team. High output fistula should be replaced by an equal volume of a balanced crystalloid fluid (e.g. Hartmann's solution).[20] Definitive surgery needs to be planned by specialists. Patients require meticulous skin care due to corrosive effects from fistula output and also require psychological support as in many instances they will be in hospital for prolonged periods following complications. Patients require regular input from the nutritional team and dietician for arrangement of parenteral nutrition and require a dedicated single lumen line for this.

Sepsis

Sepsis is defined as life-threatening organ dysfunction caused by a dysregulated host response to infection.[21]

Pathophysiology of Sepsis

A normal response to infection includes a local response which causes vasodilation, an increased permeability of capillaries to allow migration of leukocytes to site of injury. In severe infection, there is an excess of inflammatory mediators which are released.

There is increased vascular permeability and intravascular molecules leak into the extravascular space. This results in reduced circulating plasma volume causing hypotension and tachycardia. The accumulation of the extravascular fluid causes peripheral oedema and pulmonary oedema and consequently respiratory failure. There is a rise in lactate due to reduced oxygen delivery and anaerobic respiration. There is a disruption of clotting homeostasis; increased coagulation and inflammation with impaired fibrinolysis. Multi-organ failure manifests as:

- Respiratory failure: ARDS
- Cardiovascular
- Cerebral
- Acute kidney injury
  Postoperative causes of sepsis include:
- Urinary tract infection (from indwelling catheter)
- Pneumonia
- Wound infection
- Collection
- Anastomotic leak
- Prosthesis infection
- Line infection
  It is therefore important for junior doctors to know how to prevent, recognize and manage septic patients.

Septic Shock

Septic shock is a subset of sepsis in which underlying circulatory and cellular/ metabolic abnormalities are profound enough to substantially increase mortality.[21] This group of patients have refractory hypotension and inadequate tissue perfusion. They require vasopressors to maintain a mean arterial pressure (MAP) of 65 mmHg or more and have a serum lactate of more than 2 mmol/L, both in the absence of hypovolaemia. These patients require prompt critical care input.

Anastomotic Leak

An anastomotic leak is defined as a leak of luminal contents from a surgical join between two hollow viscera. If this occurs, it carries a mortality risk of up to 50%.

Risk Factors

The development of AL has modifiable and non-modifiable risk factors (Table 7.11).

Diagnosis of Anastomotic Leak

Early recognition of anastomotic leak is key.

The following can all indicate AL; none are pathognomonic but individually each should alert a clinician to the possibility of an AL:

- Tachycardia
- Pyrexia

TABLE 7.11	Table of Risk Factors for Anastomotic Leak (AL).

Modifiable Risk Factors	Non-Modifiable Risk Factors	Intraoperative Risk Factors
• Smoking • Obesity • Alcohol excess • Corticosteroids • Malnutrition • Preop short- and long-course radiotherapy	• Male gender • Age: some studies have shown that increased age is associated with AL • History of radiotherapy • Diabetes mellitus • Co-morbidity: pulmonary disease, vascular disease, renal impairment, increasing ASA grade all are associated with an increase in AL. • Emergency surgery • Distal anastomosis • Advanced tumour stage • Metastatic disease	• Contaminated surgery • Use of intraoperative inotropes • Significant blood loss • Use of blood transfusion • Prolonged surgery

ASA, American Society of Anesthesiologists.

- Raised C-Reactive protein (CRP)
- Raised WBC
- Pain out of proportion
- Arrhythmia
- Ileus
- Failure to progress
- Rectal bleeding/passage of bloody mucous

In a patient with bowel resection and anastomosis, evidence of SIRS or sepsis should be considered to mean AL until proven otherwise. When suspicion of AL arises a frequent senior surgeon review is mandatory.

Imaging for Anastomotic Leak

- Imaging is not essential if the patient is unwell, unstable and clinical suspicion is high enough to warrant a direct return to theatre.
- Otherwise, CT scanning with water-soluble contrast enema and i.v. contrast is recommended.
- Cross-sectional imaging in a patient with haemodynamic instability should not be undertaken without invasive monitoring and presence of critical care personnel.

Management of Anastomotic Leak

There are two phases to the management of AL.

Initial Management. The first phase is the initial resuscitative phase as with all cases of sepsis (care bundles vary):

- Oxygen
- Lactate check
- Drawing of blood cultures
- Blood tests: FBC
- Antibiotics
- Fluid resuscitation: intravenous crystalloid boluses
- Urinary catheter

Definitive Management. Involvement of a second senior surgeon is highly recommended. Options depending on the grade and severity of the AL include:

- Conservative
- Radiologically guided drainage +/– washout + defunctioning

- Transanal drainage: endoscopic placement of vacuum devices into presacral cavity (Endo-SPONGE)
- Return to theatre: laparotomy, washout, take down of anastomosis and creation of stoma +/– repair of stoma + diverting ileostomy.

Surgical Site Infection

Surgical site infection (SSI) can be defined as an infection that occurs after surgery in the part of the body where surgery took place. SSI can be:
- Superficial
  - Skin, e.g. wound infection
- Deep
  - Tissue under the skin
  - Organs
  - Implanted material, e.g. prosthetic joint

There are some preoperative, intraoperative and postoperative measures that can be taken to prevent SSIs (Table 7.12).[22]

Wound Infections

Surgical wounds are categorized into four classes:
- Clean
- Clean-contaminated
- Contaminated
- Dirty

See Table 7.13 for a classification of surgical wounds.

Preventative Measures for Wound Infection

Wound Management

- Healing by secondary intention: in some cases, where there has been gross contamination of the wound (for instance direct faecal contamination of laparotomy wound), it may be judged that risk of wound infection is high and the wound may be left open (and to consider delayed primary closure or allow for healing by secondary intention).
- Negative pressure for closed incisions: where patients are judged to be at high risk of wound infection (obese or

TABLE 7.12   Strategies to Prevent Surgical Site Infection.

Preoperative	Perioperative	Postoperative
Optimizing patient factors: Decolonization treatment for nasal carriers of *S. aureus* Washing with antimicrobial soap Correction of malnutrition Diabetes improvement if poorly controlled Stopping smoking Weight loss	Administration of antibiotics before incision Surgical site preparation with alcohol based antiseptic solutions based on CHG Maintaining body temperature Maintaining glucose control Hair removal should NOT be performed preoperatively	Nutrition Removing drains when not required Controlling blood sugars Aseptic technique for reviewing wounds

CHG, Chlorhexidine gluconate.

TABLE 7.13   Classification of Surgical Wounds.

Class	Definition	Examples
Clean	No inflammation No entry of respiratory, GI or GU tracts Aseptic technique maintained	Inguinal hernia repair Thyroidectomy
Clean-contaminated	Respiratory/GI/GU tracts entered but no significant spillage	Appendicectomy for mild appendicitis Cholecystectomy
Contaminated	Acute inflammation Visible contamination Open injuries <4 hours	
Dirty	Presence of pus Perforated viscus Open injuries >4 h	Laparotomy for perforated DU/small bowel/colon

DU, Duodenal ulcer; GI, gastrointestinal; GU, genitourinary.

diabetic), it may be advantageous to use negative pressure therapy for closed incisions as a preventative strategy to avoid infection.

Wound Dehiscence

Wound dehiscence of the abdominal wall can be:
- Superficial, e.g. skin
- Full thickness
Wound dehiscence may occur due to:
- Infection
- Immunosuppression
- Poor surgical technique

Signs of wound dehiscence are discharge (pus stained fluid implies infection), local cellulitis, wound coming apart.

The wound should be opened up at the affected area to allow fluid to discharge and the wound should be cleaned and packed as appropriate and left to heal by secondary intention. The facial layer should be examined gently to check that it is opposed and that there is no full thickness dehiscence which can lead to a 'burst abdomen'.

In rare instances of 'burst abdomen' where bowel is exposed, the bowel should be covered immediately with large surgical packs soaked in warm water, the surgeon on duty should be contacted and a return to theatre planned for urgent re-closure of all layers (mass closure). A burst abdomen can be heralded by discharging of haemoserous fluid.

Collection

Collections can occur after any surgery. Types of collections include:
- Haematoma
  - These will dissolve slowly and become reabsorbed but can become problematic infection ensures
- Serous/haemoserous collection: from recent surgery
- Bile, e.g. bile leak after laparoscopic cholecystectomy
- Pancreatic fluid
- Pus (intra-abdominal abscess)
  - Recent surgery: appendicitis, colectomy, repair of perforated ulcer, laparoscopic cholecystectomy

Intra-abdominal abscesses are commonly located in the pelvis or subphrenic space and can be managed:
- Conservatively with antibiotics
- IR guided drainage: usually a pig tail catheter
- Surgery

Organisms involved are usually from GI source, for example:
- Bacteroides (anaerobic)
- *Escherichia coli* (aerobic)

Prosthetic Infection

Many types of surgery require prosthesis insertion such as:
- Joint replacement
- Breast implant
- Vascular grafts
- Artificial valves
  Infection can be transmitted:
- From the skin surface
- Haematological spread from an infection at another organ
- Rarely from the operating room environment

Infection to any of these prostheses is life-threatening and disastrous for the patient and involves high-risk surgery for removal of the implant and possible revision surgery. Strategies for prevention are listed in Table 7.12. SSI prevention care bundles should be used to prevent prosthetic infections and local hospital guidelines should be followed for antibiotic prophylaxis.

Summary

The success of surgery does not simply lie with the technical abilities of the surgeon. For a patient to recover appropriately and return home after surgery demands meticulous preoperative and postoperative care. Patient recovery demands for clinicians to pre-empt clinical problems and complications to avoid disaster.

References

1. Nightingale J. *Intestinal Failure*. Cambridge: Cambridge University Press; 2001.
2. Park GR, Roe PG. *Fluid Balance and Volume Resuscitation for Beginners*. Cambridge: GMM publishing; 2000.
3. Membership of the working party: Griffiths R, Beech F, Brown A, et al. Peri-operative care of the elderly 2014. Association of Anaesthetists of Great Britain and Ireland. *Anaesthesia*. 2014. https://doi.org/10.1111/anae.12524.
4. Baker C. *Obesity Statistics. House of Commons Briefing Paper*. [online] https://commonslibrary.parliament.uk/research-briefings/sn03336/.
5. Ogden CL, Carroll MD, Fryar CD, et al. Prevalence of obesity among adults and youth: United States, 2011-2014. *NCHS Data Brief*. 2015; 11(219):1–8. https://www.cdc.gov/nchs/data/databriefs/db219.pdf. Accessed January 29, 2018.
6. Eckel RH, Grundy SM, Zimmet PZ. The metabolic syndrome. *Lancet*. 2005;365(9468):1415–1428.
7. Mutter TC, Chateau D, Moffatt M, et al. A matched cohort study of post-operative outcomes in obstructive sleep apnea. *Anesthesiology*. 2014;121:707–718.
8. Chung F, Subramanyam R, Liao P, Sasaki E, Shapiro C, Sun Y. High STOP- bang score indicates a high probability of obstructive sleep apnoea. *Br J Anaesthesia*. 2012;108:768–775.
9. Freemantle N, Holmes J, Hockey A, et al. How strong is the association between abdominal obesity and the incidence of type 2 diabetes? *Int J Clin Pract*. 2008;62(9):1391–1396. https://doi.org/10.111/j.742-241.2008.01805.x. Epub 2008 Jun 28.
10. Joint British Diabetes Societies for inpatient care: Management of adults with diabetes undergoing surgery and elective procedures: Improving standards. Summary. 2016. https://www.diabetes.org.uk/resources-s3/2017-09/Surgical%20guideline%202015%20-%20summary%20FINAL%20amended%20Mar%202016.pdf.
11. Milde AS, Bottiger BW, Morcos M. Adrenal cortex and steroids. supplementary therapy in the perioperative phase. *Anaesthesist*. 2005;54(7):639–654.
12. Wynter-Blyth V, Moorthy K. Prehabilitation: Preparing patients for surgery. *BMJ*. 2017;358:j3701. https://doi.org/10.1136/bmj.j3702.
13. Basse L, Hjort Jakobsen D, Billesbølle P, et al. A clinical pathway to accelerate recovery after colonic resection. *Ann Surg*. 2000;232(1):51–57.
14. Gustafsson UO, Hausel J, Thorell A, et al. Adherence to the enhanced recovery after surgery protocol and outcomes after colorectal cancer surgery. *Arch Surg*. 2011;146(5):571–577.
15. Gustafsson UO, Oppelstrup H, Thorell A, et al. Adherence to the ERAS protocol is associated with 5-year survival after colorectal cancer surgery: a retrospective cohort study. *World J Surg*. 2016;40:1741–1747.
16. Pucher P, Aggarwal R, Darzi A. Surgical ward round quality and impact on variable patient outcomes. *Ann Surg*. 2014;259(2):222–6.
17. Khuri SF, Henderson WG, DePalma RG, et al. Determinants of long-term survival after major surgery and the adverse effect of postoperative complications. *Ann Surg*. 2005;242:326–343.
18. Bragg D, El-Sharkawy AM, Psaltis, et al. Postoperative ileus: recent developments in pathophysiology and management. *Clin Nutri*. 2015;34:367–376.
19. Baker ML, Williams RN, Nightingale JMD. Causes and management of a high-output stoma. *Colorectal Dis*. 2011;13(2):191–197.
20. Association of Surgeons of Great Britain and Ireland (ASGBI). *The Surgical Management of Patients with Acute Intestinal Failure*. London: ASGBI; 2010. https://www.irspen.ie/wp-content/uploads/2014/10/ASGBA_The_surgical_management_of_patients_with_acute_intestinal_failure.pdf.
21. Singer M, et al. The third international consensus definitions for sepsis and septic shock (Sepsis-3). *J Am Med Assoc*. 2016;315(8):801–810. https://doi.org/10.1001/jama.2016.0287.
22. WHO. *Global Guidelines for the Prevention of Surgical Site Infection*; 2016. http://apps.who.int/iris/bitstream/10665/250680/1/9789241549882-eng.pdf?ua=1. Accessed January 30, 2018.
23. Powell-Tuck J, Gosling P, Lobo D, et al. *British Consensus Guidelines on Intravenous Fluid Therapy for Adult Surgical Patients*. GIFTASUP; 2011. http://www.bapen.org.uk/pdfs/bapen_pubs/giftasup.pdf. Accessed January 4, 2018.
24. Specialists in Obesity and B. Anaesthesia (SOBA). *The SOBA Single Sheet Guideline*; 2016. [online] https://www.sobauk.co.uk/guidelines-1.
25. Fearon KCH, Ljungqvist O, Von Meyenfeldt M, et al. Enhanced recovery after surgery: a consensus review of clinical care for patients undergoing colonic resection. *Clin Nutri*. 2005;24:466–477.
26. Metheny NM. *Fluid and Electrolyte Balance: Nursing Considerations*. 5th ed. Massachusetts: Jones and Bartlett Learning; 2012.

27. American Society of Anesthesiologists. *ASA physical status classification system*; 2014 [online] Available at: https://www.asahq.org /resources/clinical-information/asa-physical-status-classification-system. Accessed January 28, 2018.

28. American College of Surgeons. *ATLS Student Course Manual: Advanced Trauma Life Support, ATLS Ninth ed*. Chicago: American College of Surgeons; 2012.

Further Reading

ACPGBI Guidelines; *Prevention, Diagnosis and Management of Colorectal Anastomotic Leakage*; 2016. https://www.acpgbi.org.uk/content/uploads/2017/02/Prevention-diagnosis-and-management-of-colorectal-anastomotic-leakage-ASGBI-ACPGBI-2016.pdf. Accessed January 3, 2018.

Guenaga KF, Matos D, Wille-Jorgenson P. Mechanical bowel preparation for elective colorectal surgery (review). *Cochrane Databases Syst Rev*. 2011;(9):CD001544. https://doi.org/10.1002/14651858. CD001544.pub4.

Kim JT, Kumar RR. Reoperation for stoma-related complications. *Clin Colorectal Surg*. 2006;19:207–212.

Joint British Diabetes Societies for Inpatient Care. *Management of Adults with Diabetes Undergoing Surgery and Elective Procedures: Improving Standards Summary*; 2016. https://www.diabetes.org. uk/resources-s3/2017-09/Surgical%20guideline%202015%20-%20summary%20FINAL%20amended%20Mar%202016.pdf. Accessed January 31, 2018.

Lobo DN, Bostock KA, Neal KR, et al. Effect of salt and water balance on recovery of gastrointestinal function after colonic resection: a randomised controlled trial. *Lancet*. 2002;359:1812–1818.

Phillips RKS, Clark S. *Colorectal Surgery: A Companion to Specialist Surgical Practice*. 5th ed. Saunders Elsevier; 2014.

Royal College of Surgeons Website. https://www.rcseng.ac.uk/standards-and-research/gsp/domain-1/1-3-record-your-work-clearly-accurately-and-legibly/. (last accessed 28th December 2017).

Silen W. *Cope's Early Diagnosis of the Acute Abdomen*. Oxford: Oxford University Press; 2010 [chapter 23].

8

Perioperative Management and Postoperative Complications

PREOPERATIVE ASSESSMENT

Day Surgery

Background and Context

In the UK, day surgery is defined as a patient being admitted to hospital, having a planned procedure, and being discharged all in the same calendar day. The Department of Health set a target for 75% of elective surgery to be performed as day cases.[1] In a 2004 publication, the Institute for Innovation and Improvement recommended 'treat[ing] day surgery... as the norm for elective surgery' as its number 1 'High Impact Change for Service Improvement and Delivery'.[2] In other areas of the globe, such as the United States, high uptake of day surgery as a mainstay of elective surgical practice has been documented since the early 1990s.[3]

Within the elective setting, day surgery accounts for 78% of elective surgical activity.[4] Additionally, the number

of procedures suitable for day surgery has increased from 14 in the initial 'basket' published by the Audit Commission in 1990,[5] to over 200 in the British Association of Day Surgery guidelines published in June 2016.[6]

Advantages of Day Surgery and Considerations

Day surgery has benefits for patients, staff and organizations. There is some evidence that surgery in the day case setting may result in reduced infection rates,[7] particularly with respect to hospital-acquired infections.[1] Patient satisfaction following day case surgery is high, as convalescence takes place in their own home with minimum disruption to their daily lives. Finally, day surgery results in reduced hospital costs and increased efficiency, which are of clear benefit to healthcare organizations.[8]

However, the primary principles of day surgery must remain focused around appropriate patient and surgical procedure selection. A number of guidelines have been formulated within the UK to aid clinicians and hospital organizations with this process. These include:

- Guidelines for the Provision of Anaesthetic Services, Royal College of Anaesthetists, 2016
- Day Case and Short Stay Surgery, Association of Anaesthetists of Great Britain & Ireland, 2011
- Directory of Procedures (5th edition), British Association of Day Surgery, 2016
- Department of Health. Surgery Health Building Note 10-02: Day Surgery Facilities, 2007

Preoperative Assessment for Day Surgery

The preoperative assessment clinic is best placed for assessing patient suitability for day surgery. This will depend on social factors, surgical factors and an assessment of the patient's medical co-morbidities. In general, there are few absolute contraindications to day surgery.

Social Considerations

Patients must be appropriately informed, motivated and consent to day surgery where this is planned. They must have an adequate support system, access to a telephone, written postoperative care instructions and a responsible adult staying with them for at least 24 hours after surgery.

Medical Factors

The majority of medical factors do not preclude patients having day surgery. Historical limitations such as American Society of Anesthesiologists (ASA) status have not been shown to increase patient mortality after day surgery.[9] Well-controlled, chronic conditions such as epilepsy or diabetes are often better managed where there is minimal disruption to normal routine. Any pre-existing medical conditions should be fully optimized prior to day surgery where possible.

Special Considerations:

- In general, full-term infants over the age of 1 month are appropriate for day surgery. In the premature population, this age limit is generally extended to 60 weeks post-conceptual age.
- Increasing body mass index (BMI) is associated with an increased incidence of complications intraoperatively and in early recovery. These issues are often resolved by the time day surgery patients are discharged and there is no evidence that the risk of late postoperative complications increases with obesity. Conversely, obese patients often benefit from the short-duration anaesthetic techniques and the early mobilization associated with day surgery, and day case bariatric surgery is an evolving area of day surgery practice.

Anaesthetic Factors

The management of patients for day surgery is targeted towards short-duration anaesthesia with minimal side effects. Anaesthetic management of day surgery patients is targeted towards reducing the risk of postoperative nausea and vomiting (PONV) and inadequate analgesia, as these are two of the most common factors in unplanned admission for day surgery. As such, anaesthetic techniques are often multimodal and may involve local anaesthetic infiltration or nerve blocks in addition to general anaesthesia.

Surgical Factors

In general, procedures listed in the British Association of Day Surgery (BADS) Directory of Procedures are appropriate for day surgery. However, the procedure should not carry a significant risk of serious complication requiring specialist observation or care. Furthermore, anticipated postoperative symptoms must be controllable by the use of oral medications and local anaesthetic techniques where appropriate.

Preoperative Assessment

The preoperative assessment visit entails a holistic evaluation of an individual patient. This means undertaking a thorough review of their medical conditions and how well they are managed. Investigations and specialist referrals that impact anaesthetic and surgical management should be arranged in a timely manner, so as not to delay surgery. Finally, regular medications should be reviewed, and written information provided for patients who must alter their regular medications around the time of surgery.

Systems Review: Cardiovascular

Major adverse cardiac events (MACE) represent a major component of perioperative morbidity and mortality in patients undergoing non-cardiac surgery. It is essential that preoperative assessment identifies those patients at elevated risk of MACE and optimizes them appropriately.

Assessing Cardiovascular Risk for Non-Cardiac Surgery

A number of risk scoring systems for assessing the risk of MACE in non-cardiac surgery exist. Historically, this has been in the form of a Cardiac Risk Index proposed by Goldman et al. in 1977.[10] This initial 9-point scoring system was subsequently revised in 1999 by Lee et al. to generate the Revised Cardiac Risk Index[11] (RCRI) (Table 8.1).

Whilst simple predictors of cardiac risk are easy to use and remember, recent guidelines have suggested the use of more holistic surgical risk calculators to further stratify risk for individual patients. Current recommendations from the American College of Cardiology/American Heart Association (ACC/AHA) advocate the use of the NSQIP Surgical Risk Calculator developed by the American College of Surgeons.[12] Although not validated in populations outside North America, the following five factors out-performed the RCRI as predictors of perioperative myocardial infarction or cardiac arrest[13]:

- ASA class
- Dependent functional status

TABLE 8.1 Lee's Revised Cardiac Risk Index.

Revised Cardiac Risk Index

History of ischaemic heart disease
History of congestive heart failure
History of cerebrovascular disease (stroke or transient ischaemic attack)
History of diabetes requiring preoperative insulin use
Chronic kidney disease (creatinine >2 mg/dL)
Suprainguinal vascular, intraperitoneal or intrathoracic surgery

Risk for cardiac death, non-fatal MI, and non-fatal cardiac arrest:
0 predictors = 0.4%, 1 predictor = 0.9%, 2 predictors = 6.6%, ≥ 3 predictors = over 11%

MI, Myocardial infarction.

TABLE 8.2 NICE Classification of Hypertension.

Stage	Clinic Blood Pressure	Ambulatory Blood Pressure
Stage 1	140/90 mmHg or higher	135/85 mmHg or higher
Stage 2	160/100 mmHg or higher	150/95 mmHg or higher
Stage 3	180/110 mmHg or higher	N/A

From NICE Guideline CG 127. Hypertension in adults: diagnosis and management. 2011.

- Age
- Abnormal creatinine (>1.5 mg/dL)
- Type of surgery (highest odds ratio: aortic, foregut, hepatopancreatobiliary, intracranial surgeries)

Hypertension

Across England, an estimated 24% of the population have either GP-recorded or undiagnosed essential hypertension.[14] Well-controlled essential hypertension in itself is not a risk factor for MACE.[15] However, in patients with poorly controlled hypertension, a shared decision must be made regarding the risks of delaying surgery in order to optimize blood pressure control. A full review of the treatment protocols for hypertension is beyond the scope of this chapter, but it is important that clinicians are familiar with NICE guidance for identifying and treating patients with hypertension[16] (Table 8.2).

Prior to starting antihypertensive therapy, patients should have an assessment of their 10-year cardiovascular risk using a calculator such as QRISK2. Patients with stage 3 hypertension should be started on antihypertensive therapy without waiting for further ambulatory measurements in the community. It is important to assess patients for evidence of end-organ damage, such as chronic kidney disease (CKD), ischaemic heart disease and hypertensive retinopathy. In young patients, or in patients where optimization proves difficult, investigation of causes of secondary hypertension should be considered. Finally, in the preoperative setting, certain antihypertensives such as ACE-inhibitors are routinely stopped. Patients should be provided with written guidance about the use of blood pressure medication around the time of surgery.

Ischaemic Heart Disease

In 2012, cardiovascular disease accounted for 16% of all deaths in men and 10% of all deaths in women in the UK.[17] This represents a significant burden to the National Health Service and is a common risk factor in patients presenting for surgery. The main causes of death from cardiovascular causes are coronary heart disease (46%) and stroke (26%). The last 20 years have seen a significant increase in the number of percutaneous coronary interventions (PCI). However, surgical revascularization (CABG) remains the treatment of choice for patients with complex coronary lesions or severe left main coronary artery disease.

As such, patients with active cardiac conditions should have the severity of their disease assessed in order to determine whether there are options for preoperative optimization. In the elective setting, investigations are aimed at determining the aetiology of the active disease and starting appropriate management. This would include non-invasive tests such as ECG and echocardiography, but in patients with a high index of suspicion, invasive tests such as coronary angiography may be appropriate. In cancer surgery, the benefit of these tests must be weighed against the risk of delaying surgery.

In emergency situations, full investigation and preoptimization may be precluded by time constraints, but simple measures to minimize risk should be taken. These are based around the physiological principles of maintaining oxygen delivery and reducing myocardial workload. In the immediate preoperative period, this could include: blood transfusion and correction of anaemia, optimization of fluid status, control of cardiac dysrhythmias, electrolyte replenishment, adequate analgesia and maintenance of normal oxygen levels.

Recent Myocardial Infarction

Special considerations apply if patients have had recent PCI prior to surgery. Non-cardiac surgery increases the risk of stent thrombosis, myocardial infarction, and death; particularly if dual antiplatelet therapy (DAPT) is discontinued perioperatively.[18] Irrespective of antiplatelet therapy, surgery performed in the first 6 weeks after PCI is associated with a higher risk of in-stent restenosis.[19] However, bleeding in the context of surgery, and particularly surgeries on closed spaces, is not a risk to be taken lightly. A further conundrum is presented by the utilization of bare metal stents (BMS) or drug-eluting stents (DES). In general, patients who receive a DES require at least a year of DAPT prior to discontinuation, and this has significant impact on those awaiting elective non-cardiac surgery. With the introduction of newer generation DES and biomatrix stents, guidance in this area is constantly evolving, and it is important that a discussion with the cardiologist inserting the stent takes place prior to cessation of antiplatelet therapy.

Selected important recommendations from the ACC/AHA 2014 guidelines[20] suggest that:

- Preoperative PCI should not be performed unless patients demonstrate high-risk coronary anatomy (left main stem disease), unstable angina, myocardial infarction, or life-threatening arrhythmia due to ischaemia.
- Elective non-cardiac surgery should be delayed by 14 days after balloon angioplasty, 30 days after BMS implantation, and 365 days after DES implantation if DAPT must be discontinued.
- Where necessary, elective surgery after DES implantation may be considered after 180 days if the risk of further delay is greater than the risk of ischaemia or stent thrombosis.
- If emergency non-cardiac surgery is required in a patient with recent PCI, a consensus decision amongst the treating clinicians is required as to the risks of coronary ischaemia, bleeding and the implications for long-term coronary revascularization.
- If PCI is indicated and surgery is likely to occur within 1 to 12 months, then a strategy of BMS and 4–6 weeks of DAPT may be an appropriate option.

Cardiac Dysrhythmia

Atrial fibrillation is the most common atrial arrhythmia and has a prevalence of 1–2%. In the preoperative setting, it may be present in the patient history, diagnosed on clinical assessment or after an ECG. Atrial fibrillation is associated with an increased risk of stroke, thromboembolic disease and heart failure. Significant bleeding associated with anticoagulant therapy used for stroke prevention is also a significant cause of morbidity and mortality.

Current guidelines recommend transthoracic echocardiography (TTE) in patients for whom cardioversion is considered, in whom there is a high risk of underlying structural heart disease (e.g. heart failure or a murmur) and in whom risk stratification for antithrombotic therapy is needed.[21] Echocardiography may aid clinicians by excluding significant valvular heart disease, identifying regional wall motion abnormalities and quantifying left ventricular ejection fraction.

The most common issues in the perioperative setting relate to the use of medications in the treatment of atrial fibrillation and in the prevention of stroke. These will be covered at length in a subsequent section. However, treatment aims prior to surgery involve:

- Appropriate rate control
- Rhythm control by electrical or chemical cardioversion where appropriate
- Treatment of any underlying precipitating factors, such as electrolyte abnormalities or poorly controlled thyroid disease
- Assessment of thromboembolic risk and bleeding risk

TABLE 8.3 NYHA Classification of Heart Failure.

Class I	No limitation of physical activity
Class II	Slight limitation of physical activity in which ordinary physical activity leads to fatigue, palpitation, dyspnoea, or anginal pain; the person is comfortable at rest
Class III	Marked limitation of physical activity in which less than ordinary activity results in fatigue, palpitation, dyspnoea, or anginal pain; the person is comfortable at rest
Class IV	Inability to carry on any physical activity without discomfort but also symptoms of heart failure or the anginal syndrome even at rest, with increased discomfort if any physical activity is undertaken

NYHA, New York Heart Association.

Heart Failure

Heart failure has been demonstrably linked to significant perioperative complications, with complication risk linked with the degree of systolic dysfunction. Patients with a left ventricular ejection fraction (LVEF) < 35% are at highest risk.[22] However, even asymptomatic LV dysfunction is predictive for both 30-day and long-term mortality.[23,24] More recently, there has also been a focus on patients with diastolic dysfunction. This early indicator of dysfunction is thought to be a sensitive marker of ischaemia and is also predictive of increased postoperative complications.[23] Patients with diastolic dysfunction have previously been demonstrated to have a distinctive phenotype, with 35–60% of them being elderly, and more likely to be female.[25,26]

Patients with heart failure should be stratified according to their symptoms and functional capacity (Table 8.3). Common signs and symptoms include: dyspnoea, orthopnoea, or paroxysmal nocturnal dyspnoea, bilateral ankle oedema, elevated JVP and tachycardia (heart rate >120 bpm). Functional capacity is commonly stratified by using the New York Heart Association classification of heart failure.

Although routine preoperative evaluation of LV function is not recommended in asymptomatic patients, where there is previously documented dysfunction, repeat echocardiography may be considered if there has been no assessment in the last 1 year.

A Note on Pacemakers and Implantable Cardiac Devices

The number of patients presenting for surgery with cardiac implantable electronic devices (CIEDs) is increasing. CIEDs fall into three categories:

- Implanted loop recorders or cardiac monitors designed for ECG monitoring
- Cardiac pacemakers
- Implantable cardioverter defibrillators (ICD)

TABLE 8.4	GOLD Criteria for Classification of Disease Severity.

In all patients with FEV_1/FVC <0.7

	FEV_1 post-bronchodilator
Stage 1 - Mild	FEV_1 ≥80% predicted
Stage 2 - Moderate	FEV_1 50%≤ FEV_1 <80% predicted
Stage 3 - Severe	FEV_1 30%≤ FEV_1 <50% predicted
Stage 4 - Very Severe	FEV_1 <30% predicted

COPD, Chronic obstructive pulmonary disease; FEV_1, forced expiratory volume in the first second; FVC, forced vital capacity.

Electromagnetic interference when diathermy is used may lead to inappropriate device function and cessation of cardiac activity or inappropriate delivery of an electric shock. It is therefore imperative that the theatre team are aware if a patient has a CIED.

Guidelines from the British Heart Rhythm Society suggest that:

- where a CIED is identified, clear documentation should be noted including the details of the CIED, follow-up details and the date of last follow-up
- advice should be taken from the follow-up centre regarding: the need for follow-up postoperatively, the need for adjusting sensing or pacing parameters and the need for deprogramming an ICD prior to surgery
- all patients with CIEDs should have cardiac rhythm monitoring from the outset of the procedure
- where possible, surgical diathermy should be avoided
- where surgical diathermy is unavoidable, bipolar diathermy should be considered in preference to unipolar. Diathermy use should be limited to short bursts, and the site should be as far away from the pacemaker site as possible
- there should be immediately available access to external defibrillation equipment and external temporary pacing.

Systems Review: Respiratory

Chronic Obstructive Pulmonary Disease (COPD)

COPD is a chronic and progressive inflammatory respiratory condition that affects 2% of the population in the UK. It has a strong link with smoking and presents as a varied spectrum from mild to very severe disease. The diagnosis of COPD by spirometry is well-described, and severity is classified according to airflow limitation (Table 8.4).

FEV_1 in particular has been implicated as an independent predictor of postoperative morbidity and mortality, particularly in severe disease (FEV_1 <30%).[27] Preoperative assessment of patients with COPD must include assessment of patient compliance with treatment (Fig. 8.1), as well as functional capacity as this has implications for assessing the need for preoperative optimisation, as well as the postoperative rehabilitation of patients and their ability to comply with physiotherapy. Simple

assessments of functional capacity include the 6-minute walk test, or climbing a flight of stairs. Additionally, these patients require an ECG to look for evidence of right-sided heart disease, or concomitant ischaemic heart disease.

Smoking Cessation

Smoking history in the perioperative setting is extremely important. Current smokers have a two-fold increased risk of postoperative pulmonary complications (PPCs), including pneumonia, prolonged stay in intensive care and requirement for mechanical ventilation. This is attributed to the impaired ciliary function and impaired macrophage and natural killer cell activity caused by exposure to cigarette smoke. Although the risk of PPCs remains elevated up to 1 year following smoking cessation, the greatest reduction in risk occurs after stopping smoking for just 8 weeks.[28] There has been some suggestion that stopping smoking for a shorter time frame than this is associated with an increased risk of PPCs, but these data are primarily from observational data in cardiac centres, and have yet to be reproduced elsewhere.[29] Most centres advocate stopping smoking before surgery irrespective of the interval. Nicotine replacement therapy should be prescribed for patients at risk of withdrawal in the perioperative period.

Asthma

Asthma is a common respiratory condition, characterized by reversible airflow obstruction caused by bronchial smooth muscle contraction. It is a common disease that affects 7–8% of the population in the UK[30] and United States.[31] Well-controlled asthma is not a risk factor for PPCs.[32] However, poorly controlled asthma, recent symptoms and a history of tracheal intubation all put patients at increased risk for perioperative complications. Although the risk of complications is infrequent at just 2%, the overwhelming majority of closed claims relate to significant brain injury or death in the context of severe bronchospasm.[33] It is therefore necessary to consider optimization of medications and referral to specialist services if patients present to preoperative assessment with poorly controlled asthma (e.g. peak expiratory flow rate variability of >20%).

The other challenge that patients with asthma present relates to medication. Patients with severe asthma may often have concomitant steroid use which will need to be accounted for around the time of surgery, and it is important that routine anti-asthmatic medications are continued throughout surgery. Adequate analgesia is essential in the care of these patients. In particular, it is important that documentation is made of the response to non-steroidal anti-inflammatory medications. Referral to a critical care setting should be considered in patients with previous tracheal intubation for asthma or brittle disease.

Obstructive Sleep Apnoea (OSA)

Preoperative assessment should include screening for OSA. OSA is the most common type of sleep-disordered breathing, with a prevalence of 11.4% in men and 4.7% in women.[34] Obesity hypoventilation syndrome is a distinct

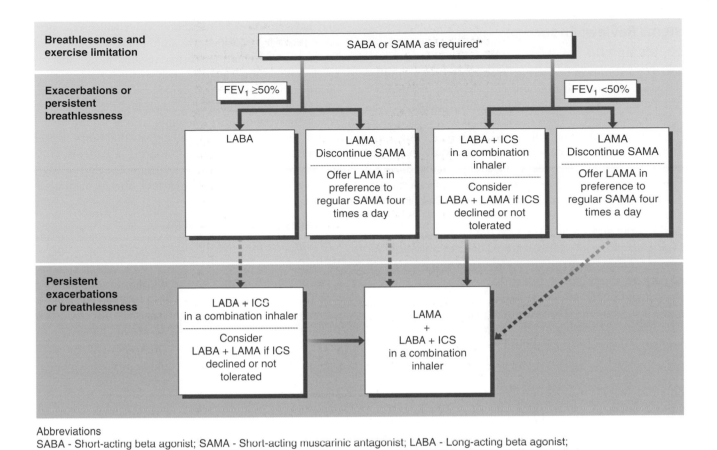

Abbreviations

SABA - Short-acting beta agonist; SAMA - Short-acting muscarinic antagonist; LABA - Long-acting beta agonist; LAMA - Long-acting muscarinic antagonist; ICS - inhaled corticosteroid; *SABA (as required) may continue at all stages

→ Offer therapy (strong evidence)   ▪▪▪▪▪▶ Consider therapy (less strong evidence)

• **Fig. 8.1** NICE Chronic Obstructive Pulmonary Disease (COPD) Guidelines

entity from OSA and requires the presence of obesity (BMI >30), awake hypercapnoea and hypoxaemia, and sleep disordered breathing. Diagnosis of OSA is based on the Apnoea-Hypopnoea Index (AHI), which is calculated after overnight polysomnography. Patients with OSA are at an increased risk of cardiovascular disease, including heart failure, hypertension and coronary artery disease. They are also more likely to develop metabolic syndrome, have a high BMI and have cerebrovascular disease as a result of low arterial oxygen levels.

A simple screening test, the STOP-BANG questionnaire, can be used for patients with a high index of suspicion for sleep disordered breathing (Table 8.5). A STOP-BANG score of 4 has a high sensitivity (87.5%) and specificity (90.5%) for identifying OSA in surgical populations.[35] Other tests that can be used include the Epworth Sleepiness Scale (ESS) and the 4-Variable screening tool.

Anaesthetic considerations in the patient with OSA presenting for surgery include:
- An assessment of cardiac function
- An assessment of awake pulmonary gas exchange
- Increased susceptibility to respiratory depressants such as opioids and benzodiazepines
- An association with obesity and difficult intubation

TABLE 8.5	STOP-BANG score for OSA screening.
S	Snoring
T	Daytime Tiredness
O	Observed cessation of breathing during sleep
P	Pressure - being treated for hypertension
B	BMI >35 kg/m2
A	Age >50
N	Neck circumference >40 cm
G	Gender: male

OSA, Obstructive sleep apnoea.

Patients with congestive heart failure or hypercapnia should receive a trial of CPAP therapy for up to 3 months preoperatively. Patients already on CPAP should continue this perioperatively, and may warrant admission to critical care for postoperative monitoring. Anaesthetic technique and analgesic regimens should be carefully titrated to minimize the use of long-acting central respiratory depressants such as morphine wherever possible.

Systems Review: Endocrine
Diabetes Mellitus

Diabetes is a common endocrine disorder that has a significant impact on morbidity and mortality in surgical patients. In the perioperative period, patients with hyperglycaemia have increased lengths of stay, as well as an increased risk of postoperative pneumonia, acute kidney injury and myocardial infarction.[36] Diabetes is also associated with increased rates of end-organ damage including cardiovascular disease, cerebrovascular disease, chronic kidney disease, retinopathy and peripheral neuropathy. The microvascular implications of diabetes also mean these patients are predisposed to poor wound healing and surgical site infections.

Guidelines from the Joint British Diabetes Societies for Inpatient Care recommend that preoperative assessment of these patients should focus on the following factors:

- Assessment of diabetic control using markers such as glycated haemoglobin (HbA1c) and fasting blood glucose.
- Optimization of diabetic control and referral to specialist services if control is poor (HbA1c >69 mmol).
- Day of surgery admission should be the 'default' position, in contrast to previously, where admission for variable rate insulin infusion on the night prior to surgery was the norm.
- Giving the patient written instructions with planned medication changes on the day of admission.
- Prioritizing list position to minimize starvation time.
- Multimodal analgesia and antiemetic therapy to aid return to normal diabetes management and minimize time spent on variable rate insulin infusions.
- Foot care is extremely important as these patients are at high risk of developing foot ulcers. Contraindications to anti-embolism stockings must be carefully considered and patients with 'at risk' feet should be clearly identified.
- At discharge, ensure patients have clear information on 'sick day rules' and instructions on what to do if they feel unwell.

Thyroid Dysfunction

Patients with thyroid dysfunction represent up to 21% of the female population and 3% of the male population,[37] with the predominant abnormality being elevated thyroid-stimulating hormone (TSH) implying reduced baseline thyroid function. Furthermore, just 60% of patients on established thyroid medication had TSH values within the normal range. Routine screening is not indicated in patients where there is a low index of suspicion of thyroid dysfunction. However, patients with known hyper- or hypothyroidism should have a TSH level included in the preoperative assessment, in order to ensure that thyroid function is optimized.[38]

In patients with known disease, abnormal thyroid function has significant impact on the cardiovascular system. Hypothyroidism is associated with diminished cardiac output and increased afterload.[39] These patients are predisposed to hypotension under anaesthesia, and they also may have an impaired respiratory drive which may predispose them to postoperative pulmonary complications.[40] Patients with hypothyroidism are also more susceptible to electrolyte abnormalities such as hyponatraemia[41] and postoperative ileus.[42] However, despite these observations, small scale observational data has found little difference in postoperative morbidity outcomes such as wound infection or mortality.[43] A 2017 review suggests that non-emergency surgery should therefore be postponed in patients who are severely hypothyroid, with serum thyroxine levels <1 µg/dL, or those with complications such as altered mentation or heart failure.[38]

Systems Review: Renal
Chronic Kidney Disease

Chronic kidney disease (CKD) is an increasingly common medical condition that affects roughly 11 to 13% of the global population.[44] It is defined as a structural or functional abnormality of the kidneys which persists for more than 3 months. This may manifest as a decreased glomerular filtration rate (GFR) or other markers of kidney damage, such as electrolyte abnormality, proteinuria or structural abnormality on imaging. In the UK, the annual incidence of new patients requiring renal replacement therapy (RRT) is 108 per million people.[45] Patients with CKD are at increased risk of cardiovascular disease and MACE.

CKD severity is classified by GFR using the Kidney Outcomes Quality Initiative (KDOQI) criteria.[46] Additionally, NICE guidelines further suggest assessing risk by quantifying albuminuria using the albumin: creatinine ratio (Fig. 8.2). It is important that patients with CKD have an informed discussion about the implications of general anaesthesia and surgery for their short-term and long-term renal function.

Patients with CKD require an assessment of their extra-renal disease. This includes:

- Cardiovascular system. Patients with CKD are at an increased risk of perioperative MACE. They may have concomitant hypertension, ischaemic heart disease, congestive cardiac failure and valvular heart disease.
- Fluid and fluid status. These may be grossly deranged in patients with CKD, particularly if they are in a low-clearance phase or are dependent on RRT. The assessment and optimization of their fluid state is important prior to surgery and will require discussion with nephrologists. Additionally, for patients who are RRT-dependent, there may be practical issues surrounding access to their usual mode of treatment.
- Vascular access issues. Patients with end-stage CKD may have had multiple vascular access attempts, including tunnelled dialysis lines, previous central access for haemofiltration and arteriovenous fistulae. It is important for the clinician to be aware of previous sites, as well as any plans for future venous access.
- Respiratory. Up to 40% of patients with CKD have pulmonary hypertension related to their cardiovascular issues. This may lead to significant right heart

GFR and ACR categories and risk of adverse outcomes			ACR categories (mg/mmol), description and range		
			<3 Normal to mildly increased	3–30 Moderately increased	>30 Severely increased
			A1	A2	A3
	≥90 Normal and high	G1	No CKD in the absence of markers of kidney damage		
	60–89 Mild reduction related to normal range for a young adult	G2			
	45–59 Mild–moderate reduction	G3a[1]			
	30–44 Moderate–severe reduction	G3b			
	15–29 Severe reduction	G4			
	<15 Kidney failure	G5			

GFR categories (ml/min.1.73m²), description and range

Increasing risk

Increasing risk

• **Fig. 8.2** Risk Stratification in Chronic Kidney Disease ACR, Albumin:creatinine ratio; CKD, chronic kidney disease; GFR, glomerular filtration rate. (Adapted with permission from Kidney Disease: Improving Global Outcomes (KDIGO) CKD Work Group, 2013. KDIGO 2012 clinical practice guideline for the evaluation and management of chronic kidney disease. Kidney International. (Suppl. 3), 1–150.)

dysfunction and needs to be assessed prior to having a general anaesthetic.

- Endocrine. Patients with long-standing renal disease may have issues with hyperparathyroidism, hypercalcaemia and vitamin D deficiency. Additionally, up to 50% of cases of established renal failure in the United States are caused by diabetes mellitus.[47]
- Clotting and coagulopathy. Platelet dysfunction is common, with an increase in prothrombotic tendencies in the early stages of renal disease. In advanced CKD, platelet adhesion and aggregation is impaired, putting patients at risk of haemorrhagic events such as gastrointestinal (GI) and intracranial bleeding. On the other end of the spectrum, data from thromboelastography also shows that patients with uraemia have hypercoagulable activity.[48] Finally, patients with stage 3 CKD or worse develop a normochromic, normocytic anaemia due to deficiency in erythropoietin, folate, iron or vitamin B_{12}.[49]
- Immunological. Patients with CKD may be on long-term immunosuppression in view of their underlying pathology or because of their transplant status. Additionally, end-stage renal disease and uraemia have widespread effects on the innate and adaptive immune systems, with altered expression of pattern recognition receptors such as Toll like receptors causing significant immunosuppression.[50]

Medications Review and Recommendations

Various guidelines exist for the management of medications in the perioperative period (Table 8.6). It is essential that patients receive written information about medication use on the day before, and the day of surgery. Over 50% of patients omit important cardiac medications on the day of surgery, whilst 33% of them have medications withheld on the day after surgery.[51]

Other Medications

Steroids

Patients receiving steroid therapy in the last three months should be treated as if they are on steroids. For patients on the equivalent of less than 10 mg of prednisolone per day, additional steroid cover is not required. For those with a significant

TABLE 8.6	Perioperative Medicine Management Recommendations.	
Medication	**Day of Surgery**	**After Surgery**
Antihypertensives		
Alpha and beta-blockers/ Calcium channel blockers	Take as usual	Continue oral medication unless hypotensive
ACE-inhibitors/ Angiotensin receptor blockers/ Diuretics	Omit on day of surgery If normally taken in the evening, omit the day before surgery	Resume when patient has re-established oral intake
Diabetic Medications		
Metformin	If taken once or twice a day: do not stop If taken three times a day: omit lunchtime dose irrespective of time of surgery	Aim to resume normal medications as soon as possible Metformin should only be recommenced if eGFR >60 mL/ min/1.73m^2
Sulphonylureas	If taken once a day: omit morning dose If taken twice a day: omit morning dose (a.m. list), or omit both doses (p.m. list)	
Thiazolidinediones DDP-IV inhibitors GLP-1 analogues	Take as normal irrespective of time of surgery	
SGLT-2 inhibitors	Omit morning dose irrespective of time of surgery	
Long-acting insulin (once daily dose)	Dose to be reduced by 20% on the day before surgery **and** the day of surgery	Patients expected to miss more than one meal should be started on a variable rate insulin infusion
Twice daily insulin	Day before surgery: no dose change Day of surgery: reduce morning dose by 50% irrespective of time of surgery Normal insulin with evening meal	Basal insulin should be continued at 80% of usual dose VRII can be discontinued when the patient is eating and drinking
3–5 daily injections	Day before surgery: no dose change Day of surgery: omit short-acting insulin when no meal is eaten (i.e. breakfast or lunch) Reduce long-acting insulin dose by 80% Normal insulin with evening meal	Give usual insulin with meal and discontinue VRII 30–60 minutes later
Anticoagulants		
Antiplatelets Aspirin Clopidogrel	Continue in minor surgery. Stop for 7 days pre-op if major surgery or high risk of bleeding. However, even if there is a high risk of bleeding, continuation should be considered if the patient is at high risk of thrombus Stop for 7 days pre-op if major surgery or high risk of bleeding	Re-start when risk of bleeding is no longer significant
Warfarin	Assessment of risk of thrombosis: Low risk: Stop 5 days before surgery High risk: Stop 5 days before surgery. Start therapeutic LMWH and continue until the day before surgery	
NOACs	Most NOACs do not need to be stopped for low bleeding risk procedures. For high bleeding risk procedures, the last dose should be 24–72 hours before surgery depending on renal function. Bridging with LMWH is not required	

ACE, Angiotensin-converting enzyme; DDP-IV, Dipeptidyl peptidase-4; eGFR, estimated glomerular filtration rate; GLP-1, glucagon-like peptide-1; LMWH, low-molecular-weight heparin; NOAC, new oral anticoagulants; SGLT-2, sodium-glucose co-transporter-2; VRII, variable rate insulin infusion.

steroid dose, additional IV hydrocortisone should be given at induction and continued after surgery for 1–3 days.

Analgesics

Patients taking medication for chronic pain can be poorly managed around the time of surgery. In general, patients should be prescribed their normal analgesics, as well as additional analgesics to account for the pain associated with surgery. Regional anaesthesia techniques may be useful in minimizing opioid requirements and providing adequate analgesia. Involving the pain team early in the management of these patients is good for continuity of care and patient management.

TABLE 8.7   Routine Investigations Recommended by NICE.

	ASA 1		ASA 2		ASA 3 or 4	
FBC	Surgery Type		Surgery Type		Surgery Type	
	Minor	Not routinely	Minor	Not routinely	Minor	Not routinely
	Intermediate	Not routinely	Intermediate	Not routinely	Intermediate	Consider
	Major/Complex	Yes	Major/Complex	Yes	Major/Complex	Yes
Clotting		Not routinely irrespective of surgery type		Not routinely irrespective of surgery type		Consider if chronic liver disease or anticoagulant therapy
Kidney Function	Surgery Type		Surgery Type		Surgery Type	
	Minor	Not routinely	Minor	Not routinely	Minor	Yes, if risk of AKI
	Intermediate	Yes, if risk of AKI	Intermediate	Yes, if risk of AKI	Intermediate	Yes
	Major/Complex	Yes, if risk of AKI	Major/Complex	Yes	Major/Complex	Yes
ECG	Surgery Type		Surgery Type		Surgery Type	
	Minor	Not routinely	Minor	Not routinely	Minor	Yes, if no ECG in last 12 months
	Intermediate	Not routinely	Intermediate	Yes if CVS disease, renal, or diabetes	Intermediate	Yes
	Major/Complex	Yes if age >65	Major/Complex	Yes	Major/Complex	Yes
Spirometry/ Arterial Blood Gas		Not routinely		Not routinely		Not routinely. Seek advice from specialist if known or suspected disease

AKI, Acute kidney injury; ASA, American Society of Anesthesiologists; CVS, cardiovascular system.

Bowel Preparation

Bowel preparation before surgery is thought to decrease the bacterial load of the colon and therefore decrease infection. Additionally, it may improve operating conditions by clearing the bowel lumen of stool and reducing intraluminal pressures whilst operating. There is currently no evidence to support the use of bowel preparation in reducing complication rates.[52] A number of preparations exist, which rely primarily on osmotic agents and laxatives that increase GI motility. Given the nature of these agents, it is important to monitor patients for significant fluid and electrolyte shifts that may occur following the use of bowel preparation agents.

Investigations

Investigations for patients should be considered in the context of their ASA grade, as well as the type of surgery they are having (Table 8.7).

Additional Tests/Recommendations (NICE UK)

All women of childbearing potential should have a pregnancy test on the day of surgery.

Do not carry out routine chest X-rays, urine dipstick analysis, or sickle cell trait testing unless indicated by history or surgery.

Resting echocardiography should be requested if a patient has: a heart murmur **and** a cardiac symptom **or** signs and symptoms of heart failure. This patient must be discussed with an anaesthetist and have an ECG prior to echocardiogram.

THE HIGH-RISK PATIENT

Increasingly, patients who present for surgery are elderly and have multiple co-morbidities. The surgery is often major or complex. These patients are often labelled 'high risk' and have a high risk of perioperative morbidity and mortality. These so-called 'high-risk' patients need to be identified; thus objective risk assessment is important in major surgery. Additionally, it may be possible to optimize their co-morbidities prior to surgery and influence their outcome in a positive manner. Shared decision making for high-risk patients is a key concept in achieving optimal outcomes in these patients.

Assessing Physiological Fitness

Physiological fitness and functional capacity are predictors of patient outcome after major surgery. Cardiopulmonary exercise testing (CPET) is an objective and reliable method of measuring cardiopulmonary reserve. Poor cardiorespiratory reserve is an independent predictor of increased postoperative complications and hospital length of stay in many forms of major abdominal surgery.[53]

CPET is usually conducted on a cycle ergometer, with the patient wearing a mouthpiece or facemask that allows the measurement of gas exchange. The patient then undergoes a ramped protocol test of increasing intensity and resistance. Patients are monitored with a 12-lead ECG, blood pressure cuff and a pulse oximeter throughout. The test is terminated on completion of the protocol (normally 8 and 12 minutes), or by patient symptoms.

Key Physiological Concepts

Muscle contraction relies on the high-energy phosphate groups found in adenosine triphosphate (ATP). ATP is supplied by the breakdown of glycogen to pyruvate, as part of normal aerobic metabolism. This process utilizes oxygen molecules. In states of stress, such as exercise, or after surgery, the body augments oxygen uptake (VO_2) to meet this need by increasing respiratory rate and tidal volume. Maximal oxygen uptake (VO_2 max or **VO_2 peak**) is a reflection of fitness and of patient motivation.

At a particular point, the body's ability to take up oxygen and produce ATP by aerobic metabolism is insufficient to meet the body's needs. Thus, in addition to generating ATP via aerobic pathways such as the glycolytic pathways, ATP is generated by anaerobic metabolism. This is a fundamentally less efficient process, producing a smaller amount of ATP per glucose molecule, as well as lactic acid. The VO_2 at which this happens is called the **anaerobic threshold**. This is defined as the point at which extra CO_2 starts to be generated and detected. Unlike VO_2 max, it is not dependent on patient motivation. In disease states, the ability of the body to cope with increased stress by increasing oxygen uptake is impaired, and the anaerobic threshold is reduced.

A final important variable in the prediction of outcome is the **ventilatory equivalent for CO_2**. This is calculated by dividing minute ventilation by VCO_2, traditionally at the anaerobic threshold. Functionally, this represents how hard the lungs need to work to remove a set quantity of CO_2, and hence is a measure of alveolar gas exchange. Lower values imply better ventilation and perfusion matching, and more efficient lungs.

The Evidence Behind CPET

The first work establishing a link between poor functional capacity and poor patient outcome was done by Older et al.

more than 20 years ago.[54] Patients were considered high risk if they had an anaerobic threshold of <11 ml/kg/min. Based on the results of CPET, high-risk patients were recovered in an intensive care setting. Additionally, patients who had anaerobic thresholds of over 11 ml/kg/min but with evidence of cardiovascular ischaemia or respiratory dysfunction were nursed in a high dependency unit postoperatively. Approximately 50% of patients were deemed low-risk and nursed on a ward postoperatively. In this study, postoperative death due to cardiorespiratory causes were seen only in the group with a reduced anaerobic threshold.

Since then, the body of evidence has expanded to assess the role of CPET in patients requiring major intra-abdominal, urological,[55] bariatric[56] and aortic vascular surgery.[57] Interestingly, anaerobic threshold has proved to be less useful[58] than peak VO_2[59] in patients having upper GI surgery such as oesophagectomies (Table 8.8).

The Elderly Patient

Elderly patients comprise an increasing percentage of patients presenting for both elective and emergency surgery. In the United States, they account for 40% of all surgical patients per year[60] and, in the UK, approximately 1.25 million people are over the age of 85.[61] Elderly people are more likely to have a major perioperative complication, such as a cardiovascular event. Despite overall low mortality rates, they are also at a greater risk of death should a complication occur.[62] Other independent predictors of morbidity and mortality include decreased functional status preoperatively, clinical signs of congestive heart failure, ASA classification, emergency surgery and intraoperative tachycardia.[63] In recent years, it has become clear that in addition to assessing physiological fitness, assessing physiological reserves by assessing frailty may contribute to decision-making for surgery.

Assessing Frailty

Frailty has been defined as a 'distinctive health state related to the ageing process in which multiple body systems gradually lose their in-built reserves' (British Geriatrics Society). Although there is clearly a lot of overlap between age, frailty, disability and long-term co-morbid conditions, these conditions are not identical, and it is important to distinguish between them. Data published by the National Surgical Quality Improvement Program has demonstrated that an intermediate to high modified frailty index score is significantly associated with an increase in the incidence of complications at 30 days.[64] Two broad models of frailty have been described in the literature.

Phenotype Model

First described by Fried et al.,[65] the phenotype model of frailty describes a clinical syndrome in which a group of patient characteristics predict a poorer outcome if present. These characteristics are:
- Unintentional weight loss
- Self-reported exhaustion

TABLE 8.8	Other Methods for Assessing Functional Status.

Subjective

METS	One metabolic equivalent (MET) is defined as the amount of oxygen consumed when sitting at rest and is roughly equal to 3.5 mL O_2/kg/min. Functional capacity is classified as excellent (>10 METs), good (7 METs to 10 METs), moderate (4 METs to 6 METs), or poor (<4 METs).[12] Perioperative and long-term cardiac risk is highest in patients who have poor functional capacity. Activities equivalent to 4 METs include walking at 2–3 mph, climbing a flight of stairs, golfing with a cart, and slow ballroom dancing.
Questionnaires	The most commonly used questionnaire is the Duke Activity Status Index (DASI). This quantifies functional capacity by using more commonly performed activities, such as housework and showering or dressing. It is recommended for use by the ACC/AHA guidelines in assessing preoperative risk.
ASA-Physical Status	This is covered in detail under ASA. ASA scores are commonly used in risk assessment as high scores are associated with poorer outcomes such as intraoperative complications, length of stay and mortality.
WHO Performance Status	The WHO performance status classification is similar to the ASA Physical status. Patients are categorised as: 0: Able to carry out all normal activity without restriction; 1: Restricted in strenuous activity but ambulatory and able to carry out light work; 2: Ambulatory and capable of all self-care but unable to carry out any work activities; up and about more than 50% of waking hours; 3: Symptomatic and in a chair or in bed for greater than 50% of the day but not bedridden; 4: Completely disabled; cannot carry out any self-care; totally confined to bed or chair.

Objective

CPET	Cardiopulmonary exercise testing is covered in detail under Assessing Physiological Fitness. It provides an objective assessment of physiological variables that are independent of patient effort; such as anaerobic threshold.
6 Minute Walk Test	The 6-minute walk or incremental shuttle walk test is a simple test that can be carried out in a clinic setting. It correlates with peak oxygen consumption in patients with cardiopulmonary disease and is a good predictor of cardiovascular fitness. However, many patients may not be able to complete this test due to other physical factors such as back pain or poor balance.

ACC/AHA, American College of Cardiology/American Heart Association; ASA, American Society of Anesthesiologists.

- Reduced muscle strength
- Reduced gait speed
- Low levels of activity or low energy expenditure

This phenotype was independently predictive of falls and worsening mobility, hospitalization and death.

Cumulative Deficit Model

This model, first published by Rockwood et al., suggests that it is the accumulation of various deficits associated with ageing that combine to give a continuous spectrum of frailty.[66] An individual's frailty index score is reflective of the cumulative number of deficits present, and a higher score reflects a higher likelihood that frailty is present (Fig. 8.3).

Identifying the Frail Patient

Although the words frail and elderly are not synonymous, there is naturally a lot of overlap between these patients. Thus, most research for identifying frail patients has been validated in the geriatric population. A useful method for identifying frailty in patients is the Edmonton Frail Scale (Fig. 8.4), a simple to use screening tool that is validated in patients over the age of 70 having surgery.[67,68] This tool can be used in the preoperative

setting. However, recent practice has moved towards incorporating proactive comprehensive geriatric assessment in the community, ideally assessing and optimizing these patients prior to their presentation to secondary care.

Cognition and Capacity

Another issue pertinent to the pre-assessment of patients who are elderly or frail is the assessment of their cognitive function and decision-making abilities. The Dementia UK: Update report published in 2014 estimated that there will be over 1 million people living with dementia by 2025. Dementia has clear implications for a patient's ability to discuss and consent to elective surgical procedures. It is the responsibility of clinicians to make a thorough assessment of a patient's capacity. Patients with dementia are also at increased risk of delirium with long-term worsening of cognition, and the implications of this should also be discussed with patients and their caregivers.

MoCA

The Montreal Cognitive Assessment (MoCA) is a one-page, 30-point test that takes approximately 10 minutes to

Clinical frailty scale*

1 Very fit – People who are robust, active, energetic and motivated. These people commonly exercise regularly. They are among the fittest for their age.

2 Well – People who have **no active disease symptoms** but are less fit than category I. Often, they exercise or are very **active occasionally**, eg. seasonally.

3 Managing well – People whose **medical problems are well controlled,** but are **not regularly active** beyond routine walking.

4 Vulnerable – While **not dependent** on others for daily help, often **symptoms limit activities.** A common complaint is being "slowed up", and/or being tired during the day.

5 Mildly frail – These people often have **more evident slowing** and need help in **high order IADLs** (finances, transportation, heavy housework, medications). Typically, mild frailty progressively impairs shopping and walking outside alone, meal preparation and housework.

6 Moderately frail – People need help with **all outside activities** and with **keeping house.** Inside, they often have problems with stairs and need **help with bathing** and might need minimal assistance (cuing, standby) with dressing.

7 Severely frail – **Completely dependent for personal care,** from whatever cause (physical or cognitive). Even so, they seem stable and not at high risk of dying (within ~ 6 months).

8 Very severely frail – Completely dependent, approaching the end of life. Typically, they could not recover even from a minor illness.

9. Terminally ill – Approaching the end of life. This category applies to people with **a life expectancy <6 months,** who are **not otherwise evidently frail.**

Scoring frailty in people with dementia

The degree of frailty corresponds to the degree of dementia. Common **symptoms in mild dementia** include forgetting the details of a recent event, though still remembering the event itself, repeating the same question/story and social withdrawal.

In **moderate dementia**, recent memory is very impaired, even though they seemingly can remember their past life events well. They can do personal care with prompting.

In **severe dementia**, they cannot do personal care without help.

* I. Canadian study on health & aging, revised 2008.
2. K. Rockwood et al. A global clinical measure of fitness and frailty in elderly people. CMAJ 2005; 173;489-495.

© 2007-2009. Version 1.2. All rights reserved. Geriatric Medicine Research Dalhousie University Halifax, Canada. Permission granted to copy for research and educational purposes only.

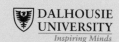

• **Fig. 8.3** The Clinical Frailty Scale (© 2007-2009 Geriatric Medicine Research, Dahlousie University, Halifax, Canada.)

administer. It assesses several domains, including memory recall, visuospatial ability, language, attention and executive function (Fig. 8.5). The MoCA has been translated into over 36 languages and dialects and has been adapted for various cultures globally.

Capacity

The concept of capacity is closely linked to the concepts of cognitive and executive function. Capacity is assessed by considering the following domains:
• Understanding of information. It is the clinician's responsibility to ensure that the information provided to the patient is in a language or format that they understand.
• Assimilation of information
• The ability to weigh up the benefits and risks of the decision given the information
• The ability to make a decision based on those risks and benefits

Comprehensive Geriatric Assessment

The Comprehensive Geriatric Assessment (CGA) is a multidisciplinary, holistic assessment of an individual patient by a number of specialists. It comprises an assessment of the following domains:

• Medical conditions: co-morbid conditions, medication review, nutritional status
• Mental health: cognition, mood, anxiety, fears
• Functional capacity: activities of daily living, gait, activity status
• Social circumstances: social network, family/friend support
• Environment: home comfort, transport facilities, accessibility to local resources

It is an established clinical approach for evaluating and optimizing issues for the older patient, and has been demonstrated to improve independence, physical function and mortality at 36 months.[69] Comprehensive geriatric assessment has been incorporated into specialist services for the perioperative care of elderly patients. There has also been a significant ethos change from 'reactive' to 'proactive' models of care.[70]

Assessing Risk

The assessment of perioperative risk is a subject that has been extensively investigated in the literature. Risk stratification is important for informed decision making by patients and clinicians, as well as for enabling meaningful comparison of surgical outcomes. Risk stratification tools are often

The Edmonton frail scale

Name : _____

d.o.b : _____   Date : _____

Frailty domain	Item	0 point	1 point	2 points
Cognition	Please imagine that this pre-drawn circle is a clock. I would like you to place the numbers in the correct positions then place the hands to indicate a time of 'ten after eleven'	No errors	Minor spacing errors	Other errors
General health status	In the past year, how many times have you been admitted to a hospital?	0	1–2	≥2
	In general, how would you describe your health?	'Excellent', 'Very good', 'Good'	'Fair'	'Poor'
Functional independence	With how many of the following activities do you require help? (meal preparation, shopping, transportation, telephone, housekeeping, laundry, managing money, taking medications)	0–1	2–4	5–8
Social support	When you need help, can you count on someone who is willing and able to meet your needs?	Always	Sometimes	Never
Medication use	Do you use five or more different prescription medications on a regular basis?	No	Yes	
	At times, do you forget to take your prescription medications?	No	Yes	
Nutrition	Have you recently lost weight such that your clothing has become looser?	No	Yes	
Mood	Do you often feel sad or depressed?	No	Yes	
Continence	Do you have a problem with losing control of urine when you don't want to?	No	Yes	
Functional performance	I would like you to sit in this chair with your back and arms resting. Then, when I say 'GO', please stand up and walk at a safe and comfortable pace to the mark on the floor (approximately 3 m away), return to the chair and sit down'	0–10 s	11–20 s	One of : >20 s , or patient unwilling, or requires assistance
Totals	Final score is the sum of column totals			

Scoring:
0 – 5 = Not frail
6 – 7 = Vulnerable
8 – 9 = Mild frailty
10 – 11 = Moderate frailty
12 – 17 = Severe frailty

Total [/17]

Administered by : _____

• **Fig. 8.4** The Edmonton Frail Scale

numerical scores, with particular levels of risk associated with each score (for example, the American Society of Anesthesiologists Physical Status Index [ASA-PS]), or individualized indices such as those published by the National Surgical Quality Improvement Program. A multitude of tools have been developed to stratify patient risk. Some are specialty-specific, and some incorporate intraoperative findings as well as physiological variables to make a prediction of risk.

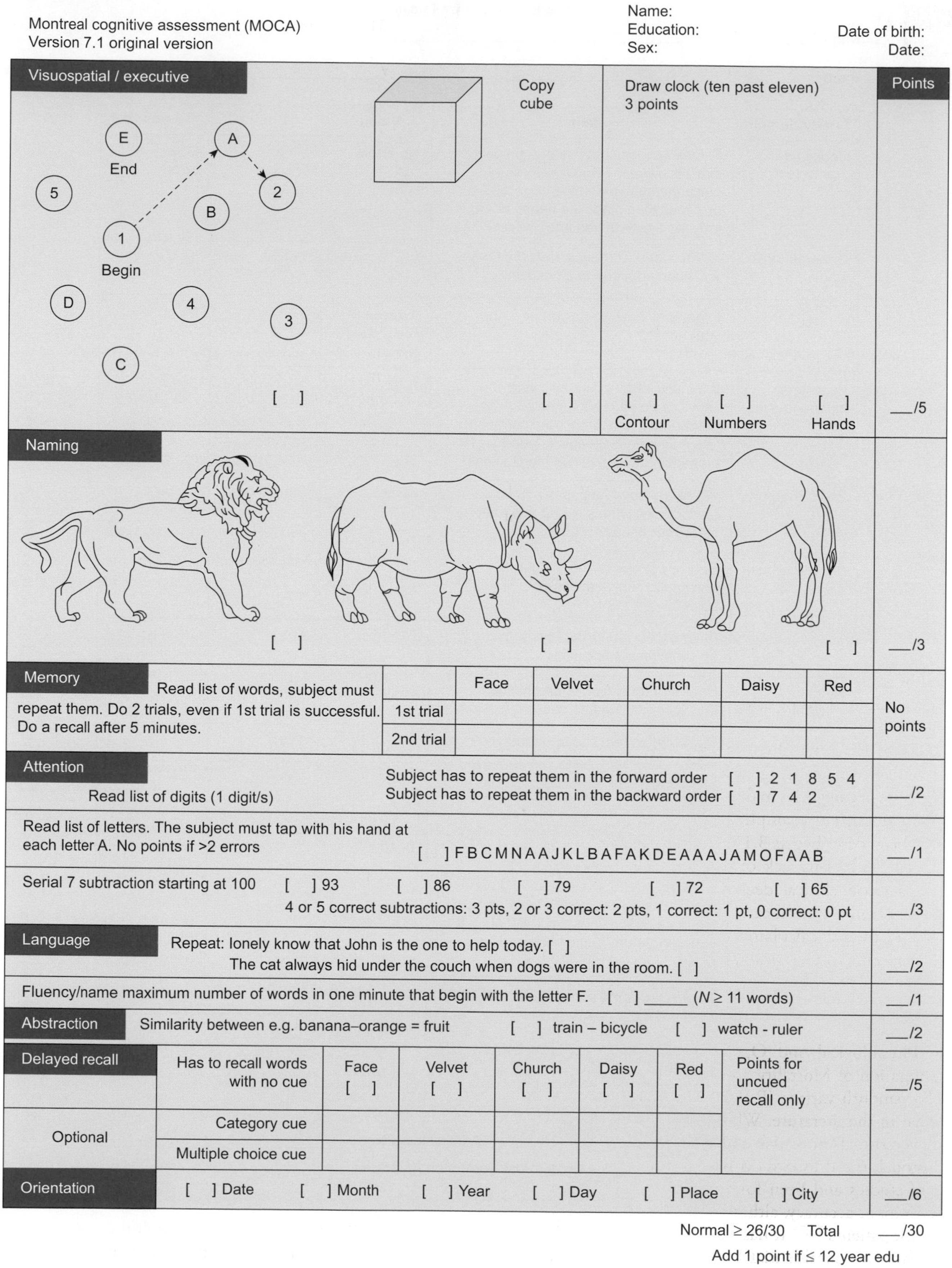

Montreal cognitive assessment (MOCA)
Version 7.1 original version

Name:
Education:
Sex:
Date of birth:
Date:

Visuospatial / executive		Points

Copy cube

Draw clock (ten past eleven)
3 points

[ ]

[ ]

[ ] Contour   [ ] Numbers   [ ] Hands

___/5

Naming

[ ]   [ ]   [ ]   ___/3

Memory Read list of words, subject must repeat them. Do 2 trials, even if 1st trial is successful. Do a recall after 5 minutes.

	Face	Velvet	Church	Daisy	Red	
1st trial						No points
2nd trial						

Attention Read list of digits (1 digit/s)

Subject has to repeat them in the forward order   [   ] 2 1 8 5 4
Subject has to repeat them in the backward order [   ] 7 4 2

___/2

Read list of letters. The subject must tap with his hand at each letter A. No points if >2 errors

[   ] F B C M N A A J K L B A F A K D E A A A J A M O F A A B

___/1

Serial 7 subtraction starting at 100   [   ] 93   [   ] 86   [   ] 79   [   ] 72   [   ] 65

4 or 5 correct subtractions: 3 pts, 2 or 3 correct: 2 pts, 1 correct: 1 pt, 0 correct: 0 pt

___/3

Language

Repeat: lonely know that John is the one to help today. [   ]
The cat always hid under the couch when dogs were in the room. [   ]

___/2

Fluency/name maximum number of words in one minute that begin with the letter F.   [   ] _____ (N ≥ 11 words)

___/1

Abstraction Similarity between e.g. banana–orange = fruit   [   ] train – bicycle   [   ] watch - ruler

___/2

Delayed recall

Has to recall words with no cue	Face	Velvet	Church	Daisy	Red	Points for uncued recall only	
	[ ]	[ ]	[ ]	[ ]	[ ]		___/5
Optional Category cue							
Multiple choice cue							

Orientation   [   ] Date   [   ] Month   [   ] Year   [   ] Day   [   ] Place   [   ] City   ___/6

Normal ≥ 26/30   Total   ___/30

Add 1 point if ≤ 12 year edu

• **Fig. 8.5** The MOCA Assessment (Copyright Z. Nasreddine, MD. Reproduced with permission. Available at http://www.mocatest.org.)

TABLE 8.9	The ASA Physical Status Index.
ASA I	A normal, healthy patient
ASA II	A patient with mild systemic disease, and without substantive functional limitations
ASA III	A patient with severe systemic disease and substantive functional limitations
ASA IV	A patient with severe, systemic disease that is a constant threat to life
ASA V	A moribund patient who is not expected to survive without the operation
ASA VI	A declared brain-dead patient whose organs are being removed for donor purposes

ASA, American Society of Anesthesiologists.
Modified from https://www.asahq.org/standards-and-guidelines/asa-physical-status-classification-system

ASA

The ASA-PS is a basic, single variable classification of risk based on clinician assessment of an individual patient (Table 8.9). As it is essentially a face evaluation of functional capacity, it was not initially designed as a tool for risk prediction. However, in recent review articles a high ASA score was found to correlate with poor clinical outcomes such as intraoperative complications, length of hospital stay and mortality.[71] ASA is also an indicator for readmission to hospital at 30 days.[72]

Other limitations of using the ASA score to predict risk include:

- Poor to fair inter-observer consistency,[73] making it an unreliable tool for surgical audit or research.
- The use of categories makes it difficult to quantify risk for individuals. For example, mortality in ASA III patients has been described as 3.1%, and that of ASA IV patients as 14.7%.[74] This lack of discrimination has significant impacts on clinical decision-making, such as planned postoperative critical care admission.
- Unlike the risk calculators that have been developed, it is not specific to a surgical discipline or patient group.

Possum

The Physiological and Operative Severity Score for the enumeration of Mortality and morbidity (POSSUM), and its Portsmouth variant (P-POSSUM) has been extensively studied in the literature. Whilst there were concerns about the overestimation of risk and adverse outcome in the initial model, the P-POSSUM has been used in a large number of studies and been found to be of moderate to high discriminant accuracy, although it still over-predicts risk in low-risk patients.[75,76] It has been adopted into guidance by the National Confidential Enquiry into Patient Outcome and Death (NCEPOD) for predicting risk in the care of patients having emergency laparotomy.

TABLE 8.10	The 6 Variables Calculated By SORT.
Severity of Operative Procedure (automatically calculated online)	
ASA Physical Status Index	
Urgency	
Thoracic, gastrointestinal, or vascular surgery	
Cancer	
Age	

ASA, American Society of Anesthesiologists.

Apart from the over-prediction of risk, other limitations of using the P-POSSUM model include:

- The inclusion of intraoperative findings and variables, which makes preoperative risk predictions unreliable.
- The large number of variables, including the interpretation of a chest radiograph, means that calculating the score can be time-consuming.

SORT

There are a multitude of preoperative surgical risk prediction calculators available for clinicians to use. The Surgical Outcome Risk Tool (SORT) is validated for use in non-neurological and non-cardiac surgery in adults with good discrimination (Table 8.10). It is a simple, 6-variable risk stratification tool designed for use after the 2011 NCEPOD study on perioperative care ('Knowing the Risk') and validated in a large general surgical population of almost 20 000 patients.[66]

Its limitations include:

- The need for online access either to the calculator or the app.
- It has thus far only been validated in the UK population.

Shared Decision Making and the Multidisciplinary Team

There has been a substantial increase in the number of elderly and high-risk patients having surgery. Increasingly, the focus of clinical questions has therefore centred on doing the right thing for the right patient, at the right time. High-risk patients in particular have posed a number of conundrums and they are the focus of a separate review by the Royal College of Surgeons. Mortality for these patients exceeds that of cardiac surgery by two- to three-fold,[77] and complication rates as high as 50% have been documented in those having emergency surgery.[78] Furthermore, this subset of patients accounts for over 80% of postoperative deaths but less than 15% of inpatient procedures.[79]

Current guidelines define those patients with a predicted hospital mortality risk of 5–10% as 'medium risk', and ≥10% as 'high risk'. In the elective setting, it is recommended that these patients are reviewed by a consultant anaesthetist. Objective assessment of functional capacity and a holistic approach are needed to guide management. It is also recommended that these patients have a clearly-defined pathway for their perioperative management, which includes admission to critical care postoperatively. The discussion and the decision to operate on a patient must therefore also incorporate a consideration of all these factors.

Shared decision making is an approach that has been described as 'the pinnacle of patient-centred care'.[80] It describes the 'use of the best available evidence to support patients in making healthcare decisions based on their own values, preferences, and beliefs'.[81] It places a focus on the patient making the decision for surgery in conjunction with information about their specific risk factors and lifestyle goals. Shared decision making has been shown to improve patient satisfaction with healthcare services[82] and improve patient engagement in their care. For example, where given an informed choice, patients with breast cancer tended to opt for more conservative therapy, and had less decisional conflict when making that choice.[83]

The preoperative assessment clinic is therefore ideally suited to ensure patients have the necessary tools to make an informed decision.

Optimization and Prehabilitation

One of the benefits of thorough preoperative assessment of patients presenting for major surgery is the chance to identify patients who would benefit from a period of preoperative optimization. This can take multiple forms.

Medication Optimization

Most commonly, preoperative optimization involves the titration of medication for co-morbid disease in the community, often with the input of specialist services. Examples of this would include titration of medication for obstructive airways disease following the results of lung function tests, or the optimization of diabetes medications for patients who present with elevated HbA1c.

More recently, there has been increasing interest in the role preoperative exercise and improvement of aerobic capacity has in improving patient outcome. There is some evidence to show that prehabilitation significantly reduces the risk of postoperative pulmonary complications. However, whilst there is a demonstrable link between exercise and aerobic fitness, systematic reviews of prehabilitation programs have yet to demonstrate a clear link between exercise and patient outcome.[84]

Another area of interest has been nutritional prehabilitation. Patients with cancer undergoing neoadjuvant therapy prior to surgery often have reduced nutritional intake which leads to cachexia, and ultimately reduced metabolic reserve. There is a clear link between malnutrition prior to major GI or cancer surgery, and poor outcomes including length of hospital stay, readmission rates and mortality.[85,86]

A perioperative nutrition screen such as the Malnutrition Universal Screening Tool, or that recently proposed by the Perioperative Quality Initiative group,[87] can be used to identify those patients at highest risk of adverse outcomes.

INTRAOPERATIVE MANAGEMENT

Safety First – The WHO Checklist and its Implications

First introduced by the WHO in 2009, the WHO Safe Surgery Checklist is part of the Safe Surgery Saves Lives initiative (Fig. 8.6). The three-part checklist has since been widely adopted globally as part of operating theatre practice. There is good evidence to show that adoption of the checklist is associated with significant reduction in mortality rates in both North America[88] and Europe.[89] Additionally, the concept of briefing and debriefing has a positive impact on theatre team attitude.[90]

Anticipated Critical Events

Blood Loss

Perioperative bleeding is a potentially catastrophic complication that results in morbidity and mortality if left untreated. A number of factors increase the risk of perioperative bleeding, including patient factors, surgical factors and issues related to the pathology (such as trauma). Conversely, the treatment of bleeding by transfusion of blood and blood products is not risk-free. Blood transfusion is associated with a number of adverse outcomes, including the predisposition to error and immunological reaction to transfusion that is reported on by the Serious Hazards of Transfusion (SHOT) committee. In 2016, over 2 million units of blood components were transfused to patients in the UK, more than half of which were red blood cells. Almost 3100 cases were included in their case report, and 87% of these adverse outcomes were associated with human error. The management of bleeding in the elective setting is therefore as much about preoperative optimization and prevention of transfusion as it is about knowledge of massive haemorrhage management.[91]

In the elective setting, all patients listed for major surgery should have their haemoglobin concentration measured.[92] If found to be anaemic (Hb <130 gL^{-1} for men, Hb <120 gL^{-1} for women), surgery should be delayed whilst investigation and treatment is instigated wherever possible. This may be with oral supplementation, such as ferrous sulphate or vitamin B supplements, or with parenteral formulations such as IV iron. Other considerations for the patient having elective surgery include:

- Cessation of anticoagulant or antiplatelet drugs wherever possible
- Discussion and arrangements for cell salvage, if appropriate

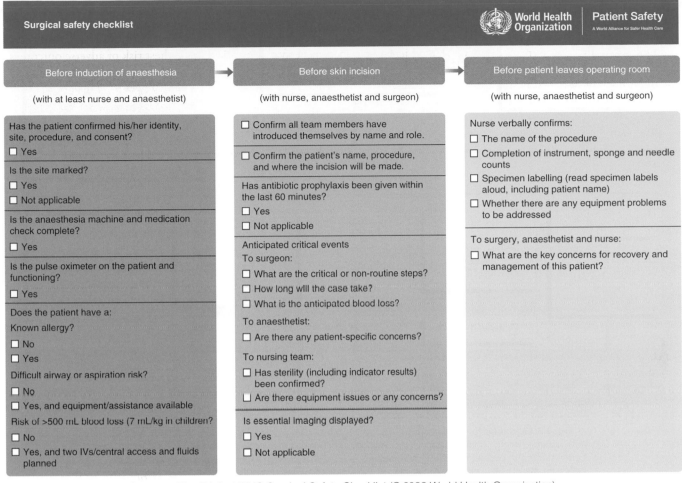

Surgical safety checklist

World Health Organization | Patient Safety
A World Alliance for Safer Health Care

Before induction of anaesthesia
(with at least nurse and anaesthetist)

Has the patient confirmed his/her identity, site, procedure, and consent?
☐ Yes

Is the site marked?
☐ Yes
☐ Not applicable

Is the anaesthesia machine and medication check complete?
☐ Yes

Is the pulse oximeter on the patient and functioning?
☐ Yes

Does the patient have a:
Known allergy?
☐ No
☐ Yes

Difficult airway or aspiration risk?
☐ No
☐ Yes, and equipment/assistance available

Risk of >500 mL blood loss (7 mL/kg in children?
☐ No
☐ Yes, and two IVs/central access and fluids planned

Before skin incision
(with nurse, anaesthetist and surgeon)

☐ Confirm all team members have introduced themselves by name and role.

☐ Confirm the patient's name, procedure, and where the incision will be made.

Has antibiotic prophylaxis been given within the last 60 minutes?
☐ Yes
☐ Not applicable

Anticipated critical events
To surgeon:
☐ What are the critical or non-routine steps?
☐ How long will the case take?
☐ What is the anticipated blood loss?

To anaesthetist:
☐ Are there any patient-specific concerns?

To nursing team:
☐ Has sterility (including indicator results) been confirmed?
☐ Are there equipment issues or any concerns?

Is essential imaging displayed?
☐ Yes
☐ Not applicable

Before patient leaves operating room
(with nurse, anaesthetist and surgeon)

Nurse verbally confirms:
☐ The name of the procedure
☐ Completion of instrument, sponge and needle counts
☐ Specimen labelling (read specimen labels aloud, including patient name)
☐ Whether there are any equipment problems to be addressed

To surgery, anaesthetist and nurse:
☐ What are the key concerns for recovery and management of this patient?

• **Fig. 8.6** The Original WHO Surgical Safety Checklist (© 2009 World Health Organization)

- The use of tranexamic acid in surgery
- Consideration of anaesthetic techniques such as hypotensive or regional anaesthesia

There has been much debate in the literature about transfusion 'triggers' and the risks and benefits of restrictive versus liberal transfusion strategics. In general, there is no evidence that 'restrictive' strategies employing transfusion thresholds of 7–8 g/L causes harm, except for in particular patient groups.[93] In patients with acute coronary syndrome, a slightly higher threshold of 80–100 g/L may be employed.[94]

Massive Haemorrhage + Blood Products

There are a number of definitions of major haemorrhage which exist in the literature. Common definitions include:

- The transfusion of ≥10 units of red blood cells (or a total blood volume) within 24 hours
- Transfusion of >4 units of red blood cells in 1 hour with a need for ongoing transfusion
- Replacement of >50% of total blood volume within 3 hours

Massive haemorrhage and transfusion occur most commonly within the disciplines of trauma and obstetric practice. In trauma settings, systolic blood pressure (SBP) is one of the most important predictors of mortality in the bleeding patient.[95] In 2013–17, haemorrhage was the second most common direct cause of maternal mortality.[96] Hospitals should have a massive transfusion protocol in place to manage these emergencies appropriately.

Management of massive haemorrhage should prioritize stabilizing the patient **and** definitive management of bleeding (generally by surgical techniques). Blood warmers and a rapid infusion device should be available and used in order to prevent the deleterious effects of hypothermia. Wherever possible, point of care (POC) testing should be used to guide transfusion practice.[97]

There has been much debate over physiological endpoints in resuscitation during massive haemorrhage. There is evidence that immediate fluid resuscitation in the hypotensive patient results in higher volumes of fluid being given in the initial and perioperative phase for trauma patients, and that these patients have worse outcomes than patients who have a 'delayed resuscitation' phase.[98] Increasing the blood pressure prior to definitive haemostasis is thought to disrupt and delay clot formation, precipitating rebleeding. The data from non-trauma patients also suggests that

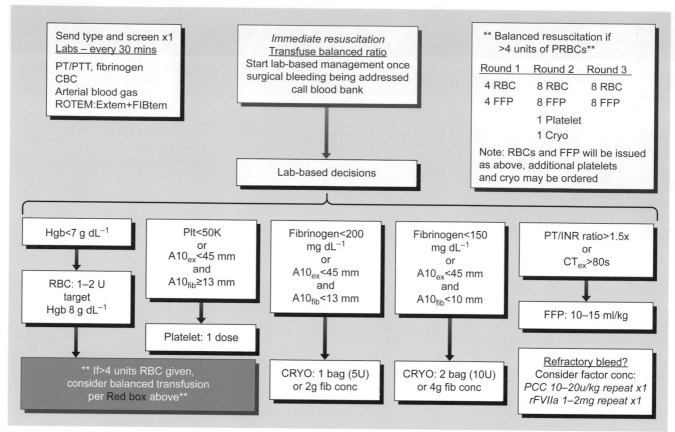

• **Fig. 8.7** Guidance for Transfusion of Blood Products CBC, Complete blood count; FFP, fresh frozen plasma; Hgb, haemoglobin; INR, international normalized ratio; PCC, prothrombin complex concentrate; Plt, platelet count; PRBCs, packed red blood cells; PT/PTT, prothrombin time/partial thromboplastin time; RBC, red blood cell; rFVIIa, recombinant factor VIIa; ROTEM, rotational thromboelastometry. (From Ghadimi K, Levy JH, Welsby IJ. Perioperative management of the bleeding patient. *Br J Anaesth*. 2016;117(3):iii18–iii30.)

permissive hypotension improves mortality by reducing rebleeding.[99,100] More recently, data has emerged to support a novel hybrid approach to resuscitation. In this approach, animals exposed to a blast injury underwent 60 minutes of initial hypotensive resuscitation (target SBP of 80 mmHg) followed by a revised normotensive resuscitation (target SBP of 110 mmHg).[101] Animals resuscitated according to the hybrid method had significantly longer survival times, prompting the adoption of hybrid resuscitation strategies in major trauma.

Choice of Blood Products

Most hospitals have massive haemorrhage policies which are activated after an initial transfusion of up to 4 units of packed red blood cells (PRBC). Subsequent requirement for products would generally include the transfusion of more PRBCs and fresh frozen plasma (FFP), followed by platelets, cryoprecipitate and PRBC as guided by POC tests of haemostasis. At this point, most hospitals would also recommend discussion with the local haematology team. Much discussion has existed in the literature over the ratio in which blood products should be transfused. Historically, data from the military in damage control resuscitation suggested that

a ratio of 1:1:1 (PRBC:FFP:platelets) was ideal for maintaining the closest approximation to reconstituted whole blood and reduce the development of coagulopathy. However, more recent data from the civilian trauma population suggests that although early transfusion of FFP is associated with improved 6-hour survival, there is no difference in mortality between patients who receive these products in a 1:1:1 ratio compared to a 2:1:1 (PRBC:FFP:platelets) ratio[102] (Fig. 8.7).

Special Equipment Requirements
Tourniquets

Tourniquets are pneumatic devices that are used for controlled arterial compression in the extremities (Table 8.11). Most often, they consist of an inflatable cuff with connective tubing and a pressure device. These cuffs may have one or two bladders that are inflated to occlude blood flow to the extremity being operated on.

Recommended standards for tourniquet include the following:
• Appropriate selection of tourniquet size, with cuffs exceeding the circumference of the limb by 7–15 cm
• Adequate exsanguination prior to cuff inflation

TABLE 8.11	Indications and Contraindications for Tourniquet Use.	
Indications for Tourniquet Use	Contraindications for Tourniquet Use	
Maintenance of a bloodless field for surgery	Open fractures	
Intravenous regional anaesthesia techniques (Bier's block) for surgery or complex regional pain syndromes	Severe crush injuries	
	Severe hypertension	
	Skin grafts	
	Peripheral arterial disease	
	Diabetes mellitus	
	Sickle cell anaemia	
Prehospital setting to minimise blood loss prior to definitive management	Compartment syndrome	
	Malignant tumours	

- Monitoring of pressure gauges before and during surgery
- Tourniquet pressures should not exceed 50 mmHg and 100 mmHg above patient's SBP for upper and lower limbs, respectively
- Adequate padding (at least 2 layers) underneath the tourniquet
- Preventing skin cleaning solution accumulating under the cuff
- Tourniquet inflation time and pressure should be documented and kept to a minimum

Physiological Implications of Tourniquet Use

- **Cardiovascular changes:** These are not normally significant in a healthy patient. However, in a patient with significant cardiovascular disease, tourniquet inflation causes a shift of the blood volume of the limb into the central venous circulation. In the lower limbs, it also causes an increase in systemic vascular resistance. These changes can have catastrophic effects on cardiovascular function and may cause circulatory overload and pulmonary oedema.
- **Metabolic effects:** Deflation of a tourniquet causes redistribution of the circulating volume back into the limb. This leads to reactive hyperaemia and the redistribution of ischaemic metabolites into the systemic circulation. This may cause lactatemia, acidaemia and hypercarbia.
- **Respiratory effects:** These relate to the metabolic effects of limb ischaemia. Tourniquet deflation usually causes a rise in end-tidal carbon dioxide concentrations, which results in an accompanying increase in respiratory rate and minute volume.
- **Neurological effects:** Mechanical compression on a nerve leads to a conduction block in motor and sensory nerves between 15 and 45 minutes after cuff inflation. Nerve injury leading to long-lasting dysfunction is the most common complication of tourniquet use.
- **Muscle effects:** Progressive tissue hypoxia following cuff inflation can result in microvascular injury. Patients develop 'post-tourniquet syndrome' with a swollen, stiff and weak limb. Rhabdomyolysis has also been documented following tourniquet use.

Positioning

Different patient positions are required to provide surgical access for a range of procedures (Table 8.12). Patient positioning is an important component of good intraoperative care. In general, patients are transferred and positioned for surgery after induction of anaesthesia. Issues related to inappropriate or unsafe positioning include:

- Nerve damage
- Ocular injuries
- Pressure sores
- Compartment syndrome
- Venous air embolism
- Raised intracranial pressure

Principles of Anaesthesia

Fig. 8.8 summarizes anaesthetic techniques.

Local Anaesthesia

Local anaesthetic (LA) infiltration is used commonly in anaesthetic practice to aid with placement of devices such as central venous catheters. In ophthalmic practice, topical LA is commonly used. The perceived advantage of LA use is the avoidance of a general or regional anaesthetic. This negates the need for starvation times and has a positive impact on list turnover times. However, LA infiltration in isolation is unlikely to be suitable for the majority of open surgical procedures. Often, the surgical field is supplied by multiple visceral or somatic nerves that may not be reliably blocked by a superficial infiltration of LA. Additionally, although a lesion may be small (for example an abscess), the success of infiltration relies on a number of other factors, including vascular supply to the tissue, and reduce efficacy in the presence of infection. Nevertheless, LA infiltration remains an important component of postoperative analgesia, as part of a multimodal regime.

Regional Anaesthesia

Regional anaesthesia can be divided into two main categories: peripheral nerve blocks (PNB) and central neuraxial techniques (Table 8.13). These techniques are employed either as sole methods of anaesthesia for surgical procedures, or as adjuncts in the multimodal approach to analgesia after surgery. In addition to acute post-surgical pain, there is good evidence to suggest that employing a regional anaesthetic technique has benefits in preventing or reducing the incidence of chronic post-surgical pain (CPSP). This is particularly true of procedures where the incidence of CPSP is high, for example after thoracotomy.[103]

In general, the duration of block depends on the technique, local anaesthetic and additives used. Most peripheral nerve blocks provide pain relief for up to 4 to 24 hours postoperatively, and can provide anaesthesia for procedures up to 2 hours long. Catheter-based techniques have also been developed for patients expected to have ongoing pain due to their pathology, for example, in rib fractures.

TABLE 8.12 **Common Positions for Surgery and Associated Concerns.**

Position	Physiological Implications	Concerns
Supine	Reduction in FRC and V/Q mismatch Aortocaval compression in pregnancy over 20/40 Increased likelihood of aspiration	Pressure on the occiput, sacrum and heels Compression of the ulnar nerve from the sides of the operating table Brachial plexus injury if arms abducted Loss of lumbar lordosis causing back pain
Lithotomy/ Lloyd Davies	Reduction in FRC and V/Q mismatch Redistribution of pooled lower limb blood initially causing potential volume overload Reduction in venous return on returning to supine position Increased likelihood of aspiration	Cephalad movement of endotracheal tube and endobronchial intubation Stretch injury to obturator and sciatic nerves Compression of the femoral, common peroneal and saphenous nerves Calf compression causing venous thromboembolism or compartment syndrome Injury to hands when table position is altered
Prone	Increased FRC and relative improvement in V/Q mismatch Higher intra-thoracic pressures Reduction in cardiac output Retinal ischaemia	Difficulty in accessing airway Ocular/conjunctival oedema Brachial plexus injury Spinal cord injury or reduced vertebral artery blood flow
Lateral	Dependent lung is relatively underventilated and overperfused Non-dependent lung is relatively overventilated and underperfused Outflow obstruction of dependent arm Increased likelihood of aspiration	Corneal abrasion Stretch or compression injury to brachial plexus Compression injury of common peroneal and saphenous nerve Inaccurate BP readings from dependent arm
Trendelenburg	Reduction in FRC and V/Q mismatch Redistribution of pooled lower limb blood initially causing potential volume overload Reduction in venous return on becoming supine Increased likelihood of aspiration Raised intracranial pressure Raised intraocular pressure + retinal ischaemia	Facial oedema Laryngeal oedema Sliding off the table if inadequately secured in steep Trendelenburg
Reverse Trendelenburg Sitting/Beach Chair	Increase in FRC and lung compliance Hypotension Improved head + neck venous drainage Reduced cerebral perfusion Reduced likelihood of passive regurgitation	Possibility of venous air embolism, particularly during craniotomy

BP, Blood pressure; FRC, functional residual capacity; V/Q, ventilation/perfusion.

Similarly, central neuraxial blockade can be used to provide anaesthesia or analgesia for surgery. Spinal anaesthesia can be used for procedures up to 2 hours long.[104] The duration of anaesthesia is extended when a combined spinal/epidural technique is used.

In patients with particularly impaired cardiorespiratory function, or in pregnancy, a regional anaesthetic technique may be the preferred method of anaesthesia in order to minimize perioperative complications associated with having a general anaesthetic. Other advantages to regional anaesthetic techniques include:

- Sparing of opioids and reduced nausea and vomiting
- Reduced blood loss
- Reduced post-operative cognitive dysfunction
- Other benefits include reduction in deep vein thrombosis (DVT) and respiratory complications

In general, regional anaesthesia is a safe technique which is widely applicable in clinical practice. However, as with any procedures, these techniques are not without risk and patients must therefore be appropriately informed and consented for these procedures (Tables 8.14, 8.15). Of all anaesthesia-related claims handled by the National Health Service Litigation Authority, 44% were related to regional anaesthesia. In general, these claims related to nerve injury, and epidurals were the most common regional technique involved.

Developments in regional anaesthesia that have improved its safety profile include:

- The use of ultrasound to guide needle or catheter placement. Using ultrasound results in more successful blocks that are performed in a shorter time.[105]
- Guidelines from the Royal College of Anaesthetists suggest a 'Stop Before You Block' check in the anaesthetic

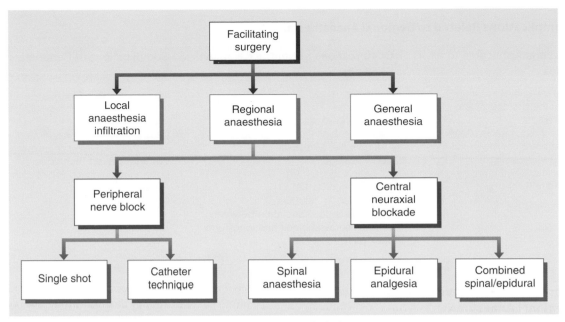

• **Fig. 8.8** Anaesthetic Techniques

TABLE 8.13	**Commonly Used Regional Anaesthetic Techniques.**	
	Central Neuraxial Blockade	**Peripheral Nerve Blocks**
Spinal Anaesthesia	Low volume local anaesthetic is injected into the intrathecal space. This results in rapid onset of anaesthesia.	Approaches to the Upper Limb/Brachial Plexus: - Interscalene block - Supraclavicular block - Infraclavicular block - Axillary block - Peripheral block of individual nerves
Epidural Anaesthesia	Local anaesthetic is injected into the epidural space (i.e. there is no breach of the dura). Epidural techniques commonly involve siting a catheter, and can be used for anaesthesia and analgesia.	Approaches to the Lower Limb: - Femoral nerve block - Fascia iliaca block - Popliteal block - Sciatic block - Ankle block
Combined Spinal Epidural	A combination of the techniques described above.	Approaches to the Thorax/Abdomen: - Serratus anterior block - Intercostal block - Paravertebral block - Transversus abdominis plane (TAP) block - Quadratus lumborum block - Ilioinguinal/Iliohypogastric

room immediately prior to nerve block placement, akin to a surgical safety checklist.

General Anaesthesia

The principles of general anaesthesia are extensively covered in other, dedicated texts and will only be covered briefly here. General anaesthesia is classically thought of as a dedicated triad of priorities, consisting of analgesia, muscle paralysis and hypnosis. Techniques involved in the induction and maintenance of anaesthesia include the use of: inhalational agents alone, intravenous agents or a combination of the two. Irrespective of the anaesthetic technique used, general anaesthetic agents have a profound depressant effect on the cardiorespiratory and central nervous system with airway management and monitoring of vital signs being mandatory. As a result of this, several factors must be considered when assessing a patient for a general anaesthetic (Table 8.16). In emergency situations, or in patients with significant co-morbidity, the administration of general anaesthesia becomes more challenging and carries a higher risk of morbidity and mortality. General anaesthesia can be administered via an inhalational or intravenous route. Commonly,

TABLE 8.14	Complications Related to Regional Anaesthesia.	
Complications Applicable to all Techniques	Complications of Central Neuraxial Blockade	Complications of Peripheral Nerve Block
Infection at the site of injection Bleeding at the site of injection Multiple attempts Failure of technique necessitating repeat attempt or conversion to general anaesthesia Local anaesthetic systemic toxicity Local anaesthetic allergy	Headache Hypotension Nausea and vomiting Inadvertent high block ('high spinal') Arachnoiditis/ Meningitis Nerve damage: -　Temporary 1: 1000 -　Permanent 1: 13 000 -　Paralysis 1: 250 000 *NB there is no association between central neuraxial block and long-term back pain	Wrong site procedure Nerve damage causing weakness or paraesthesia Damage to structures surrounding site of injection, e.g. lung or vasculature **Catheter-Based Techniques:** Looping/knotting/kinking of catheters

TABLE 8.15	Absolute and Relative Contraindications for Regional Anaesthesia.	
Absolute	**Relative**
Patient refusal Allergy to local anaesthesia Infection directly over the intended site of injection **Central Neuraxial Block:** Anatomical abnormality, e.g. spina bifida Raised intracranial pressure Acquired coagulopathy or bleeding disorder	High BMI Altered anatomy Infection distinct from the site of injection Recent use of antiplatelets or anticoagulants including low molecular weight heparin Bleeding disorder Pre-existing neuropathy Uncooperative patients

induction of anaesthesia is via the intravenous route. Anaesthesia can be maintained with inhalational anaesthetic using volatile agents, or total intravenous anaesthesia.

Analgesia

Adequate intraoperative analgesia is extremely important in reducing the sympathetic response to surgery. It should be multi-modal and incorporate the WHO recommendations for escalating pain relief. In general, analgesic regimens for surgery include:

- Non-opioid parenteral analgesia such as paracetamol +/– a non-steroidal anti-inflammatory drug (where appropriate).
- Opioid medications are commonly used intraoperatively. Short-acting opioids, such as fentanyl and alfentanil, are used at induction of anaesthesia. Longer-acting opioids, such as morphine or oxycodone, are given to provide intraoperative and immediate postoperative analgesia. For stimulating surgeries, or surgeries where hypotension is necessary to maintain a bloodless surgical field, an infusion of a very short-acting opioid such as remifentanil can be employed.
- Local anaesthetic infiltration prior to incision or at the end of surgery. Commonly used agents include levobupivacaine and ropivacaine. It is crucial that the physician performing the infiltration is aware of the maximum toxic dose of local anaesthetic, which is calculated according to body weight.
- Regional anaesthetic techniques may be employed preoperatively (such as during central neuraxial blockade) as an adjunct to analgesia. The use of regional anaesthetic techniques is opioid-sparing and is particularly useful in patients with respiratory compromise or PONV.
- Opioid therapy and catheter regional anaesthesia techniques have the added advantage of being easily extended into the postoperative setting. Patient-controlled analgesia (PCA) traditionally utilizes morphine or fentanyl. However, in some centres, PCAs using ketamine or oxycodone may be available. Patient-controlled epidural analgesia or continuous epidural infusion is also widely available. Monitoring for these modalities of analgesia must be stringent, and staff must receive adequate training in the care of these patients.
- Around the time of surgery, agents for neuropathic pain such as gabapentin may be started. The majority of evidence for this is in the field of elective orthopaedic surgery, where gabapentin and pregabalin have been demonstrated to reduce pain in the postoperative setting.[106] Additionally, single dose gabapentin is potentially of use in the management of acute postoperative pain, although its number needed to treat is high.[107]
- Other agents used in the treatment of intraoperative and postoperative pain include: ketamine, which antagonizes NMDA receptors and is used widely in the pre-hospital setting, and α_2-agonists such as clonidine or dexmedetomidine.

Monitoring Equipment and Specific Levels of Support

Non-Invasive Monitoring

Minimum standards for patient monitoring during anaesthesia as set out by the Association of Anaesthetists of Great Britain and Ireland are as follows:

- Pulse oximetry

TABLE 8.16	Implications of General Anaesthesia.	
System	**Physiological Implications**	**Considerations**
Airway	Loss of protective airway reflexes Aspiration risk: fasting status, ileus, GORD	Airway management – supraglottic airway device or definitive management with endotracheal intubation Dentition and oral hygiene Previous documented difficult intubation and need for difficult airway equipment Need for NG tube for aspiration of gastric contents or postoperative nutrition
Breathing	Impaired respiratory function resulting in potential for hypoxia and hypercarbia Impaired ciliary function leading to increased respiratory secretion load	Need for mechanical ventilation postoperatively: significant respiratory disease, high oxygen requirements, underlying infection Need for arterial blood gas monitoring to assess adequacy of gas exchange
Circulation	Impaired cardiovascular function resulting in bradycardia or hypotension Increased potential for blood loss	Fluid replacement +/– blood transfusion Invasive monitoring of haemodynamic parameters: arterial line, central venous catheter, oesophageal Doppler, pulse contour analysis device, urinary catheter Inotropic or vasopressor therapy
Disability	Postoperative cognitive dysfunction	History of previous awareness Mode of anaesthesia Intraoperative and postoperative plan for analgesia
Modality of Surgery	Laparoscopic versus open procedures Positioning of patient during procedure	Need for endotracheal intubation Need for muscle relaxation and mechanical ventilation intraoperatively
Other Considerations	Loss of thermoregulatory reflexes Hyperglycaemia Risk of surgical site infection	Need for temperature monitoring and warming Glucose monitoring +/– sliding scale Appropriate antibiotics for prophylaxis

BMI, Body mass index; GORD, gastro-oesophageal reflux disease; NG, nasogastric.

- Non-invasive blood pressure measurement
- 3-lead ECG
- Airway pressure
- Inspired and expired concentrations of oxygen, carbon dioxide and volatile anaesthetic agent (if used)
- Peripheral nerve stimulator

Other minimally invasive means of monitoring an anaesthetized patient include depth of anaesthesia monitoring using EEG analysis, and the insertion of a urinary catheter to monitor urine output. Additionally, there are standards related to temperature measurement and glucose measurement that have been discussed elsewhere in this chapter.

Invasive Monitoring

Invasive monitoring should be considered for patients with significant cardiorespiratory disease in order to guide intraoperative management. The primary aim of most invasive monitoring devices is to provide clinicians with real time input on gas exchange and cardiac function. Common devices used for invasive monitoring are shown in Table 8.17.

Cardiovascular Support and Goal Directed Fluid Therapy

One of the key issues in the perioperative care of the critically unwell or high-risk patient has been the measurement

and maintenance of cardiac output through various strategies. There has been much debate over this in the literature, with chief criticisms of the studies in the evidence base being their size and their reproducibility in every day clinical practice. Additionally, a significant amount of the literature predates modern clinical practice, and thus, questions have been raised about the validity of their conclusions when 'standard care' has made such progress as to routinely incorporate haemodynamic therapy algorithms into guidelines for best practice. Controversy has also surrounded the concept of 'supranormal' oxygen delivery and the prioritization of haemodynamic parameters over measurements of flow to the peripheral tissues.

Recently, attempts to address this issue have included the OPTIMISE trial,[108] which recruited almost 800 patients who were subsequently randomized to cardiac output guided therapy using intravenous fluid and dopexamine, or usual care. Although this trial did not show a statistically significant difference in primary outcome between the two groups, subsequent analysis suggested that the trial was possibly underpowered. A Cochrane Database Systematic Review[109] indicated that increasing perioperative blood flow using haemodynamic treatment algorithms reduced the incidence of renal failure, respiratory failure and wound infections. Patients receiving these therapies also had a

TABLE 8.17 Devices Used in Invasive Monitoring.

Device	Information Provided
Arterial Line	Beat to beat monitoring of heart rate and blood pressure Pulse contour analysis provides information about haemodynamic parameters such as cardiac index, stroke volume and systemic vascular resistance Monitoring of gas exchange in the lungs Monitoring of metabolic parameters: pH, lactate, base excess, electrolytes Monitoring of blood glucose levels
Central Venous Catheter (CVC)	Assessment of volaemic status when sited in the neck (JVP) Assessment of central venous saturations when sited in the neck
Oesophageal Doppler	Insertion of probe into the distal third of the oesophagus provides a measurement of blood flow velocity in the descending aorta. The device also measures heart rate and peak velocity Subsequent calculations and pulse contour analysis allow for the estimation of haemodynamic variables such as stroke volume, cardiac output and corrected flow time
Pulmonary Artery Flotation Catheter (PAFC)	Used primarily in cardiac surgery, this method utilizes the physical principles of thermodilution to estimate cardiac output. A catheter with a thermistor at the distal tip is placed into the SVC via an introducer (not dissimilar to a CVC). The catheter is then guided into the heart, and subsequently the pulmonary vasculature. Using a PAFC allows for continuous monitoring of cardiac output, mixed venous saturations, and right heart, pulmonary artery and pulmonary capillary pressures.

JVP, Jugular venous pressure; SVC, superior vena cava.

reduced length of stay in hospital at 1 day. It concluded that although the balance of current evidence meant that it should not be assumed that this will reduce mortality, the intervention had value and was unlikely to cause harm.

Vasopressors and Inotropes

In addition to fluid therapy, part of the treatment algorithm for treatment of haemodynamic compromise in the critically ill patient involves the use of vasoactive drugs (Table 8.18). Vasoactive drugs may cause vasoconstriction, positive ino- or chronotropy, or both. In general, they require the placement of a central venous catheter for administration.

Respiratory Support

Intraoperative Management Goals

The induction of general anaesthesia invariably results in changes to ventilation-perfusion ratios in the lungs. Atelectasis due to anaesthesia, high BMI, supine positioning, patient co-morbidities, high fractions of inspired oxygen and positive pressure ventilation can all cause changes to ventilation and worsen shunt intraoperatively.[110] This leads to the development of postoperative pulmonary complications and worsening of clinical outcome. Strategies to minimize or prevent atelectasis include using recruitment manoeuvres, supraphysiological tidal volumes or low positive end-expiratory pressure strategies in order to maximize lung inflation. Anaesthesia providers are thus faced with the challenge of preventing intraoperative atelectasis whilst bearing in mind the potential for volutrauma and barotrauma.

Intraoperatively, management goals relate to the maintenance of physiological oxygen saturations, partial pressure of oxygen and carbon dioxide, and normal pH levels. Although there is little evidence that large tidal volumes cause significant harm[111] in the short-term, anaesthetists must be aware of the potential for barotrauma and account for confounding factors such as extremes of body weight, laparoscopic surgery or reverse Trendelenburg positioning.

Assessing Ongoing Need for Ventilation

The continuation of mechanical ventilation following surgery is dependent on numerous factors. Postoperative extubation is often slightly different to weaning from mechanical ventilation in the critical care setting, although both instances involve a clinical assessment of a patient's likelihood of failing extubation. In the critical care setting, this is often formalized by a spontaneous breathing trial on minimal ventilator settings. Arterial blood gas analysis and physiological variables such as oxygen saturation and heart rate are used to determine patients' suitability for extubation. In the operating theatre, given the time constraints of an operating list and the relative fitness of patients compared with those in critical care, this is impractical and seldom required in the elective setting. Other factors must therefore aid in clinical decision making regarding extubation:

- Patient factors: Stable cardiorespiratory disease and normal respiratory and metabolic parameters. In practice, this involves sampling an arterial blood gas if there is significant concern. Patients should be normothermic, and have a low additional oxygen and vasopressor requirement.
- Surgical factors: Special scenarios such as damage-control surgery mean that a return to theatre as soon as the next

TABLE 8.18 Common Vasoactive Drugs in Anaesthesia and Intensive Care.

Drug	CVC?	Mechanism of Action	Vasoconstriction	Inotropy	Chronotropy
Ephedrine	N	Mixed effects on α and β receptors	Y	Y	Y
Metaraminol	N	Primarily via α_1 agonism. Retains some β activity	Y	N	N
Phenylephrine	N	α_1 agonist	Y	N	N
Atropine	N	Anticholinergic	N	N	Y
Noradrenaline	Y	Primarily via α_1 agonism. Retains some β activity	Y	N	N
Adrenaline	Y	β effects predominate in low dose infusion At higher doses, α_1 agonism occurs	Y	Y	Y
Vasopressin	Y	Anti-diuretic hormone; works on peripheral receptors (AVPR1A)	Y	N	N
Dopamine	Y	D_1 and D_2 agonism β effects predominate in low dose infusion At higher doses, α_1 agonism occurs	Y	Y	Y
Dobutamine	Y	B_1 effects predominate	N	Y	Y
Dopexamine	Y	Synthetic analogue of dopamine B_2 effects predominate	N	Y	Y
Milrinone	Y	Selective phosphpodiesterase III inhibition	N	Y	Y

day is expected. Partly because of the nature of surgery (e.g. laparostomy), these patients often stay intubated until the second stage of their surgery is complete. It should be noted that staged procedures are not an absolute contraindication to extubation.

- For critically unwell patients, an additional period of observation prior to extubation on intensive care should be considered. This provides some time for stabilizing and optimizing the patient.
- Anaesthetic factors: Anaesthetists are responsible for ensuring that the effects of muscle relaxants have been fully reversed prior to extubation to avoid patient awareness. Additionally, it is imperative that patients have their analgesia optimized prior to extubation.

Surgical Site Infection Bundle

Surgical site infections (SSIs) are one of the most common healthcare-associated infections, which extend patient length of stay for a considerable time.[112] A number of factors, some of which are modifiable, increase the risk of SSI (Table 8.19).

Antibiotic Prophylaxis

Antibiotic prophylaxis plays an important part in preventing SSIs. However, the indiscriminate use of antibiotics for prophylaxis has well-documented consequences such as antibiotic resistance, as well as predisposing patients to problems such as *Clostridium difficile*-related diarrhoea. NICE guidance recommends using a local antibiotic formulary to

TABLE 8.19 Risk Factors for the Development of Surgical Site Infection.

Patient	Surgical
Age	Duration of surgical scrub
Nutritional status	Preoperative shaving
Diabetes	Length of operation
Smoking	Appropriate antimicrobial
Obesity	prophylaxis
Co-existent infection at a remote body site	Operating room ventilation
Colonization with micro-organisms e.g. *Staphylococcus aureus*	Sterilization of instruments
	Foreign material in the surgical site
	Surgical drains
Immunosuppression	Surgical technique inc.
Length of preoperative stay	haemostasis, poor closure,
Coexistent severe disease which limits activity	tissue trauma
Malignancy	Postoperative hypothermia

ensure appropriate selection of antimicrobial agent, as well as duration of treatment.

In general, antibiotic prophylaxis is recommended[113] in:
- Clean surgery, which involves the placement of a prosthesis or implant;
- Clean-contaminated surgery, which involves an incision and controlled entry into the respiratory, alimentary or genitourinary tract with no contamination;
- Contaminated surgery; and
- Surgery in a dirty or infected wound.

Antibiotic prophylaxis should be optimally timed, and in the 60 minutes prior to skin incision (and ideally as close to

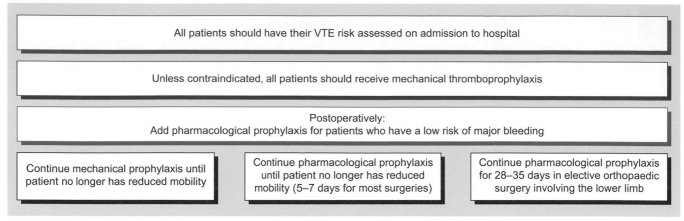

• **Fig. 8.9** Flow Chart for Venous Thromboembolism (VTE) Assessment after Admission

the time of incision as practically possible). In general, for most types of surgery, a single dose of antibiotic is sufficient for prophylaxis. For joint arthroplasties, up to 24 hours of antibiotic prophylaxis should be considered. For elective surgery lasting longer than the antibiotic half-life,[106] or cardiac surgery longer than 4 hours, an additional intraoperative dose is recommended.[114]

The choice of agent must reflect the likely spectrum of contaminating organisms. Agents should be bactericidal, non-toxic and inexpensive. For GI, genitourinary and gynaecological surgery, common pathogens are Gram-negative bacilli, enterococci and anaerobes (in the lower GI tract). As such, antibiotic prophylaxis is with an agent such as second- or third-generation cephalosporins, or amoxicillin/clavulanic acid. Where there is concern about anaerobe cover, metronidazole can be given as a second agent.

Glycaemic Control

Monitoring of blood glucose may be done by capillary blood glucose measurement, or by arterial blood gas if invasive monitoring is in place. Blood glucose should be checked before induction of anaesthesia; and at least hourly during the procedure. Target blood glucose in the anaesthetized patient should be 6–10 mmol/L, but current guidelines state that blood glucose of up to 12 mmol may be acceptable. For longer procedures, or where it is expected that a patient will miss two or more meals, the modality of choice for blood glucose control is a variable rate insulin infusion. This is of additional relevance in patients who are diabetic.

Temperature

Perioperative hypothermia is defined by a core body temperature of less than 36°C before, during and for the 24 hours after surgery. It has a significant implication on patient outcome, with issues relating to adverse cardiovascular events,[115] coagulopathy leading to haemorrhage,[116] wound infections[117] and length of patient stay.[118] Patient temperature should be measured from a site that is shown to be a direct estimate of core temperature. These include: the

distal oesophagus, sublingual, axilla, bladder or the pulmonary artery. All patients should have their risk of inadvertent hypothermia assessed. Patients with 2 or more of the following risk factors are at high risk of hypothermia[119]:
- ASA grade II to V
- Preoperative temperature below 36°C and warming is not possible
- Combined regional and general anaesthesia
- Intermediate, major or complex surgery
- At risk of cardiovascular complications

Active warming should be started before induction of anaesthesia if a patient's temperature is below 36°C. Intraoperatively, patient temperature should be measured and documented every 30 minutes until the end of surgery. Methods of preventing heat loss include: ensuring adequate ambient temperature in theatres, and minimizing the extent and length of time patients are exposed for. Methods of actively warming patients include forced air warmers, warming blankets, warm fluid/blood for IV infusion and lavage of body cavities (e.g. the abdominal cavity) with warm fluid.

VTE Prophylaxis

Venous thromboembolism (VTE) causes serious morbidity and mortality amongst hospital inpatients. An estimated 10% of deaths in hospital patients are due to pulmonary embolism (PE), and the incidence in patients having orthopaedic surgery without thromboprophylaxis is as high as one in three patients. In the general surgery population, this incidence is slightly lower, with up to one in five patients having an asymptomatic VTE.[120] It is thus essential that perioperative care includes an assessment of a patient's individual VTE risk, and that appropriate thromboprophylaxis is prescribed promptly (Fig. 8.9).

NICE guidelines recommend that surgical and trauma patients are treated as having an increased risk of VTE if they have:
- A surgical procedure with a total anaesthetic and surgical time in excess of 90 minutes (60 minutes if surgery involves the pelvis or the lower limb)

TABLE 8.20	Risk Factors for Venous Thromboembolism (VTE) and Bleeding.	
Patient Risk Factors For VTE	**Patient Risk Factors for Bleeding**
Active cancer or cancer treatment	Active bleeding
Age >60 years	Acquired bleeding disorder
Critical care admission	Concurrent use of anticoagulants
Dehydration	Lumbar puncture/epidural/ spinal anaesthesia expected in the next 12 hours
Known thrombophilia	
Obesity (BMI >30 kg/m^2)	
One or more significant medical co-morbidities (e.g. heart disease)	Lumbar puncture/epidural/ spinal anaesthesia in the last 4 hours
Personal history of VTE	Acute stroke
First-degree relative with a history of VTE	Thrombocytopaenia (platelets < 75 × 10^9/L)
Use of hormone replacement therapy	Uncontrolled systolic hypertension (BP 230/120 mmHg or higher)
Use of oestrogen-containing contraceptive therapy	Untreated inherited bleeding disorders
Varicose veins with phlebitis	

- An acute surgical admission with an inflammatory or intra-abdominal condition
- Expected reduction in mobility
- One or more patient risk factors for VTE

All patients should also have their risk of bleeding assessed prior to the prescription of pharmacological prophylaxis (Table 8.20).

Mechanical Thromboprophylaxis

NICE guidelines recommend mechanical thromboprophylaxis be started at admission. These can involve: anti-embolism stockings, foot impulse devices and intermittent pneumatic compression devices. It is important that anti-embolism stockings are not used in patients with suspected or proven arterial disease, peripheral neuropathy, previous arterial bypass grafting, severe oedema and poor skin conditions. Ill-fitting stockings contribute to skin breakdown and the development of pressure ulcers. Patients should have their legs measured and the correct size of stocking fitted. Anti-embolism stockings should provide graduated compression and a calf pressure of 14–15 mmHg.

Pharmacological Thromboprophylaxis

NICE recommends that the choice of pharmacological VTE agent be based on local policies and individual patient factors. Most trusts recommend low-molecular-weight heparins such as enoxaparin, dalteparin or tinzaparin. Other options include unfractionated heparin or oral anticoagulants such as Factor Xa inhibitors or direct thrombin inhibitors. The following patient factors should be taken into account when prescribing pharmacological prophylaxis:
- Renal impairment. Patients with severe renal impairment may require heparin thromboprophylaxis.

- Extremes of body weight
- Increased bleeding risk

POSTOPERATIVE MANAGEMENT

The Postoperative Stress Response to Surgery

Surgery in the elective or emergency setting provokes a physiological stress response in patients postoperatively. It is a complex hormonal and metabolic process which is mediated by several neuroendocrine axes. General anaesthesia, regional anaesthesia and analgesic agents modify the stress response to varying degrees.

Acute Phase Response

Tissue injury causes widespread production and activation of inflammatory cytokines, particularly IL-6. The degree of response is related to tissue damage and is reduced in minimally invasive approaches such as laparoscopy. The acute phase response results in:
- Widespread increase in cytokine levels, particularly IL-1, IL-6, IL-8, and TNF$_\alpha$
- Pyrexia
- Protein synthesis (c-reactive protein, fibrinogen, caeruloplasmin, serum amyloid A and P, complement proteins, and coagulation proteins
- Reduction in transport proteins such as transferrin and albumin
- Leucocytosis and neutrophilia
- Altered vascular permeability
- Increased muscle proteolysis
- Activation of the neuroendocrine response

Neuroendocrine Response to Surgery

Table 8.21 summarizes key hormonal changes in the stress response to surgery.

The net effect of surgery is therefore to produce a catabolic state in the patient that is related to the size of the surgical insult. Widespread sympathetic activation can have a catastrophic impact on myocardial workload and oxygen demand and delivery. The accompanying adrenal response often results in significant fluid overload and tissue oedema. Attenuating the stress response to surgery has therefore long been of interest to clinicians and researchers.

Questions have also been raised about the potential harm caused in totally obliterating the stress response. Much of this concern has come from the use of etomidate, an IV anaesthetic agent previously used in cardiac surgery for its stable haemodynamic profile. Adrenal enzyme activity is inhibited after just one dose of etomidate,[121] and concerns about adverse outcomes related to this[122] have resulted in a widespread reduction of its use.

TABLE 8.21	Key Hormonal Changes in the Stress Response.
Hormone	**Effects**
Sympathetic Nervous System	Catecholamines are released from the adrenal medulla Increase in presynaptic noradrenaline release Cardiovascular system causes tachycardia and peripheral vasoconstriction Redistribution of blood flow to essential organs Renin release stimulates the secretion of aldosterone and results in sodium and water retention Inhibition of peristalsis Bronchodilation
Hypothalamic–Pituitary–Adrenal Axis	Hypothalamic releasing factors are secreted into the hypothalamic-hypophyseal system **Anterior Pituitary:** ↑ ACTH causing increased cortisol release ↑ growth hormone: glycogenolysis and lipolysis ↑ prolactin **Posterior Pituitary:** ↑ arginine vasopressin (antidiuretic hormone) causing water retention and further ACTH release No change to TSH, LH or FSH
Cortisol	Magnitude and duration of increase correlates with insult severity Response is not abolished by the administration of corticosteroids **Net catabolism:** Protein and muscle breakdown for gluconeogenesis Lipolysis Inhibition of glucose utilization causing hyperglycaemia Sodium and water retention, potassium loss ↓ leucocyte migration and inhibit inflammatory mediator synthesis
Insulin	Anabolic hormone normally secreted in response to hyperglycaemia Secretion is reduced in the stress response due to the effect at α_2 receptors by circulating catecholamines Functional insulin deficiency causes ongoing hyperglycaemia

ACTH, Adrenocorticotrophic hormone; FSH, follicle stimulating hormone; LH, luteinising hormone; TSH, thyroid stimulating hormone.

Routine Postoperative Care

The Day Case Patient

Criteria for Discharge Following Surgery

Discharge following day surgery may be nurse- or clinician-led. Patients must be able to mobilize adequately before surgery and be supplied with clear instructions about post-operative wound care and medications, which may include antibiotics and thromboprophylaxis. Clear national guidance for suitability for discharge from day surgery exists, and most trusts will have implemented their own local protocols (Table 8.22).

The Enhanced Recovery Patient

ERAS Protocol

First introduced as 'fast-track' surgery, Enhanced Recovery After Surgery (ERAS) protocols represent a set of evidence-based interventions designed to attenuate the stress response to surgery, maintain physiological function and expedite a return to baseline function.[123] Their implementation results in reduced postoperative morbidity and mortality. Intra- and postoperative ERAS protocols vary by site, but incorporate the main principles from the ERAS society's guidelines outlined in Table 8.23.

Nutrition

Starvation, the stress response to surgery and the postoperative acute inflammatory phase have all been implicated in the metabolic response to surgery. Additionally, patients presenting for major surgery may have had neoadjuvant chemotherapy and/or a significant period of weight loss related to their pathology. Recommendations from the European Society for Clinical Nutrition and Metabolism highlight the importance of nutritional status assessment before and after surgery. Poor nutritional status impacts on both morbidity and mortality.

In general, enteral nutritional intake should not be interrupted after surgery. Patients should have their oral intake adapted according to their body habitus, daily nutritional needs and the type of surgery. Contraindications to enteral feeding include intestinal obstruction, ischaemia or haemorrhage.

If enteral intake is limited and a patient is receiving under half of their recommended energy and nutrient requirements, then parenteral nutrition (PN) should be considered. The average energy intake for a patient over 24 hours should be between 25 and 30 kcal/kg, depending on the severity of the stress response. In severe stress, protein requirements are also increased at 1.5g/kg per day. The

TABLE 8.22	Discharge Checklist for Day Surgery					
Criteria		**Yes**	**No**	**N/A**	**Initials**	**Details**
Vital signs stable						
Orientated to time, place, and person						
Passed urine (if applicable)						
Able to dress and walk (where appropriate)						
Oral fluids tolerated (if applicable)						
Minimal pain						
Minimal bleeding						
Minimal nausea/vomiting						
Cannula removed						
Responsible escort present						
Has carer for 24-h postop						
Written and verbal postop instructions						
Knows who to contact in an emergency						
Follow-up appointment						
Removal of sutures required?						
Referrals made						
Dressings supplied						
Patient copy of GP letter						
Carbon copy of consent						
Sick certificate						
Has take-home medications						
Information leaflet for tablets						
Postop phone call required						

From Tickner, C., Barkor, K., Blankc, S., 2009. Nurse Led Discharge. British Association of Day Surgery (BADS), London.

glucose:fat calorie ratio in parenteral feed should approach 60:40 or even 70:30, in order to minimize the hyperlipidaemia associated with PN.

Although there has been a lot of interest in this field, current guidelines do not support the routine use of enteral formulas enriched with immunonutrients such as omega-3-fatty acids. However, their use may be considered in cancer patients who are malnourished.

The High-Risk Patient

Postoperative Critical Care

Postoperative critical care has been a major focus of risk management for the high-risk patient in recent years. Guidance from multiple national bodies including the Royal College of Surgeons and the Royal College of Anaesthetists have all emphasized the importance of critical care and outreach in mitigating risks for these patients. Patients who are deemed to be high-risk have a mortality of greater than 5%, and should be admitted to a critical care setting postoperatively. The variability in intensive care service provision and bed availability mean that no direct randomized control trials have been done to evaluate the outcomes for patients admitted to intensive care. However, many of the interventions for which there is an evidence base, such as goal-directed fluid therapy, or organ support, are carried out almost exclusively in intensive care settings. The Intensive Care Society has defined levels of care based on several patient factors (Table 8.24).

Stepdown from Intensive Care

Wherever possible, planning should occur well ahead of the time of transfer in critical care. This includes the early identification of patients for potential discharge during the time of the morning ward round, clear communication with the receiving team and the ward and informing the patient and their relatives about the plan. Referral should be made to the Critical Care Outreach Team wherever possible, in order to ensure a review following step-down. Clear verbal and written handover must take place between the clinicians and nursing staff looking after the patient. Wherever possible, step-down transfers between 22:00 and 07:00 hours should be avoided. Finally, National Early Warning Score (NEWS) charts should be recorded on the transfer form before and after transfer.

Postoperative Complications and the Unwell Surgical Patient

Complications following an operation can be classified by whether they are related to having surgery (for example, the risk of general anaesthesia), or by complications specific to a particular surgical procedure (for example, cardiac tamponade following coronary artery bypass surgery). Complications can also be classified according to when they have occurred, i.e. immediately (during and within the first 24 hours), early (within the first week), or late. Delayed recognition and management of postoperative complications can

TABLE 8.23	Main Enhanced Recovery After Surgery (ERAS) Society Recommendations.	
Phase	**Goal**	**Practical Points**
Pre-Op	Pre-admission risk stratification	Use of scoring systems for surgery e.g. POSSUM Assess cardiac risk, functional capacity, and risk of acute kidney injury
	Optimise pre-existing health conditions	Correction of preoperative anaemia Reduction of cardiovascular risk Smoking cessation and alcohol abstinence advice
	Minimize fasting time	Clear fluids until 2 h, solids until 6 h before anaesthesia Treatment with oral carbohydrate drinks helps reduce hypoglycaemia
Intra-Op	Prevention and treatment of postoperative nausea and vomiting (PONV)	Identification of patients likely to be at high risk of PONV Reducing preoperative fasting, adequate hydration and carbohydrate loading Use of total intravenous anaesthetic techniques Opioid sparing analgesic techniques, e.g. thoracic epidural Combination antiemetic therapy for high-risk patients
	Standard anaesthetic protocol	Depth of anaesthesia and neuromuscular blockade monitoring Inspired oxygen concentration to produce normal arterial oxygen levels or saturations Normothermia and normoglycaemia Goal-directed fluid therapy
	Surgical techniques	Strong evidence for laparoscopic surgery
	Nasogastric tubes	Routine insertion of nasogastric tubes should be avoided
Post-Op	Fluid management	Maintain fluid homeostasis Encourage early oral fluids, and discontinue IV fluids once tolerated Avoid weight gain more than 2.5 kg
	Pain management	Multimodal techniques are the standard of care Thoracic epidural is of clear benefit in open surgery, or patients at risk of respiratory complications Intrathecal morphine also improves early postoperative analgesia. Slightly higher risk of pruritus, hypotension, respiratory depression and urinary retention
	Postoperative delirium	Avoid prolonged fasting, disturbances of sleep-wake cycle, and deliriogenic medications Systematic delirium screening is recommended
	Postoperative ileus	Opioid-sparing analgesia Early mobilization Laxatives Early feeding/gum chewing

contribute to significant increase in morbidity and mortality. The concept of 'failure to rescue' refers to death after a treatable complication. A number of different factors contribute to poor outcomes in the deteriorating patient, but core issues include:

- Failure to take or record observations
- Failure to recognize early signs of deterioration
- Failure to appropriately communicate or escalate concerns[124]

These concerns have also resulted in the development of courses to help team members identify and manage the critically unwell patient. The most important immediate complications are covered in the rest of this chapter.

Respiratory Complications

Respiratory failure following surgery can be due to a number of different causes (Table 8.25). It is classified into type I (hypoxaemia alone), or type II (hypercapnia with co-existent hypoxaemia). The fundamental physiological principle is the failure of the cardiorespiratory system to provide sufficient alveolar ventilation. This is generally due to issues with ventilation and/or lung perfusion, causing a mismatch between the two.

The treatment of respiratory failure involves investigating and treating the underlying cause by examination and plain radiographs in the first instance. An arterial blood gas (ABG) should be taken in order to help guide therapy. Indications for non-invasive ventilation (NIV) include[125]:

- Persistent acidaemia or hypoxia despite adequate treatment of initial cause (e.g. oxygen therapy, diuresis, antibiotics, or bronchodilator therapy)
- Hypercapnia

NIV is relatively contraindicated in patients who have significant facial deformity or burns, in severe respiratory

TABLE 8.24	Levels of Monitoring.
Level 0	Patients requiring hospitalisation. Needs can be met through normal ward care.
Level 1	Patients recently discharged from a higher level of care Patients in need of additional monitoring, clinical interventions, clinical input or advice Examples: epidural analgesia, PCA, TPN, VRII, or CPAP Patients requiring critical care outreach service support
Level 2	Patients needing preoperative optimization Patients needing extended postoperative care Patients receiving single organ support: Basic respiratory: non-invasive ventilation. FiO_2 greater than 50%. Basic cardiovascular: need for invasive monitoring (arterial line, CVC), single vasoactive agent Advanced cardiovascular: multiple vasoactive medications, continuous cardiac output monitoring Renal: acute renal replacement therapy Neurological: CNS depression sufficient to prejudice the airway and protective reflexes Dermatological: burns >30% skin area
Level 3	Patients receiving advanced respiratory support Examples: invasive mechanical ventilation with endotracheal tube, BIPAP, extracorporeal support Patients receiving a minimum of 2 or more organs supported

CNS, Central nervous system, CPAP, continuous positive airways pressure; CVC, central venous catheter; FiO_2, fraction of inspired oxygen; PCA, patient-controlled analgesia; TPN, total parenteral nutrition; VRII, variable rate insulin infusion.

TABLE 8.25	Differential Diagnoses to Consider in Respiratory Failure.	
Impaired Ventilation	**Impaired Perfusion**
Infection	Pulmonary embolus
Pulmonary oedema	Low cardiac output
Acute respiratory distress syndrome	states
Atelectasis	
Hypoventilation due to respiratory depression	
Exacerbation of underlying airways disease	

failure (pH <7.15) and in those who are somnolent or who have cognitive impairment. NIV is also not indicated in acute exacerbations of asthma or severe pneumonia. Intubation and mechanical ventilation should be considered if patients with these pathologies are deteriorating, or if there has been little improvement in respiratory parameters on repeat ABG sampling.

Cardiovascular Complications

The list of differential diagnoses for the patient with cardiovascular compromise is extensive.

Haemorrhage

The management of major haemorrhage and the use of blood products has been described earlier in this chapter. Postoperative haemorrhage should be recognized and treated promptly. Haemorrhage can sometimes be concealed, and it is important that clinicians expose and examine patients

appropriately (Table 8.26). Management of a patient with postoperative bleeding should include:
- Initial resuscitation with crystalloid or colloid unless massive haemorrhage evident
- Assessment of need for transfusion with blood and blood products
- Control of bleeding source
- Correction of coagulopathy

Sepsis

Surgical site infection (SSI) is a general complication which can be potentially life-threatening. The SSI bundle described earlier has significantly reduced the risk of SSIs in the postoperative period. These infections are classified by the CDC into: incisional, deep incisional and organ/space SSIs.[126] When considering the management of a patient with an infection, it is important to evaluate the factors listed in Table 8.27.

In addition to SSI, patients are also at risk of other hospital-acquired infections perioperatively. The risk of these increases with the length of their inpatient stay. These include lower respiratory tract infections such as hospital-acquired (or ventilator-associated) pneumonia, colonization with a resistant organism such as MRSA, or infections associated with antibiotic use, such as *C. difficile*-associated diarrhoea.

Sepsis has recently been re-defined as **a life-threatening organ dysfunction caused by a dysregulated host response to infection.**[127] Along with this, the use of the traditional inflammatory criteria (SIRS) has been re-evaluated. The majority of patients admitted to intensive care fulfil SIRS criteria as part of their disease process[128]; and 12% of patients with sepsis do not fulfil the criteria for SIRS.[129]

TABLE 8.26 **Degrees of Hypovolaemic Shock.**

	Blood Loss (%)	Blood Loss (mL)	Pulse	Pulse Pressure	Blood Pressure	Urine Output (mL/h)	Respiratory Rate	Mental State
Class I	>15%	750	<100	N	N	>30	14–20	Slight anxiety
Class II	15–30%	750–1500	>100	↓ (DBP↑)	N	15–30	20–30	Mild anxiety
Class III	30–40%	1500–2000	>120	↓	↓	5–15	30–40	Anxious/ confused
Class IV	>40%	>2000	>140	↓	↓	<5	>34	Confused/ lethargic

DBP, Diastolic blood pressure.

TABLE 8.27 **Risk Factors for Surgical Site Infection.**

Microbe-Related Risk Factors	Host-Related Risk Factors	Operation-Related Risk Factors
Staphylococcus aureus; *Streptococcus pyogenes*	Significant co-morbid disease: diabetes, cancer, morbid obesity Protein-calorie malnutrition Age Systemic infection	Duration of operation Prolonged hospital stay before surgery Tissue trauma Foreign material in the wound Poor haemostasis

TABLE 8.28 **qSOFA Criteria in Sepsis.**

H	Hypotension: SBP ≤100 mmHg
A	Altered mental status (any GCS <15)
T	Tachypnoea: RR ≥22

GCS, Glasgow Coma Score; qSOFA, quick Sepsis Organ Failure Assessment; RR, respiratory rate; SBP, systolic blood pressure.

Organ dysfunction should now be quantified by the Sepsis Organ Failure Assessment (SOFA) score. A score of 2 points or more is associated with an in-hospital mortality greater than 10%. In response to criticisms about the practicality of calculating the SOFA score, current recommendations are to use the quickSOFA (qSOFA) assessment (Table 8.28). Limitations of this method of assessment include its poor sensitivity for early risk assessment.

Investigation of the patient with sepsis includes the 'septic screen', including cultures from blood, wound sites, urine and sputum where appropriate, urinalysis, and a chest X-ray. Foci of infection such as incisions, drain sites and central venous catheters must be assessed. Resuscitative management includes the institution of the 'Sepsis 6', as advocated by the UK Sepsis Trust:

- **Administer oxygen** with the aim of keeping saturations >94% (88–92% in COPD)
- **Administer IV antibiotics** within 1 hour, considering likely source and patient allergy
- **Administer IV fluids** using a 10 mL/kg bolus of a balanced crystalloid solution
- **Take blood cultures**
- **Measure serial lactates**
- **Measure urine output**

Significantly elevated venous lactates (>4 mmol) which do not resolve on initial fluid resuscitation warrant referral to critical care. In the postoperative patient where a clear focus is identified, decisions should be made regarding the need to return to theatre and source control.

Thromboembolism and its Treatment

Prophylaxis for thromboembolic disease has been described earlier in this chapter. Significant thromboembolic disease such as a large PE can cause haemodynamic instability. Patients with a high index of suspicion for pulmonary embolus should be treated with a low-molecular-weight heparin and the investigation of choice is a contrast CT of the pulmonary arteries (CTPA). These patients should be anticoagulated on warfarin or a newer anticoagulant following diagnosis. In massive PE with circulatory collapse, patients may be too unwell for mobile imaging. Right heart dysfunction may be seen on bedside ECHO. Thrombolysis with alteplase is the first-line treatment for massive PE and may be given on clinical grounds alone if cardiac arrest is imminent.[130]

Myocardial Injury

Major adverse cardiac events after surgery must be ruled out in a patient with circulatory dysfunction. The VISION study identified that 87.1% of myocardial injury after surgery occurs within the first 2 postoperative days. These patients are at higher risk of non-fatal cardiac arrest, congestive cardiac failure and stroke.[131] Patients should have a 12-lead ECG and investigation with serial troponin measurements in addition to a full set of blood tests. They should be referred to a cardiologist urgently for further assessment. Predictors of mortality from the VISION study include: age over 75, new ST elevation or left bundle branch block, and ECG changes indicative of anterior ischaemia. The treatment of myocardial infarction will normally necessitate anticoagulation and antiplatelet therapy, and the risk of bleeding must be balanced against the risk of further injury.

Cardiac Dysrhythmia

The development of cardiac dysrhythmias such as atrial fibrillation may cause haemodynamic compromise. Common causes of arrhythmias include: electrolyte disturbances, infection, hypoxia and myocardial ischaemia. As with myocardial infarction, a full set of blood tests and a 12-lead ECG should be the baseline for all investigations. Additionally, an arterial or venous blood gas provides point of care testing to rule out electrolyte disturbances that require immediate correction. Cardiac dysrhythmias can be corrected by electrical or chemical methods, and require urgent attention if they compromise haemodynamic status.

Cognitive Dysfunction

Delirium

Delirium is defined as 'an acute and fluctuating disturbance of consciousness… accompanied by change in cognition and perceptual disturbances secondary to a general medical condition'.[132] Delirious patients are often described as confused and agitated. However, it is important to remember that 50% of patients present with hypoactive delirium, which is associated with poorer outcomes such as increased mortality and admission to long-term care.[133]

Postoperative delirium after surgery affects up to 20% of patients in the postoperative period. Independent risk factors for delirium include: age, pain, ASA score ≥3, co-morbidities, critical care admission, dehydration, polypharmacy, malnutrition and preoperative cognitive impairment.[106] The use of certain medications such as benzodiazepines and some analgesics also contribute to the development of delirium.

Delirium is associated with worse outcomes such as functional decline[134] and increased number of days in ICU and hospital.[135] Patients are more likely to be discharged to an institution, hasten pre-existing dementia, and all-cause mortality increases by 10–20% every 48 hours.[126] They must therefore be actively screened for delirium in the immediate postoperative phase, particularly if there is a high index of suspicion. A validated test is the Confusion Assessment Method,[136] which can be adapted for patients in intensive care (Table 8.29).

Delirium should be treated by identifying and treating the underlying cause. General non-pharmacological principles for the care of patients with delirium include: optimizing sleep-wake cycles, calm environments, frequent reorientation

TABLE 8.29 **Confusion Assessment Method.**

Criteria A AND	Acute onset and fluctuating course
Criteria B	Inattention (distractible, can't concentrate)
AND EITHER	
Criteria C OR	Disorganised thinking (rambling/ illogical ideas)
Criteria D	Altered consciousness (hyperalert/ drowsy)

and reassurance, and optimizing sensory impairments (e.g. hearing aids and spectacles). If pharmacological intervention is necessary, then a single agent such as haloperidol should be carefully titrated to effect. Patients who are particularly at risk should be identified and monitored perioperatively.

Acute Pain

Pain is one of the most common and treatable causes of delirium. Acute pain in the postoperative setting should be treated promptly in order to prevent this, but also to reduce the incidence of chronic pain. Analgesic regimens have been discussed elsewhere in this chapter. It is important to emphasize the need for step-wise, incremental titration of analgesia, and the need for a multi-modal approach, particularly in patients with pre-existing chronic pain. Early involvement of the acute pain team is recommended.

Fluid Management

Fluid management after surgery is complicated by the acute phase and stress response to surgery. Salt and water retention, combined with increased vascular permeability and low protein states, means that patients are likely to have a degree of fluid overload in the extravascular space, whilst remaining intravascularly depleted.

Acute Kidney Injury (AKI)

Chronic kidney disease and its implications for the development of acute renal impairment have been discussed in the preoperative section of this chapter. Postoperative AKI accounts for up to 40% of all cases of in-hospital AKI.[137] AKI should be diagnosed and staged by changes in serum creatinine or urine output (Table 8.30). Patients with abnormalities in both criteria for more than 3 days are at the greatest risk of death and renal replacement therapy.[138]

The management of AKI should involve identifying and correcting reversible causes, and contemporaneous resuscitation:

- Stop nephrotoxic medications wherever possible
- Fluid resuscitation with balanced crystalloid
- Diagnosing + relieving urinary tract obstruction
- Urinary catheter and monitoring of fluid status

TABLE 8.30	Diagnostic and Staging Criteria for Acute Kidney Injury (AKI).		
Diagnostic Criteria for AKI			
Increase of serum creatinine by more than 26.4 µmol; OR			
Increase in serum creatinine ≥1.5 × baseline level; OR			
Urine volume <0.5 mL/kg per h for 6 hours			
AKI Staging System			
Stage	Serum Creatinine Criteria		Urine Output Criteria
AKI Stage I	Increase of serum creatinine 26.4 µmol; OR Increase to 1.5–1.9 times from baseline		Urine output <0.5 mL/kg per h for 6–12 hours
AKI Stage II	Increase to 2.0–2.9 times from baseline		Urine output <0.5 mL/kg per h for ≥12 hours
AKI Stage III	Serum creatinine ≥354 µmol; OR Increase to ≥3.0 times from baseline; OR Treatment with RRT		Urine output <0.5 mL/kg per h for ≥24 hours; OR Anuria for ≥12 hours

- Regular monitoring of electrolytes and metabolic parameters

Indications for renal replacement therapy include:

- Management of fluid overload (e.g. pulmonary oedema)
- Refractory hyperkalaemia
- Metabolic acidosis
- Uraemia
- Removal of drugs by dialysis (e.g. salicylates and lithium)

Patients with a clear cause and improvement of their AKI do not need referral to nephrology. However, all other patients should be referred within 24 hours.[139] Indications for referral include:

- Criteria for renal replacement therapy met
- Patients with renal transplant
- AKI cause unclear
- AKI stage 3 or more
- Inadequate response to treatment
- CKD stage 4 or 5
- A diagnosis which needs specialist treatment (e.g. vasculitis)

Gastrointestinal Complications

The acute stress response to surgery has a number of deleterious effects on the GI system.

The Prevention of Stress Ulcers

Stress-related mucosal damage and GI bleeding is well-described in the literature and when it was first being studied, had a prevalence of up to 25%.[140] The routine use of postoperative H_2 blockers and proton pump inhibitors (PPIs) has greatly reduced the incidence of stress-related ulceration. In general, PPIs seem to be more effective in preventing clinically important or overt GI bleeding.[141] Adverse effects associated with prophylaxis include the association with ventilator-associated complications, and the potential increased

risk of colonization with *C. difficile*. Another important component in reducing stress-related mucosal damage is early enteral feeding, which is more effective at raising intra-gastric pH than pharmacological prophylaxis.[142]

Postoperative Ileus and Impaired Nutrition

The prevention of postoperative ileus has been the focus of much research. As has been discussed elsewhere in this chapter, it is one of the main aims of enhanced recovery protocols. Patients who develop a postoperative ileus are more likely to have a prolonged hospital stay and nutritional issues. Important considerations for this subset of patients include:

- The need for a nasogastric tube and mechanical decompression
- Ongoing nutritional needs. If enteral nutrition is insufficient to meet these, then parenteral nutrition must be considered
- Dehydration secondary to intraluminal fluid loss and reduced oral intake. Maintenance IV fluids should be considered in these patients
- Impaired respiratory function secondary to pain, abdominal distension and the risk of aspiration
- Increased pain requiring step-up analgesia
- Mechanical causes of obstruction that may require a return to theatre

Considerations for Discharge

Preparation for Discharge

Good postoperative care extends into discharge planning. It is important to consider the impact of major surgery on patients' long-term health and quality of life. Patients with complex disease or co-morbidities should also receive input from physiotherapy and occupational therapy in a multidisciplinary setting. It is important that changes to medication are clearly communicated to patients around the time of discharge, and this requires organization with the community pharmacy. Additionally, patients require training in specific care needs, such as colostomy care. Frail patients may leave hospital with increased care needs, resulting in a modification to their package of care in the community. These processes take time and planning should begin in the early postoperative period.

Follow-Up

Surgical patients with long-term disease require ongoing care and follow-up after discharge from hospital. This may be in the form of surgical outpatient clinics or further investigations. Patients who have been in intensive care may also attend follow-up clinics for critical care. It is essential that there is clear communication between primary and secondary care for all these patients.

References

1. Day Surgery: Operational Guide. Department of Health, London 2002.
2. 10 High Impact Changes for Service Improvement and Delivery. A Guide for NHS Leaders. NHS Modernisation Agency, 2004.
3. Claxton AR, McGuire G, Chung F, Cruise C. Evaluation of morphine versus fentanyl for postoperative analgesia after ambulatory surgical procedures. *Anesth Analg.* 1997;84:509–514.
4. NHS Reference costs 2013 to 2014. Department of Health, London, 2014.
5. Acute Hospital Portfolio – Review of National Findings. Day Surgery Audit Commission, 2001.
6. BADS. *BADS Directory of Procedures.* fifth ed. British Association of Day Surgery, London, 2016.
7. Edmonston DL, Foulkes GD. Infection rate and risk factor analysis in an orthopaedic ambulatory surgical center. *J Surg Orthop Adv.* 2010;19:174–176.
8. Healthcare Commission. *Acute Hospital Portfolio Review: Day Surgery.* Commission for Healthcare Audit and Inspection, London, 2005.
9. Ansell GL, Montgomery JE. Outcome of ASA III patients undergoing day case surgery. *Br J Anaesth.* 2004;92:71–74.
10. Goldman L, Caldera LDI, Nussbaum SR, et al. Mutlifactorial index of cardiac risk in noncardiac surgical procedures. *N Eng J Med.* 1977;297:845–850.
11. Lee TH, Marcantonio ER, Mangione CM, et al. Derivation and prospective validation of a simple index for prediction of cardiac risk of major noncardiac surgery. *Circulation* 1999;100:1043–1049.
12. Fleisher LA, Fleischmann K, Auerbach AD, Barnason SA, Beckman JA, Bozkurt B, et al. ACC/AHA Guideline on Perioperative Cardiovascular Evaluation and Management of Patients Undergoing Noncardiac Surgery. *J Am Coll Cardiol.* 2014;64(22):e77–e137.
13. Gupta PK, Gupt H, Sundaram A, et al. Development and validation of a risk calculator for prediction of cardiac risk after surgery: clinical perspective. *Circulation* 2011;124:381–387.
14. Hypertension prevalence estimates in England: Estimated from the Health Survey for England. Public Health England, 2016.
15. Weksler N, Klein M, Szendro G, et al. The dilemma of immediate preoperative hypertension: to treat and operate, or to postpone surgery? *J Clin Anaesth.* 2003;15:179–183.
16. NICE Guideline CG 127. *Hypertension in adults: diagnosis and management.* National Institute for Clinical Excellence, 2016.
17. Bhatnagar P, Wickramasinghe K, Williams J, Rayner M, Townsend N. The epidemiology of cardiovascular disease in the UK 2014. *Heart.* 2015;101:1182–1189.
18. Artang R, Dieter RS. Analysis of 36 reported cases of late thrombosis in drug-eluting stents placed in coronary arteries. *Am J Cardiol.* 2007;99:1039–1043.
19. Schouten O, Bax JJ, Damen J, Poldermans D. Coronary artery stent placement immediately before noncardiac surgery: a potential risk? *Anesthesiology* 2007;106:1067–1069.
20. 2014 ACC/AHA Guideline on perioperative cardiovascular evaluation and management of patients undergoing noncardiac surgery. *J Am Coll Cardiol.* 2014;64:22.
21. *Atrial Fibrillation: The Management of Atrial Fibrillation.* National Institute for Clinical Excellence, 2014.
22. Kazmers A, Cerqueira MD, Zierler RE. Perioperative and late outcome in patients with left ventricular ejection fraction of 35% or less who require major vascular surgery. *J Vasc Surg.* 1988;8:307–315.
23. Flu W-J, van Kuijk J-P, Hoeks SE, et al. Prognostic implications of asymptomatic left ventricular dysfunction in patients undergoing vascular surgery. *Anesthesiology.* 2010;112:1316–1324.
24. Meta-analysis Global Group in Chronic Heart Failure (MAGGIC). The survival of patients with heart failure with preserved or reduced left ventricular ejection fraction: an individual patient data meta-analysis. *Eur Heart J.* 2012;33:1750–1757.
25. Masoudi FA, Havranek EP, Smith G, Fish RH, Steiner JF, Ordin DL, et al. Gender, age, and heart failure with preserved left ventricular systolic function. *J Am Coll Cardiol.* 2003;41:217–223.
26. Phillip B, Pastor D, Bellows W, Leung JM. The prevalence of preoperative diastolic filling abnormalities in geriatric surgical patients. *Anesth Analg.* 2003;97:1214–1221.
27. Berry MF, Villamizar-Ortiz NR, Tong BC, et al. Pulmonary function tests do not predict pulmonary complications after thoracoscopic lobectomy. *Ann Thorac Surg* 2010;89:1044–1051
28. Arozullah AM, Conde MV, Lawrence VA. Preoperative evaluation for postoperative pulmonary complications. *Med Clin North Am.* 2003;87:153–173.
29. Lumb A, Biercamp C. Chronic obstructive pulmonary disease and anaesthesia. *Con Edu Anaesth Crit Care Pain* 2014;1:1–5.
30. Asthma UK Data Portal. Available from: https://www.asthma.org.uk/support-us/campaigns/data-visualisations/.
31. CDC – Asthma – Data and Surveillance – Asthma Surveillance Data. Available at: http://www.cdc.gov/asthma/asthmadata.htm.
32. Tirumalasetty J, Grammer LC. Asthma, surgery, and general anesthesia: a review. *J Asthma.* 2006;43:251–254.
33. Peterson GN, Domino KB, Caplan RA, Posner KL, Lee LA, Cheney FW. Management of the difficult airway: a closed claims analysis. *Anesthesiology.* 2005;103(1):33–39.
34. Seet E, Han T, Chung F. Perioperative clinical pathways to manage sleep-disordered breathing. *Sleep Med Clin.* 2013;8:105–120.
35. Chung F, Yang Y, Liao P. Predictive performance of the STOP-BANG Score for identifying obstructive sleep apnoea in obese patients. *Obes Surg.* 2013;23:2050–2057.

36. Frisch A, Chandra P, Smiley D, et al. Prevalence and clinical outcome of hyperglycemia in the perioperative period in non-cardiac surgery. *Diabetes Care*. 2010;33:1783–1788.

37. Canaris GJ, Manowitz NR, Mayor G, Ridgway EC. The Colorado thyroid disease prevalence study. *Arch Intern Med*. 2000;160(4):526–534.

38. Palace MR. Perioperative management of thyroid dysfunction. *Health Serv Insights*. 2017;10:1178632916689677.

39. Anthonisen P, Holst E, Thomsen AA. Determination of cardiac output and other hemodynamic data in patients with hyper- and hypothyroidism, using dye dilution technique. *Scand J Clin Lab Invest*. 1960;12:472–480.

40. Stahatos N, Wartofsky L. Perioperative management of patients with hypothyroidism. *Endocrinol Metab Clin North Am*. 2003;32:503–518.

41. DeRubertis Jr FR, Michelis MF, Bloom ME, et al. Impaired water excretion in myxedema. *Am J Med*. 1971;51:41–53.

42. Bastenie PA. Paralytic ileus in severe hypothyroidism. *Lancet*. 1946;1:413–416.

43. Ladenson PW, Levin AA, Ridgeway EC, Daniels GH. Complications of surgery in hypothyroid patients. *Am J Med*. 1984;77:261–266.

44. Hill N, Fatoba S, Oke J, et al. Global prevalence of chronic kidney disease – a systematic review and meta-analysis. *PloS One*. 2016;11(7):e0158765.

45. Craig RGR, Hunter JMJ. Recent developments in the perioperative management of adult patients with chronic kidney disease. *Br J Anaesth*. 2008;101:296–310.

46. 2012 KDIGO clinical practice guideline for the evaluation and management of CKD.

47. US Renal Data System USRDS 2007 Annual Data Report: Atlas of Chronic Kidney Disease and End-Stage Renal Disease in the United States. Bethesda, MD. National Institutes of Health, National Institute of Diabetes and Digestive and Kidney Diseases, 2007.

48. Pivalizza EG, Abramson DC, Harvey A. Perioperative hypercoagulability in uraemic patients: a viscoelastic study. *J Clin Anesth*. 1997;9:442–445.

49. Obrador GT, Pereira BJ. Systemic complications of chronic kidney disease. Pinpointing clinical manifestations and best management. *Postgrad Med*. 2002;111:115–122.

50. Kato S, Chmielewski M, Honda H, et al. Aspects of immune dysfunction in end-stage renal disease. *Clin J Am Soc Nephrol*. 2008;3(5):1526–1533.

51. Kluger MT, Gale S, Plummer JL, et al. Peri-operative drug prescribing pattern and manufacturers' guidelines. An audit. *Anaesthesia*. 1991;46(6):456–459.

52. Guenaga KF, Matos D, Castro AA, Atallah AN, Wille-Jorgensen P. Mechanical bowel preparation for elective colorectal surgery. *Cochrane Database Syst Rev*. 2003;(2):CD001544.

53. Snowden CP, Prentis JM, Anderson HL, et al. Submaximal cardiopulmonary exercise testing predicts complications and hospital length of stay in patients undergoing major elective surgery. *Ann Surg*. 2010;251:535–541.

54. Older P, Hall A, Hader R. Cardiopulmonary exercise testing as a screening test for perioperative management of major surgery in the elderly. *Chest*. 1999;116:355–362.

55. Wilson RJT, Davies S, Yates D, et al. Impaired functional capacity is associated with all-cause mortality after major elective intra-abdominal surgery. *Br J Anaesth*. 2010;205:297–303.

56. Hennis PJ, Meale PM, Hurst R, et al. Cardiopulmonary exercise testing predicts postoperative outcome in patients undergoing gastric bypass surgery. *Br J Anaesth*. 2012;109:566–571.

57. Carlisle J, Swart M. Mid-term survival after abdominal aortic aneurysm surgery predicted by cardiopulmonary exercise testing. *Br J Surg*. 2007;94:966–969.

58. Forshaw MJ, Strauss DC, Davies AR, et al. Is cardiopulmonary exercise testing a useful test before esophagectomy? *Ann Thorac Surg*. 2008;85:294–299.

59. Nagamatsu Y, Shima I, Yamana H, et al. Preoperative evaluation of cardiopulmonary reserve with the use of expired gas analysis during exercise testing in patients with squamous cell carcinoma of the thoracic esophagus. *J Thorac Cardiovasc Surg*. 2001;121:1064–1068.

60. Etzioni DA, Liu JH, Maggard MA, Ko CY. The aging population and its impact on the surgery workforce. *Ann Surg*. 2003;238:170–177.

61. Office of National Statistics. Population; Ageing; 2008. Available from http://www.statistics.gov.uk/cci/nugget.asp?id=949.

62. Hamel MB, Henderson WG, Khuri SF, et al. Surgical outcomes for patients aged 80 and older: morbidity and mortality from major noncardiac surgery. *J Am Geriatr Soc*. 2005;53:424–429.

63. Leung JM, Dzankic S. Relative importance of preoperative health status versus intraoperative factors in predicting postoperative adverse outcomes in geriatric surgical patients. *J Am Geriatr Soc*. 2001;49(8):1080–1085.

64. Selb C, Rochefor H, Chomsky-Higgins K. Association of patient frailty with increased morbidity after common ambulatory general surgery operations. *JAMA Surg*. 2017;153(2):160–168.

65. Fried LP, Tangen CM, Walston J, et al. Frailty in older adults: evidence for a phenotype. *J Gerontol Series A*. 2001;56(3):M146–156.

66. Rockwood K, Mitnitski A. Frailty in relation to the accumulation of deficits. *J Gerontol A Biol Sci Med Sci*. 2007;62(7):722–727.

67. Meyers B, Al-Shamsi H, Raks S, et al. Utility of the Edmonton Frail Scale in identifying frail elderly patients during treatment of colorectal cancer. *J Gastrointest Oncol*. 2017;8(1):32–38.

68. Dasgupta M, Rolfson DB, Stolee P, et al. Frailty is associated with postoperative complications in older adults with medical problems. *Arch Gerontol Geriatr*. 2009;48:78–83.

69. Partridge JSL, Harari D, Martin FC, et al. The impact of preoperative comprehensive geriatric assessment on postoperative outcomes in older patients undergoing scheduled surgery: a systematic review. *Anaesthesia*. 2014;69:8–16.

70. Harari D, Hopper A, Dhesi J, et al. Proactive care of older people undergoing surgery ('POPS'): designing, embedding, evaluating and funding a comprehensive geriatric assessment service for older elective surgical patients. *Age Ageing*. 2007;36:190–196.

71. Moonesinghe SR, Mythen M, Das P, et al. Risk stratification tools for predicting morbidity and mortality in adult patients undergoing major surgery. *Anesthesiology*. 2013;119:959–981.

72. Sathiyakumar V, Molina CS, Thakore RV, et al. ASA score as a predictor of 30-day perioperative readmission in patients with orthopaedic trauma injuries: an NSQIP analysis. *J Orthop Trauma*. 2015;29(3):e127–132.

73. Mak PH, Campbell RC, Irwin MG. The ASA Physical Status classification: inter-observer consistency. *Am Soc Anesthesiol Anaesth Intensive Care*. 2002;30(5):633–640.

74. Protopapa KL, Simpson JC, Smith NCE, Moonesinghe SR. Development and validation of the Surgical Outcome Risk Tool (SORT). *Br J Surg*. 2014;101:1774–1783.

75. Shuhaiber JH, Hankins M, Robless P, Whitehead SM. Comparison of POSSUM with P-POSSUM for prediction of mortality in infrarenal abdominal aortic aneurysm repair. *Annal Vascu Surg*. 2002;16(6):736–741.

76. Tekkis PP, Kessaris N, Kocher HM, Poloniecki JD, Lyttle J, Windsor AC. Evaluation of POSSUM and P-POSSUM scoring systems in patients undergoing colorectal surgery. *Br J Surg.* 2003;90(3):340–345.

77. Jhanji S, Thomas B, Ely A, Watson D, Hinds CJ, Pearse RM. Mortality and utilisation of critical care resources amongst high-risk surgical patients in a large NHS trust. *Anaesthesia.* 2008;63(7):695–700.

78. Association of Surgeons of Great Britain and Ireland. *Emergency General Surgery: The future.* A consensus statement June 2007. Available from: https://www.asgbi.org.uk/publications/consensus-statements.

79. The Higher Risk General Surgical Patient. Towards Improved Care For a Forgotten Group. The Royal College of Surgeons England, 2011. Available from: https://www.rcseng.ac.uk/library-and-publications/rcs-publications/docs/the-higher-risk-general-surgical-patient/.

80. Barry M, Edgman-Levitan S. Shared decision making- the pinnacle of patient-centred care. *N Engl J Med.* 2012;366:780–781.

81. Santhirapala R, Moonesinghe R. Primum non nocere: Is shared decision-making the answer? *Perioperat Med.* 2016;5:16.

82. Scheibler F, Janssen C, Pfaff H. Shared decision making: an overview of international research literature. *Soz Praventivmed.* 2003;48(1):11–23.

83. Whelan T, Levine M, Willan A. Effect of a decision aid on knowledge and treatment decision making for breast cancer surgery. *JAMA.* 2004;292(4):435–441.

84. Moran J, Guinan E, McCormick P, et al. The ability of prehabilitation to influence postoperative outcome after intra-abdominal operation: a systematic review and meta-analysis. *Surgery.* 2016;160(5):1189–1201.

85. West M, Wischmeyer P, Grocott M. Prehabilitation and nutritional support to improve perioperative outcomes. *Curr Anesthesiol Rep.* 2017;7:340–349.

86. Burden S, Todd C, Hill J, Lal S. Pre-operative nutrition support in patients undergoing gastrointestinal surgery. *Cochrane Database Syst Rev England.* 2012;11:CD008879.

87. Wischmeyer P, Carli F, Evans D, et al. American Society for Enhanced Recovery (ASER) and Perioperative Quality Initiative 2 (POQI 2) joint consensus statement on nutrition screening and therapy within a surgical enhanced recovery pathway. *Anesth Analg.* 2018;127(5):e95.

88. Haynes A, Weiser T, Berry W, et al. A surgical safety checklist to reduce morbidity and mortality in a global population. *N Engl J Med.* 2009;360:491–499.

89. Fudickar A, Horle K, Wiltfang J, Bein B. The effect of the WHO surgical safety checklist on complication rate and communication. *Dtsch Arztebl Int.* 2012;109(42):695–701.

90. Papaspyros SC, Javangula KC, Adluri RK, O'Regan DJ. Briefing and debriefing in the cardiac operating room. Analysis of impact on theatre team attitude and patient safety. *Interact Cardiovasc Thorac Surg.* 2010;10(1):43–47.

91. Kozek-Langenecker S, Ahmed A, Afshari A. Management of severe perioperative bleeding: guidelines from the European Society of Anaesthesiology. *Eur J Anaesthesiol.* 2017;34:332–395.

92. Klein A, Arnold PI, Bingham RM. AAGBI: use of blood components and alternatives. *Anaesthesia.* 2016;71(7):829–842.

93. Carson JL, Carless PA, Hebert PC, et al. Transfusion thresholds and other strategies for guiding allogeneic red blood cell transfusion (Review). *Cochrane Database Syst Rev.* 2012;4(4):CD002042.

94. NICE Guideline NG 24. *Blood transfusion.* National Institute for Clinical Excellence, 2015.

95. Perel P, Prieto-Merino D, Shakur H, et al. Predicting early death in patients with traumatic bleeding: development and validation of a prognostic model. *BMJ.* 2012;345:E5166.

96. Saving Lives, Improving Mothers' Care. Knight M, Nair M, Tuffnell D et al. MBRRACE-UK, December 2017.

97. American Society of Anesthesiologists Task Force on Perioperative Blood Transfusion and Adjuvant Therapies. Practice guidelines for perioperative blood transfusion and adjuvant therapies: an updated report. *Anesthesiology.* 2006;105:198–208.

98. Bickell WH, Wall Jr MJ, Pepe PE, et al. Immediate versus delayed fluid resuscitation for hypotensive patients with penetrating torso injuries. *N Engl J Med.* 1994;331:1105–1109.

99. Blair SD, Janvrin SB, McCollum CN, Greenhalgh RM. Effect of early blood transfusion on gastrointestinal haemorrhage. *Br J Surg.* 1986;73:783–785.

100. Crawford JS. Ruptured aortic aneurysm. *J Vasc Surg.* 1991;13:348–350.

101. Kirkman E, Watts S, Cooper G. Blast injury research models. *Philos Trans R Soc Lond B Biol Sci.* 2011;366:144–159.

102. Holcomb J, Tilley B, Baraniuk S, et al. Transfusion of plasma, platelets, and red blood cells in a 1:1:1 vs a 1:1:2 ratio and mortality in patients with severe trauma. The PROPPR randomized clinical trial. *JAMA.* 2015;313(5):471–482.

103. Andreae MH, Andreae DA. Regional anaesthesia to prevent chronic pain after surgery: a Cochrane systematic review and meta-analysis. *Br J Anaesth.* 2013;111(5):711–720.

104. Ankcorn C, Casey W. Spinal anaesthesia - a practical guide. Update in Anaesthesia. Accessed from http://e-safe-anaesthesia.org/e_library/07/Spinal_anaesthesia_a_practical_guide_Update_2000.pdf.

105. Abrahams MS, Aziz MF, Fu RF. Ultrasound guidance compared with electrical neurostimulation for peripheral nerve block: a systematic review and meta-analysis of randomized control trials. *Br J Anaesth.* 2009;102(3):08–17

106. Khetarpal R, Kataria A, Bajaj S, et al. Gabapentin vs pregabalin as a premedication in orthopaedic surgery under combined spinal epidural technique. *Anesth Essays Res.* 2016;10(2):262–267.

107. Straube S, Derry S, Moore RA, et al. Single dose oral gabapentin for established acute postoperative pain in adults. *Cochrane Database Syst Rev.* 2010; 2010(5);CD008183.

108. Pearse RM, Harrison DA, MacDonald N, et al. Effect of a perioperative, cardiac output-guided hemodynamic therapy algorithm on outcomes following major gastrointestinal surgery: a randomized clinical trial and systematic review. *JAMA.* 2014;311(21):2181–2190.

109. Grocott MP, Dushianthan A, Hamilton MA, et al. Perioperative increase in global blood flow to explicit defined goals and outcomes after surgery: a Cochrane Systematic Review. *Br J Anaesth.* 2013;111(4):535–548.

110. Duggan M, Kavanagh BP. Pulmonary atelectasis: a pathogenic perioperative entity. *Anesthesiology.* 2005;31:1327–1335.

111. Jaber S, Coisel Y, Chanques G, et al. A multicentre observational study of intraoperative ventilator management during general anaesthesia; tidal volumes and relation to body weight. *Anaesthesia.* 2012;67:999–1008.

112. Plowman R, Graves N, Griffin M, et al. *The socio-economic burden of hospital-acquired infection.* Public Health Laboratory Service, London, 2000.

113. NICE Guideline CG74. *Surgical site infections: prevention and treatment.* Nation Institute of Healthcare Excellence, 2008.

114. SIGN 104. *Antibiotic prophylaxis in surgery.* Scottish Intercollegiate Guidelines Network, Edinburgh 2004.
115. Frank SM, Fleisher LA, Breslow MJ, et al. Perioperative maintenance of normothermia reduces the incidence of morbid cardiac events. A randomized clinical trial. *JAMA.* 1997;277(14):1127–1134.
116. Rajagopalan S, Mascha E, Na J, et al. The effects of mild perioperative hypothermia of blood loss and transfusion requirement. *Anesthesiology.* 2008;108(1):71–77.
117. Barie PS. Surgical site infections: epidemiology and prevention. *Surg Infect (Larchmt).* 2002;S9–21.
118. Yi J, Lei YJ, Xu S, et al. Intraoperative hypothermia and its clinical outcomes in patients undergoing general anaesthesia: national study in China. *PLoS One.* 2017;12(6):e0177221.
119. NICE Guideline CG65. *Hypothermia: Prevention and Management in Adults Having Surgery.* National Institute for Clinical Excellence, 2008.
120. *Demographics, Epidemiology, and Risk of VTE.* Department of Health e-learning for Healthcare. www.e-lfh.org.uk.
121. Molenaar N, Bijkerk RM, Beishuizen A, et al. Steroidogenesis in the adrenal dysfunction of critical illness: impact of etomidate. *Crit Care.* 2012;16(4):R121.
122. Chan CM, Mitchell AL, Shorr AF. Etomidate is associated with mortality and adrenal insufficiency in sepsis: a meta-analysis. *Crit Care Med.* 2012;40(11):2945–2953.
123. Fearon KC, Ljungqvist O, Von Meyenfeldt M, et al. Enhanced recovery after surgery: a consensus review of clinical care for patients undergoing colonic resection. *Clin Nutr.* 2005;24:466–477.
124. Luettel D, Beaumont K, Healey F. *Recognising and Responding Appropriately to Early Signs of Deterioration in Hospitalised Patients.* National Patient Safety Agency, London, 2007.
125. British Thoracic Society/Intensive Care Society guidelines for the ventilator management of acute hypercapnic respiratory failure in adults. *Thorax.* 2016;71:S2.
126. Horan TC, Gaynes RP, Martone WJ, et al. CDC definitions of nosocomial surgical site infections, 1992: a modification of CDC definitions of surgical wound infections. *Infect Control Hosp Epidemiol.* 1992;13:606–608.
127. Singer M, Deutschman CS, Seymour CW, et al. The Third International Consensus definitions for sepsis and septic shock (Sepsis-3). *JAMA.* 2016;315(8):801–810.
128. Churpek MM, Zadravecz FJ, Winslow C, et al. Incidence and prognostic value of the systemic inflammatory response syndrome and organ dysfunctions in ward patients. *Am J Respir Crit Care Med.* 2015;192(8):958–964.
129. Kaukonen KM, Bailey M, Pilcher D, et al. Systemic inflammatory response syndrome criteria in defining severe sepsis. *N Engl J Med.* 2015;372(17):1629–1638.
130. British Thoracic Society guidelines for the management of suspected acute pulmonary embolism. *Thorax.* 2003;58:470–484.
131. Botto F, Alonso-Coello P, Chan MT, et al. Myocardial injury after noncardiac surgery: a large, international, prospective cohort study establishing diagnostic criteria, characteristics, predictors, and 30-day outcomes. *Anesthesiology.* 2014;120(3):564–578.
132. *Diagnostic and Statistical Manual of Mental Disorders-IV.* American Psychiatric Association, Washington, DC, 2000.
133. Hosker C. Hypoactive delirium. *BMJ.* 2017;357:j2047.
134. Rudolph JL, Inouye SK, Jones RN, et al. Delirium: an independent predictor of functional decline after cardiac surgery. *J Am Geriatr Soc.* 2010;58(4):643–649.
135. González M, Martínez G, Calderón J. Impact of delirium on short-term mortality in elderly inpatients: a prospective cohort study. *Psychosomatics.* 2009;50(3):234–238.
136. Wong CL, Holroyd-Leduc J, Simel DL. Does this patient have delirium?: value of bedside instruments. *JAMA.* 2010;304(7):779–786.
137. Thakar CV. Perioperative acute kidney injury. *Adv Chronic Kidney Dis.* 2013;20(1):67–75.
138. Kellum JA, Sileanu FE, Murugan R, et al. Classifying AKI by urine output versus serum creatinine level. *J Am Soc Nephrol.* 2015;26(9):2231–2238.
139. NICE Guideline CG 169. Acute Kidney Injury: Prevention, Detection and Management. National Institute for Clinical Excellence, 2013.
140. Hastings PR, Skillman JJ, Bushnell LS, et al. Antacid titration in the prevention of acute gastrointestinal bleeding. *N Engl J Med.* 1978;298:1041–1045.
141. Alhazzani W, Alenezi F, Jaeschke RZ, et al. Proton pump inhibitors versus histamine 2 receptor antagonists for stress ulcer prophylaxis in critically ill patients: a systematic review and meta-analysis. *Crit Care Med.* 2013;41:693–705.
142. Bonten MJ, Gaillard CA, van Tiel FH, et al. Continuous enteral feeding counteracts preventive measures for gastric colonization in intensive care unit patients. *Crit Care Med.* 1994;22(6):939–944.

9

Principles of Paediatric Surgery

CHAPTER OUTLINE

General Principles

What is Paediatric Surgery?

Paediatric surgery involves a broad range of bodily systems and is the only surgical specialty defined by the age of the patient as well as the surgical condition. Patients range from children as young as 24 weeks premature weighing only 500 g up to late adolescence.

Assessing the Paediatric Surgical Patient

As with other branches of surgery and medicine, the management of a paediatric surgical patient is fundamentally based on the ability to take an accurate history and perform a thorough clinical examination. Challenges lie in our patients who, unlike adults, are often unable and sometimes unwilling to allow such a process. History must often be extracted from those involved in the primary care of the child and examination techniques require skill and carefully applied strategies that develop with experience.

What are the Main Differences Between Adult Surgery and Paediatric Surgery?

- Surgical pathology is often related to congenital or inherited disorders as opposed to acquired conditions seen in adults, such as atherosclerosis.
- Age-dependent physiological differences such as heart rate and blood pressure must be considered during assessment.
- Individual fluid and drug regimens are necessary as they are weight-dependent.
- Children rely on the consent of others, usually parents, for permission to perform surgical procedures that they may require.
- The low incidence of many surgical conditions results in the transfer of many patients to regional centres for specialized anaesthetic and surgical management.

Approach to a Seriously Ill Child

Recognition, rapid assessment and appropriate resuscitation of the seriously ill child is an important skill for any doctor involved in the care of children. Primary assessment should follow the Airway Breathing Circulation Disability Exposure (ABCDE) approach using Advanced Paediatric Life Support principles. Resuscitation should happen concurrently during the rapid clinical assessment of airway, breathing and circulation. Intravenous fluid and pharmacotherapy is weight-based and each child must be considered on an individual basis. Once the patient's condition has been stabilized, secondary assessment and investigations looking for illness-specific pathophysiology and further treatment can be instituted.

The most common presentation to the surgical team of a seriously ill child is with an acute abdomen. Intra-abdominal pathology tends to cause non-haemorrhagic fluid loss and can result in hypovolaemic shock. Younger infants are more likely to present with shock due to rapid fluid shifts and because they have a lower physiological reserve compared to older children. Tachycardia is often the first sign of shock, occurring in order to compensate for the decreased stroke volume. Generally, children compensate well for significant fluid changes, therefore hypotension is a late sign suggestive of imminent circulatory failure. The key is to identify early warning signs and fluid resuscitate appropriately, usually starting with a 20 mL/kg fluid bolus, followed by re-assessment.

Principles of Neonatal and Paediatric Transfer to a Specialist Centre

The priorities in care during transfer are:
- temperature control
- nasogastric intubation to keep the stomach empty
- airway protection, e.g. pharyngeal suction for oesophageal atresia (see below) and assisted ventilation via endotracheal tube for respiratory insufficiency
- cardiorespiratory monitoring of pulse rate and oxygen saturation
- intravenous fluids – to provide glucose and sodium; water overload must be avoided; fluid requirements are determined by the infant's age and weight (Table 9.1)

Temperature

Hypothermia is minimized by the use of an incubator and a warming mattress and by an overhead heater in the operating theatre and anaesthetic room. The extremities are wrapped and the infant nursed in warm cotton wool covered by gauze (Gamgee), exposing only the operating field. Covering the abdomen with clear adhesive film decreases convection losses even further. Sick infants may be transferred between hospitals in a transport incubator with other support as detailed below.

Nasogastric Intubation

Whenever intestinal obstruction is suspected, a nasogastric tube large enough to keep the stomach empty (8–10 Fr) is essential to minimize the risk of aspiration of gastric contents into the respiratory tract. This should be kept on free drainage and regularly aspirated.

Cardiorespiratory Monitoring

Pulse rate and arterial oxygen saturation are sensitive indicators of how the infant is responding to the stresses of illness. Continuous records help to adjust respiratory support and fluid and electrolyte replacement.

Fluid and Electrolyte Replacement

To avoid hyponatremia, this is best given as 0.9% saline with 5–10% glucose with 10 mmol of potassium added to each 500-mL bag. Close monitoring of serum electrolytes allows for volume adjustment. Maintenance fluid of 0.45% saline is acceptable though still hypotonic and must be considered in accordance with the physiological status of the patient. If the child is within the neonatal period (<44 weeks post conception), then a more accurate calculation of daily electrolyte requirement is required according to current serum levels. Any additional losses, such as stoma or drain fluid, must also be taken into account. Babies who require phototherapy for hyperbilirubinaemia need 20% extra fluid because of increased insensible loss through the skin. The infant and older child's daily fluid requirements must also be calculated according to weight (Table 9.2).

Intravenous Nutrition

If enteral feeding is not possible within 7 days of birth, parenteral nutrition (PN) is indicated for mature babies but at a younger age for premature and small-for-dates babies as they are born with very low calorie stores of glycogen and fat.

PN should also be considered in any child where enteral feeding is not possible for a period of greater than 5 days. Peripheral administration is not suitable for the hypertonic solutions used in PN, and central venous catheters are recommended.

Principles of Vascular Access in Children

Vascular access can be divided into short-term (up to 1 month) and long-term options (more than 1 month). Types of access can also be categorized depending on whether the placement of the catheter tip is in a peripheral vein or a central vein (Table 9.3). Short-term peripheral access tends to be used for intravenous fluids or medications, whereas central access can additionally be used for PN administration, CVP monitoring, vasopressors or haemodialysis. Long-term central access

TABLE 9.1 Fluids During First Week of Life

Day of Life	Fluids (mL/kg per day)
Day 1, 2	60
Day 3, 4	90
Day 5, 6	120
Day 7+	150

TABLE 9.2 Guide to Fluid Maintenance Volume in the Infant and Child According to Weight

3–10 kg	100 mL/kg per day (4 mL/kg per h)
10–20 kg	1000 mL/day + 50 mL/weight in kg less 10/day (40 mL/h + 2 mL/weight in kg less 10/h)
>20 kg	1500 mL/day + 25 mL/weight in kg less 20/day (60 mL/h + 1 mL/weight in kg less 20/h)

TABLE 9.3 Options for Vascular Access in Children and Their Advantages and Disadvantages

Type of Access	Venous Placement	Length of Use	Advantages	Disadvantages
Cannula	Peripheral	Up to 4 days	Do not require sedation Low risk for complications	Short-term use only
Midline catheter	Peripheral	Up to 28 days	May not require sedation Low risk for complications	Can be difficult to place in infants
Non-tunnelled central venous catheter	Central	7–14 days	Can be used for caustic medications/parenteral nutrition Central monitoring	Need general anaesthetic (GA) for insertion Complications associated with insertion
Peripherally inserted central catheter (PICC)	Central	1–6 months	May not require GA Low-risk of complications at insertion	Need frequent flushes and dressing changes
Tunnelled central venous catheter	Central	1–2 years or more	No limitation on activities (except swimming) Can be double lumen	Need GA for insertion +/– removal No swimming
Implantable port-a-cath	Central	1–2 years or more	No dressings No limitation on activities	Need GA for insertion and removal Single lumen Needle to access

becomes necessary for long-term intravenous medications, PN or chemotherapy, or for repeated courses of intravenous medications, blood transfusions and blood sampling.

Achieving vascular access can be particularly challenging in children. Smaller vessels often make all types of access technically more difficult. Additionally, younger children are unlikely to tolerate procedures, other than peripheral cannula insertion, without sedation and often require general anaesthetic for central vascular access. Given these challenges, it is important to think about the need for access early during the clinical course and choose the most appropriate type depending on the specific requirement for each patient.

Complications

Vascular access in children is not without significant risk and as many as one in four devices will fail prior to completion of treatment. Complications of use include infection, displacement, blockage, extravasation and thrombosis. Additionally, insertion of centrally placed devices in the neck, especially in small infants and neonates, carries risk of pneumothorax, haemothorax and, rarely, arrhythmias and right atrial perforation.

Infection in the Newborn

Infection is a constant risk for the newborn patient and increases with prematurity. Intensive care and surgical procedures add to that risk and broad-spectrum antibiotic cover is required. Which antibiotic is often determined by the incidence of local resistance. Sepsis may be indicated from temperature instability (high or low), tachycardia or bradycardia, as well as high or low white blood cell levels. A rising C-reactive protein (CRP) is often a useful marker and microbiological cultures are routinely taken to assist in therapy.

Prenatal Diagnosis and Fetal Therapy

Evidence for the effectiveness of many fetal surgical interventions is constantly under evaluation. There are currently three methods of surgical access for a prenatally diagnosed anomaly: ultrasound-guided shunt placement into the chest or bladder of an affected fetus; open uterine surgery, which carries a high risk of abortion; and the more minimally invasive fetoscopic approach.

Fetuses with conditions such as congenital diaphragmatic hernia or bladder outflow obstruction secondary to urethral valves, which are considered to have a very poor prognosis, may undergo such interventions. The procedures require a careful evaluation of the risks to the mother and child, as well as the potential benefit to the child.

Prenatal diagnosis allows for the appropriate counselling for many surgical conditions and, in some cases, prompts further investigations such as chromosomal studies to be performed. Some conditions such as gastroschisis have been shown to have survival advantages if the mother is transferred prior to delivery to a centre with paediatric surgery on site.

Surgical Pathology in Children

Appendicitis in the Paediatric Patient

Acute appendicitis is, by far, the most common surgical cause of an acute abdomen in children, accounting for more than 80% of emergency operations performed for abdominal pain. Approximately 10% of the population will develop appendicitis during their lifetime, with the peak incidence occurring in the second decade of life.

Clinical Features

The clinical diagnosis remains challenging, with only half of patients displaying the typical clinical features of right iliac fossa pain and tenderness and gastrointestinal upset with nausea, vomiting or anorexia. The presentation varies depending on the pathological progression of the disease and the age of the child. Although appendicitis is less common in younger children, clinical assessment can be particularly challenging as young children and infants may be unable to localize the pain and can be uncooperative with clinical examination. Children aged under 5 years of age have a significantly higher risk of perforation at presentation.

Common differential diagnoses include gastroenteritis, mesenteric adenitis, lower respiratory tract infections, urinary tract infections, constipation, non-specific abdominal pain and ovarian pathology in girls.

Investigations

Useful investigations include blood tests, specifically inflammatory markers, such as C-reactive protein and white blood cell count, and radiology. Significantly raised inflammatory markers, although non-specific, increases suspicion of appendicitis. However, when normal, do not exclude appendicitis especially in the context of a short clinical history. First-line imaging is usually with ultrasound, with CT reserved for cases where diagnostic uncertainty remains due to concerns about high dose radiation in children. Ultrasound imaging is user-dependent and often equivocal. Although, ultrasound may demonstrate ancillary features suggestive of intra-abdominal pathology, such as free fluid, thickened, non-peristalsing bowel loops in the right iliac fossa and occasionally can positively identify an inflamed appendix. A normal ultrasound scan may be reassuring depending on the clinical picture.

Management

Appendicectomy remains the mainstay of management for acute appendicitis in children, along with appropriate antibiotics, similarly to adults. The approach of choice is usually laparoscopic. However, in younger children, especially those with associated small bowel dilatation secondary to ileus, this may be particularly challenging due to limited space and therefore an open approach should be considered. Current guidelines suggest that children under 5 years of age should be managed at a specialist paediatric surgery centre.

Conditions Presenting with Respiratory Distress

Oesophageal Atresia with Tracheo-Oesophageal Fistula

Oesophageal atresia affects 1 in 3000 births in the UK and is a condition where the upper and lower parts of the

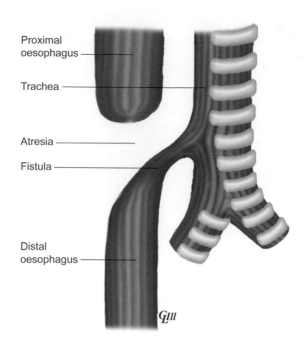

• **Fig. 9.1** Common Variant of Oesophageal Atresia and Tracheo-Oesophageal Fistula

oesophagus are not connected. Instead, the upper part of the oesophagus is blind ending and the lower part is attached to the trachea and referred to as a tracheo-oesophageal fistula (Fig. 9.1).

There are other presentations with or without the fistula which are less common. Fifty percent of infants born with this condition have other associated defects of the heart, renal or skeletal system.

Clinical Features

Prenatal polyhydramnios occurs in half of affected infants because the fetus cannot swallow the amniotic fluid. At birth, this is seen as an inability to swallow secretions and bubbling at the mouth is common.

Investigation

An inability to pass a nasogastric tube as well as a chest X-ray demonstrating the coiled tube in the upper oesophageal pouch. The presence of a fistula connecting to the stomach can be confirmed if gas is seen in the distal bowel on X-ray.

Echocardiography is usually performed on all these children preoperatively to look for cardiac defects and aortic arch position.

Management

Protection of the airway is paramount and achieved by suctioning of the upper pouch. If possible, ventilation is to be avoided. Transfer to a unit with surgical expertise can then occur.

Surgery involves ligation of the fistula and anastomosis to the upper pouch through a thoracotomy. If the gap between the two oesophageal ends is too long, then a gastrostomy is sited and a staged procedure occurs. If the gap is still too long for an oesophageal anastomosis, then a substitute of either stomach, small bowel or colon is used. A thoraco-scopic approach is also possible.

Prognosis

The long-term survival for the majority is excellent. Those born with a low birth weight and cardiac anomalies have a poor prognosis.

Complications commonly encountered are a result of scarring at the anastomosis and up to one-third of patients will require an endoscopic dilatation.

Congenital Diaphragmatic Hernia

Congenital diaphragmatic hernia occurs in 1 in 2500 births in the UK. The defect usually occurs in the left posterolateral aspect of the diaphragm, though the entire diaphragm may be missing. Bowel within the chest is often seen on the ante-natal ultrasound scan. Pulmonary hypoplasia is a common feature, as are associated anomalies such as cardiac defects.

Clinical Features

The infant often has respiratory distress at birth which requires ventilation.

Patients may also present outside of the neonatal period with recurrent chest infections, intestinal obstruction, or bowel ischaemia or necrosis following intestinal volvulus.

Investigation

A chest and abdominal X-ray usually reveal the condition (Fig. 9.2). Congenital lung cysts are a differential but excluded by the absence of gas on the abdominal X-ray. Gastrointestinal contrast studies can be used for difficult cases.

Management

The pulmonary vascular circulation is under high pressures and stability prior to any surgery is paramount. Extracorporeal membrane oxygenation may be needed in some severe cases.

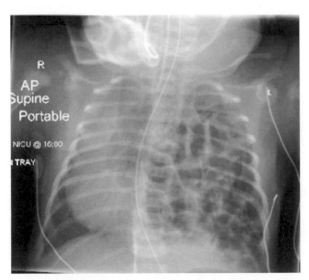

• **Fig. 9.2** Congenital Diaphragmatic Hernia

Once stable, the infant's bowel and any other viscera are reduced from the chest via a laparotomy. The defect is repaired using non-absorbable sutures primarily or by using a prosthetic patch. A thoracoscopic approach is increasingly used in many centres worldwide.

Prognosis

Overall survival for this condition is 60% but is reduced if a cardiac anomaly is present. Long-term problems are mainly related to gastro-oesophageal reflux disease and reduced pulmonary function, the latter related to the degree of pulmonary hypoplasia.

Future

In utero therapy is reserved for cases where survival is predicted as being poor. Tracheal obstruction using a small endoscopically placed intra-tracheal balloon allows for distension of the pulmonary tree and a reduced hypoplasia at birth. This technique is used in some International centres, though efficacy remains unproven.

Cervical Cystic Lymphangioma

Often referred to as cystic hygroma, this loculated lymphatic lesion can be found anywhere in the body but is often in the left posterior triangle of the neck. If large enough, it can result in tracheal compression and urgent decompression/excision is warranted. Surgery is often complex and success is reported with sclerosing these lesions if they are smaller than 5 cm.

Bilateral Choanal Atresia

This is a bony or membranous obstruction to the nasal passages at the junction of the hard and soft palates. The newborn is an obligatory nasal breather and can suffocate without the assistance of an oropharyngeal tube to maintain a patent airway.

The diagnosis is confirmed by inability to pass a nasal tube into the pharynx, and a CT scan is helpful in defining the extent of the atresia and planning operative repair, which is undertaken as soon as possible. Under a general anaesthetic, the atresia is resected transnasally using a drill. The resulting nasal airway is stented for a minimum of 6 weeks, and further resection of tissue may be required.

Micrognathia

A hypoplastic mandible causes obstruction of the pharynx by posterior prolapse of the tongue. Combination of this disorder with a cleft palate is known as the Pierre Robin syndrome. The respiratory problem is best relieved by a tracheostomy and the defects repaired at a later date.

The Newborn with Intestinal Obstruction

Unlike other surgical specialties, the clinical history of any newborn involves two people – the mother and the infant. Important features of the pregnancy such as maternal illness or polyhydramnios provide possible indicators of certain neonatal disorders.

Genetic predisposition to conditions such as Hirschsprung's disease or cystic fibrosis must also be enquired about.

Intestinal obstruction in the newborn commonly presents with either bile-stained vomiting, abdominal distension or a failure to pass stool (meconium) within 24 hours of birth. With the increasing accuracy of pre-natal ultrasound, many conditions are detected before birth. Chorionic villous sampling or amniocentesis may have been performed to look for associated chromosomal disorders.

Postnatal examination focuses on unusual or dysmorphic facial features which may indicate a chromosomal abnor-mality or a recognized syndrome, abdominal distension and tenderness, as well as normal anatomy such as the presence of a patent anus.

Duodenal Atresia/Stenosis

One in 5000 newborns has duodenal obstruction, with up to one-third having trisomy 21 (Down's syndrome), though the cause remains unknown. Theories include a failure of recanalization of the duodenum following a solid phase

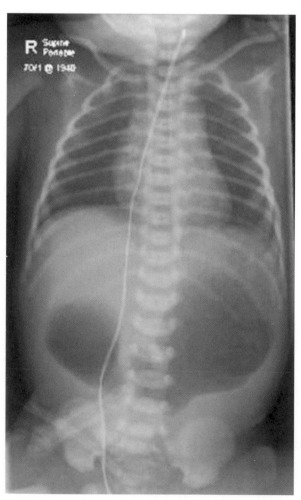

• **Fig. 9.3** 'Double bubble' X-ray

in early fetal life. Prenatally this may present with polyhy-dramnios and dilated stomach and proximal duodenum on ultrasound.

Clinical Features

Dysmorphic features may indicate the presence of trisomy 21. Obstruction may present as persistent vomiting with or without bile depending on the level of obstruction in rela-tion to the ampulla of Vater.

If a stenosis is present (a membrane with a small central opening), then the child may present later with vomiting and failure to thrive.

Investigation

Abdominal X-ray reveals two large gas-filled upper abdomi-nal structures or the 'double bubble' sign and these represent the dilated stomach and duodenum above the obstruction. The rest of the X-ray will be gasless in atresia or normal in stenosis (Fig. 9.3).

Management

Surgery involves a laparotomy to anastomose the proximal with the distal duodenum, care being taken to avoid dam-age to the ampulla. Laparoscopic repair is also feasible.

Prognosis

Feeding can take several weeks to establish in some patients but overall the prognosis is good providing no other anoma-lies are present.

Atresia of the Small and Large Bowel

More commonly seen in the ileum though can occur any-where, this interruption of intestinal continuity is thought to be due to mesenteric vascular accidents occurring dur-ing fetal life. Dilated bowel maybe seen on a prenatal ultra-sound together with polyhydramnios.

Clinical Features

Presentation depends on the level of obstruction, with infants being generally well at birth.

Investigation

Plain X-ray may reveal a 'triple bubble' sign in the case of jejunal atresia or multiple dilated bowel loops if the obstruc-tion is more distal. Contrast enema is often performed to delineate the anatomy distal to the atresia prior to any surgi-cal intervention.

Management

Laparotomy is performed with anastomosis of the proximal obstructed bowel to the distal unused segments.

Prognosis

Postoperative outcome depends on the length of bowel ana-tomically as well as functionally, with malabsorption being a significant problem for many of these children.

Malrotation with Volvulus

During fetal life, the herniated intestine is rotated clockwise through 270 degrees prior to returning to the abdominal cavity and fixing to the posterior abdominal wall. This process can be halted at any point. Disorders of rotation and fixation present numerous challenges to the paediatric surgeon.

Clinical Features

The infant often presents within the first month of life with bile-stained vomiting. The child may have a normal or scaphoid (empty) abdomen on examination. If the intestine has twisted (volvulus) and become ischaemic, the presentation is a much more urgent one with a tender distended abdomen in a shocked infant.

Investigation

Malrotation is confirmed with an upper gastrointestinal contrast study to examine the position of the duodenal-jejunal flexure. The normal position lies to the left of the midline at the level of the first lumbar vertebrae. If ischaemia is thought likely, then an urgent laparotomy is preferred with ongoing resuscitation as ischaemic changes are often irreversible after 6 hours.

Management

Laparotomy is performed to release the abnormal fixating peritoneal bands that can compress and obstruct the duodenum. The bowel is placed into a non-rotated form, thus reducing the risk of the mesentery twisting.

Prognosis

Providing sufficient bowel is maintained, prognosis is good. Long-term intravenous nutrition may be needed in severe cases.

Meconium Ileus

This condition occurs as a result of thickened impacted meconium (newborn stool) obstructing the distal ileum. It has a strong association with cystic fibrosis, which is found in up to 95% of affected infants.

Clinical Features

The terminal ileum is impacted with firm pellets of meconium, with the colon appearing very narrow and unused and often referred to as a microcolon. Prenatal perforation may take place with a sterile peritonitis and local calcification or pseudocyst formation. The infant presents with bile-stained vomiting and abdominal distension shortly after birth.

Investigation

A plain X-ray confirms distal bowel obstruction, with or without calcification from a sterile perforation. An enema using water-soluble contrast fills the empty colon and may pass through the ileocaecal valve to outline loops of ileum and the impacted meconium.

The underlying cystic fibrosis can be confirmed by the detection of one of the specific defective genes found on chromosome 7 or by the finding of elevated levels of immunoreactive trypsin in the blood.

Management

The high osmolality of the gastrografin enema may be successful in up to 50% of cases. A hydroscopic effect draws water into the bowel and assists in evacuation.

If unsuccessful, then a laparotomy, with or without a stoma, is used to decompress the ileum. The introduction of feeds postoperatively should include pancreatic enzymes to facilitate the digestion and absorption of fats.

Prognosis

Following initial impaction, further occurrences can take place throughout childhood, though usually only if compliance with medication is poor.

Hirschsprung's Disease

Congenital aganglionosis of the bowel is referred to as Hirschsprung's disease and occurs in 1 in 5000 births in the UK. Cholinergic ganglia in the myenteric plexus play an important role in the relaxation phase of normal intestinal peristalsis. The failure to relax due to the absence of ganglion cells results in a functional bowel obstruction. The aganglionic segment of bowel extends from the rectum a variable distance proximally. The cause of Hirschsprung's disease is still unclear, though is thought to be an arrest of the neural crest cell migration. A genetic role has been identified in several chromosomal disorders.

Clinical Features

Abdominal distension and failure to pass meconium within the first 24–48 hours of birth are the most common presenting features. The most frequently affected area is the rectosigmoid colon which presents as a distal bowel obstruction. Rectal examination may result in an explosive passage of stool. Death can occur if severe inflammation of the proximal bowel or enterocolitis is the presenting feature.

Investigation

Plain abdominal X-ray may reveal multiple dilated large loops of bowel and the diagnosis is confirmed with a rectal biopsy which shows increased staining for anticholinesterase throughout the muscularis mucosa and lamina propria. Contrast enema may further assist in the diagnosis. Failure of relaxation of the internal anal sphincter on manometry is diagnostic.

Management

Therapy begins with administration of broad-spectrum antibiotics and urgent decompression of the obstructed large bowel. Initially this involves regular rectal washouts. If unsuccessful, then surgical decompression is indicated in the form of stoma.

Definitive surgery involves using ganglionic bowel to replace the aganglionic segment.

Prognosis

Constipation and soiling can occur in up to one-third of children up to early adolescence but long-term outcome appears good. Early mortality occurs in up to 5–10% and is related to delayed treatment of enterocolitis.

Anorectal Anomalies

Perineal inspection at birth is an important aspect of newborn examination. The absence of a patent anus is occasionally overlooked and can result in bowel perforation.

Clinical Features

In males, this may present as a skin-covered anus or a fistula on the perineum (Fig. 9.4). Higher lesions can result in the rectum connecting to the urethra or bladder. In females, meconium may be seen to exit from the introitus or, more rarely, from the vagina.

A more severe form in females is called a cloaca (Greek for sewer) – there is a combined urogenital tract where the urethra, vagina and rectum fuse distally to form a common channel.

Investigation

Ultrasound or prone invertograms (X-ray with infant lying on its abdomen with pelvic elevation) are used by many surgeons to detect the distance of the anal canal from the perineum. Preoperative investigations such as echocardiography may also be necessary as this condition may be associated with cardiac and other defects.

Knowledge of the VACTERL (Vertebral, Anorectal, Cardiac, Tracheo-oesophageal, Esophagus, Renal and Limb) complex of associated birth defects assists in the exclusion of other often associated anomalies in these patients.

Management

Surgery involves reconstruction of the anal canal. If a high lesion is present, then a staged procedure is performed. An initial split sigmoid colostomy is fashioned (as described

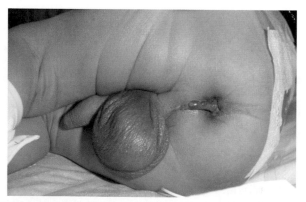

• **Fig. 9.4** Anorectal Anomaly Showing Closed Anus with a Perineal Fistula (Low Type)

by Wilkins and Pena), followed by preoperative imaging to determine any possible connection of the anal canal to the lower urinary tract. If the lesion is low, then a primary anal reconstruction is often possible.

Prognosis

This depends on the degree of continence and is ultimately related to the level of the initial defect.

Neonatal Necrotizing Enterocolitis (NEC)

Inflammation and necrosis of the intestinal wall or necrotizing enterocolitis, affecting the small or large bowel, is the most common neonatal intestinal emergency, affecting 1 in 1000 infants in the UK. The cause is not fully understood but is related to prematurity and feeding.

The risk of developing the condition decreases with increasing gestational age, suggesting an immature gut does play a role. Infection is found in up to one-third of patients, though it is unclear if this is a primary or secondary event.

Clinical Features

Systemic infection in neonates is indicated by apnoea, bradycardia, lethargy, fluctuating body temperatures and a low blood sugar together with a failure to absorb gastric feeds. These may also be the initial clinical findings in NEC. Abdominal distension then progresses to tenderness and erythema of the abdominal wall and often a passage of loose stools with blood.

Investigation

Abdominal X-ray often demonstrates dilated loops of bowel, with intramural gas (pneumatosis intestinalis) being diagnostic. Free air in the peritoneal cavity indicates a perforation, usually in gangrenous intestine. Gas shadowing over the hepatic shadow is a result of gas-forming organisms in the hepatic portal vein. Serology may reveal a thrombocytopenia and raised inflammatory markers and a metabolic acidosis.

Management

Patients are kept nil by mouth, placed onto nasogastric decompression and antimicrobial therapy commenced for sepsis using broad-spectrum antibiotics. Resuscitation includes intravenous fluids: 10% glucose in 0.18% normal saline to maintain blood sugar, and colloid or blood to expand the circulating volume and to ensure a good urine output of more than 1 mL/kg per hour. Platelet transfusions are also often required. Ventilation may be often necessary when there is respiratory failure secondary to abdominal distension, sepsis or underlying lung disease. With prompt intensive medical treatment, the majority of infants will improve but may require up to 10 days of total parenteral nutrition before reintroduction of gastric feeds. A laparotomy is indicated if:

- a perforation is obvious on X-ray or is clinically suspected
- there is failure to respond to medical management, including persistent acidosis and thrombocytopenia, which are indications of severe necrosis

Peritoneal drainage is used by some centres as management for very low birth weight infants, though randomized controlled trials have failed to show this as a significant advantage to definitive care.

At operation, gangrenous bowel is excised and either a primary anastomosis performed or the two viable ends exteriorised as stomas. If necrosis is found throughout the intestine, then either a second-look laparotomy 24–48 hours later could be performed to determine the degree of revascularization or withdrawal of treatment is undertaken following parental discussion.

Prognosis

Although the mortality rate remains high, some series have reported a 70–80% survival rate in infants surgically treated for NEC.

Longer-term complications in survivors include short-bowel syndrome or malabsorption and fibrotic strictures. With an intact ileocaecal valve, just 20 cm of small bowel can adapt to achieve adequate absorption but, without an ileocaecal valve or ileum, the jejunum has limited ability to compensate. Late strictures present as feeding difficulties or subacute obstruction and can be diagnosed by contrast studies and treated surgically with resection and anastomosis.

Congenital Abdominal Wall Defects

Gastroschisis

Gastro (belly) *schisis* (separation) is the term used to describe an evisceration of intestinal contents through a defect, usually to the right of a normally sited umbilical cord. Intestine returns to the abdominal cavity by week 13 of fetal development and failure to do so results in gastroschisis. The cause is unknown, though a vascular event is thought probable as intestinal atresias are associated in 10% of cases. Other anomalies are rare. The incidence also appears to be increasing in many parts of the developed world, including the UK.

Investigation

Antenatal ultrasound scanning has a high sensitivity in accurately diagnosing the condition.

Clinical Features

The bowel often has a very matted appearance and is seen to eviscerate through a defect in the abdominal wall that is invariably to the right of the umbilical cord.

Management

Vaginal birth is the usual mode of delivery and protection of the bowel with cling film to protect and avoid evaporation together with antibiotics and sufficient fluid resuscitation is required. Delivery of such infants in the surgical centre is preferred. Surgical treatment involves a delayed or primary reduction of the intestinal contents into the abdominal cavity. A silo or intestinal bag may be used to assist a delayed closure (Fig. 9.5).

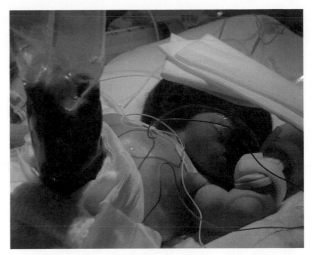

• **Fig. 9.5** Silo on a Newborn with Gastroschisis

Prognosis

Patients without atresia have an excellent prognosis, though a prolonged time to reach full feeds is expected. Patients with atresia often require long-term parenteral nutrition.

Exomphalos

Exomphalos differs from gastroschisis in that the intestinal contents are within a sac which involves the umbilical cord. The liver is also often seen in the herniated contents. Other associated defects are common such as cardiac and chromosomal abnormalities. Prenatal detection often includes analysis of cord blood or amniotic fluid for chromosomal analysis to assist in assessing prognosis.

Management

As in gastroschisis, primary closure is required and the use of a silo or prosthetic bag may also be needed. If a very large defect is present, then the sac is allowed to epithelialize initially and only skin cover is achieved. A definitive muscle closure is performed later in early childhood.

Prognosis

If no other anomalies are present, the prognosis is good and mortality low.

Bladder Exstrophy

This is a rare anomaly resulting in an exposed bladder affecting boys more frequently than girls (Fig. 9.6).

Investigation

Prenatal ultrasound can detect the lesion which, at birth, appears as a defect on the lower abdominal wall. The pubic bones are separated and the bladder mucosa is exposed.

Epispadias is when the anterior aspect of the phallus is incomplete and the urethra is exposed. Epispadias is seen alone but is also seen as part of the exstrophy anomaly.

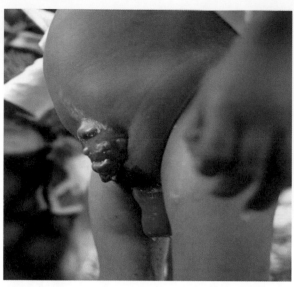

• **Fig. 9.6** Bladder Exstrophy with Rectal Prolapse in the Developing World

Management

Surgery aims to achieve continence, preserve kidney function and achieve good cosmesis. If untreated for many years, the lesion is at risk of adenocarcinoma.

Cloacal exstrophy is a more severe and even rarer condition where the exposed bladder is separated by two intestinal stomas. Most patients also have an associated exomphalos. Defining the gender is often a difficult decision as the penile shaft is very deficient.

Disorders of the Umbilicus

The umbilicus is an important part of fetal life. It allows for blood and nutrients to pass initially to and from the yolk sac to the fetus through the vitello-intestinal duct until the placenta continues that function. The umbilicus also allows for a physiological herniation of the gut during early fetal life, allowing for expansion of the fetal abdomen.

The urachus is another fetal structure that passes through the umbilicus and allows the bladder to communicate with the allantois or yolk sac diverticulum. The umbilical ring naturally regresses before birth. Problems during regression may result in a number of clinical conditions.

Umbilical Hernia

Umbilical hernia appears as a skin-covered protrusion at the umbilicus and is concerning for most parents though rarely causes symptoms. It is more common in Afro-Caribbean children and those with trisomy 21 and 18. Most surgeons would advocate monitoring of small umbilical hernias as surgery is not usually required. Defects of more than 2 cm at 3 years of age are unlikely to resolve spontaneously and are normally repaired. Incarceration is rarely reported.

Umbilical Granuloma

Clinical Features

Umbilical granuloma presents as a shiny red moist lesion described by parents as never healing following the cord disconnection. It may represent mucosa derived from the fetal intestinal connection or sepsis of the cord remnant.

Occasionally, the intestine itself does not regress completely from the umbilicus. This is a patent vitello-intestinal duct and can present with persistent leakage of meconium from the umbilicus.

If the bladder connection with the yolk sac fails to regress, this is termed a patent urachus and urine is seen to leak from the umbilicus. Any outflow obstruction to the fetal bladder can result in this condition and therefore renal tract imaging is warranted before surgical closure of the rachis.

Both persistent communications may also develop cysts which present as infected intra-abdominal masses.

Management

A simple granulated lesion can be treated with topical silver nitrate or other form of cauterization. Abdominal ultrasound may be of use in detecting a patent channel or cyst. Surgical exploration of the umbilicus with disconnection is required for both patent vitello-intestinal duct and patent urachus.

Prune Belly Syndrome

Absence of the anterior abdominal wall muscles may follow transient but severe prenatal ascites. This is a rare anomaly, seen mostly in boys, and associated with bilateral intra-abdominal testes and an abnormal urinary tract with gross dilatation and poor function. The skin lies in loose wrinkled folds, with the underlying abdominal wall muscles poorly developed and displaced laterally. The management of the urological problems and renal failure is paramount. Staged orchidopexies and surgical repair of the anterior abdominal wall should be considered.

The Inguinal Region

What is the Difference Between Inguinal Hydrocele and Inguinal Hernia?

A hydrocele is a collection of fluid within the processus vaginalis (PV) and results in a swelling in the scrotum occasionally extending into the groin.

An inguinal hernia occurs when abdominal organs protrude into the inguinal canal or scrotum. In children, inguinal hernia and hydrocele result from the same defect – failure of closure of the processus vaginalis (Fig. 9.7).

See Box 9.1 for differential diagnoses of swelling in the groin.

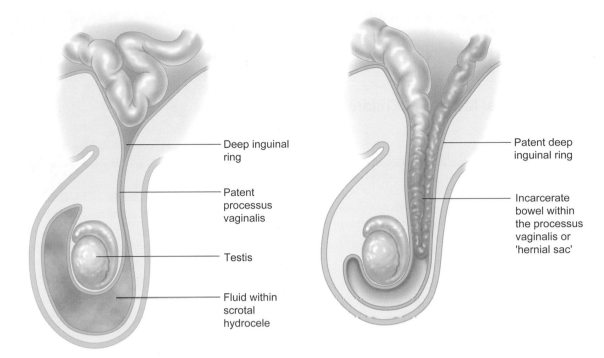

Deep inguinal ring

Patent processus vaginalis

Testis

Fluid within scrotal hydrocele

Patent deep inguinal ring

Incarcerate bowel within the processus vaginalis or 'hernial sac'

• **Fig. 9.7** Schematic Drawing Demonstrating the Difference Between Hydrocele (left) and Inguinal hernia (right)

• **BOX 9.1** **Differential Diagnoses of Swelling in the Groin**

- Inguinal hernia
- Ovary within an inguinal hernia
- Lymph node
- Undescended testicle
- Encysted hydrocele of the cord (outpouching of the patent processus)
- Tumour of spermatic cord (very rare)

Hydrocele

Clinical Features

Hydrocele is more common in the first year of life and, if still present at the age of 2 years, is unlikely to disappear. Parents report intermittent swelling, worse at the end of the day or when the child has a cough or a cold.

On examination, the swelling is fluctuant, non-tender and may extend from the scrotum to the inguinal region. It is usually irreducible, though a minority may communicate. An ability to get above the swelling differentiates it from hernia. Transillumination is often not a useful tool as hernia may also allow light to shine through as the skin and the bowel wall are so thin.

Management

A ligation of the patent tract or processus is carried out through an inguinal incision. A hydrocele in an adult is different in that surgery is performed through a scrotal approach as the aetiology is different.

Inguinal Hernia

This occurs in 1 in 100 male infants and 1 in 500 girls. Hernia is more common in premature infants. Surgery is always required as bowel incarceration can result in intestinal or testicular infarction in up to 10% of obstructed hernia. In girls it is not uncommon for an ovary to be present and be misdiagnosed as a lymph node. Incarceration can lead to ovarian torsion or infarction.

Clinical Features

A swelling is seen intermittently in the groin and may extend into the scrotum in a boy. This may be associated with pain or colic and bowel irregularity. Incarceration can present with nausea and vomiting. If obstructed, the swelling may be tender and red in appearance.

Investigation

Clinical examination is usually sufficient though ultrasound is used by some if clinical doubt exists.

Management

If possible, an attempt should be made to reduce the hernia, usually after appropriate analgesia. Once reduced an elective operation can be planned as soon as swelling in the groin has reduced. Most hernias can be reduced by experienced hands but if the hernia remains irreducible, then urgent operative reduction with or without bowel resection will be necessary.

The operation is performed through an inguinal incision with the same technique used in the hydrocele repair. The laparoscopic approach is also now feasible.

1 in 8–10 children will present clinically with a hernia on the opposite side. For this reason, laparoscopy through the hernial sac or through the umbilicus is sometimes used to detect contralateral hernias. The recurrence rate is low.

Common Abdominal Masses in Children

Pyloric Stenosis

Occurs in approximately 1 in 250 children and is more common in white northern Europeans. Gastric outlet obstruction results from hypertrophy of the circular muscle fibres of the pylorus. The cause of this condition is still largely unknown and surgery to the 'tumour' itself has remained unchanged in over a century.

Clinical Features

Children commonly present within 3–6 weeks after birth with progressive forceful vomiting and failure to thrive despite appearing hungry.

The condition is more common in males, especially first born, and is seven times more likely if there is a family history. Children are often labelled as suffering from gastro-oesophageal reflux and treated accordingly. On presentation, the infant may be below expected weight and may be dehydrated.

Investigation

Diagnosis relies largely on clinical examination but ultrasound is a highly sensitive test to confirm clinical findings.

Blood tests reveal a metabolic alkalosis. Water, hydrogen and chloride ions are all depleted with vomiting. To compensate, ion exchange occurs in the kidney. Water is brought back into the vascular compartment along with sodium and bicarbonate. This renal exchange mechanism results in a further loss of hydrogen ions in the urine, thus exacerbating the alkalosis.

Management

Treatment involves fluid resuscitation and potassium replacement. Once hydrated, metabolically stable and with a good urine output, the operation is commonly performed through a right upper quadrant or supraumbilical incision. The muscle of the pylorus is divided completely to expose the underlying mucosa. The laparoscopic approach is increasingly used in many centres and may have postoperative feeding advantages. The child is fed within hours of the operation or rested overnight and feeds slowly reintroduced. Recurrence is very rare.

Intussusception

Definition and Epidemiology

Intussusception is the invagination of one part of the intestine into an adjacent segment. In children, this occurs most commonly in the ileocaecal region (80%) (Fig. 9.8) and is secondary to inflammatory enlargement of gut lymphoid tissue following either a respiratory or gastrointestinal tract virus infection.

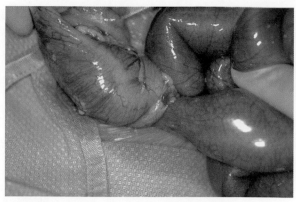

• **Fig. 9.8** Ileocolic Intussusceptions

• **BOX 9.2** **Causes of Intussusception in Children**

- Lymphoid aggregates post viral illness (most common)
- Meckel's diverticulum
- Lymphoma
- Henoch–Schönlein purpura
- Duplication cysts
- Haemangioma of the bowel
- Inspissated meconium in cystic fibrosis
- Intestinal luminal polyp
- Leukaemia
- Nephrotic syndrome

• **BOX 9.3** **Differential Diagnoses of Intussusception**

- Gastroenteritis
- Appendicitis
- Meckel's diverticulitis
- Malrotation with midgut volvulus
- Incarcerated inguinal hernia

Intussusception occurs in 1 in 250–300 children and most commonly occurs in infants between 6 months and 2 years though it can occur at any age. In older children, a pathological cause should be considered (Box 9.2 and Box 9.3).

Clinical Features

Parental history often reveals a high-pitched inconsolable cry. The child may have intermittent abdominal pain and draws up its legs during such episodes. In between spasms, the child may often appear perfectly normal or appear pale and exhausted. Finally, signs of obstruction and necrosis may result in intermittent vomiting or blood in the nappy, often described as red and jelly-like. The latter represents the intestinal mucosal sloughing as a result of ischaemia.

On examination, the child may range from appearing well to having signs of hypovolaemic shock. Careful palpation of the abdomen may reveal a right upper quadrant mass or an empty right iliac fossa (Dance's sign) with or without peritonitis. Examination of the nappy or rectal examination may reveal blood and mucus.

Investigation

Ultrasound has a near 100% sensitivity and specificity for diagnosis. Plain abdominal X-ray may reveal bowel obstruction with a paucity of gas in the right lower quadrant. Air or contrast enema is used as a therapeutic rather than a diagnostic aid.

Management

Fluid resuscitation, broad-spectrum antibiotics and, if necessary, analgesia are essential for these patients.

Pneumatic reduction is commonly used but should be performed by experienced radiologists. Operative reduction is reserved for failed air enema (20%) or those patients who are unstable with peritonitis or signs of perforation.

Air is pumped through a rectal catheter around the colon under radiological control until it enters the terminal ileum. If there is progress but incomplete reduction, the air enema can be repeated in a stable patient several hours later.

Operative reduction can be performed either by laparotomy or laparoscopically. One in 10 children will require resection. The intussusception is reduced by gently manipulating the mass back through the bowel it has invaginated. Traction is avoided as perforation may occur. Recurrence following reduction occurs in up to 5% of patients.

Appendix Mass

Appendix mass occurs usually following several days illness during which diagnoses other than acute appendicitis were considered. The omentum becomes adherent to the inflamed appendix. If peritonitis does not exist, then a trial period of conservative management with intravenous broad-spectrum antibiotics is observed. If symptoms and signs improve, then the appendix can be removed electively 6–8 weeks later to prevent recurrent attacks, which occur in up to 60% of children.

Hydronephrosis

An obstructed renal pelvis results in a build-up of urine and stagnation which, if untreated, can result in a pyonephrosis. This can lead to hypertension and loss of renal function. Causes are numerous, ranging from strictures within the ureter at the renal pelviureteric junction to external vascular compression.

Clinical Features

There may be a history of unexplained fevers or previous renal problems. Older children may show signs of hypertension.

Investigation

Urine testing may reveal infection. Ultrasound can confirm the anatomy and radioisotope studies are used to demonstrate the poor drainage and function of the infected kidney.

Management

Decompression with nephrostomy followed by pyeloplasty if sufficient renal function is present. Nephrectomy is carried out if function is poor and the other kidney is normal.

Faecaloma

A history of constipation would accompany such a clinical finding though often such children report diarrhoeal incontinence. The latter is due to overflow around the mass of liquid stool building up above the rectal faecal mass. If discovered, a rectal enema may be needed to evacuate the rectum. If this is not possible (it is very distressing to many children), then manual evacuation under general anaesthetic may be required.

Careful questioning of early bowel habit is required to eliminate Hirschsprung's disease, and it may be necessary to exclude the condition with a rectal biopsy.

Bladder Outflow Obstruction

Urinary retention is an often overlooked cause of a tender lower abdominal mass in children. Possible causes include pelvic surgery, constipation or urinary tract infection.

Tumours and the Paediatric Surgeon

Nephroblastoma (Wilms' Tumour)

This malignant renal tumour most commonly affects children and is rarely seen in adults. Approximately 40 tumours per year are diagnosed in the UK. One in five tumours are linked to abnormalities on chromosome 11.

Clinical Features

An incidental finding of an abdominal mass in a preschool child is the most common presenting symptom, though 1 in 10 may have painless haematuria. If left-sided, a scrotal varicocele may be present caused by obstruction to the left testicular vein.

Investigation

A chest X-ray and CT scan are useful to determine extent of the condition and the latter also examines the opposite kidney.

Treatment

Nephrectomy with chemotherapy with or without radiotherapy depending on the stage.

Prognosis

It is highly responsive to treatment with a greater than 90% 5-year survival rate for localized disease.

Neuroblastoma

This malignant tumour arises from either the adrenal medulla or sympathetic ganglia of the autonomic nervous system. Sites include the retroperitoneum, adrenal gland, thorax and pelvis. Approximately 100 children are diagnosed each year.

Clinical Features

Most commonly seen in children under 2 years old, neuroblastoma presents as either intra-abdominal pain with a mass or as a thoracic/cervical tumour resulting in dysphagia or respiratory compromise. A Horner's syndrome (ptosis, miosis, enophthalmos) may result from a cervical mass compressing the cervical sympathetic chain.

Non-metastatic tumour effects include hypertension from circulating catecholamines and sweating and diarrhoea from vasoactive intestinal polypeptide (VIP) production.

Investigation

High levels of urinary catecholamines are present. MRI is the imaging of choice and can identify intraspinal extension. Radioisotope studies are useful for bone invasion and tissue biopsy helps determine the likely response to different treatment modalities according to the molecular biology of the tumour.

Management

Surgery is indicated in all but the most advanced tumours. Resection may occur later in those children if an adequate response to chemo- and radiotherapy has taken place.

Survival is poor for those with advanced tumours and those diagnosed after the age of 2.

Ovarian tumour

Ovarian tumours are often detected antenatally and observed to decrease in size with increasing postnatal age. They also occur in prepubertal girls.

Clinical Features

An abdominal mass may be palpable arising from the pelvis, which often feels firm in adolescents.

Investigation

Ultrasound scan/CT/MRI may show ovarian origin. Features may include calcification or other structures suggestive of multiple cellular origins: e.g. teeth and hair.

Serology should include tumour markers such as alpha-fetoprotein, beta-hCG and CEA prior to surgery.

Management

Management is by surgical excision either by open laparotomy or laparoscopically assisted if benign nature likely. Malignant ovarian tumours are rare in childhood.

Teratomas

Terato (monstrous) *oma* (swelling) are abnormal developments of germ cells that occur in areas such as the testis, ovary or sacrococcygeum (Fig. 9.9). The tumours contain

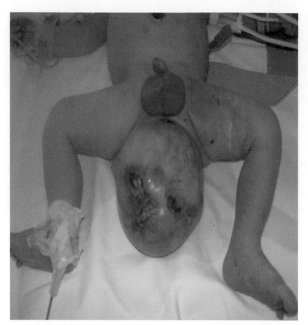

• **Fig. 9.9** Sacrococcygeal Teratoma in a Newborn

derivatives of all germ cell layers of endoderm, ectoderm and mesoderm. Most teratomas in children are benign.

Surgery usually takes place within the first few days of life. Long-term management of continence problems is often necessary after excision of sacrococcygeal tumours.

Abdominal tumours often present later in infancy and may be malignant.

Disorders of Genitalia

Undescended Testes

Epidemiology and Embryology

One in 30 males have an undescended testis at birth. This rises to nearly one in five if born prematurely. Descent may occur in the first 3 months of life in many and at 6 months the incidence overall is considerably reduced.

To understand the testis and why it fails to reach the scrotum, a basic knowledge of embryology is required. In males and females, the gonad develops on a ridge on the posterior abdominal wall early in fetal life and descends caudally reaching the inguinal canal by week 32 of fetal life. This occurs under the influence of various hormones. In the second phase of descent, the testis passes through the inguinal canal and into the scrotum under the influence of testosterone. The gubernaculum is a structure that elongates distal to the testis, creating a space for the testicle to migrate. Peritoneum elongates with the descent of the testis – referred to as the processus vaginalis. The failure of the gubernaculum to migrate is probably the most common cause of an undescended testis.

Clinical Features

Examining a child for the presence of an inguinal testicle can be difficult. It is important to have a warm room and to use distraction techniques. Gentle palpation confirms lack of a testicle in the scrotum. Gentle palpation beginning at the lateral point of the inguinal canal and passing medially has the effect of controlling the cremasteric reflex. The other hand can then palpate for the testicle from the scrotum up and laterally along the inguinal canal. If the testicle can be manipulated into the scrotum and remains there momentarily prior to retreating back into the inguinal canal, it is referred to as a retractile testis and does not require surgery. Some patients present at an older age with an impalpable testis, having previously been seen to be in the scrotum. Such patients may represent retractile testes that have 'ascended'. Monitoring on an annual basis is therefore recommended by many surgeons.

Indications for Surgery

A testicle that has failed to reach the scrotum by 6 months is unlikely to descend. Surgery is normally performed between 6 and 12 months of age. An undescended testis is associated with a number of potential problems (Box 9.4). It is hoped that operating at an early age will reduce the risk of malignant change.

Investigation

If neither testis is able to be found then a human chorionic gonadotrophin stimulation test should be performed to determine whether testicular tissue is present at all. If testosterone is measured, then laparoscopy is used to identify the intra-abdominal testes. Ultrasound and CT have limited value in location of such intra-abdominal testes.

Surgical Management

Orchdio (Greek for testicle) *pexy* (Greek for fixing together) involves a general anaesthetic but can be performed as a day case. The inguinal transverse skin incision allows exposure to the inguinal canal, which is opened and the testicle identified. The gubernaculum is transected to extract the testicle. The spermatic cord, comprising the artery and vein to the testicle, the vas deferens and the processus vaginalis all surrounded by cremasteric muscle, are then carefully mobilized from the inguinal canal. The operation then involves carefully dissecting the processus vaginalis from the vas and vessels, freeing any adhesions that are preventing the testicle from reaching the scrotum. A tunnel is then created using the surgeon's finger to create a space from the inguinal region to the scrotum. The testicle is then delivered into the scrotum and placed in a pouch

---

• BOX 9.4   Problems Associated with an Undescended Testis

- Abnormal fertility in an undescended testis
- Inability to palpate later in adult life (cancer screening)
- Cosmetic
- Increased risk of torsion
- A five-fold increased risk of malignancy if undescended at the age of 10

---

created beneath the scrotal skin and may or may not be fixed, depending on the amount of tension. Complications include testicular atrophy (1–2%) and retraction of the testicle back into the groin (1%).

Torsion of the Testis and Appendix Testis

Epidemiology

Testicular torsion can occur at any age, with peak incidences perinatally and between 10 and 20 years of age.

Aetiology

An abnormal horizontal lie of the testis indicates that there is a high attachment of the peritoneal tunica, giving the testis more mobility, and hence a possible predisposition to rotate. This is often referred to as a bell clapper testis. An inguinal testis is more likely to twist than an intrascrotal one for similar reasons.

The appendix testis is a small embryological remnant on the upper pole of the testis. This can also twist and necrose, resulting in a similar clinical picture.

Clinical Features

Perinatal torsion presents with a painless blue, often hard swelling in the scrotum, several times larger than the contralateral testis. Occasionally, incarcerated inguinal hernia can be mistaken for an acute neonatal testicular torsion.

In later childhood, torsion causes severe pain which is felt in the scrotum and lower abdomen and is usually associated with vomiting and difficulty in walking.

Examination of testicles should be routine in the investigation of abdominal pain, as the pain in the iliac fossa may divert attention from the scrotum and so delay the diagnosis. The history may reveal previous minor episodes indicating intermittent torsion.

Testicular remnant torsion may be distinguishable by the appearance of a blue dot on close examination. Conservative management with analgesics will often suffice; if there is doubt, exploration is warranted.

Investigation

The time taken to diagnose accurately torsion of the testicle only lengthens ischaemia time to the testicle. If suspected, an urgent exploration under general anaesthesia should be performed without further investigation.

Management

Through either a horizontal hemiscrotal or midline incision, the testicle is delivered and inspected. The testicle and cord are untwisted, warmed and observed for several minutes to see if colour improves. If operated on within 6 hours, a significant number will be saved and can be fixed with three non-absorbable sutures to the scrotal fascia. After 24 hours, virtually all twisted testes will need removing. Fixation of the opposite side with non-absorbable suture is usually performed to prevent a similar scenario in the future. If a torted remnant or appendix testis is found, this is also removed.

Idiopathic Scrotal Oedema

This is a form of urticarial angio-oedema of unknown cause.

Clinical Features

Bright red oedema of the scrotum or hemiscrotum is observed, which often extends posteriorly towards the anus or anteriorly over the inguinal region. The appearance resembles an acute cellulitic infection with some irritation and tenderness. However, fever and pain are not present and antibiotics do not influence the course.

The normal testis is obscured by the intense oedema of the scrotal wall.

Management

The parents are often alarmed and reassurance is necessary. There is resolution over 24–48 hours. Antihistamines and anti-inflammatory medication can speed spontaneous resolution.

Phimosis/Paraphimosis and Balanoposthitis

Phimosis of the foreskin can be considered as either congenital or acquired; or as physiological or pathological.

Removal of the foreskin or circumcision is the most commonly performed operation in the world and for centuries has been a fundamental rite of passage in many cultures.

A congenital or physiological phimosis is where the foreskin is naturally adherent to the glans penis and does not retract. This can continue to puberty without causing symptoms and up to 3% of males will still be unretractile by the age of 13.

An acquired or pathological phimosis in childhood is usually a result of balanitis xerotica obliterans (sclerotic fibrotic process of the foreskin) or due to chronic balanoposthitis. *Balano* (Greek for acorn) *itis* (inflammation) is inflammation of the glans of the penis, whereas *posthe* (Greek for foreskin) *itis* (inflammation) refers to inflammation of the skin surrounding the glans.

The only absolute indication for circumcision in childhood is a pathological phimosis. Relative indications include recurrent severe posthitis (severe inflammation of the foreskin) and paraphimosis (retraction with a tourniquet effect from the preputial ring).

Circumcision is still performed in up to 60% of males in the United States for cultural and hygienic reasons. The incidence fell dramatically in post-war England and remains at about 2% of the male population.

Recent trials in Africa suggest that circumcising males in a population with minimal use of condoms can reduce infection with HIV.

Clinical Features

A physiological foreskin, on gentle examination, will retract to reveal a spout or funnel with healthy mucosa visible. Pathological phimosis will often have a rolled pale edge with white linear radial scars. Both conditions can result in difficulty in urination, though it is much more common in a pathological phimosis.

Management

Physiological phimosis requires reassurance as well as advice on careful drying of the foreskin following urination. Drying can help in preventing dermatitis which is secondary to the concentrated ammonia found in urine being in prolonged contact with the foreskin. Topical steroids are used by many clinicians to treat the inflammation.

Circumcision is required for a pathological phimosis to prevent retraction with a tourniquet-like effect as the tight phimotic ring passes over the glans and is unable to be brought forward. This is referred to as a paraphimosis. Gentle retraction with or without a small slit dorsally is required. Circumcision is then usually offered as an elective procedure.

Hypospadias

This refers to a defect in the distal formation of the male urethra as it forms ventrally. The result is a spectrum of abnormally situated urethral openings along the course of the normal urethra. The urethral openings can be situated anywhere from above the coronal sulcus of the glans penis to the perineum in its most extreme form. The latter is often associated with chordae or fibrotic areas on the shaft, resulting in a ventral curvature.

The incidence in the UK is approximately 1 in 250 male births. The cause is thought to be an interruption in the androgenic processes required during ventral urethral formation.

Clinical Features

The disorder is usually identified at birth and rarely can be associated with other chromosomal, reproductive or endocrine anomalies. The prepuce is also incomplete and lies dorsally.

Management

Surgery usually takes place in early infancy and involves either a primary or staged procedure to tubularize a new urethra. The incomplete or hooded prepuce is often incorporated into the repair.

Principles of Paediatric Trauma

Trauma is the most common cause of death in children aged over 1 year. Different mechanisms of injury are closely associated with developmental milestones. Head injuries, either as an isolated cause or in association with other injuries, are the most common cause of death.

Thoracic, abdominal and perineal injuries are those most commonly encountered by paediatric general surgeons.

The possibility of non-accidental injury must always be considered, and if any doubt exists, the paediatric consultant with responsibility for safeguarding children should be contacted for advice. All staff treating children should undergo child protection training.

Thoracic

This accounts for the second leading cause of death in paediatric trauma with blunt trauma from road traffic accidents being mostly responsible. The paediatric chest wall is more compliant than an adult and thus fractures are less common but pulmonary contusion and pneumothorax are more common. The majority of such injuries can be managed with observation with or without chest drainage. Thoracotomy or thoracoscopy is necessary if more than 20 mL/kg of blood is required in resuscitation or if a drainage rate of >2 mL/kg/h is observed following intercostal drainage of a haemothorax.

Abdominal

If bruising is discovered on a child's abdomen following trauma, then it is likely that significant force has occurred. This may be as a direct blow or from restraint such as the seat or lap belt.

Viscera such as the liver and spleen are less protected in the infant due to nature of rib cage shape and development and a high index of suspicion for visceral injury must be maintained. Splenic injury is common in children, though the majority of intrasplenic lacerations and haemorrhage will resolve if managed conservatively with bed rest and observation for 1–2 weeks.

Deceleration injuries in road traffic accidents can affect hollow viscera such as the duodenum. CT with contrast is the preferred investigation. The mechanism of injury is the sudden visceral compression against the bony spine and shearing forces affecting retroperitoneal structures.

Assessment and Management

The ABCDE principles of resuscitation still apply to children as they do adults. Specific to the trauma setting, the primary concern is the airway together with cervical spine control. Once secured, the breathing is assessed and optimized, followed by support of the circulation. If the child is not breathing and there is no cardiac output, five rescue breaths are given prior to cardiac compression. Children require 30 chest compressions for every two breaths. Once resuscitation is successful, the neurological status of the patient is then assessed and the patient undergoes a full examination to complete the primary survey. The stabilized child can then undergo the secondary survey to look for additional injuries.

The resuscitation of children in the UK should adhere to the guidelines set out by the APLS group and this is mandatory training for all paediatric surgeons.

Safeguarding Children

Safeguarding children has been defined by the UK government as 'The process of protecting children from abuse or neglect, preventing impairment of their health and development, and ensuring they are growing up in circumstances consistent with the provision of safe and effective care that enables children to have optimum life chances and enter adulthood successfully'.

Every week a child dies as a result of non-accidental injury, usually at the hands of a parent or carer, according to the UK Home Office. Child maltreatment broadly consists of four overlapping categories of abuse: physical, emotional, sexual and neglect. Infants are at higher risk of serious injuries and these children may present to the surgical team as trauma, with multiple injuries or burns, or even with an acute abdomen.

Following the Victoria Climbié inquiry, the Every Child Matters programme aimed to improve outcomes for children in five key areas: health, safety, achievement, making a positive contribution and economic well-being. This programme led to significant changes in child protection legislation through the Children Act 2004. Multi-agency Local Safeguarding Children Boards (LSCBs), with representation from housing, health and police services, were formed to co-ordinate agency functions in relation to safeguarding and commission independent serious case reviews. The Act placed a duty on all agencies to safeguard and promote the welfare of children.

Awareness of safeguarding and child protection is a legal, moral and professional duty for all healthcare professionals. Doctors play an important role in recognizing injuries reflecting child abuse and triggering an appropriate response to prevent further harm. Additionally, medical assessment and documentation of inflicted injuries provides crucial evidence for child protection proceedings.

There are many features that may raise concerns about child maltreatment, including injuries that are not consistent with the explanation given, delay in presentation, injuries not in keeping with the developmental stage of the child, changing or conflicting history, multiple attendances and multiple injuries of different ages. More subtle features may include failure to thrive, poor hygiene or unkempt appearance, inappropriate social interactions and failure to attend medical appointments. The NICE guidelines 'When to Suspect Child Maltreatment' comprehensively details the alerting features for child abuse.

What to do if there are concerns about child maltreatment:
- Gather information from multiple sources.
- Full documentation is essential.
- Discuss the case with the named paediatrician for child protection in the trust or the on-call paediatrician.
- If in doubt, admit the child to hospital under joint care of the surgical and medical teams.
- Contact social services (there will be an emergency duty team out of hours); do not delay a referral.

Once concerns have been raised, the named safeguarding paediatrician will make a detailed assessment and make a referral to the children's and family service. Ideally, the parents should be informed of the referral unless this places the child at increased risk. The General Medical Council states that, in these situations, doctors have a responsibility to disclose confidential information to the appropriate responsible person or agency in the child's best interests and parents are not able to withhold consent for this disclosure. It is important to fully document the justification for disclosure. In the rare situation of parents refusing admission to hospital where there are significant concerns to a child's immediate safety, the police should be called to impose a police protection order ensuring the child is not removed from hospital. Local agencies will then arrange a case conference, usually attended by the paediatrician; however, a formal report may be requested from other teams involved in the child's care.

Consent for Children and Young People

In England, young people aged over 16 years are treated in the same way as adults and are presumed to have capacity to give or withhold consent for their own medical treatment.

Consent for children under 16 years of age, is usually given by an adult with parental responsibility.

Who Has Parental Responsibility?

- mother
- father, if they were married to the mother when the child was conceived or born, or they married later. Unmarried fathers have parental responsibility if they are named on the birth certificate
- legally appointed guardian
- local authority designated to care for the child
- local authority or person with an emergency protection order for the child

Parental decision to refuse consent can be overruled by the courts where treatment is felt to be in the best interest of the child. In the situation where two parents disagree on the treatment, again the decision can be made by the courts. However, healthcare professionals can choose to accept only one parent's consent and proceed with treatment if they feel that this would be in the best interests of the child. In an emergency, treatment can proceed without parental consent if obtaining consent would delay treatment and therefore put the child at increased risk.

In some situations, children under 16 years of age may be able to consent to treatment without an adult with parental responsibility, if they are deemed to be Gillick competent.

This is where the healthcare professionals believe that they have the capacity to understand the treatment and appreciate the risks and benefits. However, if they refuse consent to treatment and this might lead to significant harm, the decision can be overruled by the Court of Protection, the legal body that oversees the Mental Capacity Act (2005).

Fortunately, these difficult situations are rare, but when they do arise, it is important to discuss the situation with senior colleagues, consider discussion with the hospital's legal team and ensure thorough documentation of the discussions and decisions made.

Further Reading

General Medical Council. *0–18 Years: Guidance for all doctors*; 2007. https://www.gmc-uk.org/ethical-guidance/ethical-guidance-for-doctors/0-18-years.

HM Government. Working Together to Safeguard Children: A guide to inter-agency working to safeguard and promote the welfare of children. July 2018. https://assets.publishing.service.gov.uk/government/uploads/system/uploads/attachment_data/file/779401/Working_Together_to_Safeguard-Children.pdf.

Holcomb GW, Murphy JP. *Ashcraft's Pediatric Surgery*. 5th ed. Philadelphia: Saunders Elsevier; 2010.

NICE. Clinical guideline 89. Child maltreatment: When to suspect maltreatment in under 18s, July 2009; 2009.

Rentea RM, Peter SDS, Snyder CL. Pediatric appendicitis: state of the art review. *Pediatr Surg Int.* 2017;33:269–283. https://doi.org/10.1007/s00383-016-3990-2.

Roderick C, Davies E, Rabb L, Bowley DM. What does the surgeon need to know about safeguarding children? *Bull R Coll Surg Engl.* 2015;97(8):349–352.

Samuels M, Wieteska S. *Advanced Paediatric Life Support: A Practical Approach to Emergencies*. 6th ed. Chichester: John Wiley & Sons, Ltd; 2016.

Spitz L, Coran A. *Operative Paediatric Surgery*. London: Hodder Arnold; 2008.

Stringer MD, Oldham KT, Mouriquand PDE. *Pediatric Surgery and Urology: Long-Term Outcomes*. Cambridge: Cambridge University Press; 2006.

Thomas DFM, Duffy PG, Rickwood AMK. *Essentials of Paediatric Urology*. 2nd ed. London: Informa Healthcare; 2008.

Ullman AJ, Marsh N, Mihala G, Cooke M, Rickard CM. Complications of central venous access devices: a systematic review. *Pediatrics.* 2015;136(5):e1331–e1344. https://doi.org/10.1542/peds.2015–1507.

Wilkins S, Pena A. The role of colostomy in the management of anorectal malformations. Pediatr Surg Int. 1988:3;105–109.

10

The Older Surgical Patient

Introduction

Ageing is the most important risk factor for the development of degenerative and neoplastic surgical disease. By 2040, one in four people in the UK will be aged over 65. Persons aged over 85 are the most rapidly expanding age cohort in society. This demographic change is accompanied by evolving social attitudes and patient expectation. These factors, when combined with advances in surgical technique and anaesthesia, are leading to increasing numbers of older patients undergoing emergency and elective surgery.

Despite this, morbidity and mortality for older patients undergoing surgery remains high compared to younger patients. Ageing is complicated by multi-morbidity, loss of physiological reserve and geriatric syndromes such as cognitive impairment and frailty. These factors are independent predictors of adverse postoperative outcome, and require careful perioperative management.

Models of care characterized by collaboration between surgeons, anaesthetists and geriatricians may have evolved in the care of older patients with hip fracture, but an emerging evidence base indicates similar models may have a role across a range of surgical disciplines challenged by an ageing and multi-morbid population.

This chapter addresses the fundamental aspects of ageing relevant to surgery, and explores common perioperative issues and interventions that can be made throughout the surgical pathway to improve outcomes for older patients.

Determining Surgical Risk

Biology of Ageing and Frailty

To comprehend what it is that precisely increases the risks of surgery in older people, an understanding of the physiological changes of ageing is needed. Many physiological parameters of organ function decline with advancing age (Table 10.1). The ageing process leads to loss of physiological reserve. However, the rate of decline varies between individuals. Ageing becomes clinically relevant when physiological function has declined to such an extent that the ability of the organ to maintain function is compromised in the face of an external stressor (e.g. infection, surgery). Whilst some types of organ failure are easy to recognize clinically or with routine laboratory tests, decompensation of complex neurophysiological systems leads to delirium, immobility, falls, incontinence and failure to rehabilitate. These syndromes are characteristic of frailty.

Frailty results from progressive ageing and is an established *state of reduced physiological reserve across multiple organ systems*. This results in a reduction in ability to maintain homeostasis in the presence of acute stressors (Fig. 10.1). Approximately 10% of people aged over 65 years are considered frail, rising to 25–50% at age >85 years. Older people living with frailty are at increased risk of hospitalization, care-home admission and death. Minor physiological challenges to their health, such as infection, medication or surgery, can result in loss of organ function. Frailty is an independent predictor of perioperative mortality, morbidity, loss of independence and institutionalization. Frail patients should therefore be considered high risk even in the absence of identified organ disease.

However, frailty is a spectrum disorder with varying degrees of severity. Various scales and tools have been designed to identify frailty. The suitability of each of these models depends on clinical setting and resources available. There is currently insufficient evidence to recommend any one specific tool, though the Modified Frailty Index, Clinical Frailty Score and Edmonton Frail Scale have a building surgical evidence base. Sarcopaenia is a cardinal feature of the frailty syndrome, and there is increasing evidence that, in cancer surgery, sarcopaenia can be reliably approximated from cross-sectional psoas muscle volume. As all cancer surgery patients, and many others, undergo routine preoperative CT imaging, this may represent a pragmatic solution to the frailty screening dilemma for many surgical services.

Frailty is not just important for risk assessment: it may also be treatable. Multicomponent programmes of prehabilitation incorporating tailored comorbidity optimization, exercise, nutrition, and patient education appear to be able to reduce frailty. Early evidence also suggests these interventions may reduce surgical complications, critical care consumption, inpatient length of stay and improve patient quality of life. Further research is needed, but multimodal prehabilitation may become a new standard of preoperative care for older surgical patients in the future.

Multimorbidity

Older patients are, however, at elevated risk of adverse postoperative outcomes, not just as a result of frailty and the associated geriatric syndromes. Many overt disease states are

TABLE 10.1	Biological Changes of Ageing.
Organ System	**Effect of Ageing**
Neurological	Reduced white matter, altered neurotransmitter levels; loss of integrity of blood–brain barrier; reduced brain mass; higher cognitive effects
Cardiovascular	Reduced cardiac output; reduced vascular compliance
Respiratory	Increase in residual volume; decreased vital capacity; reduced gas exchange
Gastrointestinal	Decreased motility; reduced sphincter control; increased transit time
Renal	Reduced Glomerular Filtration rate; loss of glomeruli
Immunological	Macrophage, B-cell and T-cell function decline
Musculoskeletal	Sarcopaenia
Metabolic	Reduced body fat; reduced total body water

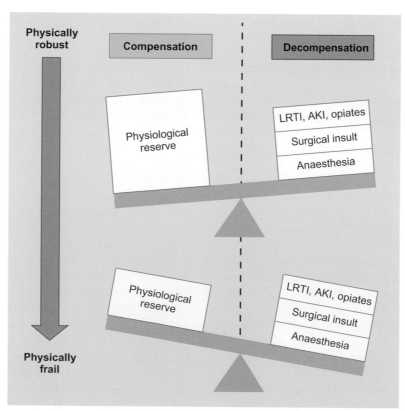

• **Fig. 10.1** Frailty and Loss of Reserve AKI, Acute kidney injury; LRTI, lower respiratory tract infection.

directly linked to advancing age, and as persons age, they typically accumulate medical pathology. Multimorbidity is defined as the coexistence of more than one chronic condition in an individual. It is associated with increased mortality, morbidity, institutionalization and poorer quality of life. Multimorbidity is highly prevalent in older people with approximately 75% of patients aged over 65 years having two or more chronic medical conditions. Multimorbidity is closely linked with polypharmacy and drug error, which is proportionally linked to the number of medications taken by a patient. It is known that each additional comorbidity adds incremental postoperative medical complications and mortality.

Risk Prediction Tools

All surgery is associated with risk. In older patients, this risk is heightened due to ageing-associated decline in end-organ function and multi-morbidity. Clinicians can utilize risk prediction scores to help guide decision making and balance risk–benefit of different treatment strategies. Accurate preoperative determination of risk is also important to enable truly informed consent for patients, particularly where non-surgical interventions may be available. There currently exist a variety of risk assessment tools. Here we present some of those most commonly used in current clinical practice:

- **ASA (American Society of Anesthesiologists) Grading** (Table 10.2) – This score uses preoperative physical status to categorize patients into five subgroups (with a sixth added for organ harvesting). It is a simple and easy to use scoring system and has been shown to correlate well with complications, admission to ICU and mortality in a wide variety of surgical specialties. Although it was never designed as a risk prediction tool, it is widely used for this purpose. The weakness of the ASA score is that most older patients fall into category 3, and there is inadequate differentiation between lower and higher risk patients within this single category.
- **Metabolic Equivalents Score (METs)** (Table 10.3) – This is a brief screening tool to estimate functional capacity as a marker of cardiovascular, pulmonary circulatory and neuromuscular status. Patients scoring <4 are at higher risk of perioperative complications, and may benefit from more detailed cardio-respiratory investigation prior to moderate-major surgery. However, the METS scale is by definition self-reported, and some studies have found that patient-reported values do not accurately correlate with objectively-measured METS at cardiopulmonary exercise testing.
- **Physiological and Operative Severity Score for the enUmeration of Mortality and Morbidity (POSSUM)** – The score was initially developed in 1991 for audit purposes and looks at 18 variables in total: 12 to assess physiological status and 6 specific to the surgical procedure. It has since been altered and several speciality specific variations have been developed. There is some evidence that

TABLE 10.2	ASA Grading.
1	Normal healthy
2	Mild systemic disease
3	Severe systemic disease
4	Severe systemic disease with constant threat to life
5	Moribund patient not expected to survive without operation
6	Declared brain dead – Organs being harvested

TABLE 10.3	Metabolic Equivalents (METs).
Activity Correlating to Measured Metabolic Equivalents	
1	Largely immobile
2	Light gardening/walking slowly
3	Vacuuming/walking at average pace
4	Mowing lawn/climbing two flights of stairs
5	Weeding garden/brisk walking
6	Moving heavy objects
7	Swimming
8–10	Running

it can over-predict mortality in low-risk planned surgery, but it is widely used across the UK. Despite incorporating parameters of major organ function (renal, cardiac, respiratory), it does not account for cognition or pre-surgical functional status. It therefore can under-appreciate risk in frail older people without established major organ pathology.

- **American College of Surgeons National Surgical Quality Improvement Program (ACS NSQIP) surgical risk calculator** – This risk calculator was built using data collected from more than 3.2 million operations from 668 hospitals participating in ACS NSQIP from 2011 to 2015. The risk calculator uses 20 patient factors and the planned procedure to predict the risk of 15 outcomes within 30-days following surgery. These outcomes include mortality, complications and, importantly, discharge to long-term rehabilitation or nursing home facilities. This can be powerful information for patients who fear functional decline and loss of independence more than death.

Role for Comprehensive Geriatric Assessment

Various perioperative risk prediction tools as described above can help to estimate perioperative morbidity and mortality. However, they remain imperfect due to their inability to identify the myriad risk factors present in frail,

TABLE 10.4	Comprehensive Geriatric Assessment.	
Component	**Tool**	**Example Intervention**
Comorbidity	Full history and itemized optimization	Optimization of cardiac, respiratory, renal disease, diabetes
Medication	Medication Review	Rationalization; STOPP-START criteria, perioperative medication plan
Nutrition	Modified MUST tool	Nutritional optimization; dietician referral
Exercise tolerance	Metabolic Equivalents Scale	Prehabilitation programme, risk assessment
Cognition	Montreal Cognitive Assessment, Modified Mini Mental State	Delirium risk reduction protocols, memory clinic referral, assessment of capacity
Frailty	Reported Edmonton Frail Scale, Clinical Frailty Scale	Multicomponent CGA intervention, PT/OT referral, gait/balance training
Mood	Depression question, global assessment, Hospital Anxiety and Depression Score	Antidepressants, referral to clinical psychology
Functional capacity	Nottingham Extended Activities of Daily Living	Social Services referral, transport
Social circumstances	Housing, support network, existing care arrangements	Social Services referral, access to local resources
Discharge plan	Identification of borough, rehabilitation facilities and access to social services support. Explanation to patient and family	Early OT and Physiotherapy referral, Social Services referral
Screening investigations (where indicated)	FBC, renal, liver, bone, thyroid profiles, haematinics, Vitamin D, ECG, CXR, BNP, HbA1c	Diagnosis of medical comorbidity and preoperative optimization

BNP, Brain natriuretic peptide; CXR, chest X-ray; ECG, electrocardiogram; FBC, full blood count; HbA1c, glycosylated haemoglobin; MUST, Malnutrition Universal Screening Tool; OT, occupational therapy; PT, physical therapy.

older surgical patients. Furthermore, they offer no intervention targets to improve surgical outcomes. Frail older patients are known to benefit from comprehensive geriatric assessment (CGA). CGA is a multidisciplinary diagnostic and treatment process that leads to the formulation of an individualized and holistic plan to address medical, social and psychological issues in the care of the older patient. It is increasingly being used in surgical settings with emerging evidence of its validity in this setting. Patients are assessed across a broad range of domains (Table 10.4) using validated tools and scales to provide information that can be used to inform surgeons, patients and relatives of a personalized risk profile and identify targets for medical intervention. Use of this methodology has been shown to reduce postoperative complications and overall length of inpatient stay. Components of CGA are illustrated in Table 10.4.

Communicating Surgical Risk

Assessing Mental Capacity

Consent is a decision-specific process that requires assessment of a patient's capacity; this includes their ability to understand, weigh up, retain and communicate information to make an informed decision (The Mental Capacity Act

2005). Importantly, mental capacity is treatment-specific, and therefore must be tested for each decision required of a patient. If a patient lacks capacity (as a result of a disorder of the brain or mind), two potential situations arise in English legal jurisdiction. Firstly, some patients may have previously awarded a relative or friend medical powers of attorney. This legally grants the attorney legal authority to make decisions on the patient's behalf in a situation in which the patient has lost mental capacity. In this situation, the attorney must be consulted and consent to proceed obtained directly from the attorney.

Secondly, where no powers of attorney have been previously awarded, responsibility for emergency decision making in a non-capacitous patient must be made in the patient's best interests by the clinicians responsible for the patient's care. Best practice would typically involve consultation with family and the wider multi-disciplinary team to determine what the patient is likely to have wanted, and what represents patient best-interests. Where no relative or friend is in a position to act as an advocate for the patient, an application for an independent mental capacity advocate (IMCA) may be required to formally determine the best interests of the patient. This legal process is not well-suited to emergency situations, where timeframes for decision making may mandate best-interest decisions to be made by the treating clinicians.

Determining Prognosis

Providing patients with adequate information about the risks of surgery lies at the heart of informed consent. Whilst risk prediction scores, such as P-POSSUM, can aid in the overall decision-making process, prognostication of what individual patients might expect in the postoperative period is important to aid decision making. Identification and quantification of frailty and cognitive impairment can help prognosticate temporary or permanent postoperative changes in functional status, dependency, cognition and mobility. These can be important factors for patients impacting upon their decision to proceed with surgery. Quality of life, rather than quantity of life, can be of greater importance to some older patients. Part of prognostication relies upon determining the natural history of disease with and without surgical intervention. This is disease-specific (e.g. inguinal hernia vs 5.5 cm aortic aneurysm vs an obstructing colorectal cancer).

Whilst age alone is not a good indicator of a patient's overall fitness for surgery, it can help to predict life expectancy. It is important to note that clinicians often underappreciate life expectancy in older persons, and this can distort the way in which risks and benefits are presented to the patient. Average life expectancy changes as we age; average life expectancy for a newborn male in the UK currently is 79 years. But a 90 year-old male, who has already surpassed the UK average, might expect to live for an additional 4 years (Fig. 10.2). It can be helpful to provide patients with information about average life expectancy to help guide individualized decisions. Life expectancy projections can be found on the Office for National Statistics website (https://www.ons.gov.uk/) and individualized calculators can be helpful (https://eprognosis.ucsf.edu/index.php). However, it should be noted that many surgical pathologies predispose the patient to frailty. As previously discussed, frailty is an important prognostic factor which means overall life expectancy at any given age may be attenuated compared

to UK national averages. Data from Clegg and colleagues (Fig. 10.3) can be useful to inform life expectancy at varying degrees of frailty.

Improving Surgical Outcomes

Risk assessment is clearly important. However, where risks are managed in accordance with modern evidence-based practice throughout the surgical pathway, they can be mitigated. This approach requires collaborative management between surgeons, physicians and anaesthetists. Preoperative optimization of the patient, prevention (and early treatment) of complications and anticipatory discharge planning in accordance with enhanced recovery principles are fundamental to high quality care of the older surgical patient.

The following sections reflect current best practice, and are derived from the most recent perioperative literature and guidelines.

Preoperative Interventions
Exercise and Prehabilitation

Exercise programmes are known to delay the onset and progression of frailty in older adults. They have also been shown to improve mortality and quality of life in the context of cardiac and lung disease. Parameters of cardio-respiratory fitness (e.g. anaerobic threshold and maximal oxygen uptake) are well-established predictors of surgical mortality. Early evidence suggests that improvements in these physiological parameters through preoperative exercise training may reduce complications and enhance recovery after surgery.

However, the exercise prehabilitation literature is currently diverse: 'prehab' has not been studied in all patient

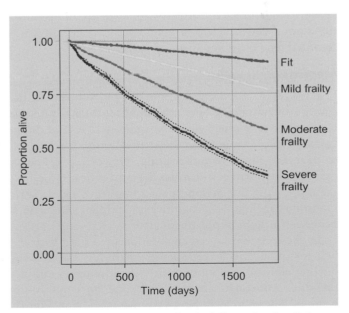

• **Fig. 10.3** 5-year Kaplan–Meier Survival Curve for the Outcome of Mortality for Categories of Fit, Mild Frailty, Moderate Frailty and Severe Frailty (Internal Validation Cohort) (Clegg A, Bates C, Young J, et al. Development and validation of an electronic frailty index using routine primary care electronic health record data. Age Ageing 2016; 45 (3): 353–360. https://doi.org/10.1093/ageing/afw039.)

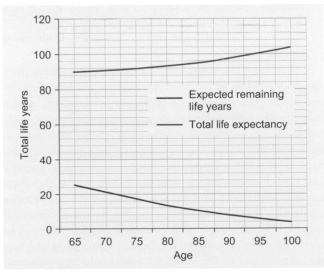

• **Fig. 10.2** UK Total Life Expectancy and Remaining Years of Life (From the Office for National Statistics, UK.)

groups, nor in all surgical disciplines. Uncertainty therefore exists as to the type, duration, intensity and frequency of exercise needed to impact on surgical outcomes. Furthermore, it remains currently unclear which patients benefit most. Early data indicate that frail older people may have most to gain from exercise programmes, and that several weeks of supervised, structured incremental exercise may be sufficient to improve their risk profile.

This is a rapidly expanding area of perioperative medicine. The most recent reports indicate the best results may be achieved by multimodal prehabilitation interventions incorporating exercise, nutrition and medical optimization.

Nutrition

Malnutrition is highly prevalent in older people and is associated with increased postoperative complications such as infection, development of pressure ulcers and delayed wound healing.

Prior to surgery, patients should be assessed for unintentional weight loss. Body mass index should be calculated using weight and height. Vitamin B_{12}, folate and iron studies may be useful in identifying treatment for correctable anaemia. Patients who are malnourished should be referred to a dietician; patients who are severely malnourished may benefit from delayed surgery until nutrition is optimized. Enteral feeding is preferable to parenteral nutrition wherever possible, as this is associated with increased risks of infection. Early enteral feeding is possible in many patients undergoing surgery and is associated with better outcomes. In patients with delayed intestinal function, postoperative parenteral feeding is unlikely to be indicated unless bowel function is not likely to return for more than 5 days. However, this period may be shorter in patients who are severely malnourished. Patients with evidence of malnutrition should have regular weights measured in hospital, a recorded food chart and dietician review.

Medication Review

Prescribing in frail older patients can be complex. In the context of advancing age and multi-morbidity, multiple medications are often clinically indicated. A medication cascade can evolve in which more medication is prescribed to treat side effects of earlier drugs. However, it is known that this polypharmacy increases the risks of drug error. Furthermore, drug interactions, poor compliance and geriatric syndromes such as falls, cognitive impairment and incontinence can arise from polypharmacy.

In these circumstances, medication prescribed with the best-intentions can become actively harmful. The anticholinergic activity of antipsychotics, antihistamines, antidepressants, anticonvulsants, opioids, and anti-muscarinics is often underestimated. Surgery presents additional physiological challenges and is often the catalyst for adverse drug-related outcomes. Hypoglycaemic drugs, anti-hypertensives and anticoagulants are prone to causing perioperative drug error. Furthermore, perioperative analgaesics, anti-emetics and antimicrobials add to a substantial preoperative anticholinergic drug burden and decompensation, commonly with delirium.

Physician preoperative medication review (as part of CGA) is advised to minimize drug burden and mitigate perioperative risk of adverse events in complex older surgical patients. Perioperative prescribing should reflect the risk profile and be supported by physicians and pharmacists with adequate experience.

Perioperative Management of Common Medical Comorbidities

Hypertension

Severe hypertension increases the risks of surgery (systolic >211 mmHg and diastolic >110 mmHg). Patients with less severe hypertension (diastolic <110 mmHg) do not appear to be at increased risk. Elective surgery should be delayed until blood pressure is adequately controlled (diastolic <110 mmHg). Continuing with anti-hypertensives is generally safe and most can be taken with small sips of water at 06:00 a.m. on the morning of surgery. Abruptly stopping some anti-hypertensives can lead to rebound hypertension (β-blockers, clonidine) and should be avoided. There is some evidence that omitting angiotensin-converting enzyme inhibitors (ACEIs)and angiotensin-receptor-blockers (ARBs) on the day of surgery reduces risk of acute kidney injury, and current guidelines advise that ACEIs and ARBs are withheld for 24 hours before surgery. Severe postoperative hypertension (systolic >180 mmHg) can be treated with i.v. labetalol or sublingual nicardipine.

Permanent Pacemakers (PPM) and Implantable Cardiac Defibrillators (ICD)

Prior to elective procedures, liaison with cardiology or pacing clinic is advised to establish make and model of the device, whether the patient is pacing-dependent and if cardiac defibrillator therapy is active. Interrogation and battery check of devices prior to surgery is recommended:
- within 6 months for ICD
- within 12 months for conventional PPM
- within 3–6 months for any cardiac resynchronization device

For surgery above the umbilicus, anti-tachycardia therapy may need to be suspended whilst pacing function can persist. In patients who are pacing-dependent, the device may need to be switched to an asynchronous pacing mode to avoid over-sensing from electromagnetic interference. In emergency surgery, a magnet can be applied to most devices to achieve suspension of anti-tachycardia therapy and asynchronous pacing. Intraoperative cardiac monitoring is essential and precautions should be taken to ensure availability of transcutaneous pacing or defibrillation if required. Reactivation of devices should be performed in the immediate postoperative period if reprogramming was performed, and device interrogation should be performed after emergency surgery that took place without any preoperative evaluation.

Heart Failure

Symptomatic heart failure should be optimized before scheduled surgery. Decision making for surgery will depend on the necessity of surgery, the severity of the heart failure syndrome and perioperative risk. Preoperative echocardiography is recommended in patients whose clinical status has changed or in whom valvular or new cardiac dysfunction is suspected. Serum BNP (brain natriuretic peptide) may be useful in those where a diagnosis of heart failure is unclear and should lead to further investigation if elevated.

Medications for heart failure should be continued perioperatively, except for ACEIs and ARBs, which should be withheld 24 hours prior to surgery. Patients with heart failure should have meticulous monitoring of their fluid balance and end organ function during the perioperative period in order to detect and prevent decompensation. High dependency care may be advisable for perioperative fluid balance in advanced disease.

Ischaemic Heart Disease

Reduced cardiovascular fitness and exercise tolerance can be common in older people; however, these factors are also important predictors of adverse postoperative cardiovascular outcomes. Exercise tolerance can be objectively assessed preoperatively using the scale of metabolic equivalents (METS). For most procedures, cardiovascular prognosis is excellent at METS 4 functional capacity, and further investigations do not change outcomes.

The patient group most likely to benefit from stress testing includes patients with both cardiovascular risk factors and functional performance <METS 4, who are due to undergo high- or intermediate-risk surgery. In older people, musculoskeletal co-morbidity can limit the value of exercise testing. In these cases, pharmacological stress testing may be helpful to establish risk of ischaemia.

Coronary angiography should be reserved for patients with high-risk features on stress imaging who are candidates for preoperative revascularization. The deployment of drug eluting or bare metal cardiac stents may mandate dual anti-platelet therapy with consequent effects on risk of perioperative bleeding. Therefore, careful decision making is required. Balloon angioplasty may be preferred in some circumstances to allow surgical intervention. Close liaison with cardiology is essential.

Antiplatelets Agents

Many patients undergoing surgery are on antiplatelet agents for primary or secondary prevention of cardiac disease. Most patients can safely stop aspirin for 5–7 days preoperatively. Patients who have previously had percutaneous coronary intervention should continue on aspirin perioperatively unless surgical risk of bleeding is high (e.g. spinal, posterior ophthalmic surgery). For patients who have had bare metal or drug eluting stent insertion, dual antiplatelets are recommended for at least 6 months from the date of deployment. Close liaison with cardiology is essential to discuss optimal timing of surgical intervention and risk associated with antiplatelet cessation. Early cessation risks in-stent thrombosis and acute ST elevation myocardial infarction. However, surgery in the context of dual antiplatelet therapy is associated with excess bleeding and need for blood transfusion. Where possible, surgery should be postponed for as long as possible up to a year after coronary intervention. In cancer or other urgent situations, this may not be possible and risk will depend upon the timing and nature of devices implanted in the coronary vasculature. The American College of Cardiology (http://www.acc.org/guidelines) and European Cardiological Society (https://www.escardio.org/Guidelines) provide up to date guidelines on perioperative management of antiplatelets, and a patient-by-patient approach is often required.

Anticoagulation

The approach to perioperative anticoagulation involves balancing the risks of surgical bleeding against those of thromboembolism. This assessment determines if and when anticoagulation should be interrupted, and whether bridging anticoagulation is indicated.

Table 10.5 below details patient factors that confer thromboembolic risk. Once procedural bleeding risk and thromboembolic risk have been estimated, then an individualized decision can be made on whether anticoagulation should be interrupted. In general, anticoagulation must be interrupted if procedural bleeding risk is high, which is the case in most types of surgery. In patients with low risk, it may be reasonable to continue anticoagulation and, in some circumstances, preferable (Table 10.6).

Patients at high/very high thromboembolic risk should have the period of interruption minimized with the use of

TABLE 10.5 Thromboembolic Risk.

Low risk	High risk
Aortic metal heart valve	Mitral metal heart valve
Xenograft heart valve	Prosthetic heart valve and atrial fibrillation
Atrial fibrillation without valvular lesion	Mitral stenosis and atrial fibrillation
>3 months following VTE	<3 months following VTE
Haemophilia syndromes (liaise with haematology)	Thrombophilia syndromes (liaise with haematology)

TABLE 10.6 Procedures Where Continuing Anticoagulation Is Preferable.

Dental procedures

Cutaneous procedure

Implantation of cardiac devices

Endovascular procedures and catheter ablation

bridging anticoagulation. If the risk of thromboembolism is transient, then it is advisable to delay surgery if possible until risk normalizes. Patients who require surgery within 4 weeks of an acute VTE who cannot be delayed and in whom anticoagulation must be interrupted can be considered for inferior vena caval filter insertion.

In most cases, warfarin should be stopped 5 days before surgery, and INR should be <1.5 before knife-to-skin. Modern direct oral anticoagulants (DOACs) should be discontinued 48–72 hours before surgery (depending on renal function). Bridging of anticoagulation with low-molecular-weight heparin should be reserved for patients usually maintained on warfarin at high risk of perioperative VTE. Bridging is rarely needed with DOACS due to the shorter washout period.

Unfractionated heparin may be required in patients with advanced renal disease where LMW heparins are contraindicated. In these cases, heparin infusions should be discontinued 4–5 hours prior to surgery.

For reversal of DOACs in the context of emergency surgery, consultation with haematology is advised, and likely to involve either prothrombin complex concentrate or monoclonal therapy. Emergency reversal of warfarin is achieved through vitamin K and prothrombin complex concentrate.

Chronic Lung Disease

Pulmonary complications are the most common medical complication of surgery. Patients with pre-existing lung disease are at increased risk of respiratory failure, though this can be complicated by other factors (Table 10.7)

Preoperative pulmonary rehabilitation in patients with underlying lung disease has been shown to improve outcome in patients undergoing cardiac, pulmonary or abdominal surgery. All patients should be advised to stop smoking preoperatively.

In patients with chronic obstructive pulmonary disease (COPD), the risk of complications is linked to severity of underling lung disease. Preoperative spirometry can highlight degree of clinical impairment (FEV_1 <50%

TABLE 10.7	Risk Factors for Developing Postoperative Respiratory Complications.	
Patient Factors	**Surgical Factors**
Underlying lung disease – asthma, COPD, bronchiectasis, fibrosis	Surgical site: thoracic + abdominal > other sites
Age	Duration of surgery
Smoking	General anaesthesia
Obesity	
Pulmonary hypertension	

severe) and ensure preoperative optimization of inhaler therapy. Patients should also be trained in deep breathing exercises; incentive spirometry should be considered. Perioperatively, patients should be closely monitored for signs of infection, receive appropriate analgesia and early physiotherapy. Supplemental oxygenation should be monitored closely, particularly due to concerns of carbon dioxide retention.

Obstructive Sleep Apnoea (OSA)

Obstructive sleep apnoea may be present in up to a quarter of adult patients undergoing surgery, but nearly 70% have no prior diagnosis. Common symptoms of snoring, excessive daytime sleepiness and episodes of apnoea should be screened for at pre-assessment. Where triggered by suspicious symptoms, Epworth and STOP-Bang scores may clarify the risk of OSA and triage to further assessment. Where possible, patients should be referred for sleep studies in advance of surgery. Stable preoperative nocturnal non-invasive ventilation may reduce perioperative complications.

The perioperative risks of OSA pertain to respiratory failure. This is exacerbated by opiate analgesics and neurosedative drugs of anaesthesia. Special anaesthetic interventions and extubation protocols may be indicated for patients with OSA. Making the diagnosis before surgery can therefore be important.

Diabetes Mellitus

Careful assessment of diabetic patients is required prior to surgery. Diabetes is associated with higher risks of postoperative infection, cardiovascular complications and adverse outcomes. Preoperative assessment should focus on modifying vascular risk and optimizing diabetic control. HbA1c should be checked within 3 months of surgery and, where indicated, optimized before surgery to improve preoperative glycaemic control.

Perioperative diabetic control aims to avoid dangerous hypoglycaemia; avoid excessive hyperglycaemia, ketoacidosis and hyperosmolar states; and maintain fluid and electrolyte status. Diabetic patients should be operated 'first on the list' to minimize time of nil by mouth disruption to their maintenance regime. Perioperative management of oral hypoglycaemics and insulin is complicated and is likely to require the support of the specialist diabetic team. Oral hypoglycaemics are mostly omitted on the day of surgery, with the exception of metformin and pioglitazone, which can be administered (assuming no use of i.v. contrast planned at surgery).

In patients anticipated to miss more than one meal, or in whom diabetic control is unstable, control of blood sugars with a variable rate insulin infusion (VRII) is required to achieve the recommended glucose range 6–10m mMol/L. VRII ('sliding scales') should be used sparingly for periods of protracted nil by mouth, or in the context of a non-functioning digestive tract.

In patients only expected to miss one meal or fewer, VRII can usually be avoided. In this context, long-acting insulins can be continued as normal. Twice daily mixed-insulin regimes are typically subject to a 50% dose reduction in the morning before surgery. Basal bolus regimes require omission of short-acting morning and lunchtime insulins with continuation of the basal long-acting insulin. Careful supervision by the diabetes team is recommended.

The VRII can be discontinued when the patient can eat and drink and revert to their standard medication. Transition off a VRII should occur when the next meal-related subcutaneous insulin is due, and this dose should be administered 30 minutes before the VRII is stopped. Dose adjustment of insulin may be indicated if oral intake is expected to be sub-maximal.

Chronic Liver Disease (CLD)

Chronic liver disease presents very specific perioperative challenges. The chief objective is to avoid decompensated CLD in the postoperative period, as this condition has a high mortality. Deranged clotting and thrombocytopaenia must be corrected prior to incision. For planned major surgery, a platelet count of <50,000/microL warrants preoperative transfusion. In surgeries in which even small volume bleeding can have catastrophic consequences (e.g. neurosurgery), a threshold of <100,000/microL is warranted. However, platelet transfusion is usually unnecessary for a minor surgery unless the count is <20,000/microL.

Preoperative anaesthetic review is essential as avoidance of neuromuscular blocking agents, halothane and older hepato-metabolized inhalational agents may be appropriate. Careful attention must be paid when prescribing to avoid hepato-metabolized drugs which may accumulate in CLD and cause encephalopathy (e.g. some opiates). High protein absorption from the upper digestive tract can precipitate hepatic decompensation. This must be avoided with prophylactic laxatives to ensure rapid transit time and bowel opening twice daily.

Ascites can accumulate following the administration of sodium-rich intravenous fluid, and should be treated with either diuresis or drainage to prevent wound dehiscence following open abdominal surgery. Low sodium diet and 20% human albumin solutions can be used to treat and prevent ascites accumulation. Nutrition is often poor and should be optimized in these patients carefully.

Hepatic decompensation typically presents with worsening jaundice, encephalopathy and ascites. Liver function tests including prothrombin time and serum bilirubin can guide management. This should be conducted in conjunction with the parent medical team. Underlying causes (e.g. medication, infection, constipation) must be aggressively treated.

Stroke

Stroke is common in older age. Furthermore, it is a well-recognized complication of major vascular and cardiac surgery with incidence as high as 10% for some types of valve surgery. For most elective non-cardiac surgery incidence is lower (1–4%).

Stroke can result in loss of cerebral auto-regulation, leaving patients susceptible to cerebral haemodynamic compromise during anaesthesia and surgery. Cessation of antiplatelet therapy can also elevate risk of stroke recurrence. It is therefore important to consider the timing of elective surgery following stroke. The highest risk of recurrence is within the first month and most elective procedures should be delayed for at least 3 months after cerebral infarction wherever possible. If significant carotid stenosis is identified, carotid artery revascularization can be performed up to 12 weeks after stroke and is usually prioritized over elective surgery. Decisions to cease antiplatelet and anticoagulant medications perioperatively should take into account the bleeding risk of surgery and risk of recurrent stroke. For patients with atrial fibrillation, the CHADSVASC score (www.chadsvasc.org) is commonly used to quantify risk of stroke in patients with atrial fibrillation; high risk patients may require bridging of anticoagulation in the perioperative period with subcutaneous heparin (see thromboembolism section).

In patients in whom a diagnosis of acute stroke is made in the postoperative period, emergent discussion with the hyperacute stroke team is required. Thrombolysis is usually contraindicated following invasive surgery (depending on type of surgical procedure), but patients may still be able to undergo interventional thrombectomy and should be considered for urgent transfer if necessary.

Parkinson's Disease

Parkinson's disease is a risk factor for inpatient falls, delirium, impaired swallow and aspiration pneumonia in the perioperative period. Ensuring effective delivery of anti-parkinsonian medications throughout the perioperative period is essential to maintain mobility and prevent complications. Liaison with neurology in advance of surgery may be necessary to allow conversion of oral medication to a Rotigotine patch for those with prolonged nil by mouth or gastric malabsorption. For low-risk procedures, oral Parkinson's medication should be given on the morning of surgery with sips of water (even if nil by mouth). Regular assessment of swallow postoperatively is essential as Parkinson's patients are particularly susceptible to swallowing impairment in the perioperative period. Nasogastric tube siting may be necessary to administer essential medication whilst nil by mouth or if swallow is decompensated. Anti-dopaminergic drugs such as metoclopramide and haloperidol are contraindicated in Parkinson's disease. Some patients have deep brain stimulators which must be turned off prior to surgery. The website www.parkinsons.org.uk provides useful advice for management of Parkinson's patients in emergencies.

Cognitive Impairment and Delirium

Cognitive impairment and dementia are underdiagnosed in older persons undergoing surgery. It is therefore important to recognize that although no formal diagnosis may

TABLE 10.8	Delirium Prevention Strategies.
Anaesthetic	• Consider depth-of-anaesthesia monitoring. Aim for values of 50–60 intraoperatively and avoid burst suppression on EEG. • Employ multi-modal analgesia to minimize opioid use. Specifically consider regional blocks, regular paracetamol and intra-op clonidine. Prescribe PRN laxatives to all these patients. • Avoid ketamine, benzodiazepines, anticholinergics and antihistamines (e.g. cyclizine). Objective neuromuscular function monitor can establish when neostigmine/glycol is not indicated. • Aim for a stable intraoperative BP. Target a systolic BP of no less than 80% pre-op baseline. Consider invasive arterial monitoring. • Avoid catheterization, drains or NG tubes unless clearly indicated.
Prevent infection	• Sit out & mobilize day 1 (unless medically contraindicated) • Remove all medical devices (e.g. CVP lines, urinary catheters, i.v. access) as soon as no longer medically indicated • Consider incentive spirometry and deep breathing exercises • Have a low threshold for chest physiotherapy
Patient orientation	• Ensure regular orientation by all staff • Optimize sleep hygiene; avoid bedrest during day • Encourage family members to visit (including overnight, if helpful) • Ensure glasses and hearing aids are available
Treat pain	• Use individualized multi-modal pain control • Ensure, if opiate is used, it is appropriate for renal function • Ensure vigilant dose titration
Review medication	• Minimize potentially inappropriate medications/psychoactive medications • Monitor for alcohol & benzodiazepine withdrawal
Avoid constipation	• Prescribe laxatives prophylactically with opiates • Use a bowel chart; monitor for constipation
Ensure nutrition	• Ensure dentures available • Resume oral diet as soon as possible • Dietician review and consider supplements for all patients at risk • Monitor fluid intake and electrolytes
Prevent falls	• Risk-assess and take preventative action

BP, Blood pressure; CVP, central venous pressure; EEG, electroencephalogram; NG, nasogastric; PRN, as needed.

previously have been made, cognitive impairment may exist nonetheless. Recognizing cognitive impairment and dementia is important, because these diagnoses may influence mental capacity to consent to surgery. It is also the most important risk factor for delirium, and various delirium prevention measures have been shown to reduce the incidence and severity of postoperative delirium (Table 10.8).

Where dementia or cognitive impairment is suspected or known to exist, formal assessment of mental capacity should be conducted. Evaluation is warranted in memory services but should not normally delay planned surgery.

Anaemia

Many types of surgery are associated with blood loss that can ensue even in the context of best surgical care. Patients with pre-surgical anaemia are at greater risk of requiring a perioperative blood transfusion. Although mitigation of bleeding risk is important, it is also mandatory to optimize anaemia prior to surgery to reduce the need for perioperative transfusions that carry inherent risks and healthcare costs. Erythropoietin and intravenous iron have a role in patients with anaemia secondary to chronic renal failure. In patients with iron deficiency anaemia or cancer, intravenous iron can improve preoperative haemoglobin and reduce the need for future transfusion. These intravenous preparations require 2–4 weeks to achieve a partial effect on haemoglobin, and 6 weeks for full efficacy; this is achievable in many existing UK surgical pathways.

Chronic Kidney Disease (CKD)

CKD is a risk factor for postoperative acute kidney injury, which is usually precipitated through renal hypoperfusion, intravenous contrast or nephrotoxic medication. To avoid acute kidney injury, meticulous attention to fluid balance is required and maintenance of perfusion blood pressure in the perioperative period. Prehydration may be required prior to surgery involving angiography, or in which the patient will be exposed to large volume contrast load. ACEIs should be discontinued 24 hours before surgery, and nephrotoxic medications avoided and/or dose adjusted for renal function throughout the admission. Close liaison with ward pharmacists is advised.

In end-stage renal failure (ESRF) patients dependent of haemodialysis, co-management with the renal team is warranted to ensure that the patient is dialysed and euvolemic at the time of surgery. Typically, this will involve preoperative dialysis the day before surgery. Express caution must be used in avoiding volume overload and excess intravenous fluids in anuric patients with ESRF.

Immunosuppression

Rheumatological disorders are common in older patients and long-term transplant survivors are increasingly numerous. These patients are often immunosuppressed with steroids and other agents. These drugs can influence the risks of postoperative infection and impair wound healing. Where chronic steroids are employed, perioperative hypoadrenal crisis must be prevented. Perioperative management of these patients is complex and co-management with specialist physicians is recommended.

Ideally, the lowest possible dose of steroids should be used in the perioperative setting. In patients requiring <5 mg prednisolone (or equivalent) daily, or who have been on any dose of steroids for <3 weeks, suppression of the adrenal–hypothalamic axis is unlikely. Dose adjustment is unlikely to be required. However, dose conversion may be required to a parenteral equivalent whilst the patient is nil by mouth. In Cushingoid patients, or those taking >20 mg prednisolone daily, suppression of the adrenal axis can be assumed. Dose supplementation and duration depends on the stress of surgery. These patients should receive 50–100 mg i.v. hydrocortisone at induction, followed by 25–50 mg hydrocortisone 8-hourly, for at least 24 hours, but, in severe surgical stress (e.g. oesophagectomy), tapered by 50% daily to their usual maintenance dose. Patients taking an intermediate dose of steroids (e.g. 10–20 mg prednisolone) should undergo preoperative assessment of their adrenal axis to avoid unnecessary administration of excess steroid.

In transplant patients, non-steroid immunosuppressants should continue at their usual dose. Parenteral administration may be required if gastrointestinal absorption will be compromised. In patients with rheumatological disease, risk assessment must be conducted to determine the risks of interrupting therapy, which may result in a disease flare compromising recovery from surgery. Existing data indicate that methotrexate, hydroxychloroquine, sulfasalazine and leflunomide are safe to continue in the perioperative period, and that continuation does not result in increased infection or complications. Furthermore, the risk of discontinuing immunosuppressants in patients with complex multi-organ disease (e.g. systemic lupus erythematosus) can be hazardous.

However, biologic disease modifying agents (DMARDs) (e.g. etanercept) should ideally be withheld for at least one treatment cycle before elective surgery (e.g. 2 weeks for etanercept). Biologic DMARDs should not be reinstated until wound healing has occurred. Perioperative liaison with the patient's treating physician is recommended. Emergency surgery should not be delayed if these drugs have been administered recently.

Anticipatory Discharge Planning

It is well-known that ensuring patient flow through the surgical bed-base requires an active approach to discharge planning. Older patients frequently decondition following surgery as a result of frailty and immobilization-induced sarcopaenia; older patients are therefore prone to increased length of stay. Although enhanced recovery programmes aim to mitigate these risks, implementation of these programmes requires leadership and teamwork from the wider multidisciplinary surgical team. Clear leadership is needed from senior surgeons on projected medical fitness for discharge. Key factors include management of patient and family expectation in the preoperative phase, setting anticipated discharge dates, early access to physical and occupational therapy and early referral to social services where needed.

Anaesthesia in the Older Person

Age-related changes in multiple organ systems render the older patient more susceptible to the adverse effects of anaesthetic agents. The central nervous system has greater pharmaco-dynamic sensitivity to all intravenous agents acting centrally, and respiratory suppression is exaggerated with opioids, benzodiazepines and volatile anaesthetic agents. Labile blood pressure is common and diastolic dysfunction makes the older heart particularly susceptible to hypotension and pulmonary oedema even with brief periods of atrial arrhythmias. Blunted autonomic responses limit the ability of the heart to maintain cardiac output in the face of hypovolaemia or vasodilatation; the requirement for inotropic agents intraoperatively is therefore much more common in older patients. Invasive blood pressure monitoring is often required for older patients.

Most intravenous drugs are metabolized more slowly due to reduced hepatic function and blood flow; low albumin can lead to higher free-drug concentrations. In addition, increased adipose tissue and reduced total body water can increase the effective concentration of induction agents such as propofol. Doses required for induction in older patients are typically reduced by 30–50%.

There is increasing evidence that depth of anaesthesia and intraoperative hypotension impact upon incidence of postoperative delirium. Intraoperative processed electroencephalogram monitoring can be used to guide depth of anaesthesia, and invasive arterial monitoring can direct maintenance of arterial blood pressure.

Poor peripheral circulation and friable skin make older patients more susceptible to nerve compression, pressure sores and compartment syndrome. Appropriate equipment must therefore be available to minimize risk.

Perioperative hypothermia is also more common in older patients and associated with delirium, coagulopathy, cardiac dysfunction and poor wound healing. Therefore regular monitoring and forced air warming or fluid warming should be available.

Perioperative neuraxial anaesthesia (e.g. epidural) and multimodal analgesia can reduce requirement for opioids with resultant benefits in delirium incidence and pulmonary complications.

Analgesia in the Older Person

The World Health Organization pain ladder is typically used as a structured guide for postoperative pain management. However, older people have altered physiology rendering them vulnerable to toxicity and delirium. Many older patients have underlying chronic kidney disease affecting excretion of opiates. Frail, sarcopaenic patients often display 'normal' serum creatinine levels, despite impaired estimated GFR (eGFR). This can lead to under-appreciation of impaired renal clearance; calculation of creatinine clearance may therefore be indicated to ensure safe prescribing.

Treatment modalities to consider include:

Patient Controlled Analgesia (PCA)

PCA should be considered in older patients in the immediate postoperative period. It is well tolerated and can even be trialled in patients with some cognitive impairment. Duration of treatment should be limited to promote mobility and functional rehabilitation.

Neuroaxial Analgesia

Epidural and spinal analgesia is generally well-tolerated and can minimize side effects of systemic analgesia and reduce infective complications. Spinal degenerative disease can limit use in some patients. Patients should be monitored for urinary retention.

Regional Nerve Block

Regional analgesia can reduce complications and opiate consumption. Fascia iliaca block is increasingly used in the management of acute neck of femur fracture patients.

Non-Steroidal Anti-Inflammatories (NSAIDS)

NSAIDS should be used with caution in older patients due to an increased incidence of kidney disease and elevated risk of peptic ulceration. If necessary, co-administration of a low dose proton pump inhibitor should be considered and duration of treatment should be limited.

Gabapentinoids

Gabapentin and pregabalin have been shown to reduce opiate consumption in the context of postoperative pain. They are neuro-sedatives and can cause delirium. They should

therefore be used with caution in the older people, though may have a short-term role in the immediate perioperative period as part of a multimodal analgesic strategy.

Opiates

Systemic opiates are the mainstay of perioperative pain control. Basic principles of use in older people include careful dose titration to pain, and avoidance of rapid escalation in dosing. However, it is important to be mindful that under-treated pain is a strong precipitant of delirium and therefore must be avoided. Opiates are highly constipating and concomitant administration of laxatives should be considered with all systemic opiate analgesics. Oxycodone or hydromorphone may be preferred in those with renal impairment.

Trauma in the Older Person

The ageing population has led to a dramatic shift over the last decade in the demographics of major trauma admissions. Patients older than 65 now make up the majority of admissions with injury severity scores >15, and the leading mechanism of injury is fall from less than 2 metres. Older patients face poorer outcomes than their younger counterparts. The reasons for this are discussed in Table 10.9.

Head Injury

Most deaths from trauma in older patients occur due to head injury. Higher prevalence of anticoagulation is partly accountable for this, but also delay in diagnosis due to co-existence of dementia or delirium. Cerebral atrophy can also mean that subacute or chronic subdural haemorrhages can take longer to cause compressive symptoms or raised intracerebral pressure.

Spinal Injury

Cervical spine injuries are common in older trauma. Pre-existing degenerative cervical spine disease, including

TABLE 10.9	Reasons for Poorer Outcomes in Older Trauma Patients.

Pre-hospital triage systems tend to focus on high-energy mechanisms of injury.

Essential hypertension and beta blockade can mask the early signs of shock. This can lead to under-appreciation of injury severity and delayed aggressive management.

Older patients are more likely to take anticoagulants. In combination with tissue fragility, higher rates of major haemorrhage are seen.

Co-morbidities, frailty and lack of physiological reserve result in higher incidence of injury-related and perioperative complications.

TABLE 10.10	Indications for Surgical Rib Fixation.

- Severe chest deformities
- Three or more consecutive rib fractures
- Flail chest (>two rib fractures in two places)

osteophytic disease, intervertebral disc degeneration, posterior ligamentous hypertrophy and pre-existing spinal canal stenosis predispose to injury and can make diagnosis more challenging. Early imaging of the cervical spine in any older patient that has endured a head injury should be strongly considered. Minor extension injuries in patients with severe degenerative disease can result in anterior or central cord syndromes.

Osteoporotic vertebral compression fractures are common in older patients and can often occur after minor falls or in the absence of defined trauma. Mid thoracic and thoracolumbar vertebrae are most commonly affected; severe pain with loss of mobility and impaired rehabilitation are common sequelae. In patients unresponsive or intolerant to analgesia, there is a mixed evidence base for kypho-vertebroplasty.

Rib Fractures

Rib fractures are prevalent in older patients with trauma. However, 50% of rib fractures are not evident on chest radiograph and are therefore commonly missed. CT imaging should be considered in any older patient with traumatic rib pain to assess the extent of injury. Prompt pain management and physiotherapy can help to prevent respiratory hypostasis, hypoxia and pneumonia, which is a common potentially fatal complication in older cohorts. Epidural analgesia or other invasive analgesic techniques (eg. serratus anterior nerve block or erector spinae nerve block) should be considered early to aid recovery. Associated pulmonary contusion, pneumothorax and haemothorax are common. These are all poorly tolerated in older patients with higher rates of respiratory failure. Close monitoring of respiratory function is essential as respiratory failure can progress abruptly in the tiring frail patient. Non-invasive or mechanical ventilation should be considered as a bridge to recovery. Surgical fixation of severe rib injuries should be considered early for those with severe injuries to help restore normal thoracic physiology and reduce long-term complications (Table 10.10).

Hip Fractures

Hip fractures are the commonest serious injury in the older people and are associated with significant morbidity and mortality. Thirty-day mortality in frail older people is around 8–10% in most UK hospitals, but in specific subgroups (e.g. patients with dementia) it may be as high as 40%. It is therefore critical that services are designed to care for these high-risk patients.

Key goals in the management of hip fracture include:
- Prompt analgesia and regular assessment; early consideration of fascia iliac blocks
- Movement of patients to specialized orthopaedic units within 4 hours of arrival
- Surgical intervention within 36 hours
- Orthogeriatric review within 72 hours
- Mobilization day one after surgery

Perioperative Service Delivery for Complex Patients

On-Call Medical Service

In the event of medical issues, ad-hoc review is requested from the on-call medical team. Disadvantages of this predominant service model are legion. Medical registrars receive little or no specific training in perioperative medicine. Furthermore, the conflicting demands of their role often leads to delay in (reactive) review and inaccessibility. The rotational nature of acute medical services leads to absent continuity of care.

Reciprocal Ward Linking

Partnering of surgical and medical teams based on location and speciality can be an effective way of providing medical support without resorting to on-call medical teams. A disadvantage of this service is that non-specialist Internal Medicine teams may lack expertise in perioperative medicine, and liaison is typically reactive rather than proactive.

Specialist Review

For a small number of patients, it is necessary to involve specialist teams closely in the perioperative period where the complexity of the patient prevents exclusive management by general physicians (e.g. transplant patients).

Anaesthetic Services

Increasingly, anaesthetists are playing a wider role in perioperative medicine. This is typically focussed on surgical pre-assessment. However, many anaesthetists lack experience in the optimization of chronic medical co-morbidity and referral to various specialist teams prior to surgery is often indicated. This can delay surgery. Postoperative anaesthetic support typically involves delivery of level 2 and 3 care to high-risk patients. Few services offer routine support for level 1 surgical patients.

Embedded Geriatric Services

In this model of care, medical support is provided by a dedicated specialist team throughout the surgical pathway. There is a clear focus on preoperative optimization, early recognition and treatment of postoperative complications, shared decision making, rehabilitation and discharge planning. This model evolved in the setting of geriatric trauma (e.g. orthogeriatrics) but also has an emerging evidence base in other surgical specialties. It promotes close collaboration between surgeons and physicians to facilitate education, training and robust governance structures. It is currently considered the gold standard and is promoted by The Royal College of Surgeons and the Department of Health.

Summary and Conclusions

As the population continues to age and the number of older patients undergoing surgery climbs, surgical and anaesthetic services must adapt to maintain quality and individualised care. Collaborative care between geriatricians, surgical and anaesthetic teams is essential to effectively manage patients. Perioperative geriatricians have a role to play throughout the surgical pathway and can contribute to case selection with personalised risk assessment, through perioperative comprehensive geriatric assessment. Proactive management of frailty, multi-morbidity and geriatric syndromes can reduce perioperative risk and improve outcomes. The recent emphasis on perioperative research in complex high-risk patients will pave the way for further advancements in the quality of care provided for surgical patients most vulnerable to adverse surgical outcomes.

11

The Dying Surgical Patient

CHAPTER OUTLINE

All of your patients will die – those you have saved from death with your skill and hard work who will go on to live their lives for many years to come, those for whom you have bought some time or perhaps an improved quality of life and the very important group in your care who are known to be dying or at considerable risk of doing so.

Just under half of all deaths take place in hospital in the UK[1] and many will die an expected death while under your care as a surgeon. This chapter seeks to provide you with the knowledge and skill to feel competent and more confident to provide care for dying patients and those they love who sit at their bedside. Many of the skills you already have and much of the knowledge you gain and the skills you acquire in compassionate care can be extended to the care of those dying in emergency situations and indeed to the care of every patient.

How Do I Review a Dying Patient?

CASE HISTORY

David is 71, married to Doris (73) with three adult children. He was admitted to the surgical ward 5 days ago and is noted to have deteriorated daily since admission. David had a diagnosis of bowel cancer 5 years ago and completed radiotherapy and chemotherapy. He was admitted to your ward to rule out bowel obstruction – this diagnosis has been ruled out and scans have demonstrated marked disease progression. David is dying with a prognosis of days. You are responsible for reviewing David today but have never met him and his family.

Before Going in to See the Patient

1. Review notes with a focus on understanding:
   a. an overview of the disease history
   b. whether there is any specific information about symptoms and any suggested management plans for those symptoms over the past days
   c. whether any specific information has been given to the patient regarding prognosis
   d. whether there have been any conversations about the patients concerns, fears, wishes and preferences
   e. who is in this person's family and close circle
   f. what information has been given to the patient's family and any concerns they raised
   g. whether a decision regarding Do Not Attempt Cardiopulmonary Resuscitation (DNACPR) has been documented and communicated with the patient and his family
   h. whether treatment escalation plans or goals of care have been clarified
   i. whether there are any comments on mental capacity
   j. whether anyone in the family holds a Lasting Power of Attorney (LPA) for health, and if so, who this is
   k. whether the patient has an advance care plan
   l. whether spiritual and religious needs have been addressed
   m. whether there has been any conversation about wishes regarding tissue donation
2. Review any recent bloods – looking particularly at the patient's renal function and hepatic function
3. Review the most recent scans
4. Review the medication chart taking particular note of whether the patient is able to swallow oral medication and whether any breakthrough medications (PRNs) have been needed in the past 24 hours

5. Check with the nurse caring for the patient as to whether s/he has any concerns

In summary, your preparation provides you with a history, recent bloods results, most recent scan, medications and the assessment of the nursing team caring for the patient – broad categories that are the same for every patient review you undertake.

Key Information to Take to the Bedside

David was diagnosed with bowel cancer 5 years ago. His admission notes recorded in the emergency department stated that his family had noticed him 'going downhill' in the 2 months prior to his admission.

David's symptoms were fatigue (sleeping most of the day and needing help to get to the bathroom) and abdominal pain. Pain is being controlled with morphine MR 30 mg bid PO and 10 mg Oramorph PRN. David usually takes 1–2 PRNs per 24-hour period. You note that the nursing records document day to day changes in David's strength. David was vomiting on admission but that has settled with metoclopramide 10 mg tds PO.

On the ward round 3 days ago, your consultant addressed David's question about prognosis – Doris and one of their children were at the bedside. Everyone agreed that they could see David deteriorating from day to day and David was not surprised to learn that the medical staff thought his prognosis was a short number of days. David's main worry was being a burden to his wife who has cardiac failure. Doris worried that David would suffer and was very sad that they would not be able to celebrate their golden wedding anniversary in 4 months' time.

The notes did not mention any concerns about capacity and abbreviated mental test score (AMTS) was normal.

There is a DNACPR decision in the notes which has been discussed with David and Doris. However, there is no information regarding the team's thoughts about how to manage David if he becomes acutely unwell and no documentation of a conversation with David discussing his views. There is no information about David's views on tissue donation. You see that David's religion is documented as Church of England.

David's eGFR is >60 mL/min. Hepatic function is abnormal – three times the upper limit of normal.

David's scan on admission showed local disease in the original tumour bed, widespread lymphadenopathy, hepatic metastases replacing >75% of his liver and small volume pulmonary metastases.

David is on 24 regular oral medications (secondary prevention of cardiovascular disease, oral hypoglycaemics, morphine and metoclopramide). David has taken four PRNs of Oramorph in the past 12 hours – his usual pattern is one or two PRNs in 24 hours.

David's nurse reports that he has had chest pain, a cough and seems much less well. There are no observations recorded as regular observations were discontinued 3 days ago.

On Entering the Room

1. Take a history from the patient and family with a focus on understanding:

- Whether the patient is well enough to answer or will you need to take the history from any family present. If the patient is unconscious or semiconscious – ask whether they do respond to those at the bedside
- The story over the last 24 hours
- Symptom check – pains and discomforts, breathlessness, nausea, bowels
- Symptom check – sleep, nightmares, confusion, hallucinations. If the patient is unconscious or semiconscious, do they pick at sheets, reach out when nothing is there or say inappropriate things?
- Any other concerns or observations noted by those at the bedside
- If the patient is unconscious or semiconscious, have the people at the bedside noted any changes in perfusion to peripheries (cold hands and feet) or changes in the rhythm or sound of breathing

2. Examine the patient:

First observations:

On approaching the patient you will see if they notice you and whether they can respond. You may see the patient open their eyes when you introduce yourself. A very ill patient may still have enough strength to flicker their eyelids or squeeze your hand gently or you may see a change in breathing rate. You may not notice any response in unconscious patients. (Continue to address patients, explaining what you are doing and briefly explaining management plans – at the very least, it conveys your respect of the patient and the life they have lived to those at the bedside.)

a. Observation:
- general colour – pallor, jaundice, cyanosis
- lying peacefully and looking comfortable or demonstrating agitation
- rate and pattern of breathing (regular or Cheyne Stokes pattern). Is the patient using their accessory muscles to aid respiration and is it effortful? Is there any vocalization or noise on expiration? Can you hear noisy, rattly breathing (often known as death rattle)?
- any evident distension, swelling or bruising?
- scan for any i.v. cannulas, other lines and the presence or absence of a catheter
- look at the person's eyes – are the corneal surfaces dry or infected
- look at the person's mouth – is there any evidence of candida infection, is the mouth dry or are there ulcers?

b. Palpation:
- to check if there is any evidence of parotid gland swelling
- to check the radial pulse (rhythm, strength and whether possible to palpate radially)
- to check circulation (temperature) and capillary refill time in the person's hands and feet
- to check for abdominal masses and for bladder distension

c. Percussion:
  - as necessary to examine the chest and abdomen
d. Auscultation:
  - to determine if cardiac failure is present (checking JVP), any signs consistent with pneumonia or pleural effusion and the presence or absence of bowel sounds
3. Personalized management plan:
  - explain what you found to those at the bedside
  - explain your management plan or the fact that you need to discuss your findings with your team and develop a plan with them
  - explain when you will come back to discuss a plan or explain when you will next review the patient
  - check that the patient and/or their family understand and are content with this plan so far

In summary, the history and examination help you develop a management plan. You manage the immediate situation to ensure patient safety and comfort as you do for every patient you review. Earlier in your career, you may wish to discuss your management plans with your surgical seniors; later in your career, you may be happy to proceed to explaining and implementing your plan.

Key Information at the Bedside

On walking to the bedside, you see that David does not respond when you introduce yourself.

Doris tells you that she is really worried about David – 'he is in pain'. Doris has observed that David is restless, moving around the bed at times and his brow is furrowed. The 10 mg of Oramorph given just after she arrived this morning helped David sleep for an hour but has worn off. In response to your enquiry, Doris tells you that David's breathing looks like very hard work; it is fast and noisy at times. Doris has observed that David was flushed and sweating for an hour but that has settled. Doris has noticed that David is reaching out – 'but there is nothing there' – and has been trying to tell her things – 'that I cannot catch'. Doris is tearful and scared. She is also very worried that David has not had anything to eat or drink today.

David is jaundiced and restless in his bed. He opens his eyes to your command but is unable to focus his attention or answer questions, though he tries to speak with you.

David's respiratory rate is 32 breaths per minute with a normal respiratory rhythm. He is using his accessory muscles of respiration but does not appear to be ventilating his right lung. There are some audible secretions in David's upper airway that are oscillating with inspiration and expiration. David's mouth is very dry.

David's hands are cold and cyanosed. It is difficult to palpate his radial artery. Capillary refill time is greater than 2 seconds. JVP is not raised. Apical pulse rate is 130 beats per minute. David has a right-sided pneumonia on examination. Abdominal examination is unremarkable apart from the fact that bowel sounds are absent. You note a urinary catheter in place.

You explain to Doris that you have found signs of pneumonia and that the pneumonia is causing a delirium (evidence of restlessness, reaching out for things and being incoherent) and making it difficult for David to regulate his breathing and circulation (evidence of tachypnoea, tachycardia, poor peripheral perfusion).

You tell Doris that you are going to arrange for an injection of morphine to help David's breathing to become more comfortable and treat any pain present, and an injection of midazolam so that he is more restful and calmer.

You explain you are going to update your senior and will be back in 30 minutes or so. You advise Doris to call their children and ask them to visit today.

On Leaving the Room

1. Ensure the patient's immediate comfort, managing the most troublesome symptoms by prescribing and/or requesting administration of PRN medication. If the patient is very ill, these PRNs need to be given parenterally, subcutaneously or, on occasion, intravenously.
2. Phone your senior, providing a clinical update in order to establish the direction of care – whether that is symptomatic management or a trial of intervention (including intravenous antibiotics) in addition to symptom management.
3. Describe the troublesome symptoms and your thoughts about how to manage those. Develop a plan with your senior, seeking advice from your palliative care service where you are both uncertain about management.
4. Prescribe PRN medications for the patient to be available in case of pain, dyspnoea, nausea and/or vomiting, agitation and delirium.
5. Prescribe a continuous subcutaneous infusion to be delivered via a syringe driver if the patient has been using PRNs in the preceding 12–24 hours.
6. Review the patient's medication chart, discontinuing all medications for secondary prevention of disease, thromboprophylaxis, laxatives and the majority of oral medications. You may wish to continue the prescription of thyroxine where the patient is able to take small amounts of food.
7. Review the local criteria for tissue donation (cornea, tissue for research purposes) in order to be able to discuss with the patient's family.
8. Discuss your plans with the nurse caring for the patient and review together whether there are any outstanding issues.

On returning to David's bedside with David's nurse, you see that he is more comfortable. His respiratory rate is now 26 breaths/min and the rhythm remains regular. David does not respond when you check his pulse – Doris says that he became more peaceful about 15 minutes after his nurse gave him the injection of the two medicines.

David and Doris's children have arrived. You invite David's family to come away from his bedside to discuss the management plan.

You and the nurse update the family that David has pneumonia and an agitated delirium. You continue on to say that David is markedly less well today and that you expect that he will die in the coming hours or short days. You fill the family in on your conversation with your senior – that it is your advice as a surgical team that treatment should be focused on symptom management. David's son comments that as a family they have seen their father deteriorate daily and they are all aware that David is dying though it is very sad and a shock just at the moment. David's nurse asks if they might like to have a side room to have some more privacy – Doris asks if the nurse could check with the other patients in the room. David loved their company and she would like him to stay in the bay but would not want to upset other people.

You discuss that David will not be able to take any medicines by mouth from now on and that you have discontinued all non-essential medicines. However, David has needed some extra medications to manage symptoms over the past 24 hours and, in order to ensure his comfort, you have prescribed an infusion of morphine (to help breathlessness and replace his regular oral morphine) and of midazolam (to help with the delirium). You explain that the infusion will be given under the skin and will take about 4 hours to build up to effective levels in David's body. An extra bolus may be necessary from time to time and those are prescribed. The boluses will be reviewed every 24 hours and the infusion adjusted if more than two boluses are needed in a 24-hour period. You enquire whether the family have any experience of syringe drivers – Doris's friend died recently and had a syringe driver at home. She died peacefully. The family do not have any concerns about syringe drivers.

You say that as David's mouth is very dry and he is breathing through his mouth, you have prescribed a gel to help ease that symptom. David's family can help with mouth care using water and the gel – David's nurse offers to come back and show the family how to do that.

You ask if David had any views on organ or tissue donation. Doris says that he always carried an organ donor card – 'surely with cancer he cannot donate anything'. You explain that you think he may be eligible to donate his corneas and you ask whether and when David's family might like to talk to the team in the hospital. They agree that they will discuss those matters after David's death. You agree to flag to the tissue donation team to be picked up in due course.

You ask if Doris and their children have any questions or concerns. They cannot think of any – you add that you do not expect that David will eat or drink again and that the surgical team sees this as a normal part of the process of dying and will not give intravenous food or fluids.

You ask if everyone who needs to know is aware that David is dying – they are. You also check whether the family might like to see a chaplain or whether David might value that.

You check with the nurse whether there is anything else to discuss, check with the family that they do not have any questions and say that you will hand over to the team on that night and will see them tomorrow.

You escort the family back to David's bedside.

You document your review, your plan and the team decision to avoid further tests and i.v. interventions.

In Conclusion

When reviewing a dying patient, gather background information before entering the room, take a history and examine the patient in the room (thinking about the patient's capacity in relation to the Mental Capacity Act, England and Wales) and develop a management plan in the room or on leaving the room.

Additional thoughts when developing an individualized management plan for a dying patient include:
- The need for a DNACPR decision and treatment (and investigation) escalation plans/ReSPECT[2]
- A low threshold for discussion of clinically assisted hydration and nutrition[3]
- Enquiring about tissue donation[4]
- Considering spiritual and religious support
- Informing the family and those who are important to the patient of deterioration and expected prognosis[5]

Considerations and Questions That Arise at the End of Life

Is This Patient Dying?

At a macro level, we know that 25–30% of inpatients on any day in an acute hospital will die of their illnesses within the subsequent 12 months.[6] The question 'is the patient dying?' is really important to ask and address as recognition of dying opens the way for essential conversations with patients and their families. It is important to ask the patient what really matters to them as that information will guide your decision making.

It can be difficult to diagnose dying no matter how experienced you are. Research has shown that nursing assistants (healthcare assistants) are the group of healthcare staff that are most accurate in terms of prognostication. Perhaps this is because they closely observe functional ability, and changes in that ability, day by day.

There are several prognostic tools available but, as yet, the tools do not help guide us as to an individual patient's prognosis.

The scales tip toward an increased likelihood of dying during this admission where there is a history of multiple admissions in the past 12 months, frequent infections, multiple co-morbid conditions especially failure of more than one major organ system, decreasing functional ability and being increasingly housebound, which all suggest increasing frailty and decreasing reserve to withstand further insults to health.

The likelihood of dying during this admission increases where there is limited or no opportunity to treat the underlying condition, e.g. the patient is on maximal management of their cardiac failure or the risks and potential adverse effects of surgery for a bowel perforation disease outweigh the benefits. The patient may also decline interventions or a trial of treatment.

Where the patient is deteriorating despite interventions (aiming to address reversible causes), it is useful to ask the patient and also their family if they see deterioration from day to day or week to week. People find this question easy to answer and it guides your ability to hone prognosis. Where you, the healthcare team and the family are noticing changes every day, then the patient is likely to die in days. It remains a good practical rule of thumb that where a patient is deteriorating:

- Day by day, they probably only have days to live
- Week by week, they probably only have weeks to live
- Month by month, they probably only have months to live[7]

Patients who have hours to short days to live often have profound muscle wasting, are very weak (being unable to sit up in bed or roll over without help), spend the majority of their time sleeping and are difficult to rouse, have limited energy and fall back to sleep during conversation, have little interest in food and possibly fluids and struggle to swallow medications. You may observe tachypnoea and tachycardia at rest, leading to altered respiratory patters including Cheyne Stokes respiration, and to altered perfusion of hands and feet (mottled, cold peripheries and it is difficult to palpate arterial pulsation).

Even very frail patients can surprise us and continue living alongside impending death day by day. This is a very difficult situation for families who are often glad to have more time with the patient, perhaps hope that they might improve but also hope that the patient's suffering ends soon. It may be helpful to acknowledge that this ambivalence is common. This is also a difficult situation for you and may leave you feeling underconfident about your diagnosis of dying. Where there are no signs of improvement, you can be confident that your patient will die, though it may take a week or 10 days. Daily review and a senior opinion are as important as they would be when managing any acutely ill patient with a reversible condition. It may be helpful to ask for a specialist palliative care review which will offer your team a second opinion.

On rare occasions, a very frail patient surprises us even more by beginning to improve against all odds. The healthcare team need to review all decisions and medications. Discussion with the patient and family needs to take place, explaining that the patient seems to be recovering – this is usually a source of relief and joy, though some will fear the thought of a further cycle of pain and suffering in the future.

Finally, listen to your accumulated experience of practice – walking away from a patient's bed thinking 'they are unlikely to survive this' or something similar is a call to action. The action needed is to define that uncertainty and communicate it to the patient and, where they do not have capacity, with their family, healthcare attorney (LPA in England and Wales) or Independent Mental Capacity Advocate (IMCA in England and Wales). Your actions enable the patient to state their view regarding whether they might/might not give consent for interventions, state their view on place of care and an creates an opportunity to speak with their families and discuss unresolved concerns.

You may be uncertain and can communicate that uncertainty – perhaps saying 'if the worst were to happen …' or 'perhaps it is best to plan for the worst and hope for the best ….'.

The Family Says 'How Long Has my Relative Got' (and Variations of That Question)?

This is an exhausting and stressful time in the life of a family – it is prudent to start your answer by checking what people have actually heard and understood and noticed during this admission. The patient's family may be seeking confirmation of what they suspect or may be very shocked that you think their relative is going to die.

Check what the family thinks about day-by-day changes and offer the observations of the team looking after the patient; e.g. 'we too see changes every day – today when I reviewed your Mum, she found it very difficult to open her eyes…'

Take time to ensure that you acknowledge that the patient is dying and acknowledge the family's sadness. It is important to name death and dying.

It may be helpful to say 'In my experience I think that we are approaching the last hours (or days) of your mother's life. It is very hard to be accurate about the time that is left but we will reassess frequently and let you know of any significant changes we see.'

Conversations About Do Not Attempt Cardiopulmonary Resuscitation (DNACPR)

The purpose of a DNACPR decision is to provide immediate guidance to those present on the best action to take (or not take) should the patient's heart stop beating. Clearly, attempted cardiopulmonary resuscitation (CPR) is contraindicated as an intervention where patients are recognized to be dying. A decision regarding the burdens and harms of the intervention weighed against the benefits of CPR needs to be made. When patients are dying, the intervention will cause burden and harms and will be unsuccessful. A DNACPR decision should be documented in the patient's records

Where possible, the patient should be involved in a discussion about the team's decision. These important conversations offer an invaluable opportunity to explore what wishes the patient holds about investigations and interventions, building a picture of what the patient's wishes would be should they lose capacity.

Where the patient has given permission, that information is shared with family members or, where the patient no longer has capacity, the team's decision should be shared with the patient's family. A decision regarding DNACPR should not be delayed until the family are available or until they next visit – rather the decision should be made and the family updated at the earliest opportunity.

In cases where the patient and/or their family disagree with the team's decision regarding DNACPR, a second opinion should be sought. Your seniors may suggest another consultant surgeon, the resuscitation team in your hospital, a palliative care opinion or alternatives.

Patients have the right to decline interventions including attempted CPR. It remains your job to weigh the benefits of all interventions against the possible harms, adverse effects and burdens. Where there is equipoise, you must discuss and weigh the decision with the patient. It is important not to assume that the patient's perceptions about benefits, harms and burdens.

Further guidance is available[8,9] from your resuscitation team.

The Family Says 'You Would Not Let a Dog Suffer Like That…'

Families are more likely than patients to state this view. There may be many reasons that they hold this view:
- Never having watched someone die and being unfamiliar with the process of dying
- Exhaustion
- Fear for their relative that they are suffering
- Lack of understanding that the patient is unconscious and unaware of the passage of time
- Wanting the waiting to finish
- Trying to hold their life in balance with visiting their dying relative
- Believing that euthanasia is needed in society

Try to understand what prompts this statement, acknowledging that this is a very difficult and stressful time in the life of a family and that it is normal to feel scared, tired and want the expected death to happen.

Explain your observations and whether you think the patient is suffering. It is a good time to review the situation and consider whether you need to ask your seniors to review the patient or whether you need to request a palliative care consultation.

Encourage families to eat and drink regularly – even if they are not hungry. Families have different styles of being with a dying relative: for some, they will undertake a vigil at the bedside; for others, they may visit once a day. It may be right to suggest that the family undertake a rota so everyone gets an opportunity to rest and sleep or you may need to give permission to families to leave their relative in the care of the staff as they take a necessary break. Encourage families to tell their GP what is happening and seek advice if they are not sleeping or feeling very anxious.

What PRNs Do I Prescribe for a Dying Patient?

PRN medication should be prescribed for every dying patient to prevent delays in symptom control if an unexpected event arises (e.g. upper GI bleed) or the patient is uncomfortable when rolled by the nurses to help manage pressure areas.

Prescribe

1. An opioid
   a. to alleviate pain and dyspnoea
   b. subcutaneously
   c. at the lowest dose that manages symptoms
   d. where the patient is opioid naïve, prescribe morphine 1.25–2.5 mg PRN 2-hourly
   e. where the patient is established on an opioid, prescribe 1/6th of the total daily dose; e.g. morphine MR 30 mg bid PO = 30 mg s.c./24 h so PRN = 5 mg s.c. 2-hourly
   f. if the patient is established on oxycodone, prescribe 1/6th of the total daily dose
   g. if the patient is on high dose opioids (>120 mg PO/24 h) or has significant renal dysfunction (eGFR <30 mL/min) or significant hepatic dysfunction (LFTs >5 times the upper limit of normal), seek advice from the palliative care team
2. An anxiolytic
   a. to alleviate anxiety and agitation at the end of life, which are very common
   b. prescribe midazolam 2.5 mg 4-hourly PRN s.c.
3. An antipsychotic
   a. to alleviate delirium at the end of life, which is very common
   b. haloperidol will help manage hyperactive delirium and also act as an anti-emetic
   c. prescribe haloperidol 0.5–1 mg 6-hourly PRN s.c.
4. An anti-emetic
   a. to alleviate nausea and address vomiting
   b. prescribe metoclopramide 10 mg 4-hourly PRN s.c. (except in Parkinson's disease)

Review the frequency and efficacy of PRNs every 24 hours in discussion with the nursing staff. They might be using PRNs to manage pain or agitation with moves. As a broad rule of thumb, if more than two PRNs are needed in a 24-hour period to manage symptoms that arise spontaneously, consider a subcutaneous infusion delivered by syringe driver.

When Do I Start a Syringe Driver?

A syringe driver is a battery operated ambulatory infusion device.

The indications for commencing a continuous subcutaneous infusion (CSCI) delivered by a battery operated syringe driver pump are:
1. More than two PRNs/24 hours which were used to manage spontaneous symptoms in dying patients
2. To replace the patient's regular opioid and prevent withdrawal reactions when the patient is too ill to take oral medicines
3. To avoid the oral route when the patient is nauseous, vomiting, has unreliable gastrointestinal absorption or has bowel obstruction

Where the patient has not been on a background opioid, calculate the dose to put in the CSCI by reviewing medication used in the previous 24 hours and rounding up to the nearest sensible dose.

Example:

Patient A had 3 × 2.5 mg Morphine s.c. in past 24 hours = 7.5 mg/24 h

Prescribe 7.5 mg/24 h by CSCI

If the patient looks uncomfortable, you might prescribe 10 mg/24 h by CSCI = 33% dose increase in analgesia per 24 hours.

Patient B had 7 × 2.5 mg morphine s.c. in past 24 hours = 17.5 mg/24 h

The patient also had midazolam 3 × 2.5 mg in past 24 hours = 7.5mg/24 h

The patient is visibly uncomfortable – frowning and restless

Prescribe 25 mg morphine (40% increase in analgesic) and midazolam 10 mg/24 h by CSCI (33% increase)

Increase the PRN doses to 5 mg morphine 2-hourly.

Remember that it takes approximately 4 hours for drug levels to rise to effective levels on commencing a subcutaneous infusion and for a new prescription to take effect. The nursing staff may need to administer PRNs in the intervening time and it helps families to know this information as they remain confident that the infusion will help.

Continue PRNs which enable good symptom management and will inform your fine-tuning of symptom management on review every 24 hours.

Should I Continue I.V. Fluids?

You should discontinue i.v. fluids if the patient has any signs of cardiac failure or has audible secretions. Patients may not be able to hold fluid in their intravascular space due to a low albumin or cardiac dysfunction in the face of protracted tachycardia and tachypnoea.

I.V. fluids are indicated in a small number of dying patients who have a high output stoma or a high bowel obstruction with considerable losses via a venting gastrostomy or by vomiting. The aim is to maintain comfort so that the patient is not thirsty or does not have symptomatic hypotension rather than aiming for accurate replacement of losses.

For all other patients, this question should be discussed and negotiated remembering that patients who are dying naturally reduce their food and fluid intake in the last week or two of their life. It is a normal part of dying that patients are only having small sips and an occasional spoonful of food. Attention to helping the patient take sips of cold water and oral hygiene is often more valuable that i.v. fluids.

Families may be particularly anxious about food and fluids. You should check that they understand the rationale, address any concerns and provide clear explanations as often as necessary.

On occasion you may agree a trial of a litre of fluid over 24 hours (i.v. or subcutaneously) to assess if it brings a dying patient benefit. Your clinical examination of the baseline and your goals of intervention should be clearly documented so that assessment against those goals is easy to undertake. It is helpful to discuss your goals with the patient and/or their family at the start of a trial of i.v. fluids so that you can work together to establish if the goals have been attained.

I Do Not Know What to Do!

It is important to recognize when you do not have the knowledge or skills to manage a situation and to seek senior support so that you receive advice and enable the patient to receive the correct care.

Your team may be able to help – the senior nursing staff on duty or your medical seniors. When your team do not have the knowledge and skills, then it is necessary and appropriate to refer to the palliative care team. Hospitals have different levels of provision. Hopefully you will be aware from induction how to request and source specialist advice including any local web-based advice.

The palliative care team will not regard any of your questions as unnecessary – they will be aware that medical undergraduate education in palliative care is limited and different across medical schools.

The palliative care team will expect you to know the history, recent blood results (especially eGFR) and to have reviewed your patient.

Where symptoms are complex, there is irreversible organ failure of two or more major organ systems or the patient or their family are suffering significant psychological distress and needing considerable support, referral to the specialist team is advised unless you and your team are feeling confident about managing this complexity.

The Patient Says 'I Want to go Home to Die'

This statement is worth exploring – perhaps asking 'Tell me more' – aiming to understand what aspirations the patient holds. Do they think that they will improve when in their own house? Do they want to see their house, garden or pet? Do they want to relieve their family of the stress of travel? Do they want to stop medicines that they worry are making them weak?

Also explore 'Have you spoken with your family about this and what do they say?' – aiming to understand whether this is an aspiration the patient holds or whether they have started to put plans in place.

Having learnt a little more about the patient's preference to be at home, the next step is determining if the patient has capacity to make this decision (Mental Capacity Act).[10] Does the patient foresee any difficulties in getting home or being at home and have they any thoughts about solutions regarding those concerns. If the patient does not have capacity in regard to this, it does not mean that they cannot return home but it does mean that the decision needs to be a 'best interests' decision.

The next important step is arranging a discussion with the patient's family. The multidisciplinary team needs to work with the patient and their family to identify risks and to put strategies in place aiming to mitigate or reduce the possible impact of those risks:

- Speaking with the patient's GP to discuss their view and check that they are happy to accept care
- Where the patient is moving to a family member's home, ensuring the patient is registered as a temporary resident with a local GP
- Speaking with the district nursing team to discuss their view and check that they are happy to accept care and to arrange a community syringe driver pump if needed
- Speaking with the Hospice at Home team or local community palliative care team to discuss what support might be available and establishing local referral criteria
- Working with Occupational Therapy colleagues to arrange a hospital bed, pressure relieving mattress, commode, wheelchair and hoist if needed
- Ensuring that the DNACPR decision and treatment escalation plans have been discussed with the patient and their family and communicated to the GP and out of hours services
- Ensuring that the patient's views on whether and in what circumstances they would want to return to acute care have been ascertained. Document those preferences and pass that information to the GP, requesting that they notify the ambulance service or out of hours provider as per local arrangements
- Reviewing the patient's current prescription. Discuss with the patient that you would prefer to deprescribe any medication for secondary prevention of disease and rationalize the medicines
- Prescribing anticipatory ('just in case') medicines to have in the patient's house, ensuring that the equipment to administer the medication is also available – needles, syringes, water for injection and a sharps box. Prescribe an analgesic, anti-emetic and sedatives to help manage delirium
- Arranging transport
- Ensuring that the patient and their family understand who to contact for help and have the numbers to hand – suggest GP practice in hours and out of hours service at other times but take account of local services
- Arranging care as needed and available to support the family in looking after the patient

At this stage, time is at a premium so it is important to plan and enact that plan quickly and thoughtfully. It is useful to say to both the patient and their family that you hope that all goes to plan and that they are comfortable and supported at home but, however, if the situation changes or a new symptom arises that needs attention, then coming in to the hospice or acute care may be the correct thing to do. It is physically and emotionally demanding to look after a dying person at home and families carry the bulk of the work and responsibility. It may not be sustainable at home and it is good to have raised this so that families do not feel that they have failed to meet the last wishes of the patient.

The Family Says 'I Want my Mother to Go Home to Die'

The first step is to establish the patient's views and whether they have capacity to make a decision regarding discharge to home. Where the patient does not have capacity, check whether a member of the patient's family has LPA for health (England and Wales). In the absence of both (capacity and LPA), then the team are establishing a 'best interests' decision.

It is not usual practice to move an actively dying patient (semi/unconscious, tachycardia, tachypnoea, disordered rhythm of breathing). It is good to discuss with your seniors and the palliative care team.

How Do I Verify a Patient's Death?

English law does not currently require that a patient is seen after death by a doctor or other healthcare practitioner. However, most hospitals have policies in place that expect staff to verify the death of a patient before they leave the ward. This is good practice in an acute setting.

The following is a pragmatic way of confirming death. It is not usually necessary to check a response to pain by trying to elicit a pain response using a trapezius squeeze or supraorbital pressure:

- Ensure the patient's records reflect that the death is expected
- Note the exact time of death where possible
- Offer your condolences to the family if present
- Explain that you are verifying that the patient has died
- Check for clinical signs of life, using a stethoscope and penlight or ophthalmoscope
- Cessation of circulatory and respiratory systems and cerebral function must be confirmed and documented. These should be checked for a minimum of 1 minute and then a second check for a minimum of 1 minute after 5 minutes have elapsed
- The following are the recognized clinical signs used when verifying death:
  1. Cessation of circulatory system
     - No carotid pulse
     - No heart sounds – verified by listening with a stethoscope for a minimum of 1 minute
  2. Cessation of respiratory systems
     - No respiratory effort
     - No chest sounds – verified by listening for a minimum of 1 minute
  3. Cessation of cerebral function
     - No eye movements
     - Pupils fixed and dilated
     - Pupils not reacting to light
     - Document your findings

How Do I Certify a Patient's Death?

Where a death is expected, then a member of the medical team providing clinical care is delegated responsibility for completing the medical certificate of cause of death (MCCD). The bereavement office in your hospital will arrange for you to access the notes and complete the certificate.

Earlier in your career, you may wish to discuss what you are planning to enter in part 1 and part 2 with your senior colleagues. The information you document is recognized to be information provided to the best of your knowledge. Your certificate provides the information needed to enable the Registrar for Births, Deaths and Marriages to complete the official death certificate. The information is also used to understand the epidemiology of disease.

When Should I Contact the Coroner's Office (England and Wales)?

If you think that the patient's death took place in violent or suspicious circumstances, establish whether you should commence CPR or whether the patient has died – you should not proceed to verify death or disturb the body or surroundings in any way. You should contact your seniors and ensure the matter is escalated to the police and that the coroner is informed. This is a highly unusual situation in a hospital.

You need to inform the coroner's office if a patient has died while being deprived of their liberty – a Deprivation of Liberty Safeguarding order is in place, the patient is a prisoner or are currently detained under the Mental Health Act.

The death may also need to be referred to the coroner – e.g. where the patient has died from an industrial disease or as a consequence of a procedure. It is wise to have checked out local arrangements as these differ. It is likely that this area has been covered in your induction. The bereavement office will be very helpful regarding local procedures.

You are not able to complete the MCCD unless the coroner's office advises that they are happy you proceed.

'But He Was on the Organ Donor Register….'

Most hospitals have a tissue donation team who will be happy to advise you. Patients who have an expected death may still be able to donate corneas, heart valves or skin in addition to donating tissue for research. The need for tissue varies – speak to your local team or review the hospital policy.

Tissue donation teams will be happy to speak with the patient and/or their family during the admission. Consider asking patients whether they are registered as an organ donor.

The Family Says 'What Do I Do After my Father Dies?'

Check your local arrangements – most hospitals have an office which administers the 'medical certificate of cause of death'. Families will need to book an appointment in office hours to collect the certificate and may be able to register the death at the same time.

The family will also need to choose a funeral director who will be responsible for collecting the patient's body and coordinating funeral arrangements.

Patients who hold a Muslim or an Orthodox Jewish faith will need certificates rapidly to enable their religious customs and practices to be observed. If you need advice, speak to the chaplain on call who will be able to guide you as to local arrangements to support families in meeting religious obligations.

Further Reading

eELCA: https://www.e-lfh.org.uk/programmes/end-of-life-care/.

This programme of over 160 modules is available as a free resource for healthcare staff. It is highly interactive and a fantastic resource.

References

1. https://popnat.hospiceuk.org/.
2. https://www.resus.org.uk/respect/.
3. https://www.gmc-uk.org/ethical-guidance/learning-materials/talking-about-end-of-life-care-clinically-assisted-nutrition-and-hydration.
4. https://www.nhsbt.nhs.uk/what-we-do/transplantation-services/tissue-and-eye-services/tissue-donation/become-a-donor/tissue-donation-after-death/.
5. https://www.gov.uk/government/uploads/system/uploads/attachment_data/file/323188/One_chance_to_get_it_right.pdf.
6. Clarke D, et al. Imminence of death among hospital inpatients: Prevalent cohort study. *Palliat. Med.* 2014;28(6):474–479.
7. Twycross R, Wilcock A. *Introducing Palliative Care.* 5th ed. London: Pharmaceutical Press; 2018:270.
8. https://www.gmc-uk.org/ethical-guidance/ethical-guidance-for-doctors/treatment-and-care-towards-the-end-of-life/cardiopulmonary-resuscitation-cpr.
9. https://www.resus.org.uk.
10. https://www.nhs.uk/conditions/social-care-and-support/mental-capacity/.

12

Organ Transplantation

CHAPTER OUTLINE

Organ Transplantation

Since the 1960s, organ transplantation has become an established surgical specialty. More than any other branch of surgery, organ transplantation requires the close cooperation of an extended multidisciplinary team of surgeons, physicians, anaesthetists, immunologists, and other allied healthcare workers to achieve a successful outcome. A synopsis of the historical landmarks of transplantation is provided in Box 12.1 and a brief summary of the range of transplants in Box 12.2.

Essential Definitions

Autograft. Free (i.e. after disconnection of the blood supply) transplantation of tissue from one part of the body to another in the same individual.

Isograft. The transfer of tissue between genetically identical individuals – in humans this is between identical twins (rejection is not a feature of auto- or isografts).

Allograft. An organ or structure transplanted from an individual of the same species. Allografts are the main class of transplant in humans at the moment.

Xenograft. The transfer of organs between dissimilar species. Presently limited to tissues that have been chemically processed to make them non-antigenic, e.g. porcine heart valves. However, this is potentially an exciting technique because, should it prove successful, the present shortage of organs for transplantation would be overcome.

Progress is being made in understanding the nature of the difficulties that form a barrier to xenografting.

Orthotopic graft. The donor organ is transplanted into the same anatomical site in the recipient. The removal of the latter is first required, e.g. liver transplantation.

Heterotopic graft. The donor organ is inserted at a site different from its normal anatomical position, e.g. kidney transplantation to the iliac fossa.

Artificial (hybrid) organ implantation. The transplantation of bio-artificial organs, which are a combination of bio-materials and living cells, e.g. a hybrid artificial pancreas. At present this technique is experimental. Success would, as with xenografting, open a new chapter in transplantation.

Cadaver graft. An organ or tissue retrieved from an individual who has been pronounced dead according to criteria which differ from one culture to another (see later). There are currently three systems of cadaveric organ donation in use: 'required request', 'opting out' and 'opting in'. These are summarized in Box 12.3; however, no matter which system is adopted, the wishes of the family of the donor are the most important factor.

Organ Donation

Organ transplantation is an accepted treatment for organ failure, but also for quality of life issues in all ages. In many

• BOX 12.1 Some Landmarks in Transplantation

Date

c. AD 300 *Cosmos and Damian:* are portrayed to have performed a leg transplant
1778 *John Hunter:* used the term transplant
1863 *Bert:* observed ingrowth of vessels into skin grafts and defined the terms autograft, allograft and xenograft
1905 *Guthrie and Carrel:* developed vascular anastomotic technique (1912 Nobel Prize)
1933 *Voronoy:* first human renal transplant – failed because of ABO incompatibility
1945 *Hume:* first short-lived functioning renal allograft
1950 *Lawler:* first long-term survivor from renal grafting (Chicago)
1954 *Murray and colleagues:* first successful kidney transplant between identical twins
1963 *Starzl:* first attempt of human liver allograft
1966 *Lillehei:* first human pancreas transplant – technical success
1967 *Lillehei:* first attempted human bowel transplant
1967 *Starzl:* first long-term survivor from liver transplantation
1967 *Barnard:* first successful heart transplant
1967–68 Acceptance of brain death concept
1981 *Shumway:* first successful heart-lung transplant
1988 *Grant:* first long-term survivor of liver and small-bowel transplant

• BOX 12.2 Major Organs and Tissue Transplanted

Thoracic Organs

- Heart (Deceased-donor only)
- Lung (Deceased-donor and Living-donor)
- En bloc Heart/Lung (Deceased-donor and Domino transplant)

Other Organs

- Kidney (Deceased-donor and Living-donor)
- Liver (Deceased-donor and Living-donor)
- Pancreas (Deceased-donor and rarely Living-donor)
- Small bowel (Deceased-donor and Living-donor)
- Multivisceral (Deceased-donor)

Tissues, Cells, Fluids

- Hand (Deceased-donor only)
- Cornea (Deceased-donor only)
- Skin graft including face transplant (almost always autograft)
- Islets of Langerhans (Pancreas islet cells) (Deceased-donor and Living-donor)
- Bone marrow/Adult stem cell (Living-Donor and Autograft)
- Blood transfusion/Blood Parts Transfusion (Living-donor and Autograft)
- Blood vessels (Autograft and Deceased-donor)
- Heart valve (Deceased-donor, Living-donor and Xenograft (Porcine/bovine))
- Bone (Deceased-donor, Living-donor and Autograft)
- Skin (Deceased-donor, Living-donor and Autograft)
- Hepatocytes (Selected donors)

• BOX 12.3 Systems Currently in Use for Organ Donation

1. *Required request:* doctors looking after the potential donor have to ask, or refer the patient to, a retrieval coordinator who will enquire about donation.
2. *Opting out or presumed consent:* all donors are presumed to have consented unless the family on approach refuse consent or the patient has previously registered his or her wish not to consent. This system produces the highest number of donors.
3. *Opting in or required consent:* Medical or nursing staff approach the family to ask about organ donation. Approximately one-third of the families refuse donation.

cases, organ transplantation is the only viable treatment option and, in the absence of effective organ support, results in the death of the patient.

- Transplantation benefits about 28,000 patients in Europe yearly.
- The availability of organs does not meet the constantly growing demand.
- According to Council of Europe data, by the end of 2015, more than 80,000 patients were waiting for a kidney, liver, heart, lung, pancreas or intestinal transplant within the EU.
- Each day, on average, 14 people die while waiting for a transplant.

The number of listed patients waiting for a transplant continues to increase in the majority of countries and the gap is widening between demand and the number of available grafts. The problems related to the availability of organs are highly complex and sensitive: they do not depend on any one single factor but result from a combination of factors including:

- Type of legislation and consent systems in place in a country
- Organization and performance of national transplant teams
- Professional organ procurement networks
- Awareness and understanding of the issues in the general population
- Ethical concerns
- Cultural and religious beliefs
- Emotional issues: most often the decision to donate organs comes at a tragic moment for family members when they are confronted with the news of their loved one's passing
- Family refusal rates vary greatly across Europe, may be as high as 50%

Diagnosis of Death – DBD and DCD Donation

It is acknowledged worldwide that the irreversible loss of the capacity for consciousness combined with the irreversible loss of the capacity to breathe equates to death.

Irreversible loss of brainstem functions produces this state. Therefore, demonstration that the functions of the brainstem have irreversibly ceased allows diagnosis of death. On the background of this principle, different legal definitions of death have been established in different countries.

In donation after brainstem death (DBD) donors, circulation and the oxygenation of peripheral tissues are maintained after death. This allows better preservation of function in the organs to be retrieved and transplanted. The range of organs suitable for transplantation is greater in DBD donation and, in general, the outcome of transplantation using DBD donor organs is better.

Donation After Brain Death (DBD)

The demonstration of the absence of all functions of the brainstem by clinical tests is adequate for the diagnosis of brainstem death (BSD), providing that severe metabolic disturbance and potential effect of drugs and hypothermia have been excluded and a cause has been established. Some countries require additional criteria such as demonstration of a lack of electrical activity on EEG or demonstration of the absence of blood flow to the brain by imaging. Criteria used to diagnose BSD in children are the same as those in adults, but the diagnosis of BSD in children under the age of 2 months is not possible. The transplant community is continually looking to maximize the deceased donor organ pool. In recent years, this has led to greater efforts to use more marginal or extended criteria donors.

Donation After Circulatory Death (DCD)

This is donation after confirming irreversible cessation of cardiac, respiratory and neurological activity by an appropriately qualified team. In practice, the irreversibility of the loss of neurological function is inferred from the length of time that breathing and circulation has been absent. Donation after circulatory death (DCD) donors are patients who have usually sustained catastrophic irrecoverable brain injury and in whom further treatment has been considered futile.

The cessation of cardiac activity is determined by the absence of pulses and heart sounds. Demonstration of asystole on ECG or the absence of blood flow on direct arterial pressure monitoring may also confirm the diagnosis. After 5 minutes of continued absence of circulation and breathing, the absence of pupillary or corneal reflex is tested to confirm cessation of neurological function. DCD has become an important source of organs.

DCD donors are classified by the Maastricht criteria. In category 1, death is declared at a site outside the hospital, and the potential donor is brought to the hospital without resuscitation. In category 2, arrest occurs unexpectedly, and resuscitation is unsuccessful. Category 3 is anticipated cardiac arrest after removal of ventilator support, and category 4 is unanticipated cardiac arrest in a brain-dead donor. Categories 1 and 2 are considered uncontrolled donation, which require maintenance of organ perfusion and rapid cooling by either postmortem cardiopulmonary resuscitation or cardiopulmonary bypass with external oxygenation. Categories 3 and 4 are considered controlled donation. The use of uncontrolled DCD allografts is rare outside Spain.

DCD is a different organ procurement technique. DCD donors experience longer warm ischemia time that begins with withdrawal of life support, proceeds through progressive hypoxia, hypoperfusion, and cardiopulmonary arrest, and ends with no organ perfusion at body temperature for the standoff period of 5 minutes. Procurement and cold preservation begins after a variable period of warm ischemia (from systolic BP <50 mmHg/O_2 saturation <80% to initiation of cold preservation). Warm ischemia followed by cold preservation exacerbates the ischemia/reperfusion injury and increases the risk for delayed graft function and primary graft non-function, and, in case of the liver, of long-term biliary complications from ischemic cholangiopathy.

Donor Type

Donors can be of different types:

- *Donor after brain death (DBD).* A donor whose heart is still beating when the brain has stopped working with the loss of brain stem function so that they cannot survive without the support of a ventilator. Organs for transplant are removed from the donor while their heart is still beating, but only after extensive tests determine that the brain cannot recover and they have been certified dead.
- *Donor after circulatory death (DCD).* A donor in whom further treatment is considered futile and medical support is withdrawn. Donation occurs after the heart stops beating and, after a further stand-off period of 5 minutes, death is certified. The organs are then removed.
- *Living donor.* A donor who is a living person and who is usually, but not always, a relative of the transplant patient. For example, a parent may donate part of their liver to their child.
- *Domino donor.* A donor with a single gene defect based in the liver that does not result in liver damage (e.g. FAP) who receives a liver transplant to treat their condition. This donor gives their liver to another recipient in a domino liver transplant, because the liver functions well for other recipients.

Evaluation of the Deceased Donor

After a brainstem-dead donor has been referred to the organ donation organization with a view to organ donation, the general suitability of the potential organ donor is carefully assessed. The medical history is checked and evidence sought of risk factors: particular care must be taken to assess the donor from the point of view of transmissible infectious agents (HIV) and malignancy. The presence of Jakob-Creutzfeldt disease is absolute contraindication to organ donation. Active systemic sepsis is also a contraindication to donation. The presence of malignancy within the past 5 years is usually a contraindication with the exception of primary tumours of the CNS, non-melanotic skin tumours and carcinoma in situ of the uterine cervix. If there are no general contradictions to organ donation, consideration is then given to organ-specific selection criteria. Donors with HIV, hepatitis B and hepatitis C may also be considered for donation in certain circumstances.

Because of the high demand for donors, there has been a progressive relaxation of the organ-specific selection criteria. The chronological age of the donor is less important than the physiological function of the organs under consideration.

The donated organs should be free from primary disease. Heart donors should have a normal electrocardiogram and, in doubtful cases, echocardiography may be necessary. For lung donors, the chest radiograph and gas exchange should be satisfactory, and bronchial aspirates should be free from fungal and bacterial infection. Potential kidney donors should have a reasonable urine output and relatively normal serum urea and creatinine levels, although acute terminal elevations are acceptable. Liver donors should not have significant hepatic disease, although impaired liver function tests are common in deceased donors and do not necessarily preclude donation. Elevation of blood glucose and serum amylase are not uncommon in deceased donors and do not preclude pancreas donation.

Acceptable donor age ranges for each of the commonly transplanted organs are:
- Kidney and liver: no age limit
- Pancreas: 10–60 years
- Heart: 1–65 years
- Lung: 5–65 years

Allocation of Organs

There are no worldwide rules or systems for organ allocation. There are different organ exchange organizations for different countries and geographical areas, including the following: NHS Blood & Transplant (NHSBT) for the UK, Eurotransplant (Germany, the Netherlands, Belgium, Luxembourg, Austria, Hungary, Slovenia and Croatia), Scandiatransplant (Sweden, Norway, Finland, Denmark and Iceland), Organizacion Nacional de Trasplantes (ONT) in Spain, North Italian Transplant (NIT) in Italy and Etablissement français des Greffes (EfG) in France. The majority of organs are allocated and transplanted within each procurement and exchange organization, but there is collaboration in case of surplus organs among these institutions.

Although there are important differences, two methods are primarily followed. Organ allocation can be patient directed (in the United States and some European countries), or centre directed, which is the case in other European countries (Spain, Scandiatransplant). An organ allocation system is based on a consensus among transplant teams, organizational structures, health authorities and patient organizations.

All systems work with two factor categories. The first category includes medical criteria such as blood group, human leukocyte antigen (HLA) compatibility (kidney transplantation), primary disease, donor and recipient matching, donor virological status, severity of recipient status and others. The second category is nonmedical criteria, which include geographical distance and resources consumed. Waiting time or cold ischemia time may appear in either category.

Most organizations have similar rules with an urgent priority group that includes, for example in the liver setting, acute hepatic failure and early re-transplantation following vascular thrombosis, or primary nonfunction of the graft.

Living Donor

Living donation transplant is common worldwide and kidney donation is most common. Liver donation has become the most common, especially in India and the East, in the absence of effective cadaveric donation. Occasionally, living donors have provided segments of pancreas, small bowel and lung for transplantation, but this is more controversial. The use of live donors for organ transplantation remains controversial. Live organ donation violates the ethical principle of non-maleficence: do no harm. Living donation involves placing living donors at risk for no direct medical benefit to themselves. The use of live liver donors has raised concern about donor safety with a mortality of 0.3% for right lobe donation. Forty percent of live donors experienced a complication (e.g., bile leak, surgical hernia, infection). As a result, the risks and benefits, the adequacy of informed consent procedures and the selection of recipients and donors remain under careful scrutiny.

There are three categories of living donors: (1) living related donors (such as parents, siblings or adult children) who are genetically related to the recipient; (2) living emotionally-related donors (such as spouses, significant others and close friends) who are genetically unrelated; and (3) living unrelated donors who are strangers to the recipient or non-directed donors: this category has also been referred to as altruistic or Good Samaritan donors.

The Living Donor Transplant Evaluation

The criteria for the evaluation of potential living donors are established. Potential risk factors for poor outcome donations include past or present significant psychiatric morbidity, substance use disorders, financial instability, lack of health insurance, desire for secondary gain, stressors and poor social support, lacking the capacity to understand risks and benefits and medical morbidity. A strained donor–recipient relationship, a history of nonadherence and lack of disclosure to family are considered relative contraindications in most living donor programs. Financial incentive is considered an absolute contraindication in the majority of centres.

Medical History. History of adherence with medical recommendations and previous surgery and chronic pain may influence outcome after donation.

Psychiatric History. In addition to screening for depression and anxiety, a history of substance abuse, physical, emotional or sexual trauma is explored.

Informed Consent. The clinician should establish that the patient is well informed about the risks and benefits of the procedure and the patient's capacity to consent to donation and the extent of their understanding of the entire process as a whole.

Coping Skills. Donors will be facing a challenging process of recovery and integration of the donation experience.

Social Support. It is vital to assess the degree of social support for the donation process, including the post-donation period.

Motivation for Donation. The motivation for donation should be investigated.

Basic Immunology of Organ Transplantation

Successful organ transplantation (with the exception of the cornea) requires the manipulation of the immunological defences of the recipient so as to overcome rejection. Because auto- and isografts do not elicit an immune response, it must be the genetic differences between the donor and the recipient that are of major importance in this process. These differences are expressed as *tissue or histocompatibility antigens*. The latter stimulate and lead the activation and proliferation of immune cells and identify cells which are the targets of the effector mechanisms induced by the immune reaction. The key cells involved in the rejection process are lymphocytes and antigen-presenting cells.

Major Histocompatibility Complex (MHC)

A large group of genes is present on the short arm of human chromosome 6 (Fig. 12.1), including those that encode the class I and class II MHC molecules which are involved in the presentation of antigens to T-cells. Class I molecules are integral membrane proteins found in all nucleated cells and platelets – the classical transplantation antigens. Class II molecules are expressed on B-cells, macrophages, monocytes, antigen-presenting cells (APCs) and some T-cells.

Human Leucocyte Antigen (HLA) Loci

There are four of these on the short arm of chromosome 6:
HLA-A – over 60 alleles have been identified
HLA-B – over 125 alleles have so far been characterized

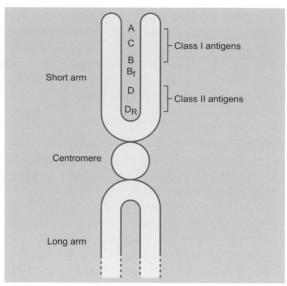

• **Fig. 12.1** Position of the Major Histocompatibility Locus on the Short Arm of Chromosome 6.

HLA-C (between A and B) – seems not to have a role in mounting the immune response

HLA-DR – appears to be clinically most important in that, if donor and recipient match for it, graft survival is improved

HLA molecules can initiate rejection and graft damage, via humoral or cellular mechanisms:

Humoral rejection mediated by recipient's AB (e.g. blood transfusion, previous transplant or pregnancy)

Cellular rejection is the more common type of rejection after organ transplants. Mediated by T lymphocytes, it results from their activation and proliferation after exposure to donor MHC molecules.

Cells Involved in the Immune Response to a Transplant

Lymphocytes

These are the key cells controlling the immune response. They specifically recognize foreign (non-self) material as different from the tissues of the body. Lymphocytes are of two main types: B-cells and T-cells.

B-cells develop in the fetal liver and subsequently in bone marrow. Mature B-cells carry surface immunoglobulins which constitute their antigen receptor. The response to an antigenic stimulus is cell division and differentiation into plasma cells under the control of cytokines released by T-cells.

T-cells develop in the thymus, which is seeded during embryonic development with lymphocytic stem cells from the bone marrow. T-cells then develop their antigen receptors and differentiate into two major peripheral subsets: one expresses the CD4 marker, and the other the CD8. T-cells have a number of functions, including:
1. Helping B-cells to make antibody (CD4+)
2. Recognizing and destroying cells infected with viruses (CD8+)
3. Activating phagocytes to destroy ingested pathogens (CD4+)

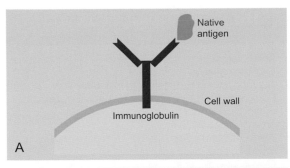

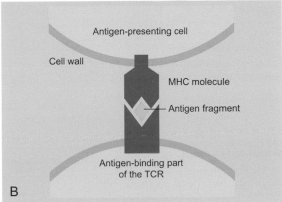

• **Fig. 12.2** (A) Antigen Handling by B-cells. (B) Antigen Handling by T-cells. TCR, T-cell receptor.

4. Controlling the level and quality of the immune response (CD8+)

Antigen-presenting cells

These are a group defined functionally by their ability to take up antigens and present them to lymphocytes in a form the latter can recognize. Some antigens are taken up by APCs in the periphery and transported to secondary lymphoid tissues. Others are intercepted as they arrive by APCs normally resident in lymph nodes and other lymphoid aggregates. B-cells recognize antigen in its native form, but T-cells recognize antigenic peptides that have been associated with self MHC molecules. In consequence, to present an antigen to a T-cell, an APC must internalize it, process it into fragments and re-express these at the cell surface in association with class II MHC molecules. In addition, many APCs provide additional stimulatory signals to lymphocytes either by direct cellular interactions or via cytokines (Fig. 12.2).

Rejection

Rejection is a destructive reaction initiated by the host to foreign HLA and other non-shared antigens. The process involves:

• antigen recognition (afferent arc)
• activation of selected clones of T-cells and the effector mechanisms (efferent arc)

Afferent arc

Two routes lead to activation:

• foreign antigen or donor antigen-presenting cells (dendritic cells) which are directly recognized by the recipient's cells

• intracellular processing of foreign antigens by host antigen-presenting cells and subsequent presentation of peptides to T-cells. Class II HLA antigens activate T helper (CD4+) cells, and class I HLA antigens activate cytotoxic (CD8+) T-cells

Efferent arc

There is proliferation and differentiation of the selected T-cell population. CD4+ cells (T helper – Th cells) produce interleukin-X (IL-10) which induces macrophages to produce IL-1, which in turn stimulates Th cells to produce IL-2 and other cytokines (e.g. IL-4, IL-5, IL-6). The latter cause B-cells to differentiate into plasma cells and to secrete antibody. Cytokines also stimulate CD8+ cells to become cytotoxic. The coating of target cells by antibody allows K cells (large granular lymphocytes), macrophages or granulocytes to recognize and destroy them through a variety of mechanisms (release of enzymes, reactive oxygen mediators and perforins).

Clinical patterns of rejection

There are three patterns of rejection:

• *Hyperacute and acute accelerated rejection* – This is the result of preformed IgG antibody and occurs within hours of exposure.
• *Acute cellular rejection* – This is infiltration by activated T-cells with recruitment of acute inflammatory cells; generally seen at 7–14 days post-transplant.
• *Chronic rejection* – This is a major cause of graft attrition and is probably antibody-mediated. There is intimal hyperplasia and endarteritis obliterans. In liver transplants, it is associated with loss of bile duct radicles. Chronic rejection is difficult to treat, but strategies that involve anti-B-cell drugs (e.g. mycophenolate mofetil) or rapamycin, which is not nephrotoxic, may have a role in the future.

Organ Matching and Retrieval

Organ Matching
ABO Blood Group Antigens Compatibility

The biological rules are the same as those which govern blood transfusion. Because ABO red cell antigens are expressed on most tissue cells, ABO-incompatible allografts undergo hyperacute rejection. The rhesus factor is expressed only on red blood cells and therefore a match for it is not required for successful transplantation.

Permissible transplants include:

• group O donor to group O, A, B or AB recipient
• group A donor to group A or AB recipient
• group B donor to group B or AB recipient
• group AB donor to group AB recipient

HLA-A, HLA-B and HLA-DR Matching

Tissue typing (identification of the A, B and DR antigens) is carried out on the donor and the recipient by the separation of lymphocytes out of heparinized whole blood and their exposure to antibodies of known HLA-A, HLA-B and

HLA-DR specificity. The influence of matching by tissue type on the successful outcome of organ transplantation is best established in renal transplantation, and its role in cardiac, liver and pancreatic transplantation is not yet clear.

Direct Cross-Matching

After a suitably matched recipient has been selected, a direct cross-match is set up because any recipient may have pre-formed circulating antibodies capable of reacting against donor cells. These antibodies may be the result of previous blood transfusion, pregnancy, viral infections or transplants. A direct cross-match incubates donor lymphocytes with the serum of the recipient in the presence of complement, to exclude cytotoxicity from circulating antibodies.

Exchange Transplantation and Desensitization Programmes

In the UK at least 500 living kidney transplants are cancelled each year because of preformed cytotoxic antibodies. In approximately half, the cause is blood group incompatibility with the remainder presenting unacceptable levels of anti-HLA antibodies. At present, there are two methods that allow these individuals to receive a transplant. One is exchange transplantation where donor A gives a kidney to recipient B and donor B donates a kidney to recipient A, thus overcoming the positive cytotoxic test. Individuals willing to exchange transplants are put onto a national register to increase the chances of finding a compatible combination. The second option is a desensitization program where, over a number of sessions using filters or antigen columns, anti-HLA antibodies are removed until their level is low enough to allow an initially incompatible transplant to proceed. There is, however, a significant risk of early rejection in these patients.

Organ Retrieval

Most organs for cadaveric transplantation come from those who have suffered irreversible structural brain damage after road traffic accidents or cerebrovascular catastrophes and have been diagnosed brain dead by agreed criteria. In most countries that accept this practice, organs are then retrieved while the heart continues to beat and the donor receives ventilatory and other support. Such conditions are absolute requirements for transplantations of heart, heart-lung and small bowel. Many centres will now accept kidneys, livers, lungs and pancreas organs from DCD.

Organ Function in Donors

Function of the organ which is to be transplanted must be established. A satisfactory past medical history and physical examination are essential. A well-perfused organ – as indicated by adequate blood pressure and normal arterial blood gas tensions – is highly desirable. See Box 12.4 for factors determining organ function after transplantation.

Heart

Requirements are normal blood pressure, ECG, chest X-ray and arterial blood gas tensions.

> **• BOX 12.4** **Factors Determining Organ Function After Transplantation**
>
> Donor characteristics
> - Extremes of age
> - Haemodynamic and metabolic instability
> - Presence of pre-existing disease in the transplanted organ
>
> Procurement-related factors
> - Warm ischaemic time
> - Type of preservation solution
> - Cold ischaemic time
>
> Recipient-related factors
> - Technical factors relating to implantation
> - Haemodynamic and metabolic stability
> - Immunological factors
> - Presence of drugs that impair transplant function
> - Comorbidities: diabetes, vascular disease

Lung and heart–lung

Requirements are negative Gram-stain on sputum and absence of pathogens on sputum culture.

Liver

Requirements are adequate liver perfusion (arterial blood pressure, blood and arterial gas tensions) and normal values for serum bilirubin, transaminase and alkaline phosphatase concentrations and a normal prothrombin time.

Kidney

Requirements are normal urine output and urinalysis (however, oliguria may be pre-renal because of dehydration) and normal serum creatinine and urea concentrations.

Pancreas

Requirements are normal serum concentrations of amylase and glucose – hyperglycaemia often develops in acute brainstem injury because of steroid administration and intravenous infusion of crystalloid-containing glucose; elevated serum glucose alone is not necessarily a contraindication.

Donor Operation

Retrieval is becoming increasingly complex because one individual may donate corneas, heart, lungs, liver, pancreas, kidneys, bone and skin. With the recent success of small-bowel transplantation, the retrieval of the small bowel and the right colon may also be included.

Retrieval Procedure

Currently, the abdominal retrieval team starts the procedure and is followed by the cardiothoracic team. The procedure for the abdominal retrieval is illustrated in outline in Fig. 12.3. Organs are cold-perfused before removal, examined after excision to ensure they are anatomically satisfactory and then cold-preserved in UW solution within double plastic bags and stored on a bed of crushed ice for transfer to the chosen transplant centre.

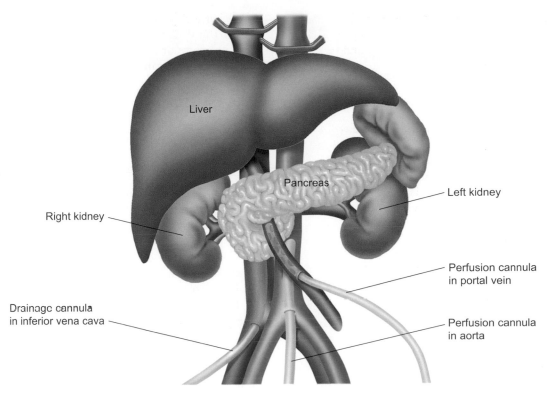

• **Fig. 12.3** Retrieval Procedure for the Abdominal Organs.

Immunosuppression in Transplantation

There is a difficult balance to achieve between the prevention or reversal of rejection and the morbidity that can result from loss of host defences against infection and also, in the long term, the development of malignant disease and kidney injury.

Immunosuppression is charged with preventing the alloimmune response against donor antigens. There are a large number of different immunosuppressant drugs available today. They inhibit one of three key signal pathways by limiting the supply of nucleotides needed for cell division or depleting one of the necessary immune cells.

1. Signal 1 blockers include calcineurin inhibitors (CNIs) such as cyclosporine and tacrolimus, as well as any anti-CD3 molecules that block the T-cell receptor complex such as OKT3 and rabbit-derived antithymocyte globulin (rATG). Signal 2 blockers include belatacept, which competitively binds the costimulatory molecule CD28, preventing it from binding CD80/CD86. Signal 3 blockers include both anti-CD25 antibodies that competitively bind the IL-2R, such as basiliximab, as well as mTOR inhibitors such as sirolimus and everolimus, which prevent any further downstream signal transduction if IL-2R becomes activated.
2. Drugs that limit the supply of purine nucleotides needed for cell division include azathioprine and mycophenolate.
3. Drugs that deplete the necessary immune cells include rATG, which depletes and lyses T-cells; OKT3, which also depletes T-cells; and alemtuzumab, an anti-CD52 molecule that lyses B-cells and T-cells.

Modern immunosuppression strategies involve using these drugs in combinations to achieve the goal of preventing alloimmune response against donor antigens, while minimizing any toxicities and side effects (Box 12.5).

Immunosuppressive Agents

Azathioprine: Metabolized in the liver to 6-mercaptopurine, this substance is a purine antagonist and reduces the synthesis of DNA and RNA in dividing cells.

Ciclosporin and tacrolimus: These act within the cell to prevent transcription of the gene for interleukin 2 (IL-2), a cytokine involved in the efferent arc of rejection.

Corticosteroids: These agents produce potent but non-specific immunosuppression and also have an anti-inflammatory action. They work by decreasing macrophage motility and phagocytic activity and also block both IL-2 release from macrophages and its generation by Th cells.

ATG: Thymoglobulin is a rabbit anti-human thymocyte immunoglobulin. It is polyclonal in nature and depletes lymphocytes in the circulation and lymphoid organs and also masks T-cell antigens non-specifically.

Monoclonal anti-CD25 antibody: Basiliximab and daclizumab are humanized monoclonal antibodies that target the IL-2 receptor. They have largely replaced ATG.

Monoclonal anti-T-cell antibody (OKT3): This is a murine antibody to the T3 antigen of human T-cells. It

• BOX 12.5 **Side Effects of Immunosuppression**

Corticosteroids

- Metabolic:
  - Glucocorticoid fat distribution, moon face, buffalo hump;
  - Mineralocorticoid hypertension, hyperkalaemia
- Endocrine:
  - Short-term diabetes, hyperlipidaemia, menstrual irregularities;
  - Long-term adrenal suppression
- Gastrointestinal: Pancreatitis, peptic ulcer disease
- Neurological/psychological: Psychosis, altered mood status, insomnia
- Musculoskeletal: Osteoporosis, avascular necrosis, vertebral fractures, femoral fractures
- Ophthalmic: Cataracts, glaucoma
- Skin: Acne, bruising, abdominal wall striae, impaired wound healing

Azathioprine

Myelosuppression, hepatotoxicity and cholestatic jaundice, acute pancreatitis

Ciclosporin

Nephrotoxicity, hepatotoxicity, neurotoxicity, gingival hypertrophy, hypertrichosis

Tacrolimus

Nephrotoxicity, hepatotoxicity, neurotoxicity, diabetes

---

produces destruction of CD3-positive T-cells which are associated with graft rejection. There are other similar monoclonal antibodies, but OKT3 is the one most widely used.

Mycophenolate mofetil (MMF): This inhibits proliferation of T- and B-lymphocytes and may prove more potent than azathioprine. It may also have a role in the prevention of chronic rejection because B-lymphocytes are thought to be important in this process, which now accounts for the majority of renal transplants lost in the long term.

Anti-IL-2 receptor antibody: This is a monoclonal antibody to the IL-2 receptor on human lymphocytes. By binding the IL-2 receptor, it blocks the pathway of activation mediated through the release of IL-2.

Monoclonal anti-CD20 antibody: Rituximab is a monoclonal antibody directed against the CD20 antigen on B-cells. It may have a role in treatment of some forms of antibody-mediated rejection.

Sirolimus and everolimus are inhibitors of mTOR that block the mTOR signal transduction pathway – a complex pathway coordinating cellular growth, proliferation and nutrition based on cellular levels of oxygen, energy, mitogenic growth factors, hormones and cellular nutrient levels. mTOR inhibitors do not inhibit calcineurin and subsequently have a very different side-effect profile to CNIs. They are used for maintenance immunosuppression and the treatment of chronic rejection.

Alemtuzumab is a recombinant DNA-derived humanized monoclonal antibody that is directed against CD52, a protein which is present on the surface of mature lymphocytes. This drug is gaining popularity for use in desensitization programs or in regimens intending to induce immune tolerance to the transplanted organ.

Clinical Regimens

These vary greatly from centre to centre but can be categorized as discussed in the following sections.

Triple Therapy

This was the most common standard induction and maintenance therapy, particularly in renal transplantation:
- Azathioprine – 2 mg/kg body weight, reduced to 1 mg/kg at the end of the first week
- Cyclosporine – 8 mg/kg body weight adjusted according to the trough (pre-dose level) of free drug in serum
- Prednisolone – 0.3 mg/kg body weight

Measuring the cyclosporine trough level is important because high levels can be nephrotoxic. Dose reductions follow satisfactory progress over 3 months. Tacrolimus has replaced cyclosporine in the majority of centres and has been associated with improved graft and patient survival after liver transplant. Many centres use MMF or azathioprine in triple therapy as a CNI sparing regime or in patients with previous significant rejection.

A standard initial maintenance immunosuppression plan for a generic recipient is as follows:
1. Tacrolimus 0.02 to 0.03 mg/kg by mouth twice a day (aiming for a serum level of 8 to 12 ng/mL)
2. MMF 1000 mg by mouth twice a day or mycophenolate sodium 720 mg by mouth twice a day
3. Prednisone taper

Over time, the doses of tacrolimus and mycophenolate should be reduced significantly and, ultimately, the mycophenolate and prednisone will be eliminated.

Polyclonal and Monoclonal Agents Against T-Cells

Basiliximab, alemtuzumab, OKT3 and ATG are agents used in some protocols for induction immunosuppression; however, ATG is useful in treating steroid-resistant rejection.

Complications of Immunosuppression

The most serious complication is an increased susceptibility to infections. Long-term immunosuppression also increases the risk of developing malignant disease, particularly squamous cell carcinoma of the skin and some forms of lymphoma. Renal damage and kidney failure is an important complication of all forms of solid organ transplant. Other complications are the outcome of the specific side effects of individual components of the suppressive regimen.

Intended immunosuppression withdrawal is still experimental and can only be considered in the setting of rigorous clinical trials under strict conditions and with intensive follow-up.

TABLE 12.1 Complications of Transplantation

Category	Nature	Possible Effects
General surgical	Wound – infection, dehiscence, incisional hernia	Occasionally life-threatening
		Further surgery required
Systemic infection	From i.v. lines, especially in liver transplantation	
	Consequent on immunosuppression	Septicaemia
Vascular suture lines	Thrombosis	Loss of graft
	Stenosis	In kidney – hypertension
Visceral suture lines	Leakage	Fistula
	Stenosis	Interference with graft function (hydronephrosis, obstructive jaundice)

General Complications of Transplantation

Apart from graft rejection and problems with drug toxicity, organ transplants of most kinds share a variety of complications which are summarized in Table 12.1. Technical problems are directly related to the quality of surgery and graft and show a decline with increasing experience (Box 12.6).

Pattern of Infection After Transplantation

Early infections (within first 4 weeks): Usually involve the urine, blood, wound or abdomen. They are most likely related to donor exposure, nosocomial pathogens and technical complications.

The usual organisms are Gram-negative enterics, *Staphylococcus* species, *Enterococcus* species, *Candida* species, and *Clostridium difficile*.

Intermediate infections (4 weeks–6 months): Period of most intensive immune suppression, usually involving the blood, intestine, lung and graft. They are most likely to be opportunistic, relapse or residual disease.

The usual organisms are herpes virus species (cytomegalovirus, herpes simplex viruses), Epstein-Barr virus, hepatitis viruses B and C, adenovirus, respiratory syncytial virus, rotavirus, *Listeria*, *Pneumocystis carinii*, and toxoplasmosis.

Long-term infections (after 6 months): Period of lower immune suppression and can involve any type of infections. If typical presentation, evaluate and treat like any other patient. If atypical presentation, always consider infection such as tuberculosis or post-transplant lymphoproliferative disease.

Monitoring the Progress of a Transplanted Organ

The monitoring methods available are as discussed in the following sections.

• BOX 12.6 Postoperative Complications

Early (<14 days):
- Vascular thrombosis or stenosis
- Primary non-function (death of patient without re-transplantation)
- Initial poor function (definition centre-dependent)
- Acute rejection
- Bleeding

Intermediate/late (>14 days):
- Acute or chronic rejection
- Abdominal infections
- Intra-abdominal abscess
- Systemic infections: Viral (e.g., cytomegalovirus (CMV) or Epstein-Barr virus (EBV)), fungal, bacterial
- Vascular complications (thrombosis/stenosis)
- Venous outflow tract obstruction
- Recurrent disease
- Malignancies (post-transplant lymphoproliferative disorders, skin cancer)

Transplant Function

- Liver – urea and electrolyte concentrations, liver function tests and measures of clotting activity
- Kidney – serum urea, electrolyte and creatinine concentrations
- Pancreas – measurement of amylase and pH in urine (if the transplanted pancreas is implanted into the bladder)

Evidence of Dysfunction

- Liver: Doppler ultrasound to eliminate technical problems such as bile duct obstruction or vascular thrombosis; biopsy if an immunological problem is suspected.
- Kidney: Doppler ultrasound examination to exclude collections around it, obstruction of the ureter and arterial or venous thrombosis. In the absence of such findings, carry out percutaneous biopsy under ultrasound guidance.
- Pancreas: The blood glucose level is not of value. Most transplants in the UK are combined kidney and pancreas,

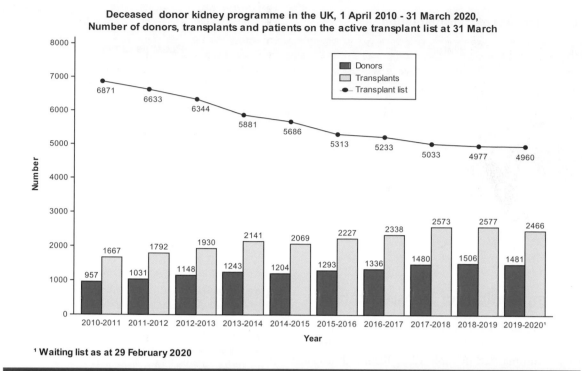

Deceased donor kidney programme in the UK, 1 April 2010 - 31 March 2020,
Number of donors, transplants and patients on the active transplant list at 31 March

¹ **Waiting list as at 29 February 2020**

Source: Transplant activity in the UK, 2019-2020, NHS Blood and Transplant

• **Fig. 12.4** Number of donor, transplants and patients active on the kidney transplant list.

and the progress of the kidney can be used to monitor the pancreas.
• Small bowel: See later.

Transplantation of Individual Organs

End-stage failure means that the organ is no longer able to sustain life.

Kidney

With increasing success, the number of allografts transplanted were increasing every year, but have now reached a plateau because of the limited availability of donors. However, more and more patients are being admitted to dialysis programs and are subsequently added to an ever-increasing list of patients waiting for a suitable allograft (Fig. 12.4).

Indications

Indication for kidney transplantation is renal failure from the following causes:
• Chronic glomerulonephritis (55%)
• Reflux nephropathy (25%)
• Polycystic disease (8%)
• Diabetic nephropathy (2%)
• Malignant hypertension (1%)
• Other causes, e.g. analgesic nephropathy (9%)

Operation

The transplant is heterotopic, with the kidney placed usually in the right iliac fossa and attached to the iliac artery and vein. The ureter is joined to the bladder to make a new ureterovesical junction (Fig. 12.5). The recipient's own kidneys are left in situ unless they are a source of sepsis.

Kidney Transplant in the UK

• In March 2017, there were 4915 adult and 80 paediatric patients on the UK active kidney transplant list.
• There were 3042 adult kidney-only transplants performed in the UK in 2016–17. Of these, 1218 were from DBD, 887 were from DCD and 937 were from living donors.
• The national rate of graft survival 5 years after first adult, deceased donor, kidney-only transplant is 87% (ranging from 77–91%). The equivalent rate after first paediatric, deceased donor, kidney-only transplant is 83% (ranging from 72–100%).
• The national rate of graft survival 5 years after first adult, living donor, kidney-only transplant is 93% (ranging from 88–97%). The equivalent rate after first paediatric, living donor, kidney-only transplant is 86% (ranging from 73–100%).
• The national rate of 10-year patient survival from listing for deceased donor, kidney-only transplants in adult

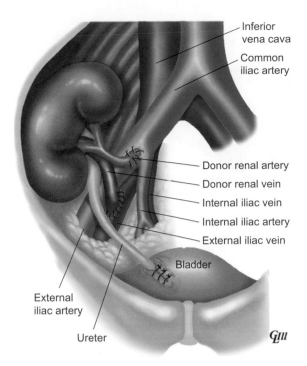

Inferior vena cava
Common iliac artery
Donor renal artery
Donor renal vein
Internal iliac vein
Internal iliac artery
External iliac vein
Bladder
External iliac artery
Ureter

• **Fig. 12.5** Completed Renal Transplant in Right Iliac Fossa.

patients is 75%. These rates vary between centres, ranging from 68% to 89%.

Liver

Approximately 6000 liver transplants are performed annually in Europe. Survival figures have improved due to ameliorations in patient selection, clinical support, organ preservation and immunosuppressive agents. In major transplant centres, a 90–95% 1-year survival is obtained. The indications are changing, with increased numbers of transplants for hepatocellular carcinoma and non-alcoholic steatohepatitis and fewer for hepatitis B and C.

Indications

Transplantation is indicated in the presence of liver failure from any of the conditions shown in Boxes 12.7 and 12.8.

Operation

The operation is a major procedure because the diseased liver may be difficult to remove and there are a number of vascular anastomoses to be made during which venous return to the heart has to be maintained (Fig. 12.6). Primary failure of function is uncommon. The morbidity and mortality of this complication is high. Survival following re-transplantation for primary non-function is less than 50%.

Results

The results of liver transplantation are rapidly improving. Currently, the majority of centres report 1-year graft survival in excess of 90%. It is of note that over 85% of patients surviving more than 6 months after liver transplantation return to active life either at school or at work.

• **BOX 12.7** **Indications for Liver Transplantation**

Indications for Adults

a) Chronic liver failure (cirrhosis) due to:
  • Chronic hepatitis B, B and D (coinfection) and C
  • Alcoholic liver disease
  • Autoimmune hepatitis
  • Cryptogenic cirrhosis
  • Congenital liver fibrosis
  • Primary and secondary biliary cirrhosis
  • Primary sclerosing cholangitis
  • Biliary atresia
  • Metabolic liver diseases: Wilson's disease, Alpha1-antitrypsin deficiency, Hemochromatosis, Protoporphyria
  • Vascular diseases
  • Budd-Chiari syndrome
b) Acute liver failure
  • Cryptogenic or non-A, non-B
  • Viral (hepatitis A, B, D (coinfection), E)
  • Intoxications (e. g. paracetamol, acetaminophen, amanita phalloides)
  • Wilson's disease
  • Extensive liver trauma
  • Budd-Chiari syndrome
c) Metabolic disorders (e.g. familial amyloid polyneuropathy, primary hyperoxaluria)
d) Liver tumours
  • Hepatocellular carcinoma: single tumours <5 cm, or up to three tumours <3 cm(Milan criteria, extended criteria centre dependent)
  • *Epithelioid haemangio-endothelioma*
  • Hepatoblastoma
  • Benign (polycystic liver disease, giant haemangioma, Caroli's disease)

Indications in Children

Biliary atresia (32%), metabolic/genetic conditions (22%), acute liver failure (11%), cirrhosis (9%), liver tumour (9%), immune-mediated liver and biliary injury (4%) and other miscellaneous conditions (13%).

• **BOX 12.8** **Contraindications for Liver Transplantation**

• Untreated systemic infections or sepsis
• Extrahepatic malignant disease
• Irreversible multiorgan failure

Rejection

The early targets of acute cellular liver transplant rejection are the bile duct epithelium and the venous endothelium. There is no consistent biochemical pattern that predicts acute cellular rejection; a non-invasive scheme of ultrasonography (to rule out vascular and bile duct pathological conditions) may need to be followed by biopsy.

There are three major histological features associated with cellular rejection:
• Endotheliitis
• Portal triads with mixed infiltrates (predominantly mononuclear but may also contain neutrophils and eosinophils)

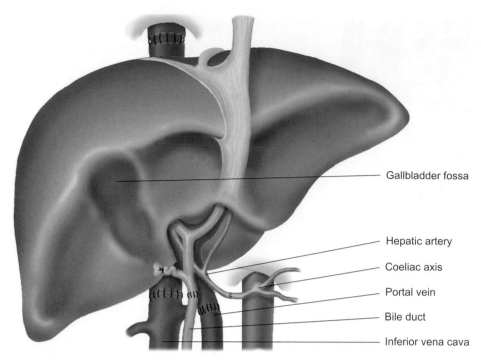

Gallbladder fossa

Hepatic artery

Coeliac axis

Portal vein

Bile duct

Inferior vena cava

• **Fig. 12.6** Completed Liver Transplant Note the numerous suture lines. The gallbladder is removed.

- Destructive or non-destructive non-suppurative cholangitis involving interlobular biliary epithelium
- CD4+ T-cells are prominent mediators of acute cellular rejection An elevated eosinophil count has a positive predictive value for acute cellular rejection of the liver, whereas a normal count generally excludes moderate or severe rejection.

The innate immune system may play a vital role in the initiation and enhancement of the immune response to organ transplantation through Toll-like receptors and subsequent cytokine production.

Operational tolerance has been demonstrated through a prospective trial of immunosuppression withdrawal.

Living Liver Donors

Living donor liver transplantation is now undertaken in a number of centres worldwide and is relatively common in some countries where deceased donation is not practised for cultural or religious reasons. The concept was first pioneered to allow children to receive the left lobe or lateral segment from an adult donor. In countries where transplantation from a heart-beating cadaveric donor is undertaken, living donor liver transplantation in children has, to a large extent, been superseded by the techniques of liver reduction or liver splitting. Split-liver transplantation, first performed by Pichlmayr in 1988, allows the liver from a deceased donor to be split in two (Fig. 12.7). The right lobe is used for an adult and the left lobe is usually used for a child, although occasionally a split liver has been used for two adults. In adult-to-adult living donor liver transplantation, the right lobe of the liver is transplanted. The donor procedure has a reported mortality rate of around 0.2% and one of the complications is bile leak.

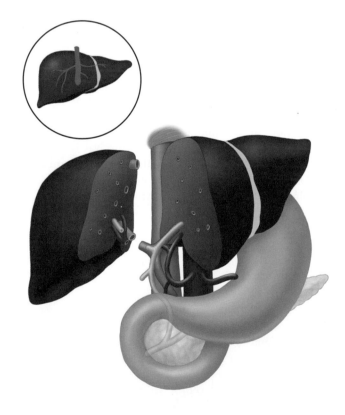

• **Fig. 12.7** Split liver transplantation, division in right and left lobe.

Auxiliary Liver Transplant

An auxiliary liver transplant involves surgically implanting a donor liver graft either orthotopically (by resecting native liver to make room) or heterotopically without removal of

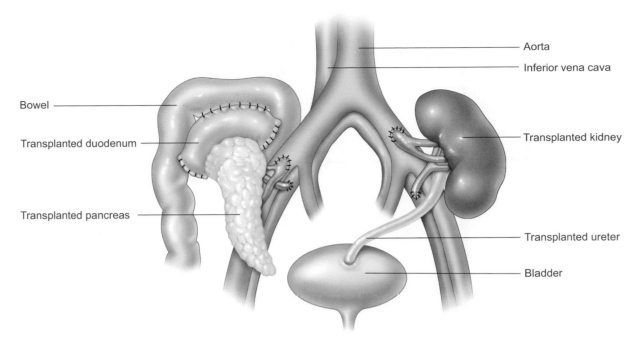

• **Fig. 12.8** Whole-Organ Pancreas Transplant.

the recipient liver. The donor liver supports the native liver until it recovers. The donor liver can then be removed or left attached. This has been used to treat acute liver failure, with the graft supporting the recipient until the native liver regenerates and immunosuppression can be withdrawn over time.

Pancreas

The large number of patients with diabetes has made transplantation of the pancreas a worthwhile goal. However, severe diabetes is often accompanied by renal disease which makes concurrent renal transplantation necessary if the patient is to be restored to health.

Indications

1. Insulin-dependent diabetes with renal failure – combined pancreas and kidney transplant
2. Pre-uraemic diabetic with severe complications, e.g. neuropathy, retinopathy and poor control of the disease – a pancreas-only transplant is needed

Operation

The technique depends on whether a whole organ or a segmental graft is to be used. The latter is removed on a pedicle of splenic artery and vein and is revascularized using the external iliac artery and vein, with the pancreatic duct drained into the urinary bladder. The whole organ is removed with the segment of duodenum that drains the pancreatic duct. Revascularization is by a similar method to the segmental graft, with the duodenal loop drained into the bladder (Fig. 12.8). The latter technique has the least complications and the highest success rate. However, as experience with pancreas transplantation has increased, many centres are changing to an enteric drainage (anastomosis of donor pancreas or duodenum to the GI tract) but complication rates are high.

Results

With increasing experience, 1- and 5-year graft survivals of 70% and 40%, respectively, are being reported.

However, transplantation of the whole pancreas is likely, in the future, to be replaced by transplantation of islet cells only.

Small Bowel

Small-bowel transplantation presents particular difficulties because:

- The transplant contains a large volume of lymphoid tissue (see graft–versus–host reaction later).
- MHC class II antigens are constitutively expressed by the bowel epithelium.
- The transplanted organ is colonized with microorganisms.

As a consequence of the last of these, there is breakdown of the intestinal barrier and the release of bacteria into the circulation (translocation), with consequent infection, as well as an increased presentation of immune signals to the recipient.

Indications

Current guidelines restrict intestinal transplantation to patients who have had significant complications from prolonged parenteral nutrition, including liver failure and repeated infections (Fig. 12.9).

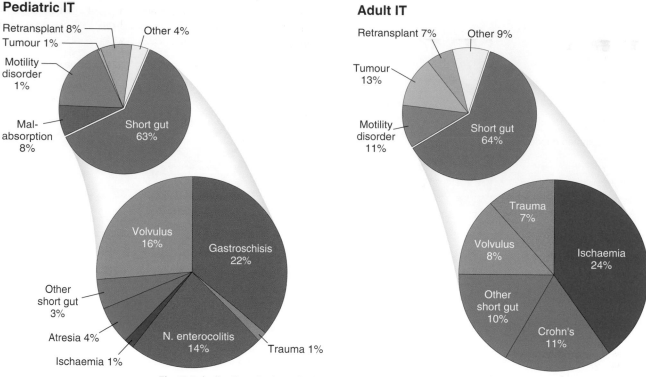

Pediatric IT

Retransplant 8%
Tumour 1%
Motility disorder 1%
Mal-absorption 8%
Other 4%
Short gut 63%

Volvulus 16%
Gastroschisis 22%
Other short gut 3%
Atresia 4%
Ischaemia 1%
N. enterocolitis 14%
Trauma 1%

Adult IT

Retransplant 7%
Tumour 13%
Motility disorder 11%
Other 9%
Short gut 64%

Trauma 7%
Volvulus 8%
Ischaemia 24%
Other short gut 10%
Crohn's 11%

• **Fig. 12.9** Indications for intestinal transplantation in adults and children.

Operation

Proximal anastomosis of the graft is to the recipient's jejunum; distally, the new gut is brought out as an end-ileostomy (Fig. 12.10).

Results

Results have continued to improve for isolated, combined with liver and multivisceral transplant (Fig. 12.11):

- In March 2017, there were 12 patients on the UK active intestine transplant list. Of those patients registered onto the transplant list in a recent 2-year period (April 2013–March 2015), 86% had received a transplant 2 years post-registration, while 4% had died, 6% were removed and 4% were still waiting.
- There were 176 intestine transplants performed in the UK in the 10-year period. 14 of these were re-transplants (8%) and 38% of the total number of transplants were in paediatric recipients, whereas 62% were in adult recipients.
- The national rates of survival after first intestine transplantation for elective adult patients were estimated at 89%, 81% and 57% at 90 days, 1 and 5 years post-transplant, respectively.
- The national rates of survival after first intestine transplantation for elective paediatric patients were estimated at 95%, 86% and 59% at 90 days, 1 and 5 years post-transplant, respectively.

Heart, Lung and Heart–Lung

This is discussed in Chapter 19.

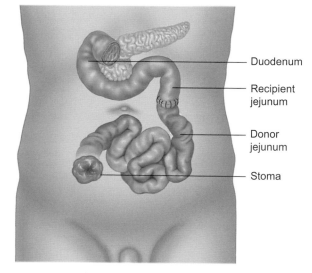

Duodenum
Recipient jejunum
Donor jejunum
Stoma

• **Fig. 12.10** Small-Bowel Transplant.

Cornea

The cornea was the first solid tissue successfully allografted in humans. In recent years, a high success rate has made corneal transplantation the most commonly performed transplant.

Indications

1. Opaque cornea from any cause
2. Thin or distorted cornea
3. Corneal loss – necrotizing ulceration or trauma

Operation

A button of the recipient's cornea is removed and replaced with a corresponding graft from the donor using very fine

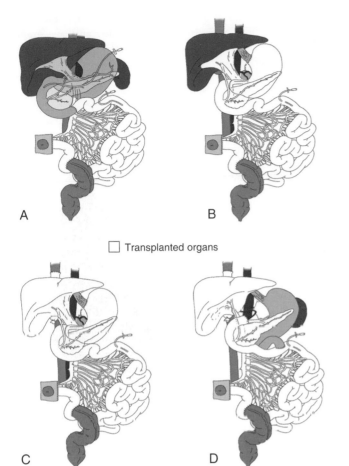

A B

☐ Transplanted organs

C D

• **Fig. 12.11** Four Types of Intestinal Transplants (A) Intestine alone. (B) Modified multivisceral transplant with exclusion of the liver. (C) Full multivisceral transplant that includes stomach, duodenum, pancreas, intestine and liver. (D) Combined liver and intestine with pancreas.

nylon sutures. Because the cornea is avascular, rejection is not a common problem unless the recipient's cornea has undergone neovascularization before the transplant takes place.

Results

Worldwide, the survival of the corneal graft is 95%, and they last long term. Close HLA matching improves the long-term result.

Transplantation in Children

In older children with a weight in excess of 20 kg, most transplant procedures are the same as for adults. The multidisciplinary team needs to specialize in the care of children. In smaller children, specialist techniques have been adapted to try to overcome donor shortage and reduce the incidence of technical complications associated with small vessels, particular in those <10 kg.

Kidney

The results of transplanting paediatric kidneys into paediatric recipients are worse than if an adult kidney is used.

Accordingly, most centres now transplant the best-matched organ, provided its size is not too discrepant; access may be modified to make the procedure feasible.

Other Organs

For liver, heart and lung, the constraints of size are more relevant, and age matching is done. However, the increasing success of using a reduced-size liver graft has overcome the problem of supply.

The Future

Future Developments in Transplantation

- Novel organ preservation/modulation
- Biomarkers for monitoring rejection, infection and tolerance
- Strategies for inducing donor-specific immunological tolerance
- Stem cell medicine and tissue engineering
- Xenotransplantation
- Manipulation of the gut microbiome

The Future of Liver Transplantation

It is likely that organ shortage will continue to be a global issue for the next 10–15 years. Optimizing surgery to avoid technical complications and medical follow up to avoid disease recurrence will reduce the need for re-transplantation. The advent of effective antiviral therapy for hepatitis B and C will impact on the global need for liver transplantation over the next 10 years. After 50 years of the use of cold preservation of organs prior to transplantation, a new era has been entered with the development of hypothermic and normothermic machine perfusion which offers the promise of ameliorating ischemia/reperfusion injury, maintaining grafts ex-vivo and modulating function prior to implantation.

In addition, the use of in situ (in the DCD cadaveric donor) regional ECMO perfusion shows early promise in improving graft quality and potentially avoiding complications such as delayed graft function or ischemic cholangiopathy. Machine perfusion and graft immunomodulation may be used in the future to reduce innate immune activation and improve survival.

The management of recipient co-morbidities in the lead up to and post-transplant will continue to be one of the main challenges going forwards. The impact of lifestyle diseases including diabetes, obesity and poly-addictions (alcohol, drugs and smoking) pose significant challenges to patient selection and long-term graft and patient survival. Managing the metabolic syndrome and, in particular, insulin resistance is central to this challenge.

The need for transparency and 'fairness' in organ allocation and monitoring centre outcomes remains a challenge worldwide. Monitoring of performance within an effective clinical governance framework will continue to develop to help patients make informed choices regarding their transplant care.

Developments in genomics and proteomics are moving towards the identification of novel biomarkers to monitor rejection, infection and tolerance. Clinical trials to wean and potentially withdraw immunosuppression are underway and are likely to improve understanding of functional tolerance.

Novel experimental therapies are being introduced into clinical practice. Gene therapy is being trialled and may be of value in non-cirrhotic inborn errors of metabolism based in the liver, e.g. Criggler-Najar type 1. Gene editing offers future promise in this field. Repopulation of organs using recipient cell through the use of organoids has been proposed. Hepatocyte transplantation is being used to repopulate failing livers and to bridge young children to organ replacement. The development of liver dialysis to sustain patients similarly to dialysis in kidney or ventricular support for the heart remains elusive at present. Experimental models of using the natural scaffold of organs reconstituted with recipient stem cells are possible within the mouse model, but not in humans.

The use of xenotransplantation, after early excitement, is slowly making progress in overcoming the obstacles posed by zoonotic infection, immunology and physiology. The use of genetically manipulated pigs for solid organ transplantations remains tantalizingly out of reach at present.

Finally, the ability to prevent or reverse disease processes damaging the liver, kidney or heart must remain central to research efforts. Reversal of fibrosis has been shown to occur with treatment of viral hepatitis with a significant number of patients being able to avoid transplantation.

However, transplantation is set to continue at an increasing rate worldwide. Access to these treatments is limited to a small minority at present. The availability and affordability of transplantation remains the greatest challenge. Lifestyle choices are increasingly implicated in organ failure and impact on graft and patient survival and have to be tackled effectively to ensure transplantation continues to be an effective treatment modality.

Further Reading

Bae C, Henry SD, Guarrera JV. Is extracorporeal hypothermic machine perfusion of the liver better than the 'good old icebox'? *Curr Opin Organ Transplant*. 2012;17:137–142.

Barker CF, Markmann JF. Historical overview of transplantation. *Cold Spring Harb Perspect Med 3*. 2013;3(4):a014977.

Benichou J, Halgrimson CG, Weil III R, et al. Canine and human liver preservation for 6 to 18 hours by cold infusion. *Transplantation*. 1977;24:407–411.

Brent LA. *History of Transplantation Immunology*. London: Academic Press; 1997.

Brockmann J, Reddy S, Coussios C, et al. Normothermic perfusion: a new paradigm for organ preservation. *Ann Surg*. 2009;250:1–6.

Broelsch CE, Emond JC, Whitington PF, et al. Application of reduced-size liver transplants as split grafts, auxiliary orthotopic grafts, and living related segmental transplants. *Ann Surg*. 1990;212:368–375.

Busuttil RW, De Carlis LG, Mihaylov PV, et al. The first report of orthotopic liver transplantation in the western world. *Am J Transplant*. 2012;12:1385–1387.

Calne RY. Early days of liver transplantation. *Am J Transplant*. 2008;8:1775–1778.

Calne RY, Sells RA, Pena JR, et al. Induction of immunological tolerance by porcine liver allografts. *Nature*. 1969;223:472–474.

Goodwin WE, Martin EC. Transplantation of the kidney. *Urol Surv*. 1963;13:229–248.

Grant D, Abu-Elmagd K, Mazariegos G, et al. Intestinal transplant registry report: global activity and trends. *Am J Transplant*. 2015;15:210–219.

Guarrera JV, Henry SD, Samstein B, et al. Hypothermic machine preservation in human liver transplantation: the first clinical series. *Am J Transplant*. 2010;10:372–381.

Gundlach M, Broering D, Topp S, et al. Split-cava technique: liver splitting for two adult recipients. *Liver Transpl*. 2000;6:703–706.

Hamilton DA. *History of Organ Transplantation: Ancient Legends to Modern Practice*. Pittsburgh: University of Pittsburgh Press; 2012:xii.

Heusler K, Pletscher A. The controversial early history of cyclosporine. *Swiss Med Wkly*. 2001;131:299–302.

Marchioro TL, Axtell HK, LaVia MF, et al. The role of adrenocortical steroids in reversing established homograft rejection. *Surgery*. 1964;55:412–417.

Marchioro TL, Porter KA, Dickinson TC, et al. Physiologic requirements for auxiliary liver homotransplantation. *Surg Gynecol Obstet*. 1965;121:17–31.

Moore FD, Wheeler HB, Demissianos HV, et al. Experimental whole organ transplantation of the liver and of the spleen. *Ann Surg*. 1960;152:374–387.

Schwartz R, Dameshek W. Drug-induced immunological tolerance. *Nature*. 1959;183:1682–1683.

Starzl TE. *The Puzzle People: Memoirs of a Transplant Surgeon*. Pittsburgh: University of Pittsburgh Press; 1992.

Starzl TE. *Experience in Renal Transplantation*. Philadelphia: WB Saunders; 1964:1–233.

Starzl TE. The long reach of liver transplantation. *Nat Med*. 2012;18:1489–1492.

Starzl TE, Fung JJ. Themes of liver transplantation. *Hepatology*. 2010;51:1869–1884.

Starzl TE, Groth CG, Terasaki PI, et al. Heterologous anti-lymphocyte globulin, histocompatibility matching, and human renal homotransplantation. *Surg Gynecol Obstet*. 1968;126:1023–1035.

Starzl TE, Hakala TR, Shaw Jr BW, et al. A procedure for multiple cadaveric organ procurement. *Surg Gynecol Obstet*. 1984;158:223–230.

Starzl TE, Klintmalm GBG, Porter KA, et al. Liver transplantation with the use of cyclosporine A and prednisone. *N Engl J Med*. 1981;305:266–269.

Starzl TE, Marchioro TL, Rowlands Jr DT, et al. Immunosuppression after experimental and clinical homotransplantation of the liver. *Ann Surg*. 1964;160:411–439.

Starzl TE, Miller C, Broznick B, et al. An improved technique for multiple organ harvesting. *Surg Gynecol Obstet*. 1987;165:343–348.

Starzl TE, Todo S, Fung J, et al. FK506 for human liver, kidney and pancreas transplantation. *Lancet*. 1989;2:1000–1004.

Starzl TE, Weil III R, Iwatsuki S, et al. The use of cyclosporin A and prednisone in cadaver kidney transplantation. *Surg Gynecol Obstet*. 1980;151:17–26.

Tzakis A, Todo S, Starzl TE. Orthotopic liver transplantation with preservation of the inferior vena cava. *Ann Surg*. 1989;210:649–652.

Vogel T, Brockman JG, Friend PJ. Ex-vivo normothermic liver perfusion: an update. *Curr Opin Organ Transplant*. 2010;15:167–172.

Wachs M, Bak T, Karrer F, et al. Adult living donor liver transplantation using a right hepatic lobe. *Transplantation*. 1998;66:1313–1316.

13

Emergency General Surgery

Introduction

Good surgical practice comes from a combination of skills, judgement and professionalism. It can also be said that in emergency general surgery (EGS) further qualities such as pragmatism, rapid problem-solving skills and meticulous communication with colleagues and patients are also much needed. This chapter reviews the management of the patient in the emergency setting and provides an overview of how high-quality emergency care should be delivered from a team perspective.

Epidemiology of Emergency General Surgery

Over 30,000 laparotomies are performed in the UK each year, with a mean length of stay of 15.6 days in 2017.[1] Since 2013, the national 30-day mortality has fallen from 11.8 to 9.5% but it still remains high. However, only 25% of patients admitted under EGS undergo an operative procedure and about 15% of patients present to EGS with a condition that is usually managed by another specialty. Referrals and regular interaction with specialties such as medicine and gynaecology are therefore critical functions of the EGS and cooperation is critical to ensuring safe and effective care.

The epidemiology of surgical pathology is further complicated by variations in social care and emergency surgical disease is greatly influenced by social behaviours such as alcohol consumption and substance abuse. For example, acute pancreatitis which is a condition with significant morbidity and mortality that is commonly triggered by alcohol excess. It is also critical to remember that alcohol is a great masker of serious pathology; a patient with traumatic intracranial bleed and low Glasgow coma score can easily be mistaken for being under the influence of alcohol. Making informed decisions about surgery and treatments is also challenging in patients who are unable to consent because of altered conscious state or mental health conditions. Increasingly, the emergency surgeon has to also deal with an ageing population; half of all laparotomies are performed in patients over the age of 70 and frailty and dementia influence pathology and raise complex issues of capacity to consent to treatment. Despite this, 77% of elderly patients undergoing a laparotomy are still not seen by a geriatrician during their in-patient stay. This has prompted the increasing adoption of multidisciplinary teams in emergency surgery, although these are not yet common practice.

The Modern Emergency Surgical Team

Historically, EGS was 'piggy backed' on to the elective practice of the consultant surgeon. Surgeons were expected to look after emergency patients while simultaneously performing elective operations and clinics. Today it is inconceivable that a team will be required to do both. Hospitals have various models but are increasingly adopting the model of a specialist emergency surgery service. During daytime hours, an EGS team typically consists of a full-time dedicated EGS consultant, specialist registrar, core trainee and one or more foundation year trainees. Although EGS is not yet a separate subspecialty to general surgery, it features prominently within the surgical curriculum with essential indicative number of operations such as emergency laparotomies and appendicectomies. Many hospitals already employ multiple EGS consultants to provide an uninterrupted service except out of hours. In the UK, these surgeons would have trained in one of the gastrointestinal subspecialties of general surgery and their numbers, in response to service demand, is increasing. This push towards sub-specialization has been driven by data from several large audits and quality improvement projects.

NCEPOD

NCEPOD stands for National Confidential Enquiry into Peri-Operative Deaths. In the 1990s, it demonstrated an increased mortality when surgery was performed at night which was independent of disease severity or patient co-morbidities. On the basis of this, formal CEPOD lists were increased during daytime hours and operations that were not required to save 'limb or life' were postponed until the morning. Furthermore, urgent operations can now be classified according to a CEPOD grading systems (Box 13.1).

Over the last 30 years the NCEPOD audit has made many reports. These can be found at https://ncepod.org.uk and a concise summary of its recommendations is below:

1. **Consultant review:** The current NHS guideline is that all patients should be seen by a consultant within 14 hours of admission to hospital. In-patients should be reviewed by specialty relevant consultants as frequently as required to plan and manage their clinical need. Consultants must ensure that lines of communication are open between them and their junior staff, particularly when the junior staff are seeing patients without them.

2. **Supervision of trainee doctors:** Consultants need to supervise junior doctors in accordance with the duty they are carrying out. If the consultant does not need to be physically present, then junior team members need to be aware of how to access them.

3. **Multidisciplinary review:** Patients should receive relevant care from multidisciplinary and multispecialty healthcare teams to treat their condition as well as any underlying co-morbidities.

4. **Documentation:** Electronic healthcare records are having a major impact in this area, but current standards for recording information in case notes should be followed. And as a minimum, every aspect of care provided and/or communicated to a patient and/or their carer must be documented in the patient's case notes legibly, stating the name, grade and specialty of the person who wrote it and when it was recorded.

5. **Monitoring and early warning scores:** Hospitals should have systems in place to undertake accurate monitoring of fluid balance in all in-patients, and act on any abnormalities. The National Early Warning Score (NEWS2 – Royal College of Physicians of London) should be used in all acute healthcare settings in the NHS to improve communication between clinicians regarding the level of a patient's deterioration. There should be agreed arrangements in place to respond to each trigger level, including:
   a) the speed of response required in each situation
   b) a clear escalation policy covering 24/7 care
   c) the seniority and clinical competencies of the responder
   d) the appropriate settings for ongoing acute care
   e) timely access to high dependency care, if required
   f) frequency of subsequent clinical monitoring.

6. **Morbidity and mortality reviews:** Multidisciplinary morbidity and mortality review should take place for all patients who die within 30 days of elective treatment or intervention and a sample of patients who die within 30 days of emergency treatment or intervention. This is consistent with the new national Learning from Deaths policy.

• BOX 13.1 CEPOD Categories with Examples from General Surgery

1 Immediate within 1 hour – ruptured AAA, major GI bleed, major trauma
2A Within 6 hours – ischaemic bowel, generalized peritonitis, perforated gut
2B Within 24 hours – appendicitis with localized peritonitis, abscesses, obstruction
3 Expedited within 2–3 days – acute cholecystectomy, reduced femoral hernia

AAA, Abdominal aortic aneurysm; CEPOD, Confidential Enquiry into Peri-Operative Deaths; GI, gastrointestinal.

7. **Critical care review:** Trusts/Health Boards should plan for and provide sufficient critical care capacity and pathways of care to meet the needs of its population including:
   a) planned postoperative admission for high risk patients
   b) emergency admissions from the community, its own hospital or any other hospital it is likely to serve
   c) when to consider step-down care to the HDU/ward
   d) transfer to community care or repatriation if appropriate.

   There should be close liaison between the medical, surgical and critical care teams when making escalation decisions. A consultant-led discussion by specialists with appropriate knowledge of what interventions are likely to be of benefit to the patient should always be undertaken when:
   a) a decision is made not to escalate a patient
   b) a decision is made to proceed with high-risk surgery when it is known there will be no critical care bed postoperatively. Such decisions should be discussed with the patient and the patient's representative (if appropriate) and documented clearly. Where there is doubt or disagreement about such decisions, the opinion of a second consultant should be sought. Step-down care or discharge from critical care should not be undertaken at night.

   Critical care outreach services should be available to patients 24-hours a day, seven days per week that include:
   a) The use of a track and trigger warning system to identify at-risk patients
   b) Rapid referral to appropriately equipped experts
   c) Timely transfer to ICU when needed
   d) Facilitation of discharge and rehabilitation of patients from critical care.

8. **Networks:** Formal networks between hospitals should be established so that every patient has access to specialist interventions, regardless of which hospital they present to and are initially offered care in. Ambulance teams should be made aware of the networks so that patients can be taken to the most appropriate hospital for the care they need. Informal or ad hoc/good-will networks should not be relied upon when referring patients for specialist review. Every hospital should have a policy that covers when to refer and/or transfer a patient for review at a specialist tertiary centre and should include repatriation protocols to ensure efficient bed utilization.

9. **Consent:** This should be taken by someone with sufficient knowledge of the proposed operation and who understands the risks involved. The grade of the person taking consent should be recorded on the consent form. However, it is accepted that in some situations (e.g. extremely urgent surgery) this may be difficult as the senior surgeon is fully occupied caring directly for the patient. In these circumstances, other senior clinicians should assist in discussions with relatives/carers where possible. All patients undergoing elective surgery should have:
   a) A deferred two-stage consent process
   b) Clearly described and written details of benefits and risks of the procedure, including death
   c) A record of the discussion and the risks clearly stated on the consent form.

   The consent process should not be undertaken in one stage on the day of operation.

   A patients' mental capacity to understand and make decisions about treatment options should be assessed in advance of taking consent. Consent should only be taken from the patient when it is certain they understand the risks and benefits of the procedure.

10. **Local policies, protocols and governance:** Trust/Health Board should have evidence-based policies, protocols and guidelines for the organization and delivery of safe care for patients in all areas of healthcare. They should be:
    a) Kept up to date
    b) Accessible to all staff
    c) Audited regularly
    d) Augmented with staff training in their use

11. **Common clinical conditions:** All patients admitted to hospital are at risk of developing other conditions due to their underlying condition, co-morbidities or treatment – the following conditions know no boundaries and should be considered in all patients:
    a) Acute kidney injury
    b) Sepsis
    c) Deterioration
    d) Mental health

The National Emergency Laparotomy Audit (NELA)

In 2012, an audit of 35 UK hospitals demonstrated a 3–40% variation in mortality from emergency laparotomy. In 2014, this precipitated NELA. The National Emergency Laparotomy Audit not only provides the data to allow clinical teams to assess and benchmark their care against national standards, but also actively encourages teams to use their own data to drive local quality improvement (QI). NELA aims to raise awareness of QI methodology to support this: for example, by sharing learning resources on the NELA website and running a series of regional workshops in England and Wales for the multidisciplinary teams working with emergency laparotomy patients. Initial data have demonstrated that adequate resuscitation, early decisions for taking a patient to theatre and intensive monitoring in HDU are key factors for improving outcomes and reducing mortality. This has demonstrated that the marginal gains of meticulous patient care with respect to sepsis management, deep-vein thrombosis (DVT) prophylaxis and ward care have a significant clinical impact. Therefore, every review of the patient must be viewed as an abbreviated clerking ending with a new differential diagnosis and a plan of management. The audit continues to evolve and has demonstrated critical insights. For example, in the UK, mortality rates are 23% at 1-year after surgery, 29% at 2 years, and 34% at 3 years following surgery, but were substantially higher in high-risk patient groups. Of all emergency laparotomy patients, 6.3% had their surgery for a complication of a recent elective procedure within the same admission, 6.0% of all emergency laparotomy patients had an unplanned return to theatre after initial emergency laparotomy and 3.4% of patients had an unplanned admission to critical care, with variation seen between hospitals. It is mandatory to complete the NELA data after each laparotomy is performed and it provides a benchmark for improving outcomes in emergency surgery.

The Medical Emergency

Medical emergencies may masquerade as a surgical emergency and vice versa (Box 13.2). The clinician must therefore keep an open mind to this and obtaining a precise history is critical. A classic example is upper GI bleeding, which is typically managed by medical specialties. A patient may have coffee ground vomiting mistakenly identified as faeculant vomiting due to bowel obstruction. A delay in diagnosis and surgery will be detrimental to patient outcome. Both lower lobe pneumonias and inferior myocardial infarction can present with significant upper abdominal pain and tenderness. An operation in these patients would be catastrophic. Many severely ill medical patients will have ileus as intestinal motility is impaired due to systemic disease and physiological and electrolyte disturbances. These patients are typically elderly, frail and multi co-morbid and thus require careful assessment.

Preoperative Work-Up of Emergency Surgery Patients

Once the decision is made to operate, communicate this with the entire team and ensure all investigations, results and consent are achieved. Be sure to book the operation in theatres and inform the anaesthetic team according to NCEPOD criteria. Consider the postoperative nursing and monitoring requirements and ensure the patient has an appropriate level of bed available. There are typically three levels of care: ward, high dependency unit and intensive care. Continue to resuscitate the patient and ensure that active treatment continues as necessary until the anaesthetist takes over in the induction room in theatre.

Anaesthetic Assessment and Perioperative Care

Unlike in elective surgery where preoperative assessment can happen some weeks before the surgery and enable investigations and optimization of the patient in preparation for the physiological insult, in emergency surgery, anaesthetic assessment often occurs just before the operation. The surgical team therefore has an added responsibility to prepare the patient for general anaesthetic. This means ensuring optimal resuscitation of the patient with adequate fluids,

---

• **BOX 13.2** **Common Medical Emergencies Presenting as Acute Abdominal Pain**

MEDICAL CAUSES OF AN ACUTE ABDOMEN FOR WHICH SURGERY IS NOT INDICATED

Endocrine and Metabolic Disorders	Infections and Inflammatory Disorders
Uraemia	Tabes dorsalis
Diabetic crisis	Herpes zoster
Addisonian crisis	Acute rheumatic fever
Acute intermittent porphyria	Henoch-Schönlein purpura
Acute hyperlipoproteinemia	Systemic lupus erythematosus
Hereditary Mediterranean fever	Polyarteritis nodosa
Hematologic Disorders	
Sickle cell crisis	Referred Pain
Acute leukaemia	Thoracic region
Other dyscrasias	Myocardial infarction
Toxins and Drugs	Acute pericarditis
Lead and other heavy metal poisoning	Pneumonia
	Pleurisy
Narcotic withdrawal	Pulmonary embolus

---

blood products are ordered, electrolyte disturbances are corrected and that co-morbidities are appropriately optimized (e.g. diabetic control and the use of a sliding scale). The surgeon needs to consider the deranged physiology of the patient before, during and after the operation. The surgeon should maintain a clear channel of communication with the anaesthetist, and modify his or her operative technique, in response to the patient's changing physiological parameters. The best example of this is in the use of damage limitation surgery in unstable patients or in the management of major haemorrhage where coagulation physiology may change suddenly.

Critical Care Outreach Teams, Rapid Response Teams or Medical Emergency Teams, depending on the geographical location, have also now become increasingly involved in sharing their expertise of critical care by reviewing and treating patients early on in their acute illness, on the ward as well as in the critical care unit, in order to prevent further deterioration and death. The benefit of Critical Care Outreach Teams has been demonstrated by a reduction in hospital morbidity and mortality. Acutely unwell surgical patients should be flagged early with the outreach teams.

Preoperative Risk Assessment

A number of preoperative risk scoring methods are commonly used in the acute setting to stratify care. This should be performed in all patients where a surgical intervention is considered. The American Society of Anesthesiology (ASA) score and the P-POSSUM (Portsmouth – Physiological and

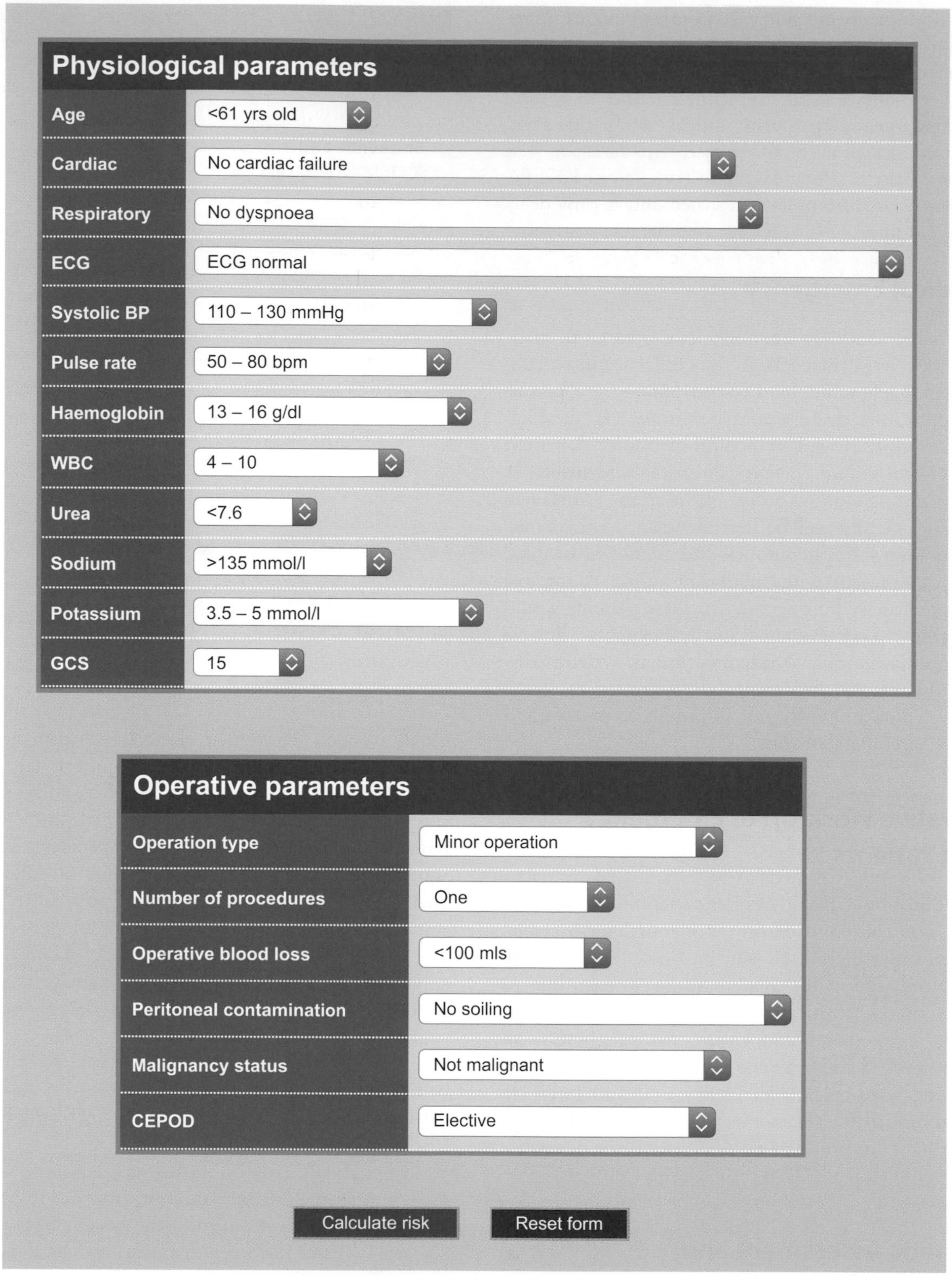

Physiological parameters

Age	<61 yrs old
Cardiac	No cardiac failure
Respiratory	No dyspnoea
ECG	ECG normal
Systolic BP	110 – 130 mmHg
Pulse rate	50 – 80 bpm
Haemoglobin	13 – 16 g/dl
WBC	4 – 10
Urea	<7.6
Sodium	>135 mmol/l
Potassium	3.5 – 5 mmol/l
GCS	15

Operative parameters

Operation type	Minor operation
Number of procedures	One
Operative blood loss	<100 mls
Peritoneal contamination	No soiling
Malignancy status	Not malignant
CEPOD	Elective

Calculate risk   Reset form

• **Fig. 13.1** P-POSSUM Score Criteria (From www.riskprediction.org.uk)

Severity Score for the Enumeration of Mortality and Morbidity) (Fig. 13.1) are commonly used. These scores are relatively accurate predictors of mortality and morbidity and they can be used for audit and quality improvement.

More recently, the NELA risk calculation tool has been developed to provide an estimate of the risk of death within 30 days of emergency laparotomy[1] and other sites such as http://sortsurgery.com also provide useful tools. All of these multivariate risk prediction scores are typically based on the retrospective analysis of large scale, patient-based databases such as NELA. They are critical for making informed decisions about surgical options and consent and for explaining risk to the patient and their family. Any mortality risk prediction above 10% should precipitate a planned ITU admission postoperatively, and those patients with a mortality risk above 5% should be considered for admission to HDU. Most risk assessment tools assume that the impact of risk factors is linear and cumulative. Therefore, the application of big data and deep learning in this field holds great promise. One example is the Predictive OpTimization Trees in Emergency surgery Risk calculator (POTTER), although this algorithm was developed using data from the American College of Surgeons National Surgical Quality Improvement Program (ACS NSQIP) for the years 2007 to 2013 with artificial intelligence to design an interactive risk calculator for emergency surgery. The data set includes more than 150 preoperative, intraoperative and postoperative variables from more than 380,000 patients. In recent work, the POTTER tool predicted the occurrence of individual postoperative complications, with moderate to extremely high accuracy. The mortality c-statistic was 0.9199, which was higher than the ASA, Emergency Surgery Score (ESS) and ACS NSQIP. Similarly, the morbidity c-statistic was higher for POTTER at 0.8511.[2] However, this is a rapidly emerging and evolving field and the true impact of artificial intelligence tools have yet to be determined.

Coagulation and DVT Prophylaxis

Bleeding tendency and hypercoagulability are two sides of the same coin in an emergency setting. Many patients present while on anticoagulants including the novel direct oral anticoagulants (DOAC); apixaban and rivaroxaban, which are non-reversible except with prothrombin factors. Luckily, this latest group of anticoagulants have a shorter half-life and a more predictable level of anticoagulation. They clear the system sufficiently 24 hours after the last dose for emergency operation to take place without unacceptably high risk of bleeding. Needless to say, surgical technique needs to be meticulous in haemostasis. Warfarin effect is measured with INR and is reversible with vitamin K or fresh frozen plasma in absolute emergency. Whereas aspirin alone is not a contraindication to surgery, dual antiplatelet therapy, often given for recently placed coronary arterial stents, is more problematic as platelet function is significantly impaired. Pooled platelet transfusion may be required for major surgery in consultation with the haematologist.

Preventing DVT requires both graduated calf compression stockings and subcutaneous heparin if not contraindicated. It must be remembered that emergency patients will often have their first dose of heparin after the operation at a time decided by the operating surgeon based on postoperative risk of bleeding, and from then on daily at the same time until discharge. Forty milligrams of Clexane is the typical prophylactic dose for a 70-kg adult. An additional technique used while the patient is asleep on theatre table is intermittent pneumatic calf compression. In high-risk patients who cannot have heparin, this should continue in the ward. Early mobilization of the patient is not only good for avoiding DVT and sarcopenia but will also reduce the time of postoperative ileus.

Human Factors in Emergency Surgery

Decision making in emergency surgery is a complex process that requires patient specific information, clinical knowledge, awareness of resource availability and a strategic overview of team capacity and function. Information in EGS is often dynamic and the team will often be placed under variable stress depending on the number of admissions it is facing. It is useful to have an overview of possible patient outcomes (Box 13.3) when making decisions as this will influence how you use available team members to efficiently manage patient flow. Using this decision tool will also foster intuitive development of decision making and facilitate discussion and feedback on patient management.

The management of emergency surgical patients is often time critical, and it can place a significant cognitive burden on the surgeon. This is exacerbated when working in an unfamiliar environment, with new or changing teams. Human factors are defined as 'Enhancing clinical performance through an understanding of the effects of teamwork, tasks, equipment, workspace, culture and organisation on human behaviour and abilities, and application of that knowledge in clinical settings'.[3] In 2007, the first UK Clinical Human Factors group (www.chfg.org) was established by Martin Bromiley and the main features are summarized in Box 13.4. He was an airline pilot whose wife died during an anaesthetic incident caused by multiple systems errors relating to human factors. Having worked in an industry where there is extensive recognition of the role of non-technical skills in safety, he questioned why the same was not adopted in healthcare at that time. Leaders for change in emergency surgery have looked to 'High Reliability Organizations' (HROs), such as the energy and aviation industries and the military, where human factors have

---

• BOX 13.3 Emergency General Surgery Patient Pathways

1. Home with no follow-up 2. Home with urgent outpatient clinic review
3. Discharge to other speciality
4. Admit for Observation/Conservative Management
5. Admit for further investigations but operation unlikely
6. Admit for further investigations – operation likely
7. Admit for surgery according to NCEPOD criteria.

• BOX 13.4 Classification of Human Factors

The Job Workplace Environment
The Individual Resilience, Decision Making, Situational Awareness
The Team Dynamics, Response to adverse events
The Organization Leadership, Safety Culture, Communication.

long been recognized to be critical to safety. In these HROs, human factors training is well-established and universal to all employees. The advent and daily utilization of checklists and standard operating procedures have been shown to reduce variation, increase familiarity and knowledge within the team and increase individual team member responsibility and sense of inclusion. The lessons learned are eminently transferrable to the emergency healthcare setting. Standardized practice reduces the individual bandwidth required to manage an emergency, at a time of peak stress and pressure. It is useful to have protocols or guidelines in place to manage critical events and medical emergencies. Training in these is crucial for optimal utilization, so that each team member is similarly aware of a plan. The concept of 10 seconds to save 10 minutes is widely taught in the pre-hospital and military fields. It allows time to step back, reassess a situation and formulate the next plan of action as a team. Taking a short time initially, to reconfigure and refocus, has been shown to save time and improve outcome in an emergency situation.

Communication in the Emergency Setting

Good communication between clinicians, the patient and their relatives is universally recognized as essential for the provision of high-quality care. Effective communication is prompt, error free and is received with clarity by the right person in a manner that is transparent. Moreover, it is data driven, and in the emergency setting, should not be impeded by social or professional hierarchy. It fosters initiative, decision making and education. Mobile communications and electronic healthcare records are radically transforming our ability to communicate. However, it is important to acknowledge that there is trade-off between time spent in front of a computer and that spent in direct contact with the patient. Although these systems have the ability for decision support and may even be used to direct therapy, direct person-to-person communication remains a critical skill for ensuring patient safety. The global adoption of mobile technologies has increased the speed of communication and bypassed the challenge of patchy hospital Wi-Fi coverage. However, their adoption in EGS must be considered in the context of data governance, security and the regulatory requirement for privacy. Both GMC and NHS England recognize the vital role mobile platforms play in patient care but urge caution with patient confidentiality, and their guidance should be closely followed (https://www.gmc-uk.org/ethical-guidance/ethical-guidance-for-doctors/doctors-use-of-social-media).

In addition to patient care–centred conversations, these applications promote group communication for the distribution of critical tasks, or for the sharing of guidelines and opportunistic educational encounters in patient care. The use of mobile messaging applications should adhere to GMC guidance, however. An exemplar methodology for their safe adoption can be found in Box 13.5.

• **BOX 13.5** **Exemplar Instructions for Mobile Messaging Use in EGS**

A. Confidentiality
   1. Password protect your screen lock with a timeout of 30 minutes maximum.
   2. Adjust the privacy settings to ensure the phone does not automatically upload photos to the cloud.
   3. When away from Emergency Surgery service, leave the group and delete all messages and photos. Rejoin the group upon return to work.
B. Escalation and Safety
   1. Provide clear instructions and commands when escalating care.
   2. Clearly define the level of help you require.
   3. If you recognize errors in information, inform the group and ensure they are corrected.
C. Photos and Data
   1. Use anonymized images only.
   2. Ask for consent as appropriate.
D. Work/Life Balance
   1. Do not message colleagues out of work hours.
   2. Group messages should stop at the end of a shift.

How to Discharge a Patient

Discharge conversations can take as long as the admission clerking with an inquisitive patient seeking reassurance. Time spent here will prevent re-admission and promote improved patient experience and economic efficiency. The upper level of readmission accepted in the UK in emergencies is 5% but it should not overly influence decision making. Patient information is critical and this can be provided verbally and in the form of a leaflet or digital content. Discharge summaries provide critical clinical information for the GP but they are also handed to patients at discharge as part of best practice. It is therefore important to limit medical jargon and make them easily understandable by the patient too (www.plainenglish.co.uk). A good discharge summary should be succinct and give clear guidance as to the expected recovery and future interventions and it should not hand over unnecessary tasks for the community team to perform. Not all patients can leave hospital once they are clinically deemed fit for discharge. It is good practice to predict this at the time of admission so planning can take place.

Pathology Presenting to the Emergency Surgeon

Acute Abdominal Pain

Urgent abdominal conditions form the bulk of the emergency activity of general surgeons. The range of causes is very wide and management often challenging. Many of the conditions are considered elsewhere in this book: intestinal obstruction, trauma, vascular emergencies, acute urological disorders, large-bowel disorders and acute lower-bowel haemorrhage. The definition of the term 'acute abdomen' is a loose one encompassing all those conditions that present with clinical features of short duration (arbitrarily less than 10 days) which might indicate a progressive intra-abdominal condition that is threatening to life or capable of causing severe morbidity. Not all patients will turn out to have such a threatening condition, but they need to be considered as being in danger until surgical evaluation has been completed. The majority of such patients have pain as their chief symptom. There are a very large number of possible causes, but most patients are found to have one of a relatively small number of common conditions. Surgical practice has for many years observed a policy of management based on 'it is better to look and see rather than to wait and see', because of the often-progressive nature of many causes of the acute abdomen. However, with the development of new technologies (e.g. laparoscopy, ultrasound and CT scanning – see below), the surgical objective has now become to reach a management decision which separates those who must have an operation to prevent dangerous progression from those who do not. Often this decision involves making an accurate diagnosis of the cause, but this is not always immediately necessary. The important matter is to classify the patient correctly into one of three categories based on the evidence available:

- operation necessary
- operation not immediately necessary; further information
- should be sought but may be followed by the need for surgery
- operation not necessary.

General Clinical Features

Pain: Abdominal pain has three origins:
- visceral
- parietal
- extra-abdominal pain

Visceral Pain

Visceral pain is generated either because of muscular contraction (colic) in organs such as the gut or ureter or because of stretching of the wall of a hollow organ (gallbladder) or the capsule of a solid one (aching pain from an enlarged liver). Organs from which such pain arises do not have a precise surface representation, so that the sensation is not accurately localized by the patient (Fig 13.2). However, pain which arises from the embryonic foregut (down to the second part of the duodenum) is usually located to the epigastrium; from the midgut (second part of the duodenum to the mid-transverse colon) to the periumbilical region; and from the hindgut to the suprapubic area (Table 13.1). Visceral pain is often severe and, in general, is central, as in bowel obstruction or biliary colic; ureteric pain is ipsilateral. In pain of visceral origin, a distinction should be made between colic, which truly comes and goes at (fairly) regular intervals, and distension, where the persistent tension on the wall or capsule of an organ produces pain of the same nature but which is more continuously present. In clinical

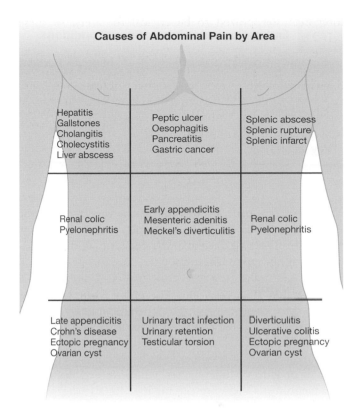

Causes of Abdominal Pain by Area

Hepatitis Gallstones Cholangitis Cholecystitis Liver abscess	Peptic ulcer Oesophagitis Pancreatitis Gastric cancer	Splenic abscess Splenic rupture Splenic infarct
Renal colic Pyelonephritis	Early appendicitis Mesenteric adenitis Meckel's diverticulitis	Renal colic Pyelonephritis
Late appendicitis Crohn's disease Ectopic pregnancy Ovarian cyst	Urinary tract infection Urinary retention Testicular torsion	Diverticulitis Ulcerative colitis Ectopic pregnancy Ovarian cyst

• **Fig. 13.2** Typical Presentation of Abdominal Pain

practice, the difference is often not appreciated, but it helps the clinician to think clearly about cause.

Parietal Pain

Parietal pain has its origin in the abdominal wall at any depth from the skin through to the peritoneum. The parietes have an accurate surface representation, so that the patient can usually indicate where exactly the pain is; examples are peritonitis and abdominal wall bruising. Sudden onset of diffuse parietal pain, associated with physical findings of peritoneal irritation, usually means perforation of a hollow viscus, rupture of an abscess into the general peritoneal cavity or bleeding. The combination of initial visceral pain and later local irritation is characteristically seen in acute appendicitis or acute cholecystitis. The initial pain of obstruction to the lumen of the organ is manifest as central colic and then, when inflammation develops, it produces localized pain at the site where the organ is in contact with the parietal peritoneum of the anterior abdominal wall. There is a potential diagnostic trap when an area of peritoneal irritation is not in contact with the anterior abdominal wall and therefore does not produce pain (see below).

Extra-Abdominal Pain

Extra-abdominal pain may take two forms:
- pain that originates from sources that share innervation with the abdominal wall – approximately T9 to

TABLE 13.1	**Embryological Origin of Some Conditions.**		
Foregut – Epigastric Pain	**Midgut – Periumbilical Pain**	**Hindgut – Suprapubic Pain**
Stomach ulcer	Small bowel	Left colon
Duodenal ulcer	Appendicitis	Sigmoid diverticulitis
Cholecystitis	Meckel's diverticulitis	Stercoral perforation
Liver	Right colonic diverticulitis	
Pancreatitis		
Splenic Infarct		

L1 – such as may occur in conditions which involve the spinal nerves
- pain from a wide variety of disorders where the mechanism is not well understood.

Apparent pain

To the three origins – visceral, parietal and extra-abdominal – should be added two clinical occurrences of apparent abdominal pain:
- Münchhausen's syndrome (so-called because it recalls the tales of Baron Münchhausen who invented marvellous adventures). There are certain individuals who present repeatedly with dramatic symptoms which often include pain as a prominent feature. There is usually a convincing story of an acute abdomen but without a cause. It is easy to be taken in by such patients, and they move from hospital to hospital undergoing needless investigation and surgery. However, it is important to take reported symptoms at face value in all cases unless there are clear records demonstrating previous episodes when no cause for pain has been found.
- Drug-dependent patients may feign pain to obtain analgesic drugs, although such patients may also develop acute abdominal conditions.

Investigation

Circumstances, particularly the patient's general condition and the localization of pain, determine the appropriate investigations. When the diagnosis remains in doubt, a wide range of investigations needs to be considered, and these are discussed under individual disorders. Provided that the condition is not judged to be life-threatening, a period of observation and review after a few hours (and preferably by the same clinician) is useful.

Routine Urine Testing

The presence of red cells or white cells can focus attention on the urinary tract as a possible cause of the problem. Other findings, such as the presence of glucose, ketone bodies and nitrites, may help in management. A pregnancy test should be performed when a fertile woman complains of abdominal pain.

Blood

Routine blood tests for full blood count, urea and electrolytes, liver function tests and C-reactive protein (CRP) are taken. It must be remembered that intra-abdominal inflammation in its early stages does not necessarily cause a raised white cell count or CRP; there is usually a delay of several hours before these acute inflammatory markers become elevated (see 'Appendicitis' below). Screening for thalassaemia and sickle cell disease should be done in Afro-Caribbean patients. Electrolyte abnormalities (such as a low potassium concentration) occur with vomiting or diarrhoea. Other blood investigations are considered under individual conditions. The serum amylase concentration must be measured in all patients with acute upper abdominal pain. A venous blood gas provides an important insight into the metabolic state of the patient and should be routinely used.

Imaging

Basic radiological tests consisting of an erect chest radiograph and a supine abdomen are often requested with initial investigations such as blood tests and urine dipstick. However, these are only helpful when gut perforation and obstruction are suspected. An erect CXR will miss up to 40% of perforations where the typical crescentic presence of air under diaphragm may be absent. AXR, on the other hand, may give clues to the level of obstruction as dilated colon will have significantly different features and distribution to dilated small bowel. Renal stones are best picked up on CT KUB (kidneys, ureters and bladder); 90% of them are radio-opaque whereas 90% of gallstones are radiolucent and will not show on AXR. Ultrasound of the abdomen is a very helpful initial investigation of the patient with abdominal pain. It is safe, low cost and it can be adopted by emergency surgeons for rapid assessment in the emergency room. It is typically used as a first-line investigation for young patients with pelvic pain to rule in gynaecological causes. Its use in ruling out appendicitis is more controversial; the appendix is frequently not seen on ultrasound in adults; however, in children, ultrasound can be a useful tool for ruling out the diagnosis. Ultrasound also has a secondary place in management of the acute abdomen either for guided biopsy or for percutaneous drainage of ascites or an abscess. In patients who are septic with overt peritonitis, it may delay definitive treatment however, particularly when a diagnostic laparoscopy is now routinely available.

In the emergency setting, the optimal cross-sectional imaging for the acute abdomen is the CT scan. Eighty-seven percent of patients undergoing laparotomy in the UK had a CT scan prior to surgery in 2017. But be aware of the patient's renal function and consider the risk of contrast nephropathy when trying to determine organ perfusion such as ischaemic bowel which is notoriously difficult to diagnose even with CT scan. CT scan is better at identifying the source of perforations or the level of obstruction. It must, however, be used with consideration of the amount of radiation it exposes the patient to and should be avoided, if possible, in children and in pregnancy.

Interventional radiology (IR) is an increasingly important modality in emergency surgery and may be deployed in the place of a laparoscopy or laparotomy. The emergency patient's physiology dictates the strategy, but, if stable, minimally invasive strategies are generally preferable. It has had particular impact in trauma and in the diagnosis and therapy of acute GI bleeding. Radiologists are now able to selectively cannulate branches of mesenteric vessels to halt bleeding from colonic angiodysplasias and diverticular bleeds. The results with gastric and duodenal ulcer bleeds are even more spectacular. In units with full IR rota, emergency surgeons seldom need to operate for gastrointestinal bleeding as IR provides another intermediate non-invasive technique should endoscopy fail.

When contacting radiology, emergency surgery teams must be fully conversant with the subtleties of the advantages and deficiencies of the previously-mentioned modalities and should defer to senior members of the team for clarification before making a request. It is often useful to formulate a question before asking for an investigation, think about how the investigation will change management and consider an investigation as a tool to confirm a suspected diagnosis rather than a trawl for many differential diagnoses.

Laparoscopy in Emergency Surgery

Laparoscopy has an important place in the assessment of patients with acute abdominal pain. It is also increasingly used for therapy (e.g. appendicectomy, closure of perforated ulcers). Laparoscopy is helpful in patients in whom the requirement for operation remains uncertain after initial assessment and investigation. For example, it is particularly useful in women with lower abdominal pain in whom the diagnosis may be either appendicitis or a number of other causes which do not require operation or in which the organ involved requires a different operative approach (Box 13.6). Laparoscopy is also useful when the clinical features in a suspected acute abdomen are atypical. Many surgeons start the procedure laparoscopically as procedures such as appendicectomy, over-sewing of a perforated ulcer and washout of diverticulitis are amenable to minimally invasive techniques. The acute 'hot' cholecystectomy has become best practice in the UK as it prevents further attacks while waiting for an elective laparoscopic cholecystectomy, and sorts the patient out during the index admission, early, reducing the recovery time from conservative management with antibiotics. This surgery is more complicated and requires further expertise in

---

• **BOX 13.6** **Causes of non-traumatic right iliac fossa pain and tenderness in young women**

- Appendicitis
- Salpingitis
- Ovarian cyst (rupture or torsion)
- Mesenteric adenitis
- Terminal ileitis (Crohn's disease, *Yersinia* infection, tuberculosis)
- Right ureteric calculus
- Urinary tract infection
- Meckel's diverticulum (inflammation, perforation or torsion)
- Cholecystitis
- Perforated duodenal ulcer

---

identifying and avoiding pitfalls compared with an elective procedure. Laparoscopy in emergency surgery is minimally disruptive to a patient's physiology. The internal milieu of the abdominal cavity is maintained at optimum body temperature and the bowel is minimally handled, avoiding adhesions. In patients with co-morbidities, it is useful in preventing postoperative respiratory infections in patients with COPD provided the anaesthetist is happy with the ventilation during the pneumoperitoneum. In heart failure patients, however, it is contraindicated as it will reduce the cardiac pre-load risking a cardiac event.

The Patient with Peritonitis

Presentation

Peritonitis is a common presentation of acute abdomen. It can be localized to a particular quadrant of the abdomen in early disease, or generalized in advanced disease with sepsis. The identification of the sick patient and prioritizing their care is the key to success. Patients with peritonitis will be dehydrated because of third space and insensible fluid loss driven by sepsis. The signs of septic shock include fever, cool peripheries, altered mental state tachycardia and tachypnoea and patients may look flushed and listless. The pain is often severe and the patient will avoid all movements that disturb the abdomen such as jumping, running, coughing and laughing. Vomiting can be a feature and is not necessarily a symptom of obstruction. Bowel habit is also an unreliable diagnostic indicator.

Past medical history is very useful. Ask if the patient has been previously affected or conservatively managed without surgery. The patient can often tell if these symptoms are similar to their previous attacks such as diverticulitis or cholecystitis. Their memory is often very reliable as the pain would have been significant. The expression 'common things are common' is used for conditions such as appendicitis, diverticulitis and cholecystitis because they can be missed in search of more exotic diagnoses. Although appendicitis is considered to be a disease of the young and diverticulitis a disease of older people, appendicitis is often diagnosed in elderly and some patients as young as 32 can have diverticulitis.

Examination of the Patient with Peritonitis

Analgesia should not be withheld from a patient with peritonitis pending examination. This is both cruel and unnecessary as signs of peritonitis are not masked easily. In fact, adequate analgesia may enable a more informative examination. The patient's vital signs are noted as these will be helpful in determining the level of sepsis. NEWS is a validated national score indicating the level of urgency and seniority required in managing the patient. As the patient is in severe pain, peritonitis should be elicited during examination carefully in a graduated manner. Examination should begin away from the site of maximal pain after interrogation of the patient and slowly proceed towards the quadrant indicated by the patient, while watching the patient's face looking for clues of distress. It is best to start with a very superficial examination and continue with a gentle percussion. If no pain is elicited, then a deeper examination with eventually a rebound test can be performed. Alternative graduated methods of eliciting peritonitis without touching the patient, particularly used in children, are asking the patient to blow up their abdomen and rapidly sucking it back in, standing up and jumping on the spot and coughing. A good way of excluding pain originating from abdominal wall is to ask the patient to perform a halfway sit up, thereby contracting the abdominal muscles, and then examining the abdomen; the tenderness should disappear in peritonitis but may persist in conditions such as rectus sheath haematoma.

Initial Management of Peritonitis

This is a surgical emergency. Attention is directed at managing sepsis and resuscitation. Surviving sepsis campaign (Box 13.7) has identified vital interventions in the first hour which make a significant contribution to survival.

The goal is early commencement of antibiotics and source control of sepsis. Despite this recommendation, the NELA audit identified that, in 2017, 76% of patients did not receive antibiotics within the appropriate time scale. These patients are often critically unwell, and critical support should be sought early and the patient should be managed in an HDU setting or a surgical ward providing

---

• BOX 13.7 The Sepsis Six

1. Give high flow oxygen via non-rebreathe bag
2. Take blood cultures and consider source control
3. Give i.v. antibiotics according to local protocol
4. Start i.v. fluid resuscitation – Hartmann's solution or equivalent
5. Check lactate
6. Monitor hourly urine output – consider catheterization

---

appropriate and experienced nursing care and monitoring. I.v. cannulas should be wide bore and in straight veins not crossing joints to avoid kinking. The patient with peritonitis may require large volume fluid resuscitation and therefore careful fluid balance is necessary with catheterization and hourly urine outputs. If a correctable surgical cause is present, surgery should not be delayed.

Surgery for Peritonitis

The operation is planned based on the most likely diagnosis and its severity. As discussed previously, liaison with ICU is required for admission if expected mortality risk is above 10%. If performed laparoscopically, early conversion to laparotomy is desirable in cases of advanced disease and surgeon's insufficient experience in emergency laparoscopy.

Postoperative Care in Peritonitis

The patient requires daily reviews on ward rounds, ideally by the same team of doctors led by a consultant. Resuscitation continues in the early postoperative period based on urine output and antibiotics are continued for a full course of 5–7 days in the presence of sepsis. A review at 48 hours with culture results may result in narrowing the spectrum of antibiotics used based on identification of the organisms. Strong opiate analgesia and PCA (patient controlled analgesia) are used if epidural was not possible due to sepsis. Ileus is expected commensurate with the severity of sepsis and its duration prior to surgery; it becomes pathological after an arbitrary duration of 5–7 days when obstruction should be suspected on rare occasions due to early adhesions or other complications. Despite the wash during surgery, bacteria can take a foothold in several spaces in the abdomen and form collections in the form of intra-abdominal abscesses. These are typically dependent areas when the patient is supine: in the pelvis, paracolic gutters, sub-phrenic and sub-hepatic spaces. If the contamination is gross, a planned return to theatre for a washout at 24–48 hours can prevent these complications. Thirty percent of laparotomy wounds will get infection and therefore require daily inspection at ward round to drain a developing abscess early before it disrupts the deeper muscular repair resulting in dehiscence or long-term incisional hernia. Other surgical complications include bleeding and ongoing leak of bowel contents requiring further surgery. Patients who undergo emergency laparotomy are susceptible to chest infections, DVT and PE and require preventative action with chest physiotherapy, adequate analgesia for painless deep breathing and DVT thrombophylaxis.

Enhanced recovery is desirable but rarely practical in a patient recovering from laparotomy for peritonitis. Initially liquids, and subsequently solids, should be gradually introduced as patient tolerates. Catheter, nasogastric (NG) tube and i.v. cannulas should be removed when they have served their purpose to avoid introduction of sepsis via these routes during recovery and to enable patient mobilization.

Acute Appendicitis

Aetiology and Pathological Features

The cause of acute appendicitis is thought to be obstruction of the appendicular lumen by either a mass of inspissated faeces (faecolith) or oedema. Distal to this, bacterial multiplication takes place and tension rises. Blood supply is then compromised and progression to gangrene is common. The appendix then ruptures and leads to a spreading peritonitis caused by enteric organisms (including Bacteroides). Alternatively, a severely inflamed appendix may be walled off by surrounding omentum and loops of bowel (an appendix mass) which will eventually contain pus (an appendix abscess). Appendicitis and many of the conditions that mimic it are commonest in the age range 2–40 years. Untreated, the condition threatens life and, although uncommon at the extremes of age, the highest mortality is in the very young and the elderly, mainly because the diagnosis is more difficult in these patients. The appendix may be in a number of different positions in relation to the caecum: medial; medial and below; extending over the pelvic brim into the pelvis; retrocaecal; or retroileal. The clinical features of inflammation are modified accordingly.

Clinical Features

Symptoms

The history typically begins with central abdominal pain of a visceral type – ill-localized and usually around the umbilicus – accompanied by a variable amount of anorexia, nausea and one or more episodes of vomiting. As the organ becomes inflamed, local peritoneal irritation, parietal pain, is felt in the right iliac fossa. Occasionally, the progression to gangrene is so rapid that these symptoms are largely absent or unrecognized by the patient, who presents with the diffuse abdominal pain of generalized peritonitis. Other variable features of the history are:

- previous similar attacks – suggestive of recurrent appendicitis
- more frequent vomiting if the appendix is retroileal
- variable urinary symptoms – frequency and dysuria – because of an inflamed appendix close to the right ureter or bladder
- mucous diarrhoea because of the formation of an appendix mass in the pelvis which irritates the wall of the rectum or sigmoid colon.

Appendicitis is most difficult to diagnose at the extremes of life, i.e. under 4 and over 70 years of age.

Physical Findings

A coated tongue and foul breath accompanied by mild pyrexia are characteristic, but absence of all three does not exclude appendicitis. Abdominal local tenderness and guarding at McBurney's point – the junction of the middle and outer thirds of a line which joins the umbilicus to the right

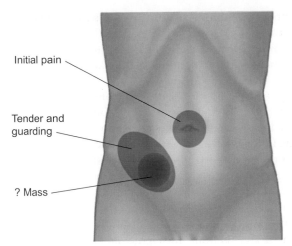

• **Fig. 13.3** Area of maximal tenderness in most cases of acute appendicitis.

anterior superior iliac spine – is present when the appendix is in its most common position, medial to the caecum (Fig. 13.3). However, these abdominal signs vary in position, are often much reduced in retroileal and, particularly, retrocaecal appendicitis and maybe absent if the organ is in the pelvis. It is often said that pressure applied in the left iliac fossa causes increased pain in the right lower quadrant (Rovsing's sign), but this is unreliable and not recommended as a diagnostic sign. Pelvic examination is especially helpful when the inflamed appendix is in the pelvis. Rectal examination is usually sufficient, but in women, where pelvic inflammatory disease and other gynaecological causes are possible, a vaginal examination is usually also done.

Investigation

When the clinical features are typical, the diagnosis is not difficult to make, but a wide variety of conditions can mimic appendicitis; in the past, up to 25% of patients submitted to operation with a provisional diagnosis of acute appendicitis did not have the condition, and few had the need for an operation. Apart from the routine investigations indicated previously, ultrasound and CT scanning and laparoscopy are all useful in diagnosis and management. Laparoscopy is most valuable in young (15–40 years) females, who may have gynaecological disease (e.g. ruptured ovarian cyst, pelvic inflammatory disease) or acute appendicitis. Ultrasonography has a place in any patient where the diagnosis is in doubt and is particularly useful in excluding ovarian disease. The finding of an enlarged appendix is highly suggestive of appendicitis, but a negative ultrasound scan does not exclude this diagnosis. CT scanning is increasingly used for diagnosis of acute appendicitis, particularly in the elderly, patients at high operative risk or those with an atypical presentation.

Management

Acute Appendicitis With or Without Peritonitis

Once the diagnosis has been made, the likelihood of progression (or the presence already of spreading inflammation) demands the removal of the organ – appendicectomy (USA: appendectomy) – which is now usually done laparoscopically, although it may also be done through a small transverse incision in the right iliac fossa. Prophylactic antibiotic therapy reduces the incidence of wound infection.

Appendix Mass

Some doubt surrounds management, and good clinical evidence is not available to resolve the issue.

Non-operative management is preferred by the majority of surgeons, with nothing by mouth, parenteral fluids, antibiotics and frequent reassessment of clinical state – the mass may resolve (the great majority), or deterioration may occur and prompt operative treatment during which the mass is explored and the appendix removed. If only an abscess is found, then it is best only to drain it laparoscopically without attempting to perform a difficult appendicectomy with possible complications. Subsequent laparoscopic interval appendicectomy is safe and avoids recurrent appendicitis.

Appendix Abscess

If it is clear, either on clinical examination or by the use of ultrasound, that an abscess has formed, this is drained, usually by an ultrasound-guided percutaneous technique or, if the IR cannot reach it safely due to overlying bowel or other vital structures, then by laparoscopic drainage as previously discussed. Rarely the abscess has progressed so far that an incision over its most prominent point would suffice on the abdominal wall.

Elective Appendicectomy

This procedure is often carried out after successful non-operative management of an appendix mass, although some surgeons do not believe this is necessary. It is also occasionally done in some patients who will be out of reach of surgical facilities should they contract appendicitis (e.g. polar scientists and technicians, astronauts). Good evidence that either of these reasons is valid is absent. Elective appendicectomy may also be recommended after recurrent attacks of appendicitis, but this is rare. Appendicectomy should not be done for vague right iliac fossa pain; the usual result is a patient who has had a surgical procedure and still has the pain.

Acute Upper GI Bleeding

The usual presentation of upper-gastrointestinal (UGI) bleeding is haematemesis – the vomiting of blood – a dramatic symptom. It is an indication of bleeding into the GI tract somewhere between the lower end of the oesophagus to the duodeno-jejunal flexure. Some blood usually passes downwards through the gut and is subject to digestion. As a result, haematemesis is usually accompanied or followed by melaena – the rectal discharge of altered dark blood. Occasionally, UGI bleeding may be so rapid that bright unaltered blood is passed per rectum. Sometimes, haematemesis may be absent in bleeding from the UGI tract and the only clinical feature is melaena.

Epidemiology and Aetiology

In the UK, UGI bleeding leads to 50–100 hospital admissions per 100,000 population each year. There are many possible causes, but only a few are common. Peptic ulcers account for more than half, and oesophageal varices, caused by portal hypertension, account for about 5–10%. In countries where liver disease is common, oesophageal varices are much more likely to be the cause of haematemesis (up to 40%), although their incidence in the UK is on the increase. In severely ill patients with renal or hepatic failure, gastroduodenal erosions are a common source of bleeding. Between a third and a half of patients who present with haematemesis are taking non-steroidal anti-inflammatory agents (NSAIDs), which can exacerbate peptic ulcer and also be associated with acute erosions. In the UK, the incidence of duodenal ulcer (DU) is much higher than that of ulcers in the stomach (gastric ulcers – GU). However, more gastric than duodenal ulcers cause haematemesis (55% GU; 45% DU), and more deaths are attributable to bleeding from GU than from DU (55% GU; 45% DU). Unusual peptic ulcers which can also bleed are those in the lower end of the oesophagus and those associated with hypergastrinaemia (Zollinger–Ellison syndrome). Gastric cancer is a relatively rare cause of haematemesis, although blood may ooze from the surface of the tumour to cause anaemia.

Mortality

UGI haemorrhage is a serious condition. Mortality rates for the common causes taken over all ages are 5–30% and have not changed much over the years. Table 13.2 gives the results of a world survey of 4431 patients who presented with UGI bleeding. In this survey, the mortality was highest for those with varices. The low mortality for bleeding peptic ulcer of 4.2% is, however, not typical; figures around 10% are common. Death depends chiefly on three factors:

- age – e.g. in peptic ulcer, it is very low in those under 50 years but very high in those over 80
- concomitant disease in the cardiorespiratory system
- cause of bleeding.

In some instances, bleeding is a terminal event in a patient already very ill or dying. In the UK, there is evidence that bleeding increasingly occurs in the old and ill. In consequence, what are real advances in management for individual patients are not reflected in an overall fall in mortality.

Clinical Features

Fresh blood may be present in the vomit. Alternatively, if it is retained for a short time in the stomach, it becomes

TABLE 13.2	Severity scale for causes of the acute abdomen		
		Grade	
Condition	<5	5	>5
Non-specific abdominal pain	•		
Ruptured abdominal aortic aneurysm			•
Ovarian cyst rupture or torsion		•	
Perforated peptic ulcer		•	
Urinary tract infection	•		
Ectopic pregnancy rupture		•	
Mesenteric adenitis	•		
Diverticulitis		•————————•	
Renal colic	•		
Appendicitis		•————————•	
Pseudo-obstruction	•		
Small-bowel obstruction		•————————•	
Fitz-Hugh–Curtis syndrome	•		
Malignancy	•		
Salpingitis	•		
Cholecystitis	•————————————————————•		
Mesenteric adenitis	•		
Intestinal ischaemia		•————————•	
Terminal ileitis	•		
Intussusception		•————————•	
Gastritis/duodenitis	•		
Volvulus of the colon		•————————•	
Gastroenteritis	•		
Inflammatory bowel disease		•————————•	
Torsion of appendices		•————————•	
Meckel's diverticulum rupture			•
Testicular torsion		•————————•	
Sickle cell crisis	•		
Referred pain from chest (myocardial infarct, pneumonia)			•
Abdominal tuberculosis	•————————————————————•		
Porphyria		•	
Irritable bowel syndrome	•		
Diabetes mellitus	•		
Dysmenorrhoea	•		

darkened by the action of acid and, when vomited, has the appearance of coffee grounds. If acute bleeding is haemodynamically significant – in excess of a blood donation (500 mL) – the patient may feel faint and show pallor. The vomit may then contain large quantities of fresh blood or clot. The Valsalva effect of vomiting may further reduce venous return to the heart and cause a vasovagal syncope (faint). With larger losses, the classical signs of haemorrhagic shock are usually present, with sweating, tachycardia and, depending on the volume lost, hypotension and air hunger. When the bleeding is severe, melaena may be an early feature. The passage of bright red blood in large quantities from the rectum indicates either a haemorrhage from below the duodeno-jejunal flexure or massive, very rapid blood loss from the upper GI tract.

Immediate diagnosis

Unless the bleeding is clearly minor, the initial history and physical examination should be brief and focused on the features essential to urgent management. There are three components to immediate diagnosis:
- Make sure that there has been acute loss of blood.
- Assess the amount and rate of bleeding – this, along with measures to restore circulating volume, is the first priority.
- Determine the cause, which often leads on to a decision as to how the episode should be treated.

Has Bleeding Occurred?

It is obviously important to establish that there has actually been a haematemesis. Measures which help are:
- Eliminate swallowed blood (e.g. from a nosebleed) as a cause.
- Examine what has been vomited – if it is not obviously fresh blood and clots are absent, test for haemoglobin; intestinal obstruction can produce what looks like coffee ground vomit.
- Do a rectal examination – fresh or altered blood gives confirmation of bleeding and can also be used in assessing the rate of loss.

Amount and Rate of Bleeding

- Make the usual observations of the circulation (pulse, blood pressure) to assess the amount of blood lost.
- In haemodynamically significant bleeding, insert a central venous catheter for measurement of central venous pressure (CVP).

Management

A cooperative multi-disciplinary approach to management is essential because it makes key decision-making easy and rapid. A team who are specialized in the management of GI bleeding has been shown to be effective in reducing

TABLE 13.3	The Rockall score for patients with upper GI bleeding			
Variable	Score 0	Score 1	Score 2	Score 3
Age	<60	60–79	>80	
Shock	No shock	Pulse >100	SBP <100	
Comorbidity	Nil major		CCF, IHD, major morbidity	Renal failure, liver failure, metastatic cancer
Diagnosis	Mallory–Weiss	All other diagnoses	GI malignancy	
Evidence of bleeding	None		Blood, adherent clot, spurting vessel	

mortality. Detailed guidance on the management of GI bleeding has been issued by the Scottish Intercollegiate Guidelines Network.[4]

Initial Management

Assessment of the Rockall risk score for upper GI bleeding[5] should be undertaken in all patients and gives an indication of the risk of mortality (see Table 13.3). The first three variables (age, shock and co-morbidity) form an initial score (pre-endoscopy assessment) and provide a guide to management. A total score of 0 predicts a mortality of less than 1%, whereas a total score of 2 gives a predicted mortality of 5.6%. The higher the total score, the greater the predicted mortality and rebleeding rate. Patients with a score of 0 may be considered for outpatient follow-up rather than admission to hospital. Those with an initial score of 1 or more should be admitted and have early endoscopy (within 24 hours). The methods of dealing with acute bleeding from any cause are followed. Frequent measurement of the CVP is not only valuable in monitoring the success of volume replacement (particularly in the elderly) but also may give early warning of further bleeding before changes in pulse rate or blood pressure have occurred.

Requirement for Blood

The objective should be to maintain a haemoglobin level greater than 10 g/dL. The quantity of blood necessary to do this and to restore a normal level of CVP is an indicator of the volume lost in the acute phase and, in bleeding from peptic ulcer, is also helpful in determining the treatment (see below). It has been shown that patients with peptic ulcer or erosive bleeding who vomit altered blood and do not have melaena and whose haemoglobin level remains above 10–12 g/dL, are unlikely to rebleed.

Diagnosis of Cause

Given that the patient has a stable circulation, either because the loss is small or because it has been corrected, further details can be obtained for both history and physical findings.

The relevant features associated with different common causes are shown in Table 13.4.

Physical Findings

Signs of chronic liver disease should be sought, including neurological features suggestive of encephalopathy. Other findings vary with the cause, e.g. the presence of supraclavicular lymph-adenopathy in bleeding from gastric carcinoma. Upper GI endoscopy is the key to achieving a diagnosis. If haemodynamic instability is present, it may be required as an emergency but can usually be deferred until the next scheduled endoscopy session. In the seriously ill, the procedure is not without some hazard, the main one being aspiration of regurgitated blood. Sedation should be kept to a minimum, particularly in the elderly. To identify a lesion does not always imply that it is the cause of the haematemesis; for example, in patients with oesophageal varices because of alcoholic liver disease, up to 40% of episodes of bleeding are from peptic ulcer or acute gastric erosions. However, precise diagnosis can be achieved in nearly all instances and is the best basis of a management plan.

Definitive Management

In any haematemesis from whatever cause, the initial definitive management is endoscopic. If this is unsuccessful, then radiological intervention or surgical treatment are considered.

Peptic ulcer

Management

Many episodes of haematemesis from ulcers are self-limiting and replacement of blood volume, withdrawal of precipitating factors (such as NSAIDs), testing for *Helicobacter pylori* infection and acid suppression therapy are all that is required. Proton pump inhibitor therapy should be started in all patients with ulcers, using high-dose intravenous therapy initially in patients at risk of rebleeding (active bleeding or a visible vessel on endoscopy). A course of *H. pylori* eradication therapy should be started if infection is confirmed.

TABLE 13.4	Salient historical features in common causes of haematemesis	
Cause	**Mechanism**	**Historical features**
Mucosal tear at cardia (Mallory–Weiss syndrome)	Forceful attempted vomiting	Acute inebriation
		Initial clear vomit
		Bright red haematemesis
Oesophageal varices	Rupture or erosion of mucosa over varix	Past liver disease
		Absence of peptic ulcer history
		Dark red haematemesis
NSAID-induced erosions	Breakdown of mucosal barrier to acid	Pain-producing associated disorder (e.g. rheumatoid arthritis)
		Intake of NSAID
Peptic ulcer	Peptic digestion of vessel in base of ulcer	Previous episodes of dyspepsia
		Diagnosed ulcer
	Fibrinoid necrosis of vessel holding lumen open	Recent worsening of symptoms
	Exacerbation of ulceration by NSAIDs	Blood of variable colour with or without clots
Angiodysplasias	Rupture or mucosal digestion of a surface lesion	No history on initial occurrence
Other causes to consider	Varies with cause	Examples:
		– History of anticoagulant intake
		– Haematological disorders

However, continued bleeding or rebleeding within a few days can occur, especially in the elderly. Factors which help to predict the likely course of the patient are:

- age – those under 40 are unlikely to bleed continuously or to rebleed and, even if they do, are better able to respond satisfactorily to any haemodynamic disturbance
- ulcer size – those with a large (greater than 1.5 cm diameter) lesion are more likely to rebleed
- endoscopic stigmas (Box 13.8)

The presence of any of these adverse factors is an indication for local control of the bleeding ulcer at the time of initial endoscopy. There are a number of methods including: adrenaline injection around the bleeding vessel, clipping of the vessel with endoscopically deployed clips and argon diathermy. These methods are often used in combination to improve success.

Radiological Embolization

Visceral angiography is usually performed via a catheter inserted into the common femoral artery. Initial injection into the coeliac axis vessels (guided by the known site of ulceration) may identify an actively bleeding site or an arterial pseudoaneurysm. If a bleeding point is found, the vessel is blocked by coils and/or haemostatic gels both proximal and distal to the bleeding point. If no definite bleeding site is seen, embolization may be guided by the endoscopically identified ulcer.

• BOX 13.8   Endoscopic stigmas which suggest the likelihood of further bleeding from peptic ulcer

- Actively bleeding vessel
- Visible vessel in ulcer base
- Adherent clot
- Black spot in ulcer base

Operations for Bleeding Peptic Ulcer

Surgery is done first and foremost to save life. The aim is to stop the bleeding and to minimize the chance of it recurring.

The ulcer is exposed and the bleeding vessel under-run with a suture. Very large gastric ulcers may require a Polya-type partial gastrectomy (Ch. 20). Limited excision of the stomach may be possible but other cases require partial gastrectomy – usually of the Billroth I type (Ch. 20). A gastric cancer may be found at operation in a patient thought to have a bleeding gastric ulcer and is dealt with by a more radical resection, although the distinction between peptic ulceration and cancer may not be easy.

Follow-up

Patients who have *Helicobacter pylori* infection should be checked for successful eradication after appropriate therapy.

Failure to eradicate should lead to second-line eradication therapy or maintenance acid suppression treatment with a proton pump inhibitor. Patients with gastric ulcers should undergo repeat endoscopy and biopsy to ensure healing and rule out carcinoma. NSAID, aspirin and anticoagulant therapy should be avoided if possible, but, if necessary, is usually covered by long-term proton pump inhibitor therapy.

Bleeding Oesophageal Varices

These are an increasingly common cause of upper GI bleeding and usually occur in patients with known liver disease or a history of alcoholism. Variceal bleeding in childhood or adolescence is the exception.

Aetiology

The varices form at the junction of portal and systemic circulations at the lower end of the oesophagus or in the cardiac part of the stomach as a consequence of portal hypertension from any cause.

Epidemiology

About 50% of those who have varices sustain a bleed, and 70% of those who bleed will do so again within a year. The mortality for each episode may be as high as 50% and is related to:
- the amount of blood lost
- ability to control the bleeding
- the severity of liver dysfunction.

Management

The treatment of bleeding varices is complex.

Lowering Portal Pressure

Lowering arterial input to the portal system, and therefore portal pressure, can be achieved by the intravenous infusion of terlipressin which should be continued for at least 48 hours. In addition, octreotide or high-dose somatostatin are given for 3–5 days. Secondary prophylaxis aimed at preventing recurrent bleeding is usually undertaken with a β-blocker such as propranolol after endoscopic variceal treatment.

Tamponade

Balloon tubes (Sengstaken–Blakemore) will nearly always arrest bleeding, but a rebleed is likely when the pressure is reduced – as it must be after 48 hours to avoid mucosal necrosis. There is a high incidence of respiratory complications. They may be used as a temporary measure to control bleeding.

Endoscopic Therapy

Oesophageal varices are treated by the endoscopic application of rubber bands. Gastric varices usually found in the cardia may also bleed and are best treated by endoscopic cyanoacrylate injection.

Radiological Portosystemic Shunt (TIPS)

If endoscopic treatment fails, patients may undergo transjugular intrahepatic portosystemic shunt (TIPS) insertion. An expanding metal stent is placed from an hepatic vein to a portal venous branch within the liver under image intensification guidance, providing an effective shunt to reduce portal hypertension. It may also be used as a prophylaxis against further variceal bleeding, particularly for gastric varices.

Gastric Erosion (Stress Ulceration)

This cause of bleeding is associated with liver failure (multiple derangements of haematological factors affecting clotting), renal failure or other multi-organ failure, particularly following trauma or severe burns. Endoscopy in severe cases always shows gastric erosions although they do not always bleed. Bleeding from erosive gastritis may often be a terminal event in the seriously ill.

Management

Initially this is non-operative, with intravenous acid suppression agents such as omeprazole or ranitidine, blood transfusion and correction of coagulopathy. Any possible cause should be corrected. Surgical intervention is rarely necessary, but gastric resection may occasionally save a seriously ill victim.

Incomplete Lower Oesophageal Tear (Mallory–Weiss Syndrome)

The mechanism is the same as that for a complete tear. The history is typically of an initial blood-free vomit followed by bright red haematemesis later. Most episodes of bleeding from this cause are usually minor and self-limiting but are occasionally severe and persistent. Endoscopic treatment is attempted if bleeding persists or active bleeding is seen. If this is unsuccessful then operation should be considered. The stomach is exposed, opened and the tear oversewn, nearly always with good results.

Dieulafoy's Lesion

A small punched-out mucosal hole erodes a vessel, usually high on the lesser curve of the stomach. The condition is uncommon and of unknown cause. Bleeding may be considerable and difficult to find either at endoscopy or at operation. Oversewing or excision at operation is the correct treatment.

Rarer Causes of Haematemesis

These include:
- arteriovenous malformations – these are rare. Angiodysplasia is the commonest, although it is seen much more frequently in the colon. Vascular ectasias are more diffuse and give streaky appearances at

endoscopy. Vascular lesions may also be part of a diffuse syndrome such as hereditary haemorrhagic telangiectasia. Management is complex and beyond the scope of this text

- bleeding via the biliary tract (haemobilia) or pancreatic-duct (haemosuccus pancreaticus)
- aorto-enteric fistula.

The Obstructed Patient

For an emergency surgeon, there are four groups of obstructed patients. The initial management is common to all of them but the speed we need to act and the need to operate or not varies according to which group the patient falls under. It is paramount for the surgeon to appreciate the clues from initial history and examination and early investigations to get this life-saving decision right. The following Table groups the common causes of obstruction accordingly (Table 13.5).

Determining Urgency

Groups C and D require rapid diagnosis, senior decision-making and operative intervention to save life. These patients are categorized as CEPOD 2A (within 6 hours). This time should be spent with quick resuscitation, organizing a CT scan, if this is not going to delay the operation unduly, and mobilizing the team for theatre. The ICU team should be alerted as the patient is likely to be at high risk of organ failure postoperatively. Risk assessment scoring with Sortsurgery or POSSUM will determine mortality. Mortality over 5% requires consideration of postoperative HDU admission and over 10% definite admission to HDU or ICU.

Group A patients have more time for investigations and preparation for theatre. The CEPOD category is 2B, which translates to maximum wait time of 24 hours. Typically, patients who arrive at night can wait until daytime hours but their diagnostics and resuscitation should continue overnight. Group B patients should not be operated on as

surgery in this group will be harmful. Often a CT scan will serve to reassure that an operation is not needed but it is not a substitute for careful history, examination and simple blood tests, which will often reveal the physiological disturbance such as hypokalaemia or renal failure. The treatment from then on is targeted at the underlying condition.

Presentation of Obstruction

The symptoms common to all obstruction are vomiting, abdominal distension and absolute constipation. The patient is often dehydrated, especially if the obstruction has been going on for a while. Pain and inflammatory response, however, are variable depending on which category the patient falls under. Severe pain is characteristic of groups C and D; the patient looks and feels very unwell with a high NEWS score and is often seen trying to convey a feeling of impending doom. Symptoms of peritonitis, such as pain on movement and breathing, are late features and the patient is often breathless due to metabolic acidosis. Urine is concentrated or very little as the patient is unable to keep anything down. Cancer rarely obstructs without an insidious past history of change in bowel habit or symptoms of pain and weight loss, and is commoner by far in the colon than in the small bowel.

Examination of the Obstructed Patient

First assess the clinical hydration state. Dry mucous membranes, thirst, loss of skin turgor, low blood pressure and tachycardia are important signs of dehydration that must not be missed. The abdomen while distended may not be particularly tender. Tenderness is a serious sign that should alert to group C or D patient. Identify obvious external hernias that are irreducible and present as hard and tender masses. Femoral hernias in elderly female patients can be easily missed if not looked for and this can be catastrophic for the patient. Abdominal scars tell the tale of past operations and can give a clue to adhesional obstruction. The more their numbers,

TABLE 13.5	**Causes of Obstruction.**		
		Mechanical	Non-Mechanical
Viable Bowel		**A**	**B**
		Adhesional small bowel obstruction	Postoperative ileus
		Incarcerated hernia	Pseudo-obstruction secondary to medical
		Tumour – primary or metastatic	conditions or surgical procedures such
		Crohn's disease	as orthopedic or gynaecological
		Gallstone ileus	Pancreatitis
		Bezoar	Drugs such as opiates
Ischaemic/Strangulated Bowel		**C**	**D**
		Adhesional small bowel obstruction	Peritonitis from all cause
		Internal hernia	Mesenteric vascular accident
		Strangulated hernia	Toxic megacolon – *Clostridium difficile* or
		Volvulus – sigmoid or caecal	ulcerative colitis
		Intussusception	

the higher the likelihood. Laparoscopic surgery generally protects the patient from adhesions except in bariatric surgery where, with the loss of weight, an internal hernia can become possible in roux-en-y gastric bypass surgery. Examining the much distended abdomen requires some imagination. Deep palpation is not possible and is uncomfortable for the patient. Percussion should reveal a tympanic abdomen and bowel sounds can be typically tinkling as liquid droplets fall into pools inside a bowel distended like a cave. This latter sound assumes peristalsis; however, in prolonged obstruction, peristalsis can cease and bowel sounds can be absent altogether. A rectal examination is mandatory to exclude a low rectal tumour. It can also reveal faecal impaction or the capacious rectum of a patient with pseudo-obstruction.

Investigations

Early investigations including blood tests and plain X-ray are mainly directed at assessing the severity of disease. A raised white cell count and CRP is an ominous sign suggesting category C and D conditions. Lactate can be deceptively normal on a venous blood gas despite presence of ischaemia, or raised despite lack of it, due to dehydration. It is nevertheless a useful investigation. Renal impairment is a sign of prolonged obstruction and gives an indication of the severity of dehydration. An abdominal obstruction is one of the few conditions causing acute abdomen in which plain abdominal X-ray is useful. The entire abdomen should be visualized for interpretation and caution should be used in over-interpreting the findings. A CT scan of the abdomen and pelvis with both intravenous and oral water soluble contrast is the gold standard investigation in most causes of bowel obstruction. If the patient has significant renal impairment with eGFR <35, i.v. contrast may result in further renal damage requiring dialysis. In a category A and B patient, it would be best to delay the CT scan until intravenous resuscitation has taken place with improvement in the eGFR.

When Do I Give Gastrograffin?

Gastrograffin is a water soluble contrast medium that can be given either as part of a series of plain radiographs of the abdomen or a CT scan. It has a dual purpose: therapeutic and diagnostic. As it has a high osmolality, it will act like an osmotic laxative when 100 mL of gastrograffin is mixed with 100 mL of water and given to the patient either orally or, better still, via the NG tube. After the NG tube is fully aspirated, the mixture is administered with a syringe and the tube is spigotted for 4 hours to enable distal passage of the contrast material. This is particularly useful in adhesional obstruction in category A and allows either early resolution of obstruction or early decision to operate if the gastrograffin fails to reach the colon in the next 24 hours with serial abdominal radiographs. If, however, adhesions are unlikely, then the decision to give the gastrograffin should be left to the radiologist as the timing of administration and the dilution method is crucial for the CT scan depending on the pathology suspected.

Laparotomy for small bowel obstruction accounted for 49% of all operations in the first NELA report. On this basis, the national small bowel audit was launched (www.acpgbi.org.uk/_userfiles/import/2017/12/NASBO-REPORT-2017.pdf). This demonstrated that over 8% of patients died in hospital and early surgery in those who ultimately needed surgery as failed conservative management, only occurred in 24% of patients. In the remaining patients, conservative management was successful in two-thirds of cases. Of these, one-half happened between 3 and 64 days, and 3% of all cases were palliative. This demonstrates the critical importance of:
1. The use of gastrograffin for early decision-making, which was only used in 21% of cases.
2. The importance of making an early decision about nutrition. Thirty-two percent were at risk of malnutrition and 49% were unable to eat for more than 5 days. Therefore, gain early input from the dietician team and consider TPN early if contemplating a conservative course.

Management

The word 'resuscitation' is frequently used in emergency surgery. It is important to appreciate what we mean by that in the context of the obstructed patient. If we are to follow the ABC, then our priority is to get a wide bore NG tube to empty the stomach in order to avoid aspiration from vomiting and decompress the small bowel somewhat to help with the abdominal distension. This will also help with breathing. Vomiting, in an obstructed patient, can be unannounced and fatal at night when the patient is asleep. Patients naturally dislike NG tubes but it is the admitting doctor's responsibility to convince the patient how important this is. Often, however, it is circulation that is the most important component of resuscitation. Rehydration with intravenous fluids to catch up with, and maintain, ongoing fluid losses, with particular attention to electrolyte disturbances, is the key to successful preparation of the patient for surgery. Like in the desert, your patient is perishing from lack of fluids!

No resuscitation is complete without monitoring of its success and progress. A urinary catheter will enable just that; aiming for minimum hourly output of 0.5 mL/kg per hour. The preoperative care is completed with good analgesia, thrombophylaxis and conversion of essential oral medication to intravenous. Time allowing, investigation and optimization of pre-morbid conditions should be performed to enable safer anaesthesia. With early surgery and restoration of intestinal continuity, function will also return early and parenteral nutrition should not be required. As in other types of surgery, use of enteral route as early as possible will prevent complications and infections.

Operative Strategies

Prevention of irreversible ischaemia, source control of sepsis, if there is a perforation of bowel, and restoration of intestinal function are the aims of surgery. Laparoscopy is increasingly used when expertise is available not only to reduce postoperative pain and hospital stay but primarily to prevent future adhesions and complications of a laparotomy wound. Eleven percent of laparotomy wounds result in incisional hernia long-term. In addition, wound infection rates are high in emergency laparotomy despite prophylactic use of antibiotics. A battery operated suction dressing is applied on most emergency laparotomy wounds to reduce wound infection rates.

GI Bleeding

From an emergency surgical perspective, there are two types of GI bleeding: upper GI where the risk of ongoing bleeding and exsanguination is high, and lower GI bleeding which, by and large, settles. There is a good reason for this. Bleeding duodenal ulcer erodes into a large named artery posteriorly, called the gastroduodenal artery, whereas colonic diverticular bleeding occurs from the small vessels perforating the bowel wall at sites of weakness that created the diverticula in the first place. Furthermore, the stomach is the most vascular part of the GI tract.

Management of GI bleeding is directed at identifying the source based on careful history and, if necessary, CT angiogram followed by early endoscopy in the form of oesophago-gastro-duodenoscopy (OGD) or colonoscopy to control the source of bleeding. If endoscopy fails, interventional radiology, if available, can deliver coils to bleeding mesenteric arterial branches and embolize the vessels showing the characteristic blush of contrast on CT angiogram. As discussed previously, surgical intervention is rare but always requires laparotomy. A bleeding duodenal ulcer can be controlled with longitudinal opening of the pylorus to reach the ulcer, which is underrun using deep stitches followed by closure of the gastrotomy transversely to avoid a stricture causing gastric outlet obstruction. For colonic bleeding, resection of the segment identified as source at CT angiogram is required with, typically, a colostomy due to patient's haemodynamic instability.

Abscesses

An abscess contains dead cells, dead and live bacteria with toxins and tissue fluid which make up the pus. It is a localized warzone between the bacteria and the host. The bacteria are protected within the abscess by inability of antibiotics and macrophages to reach the bacteria. It therefore means that, in established abscess formation, antibiotics will only work at the peripheral zone of the abscess and merely act to contain it or prevent its spread cutaneously as cellulitis. Surgical drainage is essential for resolution and the earlier the better.

Depending on its location, different bacteria will be found in abscesses and indeed the invasive nature of its drainage will alter as well. Perianal abscesses harbor intestinal anaerobes and gram negatives. Skin abscesses elsewhere mainly contain staphylococci and streptococci. Breast abscesses are drained under ultrasound guidance with needle aspiration to dryness followed by antibiotics to avoid unsightly scarring. The same consideration does not apply to the perianal region, where inadequate drainage penalizes the patient with an early recurrence due to premature closure of the wound. Culturing the pus need not be routine as antibiotics are often not required after surgical drainage. Special circumstances where culture swabs are needed are the immunocompromised patient, diabetics, patients with recurrent abscesses, patients from countries with high resistance to antibiotics, septic patients and patients on immunosuppressant drugs. The big pitfall in abscess management is missing the patient with synergistic infection causing necrotizing fasciitis. This typically occurs in the perineum but can occur anywhere in the body. The cardinal features are an acutely unwell patient in severe pain with sepsis and necrotic looking skin over and around the abscess. The infection travels regardless of fascial planes which enable the bacteria to spread rapidly. Time is of the essence once suspected and the patient requires urgent debridement to healthy bleeding tissue under general anaesthetic.

References

1. National Emergency Laparotomy Audit data. https://data.nela.org.uk/Reports/General.aspx.
2. Bertsimas D, Dunn J, Velmahos GC, Kaafarnai HMA. Surgical risk is not linear: derivation and validation of a novel, user-friendly, and machine-learning-based Predictive OpTimal Trees in Emergency surgery Risk (POTTER) calculator. *Ann Surg*. 2018;268(4): 574–558.
3. Catchpole K, McCulloch P. Human factors in critical care: towards standardized integrated human-centred systems of work. *Curr Opin Crit Care*. 2010;16(6):618–622. https://doi.org/10.1097/MCC.0b013e32833e9b4b.
4. Scottish Intercollegiate Guidelines Network, 2013. SIGN 129 Antithrombotics: indications and management. A national clinical guideline. https://www.sign.ac.uk/assets/sign129.pdf.
5. https://www.mdcalc.com/rockall-score-upper-gi-bleeding-complete.

14

Practical Procedures

Introduction

This chapter provides an introduction to the practical skills that are basic to any clinician embarking on a surgical career. We cover the use of catheters and tubes which are essential adjuncts to patient management in numerous scenarios. The principles outlined with each technique are based on the Intercollegiate Surgical Curriculum Programme (ISCP) or the Advanced Trauma Life Support (ATLS) system both of which should be familiar to all trainees in the UK.

The chapter finishes with a description of the basic principles of electrosurgery. This is the commonest energy form used in surgery and another vital adjunct to surgical practice. This energy form has become increasingly sophisticated and understanding its principles have rightly become an integral part of early surgical training in courses such as the Intercollegiate Basic Surgical Skills Course.

Preliminaries

Informed Consent

The general issue of consent is considered in Chapter 39. Informed consent based on the Montgomery ruling that must address the specific needs of the patient is required for all invasive procedures. This must be obtained in writing prior to the procedure being performed.

Explanation

The risks, benefits and alternatives to the procedure should be carefully explained and time should be given to the patient, where possible, so that questions may be asked.

Essential information that should be given to the patient includes:

- the nature of the procedure
- what is going to be removed, cut, changed or inserted
- non-specific possible complications – haematoma, infection
- specific possible complications – nerve, arterial and venous injury; cosmetic effect
- explanation of type of anaesthesia (general, local, regional) and risks involved

Additional beneficial information includes:

- the position of the scar
- what cannulas, drains and catheters will be in place after the procedure
- postoperative pain control
- when food and drink may be resumed
- what may happen during the hours or days after the procedure and for how long a period such events may last
- how long before work can be resumed

The patient should be allowed time to reflect on any information given before consenting. Best practice would also include providing patients with supplemental explanatory leaflets.

Documentation

All procedures should be recorded in the electronic or paper notes, with comments pertinent to the individual manoeuvre, e.g. the volume of residual urine found on urethral catheterization or, after a biopsy, the dispatch of a specimen to the pathological laboratory. Specific instructions for post-procedural care for nursing staff, allied health professionals or the patient should also be carefully described.

WHO and Pre-Procedure Checklist

This is discussed in Chapter 8.

Asepsis

There are varying degrees of aseptic technique (see also Ch. 5) according to the procedure and the possible subsequent effects of sepsis.

Personal Protective Equipment (PPE) for Standard Infection Control

Gloves and an impermeable disposable apron should be worn for every procedure that involves contact with a patient's secretions or blood. Non-sterile (but clean) gloves are indicated when there is a risk of contamination from patient to medical attendant (e.g. HIV, hepatitis B). Sterile gloves are part of the normal procedure to prevent access of organisms to the patient. The possibility of transmission of infection by the hands should always be maintained at a low level by keeping them clean, with short nails, everyday maintenance of hand hygiene and washing with soap or using alcohol-based gels every time a clinician is in contact with a patient. The arms should be covered by a sterile gown or exposed and clean from above the elbows.

Superficial Procedures

An example of such a procedure is superficial venous cannulation. An alcohol–chlorhexidine solution is used to clean the skin area. However, the operator requires protection against the possibility of infection from the patient. The wearing of gloves – either clean or sterile according to the circumstances – is recommended for every procedure.

Deeper and More Complicated Procedures

If the procedure is likely to leave a cannula, a drain or other device (e.g. pacemaker, central line) in situ, then sterile gloves, towels and handwashing, and full skin preparation must be used.

Immunocompromised Patients

In certain circumstances (e.g. AIDS, bone marrow transplantation, chemotherapy), immunocompromise may be present, and in such patients strict aseptic techniques should be used even for minor superficial procedures.

Handwashing and Scrubbing Up

Formal handwashing in preparation should be carried out for at least two minutes. Both the hands and forearms are placed under running water. The hands are first cleaned with an antiseptic soap. This includes using a soft brush under the nails. The palms of each hand are rubbed together and then the palms are used to wash the back of the opposite hands. Tips of the fingers are washed by flexing the fingers of each hand and rubbing the palm of the opposite hand. The space between the fingers is cleaned by interlacing the fingers of one hand over the other. The thumb is cleaned in the closed palm of the other hand.

Cleaning proceeds to each forearm working towards the elbows. The nail brush should not be used on the skin to prevent commensal bacteria from deeper layers of the skin being brought to the surface.

Rinse and allow water to drain from the skin from the hands to the elbows.

The hands and arms are each dried with a sterile towel working from the fingers down to the elbows.

Gowns are folded such that the front is within the folds of the gown. Hold the collar at arms length and let the gown unfold by gravity. Place the arms in each sleeve and ask an assistant to tie the gown.

Choose your glove size and don these using a no touch technique with both hands still within the sleeve.

Place the left glove on the palm of the left hand (still in the sleeve) with the thumb against the palm and fingers pointing towards the elbow and the thumb. Grip the opening of the glove in the left thumb and index finger on the underside and between the thumb and index finger of the right hand (still in its sleeve) on the open side. Use the right hand to sweep the opening of the glove over the opening of the left sleeve and advance the left hand into the glove. This is repeated using the right glove but with significantly more ease as the left hand and fingers are freed from their sleeve. If double gloving the second pair are donned as normal gloves.

Finally hand the paper tab on the long part of the waist tie to an assistant so it can be wound around the waist. Pull the tie from the tab and tie at the side to the shorter end.

Preparation of the Patient's Skin

The use of topical skin cleaning solutions reduces the burden of skin commensals at a procedure or operation site. The commonest types contain chlorhexidine or iodine and may be aqueous or alcoholic preparations. Local hospital guidelines often exist and should be followed. Patients allergic to iodine should have chlorhexidine solutions applied.

It is customary to apply two coats of the cleaning solution using either a swab mounted on a sponge holder or purpose made applicator. On the abdomen particular attention should be paid to the groins and umbilicus. Care should be taken when applying these solutions close to the eyes.

Cleaning fluid should not be permitted to wash onto the patient plate used for monopolar electrosurgery as this will change its conductivity. Flammable alcoholic solutions should be given at least 45 seconds for the alchohol to evaporate before applying drapes otherwise the vapours that accumulate under the drapes could be ignited when using electrosurgery.

Isolation of the Operative Field

Once the skin cleaning agent has been applied the operation site is isolated by the use of drapes applied around the cleaned area. The cleaned area should overlap the edge of the drapes that are either held in place with blunt tipped towel clips or adhesive strips that are integral to the drape.

The drapes should cover an area sufficient to allow the surgeon to operate without desterilising instruments, trolleys or the sterile gowns of the operating team.

Drapes may be simple sterile sheets or purpose designed barriers used in specific operations. Smaller adhesive drapes with a precut opening are available for minor local anaesthetic surgery.

Anaesthesia

Nearly all small procedures can be undertaken with local anaesthesia (LA). If general or regional anaesthesia (see Ch. 2) is a possible alternative, two factors will determine which is chosen: the relative risks (regional anaesthesia usually has a marginally higher risk) and patient preference.

General features relating to the pain of administration of LA are summarized below:

- The initial needle prick is painful but, especially in children, can be lessened by the use of topical local anaesthetic creams or sprays.

- Rapid injection causes pain from increased pressure in the tissues; the slower the injection, the less pain there will be. Injection into dense tissue (such as the fibrous tissue of the sole of the foot) should always be slow.
- The smaller the needle (preferably 25- or 27-G), the less pain the patient will feel upon insertion and also the slower will be the rate of injection; fine needles are often short but long ones are also available e.g. a fine spinal needle.
- The elderly often experience less pain on the injection of local anaesthetic, probably because of the laxity of their tissue.

Choice of Local Anaesthesia

Ethyl chloride spray can be used to numb the skin before a limited lance for a small abscess or for initial injections of LA. Local-anaesthetic creams, e.g. EMLA cream (a mixture of the un-ionized base forms of lidocaine and prilocaine) or Ametop cream (tetracaine 4%), are useful for paediatric venepuncture and for adults who have a phobia about needles, although it should be noted that they take up to an hour to become effective.

Commonly used local anaesthetics – with their maximum safe dose – are:
- lidocaine – 3 mg/kg to a maximum of 200 mg
- bupivacaine – 2.5–5 mg/kg to a maximum of 150 mg (it is two to four times more potent than lidocaine) (Table 14.1)
- prilocaine – 5 mg/kg to a maximum of 80 mg
- cocaine – used in ENT surgery for its local vasoconstrictor action – 1.5 mg/kg as 10% topical cocaine hydrochloride in fit adults

Addition of Epinephrine (Adrenaline)

Epinephrine (adrenaline) – a potent vasoconstrictor – added to a local anaesthetic slows the rate of absorption into the systemic circulation, reduces systemic toxicity and therefore prolongs the duration of action and may result in a more profound block. For this reason, the dose of lidocaine quoted above can be increased if 1 in 200,000 epinephrine is added to the solution (e.g. lidocaine 5 mg/kg to a maximum of 500 mg). The dose of bupivacaine should not be increased when epinephrine is used (see also Ch. 2).

TABLE 14.1	Concentration of Bupivacaine for Local and Regional Anaesthesia
Procedure	**Concentration**
Skin infiltration	0.5%
Minor nerve block	1%
Brachial plexus block	1–1.5%
Sciatic/femoral block	1–1.5%
Epidural	1.5–2%
Spinal	2–5%

Contraindications to Use of Epinephrine (Adrenaline) with Local Anaesthetic

- When the injection is close to end arteries
- Ring block of the digits (fingers and toes) and of the penis
- Intravenous regional anaesthesia (so-called Bier's block) which reduces venous drainage by the use of a tourniquet and so generates a high concentration of local anaesthetic; there is an unacceptable risk of ischaemia and of the escape of large concentrations of agent into the general circulation

If the patient has cardiac disease or is elderly, epinephrine needs to be used with caution as the patient may develop a tachyarrhythmia.

There are, however, absolute contraindications to the use of epinephrine with local anaesthetic agents, as listed in Box 14.1.

VENOUS ACCESS

Choosing the site

The ideal area for injection and short-term cannulation is the forearm. However, if the patient is obese, there can be difficulties with this. Some sites may be unsuitable for the following reasons:

- The dominant arm is avoided if possible.
- The arm which carries an arteriovenous (AV) fistula for renal dialysis is never used.
- Poor venous or lymphatic drainage in a limb (e.g. after an axillary lymph node clearance) carries a higher incidence of infected lymphangitis, and such limbs must not be used.
- Avoid foot veins whenever possible because they thrombose easily and are prone to infection.
- A skin fold which crosses a joint should be avoided, although the antecubital fossa can be used for diagnostic venepuncture.

Choice of Vein (Fig. 14.1)

Look where veins commonly occur; there is often a large vein running along the radial aspect of the forearm. Veins can sometimes only be felt rather than seen, even after the application of a tourniquet. **NB: The aim of the tourniquet used for venepuncture is that there is arterial inflow into the vein but no venous outflow.** Should there be uncertainty as to whether the structure is a vein, the tourniquet should be released. If the structure becomes impalpable, it is almost certainly a patent vein – arteries or thrombosed veins do not change shape or size when a tourniquet is removed.

To insert a cannula, the vein should be immobilized by stretching the skin, which includes positioning the adjacent joints. If the veins are difficult to cannulate because of

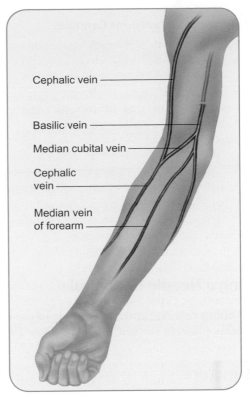

Cephalic vein

Basilic vein

Median cubital vein

Cephalic vein

Median vein of forearm

• **Fig. 14.1** Common Sites in the Arm for Venous Access.

CLINICAL BOX 14.1 AIDS TO LOCATION OF A VEIN

- Use a sphygmomanometer and inflate it to below diastolic pressure to allow arterial inflow but not venous escape of blood
- Hang the patient's arm over the edge of the bed or couch and tap (not slap) the back of the hand to cause venodilatation
- Immerse the forearm in a bowl of warm water for 2 minutes and place the tourniquet before removing the hand from the bowl
- Ask the patient to pump their fist to encourage venous filling

Additional Hint

In paediatrics or for anxious adults, EMLA cream can be helpful: apply over selected veins and cover with an occlusive dressing; wipe off after 45–60 minutes. After EMLA cream has been applied, veins do not distend as easily

mobility, then placing the cannula at a point of junction of two veins can help. If there is substantial subcutaneous fat, then often the dorsum of the hand may be the only suitable place; this area is not particularly convenient for the patient and can be painful during insertion. The antecubital fossa is also not particularly convenient for the patient, but for emergencies it is ideal as there are large, reasonably accessible veins which can take large cannulae.

There are methods which can be used to help locate a vein; these are listed in Clinical Box 14.1.

TABLE 14.2 Types of Intravenous Cannula

Size	Colour	Use
22 G	Blue	Children, small fragile veins
20 G	Pink	Low-flow intravenous infusions such as analgesia, sedation
18 G	Green	Intravenous fluids and drugs
16 G	Yellow	Blood transfusions
14 G	Grey	Rapid fluid administration – shock, major trauma and GI bleeding
12 G	Brown	Rapid fluid administration – shock, major trauma and GI bleeding

Choosing a Needle or Cannula

The types of intravenous cannulae available in the UK (and in many other places in the world) are shown in Table 14.2.

Venepuncture

Equipment

Equipment required:
- clean gloves
- tourniquet – specifically designed tourniquets with a quick release mechanism are available in most clinical areas for this purpose. However, alternatives include a sphygmomanometer or latex tubing.
- appropriate needle or cannula (see Table 14.2) (have more than one to hand in case of difficulties)
- adhesive tape and a dressing to hold the cannula in place
- 5 mL syringe
- 0.9% saline flush
- occasionally, cotton wool and adhesive tape to secure the site of unsuccessful cannulation
- bandage and tape for the same reason

Procedure

- Choose the preferred site.
- Place the tourniquet above the site of insertion.
- Swab the intended insertion area with antiseptic solution (allow alcohol to dry).
- Advance the needle or cannula-and-needle combination into the vein until a flashback of blood into the base of the cannula is seen.
- Advance the plastic cannula into the vein over the needle ensuring that the needle remains in the same position and is not pushed further into or through the vein (Fig. 14.2).
- Remove the tourniquet.
- When venepuncture alone has been done, elevate the arm above the right atrium, remove the needle and apply a small stabilizing dressing.

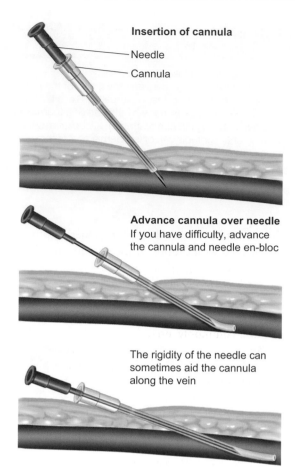

Insertion of cannula
- Needle
- Cannula

Advance cannula over needle
If you have difficulty, advance the cannula and needle en-bloc

The rigidity of the needle can sometimes aid the cannula along the vein

• **Fig. 14.2** Technique for Venous Cannulation.

- For a cannulation, occlude the end or connect the infusion immediately.

Sharps Safety

To avoid a sharps injury to yourself or an assistant, needles should not be transferred hand to hand. Always use a sharps tray or receiver. Once used a sharp should be placed directly into a sharps bin or onto the receiver before transfer to a sharps bin. Once used a needle should never be resheathed with its original cover. Many needles used in venepuncture and cannulation have a separate integral shield that covers the needle after use which should be used to prevent inadvertent injury.

Complications
Thrombophlebitis

Inflammation at a peripheral site of cannulation is manifest by pain, tenderness and a red line which spreads proximally. The cannula must be removed immediately. There is some evidence that small amounts of heparin added to the infusion can also help to prevent this complication.

Blockage

Sometimes patency can be restored with a flush of normal or heparinized saline (2–5 mL). The smaller the diameter of the syringe, the higher the pressure that can be attained (use a 5 mL rather than a 10 mL syringe).

Infection/Sepsis

Venous cannulas can be a source of local infection and sepsis. The incidence increases with time and cannulas should be removed and resited every three to five days. Best practice is to record the date of insertion of the cannula in the patient notes and on the dressing using a permanent marker as a visual check to anyone using the cannula.

Venous Cut-Down

Venous cut-down is the open exposure and cannulation of a subcutaneous vein. It is used when venous access cannot be obtained by percutaneous puncture (see previously) and is an alternative to central venous catheterization (see later) in some patients.

The most commonly used sites for this procedure are (Fig. 14.3):
- basilic vein – approximately 2.5 cm lateral to the medial epicondyle of the humerus at the flexion crease of the elbow
- saphenous vein – either at the saphenofemoral junction (2.5 cm lateral and inferior to the pubic tubercle) or 2 cm anterior and superior to the medial malleolus at the ankle. Other sites include the cephalic vein at the wrist and the external jugular (see Fig. 14.3).

Equipment

Equipment required:
- sterile towels
- orange needle (25 G)
- scalpel (10 blade)
- fine scissors
- artery forceps
- two ties (4/0 vicryl)
- cannula 12 G or 14 G
- skin sutures (Prolene or silk 3/0)
- dressing

Procedure (Fig. 14.4)

- Prepare the skin with antiseptic solution.
- Drape the area.
- Infiltrate the skin over the vein with 0.5% lidocaine, but take care not to inject local anaesthetic into the vein.
- Make a transverse full-thickness skin incision (2.5 cm) through the infiltrated area.
- By blunt dissection with the tip of an artery forceps, identify the vein and release it from any fat and fibrous tissue.
- Free the vein for at least 2 cm.
- Ligate the mobilized vein at its most distal exposed part and leave the tie attached for traction.
- Place a tie around the vein proximally but do not tighten this.
- Make a small transverse incision with scissors into the vein sufficient to accept the cannula, and dilate this opening with the tip of an artery forceps.
- Introduce a large plastic grey (14 G) or brown (12 G) cannula which has, if necessary, been separated from its needle.
- Tighten the proximal tie around the vein and the cannula firmly but be careful not to constrict the lumen of the cannula.
- Attach the intravenous apparatus and check that flow takes place.
- Close the wound with interrupted sutures and apply further antiseptic solution and a securing dressing.

Complications

Complications include:
- perforation of the posterior wall of the vein
- haematoma
- phlebitis
- cellulitis
- venous thrombosis
- transection of a neighbouring nerve (e.g. saphenous nerve at the medial malleolus)
- mistaking an artery for a vein and arterial transection
- sepsis

Central Venous Catheterization

The objective of central venous catheterization is to insert a hollow line into the proximal (usually superior) vena cava. The Seldinger technique is often used, in which a needle is placed in the vessel and an internal guide wire inserted into the vein first. The needle is then removed, the track into the vessel dilated and the cannula threaded along the wire into the lumen.

Indications

Indications include:
- measurement of central venous pressure
- infusion of certain drugs, e.g. inotropes, high concentrations of potassium (greater than 40 mmol/L)
- total parenteral nutrition (see Ch. 7)
- insertion of a Swan–Ganz catheter (see later) or cardiac pacing wires
- inability to achieve peripheral venous access, e.g. intravenous drug use with extensive previous venous thrombosis

Common Sites

Common sites include:
- internal jugular and subclavian (usually on the right)
- femoral in the groin
- median basilic vein at the elbow

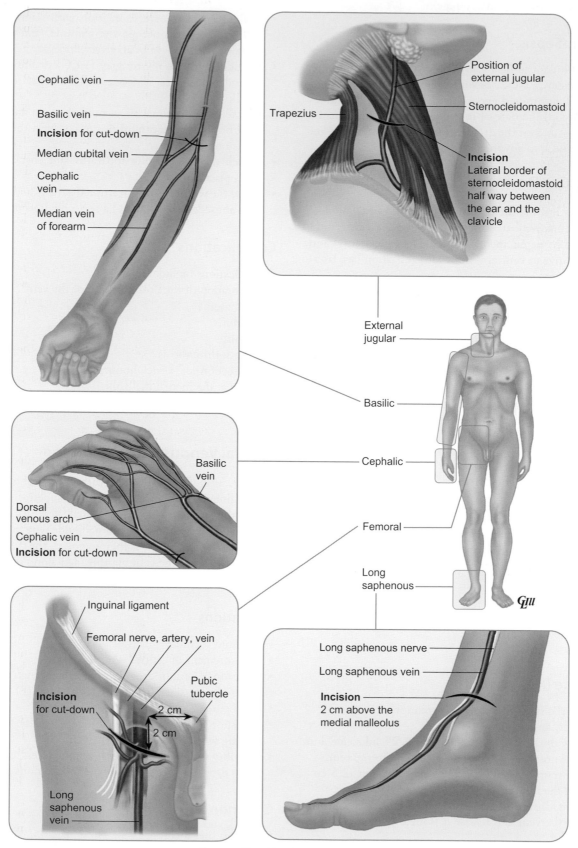

• **Fig. 14.3** Sites Used for Venous Access.

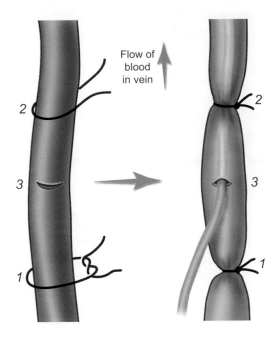

Flow of blood in vein

• **Fig. 14.4** Technique for Venous Cut-Down.

Equipment

Equipment required:
• fine scalpel blade
• orange (25 G) and green (21 G) needles
• two syringes (preferably of differing sizes, 5 and 10 mL) – one for local anaesthesia, the other for heparinized saline
• heparinized saline flush (10 mL)
• central line infusion equipment
• suture material (2/0 or 3/0 silk or Prolene)
• transparent occlusive dressing
• 1 L bag of 0.9% saline and a giving set

Prepackaged central line sets often contain not only the infusion apparatus but also many of the items mentioned above; check before looking for the rest of the materials.

Procedure

Many patients who require a central line are seriously ill and cannot easily tolerate lying flat. Therefore all the equipment must be ready before placing them in the best position for the procedure. If the patient is known to be short of intravascular volume, 500 mL of colloid or crystalline solution given through a peripheral infusion just before the procedure is often helpful to increase the diameter of the vein to be used.

The patient should be positioned in a supine position with no pillows, or with no more than one pillow. The bed should preferably be in a 15-degree, head-down tilt at the moment of puncture of the vein. The patient's arms should be placed at the side of the trunk. For subclavian vein cannulation, an assistant holding the arm on the side of the proposed cannulation, with downward traction, opens the space between the clavicle and the first rib; again, this should be done at the moment of puncture.

The procedure for cannulation is now as follows:
• It is UK national guidance that central venous puncture is performed using ultrasound scanning to locate the internal jugular or subclavian vein and guide venous puncture.
• Use an orange needle (see Table 14.2) to insert local anaesthetic over the proposed point of entry into the skin and infiltrate the proposed route towards the vein with a larger (green) needle.
• While allowing the anaesthetic to take effect, prepare the central line: all ports of entry on the apparatus are flushed through with heparinized saline and tested for patency; all are then closed either with a bung or a tap that is switched off, except for the distal one (usually labelled and in the centre of the cannula), which is left open.
• The guide wire should be prepared by checking that the end is hidden in the introducer and that it can be easily advanced (practise beforehand). Often the introducer has to be released from the sheath in which the wire is coiled.
• Flush the needle and syringe to be used to identify and cannulate the vein with heparinized saline to ensure fluid runs freely.
• Make a small (5 mm) incision through the skin at the proposed entry site.
• Insert the needle and, once deep to the skin, aspirate with the syringe and advance it under ultrasound guidance until venous blood is easily aspirated.
• Detach the syringe and ensure that blood flows freely out of the needle.
• Insert the wire and its introducer (if present – depends on the type of apparatus) into the end of the needle while grasping it to ensure that it does not move as the wire is advanced. The wire should be easily introduced without force (which should never be applied); sometimes rotation can help in that many of the wires have curled ends (if the wire does not have a pigtail end, then the soft end of the wire should be introduced – the rigid end can perforate the vein).
• Once the wire is inserted to approximately 50% of its length, the needle and introducer are removed.
• The track is dilated by the introduction of the dilator over the wire, pushing it in until it is well inside the vein.
• Remove the dilator; this is usually associated with an increase in bleeding from the entry site – a good sign as it implies that the track is well dilated.
• The central line is introduced over the wire while this is held steady; often the wire must be pulled back slightly to allow it to come out of the end of the distal port. Again, the wire must be grasped before the cannula is further advanced; otherwise it can be lost into the right side of the heart.
• Push the central venous line in; the tip should ideally lie in the superior vena cava, judged according to the size and shape of the patient.
• Aspirate the line with a syringe to ensure that its position is truly in the vein as indicated by free flow of blood. If

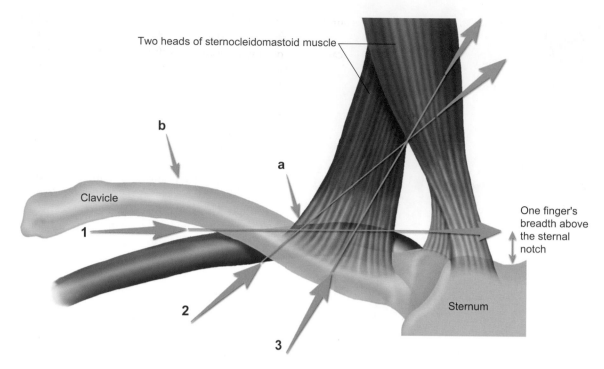

Two heads of sternocleidomastoid muscle

b

a

Clavicle

1

2

3

One finger's breadth above the sternal notch

Sternum

• **Fig. 14.5** The Approach Used for Lateral (1) and Medial (2 or 3) Cannulation of the Subclavian Vein.

there is uncertainty, an infusion of 0.9% saline can be connected and checked to see if flow is free.

- Suture the line in place, if necessary, after infiltrating further local anaesthetic.

Use of the Subclavian Vein

There are numerous techniques for cannulation of this vessel, which differ in detail, but all insertions start in the area 1 cm below the clavicle between its medial and lateral thirds (points *a* to *b* in Fig. 14.5) and the aim is to cannulate the vein as it passes over the first rib. Ultrasound location of the vein should preceed any attempted insertion. Two differing approaches are described: the lateral and the medial.

Lateral

This is carried out at the point at which the lateral third and medial two-thirds of the clavicle intersect. The needle should be aimed at a point 2 cm above the suprasternal notch and towards the opposite shoulder; it then runs in a straight line from the insertion point, passes just inferior to the clavicle and flat to the skin. If the needle is felt to bend away from this path, the usual reason is that the tip is below the first rib and towards the apex of the pleura; in this case, the advice is to withdraw and start again, using a slightly higher angle.

Medial

This is carried out at the point of intersection of the medial third and lateral two-thirds. The needle goes in initially at right angles to the clavicle, just inferior to it and towards the division of the two heads of the sternocleidomastoid muscle (see Fig. 14.5). Once the vein is punctured, the cannula is advanced into the vein at the angle used for the 'lateral' technique. The medial method may have a reduced risk of pneumothorax.

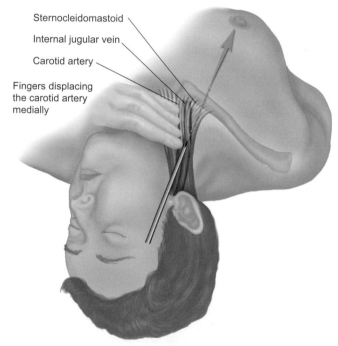

Sternocleidomastoid

Internal jugular vein

Carotid artery

Fingers displacing the carotid artery medially

• **Fig. 14.6** The Approach Used for Cannulation of the Internal Jugular Vein.

Use of the Right Internal Jugular Vein (Fig. 14.6)

Procedure

- Feel for the pulse of the carotid artery on the right side with the right hand (right-handed operators) or left hand (left-handed operators).
- Infiltrate a small area lateral to the carotid pulse at the level of the thyroid cartilage with local anaesthetic. If you attempt a lower insertion, there is an increased risk

of pneumothorax. Localize the vein with ultrasound scanning.

- Holding the ultrasound probe in the left hand to locate the vein, insert the needle at a 45-degree angle to the neck and pointing towards the nipple in the male or the anterior superior iliac spine in both males and females. Advance the needle slowly, under ultrasound guidance, while applying negative pressure with a syringe. If there is no flashback of venous blood, withdraw the needle slowly. This is sometimes successful because compression has flattened the vein. Should the carotid artery be punctured, withdraw the needle immediately and apply digital pressure for at least 5 minutes.

Post-Cannulation Checks

After all central cannulations, the radial pulse should be checked. If there are frequent ectopic beats, then it is likely that the line is in the right ventricle. A chest X-ray should be performed to verify the position of the tip of the line, which should be in the superior vena cava, and to check for complications (especially pneumothorax and haemothorax). If the line is not correctly placed, then adjustment is most easily performed under radiological control. Other means of ensuring that the line is within the vein are:

- Check easy aspiration of venous blood from all ports.
- Place the connected 0.9% saline bag and tubing beneath the patient with the tap open; blood should track back easily even if the patient has a low central pressure.
- If the blood travels up the line while above the place of insertion, it is likely you are within the artery.
- If you are uncertain, then a pressure-transducing device can be attached to the line.
- Sometimes the distal opening rests on a valve and therefore blood cannot be aspirated. If the line is pulled backwards a few centimetres, blood should then be easily aspirated.

Subcutaneous Tunnelling

Temporary lines inserted as described previously are, as time goes by, increasingly difficult to protect from the entry of bacteria. Sepsis is likely after 5–10 days, although careful care and strict asepsis decrease the incidence. However, some intensive care units judge it wise to change all central lines every 5 days. If the line is needed for long-term therapy (e.g. chemotherapy or TPN), then a subcutaneously tunnelled line should be used e.g. Hickman, Leonard or Broviac catheters (Fig. 14.7). An alternative for intermittent therapy is to place a port with venous access subcutaneously (Portacath).

The number of lumens available per line ranges from one to four. Tunnelled central lines often have an integral dacron cuff that integrates with the subcutaneous tissue to prevent microbial ingress from the entry point. The catheter is tunnelled subcutaneously from a point on the chest wall to a second incision used to place the catheter in the vein. After ensuring the dacron cuff is positioned within the tunnel the catheter is cut to length and inserted into the vein either using an ultrasound-guided seldinger technique with a guidewire, dilator and splitting sheath or by direct cut down onto the cephalic vein for a subclavian approach or the internal jugular vein. Correct positioning of the catheter is determined with fluroscopy. The second wound is then closed with a suture, ensuring the catheter is not punctured or occluded. The external catheter can be secured with a retaining suture to the chest wall.

Complications of Central Line Insertion

Complications include:
- haematoma
- cellulitis
- line infection (bacteraemia, sepsis)
- thrombosis
- phlebitis
- nerve damage including transection

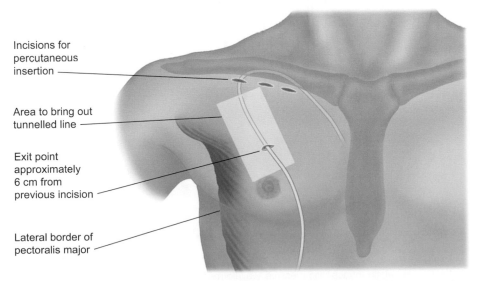

Incisions for percutaneous insertion

Area to bring out tunnelled line

Exit point approximately 6 cm from previous incision

Lateral border of pectoralis major

• **Fig. 14.7** Subcutaneous Tunnelling of an Intravenous Catheter.

- arterial puncture – more common in the internal jugular approach
- pneumothorax – more common in thin patients and if the subclavian approach is used
- haemothorax
- chylothorax
- arteriovenous fistula
- peripheral neuropathy
- lost wires or catheter in the venous system
- improperly placed catheters

Swan–Ganz Catheter

Uses

The Swan–Ganz catheter is a pulmonary artery flotation catheter which can be used to measure directly a number of cardiovascular parameters. Its use has diminished as less invasive methods of measuring cardiac output are now available – for example, transoesophageal Doppler probes – and its value has been disputed. The parameters that can be measured with a Swan–Ganz catheter include (normal range of values is shown in parentheses):

- pulmonary artery wedge pressure (12–20 mmHg)
- blood pressure
- central venous pressure (5–10 mmHg)
- cardiac output (4–8 L/min)

and to derive the following parameters:

- mean arterial pressure (70–90 mmHg)
- cardiac index (2.5–4.2 L/min per m^2)
- systemic vascular resistance (900–1600 dyne-s/cm^5)
- pulmonary vascular resistance (20–120 dyne-s/cm^5)

Measurement of Cardiac Output. Cardiac output is stroke volume × heart rate. It is measured using the thermodilution method. The change in temperature of 10 mL of 5% glucose between two given points on the catheter (CVP lumen and the tip of the catheter) is measured and cardiac output subsequently calculated.

Insertion

Insertion is as for a central venous catheter in the neck. The catheter is passed through the subclavian vein, right atrium, right ventricle and wedged in the pulmonary artery (Fig. 14.8), and then unwedged to lie in the pulmonary artery while other parameters are measured.

Pulse-Induced Contour Cardiac Output (PiCCO) Measurement

PiCCO is a technique used in the ICU to measure cardiac output and the other parameters mentioned in the previous subsection.

Principles

Measurement requires the insertion of both a central venous catheter and an arterial catheter (see the next section). A large artery is needed, usually femoral or brachial.

The arterial catheter outputs an arterial waveform, the pressures of which are known. One thermodilution assessment is first performed and then, using volumetric assessments of the arterial waveform, the transpulmonary cardiac output can be continuously monitored.

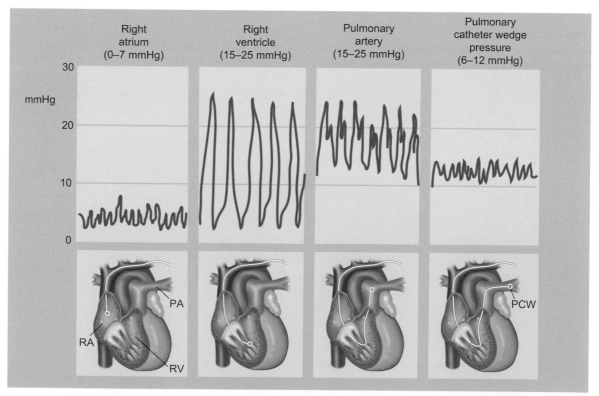

• **Fig. 14.8** Characteristic Intracardiac Pressure Waveforms of a Swan–Ganz Catheter During Passage Through the Heart PA, Pulmonary artery; PCW, pulmonary capillary wedge; RA, right atrium; RV, right ventricle.

Arterial Blood Sampling

Choice and Localization of Arteries for Puncture

Vessels of choice, in order of preference (unless there is a specific contraindication), are the radial, femoral and brachial arteries.

Radial Artery

This artery (Fig. 14.9) can be found medial to the styloid process of the radius at the wrist. Before it is used for a sample, the ulnar collateral supply should be checked using the modified Allen Test (especially if there is a history of previous wrist trauma); this is done by asking the patient to repeatedly make a tight fist while occlusive pressure is applied over the radial artery and ulnar artery. The ulnar artery occlusion is then released. The hand is then relaxed and, if it remains white for 10 seconds or more, collateral refill is inadequate and the other hand should be used (provided the same test is also negative).

Isolation is best achieved between the operator's index and middle fingers of the non-dominant hand, both fingers feeling the pulse over the tips of their palmar surfaces.

Femoral Artery

The artery is at the mid-inguinal point (a point on the inguinal ligament halfway between the pubic symphysis and the anterior superior iliac spine). It is best isolated with the index and middle fingers of the non-dominant hand on either side of the artery just below the inguinal ligament, to prevent puncture of either the femoral vein (medially) or the femoral nerve (laterally) (Fig. 14.10).

Brachial Artery

The brachial artery (Fig. 14.11) is only used if all other punctures are impossible or have failed. There is a risk of injury which could lead to peripheral ischaemia or damage to the median nerve which lies on the medial side.

Equipment

Equipment required is:
- syringe, 2 mL – a special syringe is often available
- 22 G needle (blue) or smaller
- heparin 1000 U/mL (1 mL) – standard in many hospitals
- alcohol swab
- sterile cotton wool balls/gauze swabs
- syringe cap
- plastic bag full of ice

Procedure

- Draw up 0.5 mL of heparin into the 2 mL syringe, withdrawing the plunger fully to coat the syringe walls – or use a special pre-heparinized syringe.
- The heparin in both the pre-prepared and self-heparinized syringes must be expelled completely to leave the plunger just moistened; large amounts of heparin in the

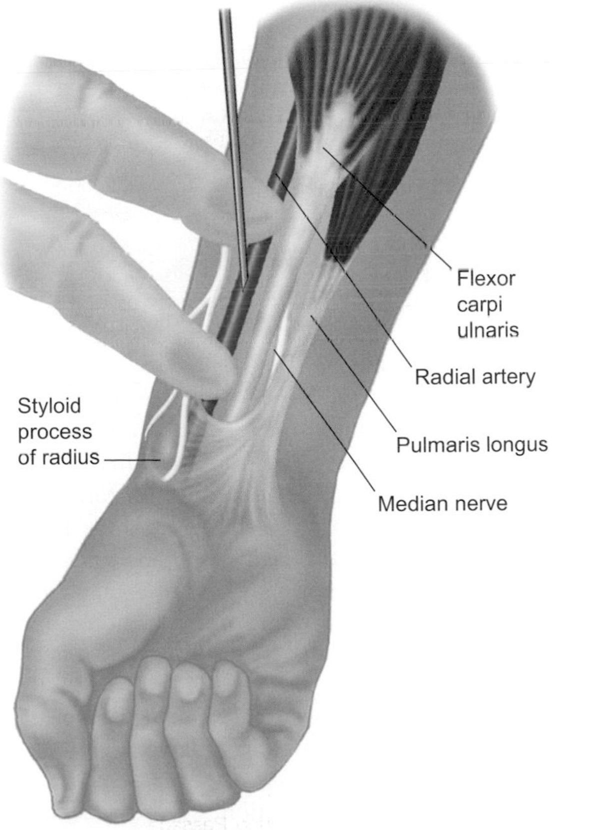

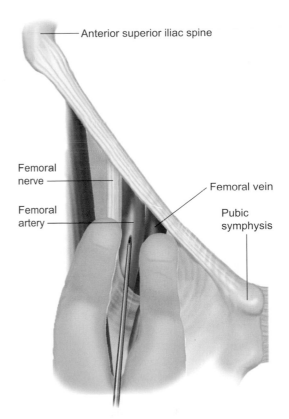

• **Fig. 14.9** The Position of the Radial Artery at the Wrist.

Flexor carpi ulnaris

Radial artery

Pulmaris longus

Median nerve

Styloid process of radius

Anterior superior iliac spine

Femoral nerve

Femoral artery

Femoral vein

Pubic symphysis

• **Fig. 14.10** The Position of the Femoral Artery in the Groin.

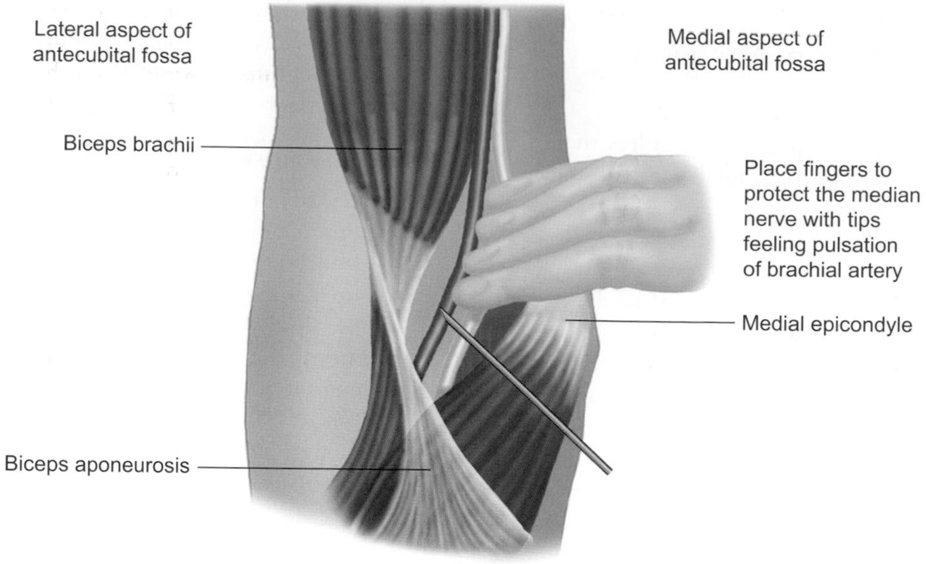

Lateral aspect of antecubital fossa

Medial aspect of antecubital fossa

Biceps brachii

Place fingers to protect the median nerve with tips feeling pulsation of brachial artery

Medial epicondyle

Biceps aponeurosis

• **Fig. 14.11** The Site for Puncture of The Brachial Artery.

syringe affect the pH of a sample taken for the determination of blood gas tension.

- Hold the syringe at a 60–90-degree angle to the skin and slowly advance the needle, maintaining a very slight negative pressure. When a flush of blood occurs, release the negative pressure; if the syringe then fills spontaneously, the artery has been entered.
- Once 2 mL of blood have been obtained, remove the syringe and needle and immediately apply pressure for at least 3 minutes.
- Tap bubbles to the needle end and expel all air that may have accumulated. Then, either take the sample immediately to the arterial blood gas analyser or place it on ice to slow down cellular use of oxygen in the sample (maximum 1 hour for reliable readings).
- If puncture fails, this may be because the artery has been transfixed; slow withdrawal of the needle sometimes yields free flow of arterial blood. If success does not follow, the arterial pulse is repalpated and a fresh attempt is made, preferably without coming out of the skin.

Understanding Arterial Blood Gas Results

Preliminaries

The percentage concentration of oxygen in the inspired air (e.g. 21% if the patient is inhaling air only) should be noted. It may take up to 20 minutes for the arterial blood gases to equilibrate after an adjustment to the oxygen supply. There may sometimes be difficulty in distinguishing between an arterial and venous sample: if the oxygen saturation (derived from the P_aO_2) is less than 50%, the blood is probably venous; 80% or above is certainly arterial. All indices should be considered together, i.e. P_aO_2, P_aCO_2, pH, base excess and H_2CO_3 (normal values are given in Table 14.3).

P_aO_2

Low Values. The patient's usual level should be known – those with chronic respiratory disease can have a P_aO_2 as low as 7.5 kPa. A common cause of a truly low P_aO_2 in

TABLE 14.3	Normal Arterial Blood Gas Values on Room Air	
Measurement	**Units**	**Level**
pH	$-\log_{10}$ concentration hydrogen ion	7.35–7.45
P_aCO_2	kPa	4.3–6.0
	mmHg	32–45
P_aO_2	kPa	10.5–14
	mmHg	79–105
H_2CO_3	mmol/L	22–26
O_2 saturation	Percentage	95–100
Base excess	mmol/L	±2

a surgical patient is a right-to-left shunt of blood through collapsed or consolidated lung tissue, in which instance the highly diffusible CO_2 is also low because of hypoxia-induced tachypnoea and hyperventilation. However, if the associated P_aCO_2 is high, there is chronic respiratory disease and/or acute respiratory failure (inability to ventilate). Those with known chronic respiratory disease who need oxygen to correct hypoxia must be given it carefully, starting with 24% O_2 and measuring the blood gases after 30 minutes to ensure that respiratory drive is maintained and that the P_aCO_2 does not rise. It should be noted that those with chronic respiratory disease can tolerate a much higher P_aCO_2 than normal.

The oxyhaemoglobin dissociation curve means that small changes in P_aO_2 may have a large effect on oxygen saturation.

High Values. Hyperventilation without added oxygen cannot significantly increase the P_aO_2. The much more likely cause is that there is too high a concentration in the inspired air, and this should be adjusted provided the P_aCO_2 is normal.

P_aCO_2

Low Values. The patient is usually hyperventilating. The causes are:

- hypoxia
- anxiety – there is an accompanying respiratory alkalosis
- compensation for a lowered pH – metabolic acidosis

Hyperventilation from anxiety leads to a respiratory alkalosis (increased pH). If there is obvious hyperventilation, then a paper bag over the patient's mouth and a suggestion that respiratory rate is reduced is usually effective, as may be an instruction to hold the breath.

If the clinical state is a compensation for a metabolic acidosis, then the pH will be either normal or low and there will be a negative base excess.

High Values. There is retention of CO_2 because of hypoventilation from one of the following:

- chronic respiratory failure (often with an associated low P_aO_2 and normal pH – chronically compensated)
- respiratory suppression from drugs (often opioids)
- exhaustion of the respiratory muscles (associated with a low P_aO_2 and inappropriately reduced respiratory rate) – the chief cause of acute respiratory failure in surgical patients
- brainstem malfunction, often with varied rates of ventilation; conscious level is decreased

Respiratory support, such as ventilation, needs to be considered in acute respiratory failure:

- if the respiratory rate is either very high (greater than 25) or very low (less than 8) on maximum supplementary oxygen from a mask and the patient is not maintaining P_aO_2 of 10 kPa
- in a previously normal patient if the P_aCO_2 is greater than 8 kPa

pH and Base Excess

If the pH is less than 7.35, there is acidosis; if greater than 7.45, there is an alkalosis. It is necessary to decide if either is metabolic or respiratory in origin and whether compensation is present. Compensation suggests a more chronic disease process (days or weeks), whereas an uncompensated disorder suggests an acute disease process. Compensation usually occurs by a change in the respiratory rate (e.g. in a metabolic acidosis, hyperpnoea causes increased excretion of CO_2) or by renal regulation of the amount of HCO_3 that is excreted.

INSERTION OF A NASOGASTRIC TUBE

Indications

Indications include:

- vomiting from small-bowel obstruction or pyloric stenosis
- acute gastric dilatation
- the prevention of gastro-oesophageal reflux which could cause aspiration in patients with impaired gastric emptying
- enteric feeding (a nasojejunal tube may also be used)
- possible protection of an anastomosis distal to the pharynx – usually in the oesophagus (nasogastric tube usually positioned at operation)

Equipment

Equipment required:

- non-sterile gloves
- nasogastric tube size 10 (small) to 16 (large)
- catheter drainage bag
- lubricant
- glass of water

Procedure

- Inform the patient what is planned and how cooperation can help. Verbal consent is obtained.
- Sit the patient upright with the chin on the chest; if this is not possible, then the alternative is on the side with the head propped up.
- Lubricate the tube and insert into one nostril directly backward towards the occiput – a patient may be aware which side is more likely to be successful. Gently advance the tube.
- If you are unable to advance, try the other nostril or reposition the patient.
- When the patient feels the tip in the pharynx, ask for a swallow and, as the tube moves, its advance is continued. Swallowing may be helped if a sip of water is given but there must not be any chance of aspiration because of an inactive gag reflex.
- Should the patient cough or becomes cyanotic, it is probably because the tube is astride the larynx or trachea. Withdraw quickly, into the hypopharynx, let the patient settle and try again (unfortunately the tube is often then pulled out completely because of a feeling of impending suffocation).
- After apparently successful insertion, check that the tube is not simply curled up in the back of the mouth. To do this, attach a 20 mL syringe to the proximal end and, with a stethoscope bell just below the left costal margin, quickly inject air; a loud borborygmus confirms that the tube is in the stomach.
- If fluid can be aspirated from the nasogastric tube, it can be tested with pH indicator paper (not litmus paper). It should be acidic (pH <5.5).
- Secure the tube to the nose with strong adhesive tape.
- If there is any doubt, the position of the tube should be checked by X-ray.
- If the catheter is to be used for enteral feeding the position should always be checked with a chest X-ray before feeding is commenced.
- Most hospitals have local policies on confirmation of tube placement and these should be consulted and followed.

Extra Hints

- A cold tube (one that has been in a refrigerator for at least 30 minutes) is stiffer and easier to direct down the oesophagus.
- A change in the position of the patient – as indicated above – can sometimes secure success.
- If the patient has a poor gag reflex, then sometimes a laryngoscope and Magill's forceps can be used to direct the tube into the oesophagus.

Fine-bore tubes for enteric feeding may be easier to insert because they are of smaller diameter and are equipped with a guide wire. However, their rigidity may, if they are forced down against resistance, lead to an abrasion or, rarely, perforation of the oesophagus. Furthermore, in an unconscious patient, it is easy to insert them into the trachea and bronchi. The final position of the tube should always be confirmed by a chest X-ray.

URINARY CATHETERIZATION

Material

Urinary catheters are usually made of either latex or silicone rubber. Silicone is less irritant and should be used if the catheter is to be left indwelling for some days or weeks. However, silicone catheters are stiffer than latex and require greater care on insertion to avoid trauma, particularly to the prostatic urethra.

Special Catheters

A Foley catheter is self-retaining because of an inflatable balloon (Fig. 14.12) and is usually but not invariably made of latex.

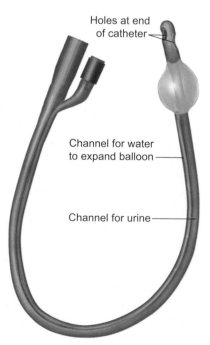

Holes at end of catheter

Channel for water to expand balloon

Channel for urine

• **Fig. 14.12** A Foley Urinary Catheter.

Three-way catheters are used for irrigation of the bladder, e.g. after prostatectomy.

Size

- 8–10 F: children and adults with tight urethral stricture
- 12–14 F: normal urethra or in the presence of mild prostatic hypertrophy
- 16–18 F: moderate prostatic hypertrophy
- 20–24 F: after prostatectomy for free drainage and in other circumstances where bladder irrigation is required with the use of a three-way catheter

The smallest size feasible should always be used.

Male Catheterization (Fig. 14.13)

Indications

Indications include:
- urinary retention
- to assess hourly urinary output
- incontinence
- after spinal or epidural anaesthesia

Equipment

Equipment required:
- urinary catheter
- sterile gloves
- lidocaine gel 0.5%
- bland antiseptic solution (e.g. cetyl trimethyl ammonium bromide) or sterile 0.9% saline
- pre-prepared catheterization pack – kidney dish, gauze swabs, sterile towels
- 10 mL syringe and 10 mL of sterile water
- urine drainage bag

Procedure

- Wash hands and don sterile gloves.
- Open out everything that is needed onto a sterile towel, usually on a trolley.
- Lay the patient flat – the more supine the position, the easier is the catheterization.
- Drape the sterile towels or paper sheets to leave the penis exposed (a self-made hole in the centre of the paper sheet is often an easy way to expose just the penis).
- If right-handed, hold the penis with a sterile gauze swab with the left hand to prevent the penis from slipping; then retract the foreskin and clean the urethral opening with a swab.
- Gently squeeze the contents of a tube of lidocaine jelly into the urethra; in anyone of age less than 50, the sensitivity of the urethra often requires the content of two tubes.
- Open the plastic sheath which contains the catheter at the tip with the right hand and place a kidney bowl just below the urethral orifice of the penis.

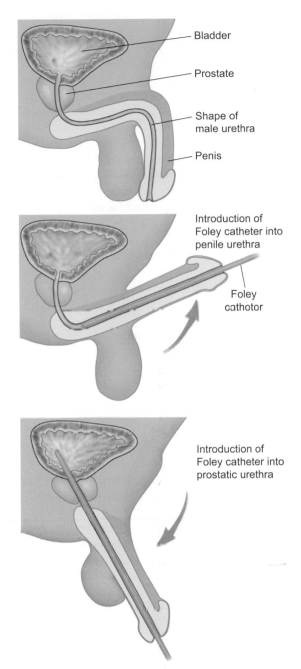

- • Fig. 14.13 Technique for Male Catheterization.

- Hold the penis in the left hand and gently insert the catheter into the urethra using the right hand while withdrawing the plastic covering; ideally the catheter remains untouched, but this almost always proves impossible and the catheter has to be advanced without its plastic covering using the clean right hand. During insertion, the external end of the catheter remains in the kidney bowl because, when the bladder is entered, urine usually spills out.
- If resistance is felt along the penile urethra or before the prostatic urethra has been traversed, pulling the penis gently upwards can help.

- Most often, resistance is found within the prostatic urethra, and pulling the penis downwards at this point can assist. Sometimes the cause is failure of relaxation of the external sphincter and, if the tip of the catheter is held at this point of resistance for 10 seconds, this is often enough to allow the sphincter to relax spontaneously.
- Force must not be used because a false passage through the wall of the urethra can be made.
- A Foley catheter should be inserted fully to ensure that the balloon is within the bladder before inflation.
- Check the capacity of the balloon – it is usually 5–10 mL but for most three-way catheters, it is 30 mL. Usually only 5–10 mL capacity is needed; if the patient has just had a prostatectomy, then 20–30 mL is required so that the catheter can sit at the bladder neck and not move into the resected prostatic cavity.
- Either squeeze the already dilated water-filled area at the distal end of the catheter (after removing the clip) or insert the 5–10 mL of sterile water gently into the injection port for the balloon. If this generates pain or discomfort, stop at once, withdraw any water and advance the catheter further into the bladder.
- Once the balloon is inflated, the catheter is withdrawn until resistance is felt as the balloon lodges against the bladder neck.
- Replace the foreskin over the glans to avoid the possibility of a paraphimosis.
- Attach the catheter to the drainage apparatus.
- Send a urine sample for microscopy and culture if indicated.

If the catheter is to be in place for a considerable time – several days or more – the smallest diameter and the minimal amount of water in the balloon (5 mL) both help to decrease the likelihood of bladder spasm.

Extra Hints

- If the catheter is in the bladder but urine does not flow, blockage by the lubrication jelly is a possibility. Aspiration with a 50 mL catheter syringe and/or injection of sterile water or 0.9% saline usually unblocks the catheter.
- If a stricture is encountered in either the penile or prostatic urethra, a narrower catheter (10–12 F) should be used.
- In a patient beyond 55 years with a history suggestive of benign prostatic hypertrophy, a larger-diameter catheter is paradoxically more likely to succeed.
- If the catheterization fails, no more than two attempts should be made before more experienced help is sought. For the second, try to use a different-sized catheter (depending on the probable cause of difficulty) and extra lidocaine gel. Further failure should lead to consideration of suprapubic drainage (see later).
- If the patient bleeds from the urethra, abandon the procedure and summon help to decide how to proceed, which may mean the use of suprapubic catheterization.

- If phimosis makes the external meatus difficult to find, gently dilate the narrow opening in the foreskin with the nozzle of the tube which contains the lidocaine jelly.

Removal of a Urethral Catheter

This is usually done by nursing staff. Failure to decompress the balloon calls for special manoeuvres.

Faulty Valve

Sometimes the valve end can be cut off. If this fails, a needle inserted into the valve channel and aspirated may release obstruction.

Persistent Impaction

Ultrasound identifies the balloon in the bladder, which can then be punctured with a fine spinal needle passed percutaneously under image control.

Catheterization in Relation to Prostatic Hypertrophy and Prostatectomy

Size of Catheter

As mentioned above, the prostatic urethra may, in the presence of prostatic hypertrophy, be more easily negotiated with a larger rather than a smaller catheter.

Bleeding

Initial rapid decompression of a dilated bladder may lead to rupture of distended veins at the bladder neck. A three-way irrigation system may be necessary until the condition settles, which it usually does.

Chronic Retention

The presence of chronic retention with a considerably distended bladder before prostatectomy makes the necessity of prolonged drainage extremely likely; a 12–14 F silicone catheter, which can be left in place for 6–8 weeks, allows the bladder to recover tone. Long-standing obstruction at the bladder neck without acute retention leads to back pressure on the kidney and a presentation with features of chronic renal failure and creatinine levels in excess of 1000 μmol/L, although the electrolyte levels are remarkably normal when there is only an obstructive cause. Catheterization in such circumstances means that there is the likelihood of the development of a polyuric phase because damage to the kidneys' distal tubules results in an inability to concentrate urine. Some 200–400 mL of urine an hour can be passed, and dehydration develops quite rapidly. The most practical way to adjust fluid balance to compensate for the polyuria is to give the amount of fluid passed out in 1 hour back intravenously over the next hour. Such polyuria may be accompanied by hyponatraemia and hypokalaemia, and replacement must be adjusted accordingly. The polyuric phase usually lasts for about 12–24 hours; continuation beyond this may mean over-replacement, with a vicious circle of water and electrolyte-induced diuresis. The hour-on-hour replacement of urinary losses is discontinued and the situation reassessed.

Post-Prostatectomy Failure of Micturition

Withdrawal of the initial drainage catheter after transurethral prostatectomy may not be followed by micturition. In such circumstances, first check the fluid balance chart – the bladder may not be sufficiently full to initiate micturition. Also, pain and the feeling of inability to micturate are not always caused by an overfull bladder; severe pain is often the consequence of detrusor muscle spasm within the bladder and is best treated not by catheterization but with a smooth muscle relaxant such as oxybutynin. If the patient has been bleeding significantly and the bladder is truly distended, this may be the result of clot retention. Catheterization with a large-bore, three-way catheter and irrigation with 0.9% saline are necessary.

At transurethral prostatectomy, it is relatively easy to dissect under the bladder neck and therefore possible to make a false passage on re-catheterization. If the catheter easily advances its full length, then this is unlikely; a check can be done by the insertion of 50 mL of water, which should readily be re-aspirated.

Female Catheterization

Anatomy

The female has a more easily traversed urinary tract than has the male. Only the muscles of the pelvic floor control access, and once the external meatus has been identified, the short urethra is straight (Fig. 14.14).

Equipment

The equipment is the same as for male catheterization. Female catheterization is often performed by the nursing staff, and doctors are asked to assist only when nursing staff have been unsuccessful. Short, ballooned catheters previously advocated for female catheterization should no longer be stocked to avoid their inadvertent use in male patients.

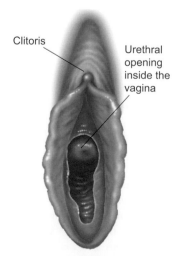

• **Fig. 14.14** Technique for Female Catheterization.

Procedure

- Collect all equipment and set up the trolley.
- Position the patient as for a vaginal examination – flat on the back with the heels together and the knees apart (hips in abduction and external rotation).
- Put on sterile gloves.
- Part the labia minora and majora with the non-dominant hand and, using the dominant hand, clean the area with a cotton wool ball soaked in sterile 0.9% saline or a bland antiseptic solution.
- Locate the urethral opening (see Fig. 14.14) behind and below the clitoris and introduce a well-lubricated catheter tip; a small amount of lidocaine jelly applied around the opening can aid entry.
- Successful catheterization is followed by the procedures listed above for male catheterization.

Difficulty

If catheterization has not been achieved, this is usually because the urethral opening has not been identified and the vagina has been catheterized instead. The labia minora must be opened generously and usually the urethral opening can be seen pouting on the anterior aspect of the vaginal wall. A focused light and lying the patient on the side can both help, as can, occasionally, a vaginal speculum. This can sometimes be a particular problem in obese patients or in patients with arthritis of the hip joints. Under these circumstances an assistant may be useful.

Suprapubic Bladder Drainage

Indication

Suprapubic bladder drainage is required when urethral catheterization has failed and the patient has a full bladder.

Equipment

Equipment required:
- sterile towels
- catheterization pack – gauze, cotton wool balls
- skin preparation
- suprapubic catheter
- needles – orange, green and white
- 1% lidocaine 10–20 mL
- 10- and 20-mL syringes
- blade or knife
- suture to tie the catheter to the abdominal wall – 3/0 or stronger
- catheter bag

Procedure

- Place the patient supine and make sure that the bladder is distended by percussion from the umbilicus downwards in the midline or by ultrasound scanning.
- Open the pack and all the equipment; if a Foley catheter is to be used, check the balloon. Use another type only if familiar with its mechanism of insertion.
- Clean the area in the midline between the umbilicus and symphysis pubis.
- Arrange the sterile towels around this area.
- Infiltrate the skin in the midline 2 cm above the pubic symphysis using the local anaesthetic and an orange needle and continue this through the layers of abdominal wall (the subcutaneous tissue and linea alba only) with the larger (green) needle.
- At the completion of infiltration, the needle is passed into the distended bladder and urine is aspirated; occasionally, the longest (white) needle is required to achieve this (urine must be aspirated before suprapubic catheterization is attempted).
- Make a stab incision in the skin large enough to take the chosen catheter.
- Insert the suprapubic trochar directly posteriorly in the same direction as that used for the final aspiration of urine.
- Once urine is obtained, advance the catheter over the trochar.
- Remove the trochar and advance the catheter further to the indicated marker; ensure that easy aspiration of urine occurs and that the patient is free from pain.
- Clean and dry the entry point and then secure the catheter – preferably at more than one point.

If the catheter falls out before 2 weeks have elapsed and the patient needs re-catheterization, this must be done within 8 hours, otherwise the track will have closed. After 2 weeks, the track will have become lined with epithelium and therefore a new catheter (often a simple silicone-covered urethral catheter) can be easily inserted.

CHEST PROCEDURES

Pleural Drainage (Air and/or Fluid)

For all chest drainage procedures:
- First check the clinical signs and the X-rays.
- Ensure that the upper level of the pleural effusion is clearly established by percussion and mark this on the chest wall.
- Position the patient comfortably in a sitting position leaning slightly forward either in bed or on a chair. Ideally a table should be placed in front with a pillow or blanket to rest on, elevated to the level of the axilla (Fig. 14.15).
- Usually, a site for aspiration/drainage is identified by ultrasound scanning.

Diagnostic Aspiration

Indications

Indications include:
- infection
- malignancy

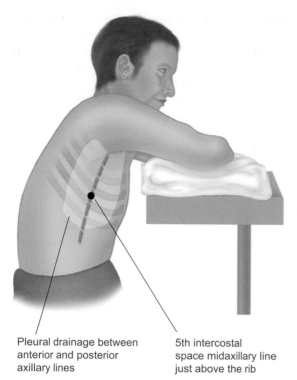

Pleural drainage between
anterior and posterior
axillary lines

5th intercostal
space midaxillary line
just above the rib

• **Fig. 14.15** The Position of a Patient During Pleural Drainage/Chest Drain.

Equipment

Equipment required:
- dressing pack
- sterile gloves
- 20 mL syringe
- orange (25 G) and green (21 G) needles
- 1% lidocaine, 10 mL
- three sterile specimen bottles

Procedure

- Confirm the signs and X-ray findings.
- Select the insertion site by ultrasound scanning or percussing out an effusion and mark the point of dullness – ideally done between the midaxillary and posterior axillary lines and at a point three fingerbreadths below the tip of the scapula.
- Infiltrate the skin over the chosen point with local anaesthetic using an orange needle and then infiltrate deeper with a green needle; the needle should pass just superior to the rib to avoid the neurovascular bundle. Always withdraw before inserting local anaesthetic. On average, fluid should be aspirated at the full depth of a green needle, but a longer needle may be required for larger or more obese individuals.
- Attach the 20 mL syringe to the appropriately sized needle and insert it through the area that has already been anaesthetized while aspirating as the needle is advanced. When flashback of fluid occurs, gently aspirate 20 mL to send for laboratory analysis: culture and sensitivity, auramine stain and TB culture; protein, glucose and amylase;

and cytology. When aspirating for cytological examination, the more fluid there is, the better (>40 mL).

Therapeutic Aspiration

Indications

Indications include:
- relief of shortness of breath from a pleural effusion
- removal of a small pneumothorax

Equipment

Equipment is as for diagnostic aspiration, plus the following additional items:
- large-bore i.v. cannula (brown or grey)
- a three-way tap
- 50 mL syringe
- i.v. giving set and an empty sterile bowel or saline bag

Procedure

Fluid

- Larger cannulae need a small incision in the skin before their insertion.
- Attach the 50 mL syringe to the cannula and aspirate on insertion. After flashback, advance the cannula over the needle and then withdraw the needle, to leave the flexible cannula in place; as this is done, the patient should breathe out and the thumb is placed over the cannula hub to prevent air being sucked in.
- A closed three-way tap is quickly attached to the hub.
- Attach the 50 mL syringe to one hub of the tap and the empty saline bag to the other.
- Aspirate 50 mL at a time, switching the three-way tap settings to allow the syringe to empty into the saline bag.
- Withdraw the cannula while the patient breathes out.
- Apply an occlusive dressing to the site of puncture.

Air

- The position of insertion of the cannula should be either in the 2nd intercostal space in the midclavicular line (see Ch. 19) or in the midaxillary line in the 5th intercostal space.
- Infiltrate as already indicated just superior to the rib and ensure aspiration of air.
- Make a small incision in the skin and insert the needle/cannula through the infiltrated area. On aspiration of air through the needle, advance the cannula quickly while the patient breathes out.
- Remove the needle immediately and, with the thumb, occlude the hub until a closed three-way tap is attached.
- Air is aspirated 50 mL at a time and expelled through the spare exit on the tap. Care must be taken to avoid the open tap coming into direct communication with the chest cavity.
- Once there is resistance to further aspiration, withdraw the cannula slightly to see if there is still residual air. It is important never to force aspiration because to do so may suck lung tissue against the end of the cannula.
- Withdraw the cannula and apply an occlusive dressing.

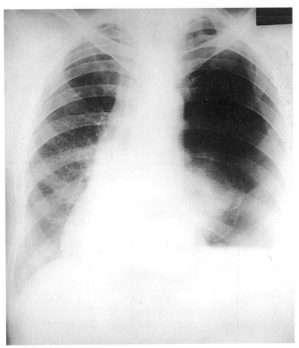

• **Fig. 14.16** Left-Sided Tension Pneumothorax with Mediastinal Shift and Complete Collapse of Left Lung.

For a therapeutic aspiration, it is advisable to halt the procedure after 1000 mL of air or fluid has been withdrawn to avoid rapid shift of the mediastinum. If cardiorespiratory signs are absent, removal of air or fluid is resumed after an hour. Failure of a chest aspiration is usually the result of a localized effusion or empyema. Ultrasound scanning and guided aspiration should be used.

Relief of Tension Pneumothorax

The causes and mechanisms are discussed in Chapter 19. The diagnosis is clinical rather than radiological (Fig. 14.16), and urgent decompression is required.

Equipment

Equipment required:
• large-bore needle or needle/cannula
• 20 mL syringe

Procedure

• Assess the patient's chest and respiratory function.
• Administer oxygen at 12 L/min by mask.
• Identify the 2nd intercostal space in the midclavicular line on the side of the pneumothorax.
• If the patient is conscious and time permits, introduce local anaesthetic with an orange needle.
• Insert the needle with the 20 mL syringe attached – a small incision in the skin makes the insertion of a needle or cannula easier.

• Aspiration of air confirms the diagnosis: the syringe is removed and, in tension pneumothorax, a hissing sound is usually heard as the air is rapidly expelled; a hand held 5 cm from the needle or cannula can detect this rush of air.

The urgent procedure described converts a tension pneumothorax into an ordinary one. If air starts to enter the thorax, a three-way tap should be placed on the needle or cannula hub and sealed, which then enables further release of air before a chest drain is inserted – this is always done.

Insertion of a Chest Drain

Indications

Indications include:
• large pneumothorax and after urgent release of a tension pneumothorax
• spreading surgical emphysema – sometimes an X-ray shows no sign of a pneumothorax, but a chest drain should be inserted on the assumption that there is a continuing leak of air into the pleural space
• large haemothorax with a possible continued source of bleeding
• large pleural effusion
• empyema

Equipment

Equipment required:
• chest drain between 22 F and 32 F but *without* an integral trochar
• 0.5% lidocaine, 20 mL
• underwater seal apparatus including bottle
• sterile water
• surgical blade
• small and large artery forceps
• heavy suture, e.g. silk 0
• adhesive tape – a waterproof variety is best

Position

The position for insertion is the 5th intercostal space in the midaxillary line on the affected side – usually approximately at the level of the nipple in a male. This site is suitable for drainage of both a pneumothorax and a haemothorax and should always be used in trauma. Drainage of a pleural effusion or an empyema may need to be slightly lower, but the site should be carefully checked against the available imaging, with particular attention to the possibility of the dome of the diaphragm being raised. The distance between adjacent ribs determines the size of the intercostal drain tube; the largest drain possible is advisable, particularly in trauma.

Procedure

• Position the patient as for pleural aspiration.
• Make a final check of the clinical signs and the chest X-ray.
• Mark the proposed site of insertion.

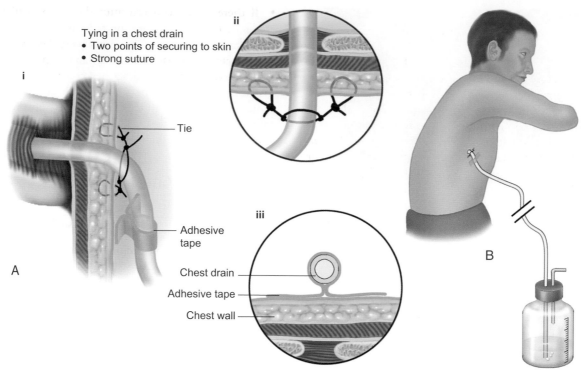

• **Fig. 14.17** (A) Technique for securing of a chest drain. i. Correct insertion of chest drain; ii. Securely sutured chest drain; iii. Secure taping of the chest drain to the skin. (B) Chest drain in position with underwater drainage.

- Prepare an area over two to three ribs in the midaxillary line and drape it.
- Anaesthetize the skin and the tissues down to the upper border of the chosen rib – not all the allocated lidocaine is used because more is often needed later.
- Make a 2–3-cm transverse incision over the proposed site of insertion.
- Use the artery forceps to dissect bluntly through the subcutaneous tissues, going down onto the superior margin of the rib and dissecting through the intercostal muscles and then the parietal pleura (Fig. 14.17A) – this is where more local anaesthetic may be required.
- When the parietal pleura is punctured with the tip of the artery forceps, there is usually the escape of fluid and/or air. Sweep the gloved index finger down the line of blunt dissection to free any adhesions within the pleural space so that injury to the lung is avoided.
- Grasp the drainage tube at its tip with artery forceps and guide it down the track with the index finger. Once the drain is within the pleural cavity, remove the forceps and advance the drain gently in a cranial direction to remove air or caudally to remove fluid.
- Attach the outer end of the drain to an underwater seal drainage apparatus.
- Close the incision with interrupted sutures and a tight tie around the drain itself – there should not be leakage around the tube or through the incision.
- Insert a purse string suture around the drain or two interrupted sutures across the tube site, leaving the ends untied for final air-tight closure when the drain is removed.
- Check that the drain is working – fluid or air according to circumstances – or that the water is rising into the tube above the level in the bottle (swinging) with respiration; failure to swing may mean that the tube is misplaced or blocked.
- Secure the connection between the drain and the underwater seal with strong adhesive tape and, after wiping dry around the insertion site and applying a sterile dressing, tape the drain to the chest wall (see Fig. 14.17B).
- Check the position of the drain by chest X-ray.

Complications

Complications include:
- damage to an intercostal artery or vein which causes either continued bleeding at the site of insertion or a haemothorax
- damage to an intercostal nerve which may cause later intercostal neuritis/neuralgia
- pleural empyema
- laceration or puncture of intrathoracic and/or abdominal organs – prevented by using blunt dissection
- local cellulitis
- local haematoma
- mediastinal emphysema
- subcutaneous emphysema
- winging of the scapula caused by injury to the long thoracic nerve (of Bell)

Further Hints

- Strong and long dissecting artery forceps are extremely useful.
- Do not use any trochar supplied with a drain – it is a common cause of injury to deep structures.
- The more subcutaneous fat that is present, the bigger the incision that is required; a good guide is that the incision needs to be as long as the subcutaneous fat is deep and at least wide enough to admit an index finger.

If the first drain does not resolve the pneumothorax or there is a large and continuing leak, further drains may well be required. The same applies if surgical emphysema continues to spread after the insertion of a chest drain.

If, after pleural drainage for acute haemothorax, more than 200 mL of blood (as distinct from bloodstained pleural effusion) drains every hour, thoracotomy may be indicated for control of bleeding.

Removal of Chest Drain

The chest drain does not have a continued role if it fails to swing with breathing or is not draining any fluid; these are the chief indications for its removal. Before this is done, the patient should be asked to cough and, if the drain does not bubble, then any leak from a hole in the lung has almost certainly been sealed; however, for certainty, the test should be repeated after 12 hours. A check X-ray before removal will confirm that the lung is completely re-expanded and that any pleural effusion has been fully drained.

Large pleural effusions should be drained over several days. The maximum should be 1 L per hour and not more than 4 L per day, otherwise there is a risk of reflex pulmonary oedema.

Equipment

Equipment required:
- sterile gloves
- suture cutters
- local anaesthetic and, if occluding sutures have not been pre-inserted, a closure suture
- occlusive dressing

Procedure

Ideally this should be done with two people: one to tie the suture and the other to remove the drain. Local anaesthetic and a standby suture should be available.
- Undo the adhesive dressing and check whether there is a purse string suture in situ; if there is, release the suture and place a half knot.
- Release the suture holding the drain.
- Ask the patient to take two large inhalations and then momentarily to hold the breath in expiration (Valsalva manoeuvre to raise intrathoracic pressure); now pull the drain out quickly.
- Tie the purse string immediately and cover the site with a sterile dressing and occlusive tape.

- If there is any concern after the removal of the chest drain, a chest X-ray is indicated.
- If the occluding suture is ineffective, then gauze should be available to place over the hole and prevent a sucking chest wound.

Pericardial Paracentesis

Indications

This procedure is used to relieve cardiac tamponade (see Ch. 19), which most commonly occurs after penetrating injuries to the chest, although a blunt injury – such as a steering wheel – can also be responsible. The removal of a small amount of blood or fluid can make a dramatic difference to the cardiac output and the patient's condition. Also, rarely in surgical practice, a chronic effusion may require aspiration. The pericardial sac is a fixed fibrous structure which, distended by only a small amount of blood, restricts cardiac filling. The removal of 15–20 mL of effusion – blood or other fluid – may save the patient's life.

Equipment

Equipment required:
- long plastic-sheathed needle 16–18 G – a single-lumen central line cannula is ideal; if this is unavailable then a needle is sufficient, but if repeated aspiration is required the procedure has to be repeated rather than re-aspirating from a cannula that remains in situ
- three-way tap
- 20-mL syringe
- small scalpel blade (if a cannula/needle is to be used)

Procedure (Fig. 14.18)

- Ideally this should be done under ultrasound guidance; however, circumstances and time in the emergency setting may make this impossible.
- Continuous recording of blood pressure, pulse rate, central venous pressure and ECG throughout the procedure is ideal, but in the urgent circumstances usually encountered this can be omitted.
- If time allows, prepare the xiphoid and subxiphoid areas.
- Attach the syringe to the three-way tap and needle/cannula.
- Feel for the apex beat to ensure that there has been no marked mediastinal shift; this may be difficult or impossible when there is cardiac tamponade.
- Anaesthetize the area and incise the skin over a point 1–2 cm inferior to the left of the xiphochondral junction at a 45-degree angle to the skin.
- Advance a long needle and cannula towards the head, aiming towards the tip of the scapula or shoulder. Aspirate as the needle is advanced and watch the ECG continuously in case needling the myocardium causes any irregularities, including an injury pattern, e.g. extreme

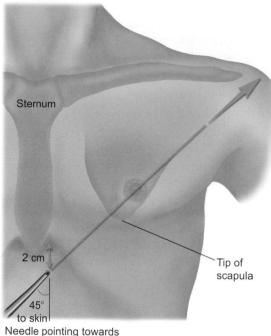

• **Fig. 14.18** Technique for Pericardial Aspiration.

ST changes or a widened and enlarged QRS complex. Premature ventricular contractions may also occur, secondary to irritation of the myocardium.

- When the needle enters the blood-filled pericardial sac, withdraw as much non-clotted blood as is possible, although it must be remembered that the epicardium will approach the inner aspect of the pericardial sac, and ECG changes may then occur.
- After aspiration is complete, slide the cannula over the needle and reattach the three-way tap, closing it off. Secure a catheter in place with adhesive tape.
- If the symptoms of cardiac tamponade persist, reaspiration or a thoracotomy may be needed.

Complications

Possible complications are:
- aspiration of ventricular blood
- laceration of coronary artery or vein
- pericarditis
- cardiac arrhythmias – ventricular fibrillation, tachycardia
- puncture of aorta, inferior vena cava, oesophagus

PERITONEAL LAVAGE

Indications

Peritoneal lavage may be useful in a patient with multiple injuries if:
- abdominal examination is equivocal because other injuries (fractures of ribs, pelvis and lumbar spine) may be obscuring physical findings

- abdominal examination is unreliable because of severe head injury, endotracheal intubation, intoxicants or paraplegia
- there is unexplained hypotension and/or blood loss

However, urgent CT scanning is now often available and has reduced the need for peritoneal lavage.

Equipment

Equipment required:
- peritoneal dialysis or peritoneal lavage catheter
- 1 L of 0.9% saline
- intravenous giving set
- scalpel
- local anaesthetic – 1% lidocaine with adrenaline 10 mL
- skin cleaner
- dressing pack and sterile towels
- instruments – tissue forceps, Allis clamps, arterial forceps

Procedure (Fig. 14.19)

- Decompress the bladder by the passage of a urinary catheter.
- Prepare the area around the umbilicus (15 × 15 cm).
- Infiltrate local anaesthetic just inferior to the umbilicus and along the midline for approximately 2–5 cm, depending on the amount of subcutaneous tissue. Create a midline incision with a broad blade sufficiently long to visualize the linea alba. Continue dissection through the linea alba and grasp its edges with the Allis forceps or arterial forceps so as to provide countertraction.
- Expose the peritoneum and pick it up with arterial forceps. Pinch the peritoneum to ensure no bowel has been caught by the arterial forceps then open the peritoneum with the belly of the blade.
- Insert the peritoneal dialysis catheter into the peritoneal cavity, advancing it towards the pelvis.
- Connect the catheter to a syringe and aspirate.
- If gross blood is not aspirated, use the i.v. apparatus to instil 500–1000 mL of warmed saline.
- Given the patient is haemodynamically stable, allow the fluid to remain in the abdomen for 5–10 minutes before siphoning it off by putting the empty 0.9% saline container on the floor and allowing the peritoneal fluid to drain from the abdomen (which can take up to 20–30 minutes). A suture secures the catheter if some time elapses before the fluid is removed and it is necessary to make sure the container is vented to allow free flow.
- After return of the fluid, remove the peritoneal catheter and repair the fascia with interrupted sutures (e.g. Prolene 0 on a J needle) and the skin (e.g. Ethilon 3/0).

Indications for Laparotomy After Peritoneal Lavage

Indications include:
- aspiration of more than 5 mL of obvious blood
- aspiration of enteric contents
- laboratory analysis of the peritoneal lavage fluid: >10,000 red blood cells/mm^3; >500 white blood cells/mm^3, bacteria and vegetable matter (usually associated with a raised WBC count)

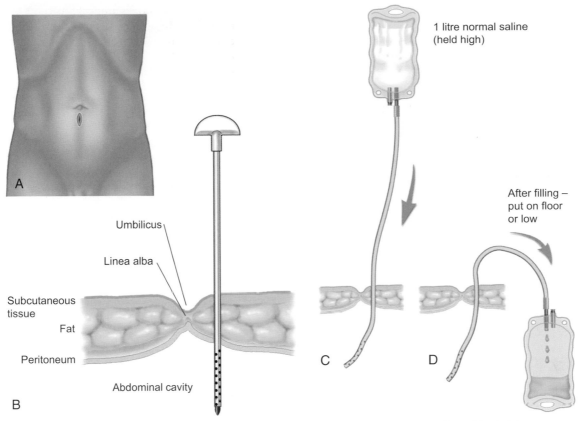

• **Fig. 14.19** Technique for Peritoneal Lavage. (A) Anterior abdominal wall showing position of the incision. (B) Transverse section of the abdominal wall with peritoneal lavage catheter and trocar. (C) Instillation of warm normal saline from a height. (D) Drop the infusion bag below the level of the abdomen to syphon fluid back into the bag.

False-negative results are obtained in 2% of peritoneal lavages, usually the consequence of isolated injury to retroperitoneal organs such as the pancreas, duodenum, diaphragm, small bowel and bladder.

AIRWAY MANAGEMENT

Any patient who is semi-conscious or unconscious must have an adequate assessment of the airway:

- Look for agitation, cyanosis, difficulty in respiratory effort and choking motions.
- Listen for snoring, gurgling, stridor and gargling sounds.
- Feel with the back of the hand for the exit of air with respiratory effort or see fogging of the oxygen mask on expiration.

Simple Management

Blood secretions should be removed from the nose and mouth with a rigid suction device. A cribriform plate fracture must be considered, and gentleness is essential.

Chin Lift

First, complete clearance of the mouth, if indicated, by sweeping a finger between the tongue and the upper palate; be wary of the tendency of a semi-conscious patient to bite. Chin lift (Fig. 14.20) is a simple procedure which can be

done on any patient without interfering with the cervical spine: the fingers of one hand are placed under the mandible in the midline, and are then lifted gently upwards to bring the chin forwards.

Jaw Thrust

The angles of the lower jaw are grasped and the mandible displaced forwards. This is the method used with a mouth-to-face mask with a good seal.

Oropharyngeal Airway

A semi-conscious or agitated patient may cause difficulty, but an unconscious one usually accepts an oral airway. This should be inserted upside down with the concavity directed upwards until the soft palate is encountered. Rotation through 180 degrees is then done, which places the concavity downwards and around the back of the tongue.

Nasopharyngeal Airway

This is useful when a patient has an upper airway obstruction but is unable to tolerate an oropharyngeal airway. The nasal airway is inserted into one nostril. It needs first to be lubricated and then inserted into the less obstructed nostril (often it is easier to insert through one or other nostril). If difficulty is encountered with one nostril, the other is used.

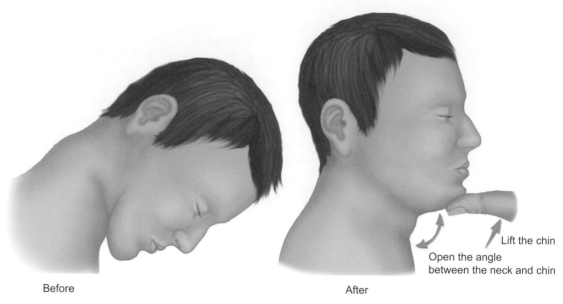

Lift the chin

Open the angle
between the neck and chin

Before

After

• **Fig. 14.20** Chin Lift.

The turbinates are often felt to fracture as the catheter is inserted, but little force is needed for this to occur and fracture is usual. If there is a suspicion of a base of skull fracture, a nasopharyngeal tube should not be used.

Surgical Airway

Indications

A surgical airway is preferred for prolonged intubation in ITU patients and essential when it is not possible to intubate the trachea. The latter can occur for various reasons:

- oedema of the epiglottis
- fracture of the larynx
- severe oropharyngeal haemorrhage
- when an endotracheal tube cannot be placed through the cords

Cricothyroidotomy

Anatomy (Fig. 14.21)

This technique is used for emergency access to the airway.

The cricoid cartilage is the only circumferential support to the upper trachea in children and therefore surgical cricothyroidotomy is not recommended in children under 12 years. A 14-gauge needle/cannula can be used instead and is inserted through the cricothyroid membrane with intermittent oxygen jet insufflation. This method can lead to carbon dioxide retention and therefore should not be used for more than 40 minutes.

Equipment

Equipment required:

- cricothyroidotomy set – often easily available in most resuscitation areas

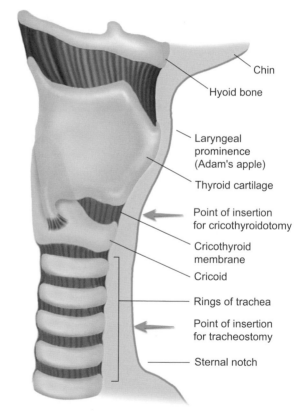

Chin

Hyoid bone

Laryngeal prominence (Adam's apple)

Thyroid cartilage

Point of insertion for cricothyroidotomy

Cricothyroid membrane

Cricoid

Rings of trachea

Point of insertion for tracheostomy

Sternal notch

• **Fig. 14.21** Cricothyroidotomy and Tracheostomy Incision Points.

- surgical blade
- curved arterial forceps and tracheal dilators
- small endotracheal tube of internal diameter 5–7 mm; if not available, then use any type of tube – metal, rubber or plastic

Procedure

- Feel for the laryngeal prominence of the thyroid cartilage (Adam's apple) – more prominent in men than women. If it is difficult to be certain, then identify the hyoid bone and work the finger downwards; if it is still impossible to identify anything above what is thought to be the thyroid cartilage, it is possible that what was thought to be the thyroid cartilage is in fact the hyoid. As the finger descends in the midline, there is a palpable gap between the thyroid cartilage and the cricoid. It is through this window that emergency cricothyroidotomy is carried out (Fig. 14.21). (Beneath the cricoid ring, it is sometimes possible to feel the rings of the trachea but this depends on how much subcutaneous tissue is present.)
- If time permits and the patient is conscious, insert local anaesthetic into the skin and subcutaneous tissues.
- Make a small transverse incision through the skin and extend this through the cricothyroid membrane; a hissing sound is audible once the trachea is penetrated. Alternatively, a Seldinger technique can be used.
- Use tracheal dilators and/or arterial forceps to expand the hole by separating the cricothyroid fibres (cricothyroidotomy set has appropriate instruments).
- Insert a small endotracheal tube (5–7-mm internal diameter) or any other appropriate tube that is available (normal tube sizes for adults are 8–8.5 mm for women and 9–10 mm for men).

Tracheostomy

This may be:
- emergency or elective
- percutaneous or open

Indications

Indications include:
- airway obstruction
- head and neck surgery
- laryngeal trauma
- failed endotracheal intubation
- prolonged tracheal intubation
- prevention of pulmonary aspiration

Emergency Tracheostomy

This is rare because cricothyroidotomy is the preferred emergency procedure. If the larynx has been completely disrupted by injury and the cricothyroid membrane is not intact, then an emergency tracheostomy is indicated. The tracheostomy procedure is the same as for an elective procedure except where indicated.

Elective Tracheostomy

It is preferable to relieve acute airways obstruction by endotracheal intubation or cricothyroidotomy and then to do an elective tracheostomy.

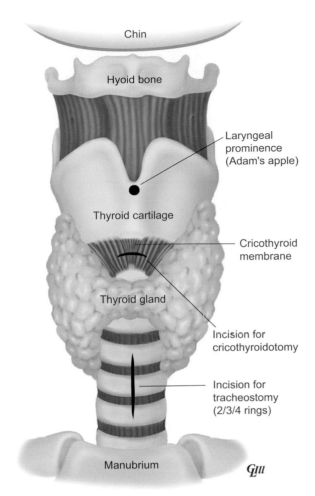

• **Fig. 14.22** Tracheostomy Technique.

Open Tracheostomy (Emergency or Elective)

Equipment Required.
- Tracheostomy set – usually obtained or used in the operating room (an operating room scrub nurse usually comes with the set).
- Tracheal tubes of internal diameter 8–8.5 mm for women and 9–10 mm for men. If the neck is very large in diameter and the tracheal rings almost retrosternal, then a long tracheal tube should be considered.

Procedure (Fig. 14.22). The procedure can be done under general or local anaesthetic and should be performed by an experienced surgeon:
- Ensure the patient's neck is extended as far as possible (in trauma, the possibility of injury to the cervical spine must be remembered and ideally an assistant should keep the head and neck central).
- Oxygen should always be given to the patient even if you think the airway is completely obstructed, because sometimes this gives the patient a few extra minutes without severe hypoxia.
- Make a transverse incision halfway between the cricoid and the suprasternal notch and between the medial borders of sternomastoid muscles. In an emergency, if the anatomy is unclear, a vertical incision can be made from

the laryngeal prominence of the thyroid cartilage to the suprasternal notch.

- Separate the strap muscles vertically in the midline through the investing fascia.
- Identify the thyroid isthmus, although it rarely needs to be divided in the adult and can usually be retracted upwards; in the child it is more likely to require division and ligation.
- Find the second, third and fourth tracheal rings.
- Incise the trachea vertically through the second, third and fourth rings; dilate the opening with either tracheal dilators or arterial forceps and insert an endotracheal tube (ideally 7–8-mm internal diameter) and attach the oxygen supply immediately.

  In an Emergency.
- After the insertion of the tracheostomy tube, bleeding is controlled with artery forceps and ties; often, the anterior jugular vein bleeds as well as the divided thyroid isthmus.
- Use a fine-bore suction tube to suck out the trachea.

  Elective and Semi-Elective Open Tracheostomy.
- Before the incision into the trachea is made, check the tracheostomy tube: inflate the cuff and make sure there are no leaks; deflate the cuff and then gently lubricate the cuff and tube with lubricating jelly. Check that the connector is compatible with the anaesthetic tube and oxygen supply.
- Insert the tube at the same time as the endotracheal tube is withdrawn; make an immediate connection to the oxygen supply.
- Do not allow anyone to remove the endotracheal tube completely until you are certain your tracheostomy tube is in the correct position.
- In a child, no part of the trachea should be excised, as there is a high risk of subsequent stenosis. Therefore, a vertical incision is made over the second, third and fourth tracheal rings and a heavy suture is inserted through each side of the tracheal incision; this aids dilatation with the tracheal dilators and allows the tube to be inserted. The ends of the sutures should be left long so that they protrude through the incision to facilitate re-intubation should the tracheostomy be accidentally removed.

The same method can be used with advantage in adults. Some surgeons excise a circular piece of trachea anteriorly and others use a distally based flap. Subsequent stenosis is less likely in the adult, whichever method is adopted.

Percutaneous Tracheostomy

Techniques. Techniques include:
- serial dilatation
- single tapered dilator
- guidewire dilatation
- forceps or screw

Indication. Percutaneous tracheostomy is indicated for prolonged endotracheal intubation to facilitate weaning and nursing care.

Equipment. Equipment required is:
- bronchoscope
- 100% O_2
- sedation

- analgesia
- neuromuscular blockade

  Procedure.
- Same position as for open tracheostomy.
- Infiltrate with lidocaine with adrenaline (epinephrine) over the incision site (1st and 2nd tracheal rings).
- Dissect down to trachea.
- Puncture trachea and insert guide wire or introducer.
- Check position of introducer/guide wire bronchoscopically.
- Dilate tract and introduce tracheostomy tube.

Complications of Tracheostomy

Potential complications include:
- loss of airway
- malposition or displacement of tube
- haemorrhage
- bacteraemia
- surgical emphysema
- pneumothorax
- occlusion of tube
- oesophageal injury
- tracheal injury

THE BASICS OF ELECTROSURGERY

Introduction

Electrosurgery is the art and science of converting electrical energy into clinically useable heat. In the UK it is often called diathermy. It is the commonest form of energy used in the operating theatre. In its historic and commonest forms, it is used for small vessel haemostasis or dividing tissue. More recently it has been modified to include larger-vessel sealing and tissue ablation.

Electrosurgery involves placing an electrical current across a patient to achieve its effect. The current is either applied between the ends of two electrodes such as forceps (bipolar electrosurgery), or between two widely separated electrodes in which there is one larger plate electrode and a second surgical instrument (monopolar electrosurgery).

In both cases, the electrical current, or electron flow, is delivered by a generator driven by a voltage and resisted by the impedance of body tissues. The effect is to deliver energy to tissue which then heats and denatures achieving the desired effect.

There are four basic concepts that underlie the understanding of electrosurgery. These ensure patient safety and an effective surgical effect. They are more apparent in monopolar electrosurgery.

1. The Patient is Part of an Electrical Circuit

By applying electricity to the body, all the factors that affect flow of electrons in a circuit will apply. In bipolar electrosurgery, the volume of tissue between the two electrodes is small. The impedance is therefore low and, in consequence, the voltage can be reduced to deliver the required energy. It is therefore inherently safer than monopolar electrosurgery, although less versatile. In monopolar electrosurgery, voltages are higher to drive the flow of electrons across a large percentage of the body. In consequence, a surgical plate placed closer to the operating site creates a safer and more efficient circuit by reducing the voltage required and improving the efficiency of the surgical instrument.

In addition, with monopolar electrosurgery there are a variable number of electrical paths between the surgical instrument and plate electrode. In general, the current will take the path of least impedance. This is important if the pathway includes a metal prosthesis or implant with which it may interact adversely. Similarly, if a plate electrode is placed over a bony prominence or scar, this may increase impedance, slow the flow of electrons and reduce the surgical effect.

2. The Electrical Current is High Frequency

The frequency of domestic alternating currents across the world are between 50 and 60 cycles per second (Hertz [Hz]). When applied to the human body, this can cause fatal electrocution even at relatively low voltages of 230 V (Europe) or 120 V (USA). Electrosurgical currents are also alternating currents delivered by a specialist generator but at frequencies of between 300,000 and 3,000,000 Hz (300 KHz and 3 MHz). At these frequencies, the current does not depolarize electrolytically active tissue such as the myocardium and electrocution does not occur even at voltages of 1000 to 10,000 V used in monopolar electrosurgery. In general, alternating circuits with frequencies over 100,000 Hz will not cause electrocution.

Observers of electrosurgery, however, will have noticed that muscle will twitch if the current is applied to its surface or in the close vicinity of a motor nerve. This activation is the result of galvanic stimulation, injury from the electrosurgical effect or lower frequency eddy currents generated by the electrosurgical effect.

3. The Surgical Effect Changes with Surface Area

As monopolar surgical circuits are alternating currents, both the patient plate and surgical instruments are 'active' and can generate heat. However, the ability of each of these electrodes to create heat is influenced by the surface area through which the current is applied. This physical property of high frequency alternating currents is termed energy density, current density or power density.

As the surface area of the current application reduces, temperature increases at an inversely proportional rate. Therefore, heating is greater and faster with small electrodes such as points, lower and slower with larger electrodes such as forceps or a blade and negligible at the plate electrode, which has an electrical transfer delivering less than 2.5 watts of power per cm^2. In this way, patient burns at the plate electrode can be avoided whilst achieving a tissue effect at the surgical electrode.

However, should a plate electrode become effectively reduced in surface area, unwanted heating and burns can occur. This happens when the plate conductivity is changed by skin preparation fluids, scars or the plate becomes detached. Fortunately, most modern generators are equipped to detect such changes and turn off the monopolar circuit to prevent burns. The patient plate should not be considered as neutral.

This effect can occur at any point along a monopolar circuit and result in unwanted heating where the current path narrows. It is responsible for unwanted coagulation of pedicles, adhesions to the bowel wall, digits, penis, spermatic cord or under ligatures and clips.

4. The Electrosurgical Circuit is a Source of Electromagnetic Induction

Any electrical circuit generates a magnetic field perpendicular to the flow of electrodes. In alternating currents, this magnetic field alternates at the same frequency as the electrical current. When a second conductor is placed in this alternating magnetic field, it will induce electron flow in this secondary conductor. Such induction can create unwanted secondary currents. An obvious manifestation of this effect is interference with a radio if playing at the same time as operating. This has led to the term radiofrequency electrosurgery.

Modern plate electrodes use this effect. The metal of the plate is separated from the skin by an adhesive gel and current is induced across the adhesive to the skin.

However, unwanted effects are seen when cables are wrapped around a towel clip to secure them or to a metal laparoscopic cannula, the latter being termed capacitive coupling.

Surgical Effects

1. Monopolar Electrosurgery

There are four basic techniques that can be achieved using monopolar electrosurgery:
- Cutting (also called pure cut)
- Cutting with edge haemostasis (also called blended cutting)
- Coagulation (also called desiccation or soft coagulation)
- Fulguration (including spray coagulation)

These different effects are achieved by changing the current output from the generator, the type of surgical electrode used at the operating site and how the electrons are delivered to the tissue at the surgical electrode.

The generator output is controlled by switches and subswitches often coloured yellow for Cut and Blended Cut or blue for Coagulation and Fulguration. These can be controlled by increasing or decreasing the power for each setting. All of these are in the control of and are the responsibility of the operating surgeon.

Cutting

This technique requires an output from the generator that delivers a continuous alternating current. It is delivered to the patient with an electrode that has a high energy density, such as a point or the edge of a blade. The current should be turned on prior to approaching the tissue. This open circuit increases the voltage, and within a few millimetres of the tissue a series of micro-sparks pass from the electrode to the tissue. It is these sparks that create the cut by causing cellular water to vaporize and cell destruction. Allowing the electrode to contact the tissue directly will therefore reduce the effectiveness of the cutting effect. Therefore, separating the edges of the cut with the fingers or by traction will assist in creating the cut.

By increasing or reducing power output, the surgeon can adjust the cutting effect to their own natural speed of working.

Cutting with Edge Haemostasis

When the sub-switch for blended cut is selected, the generator output is changed from a continuous alternating output to one that is broken into bursts of alternating current separated by an off time – an attenuated alternating current. This causes slightly deeper heat penetration than the cut edge, causing capillary haemostasis.

As attenuated currents contain a period in which there is no electron flow, voltage is higher to achieve the same energy delivery at any given power setting on the generator.

In all other respects this technique is identical to the pure cut technique.

Coagulation

This technique is used for small vessel haemostasis. It is suitable for vessels up to 2 mm in diameter. Current is applied to the vessel to slowly heat and occlude it by coaptation.

The technique uses the coagulation switch on the generator although, in practice, the output is an attenuated current similar or identical to that for blended cut.

A lower energy density surgical electrode is required such as a pair of forceps, the flat of a blade or a ball electrode. The electrode is applied to the tissue before applying the current. This avoids sparking and the higher surface area creates slower heating.

Over-applying current may cause charring and sticking to the electrode.

Fulguration

This technique creates a surface coagulation that is useful for oozing capillary beds. The sub-switch for this technique changes the generator output to an attenuated output with a long off time and therefore a high voltage.

The type of electrode is unimportant in this technique but most easily achieved with a blade or point. The current is turned on whilst approaching the tissue and within a few millimetres a rain of large sparks is formed. These are played across the tissue, creating a surface drying effect that penetrates for only a few microns into the tissue.

The technique relies on the reduced impendence offered by a bleeding capillary compared to surrounding tissue preferentially attracting the spark rain. It is therefore improved by swabbing the tissue before fulgurating.

Spray is a specialist form of fulguration in which the current voltage is rapidly and randomly changed such that sparks will vary in their conductivity. This improves the extent that the tissue is evenly covered by the spark rain.

Delivery systems that also use Argon to deliver the electrosurgical current make fulguration even more efficient and effective. It is often used in hepatic and splenic surgery.

2. Bipolar Electrosurgery

The bipolar electrosurgical current is applied to the patient through two electrodes, isolated from each other, in the same instrument. The tissue volume is smaller than in monopolar and the effect is local to the instrument as there is no long current path compared to monopolar. As impedance is lower, circuit voltage is lower. Bipolar currents are delivered from a separate output on the generator and a unique switch. The current is a continuous output in both bipolar coagulation and cutting.

Bipolar Coagulation

This technique is used for small vessel haemostasis. To achieve bipolar coagulation, the forceps are applied to the tissue across the vessel and the current applied until coagulation is achieved. It is important to keep the two ends of the instrument slightly separated to prevent current bypassing the tissue if the tips contact each other. Over-coagulation can lead to tissue sticking to the instrument which may tear the tissue on withdrawal of the instrument, and lead to further bleeding.

Although there is no current path along which heating may occur as in monopolar electrosurgery, heat may spread away from the contact point by conduction. Temperatures sufficient to cause tissue damage have been detected up to 2 cm from the point of contact. This effect is reduced by applying cool saline whilst coagulating, a technique used when coagulating close to delicate structures.

Bipolar Cutting

Historically, bipolar cutting has been difficult and clumsy due to the configuration of instruments and the difficulty in generating micro-sparks. However, with changes to the current and instruments, it has been introduced with good results into urology for prostatic resection alongside conventional monopolar resection. The technique requires higher voltages than coagulation and instruments are equipped with a second dragging electrode isolated from the resection loop. The technique is identical to monopolar cutting.

Monopolar Electrosurgery Safety

1. General Considerations

High-voltage waveforms and higher power settings are associated with a greater chance of all monopolar complications. As a general principle, keeping power setting to the lowest required to perform a task and using a lower-voltage output will minimize the possibility of all complications from monopolar electrosurgery.

If, during an operation, there is a decrease in the electrosurgical effect such that the power has to be turned up to achieve a similar effect, this should alert the surgeon to a problem in the circuit and instruments, cables and connections should be checked.

Monopolar generators are equipped with tones and alarms that are designed to sound when the main current is active or there is a malfunction. Turning these down means that members of the operating staff may be less aware of an impending complication and would not be advisable.

2. Patient Plates

Burns under patient plates comprise the commonest group of complications in electrosurgery.

Plates should be compatible with the generator being used, previously unopened, placed close to the operating field, on non-hairy or shaved skin, over a muscle bulk with the cable dependant to prevent its weight peeling the plate from the skin.

The plate conductivity is dependent upon the adhesion of the plate to the skin and anything that reduces this will create hot spots within the plate. This includes preparation fluid that infiltrates the adhesive, hairy skin that may lift the plate, high impedance scar or bony prominence underneath the plate and pressure on the plate from the opening of anti-DVT stockings.

Any effective reduction in the surface area of the patient plate will increase current density across the plate and the possibility of a burn.

Most modern electrosurgical generators are equipped with electronics that monitor patient plate conductivity and adhesion. These plates are split into two areas. A small interrogation current is passed between the two sides of the plate and any change in the resistance of this current triggers the generator to cut off the main electrosurgical circuit.

Where large reusable capacitive plates that lie behind the entire patient are used, these should be dry, free from debris and not come into contact with metal jewellery, all of which may create hot spots and burns. These plates bypass plate monitoring systems which will not alarm.

3. Current Channelling

The phenomenon of current density is applicable across an entire monopolar electrical circuit within the patient. If that path includes a narrow channel or a single (low-impedance)

artery, the cross section may be sufficient to cause coagulation at the site of narrowing and infarction at that point. This is thought to be the cause of necrosis of the bowel wall when coagulating bowel adhesions, infarction of the penis when using monopolar electrosurgery for circumcision, and infarction when used on an isolated testis or for finger and toe surgery. It may also be responsible for rare caecal fistulas from coagulating a ligated appendix stump or bile duct strictures following cholecystectomy if monopolar electrosurgery is used on the cystic duct.

Orthopaedic prostheses present a specific issue of current channelling because metal is of low impendence. The electrosurgical current will take a low impendence path preferentially and any heating effect between the prothesis and the bone has the potential to weaken bonding.

In general, the patient plate should be placed such that a metal prosthesis is excluded from the current path.

4. Cardiac Devices

Cardiac devices include implantable pacemakers, defibrillators and long-term ECG storage media.

Each of these are a metal implant and have the same interaction as an orthopaedic prosthesis. Both the pacemaker and defibrillator have cables that impact upon the endocardium at small contact points. This creates a potential high energy density area and an endocardial burn may interfere with the ability for the device to monitor cardiac rhythm.

Defibrillators recognize the radiofrequency current as a life-threatening cardiac rhythm and recording devices will fill its data banks with electrical noise.

In general, a cardiac device should not be included in the current path of a monopolar circuit and cables should be kept away from the device. If possible, bipolar electrosurgery should be used.

If electrosurgery is to be used during surgery, pacemakers are best turned to demand pacing only, defibrillators should be turned off for the duration of surgery and data recorders downloaded before and after surgery, discarding data from during the operation.

All operations, whether under local or general anaesthetic, should be performed with cardiac monitoring.

5. Glove Burns

Glove burns represent a clinical situation in which the operator or an assistant has become part of the electrosurgical circuit. This is most common when voltages and power settings are high, and gowns and drapes are wet from body or irrigation fluids, increasing conductivity between patient and the surgical team.

In general, surgical gloves do not conduct electricity so it is usually assumed that a burn from electrosurgery sustained by an operator is due to a glove puncture. This, however, is not the usual cause. Surgical gloves form a minimal barrier to radiofrequency currents, which can readily pass to an operator's hand by electromagnetic induction in situations where there is a preferential path through the surgeon.

Glove burns occur most frequently when the surgeon transfers the electrical current from a hand held electrode to forceps or a haemostat held in another hand or by an assistant. If a coagulation or fulguration current is being used and the operator turns on the current before touching the forceps, the current flow may be sufficient to pass through the operator rather than the patient. Similarly if the forceps are removed from the patient before the current is turned off, the preferential pathway is through the person holding the forceps. Where contact between and forceps is small the energy density is sufficient to melt the glove and cause a burn. In general, if low voltage outputs are used, power settings are kept low, forceps are held over a broad area, care is taken with wet drapes and care is taken applying and withdrawing the surgical electrode, such burns should not occur.

6. Laparoscopy

During laparoscopic surgery, the electrosurgical current is delivered to a patient using long instruments, with thin insulation, along cannulas that may conduct electricity, and used in a narrow field of view.

This creates the possibility of inadvertent injury from three mechanisms:

a. Direct Coupling

If electrosurgical current passes from the surgical electrode to any other metal instrument, cannula or retractor, this creates an alternate current path with the potential for a burn outside the field of view.

b. Insulation Failure

The insulation along many laparoscopic instruments may be only a few microns thick and susceptible to damage from repeated use. They should be inspected regularly, repaired or discarded when worn and single use instruments used only once. Denuded insulation from the tip or an instrument, such as a hook, exposes more of the metal tip to adjacent tissue and cracked insulation on the shaft allows for sparking to anything in contact with the instrument, especially when high voltage outputs are used.

c. Capacitive Coupling

Electromagnetic induction may occur in the laparoscopic setting either to metal cannulas or directly to tissue in contact with the shaft of the instrument. Metal, narrow, long cannulas will generate stronger currents with a greater potential for injury. This increases with high voltages and using electrosurgery in open circuit.

When a metal cannula is isolated from the abdominal wall with a non-conducting retention screw, currents will more readily pass to structures in contact with the cannula and this arrangement should not be used with electrosurgery.

The Laparoscopic Hook

The hook is a common electrosurgical electrode used in laparoscopy. It is a high energy density electrode that can be used to divide tissue using a cut technique against the heel of the hook or coagulate by direct contact, after which tissue is often divided by traction. Effective use of a laparoscopic hook for these two surgical effects requires the surgeon to apply a number of the principles already described above: contact and non-contact modes, changes in energy density at the tip and different generator outputs.

7. Technology

Over the years, generator manufacturers have changed and improved their products to improve patient safety and efficiency of the surgical effect.

Isolation of the electrosurgical circuit from earth by the use of a transformer between the socket and the generator has largely eliminated burns caused by contact between the patient and the metal of the operating table.

Monitoring of the patient plate has reduced the likelihood of burns at this site and this technology is used in some generators to also limit maximum powers in patients who have a low mass (e.g. children, the emaciated).

Recently, generators have been manufactured to measure the actual voltage and current being delivered during use. These generators ensure constant power across all tissues irrespective of impedance and deliver an improved surgical effect.

8. Fire and Ignition

Patient and operating fires require three components: fuel, an ignition source and oxygen.

In the operating environment, fuels can be found in drapes, alcoholic solutions, tubes, bowel gas and body hair. High dose oxygen is delivered by the anaesthetist or through nasal cannulas in some local anaesthetic operations, creating a high oxygen environment around the mouth and face. The surgical electrode is a potent ignition source.

In general, alcoholic solutions should be allowed to evaporate before placing drapes, care should be used around the face and mouth in local anaesthetic, ENT and oral surgery and when opening the abdomen in emergency conditions or opening the colon.

Vessel Sealing

Haemostasis using conventional electrosurgery can be used to control vessels of 2 mm or less. However, electrosurgical devices designed specifically to seal vessels can be used on arteries up to 7 mm.

There are three components to such systems: a set pressure across the vessel, a modified bipolar current, and closed loop monitoring of the current to ensure optimal sealing.

Vessel sealing causes collagen to denature and meld while leaving elastin unchanged. This creates a seal that closes the vessel lumen without making it susceptible to bursting under systolic pressure.

These systems are ineffective on calcified vessels and less effective on larger veins.

Plasma Electrosurgery

Plasma has been called the fourth state of matter and consists of a highly charged gas. Such plasmas can be created from radiofrequency current. Surgical instruments have recently been developed that can harness the energy of plasma and have been used to evaporate tissue or create a cut with minimal bleeding. These have been effectively demonstrated in plasma resection or contact plasma evaporation of the prostate using enhanced bipolar electrosurgery.

Another bipolar device designed for open and laparoscopic surgery creates a plasma that can be accelerated from an instrument tip as a beam which is focused or defocused on tissue for cutting, surface coagulation or ablation.

A further monopolar device uses a handheld blade to generate the plasma and creates a cut with reduced heat penetration into the skin compared to conventional cutting and is licenced for cosmetic and orofacial surgery.

These technologies are pushing at the boundaries of energy use in surgery.

Training and Credentialing

Since the development of the first commercial electrosurgical generator by William Bovie and first used in modern surgery by Harvey Cushing in 1926, the technology has changed and been modified beyond all recognition.

Modern generators are digital devices that may replicate some of the features of the original currents of the first 'Bovie' but have incorporated technologies that have enhanced patient safety and surgical use.

Many of the techniques and devices now associated with electrosurgery require specific techniques to make them effective and safe. Despite this, basic understanding and training in this field remains poor. Organizations such as SAGES and the Royal Colleges of Surgeons are addressing this through focused training programmes for trainees. However, as sophistication increases there are some who are calling for credentialing in the use of all forms of surgical energy.

15

An Introduction to Radiology and Diagnostic Imaging

CHAPTER OUTLINE

Introduction

There is no doubt that the practice of surgery was irrevocably changed by the discovery of X-rays in 1895 by Wilhelm Rontgen. Within months, systems were being devised to use X-rays for diagnosis and radiological equipment was even used in field hospitals during World War I. The development of imaging techniques led to the growth in the equally complex science of image interpretation and to the creation of the specialism of radiology. The development of cross-sectional computed tomography in the 1970s not only changed the management of acutely unwell patients, but also the diagnosis and treatment of cancer and chronic diseases. Imaging also plays a role in prevention of disease through the advent of screening programs that capitalized on specialized radiographic techniques such as mammography. Imaging now plays an increasingly important role in the direct treatment of vascular pathology and it has an application in the majority of surgical specialties. Interventional radiology is a rapidly advancing field where large laparotomy scars are being replaced with small incisions and a reduced morbidity.

In addition to ionizing techniques, non-ionizing techniques such as ultrasound and magnetic resonance imaging (MRI) have greatly contributed to the diagnosis and management of patients. The role of artificial intelligence technology and their application and interpretation is set to be the next revolution facing modern medicine.

This chapter will give surgeons a framework with which to understand the techniques and risks associated with various radiology imaging techniques and interventional procedures.

Requesting Imaging

Communication with the radiology team is critical for ensuring safe and effective diagnostic and interventional imaging. A request for diagnostic imaging requires accurate clinical information for scheduling of the appropriate test and for the precise interpretation of the subsequent result. Providing incomplete or inaccurate details can lead to delays in addition to a less clinically useful imaging report. As well as containing the clinical indication for the test and the minimum details required to accurately identify the patient, for example name, date of birth and a medical record number, the request must also contain details of how the patient will be attending the appointment and how to contact them to arrange this. It is essential that details of the requesting clinician's contact details, to clarify any particulars of the request and to feed back any critical or unexpected findings, as well as the details of the lead clinician, consultant or GP responsible for the patient are also included with the request. With the advent of electronic order communications these details are automatically shared when the request has been submitted via the electronic patient record (Fig. 15.1). It is a legal requirement that any request involving ionizing radiation is justified and requests without sufficient justification will be rejected or delayed when submitted to the imaging department.

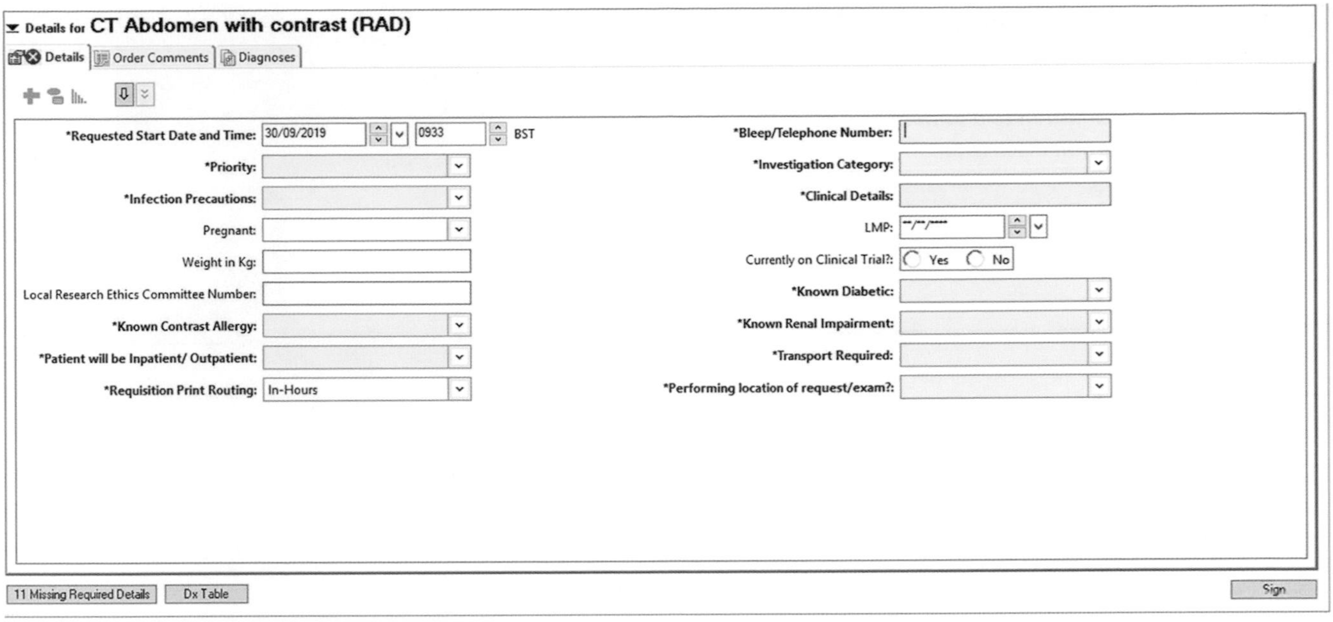
Details for CT Abdomen with contrast (RAD)

Details | Order Comments | Diagnoses

*Requested Start Date and Time: 30/09/2019 0933 BST

*Priority:

*Infection Precautions:

Pregnant:

Weight in Kg:

Local Research Ethics Committee Number:

*Known Contrast Allergy:

*Patient will be Inpatient/ Outpatient:

*Requisition Print Routing: In-Hours

*Bleep/Telephone Number:

*Investigation Category:

*Clinical Details:

LMP: **/**/****

Currently on Clinical Trial?: Yes No

*Known Diabetic:

*Known Renal Impairment:

*Transport Required:

*Performing location of request/exam?:

11 Missing Required Details | Dx Table | Sign

• **Fig. 15.1** An example order entry form for a CT Abdomen with contrast. This electronic order entry form contains important information related to the indication for the investigation for the patient. The essential items are highlighted in yellow. This includes the priority of the study and the risk factors for contrast-related nephropathy such as diabetic status and renal function. (© Cerner Corporation and/or its affiliates.)

When requesting a radiological examination, the clinical team must be aware of the patient's requirements for the mode of investigation and the contraindications and risks associated with the investigation. Any imaging investigation request must be discussed with the patient, who should be made aware of the risks, alternatives and reason for having the test. This chapter will cover most regular imaging investigations so the reader will be confident in the method, indications, contraindications and risks associated with these investigations.

Risks of Radiation Exposure

It is generally accepted that the overall exposure of the public to radiation is increasing from medical examinations. The effects of ionizing radiation can be split into those increasing the risk of cancer (stochastic) and those causing immediate cell death and tissue damage (deterministic). The deterministic effects are seen at much higher doses and these effects are the principles upon which radiotherapy treatments are based. Estimation of the risk of radiation exposure is based on data taken from studies of nuclear fallout, largely from the atomic bombs at Hiroshima and Nagasaki as well as environmental exposure at Chernobyl. The derived SI unit of Sievert (Sv) is intended to represent the stochastic risk of radiation exposure and is readily used to compare exposure to radiation. This takes into account the tissue being irradiated as well as the energy being absorbed. For example, organs such as the liver undergo more cell replication and are therefore more susceptible to stochastic effects. The Food and Drug Administration (FDA) estimates that a CT examination with an effective dose of 10 mSv is associated with 1 in 2000 risk of developing a fatal cancer. For reference, the UK's annual average radiation dose is 2.7 mSv.

Several protective steps are typically taken to limit radiation exposure:

1. Justification of the procedure. The Ionising Radiation (Medical Exposure) Regulations 2017 (IRMER2017) require every examination to be justified by a 'practitioner', which for most purposes is a radiologist. It is accepted practice for other doctors to be certified as practitioners, for example to justify fluoroscopy in theatre. Some order communications systems now have a clinical decision support built into their requesting systems to aid the referring physician by making the latest information available to them.
2. As Low As Reasonably Practicable (ALARP) protocol. This is used when deciding the imaging modality for the investigation. For example, a request for CT abdomen and pelvis for suspected appendicitis could be changed to an ultrasound abdomen and pelvis in a younger patient to reduce the radiation dose but still result in an actionable result from the imaging investigation.
3. Use of national Diagnostic Reference Levels (DRLs.) Each imaging department has a medical physics department which will monitor ionizing radiation equipment to make sure dose levels do not exceed safe levels (Table 15.1).

Radiography

Physics

Whilst in the imaging department, please refer to the images produced by X-ray radiation as radiographs and not X-rays

TABLE 15.1	Summary of Radiation Doses for Radiological Investigations, Lifestyle and Accidental Exposures: *This can be useful when explaining the risks of radiation to a patient as part of the pre-investigation discussion.*

Source of Exposure	Dose
Dental X-ray	0.005 mSv
100 g of Brazil nuts	0.01 mSv
Chest X-ray	0.014 mSv
Transatlantic flight	0.08 mSv
Nuclear power station worker average annual occupational exposure (2010)	0.18 mSv
UK annual average radon dose	1.3 mSv
CT scan of the head	1.4 mSv
UK average annual radiation dose	2.7 mSv
USA average annual radiation dose	6.2 mSv
CT scan of the chest	6.6 mSv
Average annual radon dose to people in Cornwall	6.9 mSv
CT scan of the whole spine	10 mSv
Annual exposure limit for nuclear industry employees	20 mSv
Level at which changes in blood cells can be readily observed	100 mSv
Acute radiation effects including nausea and a reduction in white blood cell count	1000 mSv
Dose of radiation which would kill about half of those receiving it in a month	5000 mSv

From https://www.gov.uk/government/publications/ionising-radiation-dose-comparisons/ionising-radiation-dose-comparisons

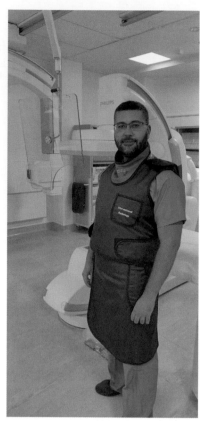

• **Fig. 15.2** This interventional radiologist is wearing a protective 'lead' apron. Note there are separate sections for his torso and body to improve comfort and coverage. Also note a separate thyroid shield. In the background of the picture, there is a protective glass shield to limit exposure from scatter rays.

as this term refers to the invisible photons that produced the images.

These are produced in a cathode ray tube in a similar fashion to an old television. The electrons bombard the anode from the cathode and are mostly converted to heat. However, a tiny percentage are slowed down by the metal atoms or collide with a 'bound' electron, shifting it into a lower energy state; the difference in this energy state is released by the emission of a photon of a specific energy. The composition of the anode depicts the characteristics of the energies or wavelengths of the emitted photons or X-rays. Most modern equipment uses tungsten or molybdenum as an anode as the range of energy is best suited for imaging biological tissue. The lower the energy of the X-ray photon, the more likely it is to be absorbed or attenuated by the subject's body. These photons do not help with imaging and only increase the patient's dose; therefore, a filter is used to remove the lower energy photons that are emitted. When an X-ray photon passes through the body, it can be attenuated by a number of interactions. The most important for dose consideration is called 'Compton scattering' where the interaction of a photon with an electron results in a photon of a different energy and direction. It is these scattered photons which are responsible to the dose to the patient and operator. This is why when taking an exposure, a shield or lead gown is used by the operator (Fig. 15.2).

X-ray detectors convert the transmitted photons into images either using a photographic plate or, more recently, using digital detectors. Live images such as those used in fluoroscopy combine an X-ray source and an image intensifier, which converts the X-ray photons into light, and these are then projected onto a TV screen. Most modern systems now use flat panel detectors, or FPDs, that directly convert the X-ray photons to digital signals and have greatly reduced dose as a consequence.

Clinical Applications of Radiography

The risks and benefits associated with radiation exposure need to be taken in context (Box 15.1). The interpretation of plain radiography is outside the scope of this chapter. Reporting these images is a complex skill and requires appreciation of technique, anatomy and disease processes. However, as a simple guide, consider that a radiograph is no different to a photograph where contrast and projection can affect the density of any projected image. For example, Fig. 15.3 shows how density can be affected by the projection. The clear distinction between two densities is a useful sign and, when combined with anatomical knowledge, can help clinch a diagnosis. This is particularly useful when looking for free gas in suspected perforations (Fig. 15.4).

Radio-Opaque Contrast

Technique

Standard radiographic techniques are often supplemented with the addition of a contrast agent to increase the desired contrast between a specific tissue and an anatomical space to answer a specific clinical question. A contrast swallow is a good example of this technique where a patient swallows a radio-dense contrast agent to produce an image of the oesophagus. With the advent of computed tomography, intravenous contrast agents are used on a regular basis.

• BOX 15.1   Summary of Radiograph Use

Advantages

1. Ubiquitous technique available almost anywhere
2. Easy follow-up
3. Tolerated by most patients
4. Quick
5. Simple interpretation possible without complex equipment
6. Non-invasive

Disadvantages

1. Requires skill and experience for complex interpretation
2. Minor radiation dose with increased risk of cancer, increased for children
3. Its use is limited in several conditions, for example back pain

---

Iodine-based contrast agents are divided by osmolarity (high, low or iso), ionicity (ionic or non-ionic), and the number of benzene rings (monomer or dimer). The enteric contrast agents can be broken down broadly into water-soluble and insoluble. Water-soluble agents include intravenous contrast such as Omnipaque and oral contrast agents such as Gastrografin or Gastromiro. Insoluble contrast agents are mainly barium salts. Excretion of the iodinated contrast agents is predominantly via renal excretion; however, in conditions such as renal failure, there is delayed excretion via the hepatobiliary system, hence contrast opacification can sometimes be demonstrated in the gallbladder in patients with extra-renal excretion.

Risk

It is important to add that most radiographic contrast agents are safe and there are very few adverse events. Fatal reactions to contrast media are rare, with an incidence of one in 170 000 injections. Obtaining consent for the injection of iodinated contrast material is usually not performed as it is considered to be safe; however, most imaging departments identify the patient's risk factors prior to the examination (Box 15.2).

It is not necessary to check creatinine for every patient; however, an estimated GFR should be obtained for all patients with increased risk. Although it is accepted dogma that contrast agents can cause an associated nephropathy, recent data, that corrects for confounding factors, does not support the increased risk of renal kidney injury after contrast administration. With this regard, severe renal impairment or actively deteriorating renal impairment should not be regarded as an absolute contraindication to medically indicated contrast administration. It is also well-established that there is no link between shellfish allergy over and above the threefold increased risk with food allergy.

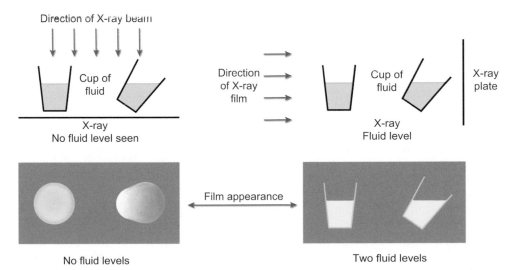

• **Fig. 15.3** For any 'silhouette' to be shown on a film, the direction of the X-ray beam must be parallel to the interface being depicted. In the case of fluid, the beam must always be horizontal regardless of the position of the patient.

A

B

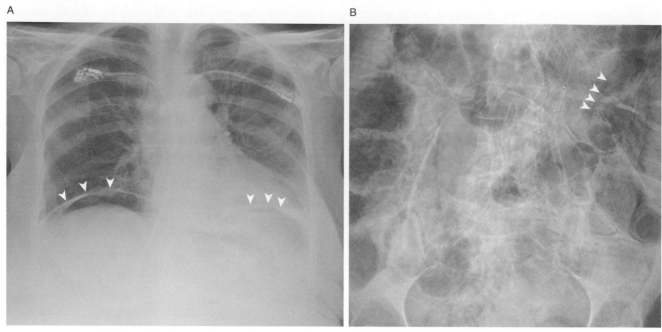

• **Fig. 15.4** (A) In this erect chest radiograph, the diaphragm is clearly depicted by the contrast of gas both superior and inferior to the diaphragm indicating a visceral perforation has occurred *(arrowheads)*. (B) In this supine abdominal radiograph, it is more difficult to appreciate the free peritoneal gas; however, the gas between the bowel wall and peritoneum depicts a silhouette of the large bowel indicating a visceral perforation *(arrowheads)*.

• **BOX 15.2** | **Risk Factors for Contrast Use**

- Previous reaction to contrast agents
- All severe reactions to medications or food
- History of atopy, asthma or bronchospasm (3–6-fold increased risk of reaction); suggest using non-ionic agents
- History of renal failure or cardiac disease
- Metformin therapy or diabetes

Contrast extravasation occurs when injected contrast no longer remains within the lumen where it was injected. This mainly occurs within the venous system via an indwelling venous catheter; however, it can also occur, for example when contrast leaks from a joint when injected for an arthrogram. Generally, intravenous contrast agents are non-toxic and the complications are mainly related to volume and a form of compartment syndrome which can occur. However, skin ulceration and tissue necrosis are also reported with very few requiring surgical intervention (Box 15.3).

Computed Tomography

Tomogram comes from the Greek words τόμος (tomos) which means slice or section and γράφω (grapho) which means to write. A tomogram is an image of a section or slice and was previously performed by rotating the moving X-ray beam and film in such a way so as to amplify the attenuation of the X-ray beam from a section of the subject being imaged, such as an orthopantomogram (OPG.) The first clinical X-ray CT scan was made by British engineer

---

• **BOX 15.3** | **Initial Management of Contrast Extravasation**

Initial Management of Contrast Extravasation (please refer to local hospital policy)
Elevate
Cold compress
Massage
Observe for worsening pain, tissue perfusion, skin blistering and change in sensation
Persistent symptoms at 2 hours or any of above – refer for plastic surgical opinion

---

Godfrey Hounsfield of EMI Laboratories, of Beatles fame. Hounsfield was later awarded the Nobel Prize in Physiology or Medicine for his discovery. A CT scanner uses an X-ray source and a detector rotating around a subject. Using the information from each position of the detector as it is rotated around a subject, it is possible to calculate the relative attenuation of a volume of tissue. The level of attenuation is measured in the Hounsfield unit (HU.) Traditionally, the HU is calibrated with water = 0 and the higher the Hounsfield unit, the higher the attenuation of the material. Each volume of tissue in a slice is represented as a pixel with its brightness corresponding to the HU. The ability for the eye to appreciate difference in grey scale contrast is exceeded by the range of HU (contrast resolution) produced by this technique. For this reason, studies are 'windowed' to allow appreciation of different ranges of contrast. For instance, lung windows allow depiction of airways and lung parenchyma all of a low HU range, whereas bone windows allow for depiction of bone quality using a high HU range.

Advances

With the advent of slip-ring technology, modern scanners are able to continuously rotate; previously, they had to de-rotate to stop cables getting stuck. This rotation can be achieved whilst moving the patient in a spiral fashion, allowing scans to be performed in a matter of seconds (Fig. 15.5). In modern scanners it is unusual to acquire images as individual 'axial tomograms' or slices; however, these still provide less noise as there is less scatter of radiation when used in this way. Multidetector arrays are used and are able to acquire up to 512 slices in one half rotation. With this technology, it is now possible to acquire a volume acquisition of the entire heart during diastole without any artefact from movement. With the advent of volume acquisition, it is also possible to produce an accurate three-dimensional (3D) representation of structures. This is very useful for surgical planning and visualization of, for example, fracture configuration (Fig. 15. 6).

Dual energy CT using either filtered or different X-ray sources allows for some tissue characterization and correction for artefacts. This has been shown to be useful in the assessment of gout, as well as optimizing metallic artefact.

With the advent of advanced photon detectors, such as those used in the large hadron collider, using photon counting technology will allow more specific tissue typing using

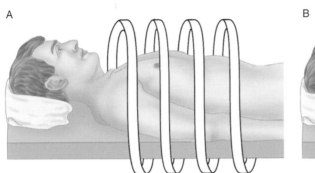
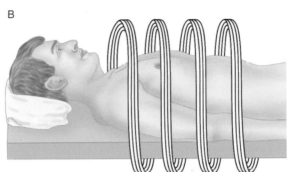

• **Fig. 15.5** (A) Diagrammatic representation of a single-slice spiral scanner in acquisition of data. The spiral is more stretched out (increased pitch) and thicker (greater collimation) than in real practice. Normally, the pitch is less than 2 (when the gap between the rings of the spiral is equal to the width or collimation) but greater or equal to 1 (when the rings of the spiral are contiguous but do not overlap). (B) The same scan with a four-slice scanner. The original width of the beam is now taken up by four separate beams, all a quarter of the original width. The multislice scanner can cover the same length of scan with thinner collimation, or utilize the same collimation to image a greater length of the subject in the same time, or a combination of both of these.

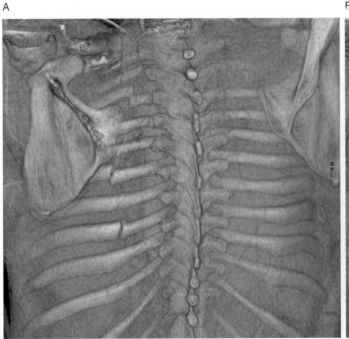
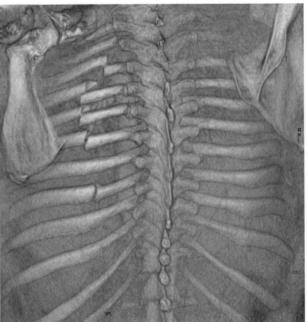

• **Fig. 15.6** (A) Soft tissue reconstruction of posterior rib fractures of a multi-trauma patient using a posterior projection. (B) For better visualization of the posterior upper rib fractures, the scapula was removed from the image using post processing software.

advanced spectral analysis and higher resolution images with reduced metal artefact (Fig. 15.7).

Novel reconstruction algorithms have been utilized to reduce patient dose using techniques such as iterative reconstruction, with some manufacturers also exploring convolutional neural networks as a method for dose reduction. However, this method still requires clinical validation.

Special Use Virtual Colonography

Double contrast barium enemas have been almost completely replaced by CT colonography as a non-invasive technique to assess the large bowel. They have been shown to be accurate, safe and better tolerated with a similar detection rate to colonoscopy (SIGGAR trial.) This technique is useful, for example, when colonoscopy is incomplete or the patient is not suitable for colonoscopy and, in the case of the former, it could be performed the same day in some centres. The bowel is emptied with a laxative preparation taken by the patient days before the procedure similar to colonoscopy. Residual faeces are 'tagged' by the timed ingestion of oral contrast. With the patient prone, the large bowel is inflated via a rectal tube with carbon dioxide to give what is called negative contrast to aid depiction of polyps. A virtual colonoscopy is performed using a computer workstation to 'fly' through the 3D-reconstructed CT images to identify polyps in a similar fashion to colonoscopy. Indeed, there are now computer-aided detection systems that have advanced to a level where polyps can be automatically identified and highlighted during the 'flythrough' (Fig. 15.8).

Nuclear Medicine

Physics

Nuclear medicine combines the ionizing radiation emitted from radioisotopes to the pharmacological properties of these isotopes and their derivatives to create specific physiological imaging information. The technique is unique as it has the ability to bind a radioactive isotope to a wide variety of molecules to produce a 'radio-ligand'. These molecules are designed to target a particular physiological property and, in this way, it is possible to combine imaging and pharmacology to produce a specific imaging technique for a specific disease process. The radioisotopes produce gamma rays, photons between energies of 50 eV to 150 eV, emitted during the radioactive decay of a radio nucleotide. Unlike CT or radiographs, the number of photons is very small and hence the imaging data contains a lot of noise. These photons are detected using gamma cameras specifically designed to amplify the detected gamma radiation. Many different radioisotopes are made in nuclear reactors, some in cyclotrons. The radioisotopes, especially the neutron-depleted isotopes from cyclotrons, have limited half-lives and nuclear medicine centres therefore tend to be near sources of isotopes.

Tomographic techniques using rotating gamma cameras are used in what is called 'single photon emission computed tomography' or SPECT. Combing gamma cameras and X-ray CT in one machine makes it is possible to use the CT data to correct for the attenuation of the emitted photons and also use the anatomical CT imaging data to fuse the functional and anatomical imaging (see Fig. 15.7). This hybrid technique has been shown to be very powerful for localizing disease, particularly in the skeletal system; for instance, when metal work is already in situ (Fig. 15.9).

The main other technique is 'positron emission tomography' or PET. This uses the unique physical property of positron emission, which produces two gamma rays of consistent energy (511 eV) at exactly opposite orientation to each other. Using this property, it is possible to calculate where the emission of the positron came from and to use this information to produce a more accurate 3D representation of the location of the radio-ligand. Combined with CT in the form of PET/CT, not only

A   B

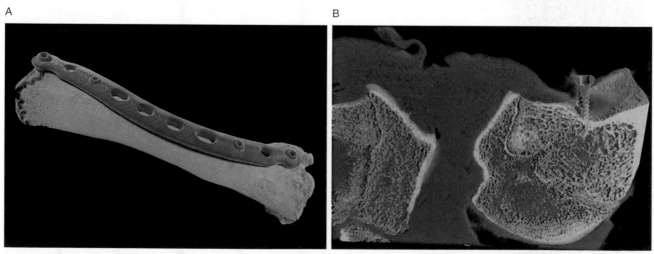

• **Fig. 15.7** A 3D volume reconstructed image of a spectral CT image of (A) a sheep's clavicle with titanium plate fixation and (B) a sheep's knee with femoral titanium screw in situ. Note the absence of streak artifact from the metal plate and screw and soft tissue differentiation. (Image credit to MARS Bioimaging Ltd.)

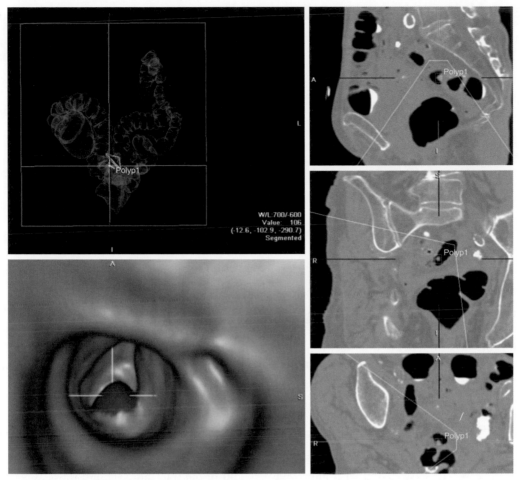

• **Fig. 15.8 Virtual Colonoscopy.** This image shows a 5 – up image view. In the left lower image, there is a computer-generated virtual colonoscopy image showing a highlighted polyp (marked *red*). The corresponding sagittal, coronal and axial images are identified in the right-hand column with a segmented colonoscopy projection in the left upper image indicating the position in the mid transverse colon.

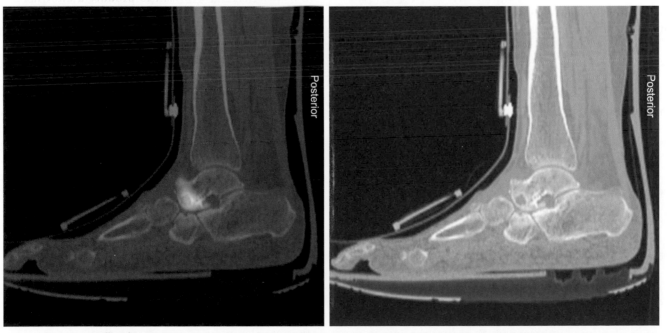

• **Fig. 15.9** SPECT/CT technetium demonstrating increased activity at the talonavicular joint where there is a subchondral cyst in the head of the talus. *SPECT,* Single photon emission computed tomography.

• BOX 15.4 | Indications for FDG PET/CT

Differentiation of benign from malignant lesions.
Searching for an unknown primary tumour when metastatic disease is discovered as the first manifestation of cancer or when the patient presents with a paraneoplastic syndrome.
Staging patients with known malignancies.
Monitoring the effect of therapy on known malignancies.
Determining whether residual abnormalities detected on physical examination or on other imaging studies following treatment represent tumour or post treatment fibrosis or necrosis.
Detecting tumour recurrence, especially in the presence of elevated tumour markers.
Selection of the region of tumour most likely to yield diagnostic information for biopsy.
Guiding radiation therapy planning.

Adapted from EANM guidelines 2015. https://www.eanm.org/publications/guidelines/2015_GL_PET_CT_TumorImaging_V2.pdf

TABLE 15.2 | Summary of Isotopes Used in Nuclear Imaging

Isotope	Symbol	Technique	Disease
fluorine-18	^{18}F	PET	Oncology
gallium-67	^{67}Ga	SPECT	Lymphoma/ infection
technetium-99m	^{99m}Tc	SPECT	Bone disease/ bleeding
thallium-201	^{201}Tl	SPECT	Cardiac
indium-111	^{111}In	SPECT	Infarction
krypton-81m	^{81m}Kr	SPECT	Ventilation

PET, Positron emission tomography; *SPECT,* single photon emission computed tomography.

is the attenuation of the gamma rays possible, it is now also possible to combine the physiological information with the anatomical information. The most commonly used radio-ligand in PET-CT is 2-deoxy-2-[fluorine-18] fluoro-D-glucose, or 18F-FDG. This is an analogue of glucose and identifies increased glucose uptake and glycolysis of cancer cells in the investigation of cancer. As a consequence, PET-CT permits precision staging of cancer and, in some cases, it is associated with improved treatment outcomes. Box 15.4 describes some indications for FDG PET/CT.

In addition to diagnostic use, nuclear medicine also has a therapeutic use. Indeed, several isotopes are used to treat cancer using radiopharmaceuticals to target tissue (Table 15.2). A well-understood example of this is using radioiodine (I-131) in thyrotoxicosis.

Risk

As with other ionizing techniques, the accuracy of nuclear medicine depends on the dose of the radioisotope used (see Table 15.1). As the typical radiation dose is one to two times the annual natural background radiation levels, this is low. This imaging technique is unique in that the patient is the source of gamma rays after the imaging has been performed, so they will continue to emit gamma rays. For this reason, special care is taken in patients who are pregnant to make sure there are strong clinical justifications and effort has been made to explore alternatives. In patients who are breastfeeding, the breast milk is discarded after administration until the patient is no longer emitting significant gamma rays. Some techniques do have a lower dose than their CT counterparts. For instance, a half dose VQ scan, used for the investigation of pulmonary embolism, is often used in pregnancy to reduce the dose to the mother and child.

Sonography

Physics

Ultrasound uses high frequency sound waves to interrogate tissue. A modern ultrasound machine uses a piezoelectric crystal to both generate and receive sound wave energy. These crystals sit in the head of the ultrasound probe or transducer. The speed of sound in tissues denotes the behaviour of the transmitted sound wave. When the transmitted sound waves interface with tissue with a different physical property and hence different inherent speed of sound, these waves are reflected, and the waves are then called echoes. The time taken for a sound wave to travel through tissue and to be reflected and returned to the transducer can be used to calculate the distance from the transducer to the anatomical structure of interest. The time and the amplitude of the echo can then be combined to produce amplitude or 'A-mode' images. Multiple waves may also be combined to generate brightness or 'B-mode' images (Fig. 15.10).

The frequency of the sound wave is a major contributor to the spatial resolution of the image. Generally, the higher the frequency, the higher the potential resolution of the image. However, it is important to note that an ultrasound wave is attenuated as it moves through tissue, and this effect is proportional to the frequency of the wave squared. Hence higher frequencies demonstrate a proportional reduction in the penetration of the ultrasound wave. Generally, a transducer with a frequency of 3 to 5 MHz is adequate to image most adult abdomens and a higher frequency probe (7–15 MHz) can be used for smaller structures such as the scrotum, neck, extremities and breast.

Doppler

The Doppler effect is named after the Austrian scientist Christian Doppler who described the phenomenon in

1842. When an ultrasound wave is reflected off tissue moving relative to the transducer, the reflected wave is changed in frequency. This frequency change is dependent on the relative movement towards or away from the transducer. In colour Doppler, red and blue are used to indicate movement towards or away from the probe. In the case of blood flowing in a vessel, the change in frequency is proportional to the cosine of the direction of movement relative to the direction of the ultrasound wave propagation. For maximum effect, a vessel would be scanned so that both the direction of the ultrasound waves and blood flow are in the same direction. In practice this is difficult, so the beam is angled to reduce the incident angle as much as possible and obtain better Doppler signal. The velocity of flow is calculated using the angle of flow to the ultrasound wave (Fig. 15.11). In addition to colour Doppler, power Doppler is another technique that uses the change in amplitude associated with the Doppler effect to depict flow. The advantage is that the signal is not dependent on direction and is very useful in the depiction of flow in smaller vessels with flow in multiple directions, such as synovitis, or detecting microvascular flow in organs.

Indications

Ultrasound is indicated in the evaluation of most visceral or soft tissue disease. In addition, the use of Doppler in vascular ultrasound can diagnose stenosis and occlusions within both the venous and arterial systems. Osseous conditions are generally not well appreciated; however, ultrasound can be used to diagnose joint effusions, periosteal collections and, using power Doppler ultrasound, the associated synovitis in an active inflammatory arthritis. Ultrasound is used in trauma screening in the form of a focused assessment with sonography in trauma (FAST) scan. This procedure is performed by trained clinicians with the clinical aim of finding free fluid to diagnose active bleeding in the context of trauma. Ultrasound is generally well tolerated by patients and, as a portable device, can be performed in clinic or on the ward, making it rapidly accessible. One of the drawbacks with ultrasound is that it is generally operator dependent. However, there is ongoing work to use machine learning to support non-expert users to improve diagnostic ability.

Risks

There is little evidence of risk associated with ultrasound; however, there is a theoretical risk of cavitation whereby

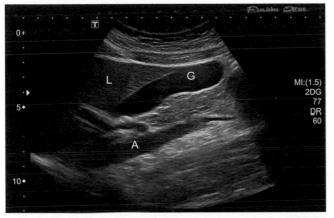

• **Fig. 15.10** Ultrasound B-mode image showing liver *(L)*, gallbladder *(G)*, and aorta *(A)*.

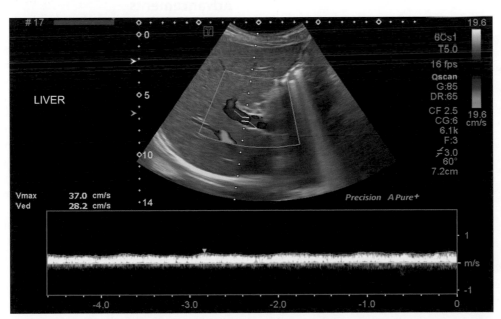

• **Fig. 15.11** Ultrasound doppler image superimposed on B-mode image of the portal vein. The red colour indicates flow towards the probe and therefore towards the liver and a graph depicting the speed of flow is shown below the main B-mode image using a marker angled to the direction of flow.

the sound waves can cause heating due to the collapse of bubbles generated by ultrasound wave energy.

Interpretation

The B-mode image splits tissues into echogenic (bright on B-mode) or hypo-echoic (dark on b-mode). Ultrasound is an excellent tool for defining tissue boundaries between different structures (Fig. 15.12). Indeed, if a structure is very reflective and attenuating such that sound waves fail to pass through, a phenomenon known as posterior acoustic shadowing occurs. This is often seen in renal or gallbladder calculi where crystals reflect the majority of ultrasound waves causing this shadow (Fig. 15.13). Remember this effect makes ultrasound a poor imaging technique for regular assessment of gas-filled structures such as the bowel. Similarly, the

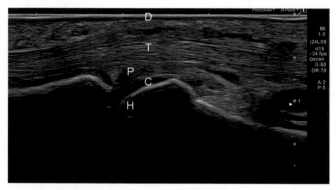

• **Fig. 15.12** B-Mode Sagittal Image of the Index Finger. This sagittal image through the index finger shows linear areas of increased echogenicity at tissue boundaries. The first layer is marked dermis (D). The tendon (T) demonstrates multiple linear echogenic lines depicting the multiple tendon fibres. The next layers depict the palmar plate (P), cartilage (C) and metacarpal head (H).

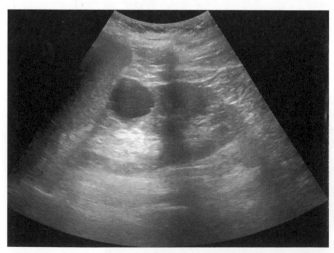

• **Fig. 15.13** B-Mode Ultrasound Image of the Left Kidney and Inferior Margin of the Spleen. This image depicts posterior acoustic enhancement caused by a large upper pole renal cyst. The tissues posterior to the renal cyst appear brighter than those at the same depth. Just to the right of this, there is an example of posterior acoustic shadowing caused by the overlying 11th rib.

opposite effect of 'posterior acoustic' enhancement occurs when a structure does not attenuate the ultrasound wave compared to the surrounding tissue, thus giving an apparent amplifying effect to the tissue posterior to this structure. This effect can be used as an acoustic window, for instance using a full bladder for the evaluation of a patient's pelvis.

Preparation

Most patients do not require significant preparation for an ultrasound study; however, it is commonplace that patients requiring a gallbladder assessment should be fasted to stop the gallbladder from contracting. A full urinary bladder is also required for a bladder scan and for transabdominal pelvic ultrasounds to provide an acoustic window through which the uterus and ovaries may be viewed unobscured by bowel gas.

Ultrasound Contrast

Contrast ultrasound is a relatively new technique. These techniques use microbubble technology to cause reflectivity. The injected microbubbles work by resonating in an ultrasound beam, rapidly contracting and expanding in response to the pressure changes of the sound wave. The size of the microbubbles mean they vibrate particularly strongly at the high frequencies used for diagnostic ultrasound imaging making them several thousand times more reflective than normal body tissues. Not only can this technique be used for diagnosis but also, by selective excitation, the microbubbles can be destroyed and potentially be used as a selective drug delivery device.

Advancements

The miniaturization of ultrasound transducers has allowed imaging of very small structures to high degrees of spatial resolution. For example, intravascular ultrasound allows the depiction of carotid or coronary vessels, allowing depiction of atheroma size, lumen and arterial wall to 100s of micrometres. This tool can be used to understand complex arterial anatomy and atheroma burden useful for identifying vulnerable plaque that may not be depicted by standard angiography. Other uses include endoscopic ultrasound, useful, for example, in the identification of enlarged lymph nodes for transbronchial biopsy.

Other advancements include the use of ultrasound elastography where mechanical deformation of tissue is performed either by manual pressure or by a sonographically produced shear wave causing tissue deformation detected by high temporal resolution ultrasound waves and converted into a sonoelastogram. This has been shown to be useful in the predication of malignancy in breast lesions and in the assessment of liver cirrhosis.

| TABLE 15.3 | Tissue Characteristics in MRI Sequences | | | | | | |

Biology	T1-weighted (Spin Echo)	T2-weighted (Spin Echo)	Proton Density (Spin Echo)	Diffusion Weighted (DWI)	Apparent Diffusion Coefficient (ADC)	Susceptibility Weighted (SWI)	Fluid-Attenuated Inversion Recovery (FLAIR)
Fat	Hyperintense	Hyperintense	Hyperintense	Hypointense	Hypointense	Hypointense	Hypointense
Acute haemorrhage	Isointense	Hypointense	Hypointense to Hyperintense	Hypointense	Hypointense	Hypointense	Hypointense
Water	Hypointense	Hyperintense	Hyperintense	Hyperintense to Hypointense	Hyperintense	Hypointense	Hypointense
Paramagnetic (Gadolinium contrast)	Hyperintense	Hypointense	Hypointense	Hypointense	Hypointense	Hyperintense	Hypointense
Oedema	Hypointense	Hyperintense	Hyperintense	Hyperintense to Hypointense	Hyperintense	N/A	Hyperintense
Tumour	Hypointense	Hyperintense	Hyperintense	Hyperintense	Hypointense	N/A	Hyperintense

Magnetic Resonance Imaging

Physics

Magnetic resonance imaging (MRI) uses the principle of nuclear magnetic resonance to interrogate the human body without ionizing radiation to produce images reflecting the underlying anatomy, chemical composition and physiology. In 2003, Paul Lauterbur and Peter Mansfield were awarded a Nobel Prize for their work which made the development of MRI possible, 26 years after the first human MRI images were produced by Dr Raymond Damadian using the first full body MRI scanner. Certain nuclei, such as protons in hydrogen atoms, possess a 'nuclear spin' based on the ratio of protons to neutrons. This nuclear spin absorbs or emits energy in the form of electromagnetic energy. Hydrogen atoms in water molecules (found in all human tissue) become aligned in the strong magnetic field of the bore of an MRI scanner. The frequency of the electromagnetic radiation released as these molecules align can be predicted by the strength of the magnetic field. This is given by the Larmor equation:

$$f_o = \gamma \, Bo$$

where f_o is the precession frequency, B_0 reflects the strength of the externally applied magnetic field in Teslas and γ is a gyromagnetic ratio giving a constant specific to each nucleus involved, in this case protons. When a patient is placed in the strong magnetic field of an MRI scanner, B_0, the nuclear spins of their protons are aligned to the main field. Once this is achieved, an electromagnetic radio frequency (RF) pulse is applied, causing the protons to absorb energy and to alter their nuclear spin alignment. As these protons return to equilibrium, energy is emitted as given by the Larmor equation

described previously. By applying additional magnetic fields called gradients that vary linearly in space, for example from head to toe, a specific section of the body can be selected to be imaged. The knocking sounds heard during an MRI scan are the result of these gradient coils experiencing a repulsive force due to the main magnetic field and hence the coils are often enclosed in concrete. These sounds can be very unnerving to the patient and often music is used to distract the patient. In addition, the bore of the MRI scanner can be very narrow, making it difficult for claustrophobic patients to tolerate. The main contrast effect in MRI imaging is based on the time for a proton to return to an aligned spin. This is influenced by two phenomena: (1) spin-spin and (2) spin lattice, described as T1 and T2 weighting, respectively. An MRI sequence is used to weight a particular image to one of these effects, hence the term T1 or T2 weighting (Table 15.3).

Contrast

The main contrast agent used in MRI is the heavy metal gadolinium, which is bound in a complex molecule. This may be injected intravenously to increase the contrast of blood vessels, tumours or differentiate between inflammation and infection. Very dilute contrast agents may also be directly injected into a joint in the case of MRI arthrograms.

Risks

As there is no ionizing radiation, MRI scans are generally considered to be safe. However, there is a risk associated with the high magnetic field. Until recently, patients with metal in their body would be at risk from heating and the movement of metal; this includes the iron oxide in tattoos.

Modern pacemaker devices are often MRI compatible but any patient with a pacemaker or other device should be discussed with the local MRI provider for suitability (Box 15.5).

Gadolinium contrast agents must also be carefully used in the context of renal failure where there is a risk of retroperitoneal fibrosis and gadolinium deposition. The European Medicine Agency (EMA) recently restricted the intravenous use of linear agents such as gadoxetic acid due to the risk of brain deposition. The risks of MRI in pregnancy are unknown; however, these appear much less in the second and third trimester. In these circumstances, it is advised that MRI procedures should be used for pregnant patients only after critical risk/benefit analysis, in particular in the first trimester, to investigate important clinical problems or to manage potential complications for the patient or fetus. Most units will have an information leaflet and a consent process for MRIs in pregnancy.

Interpretation

MRI interpretation is based predominately on tissue contrast. As previously described, the main contrast T2 and T1 and proton density are used to characterize lesions and differentiate anatomy (Fig. 15.14). However, several other techniques are used to increase contrast based on the properties of the desired tissue. Some examples of this are short-tau inversion recovery (STIR) and fluid-attenuated inversion recovery (FLAIR) where the timing of the realigning RF pulse is used to reduce the signal characteristics of fat and water, respectively. There are other techniques such as fat suppression where the inherent signal from fat is reduced using a variety of techniques. In addition, newer functional techniques such as diffusion imaging use the properties of water molecules diffusing in a restricted manner in cells compared to free diffusion outside of cells to infer cellularity of tissue (Fig. 15.15). As well as protons, MRI can be used to identify complex molecules using spectroscopy and infer information about the constituents of tissue and cell type prior to biopsy. In the future, many of these techniques will be combined into complex sequences that will be used to characterize tissue. The techniques of

> ### • BOX 15.5 | MRI Safety
> *Patient safety information that could preclude an MRI investigation and educates the patient to remove any removable metal objects.*

Risk

Pacemaker, pacing wires or heart monitor
Aneurysm clip
Deep brain stimulator, neurostimulator or cochlear implant
Programmable shunt
Heart valve/coronary stent
Medicinal patch
Artificial limb
Hearing aid
Pregnancy
Shrapnel or metal fragments in body or eyes
Dentures including dental plate or brace

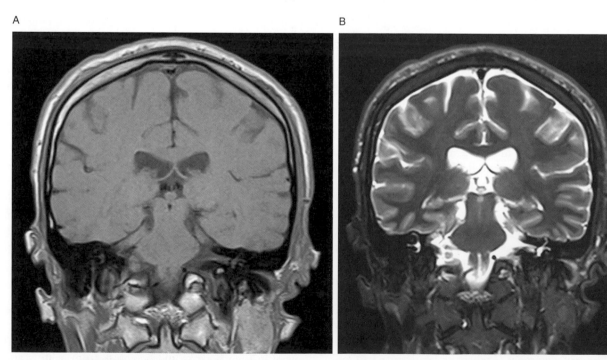

• **Fig. 15.14** (A) Coronal T1 image of the brain and neck. Note the cerebral spinal fluid spaces are low signal intensity. (B) Coronal T2 STIR coronal image. Note the previously low signal intensity fluid spaces are bright. *STIR,* Short-tau inversion recovery.

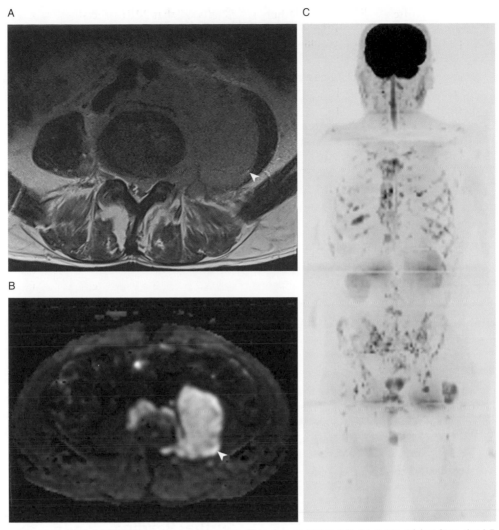

• **Fig. 15.15** (A) Axial T2 MRI on the lumbar spine. This demonstrates a large mass arising from the L5 vertebral body and extends into the left psoas major muscle group (arrowhead). The fat is depicted as bright on T2. The tumour is depicted in increased T2 signal intensity relative to muscle. (B) Axial diffusion weighted imaging (DWI) B1000 MRI image shows the same axial slice through the L5 vertebral body. The tumour demonstrates markedly increased signal intensity on diffusion weighted sequences depicting cellularity in keeping with a hypercellular tumour (arrowhead). (C) Maximum intensity projection of a DWI of a patient with multiple myeloma depicting multiple lesions in the skeleton, particularly in the ribs, pelvis and left greater trochanter.

synthetic MRI and MRI fingerprinting will transform both the acquisition and interpretation of MRI (Table 15.4).

Artificial Intelligence and the Future of Radiology

The term artificial intelligence, machine learning, deep learning and big data have recently been suggested as a panacea for modern medicine's workforce crisis. In 2016, the world economic forum suggested that healthcare's failure to embrace automation and a focus on expert labour had led to spiralling costs without the associated improvement in outcomes.

For several reasons, imaging lends itself to automation – the majority of the information is already digital, with most hospitals having a picture archiving and communication system, and radiologists are in short supply as a skilled workforce, taking many years to train.

Potentially, there are clear benefits in terms of safety and efficiency: an algorithm does not need to sleep, take breaks, and works consistently at any time of the day. Indeed, there are already clinically approved algorithms that can identify pulmonary emboli on CT scans and cervical fractures on plain radiographs. At the time of publication, there is evidence that an algorithm performing screening mammography outperforms human expert analysis. This degree of precision can improve the efficiency of a screening

TABLE 15.4	MRI Sequences, Tissue Contrast and Examples of When to Use Them	
Sequence	**Contrast**	**Example**
T1-weighted	Anatomical, bone marrow evaluation	Identify osteomyelitis in diabetic feet
T2-weighted	Tumours, oedema, fluid	Identify fistula
Proton density (PD)	Cartilage imaging	Identify cartilage defect
STIR	Bone marrow oedema	Stress fracture
FLAIR	Suppresses CSF signal in brain imaging	Identify multiple sclerosis lesion in the brain
In-phase and Out-of-phase	Fat content	Identify benign adrenal lesions
Diffusion weighted imaging	Identifies intra-cellular water molecules	Differentiate between cell death and oedema in stroke
Susceptibility weighted imaging	Calcium or blood products	Differentiate between blood or calcium in the brain

CSF, Cerebrospinal fluid; *FLAIR,* fluid-attenuated inversion recovery; *STIR,* short-tau inversion recovery.

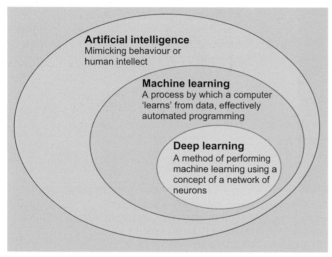

• **Fig. 15.16** Venn diagram showing the relationship between artificial intelligence, machine learning and deep learning.

programme, reducing unnecessary recalls and induced anxiety as well as improving the false negative rate and improving outcomes from cancer screening programs.

The success of deep learning or neural networks, an emulation of the interconnected neurons in a brain, in image processing has primarily led to recent successes in applying machine learning to medical imaging. It is important to recognize that deep learning is a form of machine learning which forms the basis of artificial intelligence (Fig. 15.16).

This is clearly a big area of change, similar to the rapid expansion of imaging after the discovery of X-rays mentioned at the beginning of this chapter, and with this, the job of a radiologist is going to change significantly, perhaps becoming more of a data scientist. Wherever this future lies, we must be mindful that all new technology must be proven to be safe and effective and that improving patients' safety and outcomes are the first priority. How these techniques are validated, monitored and regulated is an important consideration.

Further Reading

Adam A, Dixon A, Gillard J, Schaefer-Prokop C. *Grainger and Allison's Diagnostic Radiology A Textbook of Medical Imaging.* 7th ed. Elsevier; 2021.

Allisy-Roberts P, Williams JR. *Farr's Physics for Medical Imaging.* 2nd ed. Philadelphia: Saunders; 2007.

Brant WE, Helms CA. *Fundamentals of Diagnostic Radiology.* 5th ed. Philadelphia: Lippincott Williams and Wilkins; 2018.

de Lacey G, Morley S, Berman L. *The Chest X-Ray: A Survival Guide.* Philadelphia: Saunders; 2008.

McRobbie DW. *MRI from Picture to Proton.* 3rd ed. Cambridge: Cambridge University Press; 2017.

MHRA. *Safety Guidelines for Magnetic Resonance Imaging Equipment in Clinical Use.* 2021, https://www.gov.uk/government/publications/safety-guidelines-for-magnetic-resonance-imaging-equipment-in-clinical-use.

Raby N, Berman L, Morley S, de Lacey G. *Accident & Emergency Radiology: A Survival Guide.* 3rd ed. Philadelphia: Saunders; 2014.

16
Interventional Radiology

CHAPTER OUTLINE

Introduction

Interventional radiology (IR) is an innovative and rapidly evolving specialty. Image-guided minimally invasive procedures have increased the treatment options for patients as either adjuncts or alternatives to surgery. Some IR procedures have opened up options for patients deemed not fit for surgery, due to their low morbidity and fast recovery rates, e.g. ablation and irreversible electroporation (IRE) of liver tumours. Standard imaging modalities utilized in IR include: ultrasound, fluoroscopy, digital subtraction angiography, cone-beam computed tomography (CT), multi-detector CT and magnetic resonance imaging (MRI). These are utilized in an extensive number of procedures performed on patients from all surgical specialities. An exhaustive description of IR procedures is beyond the scope of this chapter. However, the modern surgeon must have a strong understanding of the basic principles of interventional radiology and its risks and benefits for specific surgical situations.

The Interventional Radiology Department

IR is now a recognized subspecialty of clinical radiology. To ensure patient safety, all hospital trusts should have access to a 24/7 interventional on-call service, and this level of service provision is now being widely adopted. Many interventional radiologists can perform procedures across the spectrum of IR. However, subspecialist radiologists may perform selected procedures, for example, a musculoskeletal radiologist with expertise in bone biopsies and joint injections. The IR team consists of interventional radiologists supported by radiographers and radiology nurses. The IR department is commonly within the radiology department of the hospital but may occasionally be partly sited in theatres. It will contain one or more IR suites (Fig. 16.1), a control area and a recovery area. An IR department will typically use imaging modalities outlined in Box 16.1.

The Hybrid Operating Room

A hybrid operating room (OR) combines a conventional operating room with an interventional radiology suite. Advanced imaging equipment, such as an angiography system, CT scanner or MRI scanner, is located within the operating room. This allows an operation which necessitates both open surgery and image-guided intervention to take place without moving the patient. Examples include fenestrated endovascular aneurysm repair and transcatheter aortic valve replacement. Cardiologists, vascular, neuro and orthopaedic surgeons make use of these ORs.

General Principles of IR

Pre-Procedure Planning

Requests for procedures are made to interventional radiology and some of these will have already been discussed at a multidisciplinary meeting (MDT). The requests are vetted by the IR department and often further discussion with the referring surgical team takes place. The extent of discussion with the surgeon depends on the type of intervention requested, patient factors, risks involved and requirement for additional support, e.g. anaesthetic support. Patients may be reviewed by interventional radiologists in clinic and procedures are usually

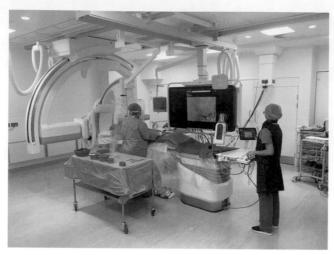

• **Fig. 16.1** An IR Suite

• **BOX 16.1** **Imaging Modalities Typically Utilized in Interventional Radiology**

1. Fluoroscopy: X-rays are used to obtain real time still images or videos, allowing visualization of iodinated contrast within the patient. Fluoroscopy systems will usually consist of a digital flat-panel detector which also has cone-beam CT capabilities.
2. Digital subtraction angiography (DSA): Only the iodinated contrast is visualized. A mask or control image is taken before the injection of contrast, and digitally subtracted from all the subsequent images. This allows detailed visualization of the injected contrast within blood vessels.
3. Ultrasound
4. Conventional multi-detector CT scanners
5. Cone-beam CT: Enables the three-dimensional characterization of vessels and adjacent structures without having to move the patient to a conventional multi-detector CT scanner, outside the IR suite. Cone-beam CT acquires information using a cone-shaped X-ray beam and high-resolution two-dimensional detector during a single rotation around the patient. A field of view of approximately 25 cm is achieved.
6. MRI
7. Neuroradiology suites in addition will have bi-planar imaging, allowing simultaneous imaging from two orthogonal planes.

---

planned following non-invasive imaging such as ultrasound, CT or MRI. The review of any imaging prior to a procedure is essential and allows the procedure time to be reduced, and therefore the radiation exposure to the patient and interventional radiologist is also reduced.

Haemostasis Considerations

IR procedures can be divided into low-, medium- and high-risk for haemorrhage. Table 16.1 summarizes these categories according to the Society of Interventional Radiology (SIR) consensus guidelines for periprocedural management of coagulation status and haemostasis risk in percutaneous image-guided

TABLE 16.1	CONSENSUS GUIDELINES FOR PERIPROCEDURAL MANAGEMENT OF COAGULATION STATUS AND HAEMOSTASIS RISK IN PERCUTANEOUS IMAGE-GUIDED INTERVENTIONS.

Low Risk of Haemorrhage

Dialysis access interventions
Venography
Central line removal
IVC filter placement
PICC placement
Drainage catheter exchange
Thoracentesis
Paracentesis
Superficial aspiration and biopsy

Medium Risk of Haemorrhage

Arterial intervention with access size up to 7F
Venous interventions
Chemoembolization/Radioembolization
Uterine artery embolization
Transjugular liver biopsy
Tunnelled central venous catheter
Subcutaneous port insertion
Intra-abdominal, chest wall or retroperitoneal abscess drainage or biopsy
Lung biopsy
Transabdominal liver core biopsy
Percutaneous cholecystostomy
Gastrostomy insertion
Spinal procedures

High Risk of Haemorrhage

TIPS
Renal biopsy
Nephrostomy tube insertion
Biliary interventions (new tract)
Radiofrequency ablation

IVC, Inferior vena cava; PICC, peripherally inserted central catheter; TIPS, transjugular intrahepatic portosystemic shunt.
From Patel, I.J., et al., Consensus guidelines for periprocedural management of coagulation status and hemostasis risk in percutaneous image-guided interventions. J Vasc Interv Radiol. 2012; 23, 727–736.

---

interventions, although local guidelines will vary and should be consulted. Needles and catheters are passed into the body without direct visualization of small vessels and without the ability to control them with vessel ligation. Therefore, certain parameters are checked prior to undertaking the IR procedure. The patient's haemoglobin, platelet count and clotting are checked and should be corrected if not within accepted limits. Anticoagulant medication should be appropriately stopped or reversed sufficiently. It is considered acceptable to continue aspirin but other antiplatelet medications such as clopidogrel should be stopped 5 days prior to most procedures. These guidelines are summarized in the addendum of newer anticoagulants to the SIR consensus guideline.[1]

Local Anaesthesia and Conscious Sedation

Minimally invasive procedures can often be performed under local anaesthesia. Conscious sedation, using a combination of short acting benzodiazepines and opioids, is used for more invasive procedures or where the procedure has a longer duration. Typically, this consists of intravenous opiate analgesia (e.g. fentanyl) and a short-acting sedative (e.g. midazolam) used in titrated doses with patient oxygen and monitoring. A typical starting dose is 25–50 µg of fentanyl and 1 mg of midazolam. Patients should have the capacity to consent to the procedure and they will need to be able to lie still for the duration of the interventional procedure. General anaesthesia is required only when patients are unable to lie still, or in selected interventional cases which are painful, long or where the patient is unstable. As a general guide, patients should fast for 6 hours prior to an IR procedure that requires sedation, although this may vary according to the procedure or local policy.

Informed Consent and WHO Checklist

Informed consent is obtained by the interventional radiologist prior to any interventional procedure. The World Health Organization (WHO) surgical safety checklist is used for all IR procedures. An example is shown in Fig. 16.2.

Biopsy

Image-guided core biopsy and fine needle aspiration cytology (FNAC) are commonly performed to confirm the tissue

diagnosis, or to stratify the risk of malignancy in the case of cytology, prior to surgical extirpation. Core biopsy needles obtain a tissue specimen of approximately 1 mm by 20 mm. The needle consists of an inner stylet with a specimen notch, into which the tissue prolapses, and an outer cutting needle which cuts the tissue when advanced over the inner stylet (Fig. 16.3). Typically, at least two adequate cores of tissue are taken and placed in formalin or saline as appropriate. FNAC consists of passing a small needle (often 21 gauge) multiple times through the lesion with or without suction applied with a syringe. The contents are gently ejected onto cytology slides and a cytology fixing agent may be added, or, alternatively, a system such as ThinPrep may be used according to the centre.

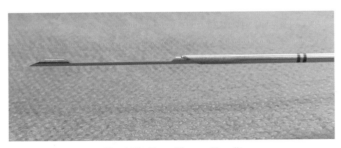

• **Fig. 16.3** Core Biopsy Needle

WHO surgical safety checklist for radiological interventions ONLY
Imaging directorate

☐ HH   ☐ SMH   ☐ CXH

Imperial College Healthcare NHS
NHS Trust

SIGN IN (to be read out loud) ⟶

Before induction of LOCAL (In recovery)
OR
Before induction of GA (in IR room)
RESPONSIBILITY INTERVENTIONAL RADIOLOGIST and if present ANAESTHETIST

Patient identity confirmed and consent form signed?
☐ Yes

Procedure *site* or/and *side* marked?
☐ Yes   ☐ N/A

Any allergies (including contrast media)?
☐ Yes   ☐ No

Risk of >500ml blood loss (7ml/kg in children)?
☐ No   ☐ Yes (adequate IV access/bloods)

Blood result (incl renal/Coag):
☐ Checked   ☐ N/A
☐ Normal   ☐ Abnormal–what measures taken?

Is the patient anti-coagulated?
☐ Yes   ☐ No

FOR SEDATION and GA CASES   YES ☐   N/A ☐
Aspiration risk? (NBM/loose dentures)
☐ No
☐ Yes, measures taken and equipment/assistance available
Has the appropriate medication been prescribed prior to the procedure?
Yes ☐   N/A ☐

FOR GA CASES ONLY   YES ☐   N/A ☐
Anaesthetic machine and monitoring equipment check complete?
☐ Yes   ☐ No

RADIOGRAPHER
IRMER requirements (incl. LMP)? ☐ Yes

RESPONSIBLE RADIOLOGIST	ANAESTHETIST
Name:	
Position: Consultant IR / IR fellow/ Rad SPR	Consultant/SPR/ fellow
Signature:	
Date:	

THE CHECKLIST IS FOR RADIOLOGY INTERVENTIONS ONLY

TIME OUT (to be read out loud) ⟶

Before start of radiological intervention (before scrubbing up)- IN THE IR ROOM
RESPONSIBILITY OF INTERVENTIONAL RADIOLOGIST
ALL team members to be present

Team members introduce themselves by name/role? ☐ Yes

Patient's name?   ☐ Yes
Procedure, site and position?   ☐ Yes
Radiologist:
• Any critical steps in this case?   ☐ Yes   ☐ No
• Specific equipment required?   ☐ Yes   ☐ No
• Essential imaging reviewed and/or displayed?
                                      ☐ Yes   ☐ N/A
• VTE prophylaxis required?   ☐ Yes   ☐ No

Anaesthetist: Present ☐   N/A ☐
• Any patient specific concerns?   ☐ Yes   ☐ No
• ASA grade?   ☐ Yes
• Monitoring equipment and additional levels of support needed?   ☐ Yes   ☐ No

Nurse:
• Monitoring equipment check complete?   ☐ Yes
• Any issues or concerns?   ☐ Yes   ☐ No

Has the surgical site infection (SSI) bundle been undertaken?   ☐ Yes   ☐ N/A
• Antibiotic prophylaxis within the last 60 minutes
• Patient warming/ hair removal
• Glycaemic control

RESPONSIBLE RADIOLOGIST
Name:
Position: Consultant IR / IR fellow/ Rad SPR
Signature:
Date:
PATIENT DETAILS
Last name:
First name:
DOB
MRN

SIGN OUT (to be read out loud) ⟶

Before any member of the team leaves the interventional radiology suite
RESPONSIBILITY OF INTERVENTIONAL RADIOLOGIST

Name of procedure recorded?
☐ Yes

Instruments, swabs and sharp counts complete?
☐ Yes

Implanted devices recorded?
☐ Yes   ☐ N/A

Specimens labelled?
☐ Yes   ☐ N/A

Equipment problems identified?
☐ Yes   ☐ No

All cannulae have been identified and /or removed or adequately flushed.
☐ Yes   ☐ N/A

All IV administration sets and extension sets without active flow have been removed.
☐ Yes   ☐ N/A

Radiologist, anaesthetist and registered practitioner:

Any key concerns for recovery/management of this patient?   ☐ Yes   ☐ No
Post-op instructions?
☐ Yes
  ○ Obs:
  ○ Medications: Antibiotics/dual platelet therapy
  ○ Bed rest duration :

RESPONSIBLE RADIOLOGIST
Name:
Position
Signature:
Date

Remember to scan COMPLETED WHO checklist onto Soliton

This modified checklist should not be used for other surgical procedures. This checklist contains the core content for England and Wales (V15)

• **Fig. 16.2** WHO Checklist (Courtesy Imperial College Healthcare NHS Trust)

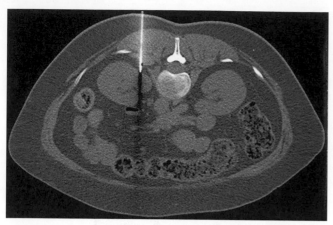

• **Fig. 16.4** CT-Guided Biopsy Case Demonstrates a Small Medial Renal Lesion with a Co-Axial Needle Inserted to the Edge of the Lesion

---

• BOX 16.2 Seldinger Technique

1. The intended vessel, organ or fluid collection is punctured with a sharp hollow needle.
2. A wire is passed through the needle.
3. The needle is removed over the wire.
4. A catheter, drain or sheath is inserted over the wire and into the intended location.

Ultrasound does not use ionizing radiation and is used as the first choice because ultrasound enables real-time imaging to guide the biopsy or FNAC needle placement into the lesion. If the target to be biopsied cannot be visualized adequately with ultrasound, CT guidance may be used. Fig. 16.4 demonstrates an axial CT image with the patient lying prone. There is a small medial renal lesion with a co-axial needle inserted to the edge of the lesion. Once CT confirms correct position of the co-axial needle, the biopsy needle is inserted through the co-axial needle and core biopsies taken.

Seldinger Technique and Drain Insertion

Dr Sven Ivar Seldinger, a Swedish radiologist, introduced the Seldinger technique in 1953 in order to achieve safe access into blood vessels. The modified Seldinger technique (Box 16.2; Fig. 16.5) is now utilized to achieve safe access into vessels and hollow organs. This technique is used in numerous IR procedures, from the drainage of postoperative collections and nephrostomy insertion to arterial and venous access.

Embolization

Embolization is the intentional occlusion of blood vessels and is usually performed to stop haemorrhage or in the treatment of some benign and malignant tumours. Examples of embolization procedures will be described in the following sections. Digital subtraction angiography is used to delineate

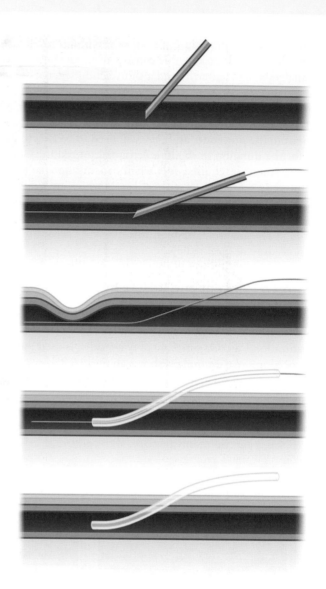

• **Fig. 16.5** Modified Seldinger Technique Diagram

the vessel anatomy and the path that the interventional radiologist must negotiate with wires and catheters in order to select the target vessel or vessels as selectively as possible. Wires and catheters come in a wide range of shapes and sizes. A variety of embolic agents is available and used in different procedures: particulate agents (e.g. polyvinyl alcohol (PVA), gelatin foam), liquid agents (e.g. cyanoacrylate (glue), ethylene vinyl alcohol copolymer (Onyx), sclerosants), mechanical occlusion devices (e.g. coils, detachable plugs, balloons).

SUBSPECIALIST IR PROCEDURES

Urology

Nephrostomy Insertion and Ureteric Stenting

A nephrostomy is a percutaneous drain in the renal pelvis (Fig. 16.6). Indications include obstructive uropathy due

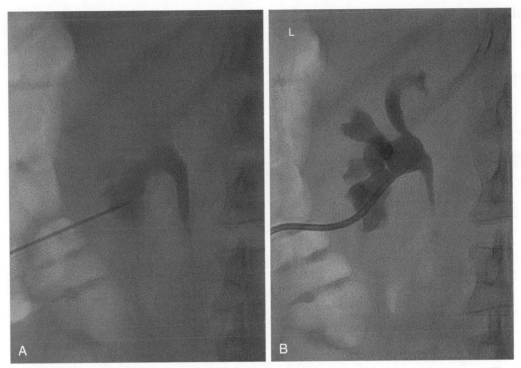

• **Fig. 16.6** (A) Contrast injected through an insertion needle within the lower pole calyx of a kidney. (B) Contrast injected through a pigtail nephrostomy catheter within the renal pelvis.

to an intraluminal calculus or tumour, or extrinsic compression from tumour or inflammation; urinary diversion to treat a urine leak; access for antegrade ureteric stent insertion; and access for percutaneous nephrolithotomy (PCNL). In the acute setting of obstructive uropathy and urinary tract infection, a nephrostomy is often chosen over retrograde ureteric stenting by the urologist. However, trials have not demonstrated superiority of one modality of decompression over the other in the presence of infection. A nephrostomy is performed with the patient under conscious sedation. Intravenous antibiotics are administered prophylactically, typically a cephalosporin +/- gentamicin. The patient is positioned so that the kidney can be imaged by ultrasound, normally in the prone or semi-prone position. Needle access is preferentially into a lower pole calyx as this typically avoids major renal artery branches. A locking pigtail drainage catheter is inserted using Seldinger technique and attached to a drainage bag in order to drain freely. Once the urinary system is free of infection, the nephrostomy can be converted to a ureteric stent under fluoroscopic guidance. Injection of iodinated contrast through the nephrostomy (nephrostogram) can characterize the ureteric stricture or obstruction and a wire and catheter are used to negotiate past the stricture under fluoroscopic guidance and into the bladder. A double-J ureteric stent can then be inserted antegrade through the nephrostomy access.

Embolization of Renal Tumours

Indications for renal tumour embolization include palliation for advanced stage renal cell carcinoma (RCC), preoperative embolization before nephrectomy, an adjunctive technique to thermal ablation and treatment for angiomyolipoma (AML). AMLs are considered for embolization if symptomatic due to haemorrhage, flank pain or mass effect. AMLs larger than 4 cm have an increased rate of haemorrhage and symptoms, so are considered for prophylactic embolization (Fig. 16.7). RCCs are sometimes preoperatively embolized with particulate agents, e.g. PVA and gelfoam, or alcohol in order to reduce blood loss during nephrectomy, although this practice varies between centres.

Varicocoele Embolization

Varicocoeles are dilated pampiniform plexus veins in the scrotum which develop secondary to incompetent draining testicular veins. Varicocoele occurs in approximately 15% of men and can cause discomfort. Men who are infertile or sub-fertile have been found to have a higher incidence of varicocoele. Varicocoele embolization is an alternative to surgery and can be performed as an outpatient procedure. Access is via the common femoral veins or internal jugular veins. The left testicular vein drains to the left renal vein and is more commonly affected. The right testicular vein has a variable drainage to the inferior vena cava (IVC) or right renal vein. The testicular veins can be catheterized selectively and embolized with coils +/- a sclerosant.

Prostate Artery Embolization

A more recent procedure which has demonstrated a significant improvement in symptoms and quality of life is

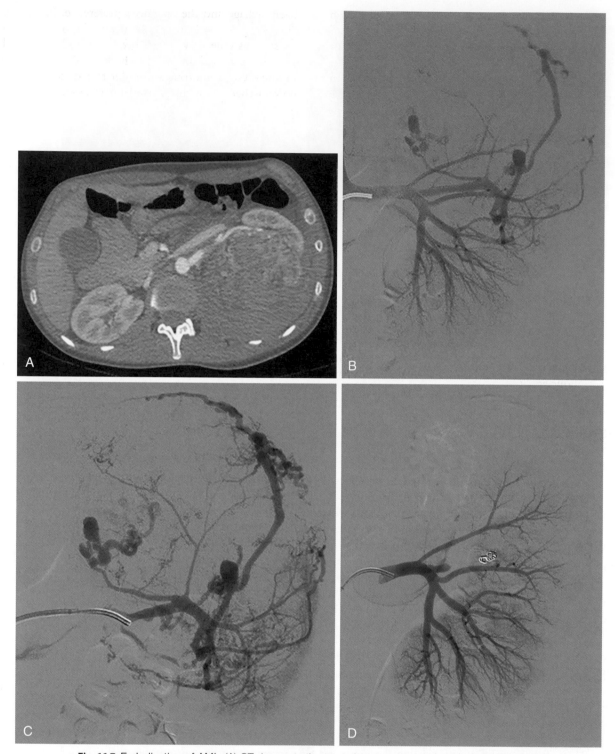

• **Fig. 16.7** Embolization of AML (A) CT demonstrating acute haematoma surrounding an AML. (B) DSA images demonstrating the renal artery angiogram. (C) Selective angiogram of the AML. (D) Renal angiogram post-embolization of the AML with PVA particles and coils and preserved normal renal parenchyma. *AML,* Angiomyolipoma; *CT,* computed tomography; *DSA,* digital subtraction angiography; *PVA,* polyvinyl alcohol.

prostate artery embolization for benign prostatic hyperplasia (BPH). This can be challenging because of the often-atherosclerotic arteries and careful preprocedural planning and imaging with arterial phase contrast-enhanced CT is performed.

Upper and Lower GI

Embolization for GI Haemorrhage

Angiography and embolization are part of the treatment algorithm for non-variceal GI haemorrhage. For upper GI bleeding (Box 16.3), endoscopy remains the intervention of choice as this enables both diagnosis and treatment of haemorrhage in the majority of cases. If unsuccessful, or in cases of lower GI haemorrhage when endoscopy is more difficult, a CT angiogram and percutaneous embolization may be performed. A triple-phase contrast-enhanced CT scan can accurately locate the site of haemorrhage. The non-contrast scan gives a baseline. For active haemorrhage to be diagnosed, there should be an increase in the amount of contrast within the bowel demonstrated between the arterial and portal-venous phase scans (Fig. 16.8). CT can detect haemorrhage at a rate of 0.3 mL/min and is more sensitive than angiography (0.5 to 1.0 mL/min). CT prior to embolization is not always required, for example, if the site has been clipped at endoscopy, which has failed to control the haemorrhage. Prior to and at the time of embolization, patients should be adequately resuscitated, correcting hypotension and coagulopathy. Embolic agents are less effective in the coagulopathic patient. Arterial access is usually via the common femoral artery. Selective angiograms using digital subtraction angiography (DSA) are performed and the site of arterial extravasation can be identified. That artery is then selected using catheters, wires and microcatheters as necessary. The embolic agent of choice will depend on the site of

haemorrhage and the operator's preference. Particle embolization with gelatin foam, PVA particles or liquid embolics such as glue may be used for upper GI haemorrhage. Coils are also used throughout the GI tract, and particularly in lower GI haemorrhage in order to reduce the chance of bowel ischaemia by distal arterial occlusion.

Gastrostomy

Radiologically inserted gastrostomy (RIG) is an alternative to percutaneous endoscopic gastrostomy (PEG). Both RIG and PEG have replaced surgical gastrostomy in the majority of instances. Gastrostomy is indicated when patients have inadequate nutritional intake because of dysphagia caused by neurological disorders, surgery and radiation for head and neck cancers, or oesophageal obstruction. Gastrostomy is also inserted for gastric decompression. RIG involves insertion of a wire and sheath through the anterior abdominal wall and into the stomach using fluoroscopic guidance and Seldinger technique. A balloon-retained or pigtail catheter can then be inserted. Alternatively, the same tube as used for PEG can be inserted by first negotiating the wire up the oesophagus and out through the mouth, then the gastrostomy tube is inserted over this wire and pulled out through the anterior abdominal wall with the disc bumper remaining in the stomach. Contraindications to RIG include sepsis, haemodynamic instability, total gastrectomy, active peritonitis, bowel ischaemia and gastric varices. Relative contraindications, due to the higher complication rates, include ventriculoperitoneal shunt, ascites, partial gastrectomy, oesophagectomy with gastric pull-through, colonic interposition and patients on long-term steroids or immunosuppression. Risks of the procedure and post procedure

---

• BOX 16.3 Upper GI Bleeding

- Resuscitation of patient
- Endoscopy +/– treatment
- CT angiogram (triple phase) and/or catheter angiography +/– embolization

---

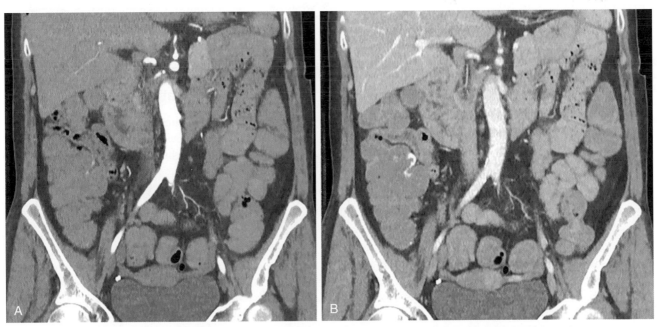

• Fig. 16.8 Post Polypectomy During Colonoscopy Coronal CT images in the (A) arterial phase followed by the (B) portal venous phase depicting an increase in contrast extravasation into the lumen of the ascending colon consistent with active lower GI haemorrhage.

include haemorrhage, infection, peritonitis and displacement and blockage of the gastrostomy tube.

Oesophageal, Duodenal and Colonic Stenting

Uncovered and covered expandable metal stents can be inserted using fluoroscopic guidance instead of, or in combination with, endoscopy. Indications include inoperable oesophageal, gastric and descending or sigmoid colon tumours. Oesophageal stents are mostly covered and are used to palliate dysphagia. They can also be used in selected cases of oesophageal fistula, perforation and benign strictures refractory to balloon dilatation. Oesophageal stents are available with a one-way valve to prevent reflux. Duodenal stents are placed for gastric outlet obstruction and are usually inserted via the mouth, but can be inserted by creating a gastrostomy in difficult cases. Left-sided colonic obstruction due to malignancy can be palliated with colonic stent insertion. These are often performed in conjunction with an endoscopist. Meta-analyses comparing colonic stent insertion with emergency surgery as palliation demonstrated lower postoperative mortality, reduced hospital stay and earlier commencement of chemotherapy.[2,3] Stent migration is less likely with the newer stents but oesophageal or bowel perforation is a risk, and therefore stents should not be post-dilated with a balloon.

Hepatobiliary

Interventional oncology is a fast-evolving field of IR and has had a huge impact in the management of hepatic malignancies. Hepatic malignancies include hepatocellular carcinoma (HCC), primary intrahepatic cholangiocarcinoma and colonic and neuroendocrine metastases, as well as metastases from numerous other primaries. Some of these procedures are detailed below.

Portal Vein Embolization

For patients with primary hepatic malignances or metastases who are considered candidates for major liver resection, the remnant liver volume must be adequate for hepatic function. Once the extent of liver resection has been determined, the future liver remnant (FLR) can be estimated from the CT. This is usually in patients undergoing a right hepatectomy or extended right hepatectomy (resection of the right liver and segment four). In patients with healthy underlying liver, if the FLR is less than 20% of its total volume, portal vein embolization (PVE) should be performed approximately 4 to 6 weeks prior to surgical resection to reduce rates of postoperative liver insufficiency. The main blood supply to the liver is from the portal vein. PVE redirects portal vein flow and improves the function and hypertrophies the non-embolized or FLR. Cirrhotic livers will require a larger FLR compared to healthy underlying livers, and PVE is recommended in those with a FLR of less than 40%. CT imaging is performed 4 weeks post-PVE to assess for any adverse features such as an increase in tumour size or complications following PVE resulting in unresectability. Liver resection is then performed 4 to 6 weeks following PVE.

Ablation

Image-guided ablation is indicated in certain patients with HCC or metastases when surgical resection is precluded, and can also be used as a bridge treatment to transplantation in patients with HCC. Chemical ablation with percutaneous ethanol injection (PEI) does not always achieve complete tumour ablation and has largely been superseded by thermal ablation. Thermal ablation includes radiofrequency ablation (RFA), microwave ablation or cryoablation. Patients with up to three HCCs of less than 3 cm are considered for thermal ablation depending on their Child Pugh score. These criteria follow guidelines proposed by the European Association of Study of Liver (EASL)[4] and the American Association of Study of Liver Disease (AASLD)[5] based on clinical studies which demonstrate a long-term survival benefit in patients with HCC.

Microwave ablation uses a needle-like antenna which is placed centrally within the tumour under image guidance with ultrasound, CT or MRI. High frequency microwave energy causes frictional heating of the surrounding tissue and causes coagulative necrosis of the tumour and a margin of at least 5–10 mm. The minimal invasiveness of the procedure is the key advantage, particularly in patients with poor liver function. Although it is considered safer than surgical resection, complications include haemorrhage, abscess formation, biliary tract damage and liver failure. Five percent dextrose or air can be introduced to separate peripheral tumours from surrounding structures, such as colon, and allow a safe ablation zone. The location of some tumours, for example, adjacent to a main biliary duct or too eccentric to allow traversal of non-tumour liver tissue with the antenna, increase the rate of complication and may not be suitable for ablation.

TACE/Radioembolization

For unresectable liver tumours, a cytotoxic agent, either chemoembolization or radioembolization, can be delivered intra-arterially. These techniques have been shown to prolong survival and improve time to progression of disease. Transcatheter arterial chemoembolization (TACE) increases the concentration of chemotherapy agent delivered directly to the arterial supply of the hepatic tumours while reducing systemic toxicity. The chemotherapy agent is either delivered with ethiodized oil or, more recently, with drug-eluting beads (DEB-TACE). During radioembolization, glass or resin particles impregnated with the isotope yttrium-90 are infused directly into the selected hepatic artery. Prior work-up with hepatic angiography and nuclear medicine shunt studies are required to ensure that the beta-emitting isotope is delivered only to the tumours and not to other organs such as the stomach.

Percutaneous Biliary Drainage

Percutaneous transhepatic cholangiography and drainage (PTCD) is indicated when there is biliary obstruction and endoscopic retrograde cholangiopancreatography (ERCP) is not possible or has failed. Obstruction due to cholangiocarcinoma, particularly if involving right- and left-sided ducts, should be drained percutaneously. The procedure is performed under conscious sedation and prophylactic antibiotics. An externally draining catheter can be initially inserted if the obstruction or stricture cannot be bypassed. Once the obstruction is bypassed, an external–internal drain is inserted, allowing drainage of bile into the duodenum and restoring the normal anatomical drainage of bile. Non-operative malignant strictures can be stented with self-expanding metal stents.

Cholecystostomy

Drain insertion into the gallbladder (cholecystostomy) is indicated to drain an infected gallbladder in critically ill patients or those unsuitable for surgery or ERCP. Once a drain has been inserted, it typically remains in situ for 6 weeks in order to allow a mature fistula tract to form so that bile does not leak into the peritoneal cavity upon removal. Prior to removal, a tubogram is performed to ensure the absence of distal obstruction or complication from the drain insertion. The patient can then proceed to cholecystectomy if indicated.

Vascular

Dotter

Charles Theodore Dotter, a US vascular radiologist, is described as the 'father of interventional radiology'. A pioneer in multiple IR procedures, he performed the first angioplasty in 1964 on an 82-year-old woman with critical limb ischaemia who refused amputation. He opened up a severe stenosis in the superficial femoral artery using Teflon catheters and her ulcer healed.

Angiography, Angioplasty and Stenting

Peripheral arterial disease is a systemic disease that affects 10% of the population. Atherosclerosis accounts for >95% of cases. Patients are treated with risk factor modification and best medical therapy with anti-platelet therapy, statins, ACE inhibitors and antihypertensives. Short distance claudication and critical limb ischaemia are indications for surgical or percutaneous endovascular revascularization. Most patients have non-invasive imaging prior to intervention either by duplex ultrasound, CT or MRI. The Trans-Atlantic Inter-Society Consensus Document on Management of Peripheral Arterial disease (TASC) II guidelines[6] indicate which lesions should be considered for surgical treatment versus endovascular. Given the advancement in endovascular techniques and equipment since these guidelines were published, there has been an increase in the proportion

undergoing endovascular treatment. The co-morbidities of the patient are also considered and many patients who are unfit for surgery are able to undergo revascularization and avoid amputation. Endovascular revascularization has lower morbidity and mortality and shorter hospital stays than surgical bypass. Patency rates are, in general, lower than surgery. However, endovascular revascularization is often attempted first and does not preclude future surgery. The access is usually via the common femoral artery but can also be via the radial, brachial, popliteal or pedal arteries. Ultrasound is often used to guide needle access into the access artery, using Seldinger technique as described previously. Once the artery has been accessed with a wire, a vascular sheath is inserted, which secures access and allows the passage of catheters through it. Stenoses and occlusions are crossed with wires and catheters. If one is unable to cross intra-luminally, a sub-intimal channel can be created. A non-compliant angioplasty balloon is then inflated across the lesion and, if the artery has not sufficiently opened up (>30% residual stenosis), a nitinol stent can be inserted (Fig. 16.9). Drug-eluting balloons and stents (DES) release an anti-proliferative drug into the vessel wall, thereby reducing intimal hyperplasia and reducing the restenosis rates. These were widely adopted but following a meta-analysis which demonstrated increased mortality rates at two and five years after the use of paclitaxel coated DEB/DES, further research is awaited. They are now used in selected cases following appropriate discussion and consent of the patient. Angioplasty and stenting are also used to unblock vessels throughout the body including the carotid artery, mesenteric arteries and deep veins.

Thrombolysis

Acute thrombosis of peripheral arteries or veins can be treated percutaneously with pharmacological or mechanical thrombolysis. It also allows treatment of a causative underlying stenosis with balloon angioplasty or stenting.

Endovascular Aneurysm Repair

Endovascular aneurysm repair (EVAR) is currently more frequently performed than open surgical repair of abdominal aortic aneurysm (AAA). This is due to the less invasive nature, quicker recovery and lower 30-day mortality of EVAR. EVAR uses stent grafts (material-covered stents) to cover the aneurysmal section of the aorta and iliac arteries. AAA are defined as measuring >3 cm diameter and over 90% arise infra-renal. The rupture risk increases as the diameter of the aneurysm increases. Indications for AAA repair are aneurysm size greater than 5.5 cm; rapid aneurysm growth of more than 1 cm per year; symptomatic or ruptured aneurysms; and saccular aneurysms. CT is performed to assess anatomical suitability for infra-renal EVAR. If the neck of the aneurysm is not suitable for infra-renal EVAR or the aneurysm commences in the thoracic aorta, custom-made grafts which allow the visceral vessels to be perfused can be

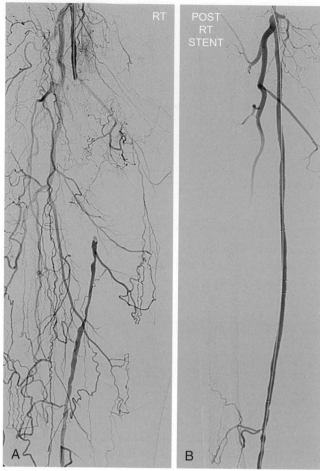

• **Fig. 16.9** (A) DSA demonstrating occlusion of the superficial femoral artery with collateral arteries and (B) after sub-intimal recanalization, angioplasty and stent insertion. DSA, Digital subtraction angiography.

inserted (fenestrated or branched EVAR). EVAR requires lifelong follow-up imaging due to the risk of endoleak (persistence of perfusion of the aneurysm sac) and therefore risk of rupture. Thoracic EVAR is also used in selected cases of aortic dissection, either because of malperfusion of the abdominal organs, bowel and legs or due to subsequent aneurysmal dilatation. Stent grafts are also used to exclude aneurysms in many smaller arteries, for example, mesenteric arteries and popliteal arteries. Significant changes in the status and training of vascular surgeons have occurred in the last few years and some endovascular competencies are included in their curriculum.

Interventional Neuroradiology

Cerebral Aneurysms

In most centres across the UK, neuro-interventional radiology procedures are performed by dedicated neuroradiologists who specialize in neurointervention. A common IR procedure for neuroradiologists is endovascular coil embolization of cerebral saccular (berry) aneurysms. This may be performed electively or in the acute setting of a ruptured aneurysm causing subarachnoid haemorrhage (SAH). Patient characteristics and the aneurysm anatomy are assessed when deciding whether the patient should undergo treatment by coil embolization or surgical clipping. Cerebral angiography is performed and the aneurysm size, aneurysm neck width, location and whether branches arise from the aneurysm, as well as the presence of other aneurysms, are assessed. During embolization, detachable microcoils are introduced through a microcatheter placed in the aneurysm. Coil embolization has a lower risk of short-term complications than surgical clipping but may require a repeat procedure. A meta-analysis of prospective trials concluded that patients had a significantly lower rate of poor outcome at 1 year with coil embolization than with surgical clipping for ruptured aneurysms amenable to treatment by either therapeutic technique.[7]

Epistaxis

Epistaxis is usually idiopathic or related to risk factors such as hypertension, anticoagulation, digit trauma and old age. Epistaxis may be caused by blunt force trauma, tumours or hereditary haemorrhagic telangiectasia. Patients with recalcitrant epistaxis unresponsive to adequate nasal cautery and packing, can be considered for endovascular embolization as an alternative to sphenopalatine artery ligation. Pre-embolization angiograms of the internal and external carotid arteries are performed to delineate important anastomoses that could increase the risk of complications such as stroke or blindness during embolization. The terminal branch of the internal maxillary artery, the sphenopalatine artery, provides the dominant supply to the nasal cavity. Embolization has similar success rates to surgical ligation, but requires there to be ongoing bleeding at the time of the procedure.

Trauma

Trauma patients are assessed for surgical or non-surgical management by the trauma team, which will include a radiologist. CT scanning is performed in the arterial and portal venous phases. The decision depends on the site of the injury or injuries and the haemodynamic status of the patient. Haemodynamically unstable patients require surgical exploration, whereas stable patients may undergo endovascular embolization for haemorrhage. Common sites of injury which may be treated with endovascular embolization are splenic lacerations, renal and liver lacerations and pelvic fractures causing arterial haemorrhage.

Splenic Artery Embolization

Injury to the spleen, as defined by the American Association for the Surgery of Trauma (AAST) splenic injury scale, can be non-surgically managed by splenic artery embolization (SAE). This negates the need for splenectomy and aims to retain some or most of the function of the spleen. Post-splenectomy prophylactic vaccine and antibiotic guidelines are still implemented. There is controversy over the indications for SAE. Haemodynamically stable patients with evidence of active extravasation on CT, AAST grades III–V (www.aast. org), large haemoperitoneum or a dropping haematocrit in the absence of another source of haemorrhage are considered for SAE. Embolizing the proximal splenic artery reduces the perfusion pressure sufficiently to arrest haemorrhage but also allows perfusion of the spleen through collateral arteries through the pancreas. Alternatively, selective embolization of distal splenic artery branches can be performed for active extravasation or pseudoaneurysm. At our institution, we perform a follow-up CT scan 48 hours post injury in order to detect latent pseudoaneurysms. 4 hours of bedrest is implemented post-procedure and, if required, anticoagulation can be commenced 48 hours after treatment of haemorrhage.

Inferior Vena Cava Filters

Patients who are at risk of pulmonary embolism (PE) or who have had deep venous thrombosis (DVT) or PE are treated with anticoagulants. There are several accepted indications for IVC filter insertion. Indications in surgical patients include those who have a contraindication to anticoagulation such as undergoing a surgical procedure or untreated subarachnoid haemorrhage and multi-trauma patients. An IVC filter is inserted via the femoral vein or jugular vein into the IVC below the renal veins. Almost all filters now inserted are retrievable and should be removed as soon as the patient is able to start anticoagulation (Fig. 16.10).

Haemodialysis Fistulae and Renal Transplants

Haemodialysis arteriovenous (AV) fistulae are formed by surgically anastomosing an artery to a vein, predominantly in the arm, arterializing the vein and allowing haemodialysis. The artery and vein are most commonly anastomosed side-to-side and creation of a radio-cephalic fistula at the wrist is the preferred first choice. If this is not possible due to small or diseased arteries or veins, then the next choice is the brachiocephalic fistula above the elbow. If the anatomy is unsuitable, a tube graft can be used between the artery and vein to create a communication. A number will fail to mature into useable fistulae. Mature fistulae or grafts can also develop stenoses, which reduce the blood flow through the fistulae and dialysis is difficult or not possible to achieve. These were historically treated by surgical revision, but most cases are now treated with percutaneous balloon angioplasty of the stenosis. If the fistula clots (thromboses), it can be treated percutaneously with mechanical thrombectomy and, occasionally, using thrombolysis with tissue plasminogen activator (tPA). Percutaneous treatment prolongs the patency of fistulae and reduces morbidity. Percutaneous AV fistula creation between the ulnar artery and vein using a radiofrequency magnetic catheter based system has demonstrated encouraging short-term outcomes. It may become a

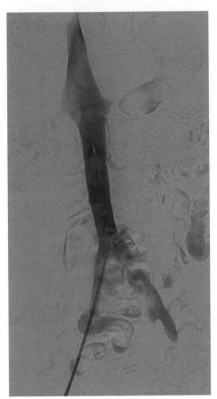

• **Fig. 16.10** DSA Demonstrating a Retrievable Inferior Vena Cava (IVC) Filter. DSA, Digital subtraction angiography.

viable alternative to open surgery in patients with suitable anatomy. Occasionally, a stenosis occurs at the anastomosis of the transplanted renal artery to the native iliac artery. This endangers the renal transplant, and percutaneous balloon angioplasty and stent insertion can be performed, removing the need for revision surgery.

Breast Surgery

Breast radiologists are key members of the breast clinic and multidisciplinary team. They perform image-guided biopsies of breast lesions in the outpatient setting. Ultrasound-guided large core biopsies are performed if the lesion is visible with ultrasound. Breast microcalcifications and small solid masses, which are not visible by ultrasound, are sampled by mammographic stereotactic biopsy. During stereotactic biopsy, a vacuum-assisted core biopsy needle or mechanical rotating biopsy device are used which allow larger samples to be taken. For abnormal breast lesions which cannot be palpated, image-guided wire localization is performed prior to surgery.

Musculoskeletal

Using a multimodality approach, it is possible to aid the diagnosis of several musculoskeletal problems. Image-guided soft tissue and bone biopsies are very useful in the diagnosis of malignancies affecting the musculoskeletal system. In addition, it is now accepted practice to treat some bone disorders such as osteoid osteomas with image-guided

RFA. Image-guided injections of local anaesthetic and steroid preparations can reduce pain and help with symptom control for several musculoskeletal conditions.

Future of IR

Training as an interventional radiologist follows a defined curriculum, culminating in a certificate of completion of training in Clinical Radiology with Interventional Radiology sub-specialization. Following foundation training and often core surgical or medical training, IR training extends over 6 years. The first 3 years focus on general radiology training as well as acquiring core interventional skills. The last 3 years focus on developing advanced interventional skills as well as maintaining competencies in general radiology. In the future IR may become a specialty in the UK, as it has become in the USA. This will allow further refinement of training and better workforce planning.

Given the pace of innovation and adoption of new procedures into clinical practice, procedures currently in their research phase will be in use in the near future. For example, gastric artery embolization has demonstrated promising results in the treatment of obesity. Advancements in technology are constantly pushing the boundaries of what we are able to achieve in interventional radiology.

References

1. Patel IJ, Davidson JC, Nikolic B, et al. Addendum of newer anticoagulants to the SIR consensus guideline. *J Vasc Interv Radiol.* 2013;24:641–645.
2. Liang TW, et al. Palliative treatment of malignant colorectal obstruction caused by advanced malignancy: a self-expanding metallic stent or surgery? A system review and meta-analysis. *Surg Today.* 2014;44:22–33.
3. Zhao XD, et al. Palliative treatment for incurable malignant colorectal obstructions: a meta-analysis. *World J Gastroenterol.* 2013;19(33):5565–5574.
4. European Association for the Study of the Liver. EASL Clinical Practice Guidelines: management of hepatocellular carcinoma. *J Hepatol.* 2018;69:182–236.
5. Marrero J, et al. Diagnosis, staging, and management of hepatocellular carcinoma: 2018 Practice Guidance by the American Association for the Study of Liver Diseases. *Hepatology.* 2018;68:723–750.
6. Norgren L, et al. Inter-society Consensus for the Management of Peripheral Arterial Disease (TASC II). *J Vasc Surg.* 2007;45:S5–S67.
7. Lanzino G, Murad MH, d'Urso PI, Rabinstein AA. Coil embolization versus clipping for ruptured intracranial aneurysms: a meta-analysis of prospective controlled published studies. *AJNR.* 2013;34(9):1764–1768.

Further Reading

Geschwind J-F H, Dake M. *Abrams' Angiography Interventional Radiology.* 3rd ed. Philadelphia: Lippincott, Williams & Wilkins; 2013.

Kandarpa K, Machan L, Durham J. *Handbook of Interventional Radiologic Procedures.* 5th ed. Wolters Kluwer; 2016.

Kessel D, Robertson I. *Interventional Radiology: A Survival Guide.* 4th ed. Elsevier; 2016.

17

Surgical Technology and Innovation

CHAPTER OUTLINE

Introduction

The phenomenal advances witnessed in surgery, particularly over the last three decades, owe their existence primarily to the unprecedented rate at which technology has evolved. This has led to improved outcomes, reduced morbidity and enhanced patient safety. For example, minimally invasive surgery would not have existed without the advent of the endoscope and a number of technologies that rapidly ensued to address limitations relating to access and ergonomics.[1] This chapter provides an overview of the key technologies that have had a major impact on modern surgical practice including a variety of novel medical devices, minimally invasive and robotic surgery and technologies employed in modern surgical education. Despite these impressive technological advances, it is important to remember that surgical technology augments but does not replace the surgeon's capabilities. There is no technology (including artificial intelligence) that can act as a substitute for surgical experience and volume or the fundamental attributes that define a surgeon such as manual dexterity, visuospatial awareness, organizational ability, emotional resilience, physical stamina, communication skills and the ability to lead and manage a team effectively.[2] As such, when referring to safety and comparative effectiveness of different surgical technologies in this chapter, it is important to understand that these only apply when 'in the right hands'. Similarly, in the context of surgical education, the numerous innovations and technological tools available (including virtual reality simulation) should not be regarded as a replacement for real life-world, experiential learning but as adjuncts developed to enhance learning in the context of restrictions imposed on the number of working hours for surgical trainees and the limited availability of animal and cadaveric models traditionally used for learning anatomy and practising surgical operations in a safe and controlled environment.

Medical Devices in Surgery

A medical device is defined as 'an instrument, apparatus, implement, machine, contrivance, implant, *in vitro* reagent, or other similar or related article, including a component part, or accessory which is:

- recognized by the official national body (e.g. MHRA for UK and FDA for US)
- intended for use in the diagnosis of disease or other conditions, or in the cure, mitigation, treatment, or prevention of disease, in man or other animals, or
- intended to affect the structure or any function of the body of man or other animals, and which does not achieve any of its primary intended purposes through chemical action within or on the body of man or other animals and which is not dependent upon being metabolized for the achievement of any of its primary intended purposes.'[3–5]

A plethora of medical devices are used on a daily basis in surgery. The most innovative ones shaping modern surgical practice are discussed below.

Energy Devices

Energy devices have revolutionized modern surgical practice. Their ability to seal, coagulate, and transect tissues

TABLE 17.1	The Different Types of Energy Devices.[8]					
Energy Devices						
Energy used	Maximum vessel diameter (mm)	Temperature generated (°C)	Lateral thermal spread (mm)	Average cutting time (s) (for 7-mm vessel)	Average burst pressure (mmHg) (for 7 mm vessel)	Examples
Ultrasonic	5–7	50–100	1–3	18.8	1878	Harmonic scalpel (Ethicon)
Advanced bipolar technology	5–7	60–95	2	26.9	1224	Ligasure (Medtronic)
Combination of above	7	<100	<1	10.7	1780	Thunderbeat (Olympus)

(including blood vessels) has considerably enhanced patient safety and paved the way for the introduction of minimally invasive surgery techniques including laparoscopic surgery.[6] In addition to reducing blood loss and operative time, a bloodless operative field ensures optimal visualization not only of the target organ(s), but also of adjacent critical structures (such as vessels and nerves) thus facilitating their identification and preservation.[7] The main types of energy devices relate to the type of energy used and can be classified into those using ultrasonic energy, advanced bipolar technology or a combination of both (Table 17.1).

The most commonly employed ultrasonic device is the harmonic scalpel (Ethicon Endo-Surgery, Inc., Johnson & Johnson, Cincinnati, OH) (Fig. 17.1). Harmonic technology works on the principle of delivering ultrasonic energy (at a frequency of 55.5 kHz) to simultaneously cut and coagulate tissue. The temperatures reached by ultrasonic vibrations are much lower (50–100°C) than those reached by conventional bipolar electrocoagulation (150–400°C).[9] This, combined with the lateral thermal spread, which for ultrasonic coagulation is limited to 1–3 mm, makes the harmonic scalpel safe (in the right hands).[10] Ultrasonic coagulation has been shown to seal reliably blood vessels of up to 5–7 mm in diameter.[11]

Its unique properties, combined with the fact that it comes in a variety of tip shapes (including shear, blade and hook) and lengths render the harmonic scalpel a well-suited instrument for a broad range of surgical procedures, both open and laparoscopic, including endocrine, head and neck, thoracic, hepato-pancreato-biliary, colorectal, urological and gynaecological.[12] The harmonic scalpel can be mounted on one of the robotic arms of the da Vinci surgical robotic system (Intuitive Surgical Inc., Sunnyvale, CA) and thus is also commonly used in robotic surgery.[13–15]

There is level I evidence to support not only the safety of the harmonic scalpel but also its superiority over conventional haemostatic techniques (such as ligatures, titanium vessel clips and staples) across a range of surgical procedures.

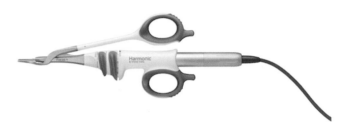

• Fig. 17.1 HARMONIC FOCUS+ Shears. (©Ethicon, Inc-HARMONIC FOCUS®+ Shears).

The advantages most commonly reported relate to operative time, blood loss, drain output, length of hospital stay and cost-effectiveness.[16–18] This evidence relates primarily to laparoscopic surgery.[19]

The other type of energy device that is widely used is Ligasure (Covidien Products, Medtronic, Inc., Minneapolis, MN) (Fig. 17.2). It also comes in a range of tip shapes and lengths to accommodate the needs for open and endoscopic surgery across various body parts including the head and neck, thorax, abdomen and pelvis.[20] Ligasure works through a combination of pressure and energy to seal vessels and its most recent version (Ligasure Small Jaw) includes an integrated cutting blade for dividing tissues. Ligasure employs advanced bipolar technology, which limits the risk of thermal injury through a negative feedback loop. Similar to the harmonic scalpel, Ligasure can also seal blood vessels of up to 5–7 mm in diameter.[21]

There is level I evidence to support not only the safety of Ligasure but also its superiority over conventional haemostasis in relation to operative time, intraoperative blood loss and cost.[22–24] However, similar to the harmonic scalpel, this advantage primarily relates to laparoscopic surgery and has not been replicated in randomized controlled trials (RCTs) evaluating its role in open surgery.[25]

Despite the plethora of RCTs comparing the harmonic scalpel or Ligasure to conventional haemostasis, there is a paucity of studies conducting direct comparisons between the two.[26] This avoidance of head-to-head comparisons

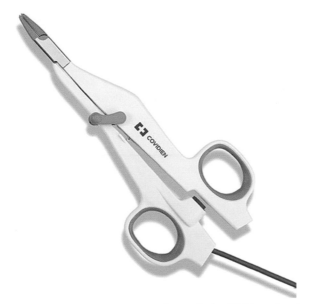

• **Fig. 17.2** Ligasure Small Jaw Open Sealer/Divider. (Courtesy Covidien Products, Medtronic, Inc., Minneapolis, MN).

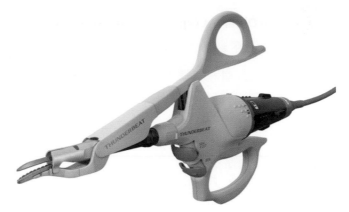

• **Fig. 17.3** Thunderbeat. (Courtesy Olympus Medical Systems Corp., Tokyo, Japan).

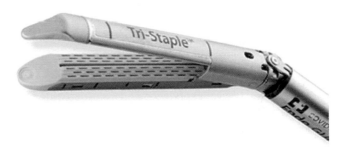

• **Fig. 17.4** Endo GIA 30 mm Reload with Tri-Staple Technology Curved Tip. (Courtesy Medtronic, Inc., Minneapolis, MN).

represents a well-described bias in research known as the 'straw man effect' where novel interventions tend to be preferentially compared against older ones (that are more likely to be inferior) rather than concurrent ones in an attempt to demonstrate superiority.[27] This limitation can be overcome through network meta-analysis, a novel evidence synthesis technique allowing for indirect pair-wise comparisons.[28]

In a recent network meta-analysis in thyroid surgery, the comparative effectiveness of the harmonic scalpel was demonstrated over both clamp-and-tie haemostasis and Ligasure with the important exception of recurrent laryngeal nerve injury, where the safest mode was clamp-and-tie haemostasis followed by Ligasure and then the harmonic scalpel.[7] This finding emphasizes a very important point relating to the fact that any medical device, no matter how safe or innovative it may be considered, cannot act as a substitute for surgical experience and volume.[29]

A number of other energy devices are also available such as ENSEAL (Ethicon Endo-Surgery) and Thunderbeat (Olympus Medical Systems Corp., Tokyo, Japan) (Fig. 17.3). ENSEAL uses advanced bipolar technology whilst Thunderbeat is the first energy device to integrate ultrasonic coagulation and advanced bipolar technology in one instrument.[6,30] Thunderbeat can be used to securely cut and seal blood vessels of up to 7 mm in diameter with clinical studies reporting it to be equivalent to the harmonic scalpel, Ligasure and ENSEAL in terms of both safety and cost-effectiveness.[31,32]

Stapling Devices

Stapling devices constitute one of the most important advents in modern surgery (Fig. 17.4). In addition to their role in open surgery, stapling devices have revolutionized minimally invasive surgery. By providing the ability to perform technically demanding procedures such as colorectal resection and intracorporeal anastomosis in a safe and rapid manner without the need for laparotomy, stapling devices have paved the way for a number of newly enabled minimally invasive procedures. Examples include laparoscopic colorectal and bariatric surgery, thoracoscopic surgery for lung cancer and transoral surgery for upper aerodigestive tract malignancies.[33]

The portfolio of stapling devices is wide. These can be broadly categorized based on their tip shape (and length), which can vary depending on the anatomic region and procedure they are designed for (Table 17.2).

Stapling devices have been shown to be associated with reduced operative time and an equivalent safety and effectiveness to hand-sewn anastomosis for a variety of procedures. In colorectal surgery, there is level I evidence demonstrating the reduced risk of anastomotic leak with staplers for ileocolic anastomosis.[34] When comparing techniques for closure of loop ileostomy, stapled closure appears superior to hand-sewn anastomosis with regards to bowel obstruction rate and operative time and equivalent in terms of the risk for anastomotic leak.[35]

Despite overall superiority, the number of times a stapling device is fired during laparoscopic anterior resection for rectal cancer has been shown to have a negative impact on outcomes; with three or more firings significantly increasing the risk of anastomotic leak.[36] This reiterates the point discussed in the introduction about the critical

TABLE 17.2	The Different Types of Stapling Devices According to Tip Shape.

		Stapling Devices	
Tip shape	**Applications**	**Advantages**	**Examples**
Linear	• Colorectal • Gastric • Head & Neck • Thoracic • General	Simultaneous cutting and stapling achieved (e.g. transoral stapling of Zenker diverticulum, laparoscopic sleeve gastrectomy)	• Ethicon Linear Cutter (Ethicon) • Endo GIA (Medtronic)
Curved	• Colorectal • General • Thoracic	Facilitates instrumentation in difficult-to-access areas (e.g. deep pelvis for laparoscopic-assisted low anterior resection, division of hilar or segmental vascular and bronchial structures during VATS)	• CONTOUR (Ethicon) • Endo GIA Curved Tip (Medtronic)
Circular	• Bariatric • Colorectal • Head & Neck • General	Designed for intraluminal end-to-end anastomosis (e.g. jejuno-oesophageal anastomosis following pharyngolaryngectomy and jejunal free flap reconstruction or colonic anastomosis following laparoscopic resection)	• ECHELON CIRCULAR Powered Stapler (Ethicon) • DST Series EEA Stapler (Medtronic)

VATS, Video-assisted thoracic surgery.

importance of surgical experience and volume (with which comes economy of movement).[37]

For anastomosis following oesophagectomy, there is level II evidence to support stapling devices in terms of reduced operative time and blood loss with equivalent complication rates, including anastomotic leak, compared to hand-sewn anastomosis.[38] However, the risk of benign stricture formation is higher when using a stapling device.[38] Finally, in terms of gastric surgery, there is level I evidence to support the use stapling devices for the formation of gastroenteric anastomosis following distal gastrectomy for gastric cancer and Roux-en-Y gastric bypass in bariatric surgery.[39,40] Mechanical stapling was shown to be quicker with equivalent safety and effectiveness to hand-sewn anastomosis.[40]

The development of new stapling devices that can be mounted to the robotic arms of the da Vinci robot has further expanded their role in minimally invasive surgery. The EndoWrist stapler system (Intuitive Surgical), in addition to allowing the performance of technically demanding procedures such as intracorporeal anastomosis robotically, has also facilitated the development of robotic surgery for lung cancer.[41] Other advances in the field include powered stapling devices in which the staples and knife blade are driven by a power source (as opposed to manual force) to enhance stability and precision, and sensing stapling devices.[42,43]

Surgical Navigation Technology

Surgical navigation encompasses a variety of computerized technologies designed to improve surgical accuracy by enhancing the visual input of the surgeon in real time. This technology is especially valuable in minimally invasive surgery for difficult-to-access, anatomically complex areas that contain numerous critical structures constrained in a narrow space. Such areas include the skull base, inner ear and

paranasal sinuses, making otorhinolaryngology–head and neck surgery and neurosurgery the two surgical specialties where intraoperative navigation is most widely used. The presence of multiple bony landmarks in the skull adds to its anatomic complexity but at the same time serves as an advantage when it comes to three-dimensional (3D) registration, as those landmarks remain fixed.[44]

There are two types of navigation systems, optical and electromagnetic. Optical navigation systems track the position of instruments intracorporeally through the triangulation of light-emitting diodes (LED) or reflective spheres attached to these, whilst electromagnetic systems detect the position of copper coils attached to the instruments by detecting changes in the electromagnetic field generated by the system's emitter. Each system has its own advantages and disadvantages but in practice they have been shown to be equivalent in terms of accuracy.[45] The use of intraoperative navigation has been associated with reduced complication rates in endoscopic sinus surgery.[46] Recently, stereotactic navigation has been experimented in cadavers for rectal surgery as, similar to the skull, the pelvis represents a bony cage providing fixed, non-deformable landmarks for 3D registration.[47]

It is important to remember that at present, all commercially available navigation systems are limited in terms of their accuracy by a target registration error (TRE) ranging between 1.5 mm and 2.0 mm, and often even exceeding 2.0 mm. As such, no existing navigation system can be fully trusted and the surgeon's clinical acumen should always take priority.[44]

In laparoscopic surgery, where there is a paucity of fixed bony landmarks, augmented reality (AR) has been proposed as a possible navigation technology, often combined with intraoperative ultrasound or other imaging modalities. Through AR, computer-generated images are projected to

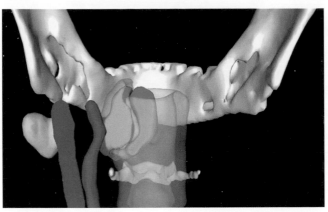

• **Fig. 17.5** Augmented Reality (AR) view of a left oropharyngeal tumour with a superimposed view of the great vessels of the neck to alert the surgeon of their close proximity to the tumour.

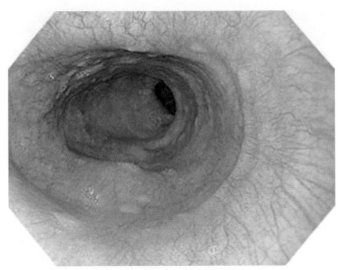

• **Fig. 17.6** Narrow Band Imaging (NBI) of the Colon. (Courtesy Olympus Medical Systems Corp., Tokyo, Japan).

the real environment. These images display important structures such as neurovascular bundles, which, through the use of 'smart glasses', are superimposed to the surgeon's view (Fig. 17.5). Real-time data based on preoperative 3D reconstruction is continuously inputted and can be adjusted (e.g. in terms of opacity) to enhance safety and reduce operative time.[48]

Beyond pre-clinical studies, AR has been applied in a variety of operations including minimally invasive (laparoscopic or robotic-assisted) hepatectomy,[49] splenectomy,[50] pancreatectomy,[51] nephrectomy[52] and myomectomy.[53] However, these are all limited to case reports (or at best small case series) thus making the use of AR in surgery experimental at present. This is likely to change, however, with AR playing an increasingly important role.

In summary, surgical navigation technology incorporates a multitude of different technologies. Some are already established, as there is evidence that they enhance patient safety and clinical outcomes. Others, more recently developed, are still in the pre-clinical stages of development, yet appear very promising. It is likely that in the near future, surgical navigation will form a core part of standard surgical practice.

Intra-Operative Tissue Sensing Using Mass Spectrometry (The iKnife)

The intelligent knife (iKnife) works by aspirating smoke plumes from monopolar diathermy into a mass spectrometer for real time chemical analysis of tissues.[54] Machine learning tools are applied to the raw data to search for patterns of molecules against large databases of previously validated spectra. This can be achieved very quickly (in a few hundredths of a second) and the resulting mass spectrometric profiles are highly specific to the type of tissue analysed, allowing for tissue identification as well as characterization on a level comparable with histopathological analysis. This analytical coupling creates new chemical information sets that describe the tissue and its associated pathology.[55] It is highly accurate (e.g. it has >95% diagnostic accuracy for the

detection of breast cancer).[56] This technology is currently undergoing clinical trials to evaluate its ability to detect cancer margin involvement during wide local excision of breast cancer and in the endoscopic treatment of complex colonic polyps.

In Vivo Optical Imaging

Beyond the adaptation of established imaging modalities for intraoperative use (e.g. ultrasound in laparoscopic surgery[57] and MRI in neurosurgery[58]) and the injection of dyes (e.g. indocyanine green) for in vivo fluorescence (molecular) imaging in surgical oncology[59] (e.g. to identify sentinel lymph nodes[60] or neurovascular bundles[61]), the most recent innovation in the field relates to optical imaging.

Optical imaging is an umbrella term incorporating a number of different technologies. These are distinguished by the frequency of light they use (e.g. infrared or ultraviolet). The three most applicable to minimally invasive surgery are narrow band imaging, optical coherence tomography and confocal laser endomicroscopy.[62]

Narrow band imaging (NBI) technology (Olympus Medical Systems) is based on selectively filtering longer wavelength (red) light from the illumination source.[62,63] This causes a reduction in the spectral bandwidth of shorter wavelength (blue and green) light (from 415 nm and 540 nm, to 50–70 nm and 20–30 nm, respectively).[62,63] The resulting light beam consisting of lower wavelengths is less able to penetrate tissues. This, combined with the fact that the optical absorbance of haemoglobin peaks at 415 nm, makes mucosal and submucosal structures containing haemoglobin (i.e. blood vessels) 'light up' with NBI (Fig. 17.6).[62,63]

Thus, NBI represents a very useful technique when evaluating mucosal lesions for their malignant potential – as angiogenesis represents a core feature of cancer.[64] Clinical applications of NBI include in vivo evaluation of colorectal polyps,[64] oral, oropharyngeal and hypopharyngeal lesions

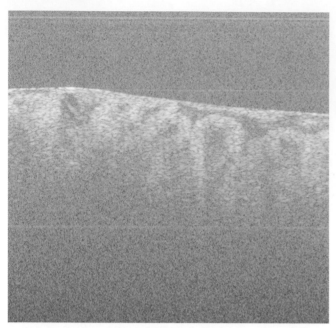

• **Fig. 17.7** Optical Coherence Tomography (OCT) of Gastric Mucosa.

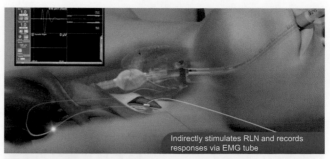

Indirectly stimulates RLN and records responses via EMG tube

• **Fig. 17.8** Automatic Periodic Stimulation (APS) of the Vagus Nerve During Thyroid and Parathyroid Surgery. (Courtesy Medtronic, Inc., Minneapolis, MN).

(e.g. raised lesions, leukoplakia, ulcers)[65] and oesophageal pathology (including early squamous cell carcinoma).[66] In addition to allowing more targeted biopsies and potentially earlier diagnosis of cancer, NBI can also be used for the intraoperative determination of surgical margins.[67]

On the other hand, optical coherence tomography (OCT) uses light at the infrared bandwidth to produce cross-sectional tissue images.[68] Though it constitutes an optical technology, OCT more resembles ultrasound. The two are based on the same principle of emitting waves and producing images based on the differential absorption and reflection characteristics of individual tissues. The difference is that OCT uses light waves (as opposed to sound waves used in ultrasound). However, due to the difference in wavelengths, the resolution achieved with OCT is much higher than that of ultrasound.[69]

The resolution obtained with OCT is so high (10–20 μm range) that it is comparable to that of histology.[69] This, combined with the fact that OCT probes can be mounted on conventional endoscopes, has introduced the concept of 'optical biopsy'.[68] OCT can be utilized in a variety of anatomical areas to 'biopsy' lesions down to a depth of 1.5–2 mm (Fig. 17.7).[70] Examples include the evaluation of oesophageal pathology (including Barrett's oesophagus, dysplasia and cancer),[69] oral[70] and laryngeal lesions.[71] Though still in its early days, OCT is likely to become increasingly important in clinical practice, particularly as a screening tool for upper aerodigestive tract malignancies.

Finally, confocal laser endomicroscopy (CLE) involves the combination of confocal microscopy and optical endoscopy.[72] By doing so, 1,000-fold magnification is achieved, thus providing imaging at cellular and subcellular levels, down to a depth of 250 μm.[73] Through the use of dyes (e.g. fluorescein), CLE allows 'real-time in vivo histology'.[72]

Current applications for CLE involve the endoscopic evaluation of mucosal lesions of the gastrointestinal tract,[72] larynx[74] and bladder.[75] Real-time in vivo mucosal microscopic imaging is also feasible with endocytoscopy, which (in contrast to CLE) is based exclusively on high-level magnification obtained through optical lenses integrated within the endoscope.[76]

The aforementioned optical imaging modalities are of special importance as they allow the intraoperative in vivo evaluation of lesions in real time, including (in certain cases) the potential of distinguishing between benign and malignant lesions, thus enhancing surgical precision. However, it is equally important to reiterate that histology remains the gold standard for definitive diagnosis.

Intraoperative Nerve Monitoring

Intermittent IntraOperative Nerve Monitoring (IONM) to assess the functional integrity of nerves such as of the recurrent laryngeal nerve (RLN) during thyroid surgery is not a new concept.[77] However, there have recently been several important advances in the field of IONM.

The use of IONM has expanded to various other surgical operations, particularly in the head and neck. Examples include facial nerve monitoring in parotid and mastoid surgery where, having been shown to reduce the incidence of postoperative facial weakness, it now constitutes standard surgical practice.[78–80] More recently, there have been animal studies evaluating the role of facial nerve monitoring during image-guided robotic cochlear implantation.[81]

The most clinically impactful innovation in the field of IONM relates to continuous IONM (CIONM). Contrary to intermittent IONM in thyroid surgery where the RLN and external branch of the superior laryngeal nerve (EBSLN) are intermittently stimulated by the surgeon, in CIONM, there is automatic periodic stimulation (APS) of the vagus nerve through the placement of an electrode probe directly on the vagus nerve (APS Electrode, Medtronic).[82]

There are several advantages to CIONM over intermittent IONM. The most important relates to the fact that CIONM provides the surgeon with continuous real-time feedback on the status of the nerve monitored (Fig. 17.8).[83] Thus, CIONM can provide warning for an impending nerve injury, which can be prevented by adapting surgical strategy.[84] This may involve modifying surgical manoeuvres associated with electrophysiologic events to release tension from the nerve or, in cases where there is loss of signal on the first side, conversion to a two-stage thyroidectomy.[84] CIONM is, however, still novel and more time will be needed to establish its role and limitations.

3D Printing

This innovation has proven revolutionary in terms of optimizing preoperative planning and surgical training.[85] Despite its recent introduction in surgery, there are numerous specialties already benefiting from this technology. Examples include preoperative planning and patient education in congenital and structural cardiac surgery to enhance the spatial understanding of structurally complex anomalies.[86] Similarly, 3D printing is widely used in otorhinolaryngology–head and neck surgery and plastic surgery to plan osteotomies for free flap mandibular and maxillary reconstruction,[87] as well as the design and manufacturing of prostheses including dental implants.[88]

Other applications include the production of 3D kidney graft and pelvic cavity models for the personalized planning of renal transplantation,[89] 3D skull models in craniosynostosis surgery[90] and 3D models of liver vessels and tumours in hepatectomy.[91] Finally, 3D printing has been shown to provide an important adjunct to cadaveric models for surgical training.[92]

Implantable Devices

Implantable devices represent another important group of surgical technologies. In certain surgical specialties, implantation has had such an important role in transforming patient outcomes that it has led to the development of entirely new subspecialties. Examples include functional neurosurgery and auditory implantation. The most recent developments are discussed.

Despite cochlear implants having been around for over 40 years and having revolutionized the treatment of profound deafness in both paediatric and adult patient groups, there are still certain groups of patients where cochlear implantation is either not possible or has no role. This relates to patients with retrocochlear hearing loss, such as those with cochlear ossification (e.g. post-meningitis) or severe malformations, and those where the cochlear nerve itself is either congenitally absent or non-functional as a result of trauma, tumour (e.g. vestibular schwannoma) or surgery.[93] This is where the novel technology of auditory brainstem implants (ABIs) comes into play.

ABIs involve the surgical placement of electrodes directly on the brainstem over the cochlear nucleus complex. Preliminary studies in patients with neurofibromatosis type 2 (NF2) – 90% of whom develop bilateral vestibular schwannomas – have shown positive outcomes in terms of open-set speech recognition in pure auditory mode.[94] The expansion of ABIs in other patient groups, particularly congenitally deaf paediatric patients with cochlear malformations or absence of the cochlear nerve(s) as well as post-lingually deafened (non-NF2) adults, represent two areas currently under research where ABI may prove revolutionary.[95]

Another recent and very important application of surgical implants involves upper airway stimulation for obstructive sleep apnoea (OSA), an increasingly common disease with substantial morbidity and mortality when untreated.[96] Though existing treatment in the form of continuous positive airway pressure (CPAP) is highly effective, adherence falls below 50% necessitating the need for alternative treatments.[97]

A number of surgical treatments have been recently developed for OSA including transoral robotic surgery (TORS).[13,98] Following research illustrating a strong correlation between activation of the genioglossus muscle and patency of the upper airway, the most recently proposed surgical treatment for OSA involves the unilateral implantation of a stimulating device on the main trunk of the hypoglossal nerve designed to deliver electrical stimuli in a synchronized manner along the inspiratory phase of the patient's respiratory cycle.[99] Following initial small studies with the Inspire (Medtronic) device,[99] other neurostimulation systems have been utilized in larger studies confirming its promising role in the treatment of OSA.[100] Most recently, results of RCTs are emerging confirming the value of hypoglossal nerve stimulation for the treatment of OSA in patients intolerant of CPAP.[101,102]

Implantable stimulating devices are also increasingly used in the management of neurological conditions refractory to pharmacological treatment where they are gradually replacing previous destructive procedures (e.g. thalamotomy for controlling Parkinsonian tremor or temporal lobectomy for intractable epilepsy).[103,104] These include deep brain stimulation (DBS) for drug-resistant Parkinson's disease and vagus nerve stimulation for epilepsy that is not controlled by medication alone.[104,105]

In general surgery, examples of implantable devices include gastric pacemakers for the treatment of morbid obesity and gastroparesis,[106] the Alfapump system (Sequana Medical AG, Zurich, Switzerland), an innovative subcutaneous device for patients with cirrhosis that continuously diverts ascitic fluid to the urinary bladder[107] and, more recently, an implantable batteryless pump for real-time glucose-responsive pulsatile insulin administration.[108]

The most recently emerging technology in the field of implantable devices relates to biosensors. The term refers to miniaturized in vivo sensors designed for the continued monitoring of target analytes.[109] Biosensors are likely to greatly enhance personalized healthcare, reduce unnecessary physician appointments and facilitate big data collection for a number of diseases. As such, biosensors are likely to dominate clinical practice in the near future, though this is not yet the case as a result of a combination of technological, cost-related and ethical barriers (including concerns expressed over the ownership and use of individual patient data).[109]

TABLE
17.3   **Examples of Procedures Performed Using Minimally Invasive Surgical Techniques.**

Surgical Specialty	Procedure
Upper Gastrointestinal Surgery	• Oesophagectomy • Gastrectomy • Gastrostomy
Lower Gastrointestinal Surgery	• Appendicectomy • Colorectal resection
Hepato-pancreato-biliary Surgery	• Cholecystectomy • Partial hepatic resection • Partial pancreatic resection
Endocrine Surgery	• Thyroidectomy • Parathyroidectomy • Adrenalectomy
Bariatric Surgery	• Gastric banding • Roux-en-Y gastric bypass • Sleeve gastrectomy
Vascular Surgery	• Aortofemoral bypass • Endovascular Aortic Aneurysm Repair (EVAR)
Urology	• Prostatectomy • Nephrectomy • Cystoprostatectomy • Percutaneous and transurethral nephrolithotomy • High-Intensity Focused Ultrasound (HIFU) of prostate
ENT – Head and Neck Surgery	• Transoral LASER Microsurgery (TLM) • TransOral Robotic Surgery (TORS) • TransOral UltraSonic Surgery (TOUSS) • Minimal access cochlear implantation • Endoscopic thyroid and parathyroid surgery • Endoscopic transsphenoidal hypophysectomy • Extended endoscopic endonasal skull base surgery
Cardiothoracic Surgery	• Endoscopic Coronary Artery Bypass Grafting (CABG) • Transapical aortic valve implantation • Minimally invasive aortic valve repair • Minimally invasive mitral valve repair • Video-Assisted Thoracic Surgery (VATS)
Orthopaedic Surgery	• Arthroscopic surgery • Minimally invasive arthroplasty • Endoscopic carpal tunnel decompression
Neurosurgery	• Endoscopic third ventriculostomy • Gamma knife stereotactic radiosurgery • Endovascular treatment of Berry aneurysms • Percutaneous vertebroplasty and kyphoplasty

Minimally Invasive and Robotic Surgery

Minimally Invasive Surgery (MIS)

The term 'minimally invasive surgery' was first used by John Wicker, an English urologist, who established a department for MIS at the Institute for Urological Surgery in 1983.[110] Many conventional open surgical procedures have now been replaced by minimally invasive ones, which have been shown to offer increased safety, lower rates of postoperative morbidity, shorter hospitalization and improved cosmetic results.[111,112] Advances in surgical skills and the technology

for MIS have allowed its application to all surgical specialties to some degree (Table 17.3).

Robotic Surgery

The word 'robot' was first coined by the Czech playwright Karel Capek in 1921.[113] Robots have been extensively used in other industries to perform precise, repetitive and hazardous tasks, and are now increasingly adopted in healthcare, with the increasing demand for technological innovation in surgery.[114] Robotic surgery ultimately arose to address the

TABLE 17.4	The Advantages and Disadvantages of Laparoscopic Versus Robotic Surgery.[124]	
	Laparoscopic	**Robotic**
Advantages	• Well-developed technology • Widely available • Relatively affordable • Effective	• Three-dimensional views • Improved dexterity • 7 degrees of freedom • No fulcrum effect • Tremor filtering • Telesurgery possible • Ergonomics • Complex/micro surgery
Disadvantages	• Reduced haptic feedback • Two-dimensional view • Compromised dexterity • Reduced degrees of freedom • Fulcrum effect • Increased tremor transmission	• Lack of haptic feedback • Expensive • Limited evidence base • Large size and footprint

limitations associated with laparoscopic procedures, including the lack of natural hand-eye coordination, the limitations of two-dimensional views, fewer degrees of freedom and the need to improve accuracy and precision.

Robotic surgery is extensively used across the spectrum of surgical specialties and subspecialties. In otorhinolaryngology–head and neck surgery, its minimally invasive nature offers significant advantages over open surgery, which is commonly associated with significant morbidity (e.g. mandibulotomy and/or pharyngotomy performed solely for accessing tumours located in difficult-to-access areas, e.g. at the base of tongue).[115] In neurosurgery, robotic surgery achieved the completion of complex procedures at microscopic scale, something extremely challenging in the absence of robotic assistance even when the operative microscope is employed.[116] Robotic technology is also being applied in cardiothoracic surgery, obviating the need for median sternotomy for procedures, including coronary artery bypass grafting and mitral valve surgery.[117] In gastrointestinal surgery, a number of procedures are now commonly performed robotically, including gastrectomy for gastric cancer, gastric banding and gastric bypass for morbid obesity and Nissen fundoplication for severe gastroesophageal reflux disease.[116] However, the field where robotic technology is currently most widely implemented is that of urological surgery, where the depth of the pelvis and size of anatomical structures makes surgery challenging, particularly when using rigid laparoscopic instruments.[118]

The Advantages and Disadvantages of Robotic Surgery

The development of robotic surgery arose to counter the limitations associated with traditional laparoscopic surgery. Laparoscopy is associated with limitations in terms of the technical and mechanical nature of the equipment, which include limitations relating to hand-eye coordination (i.e. to move an instrument in one direction, the surgeon's hand must move in the opposite direction to the target visualized on the monitor), the Fulcrum effect, enhancement of transmitted tremor and reduction in dexterity (i.e. restriction on the degrees of freedom as a result of the rigidity of traditional laparoscopic instruments, resulting in fewer than the seven degrees of freedom achievable by the human wrist). Robotic surgery therefore offers significant advantages over laparoscopic surgery addressing all of the above limitations (Table 17.4).[114,119–123]

Robotic systems enhance dexterity through use of instruments with increased degrees of freedom, allowing for better tissue manipulation[124]; additionally, hardware and software filters reduce tremor and scale movement from larger movements with the control grips to smaller micromovements inside the patient.[125] These aspects of the system also offer advantages over open surgery.[124] Where humans have limited dexterity outside natural scale and have limitations on geometric accuracy, robotic surgery allows motion scaling to enhance surgical precision. Furthermore, where humans are prone to tremor and fatigue, robotic systems are stable and untiring. However, at present, robotic systems lack haptic feedback.

The system allows for fine hand-eye coordination and eliminates the fulcrum effect. The ability to sit at an ergonomically designed console prevents the surgeon from having to perform awkward movements and adopt uncomfortable positions in order to move the instruments or improve visualization. The surgeon's view is further enhanced at the console by offering a magnified high definition (HD) view with depth perception (3D), as well as a stable view controlled via the robot (Fig. 17.9).

Robots offer stability, accuracy, integration with modern imaging technology, great range of motion and the ability for telesurgery.[116] Additionally, robotic surgery has been shown to be easier to learn, including the translation of open surgical skills to the robotic interface.[126,127] Therefore, where laparoscopy had not been adopted by many surgical specialties due to the difficulty of developing proficiency

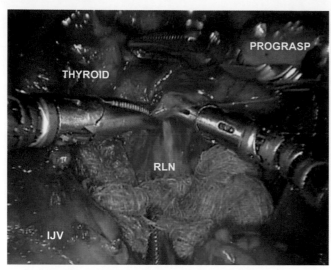

• **Fig. 17.9** Intraoperative Robotic Console Surgery View of the Recurrent Laryngeal Nerve (RLN) and Internal Jugular Vein (IJV) During Robotic Parathyroidectomy.

and a prolonged learning curve (compared to open surgery) for certain procedures, robotic surgery eliminates this challenge. It also offers significant benefits to the patient including improved cosmetic outcomes, shorter hospital stay and decreased postoperative complications. As such, robotic surgery has high levels of patient acceptability and an increasing demand.[128–130]

This, of course, comes at an increased cost, which at present represents the largest barrier to the adoption of robotic surgery. Costs include acquisition of the robotic system, maintenance, consumables and training for robotic surgeons and their theatre teams.[114] However, with the upcoming expiry of patents currently held by Intuitive Surgical Inc. (Sunnyvale, CA) and the imminent market entry of several multinational medical device corporations, these costs are likely to drop significantly in the near future. Examples of novel robotic surgical platforms and their manufacturers include those currently been developed by Medtronic, Inc. (Minneapolis, MN), Johnson & Johnson, Inc. (New Brunswick, NJ) in collaboration with Google LLC (Mountain View, CA), Cambridge Medical Robotics, CMR Surgical, Ltd. (Cambridge, UK) with the Versius robot and Titan Medical, Inc. (Toronto, ON) with the SPORT robot. Their market entry will introduce the much-awaited competition to drive down costs, thus making robotic surgery more widely available.[115,117,131]

Needlescopic Surgery

Needlescopic surgery is an alternative to laparoscopy, reducing access trauma even further. This technique involves using instruments and ports that are smaller than 3 mm in diameter.[132] In RCTs comparing needlescopic and conventional laparoscopic cholecystectomy, there were no significant differences between open conversion, postoperative pain and recovery time, though there was a significant difference in the perceived cosmetic outcome.[133,134]

Single Incision Laparoscopic Surgery (SILS)

Laparoscopy is also possible through a single incision, known as SILS.[135] It uses the same instruments as conventional laparoscopic surgery, and has been applied for performing cholecystectomy, appendicectomy, sleeve gastrectomy and splenectomy.[135–137] However, concerns have been reported relating to an increased incidence of biliary complications and incisional hernias.[138–140]

Natural Orifice Transluminal Endoscopic Surgery (NOTES)

Common to all procedures discussed in this chapter is the desire to reduce invasiveness and improve efficiency. Natural orifice transluminal endoscopic surgery, or NOTES, inserts surgical instruments through a natural orifice, for example the mouth, anus, vagina or urethra,[141,142] thus eliminating the need for external incisions, though internal ones may still be necessary for access. This is considered a logical evolutionary step in the advancement of minimally invasive surgery. NOTES has the advantage of reducing trauma and infection, and enhancing recovery time as a result of a reduction in pain, as well as reducing the potential for adhesion formation following abdominal surgery.[141,143,144] It is therefore likely to be increasingly accepted by patients; in addition, since many endoscopic procedures can be performed under sedation only, in can be postulated that certain NOTES procedures may also be performed without the need for general anaesthesia and intubation.[144]

Long before the concept of NOTES was formally described, procedures performed through natural orifices were being performed. In 1813, the first colpotomy with transvaginal approach in hysterectomy was described.[145] In the 1940s, gynaecologists used a flexible endoscope passed through the recto-uterine pouch to view the pelvic organs and perform sterilization.[145] The first case of a trans-oral cholecystectomy was published in 2007 and this has since been followed by case series of appendicectomy, sleeve gastrectomy, splenectomy and other procedures.[135] The most commonly discussed procedure is the transvaginal cholecystectomy[142]; the most popular routes are transvaginal and transgastric, with the most popular procedure being cholecystectomy. The transvaginal route's popularity is likely linked to the ease of and knowledge surrounding a standard closure method for colpotomy, which have been performed by gynaecologists for many years. Despite this, many patients are concerned about the fertility and sexuality implications of this route and, of course, it is only feasible in female patients.[142]

Key challenges in NOTES include instrument introduction and advancement, manoeuvrability, adequate visualization and haptic feedback.[141] In particular, the use of current flexible endoscopes, which are designed for use in the gastrointestinal tract, have some limitations when used in the peritoneal cavity[144,146]; these concerns relate to the stability of the endoscope and the size of the instrument channel.

This may be overcome with the development of innovative devices or through hybrid approaches that combine laparoscopy and NOTES.[144] Additionally, hybrid NOTES facilitates standard closures of visceral incisions, leak testing and improved visibility.[142] For optimal function in NOTES, endoscopes require miniaturization and redesign to improve conduit access and flexibility; novel assist devices and devices for closure following NOTES are also needed.[147]

The Future of Minimally Invasive Surgery

The initial evolution and development of minimally invasive surgery and, specifically, robotic technology, was largely born from the limitations of laparoscopy.[114] The future of minimally invasive surgery lies in identifying and exploring the creative possibilities of the technology we have developed to date.

Imaging

One possibility for expanding the future of robotic surgery is the concurrent use of preoperative and intraoperative imaging (CT and MRI)[124]; the aim of this would be to guide the surgeon in surgical planes and pathology identification. Additionally, this would allow rehearsal of surgical procedures with simulators.

Telesurgery

Owing to the nature of robotic systems, with the surgeon remote to the patient within the operating room, it is possible for the surgeon to be located at a long-distance location from the patient.[124] With this arrangement, surgeons could provide consultation, guidance, teaching and assessment. In 2001, a surgeon in New York city successfully completed a robot-assisted laparoscopic cholecystectomy on a patient in Paris, France, using the ZEUS system.[148] The da Vinci theoretically allows for telesurgery; however, the communication system uses a short distance communication relay. Animal studies have shown that telesurgery is feasible, but that there are challenges posed by the distance and the latency between the action and reaction, which could impact on patient outcome.[149] Similar studies using public internet reduced this latency, and demonstrated feasibility of this concept.[150]

Tactile Feedback

A major limitation of robotic surgery is the lack of tactile or haptic feedback.[124,151] Future advancements in robotic surgery will include the development of systems that relay touch sensations including temperature, pressure, tension and vibration. Some laboratories are already focused on developing this.[152–157]

In Vivo Robots

In vivo robots have been discussed as an alternative to endoscopy, or as an extension to the concept of NOTES. Though this concept is still in its infancy, current examples include inchworm robotic systems,[158] rolling stents[159] and intra-abdominal robots.[160–162] Micro- and nanorobotic systems are also being envisioned which may be small enough to enter the bloodstream through microscopic incisions as a means of enhanced tissue preservation.[163]

Automation and Artificial Intelligence

The concept of robots is often linked to automation and artificial intelligence.[124,151] Currently, the robotic system relies on the surgeon (master) controlling the robot (slave); however, it is conceivable that the robotic system may be programmed to perform an operation or a specific task involved within certain boundaries under the mere supervision of the surgeon. This may include programming the robot to avoid certain 'danger areas' and thus prevent surgeon error or even extend to adding an intelligent component that allows the robot to identify the target area and perform a task independently.[164]

Data-Driven and Digital Surgery

As part of the move towards personalized, evidence-based medicine, data intelligence is likely to shape the future of surgery. The rise of big clinical databases offers a unique opportunity for data-driven surgery aimed at improving the quality and value of surgical healthcare through the automated collection, processing, linkage and analysis of large, complex datasets to measure innovation in surgery.[165,166] The first two metrics for measuring diffusion and evidence-based value of surgical innovations have recently been introduced and validated.[167] This represents a crucial step towards the transition to a data-driven surgery era, where surgical innovation metrics will assist in informing policy and guide surgical decision-making on an personalized patient basis.[168] At the same time, data intelligence has enabled the development of digital surgery, with digital tools such as Digital Surgery and Touch Surgery (both from Touch Surgery Labs, London, UK) proving increasingly important in promoting 'data-driven, human-centric surgery' and surgical education respectively.[169,170] These are discussed in greater detail in the following section.

Technological Advances in Surgical Education

The reliance of surgical education on technological innovation has become more apparent in recent years as various political reforms have come into place, which have transformed the training landscape. A prominent example relates to the European Working Time Directive (EWTD), which has been estimated to have decreased the training opportunities for junior doctors by up to 40% as a direct result of reduced training time and a shift-work pattern,[171] leaving many trainees feeling that the quality of their training and operative competence has declined since implementation of the directive.[172–175]

In his book *Outliers*, Malcolm Gladwell popularized the '10,000-hour rule' which states that to become an expert in a given field 10,000 hours of practice is required.[176] In a craft-based specialty such as surgery in which practice is required to achieve technical competence, the political influences described above conspire to diminish training opportunities, which can potentially have a huge effect on the operative ability of a young surgeon completing their training programme. Indeed, some reports suggest that total surgical training time has reduced from 30,000 hours to around 8000 hours.[177] As a result, surgical education is becoming more dependent on technology in order to bridge the gap caused by the decline in training time. This section describes some of the technological advances which have supplemented surgical training by enhancing skill acquisition and assessment, and ensuring trainees are ready for independent practice by the time they reach the end of their training.

Online Learning

Online learning, also referred to as e-learning or web-based learning, is the use of internet resources to enhance learning and encompasses a range of educational interventions. Early use of online learning involved simply uploading lecture slides and accompanying notes onto a website without any active participation on the part of the trainee. However, with development of Web 2.0, web-based learning has progressed to include online tutorials, synchronous or asynchronous interactions, virtual patients and multimedia capabilities such as webinars.[178] Many of these strategies are administered using a virtual learning environment (VLE) which represents an online interface allowing learners to access learning material and interact with their peers.[179]

Theoretical Aspects

Many of the advantages of web-based learning are rooted in pedagogical theory. For instance, *constructivism* is the notion that learners actively construct knowledge and ideas by a process of assimilation and accommodation, allowing one to give meaning to what is learnt.[180] *Social constructivism*, pioneered by Lev Vygotsky, refers to how this process of constructing knowledge occurs as a result of interactions between the learner and those around them, reinforcing the social nature of learning and understanding.[181] Online learning can involve interaction between the learner and the trainer, as well as with other learners, through the use of discussion boards and chat rooms. The exchange of ideas that arises from this interaction allows co-construction of knowledge for all involved,[182] as well as self-reflection and critical awareness.[179]

The General Medical Council (GMC) Good Medical Practice guidelines state that 'You must keep your professional knowledge and skills up to date'.[183] For trainees to keep pace with the ever-expanding pool of knowledge and evidence upon which their practice relies, they must engage in self-directed learning, which online learning can facilitate. The nature of web-based learning allows trainees to access educational resources in their own time and at their own pace, enabling them to schedule it around their work commitments. Web-based instruction also allows trainees to have control of their learning by allowing them to access the material in the sequence in which they desire.[182] Furthermore, autodidaxy – the independent pursuit of learning outside the formal institutional setting – is encouraged with the use of hyperlinks to other resources such as journals and websites which enables users to access further learning material that is formally provided outwith.

Lave and Wenger introduced the concept of communities of practice (CoP) which proposes that learning occurs through informal discussions with peers during which experiences are shared.[184] CoP are based on the idea that people learn and develop through social interaction rather than by just simple knowledge acquisition in a classroom.[185] Lave and Wenger also described the idea of legitimate peripheral participation (LPP), the notion that a newcomer to a CoP is initially positioned at the periphery of the group but as they spend more time engaging with other members and acquire more knowledge, they gradually move to a more central position and make a greater contribution to the group's activity.[184] Virtual CoP have been proposed as a facet of online learning.[186] For example, web-based discussion groups can be formed based on clinical cases and new members of the group will initially be at the periphery. As they spend more time interacting with others and acquire the group's tacit knowledge, they move to a more central position and contribute further to the online discourse.[182]

Flexibility

Online learning material can be widely distributed over a large geographic area such that all trainees can access the same resources. This is particularly advantageous if expertise among trainers varies within a region.[178] Web-based learning, including asynchronous discussions, also offers flexibility in the timing of trainee participation in contrast to traditional lectures, which are delivered at a fixed time and place.[187] With the restraints of the EWTD, such flexibility ensures that all trainees are given the opportunity to participate. For example, the *eSurgery* course developed by Health Education England (HEE) and the Royal College of Surgeons of England is a free online resource in which modules are mapped to the Intercollegiate Surgical Curriculum Programme (ISCP).[188] The modules are accessible at any time to allow trainees to fit them in around their busy clinical jobs.

Individualized Learning

Web-based learning allows trainees to complete online modules in an order and pace of their choosing. Trainees who struggle with a particular topic can spend longer on the related module but can progress rapidly through modules with which they are more familiar, as opposed to lecture-based education where the pace and depth is determined by the faculty.

Multiple Instructional Methods

Online learning allows learners to engage in multiple instructional methods which would otherwise be difficult to administer in a traditional face-to-face setting.[189] For example, virtual patient scenarios enable learners to encounter a wide variety of medical conditions, and the iterative nature of these scenarios facilitates learning by deliberate practice.[190] Interactive models and use of multimedia can enrich learning material in ways that are not possible in a lecture theatre or textbook resulting in greater learner engagement.[178] For example, Touch Surgery (Touch Surgery Labs) is an application which uses digital technology to provide interactive surgical simulations which are accessible on smartphones and computers, along with step-by-step multimedia narrative guides for each procedure.[191] Asynchronous interactions allow trainees to consider the concept under discussion before responding, in contrast to face-to-face encounters in which conversations move quickly and can impede critical thinking.[178,192]

Disadvantages of Online Learning

Social Isolation and Interpersonal Skills

Although web-based learning offers flexibility in time and place that learning can occur, users will usually engage with online material alone in their private time which can lead to social isolation.[178] Furthermore, the social organization of a virtual interaction differs distinctly from the real world and therefore the appropriate team-working and communication skills required in clinical practice may not be adequately fostered.[178] Virtual interactions use the written word as a medium for communication, which does not allow the learner to use or recognize non-verbal cues that are intrinsic to face-to-face encounters.[193] However, use of web-based video communication platforms during online discussion may help to overcome these limitations.

Practical Skills Acquisition

Peyton's four-step approach to learning a practical skill involves close interaction between the learner and trainer while simultaneously performing the skill.[194] This model is less readily applied during online instruction compared with face-to-face practical skills sessions. Although websites can make use of multimedia platforms to demonstrate surgical tasks and help trainees conceptually appreciate a procedure, the inability for a trainee to obtain hands-on experience and practise the skill with verbal expert feedback remains a major drawback.[195]

In sum, trainee surgeons can benefit from online learning provided it does not replace more traditional methods of instruction in which face-to-face encounters confer an advantage in some settings. Instead, web-based learning should be used to supplement traditional approaches as part of a blended curriculum. If utilized in this way, a greater variety of learner styles can be accommodated for and surgical trainees can reap its potential benefits.

Social Media and Surgical Education

The use of social media to complement traditional models of surgical education has gained traction in recent years due to the expanding role social media play in our personal and professional lives. The evolution of Web 2.0 technology has radically altered the way in which individuals engage with one another and has provided a more dynamic way for users to interact, communicate and share information compared with more traditional methods of learning. Recent data from the UK show that 90% of households have internet access and that over 40 million people use social media.[196] Accordingly, surgical education is capitalizing on social media to facilitate knowledge sharing and online discussions, and to help create virtual communities of practice for a new generation of learners.

In order to help us understand how social media enhances the learning experience for surgeons, established learning theories have evolved from traditional behaviourist and constructivist paradigms to connectivist models. Introduced by Siemens and Downes, connectivism explains how learning is facilitated through online communication and sharing information over the internet.[197,198] Learners can more easily maintain an up-to-date knowledge base due to the instantaneous flow of information between users distributed over a wide geographic area. Moreover, social media can help fill the education gaps arising from the current climate of restricted working hours and diminished operative exposure. In line with andragogical principles, social media can also empower trainees to engage in self-directed learning and construct their own knowledge frameworks.[199] Even if trainees favour more traditional learning methods, many textbooks and lectures are freely available online that can be shared and discussed on social media platforms. Empirical evidence shows that social media improves knowledge acquisition, skills learning, and professional attitudes,[200] qualities which are lauded by the ISCP in the UK.[201] Despite these advantages, the challenges of implementing social media-based educational campaigns include concerns about online security and privacy, technical issues and variable user engagement.[200] In addition, the GMC has issued specific guidance regarding doctors' use of social media platforms and highlights the importance of preserving professional boundaries, maintaining patient confidentiality and respecting colleagues.[202]

There are a variety of social media platforms available for surgical trainees that may help enhance their learning experience. These include social networks such as Facebook and Twitter, online blogs, video-sharing sites and podcasts, all of which can provide a novel dimension to the educational journey (Table 17.5).

Blogs

Blogs are websites managed by individuals or organizations that allow users to post public comments and replies in response to a specific subject. Blogs can be created using online publishing platforms such as Wordpress (www.wordpress.com) and can be used to share and discuss interesting articles or topics. Such exchanges are analogous to those that occur at surgical conferences or society meetings; however, with the advent of mobile internet technology,

<table>
<tr><td>TABLE 17.5</td><td colspan="2">Social Media Platforms with Valuable Examples for Surgical Training.</td></tr>
</table>

Social Media Platform	Valuable Examples for Surgical Training
Video channels	<ul><li>YouTube (https://www.youtube.com)</li><li>Vimeo (https://vimeo.com)</li><li>CSurgeries (https://www.csurgeries.com)</li><li>WebSurg (https://www.websurg.com)</li></ul>
Facebook groups	<ul><li>The Royal College of Surgeons of England (https://www.facebook.com/royalcollegeofsurgeons)</li><li>SAGES (https://www.facebook.com/SAGESSurgery)</li><li>Clinical Anatomy & Operative Surgery (https://www.facebook.com/ClinAnat.OperSurg)</li><li>Society of Robotic Surgery (https://www.facebook.com/Society-of-Robotic-Surgery)</li></ul>
Twitter hashtags	<ul><li>#Surgery</li><li>#SurgEd</li><li>#Academicsurgery</li><li>#ASGBI</li><li>#ACSCC18</li></ul>
Blogs	<ul><li>Inside Surgery (www.insidesurgery.com)</li><li>Images of Surgery (http://imageofsurgery.com)</li><li>OpNotes (http://opnotes.com)</li></ul>
Webinars	<ul><li>The Royal College of Surgeons of England webinars (https://www.rcseng.ac.uk/news-and-events/events/webinars)</li><li>Cleveland Clinic Center for Continuing Education (http://www.clevelandclinicmeded.com/online/webcast)</li></ul>
Podcasts	<ul><li>Surgery 101 (http://surgery101.org)</li><li>Behind The Knife (https://behindtheknife.libsyn.com)</li></ul>

blogs allow interactions to occur at times and locations that are flexible and more suitable to the user. In addition to providing a platform to share and discuss topical subjects, blogs also allow users to post interesting anecdotes and share their personal experiences about a particular case or surgical technique. Inside Surgery (www.insidesurgery.com) is an example of a surgical blogging site that contains a wealth of information about a wide range of surgical topics, and gives trainees the opportunity to learn from surgeons from around the world.

Microblogs

In contrast to traditional blogs, microblogs allow a faster and sometimes more convenient way of sharing information. The most popular microblogging site is Twitter, which allows users to share tweets of up to 280 characters. Many individuals and surgical societies use Twitter to disseminate information and share ideas with 'followers', including journal articles, videos and details of upcoming conferences. Twitter provides a way for trainees to interact with and learn from experts in their field, some of whom actively tweet or re-tweet about a range of topics. The use of Twitter handles such as #Surgery, #SurgEd or #Academicsurgery unifies users that are posting about the same topic and facilitates greater connectivity between spatially disparate learners. In a study by Brady et al., a 6-month Twitter campaign using the hashtag #Colorectalsurgery was launched in order to bring together discussions and posts of interest to a global community of colorectal surgeons.[203] The hashtag was used

in 15,708 tweets resulting in over 65 million impressions, with peak use of the hashtag coinciding with major colorectal conferences.[203] Surgical conferences are now using meeting hashtags, such as #ACSCC18 (American College of Surgeons) and #ASGBI (Association of Surgeons of Great Britain and Ireland), to disseminate conference content to a virtual audience, enabling individuals not physically present at the meeting to participate in relevant discussions.

Video Channels

Video sharing sites such as YouTube and Vimeo can be extremely valuable teaching tools for surgeons. Although watching videos cannot provide the tactile experience of performing a procedure in real-life, it does allow users to learn a procedure in a stepwise approach at a pace of their choosing. Trainees can rewind videos and revisit specific steps of an operation until they are fully understood and ingrained without the time pressures associated with a real operating theatre. Video channels are more interactive than textbook learning and more accessible than training with an expert. In a survey of medical students, residents and faculty, 90% of respondents reported using videos as preparation prior to surgery, with YouTube being the most preferred source.[204] Links to videos can also be shared on other social media platforms, which can increase the impact of video-based learning. One of the limitations of using openly available online videos as educational tools is the lack of peer-review and the ambiguity of data sources.[205] However, some websites (e.g. www.csurgeries.com and www.websurg.com) are

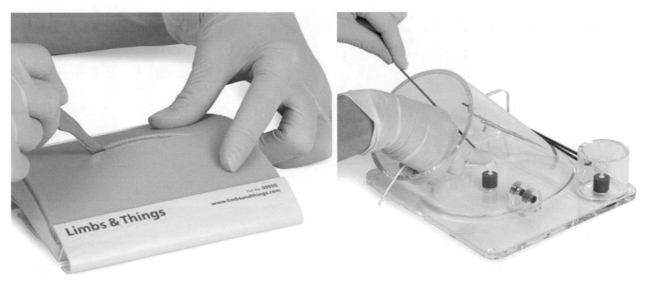

• **Fig. 17.10** Synthetic models used for practising basic surgical skills including skin pad jigs (left) and tonsillectomy knot tying trainers (right). (Courtesy limbsandthings.com).

now offering peer-reviewed videos for learners with content provided by world-leading experts.

Podcasts

Podcasts are pre-recorded discussions or lectures made available online which can be downloaded and listened to anytime and anywhere. With the widespread use of mobile internet technology, the use of podcasts in surgical education has become increasingly popular. Examples of podcast providers for surgical education include Surgery 101, which provides short episodes covering core topics in general surgery and is aimed at medical undergraduates as well as junior surgical trainees. The Behind the Knife podcast includes interviews of leaders from a range of surgical specialties, imparting a 'behind the scenes' insight into interesting and controversial areas of surgical practice. It also offers educational material to assist listeners sitting the American Board of Surgery examinations.

The use of social media in surgical education is still in its early stages but is set to increase in popularity as websites offer improved connectivity and communication. The flexibility in time and location of learning in the context of working time restrictions and shift-based working patterns, its ease of use and accessibility makes social media-based learning an attractive adjunct to traditional educational tools.

Surgical Simulation

Surgical simulators have evolved considerably over the last few years and are now widely used in surgical training to facilitate acquisition, refinement and automaticity of visuospatial and motor skills in a safe, risk-free environment outside the operating theatre.[206,207] They comprise a range of different devices which vary considerably with respect to their degree of fidelity, and which can be categorized as 'organic' (e.g. cadaveric and animal models) or 'inorganic' (e.g. bench-top box trainers or virtual reality simulators).[208] Whilst organic models

provide a greater sense of anatomical realism, limited supply, strict regulation (e.g. the Human Tissue Act 2004, United Kingdom) and high storage costs precludes widespread adoption.[209,210] Conversely, lower fidelity inorganic simulators are less expensive, portable and can be used multiple times.[209,210]

Cadaveric Models

Human cadavers have traditionally been used during dissecting room training and the high degree of realism enables trainees to acquire a detailed understanding of anatomical relationships, tissue handling and disease processes. Cadaveric training is used for a wide variety of procedures, such as laparoscopy,[211] vascular surgery,[212] surgical oncology[213] and robotic surgery.[214] However, despite being highly regarded by surgical trainees, there is currently limited evidence demonstrating that skills acquired during cadaveric training are transferable to the operating theatre.[215]

Synthetic Models and Box Trainers

Synthetic models are usually made of latex, plastic or rubber and are particularly useful for learning basic technical skills such as knot tying or suturing. Commercially available models include knot-tying trainers, skin pad jigs and tendon repair trainers (Limbs and Things Ltd., Bristol, UK) (Fig. 17.10). In addition to being cost-effective,[216] evidence has shown that skills learnt on bench-top models are transferable to human cadaveric models,[217] and that assessment on bench-top simulators predicts performance in the operating theatre.[218,219] This would suggest that individual steps of a complex procedure can be practised and mastered separately using inanimate models before performing the complete operation.[220] Synthetic models have been widely used in basic surgical skills (BSS) courses, such as those delivered by the Royal College of Surgeons of England,[221] and are often combined with laparoscopic box trainers so that the requisite hand-eye coordination and motor skills can be

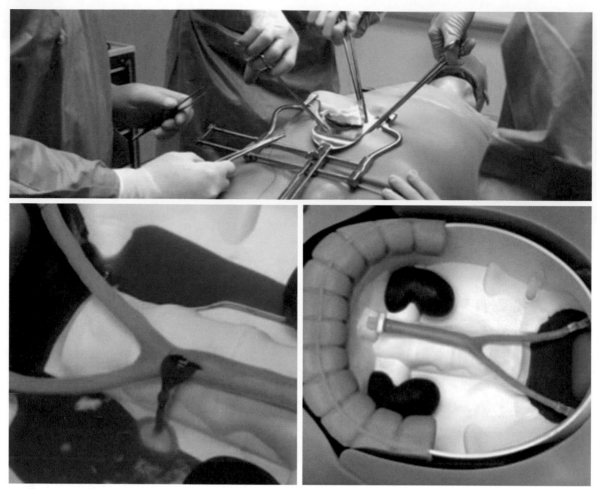

• **Fig. 17.11** The TraumaMan Surgical Abdomen Team Training System includes an anatomically complete abdominal cavity and adjustable blood flow to enable practising management of surgical crises. (Courtesy Simulab, Seattle, WA).

developed for basic minimally invasive tasks. Higher-fidelity synthetic models are also available which enable trainees to practise performing more complex procedures. For example, the TraumaMan Surgical Abdomen Team Training System (Simulab, Seattle, WA) provides an anatomically complete abdominal cavity, including adjustable blood flow, to enable team training in the management of catastrophic surgical events (Fig. 17.11). Furthermore, integration of such high-fidelity models within a fully-equipped and fully-staffed simulated operating suite allows non-technical skills such as leadership, teamwork and judgement to be fostered during a surgical crisis in a realistic working environment without jeopardizing patient safety.[222]

Virtual Reality (VR) Simulators

Advances in technology has made VR simulation increasingly popular in surgical training due to the 3D vision, a greater degree of realism and haptic feedback (Fig. 17.12).[223] VR simulators create computer-generated 3D images of the operating field, allowing trainees to manipulate the recreated tissue and receive immediate objective feedback on technical performance (Fig. 17.13). Specifically, the simulators provide comprehensive performance

reports, which include metrics such as instrument path length, number of errors and economy of movement, which can be tracked over a period of time to map a trainee's learning curve. Most VR simulators allow trainees to practise the critical steps of a complete procedure, such as dissection of Calot's triangle during a laparoscopic cholecystectomy, and also include modules that allow trainees to encounter difficult cases or practise controlling complications in a safe environment. A widely used platform is LAPMentor (3D Systems Simbionix), which, in addition to procedure modules, offers didactic education aids such as 3D anatomical maps, text-based instructions, videos of real-life procedures and visual guidance. Further developments in VR technology include a virtual operating room in which the trainee wears a VR headset allowing them to be fully immersed in the operating environment in which they can interact with a virtual team and patient, and experience realistic intraoperative distractions in order to also develop human factors skills.

There are numerous studies investigating the effectiveness of VR training in surgical skill acquisition and substantial evidence to support the use of VR simulation in laparoscopic training.[224] In trainees with limited

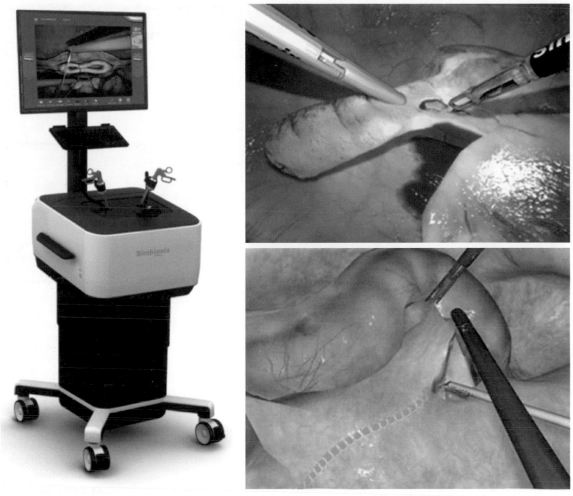

• **Fig. 17.12** Left: The Simbionix LAP Mentor simulation platform. Top right: High-fidelity simulation of a laparoscopic appendectomy. Bottom right: Intraoperative guidance demonstrating line of dissection during a colectomy. (Courtesy of 3D Systems, Simbionix simulators, Littleton, CO).

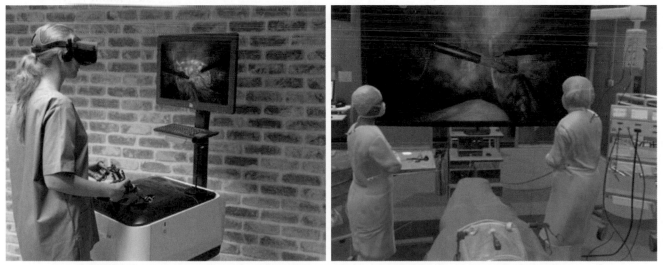

• **Fig. 17.13** Virtual Operating Suite. Left: Surgical trainee wearing a virtual reality (VR) headset while performing a simulated procedure on a VR platform, allowing them to become fully immersed in the operating room environment. Right: View from the perspective of the trainee during a laparoscopic procedure. (Courtesy of 3D Systems, Simbionix LAP Mentor simulator, Littleton, CO).

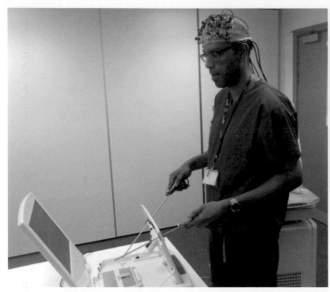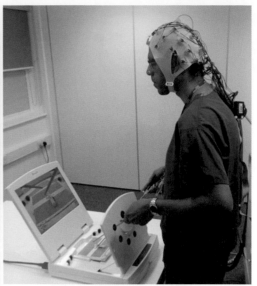

• **Fig. 17.14** The Use of Neuroimaging to Assess Surgical Skill Acquisition. Left: Functional near-infrared spectroscopy (fNIRS) measures brain activation indirectly by measuring changes in oxy- and deoxyhae-moglobin concentration in the cerebral cortex of a surgical trainee. Right: Electroencephalography (EEG) measures brain function in a surgical trainee by recording changes in electrical signals.

laparoscopic experience, VR training appears to decrease operating time and improve technical performance compared with no training or box-trainer training.[225] Additionally, RCTs have demonstrated that VR training results in faster acquisition of laparoscopic skills, as well as improved performance in the operating theatre compared to conventional clinical training.[226–229] Although the emphasis of VR simulation is on laparoscopic surgery, evidence shows that this form of simulation is also effective in training endoscopic procedures such as upper gastrointestinal endoscopy and colonoscopy.[230,231] Interestingly, there is also evidence to suggest that skills acquired with VR training are not task-specific and can be transferred when performing unrelated procedures.[232] Although the expense of high-fidelity VR simulation technology may seem prohibitive to its uptake in some training programmes, the long-term benefits of shorter learning curves and improved skill acquisition may justify the initial outlay costs.

Technology and Surgical Assessment

The development of valid and reliable methods of assessing surgical skill is crucial in current surgical training programmes given the need to achieve proficiency within the context of a shortened training time. Previously, surgical assessment was based on an apprenticeship model of informal training and skill acquisition but there is now an assortment of objective assessment tools available to trainers, many of which exploit recent advances in technology. In addition to the in-built performance assessment provided by VR simulators, a number of other technological innovations have been developed to objectively measure surgical competency.

Dexterity Analysis: Imperial College Surgical Assessment Device (ICSAD)

The ICSAD uses an electromagnetic (EM) tracking system consisting of an EM field generator and sensors attached to the dorsum of the operator's hands. The 3D Cartesian coordinates of each sensor are captured in real time with a spatial resolution of 1 mm and sampling frequency of 20 Hz. Bespoke software is used to convert the positional data into dexterity metrics that provide an assessment of movement efficiency and comprise time taken to complete the task, distance travelled (total path length), and number of movements of both hands.[233] As ICSAD is minimally intrusive, it can be used in both a simulated setting as well as in a live operating theatre. Construct, concurrent and face validity of ICSAD has been established in open[234] and laparoscopic surgery,[235–237] as well as for anaesthetic procedures.[238,239]

Brain Imaging and Skills Assessment

Developments in functional neuroimaging techniques, such as functional magnetic resonance imaging (fMRI), electroencephalography (EEG) and functional near-infrared spectroscopy (fNIRS), have made measuring surgeons' brain function to assess skill acquisition in natural operating environments possible (Fig. 17.14).[240] A number of studies have used neuroimaging techniques to assess acquisition of technical skills in surgery,[241] and have demonstrated that activity in specific brain regions varies with the extent to which surgical trainees have learnt a motor skill. Specifically, activation in the prefrontal cortex (PFC) – an area of the cortex that plays an important role in executive function – is greater in novice compared to expert surgeons during task performance due to greater attentional demands in the early stages of skill learning.[242–244] However, with repeated practice and development of skill automaticity, PFC activation

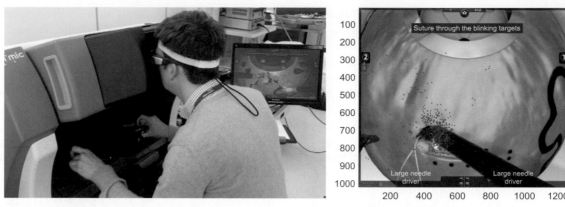

• **Fig. 17.15** Eye Tracking Technology for Assessment of Surgical Skills. Left: Surgical trainee wearing eye tracking glasses while performing robotic surgery on a virtual reality (VR) simulator. Right: Analysis of gaze behaviour demonstrates the surgical trainee's focus of attention in the field of view (red dots).

attenuates as the skill becomes ingrained and expertise develops.[243][245] Interestingly, studies have shown that early improvements in laparoscopic performance do not necessarily correlate with early attenuation in PFC activation, which occur only after months of skill refinement.[246] This would suggest that assessment of brain activation might be a more accurate reflection of skill acquisition and more sensitive to expertise differences than technical proficiency metrics.[241]

Other studies have interrogated patterns of activation in motor areas of the brain during surgical task performance.[247–249] The primary motor cortex, the supplementary motor area and the premotor area are all responsible for planning and execution of voluntary movements.[250] Neuroimaging data recorded during open[247] and laparoscopic[248,249] tasks show that there is less activation in these regions among expert surgeons compared to novices, which suggests that movement efficiency observed in experts is mirrored by efficiencies in motor regions of the brain.

The changes in activation responses observed in the prefrontal and motor areas suggest that these brain regions function as a 'scaffold' during early stages of skill learning, which is then phased out as expertise develops.[251] In terms of skills assessment, diminished responses in prefrontal and motor regions during task execution would imply that a certain degree of expertise has been achieved, whereas sustained activation might help to identify trainees in need of further training.[252]

In addition to technical skills assessment, brain imaging technology has also been employed to assess non-technical skills such as intraoperative decision-making[253] and stress-coping ability.[254] Assessment of decision-making expertise is challenging because the internal thought process in which decisions are rooted does not have measurable behavioural correlates; thus neuroimaging may offer a novel approach to objectively assess decision-making processes. Evidence shows that novices exhibit substantial prefrontal activation when faced with uncertainty during a surgical procedure, suggesting implementation of goal-directed effortful decision-making processes that demand attention and concentration.[253] In contrast, expert surgeons utilize habitual intuitive decision-making mechanisms during which solutions are selected from a repertoire of implicit knowledge, and which is reflected by reduced prefrontal responses.[253] For the purposes of assessment, excessive prefrontal responses would characterize an inexperienced decision-maker, whereas attenuated responses would indicate decision-making expertise.[253]

Unexpected intraoperative events can place excessive mental demands on the surgeon, increasing their cognitive workload and potentially jeopardizing patient outcomes.[255,256] A hallmark of surgical expertise is the ability to maintain stable operative performance during times of escalating mental demand. Neuroimaging techniques have been utilized to delineate the neural mechanisms that underpin stress-coping ability among surgeons. Senior surgical trainees have been shown to cope better with intraoperative mental demands and are able to stabilize their performance under pressure due to enhanced prefrontal recruitment and task engagement.[254] In contrast, junior surgical trainees show a reduction of prefrontal activation under stressful conditions, coupled with a deterioration in their technical performance.[254]

Eye Tracking Technology

Eye tracking technology has been proffered as a novel tool for assessing surgical skill acquisition[257] and involves recording eye movements using cameras that are either fixed or integrated into eyeglasses. The reflection of infrared light on the cornea is recorded in order to track pupil position and map the subject's focus of attention on videos of the field of view (Fig. 17.15).[258] Eye tracking technology can also capture metrics such as fixation frequency and duration, as well as pupil diameter.[257] Studies have suggested that differences in these metrics between subjects of varying expertise can be exploited as a means to assessing surgical ability.[259–261] For example, Khan et al. recorded gaze behaviour of two expert surgeons performing a laparoscopic cholecystectomy and replayed the videos to groups of experts and novices whilst capturing their gaze behaviour.[259] The experts watching the videos had significantly greater overlap with the expert subjects in terms of their patterns of gaze behaviour compared to novices.[259] Wilson et al. found that experienced surgeons spend significantly more time fixating on an area of interest during a basic laparoscopic task compared to novices, who spent more time focusing on the laparoscopic instruments.[261] Although eye tracking is still in the early stages of research in terms of its incorporation in the surgical training curriculum, there is a growing pool of evidence to support its use as an assessment tool. Furthermore, its portability, ease of use, and ability to provide objective data makes eye tracking suitable for skills assessment during surgical tasks.

Real Life, Experiential Learning Remains the Gold Standard in Surgical Education

With the advent of restricted working hours and subsequent reduced training opportunities, there has been a departure from the traditional apprenticeship model of training, which is rooted in the principles of workplace-based learning. As a result, surgical education is now more dependent than ever on technological innovations to shorten learning curves, facilitate skill acquisition, and aid assessment of surgical proficiency. Although there is an increasing variety of devices and innovations at the disposal of the surgical community for this purpose, it is important to understand that these tools cannot replace experiential learning in a real life operating theatre but simply supplement intraoperative experience.

Summary and Future Considerations

The numerous surgical technologies discussed in this chapter will undoubtedly continue to improve whilst new ones are introduced in parallel to further enhance patient safety, clinical outcomes and surgical training. Technology is also likely to be increasingly used in the provision of surgical services, a notable example being virtual clinics.[262]

In contrast to the aforementioned surgical innovations that are all incremental in nature, the technology that will most likely prove disruptive to the surgical innovation landscape over the next decade is data intelligence.[167] Through its ability to automate the categorization, linkage and analysis of previously unstructured big data, a new era of personalized, evidence-based surgery is emerging.[263] The power of deep learning in revolutionizing cancer care is becoming increasingly apparent. Neural networks can not only process unlimited genomic data obtained from liquid biopsies and link these to individual patients in real time, but can also 'learn' from the process and 'predict' in a fashion similar to how the human brain functions.[264] This will segue into precision surgery where cancer patients will be matched to the most appropriate treatment(s) based on their individual '-omics' profile, further reinforcing surgery's role as the centrepiece in the multidisciplinary treatment for virtually all solid organ neoplasms.[265] At the same time, biosensors are likely to greatly enhance personalized healthcare, reduce unnecessary follow-up appointments and facilitate big data collection in surgery, also through data intelligence.[109]

Finally, artificial intelligence is playing an increasingly important role is surgical oncology. IBM, Inc. has recently introduced IBM Watson for Oncology, a predictive algorithm trained by Memorial Sloan Kettering Cancer Center physicians to assist in the decision-making of the tumour board.[107] Although it is not possible to predict the future, it is highly likely that the exceptional abilities that come with data intelligence will earmark these emerging fields as the most dominant areas in surgical technology over the next decade.

References

1. Mack MJ. Minimally invasive and robotic surgery. *J Am Med Assoc.* 2001;285(5):568–572.
2. NHS England. *Entry Requirements, Skills and Interests (General Surgery)*; 2018. https://www.healthcareers.nhs.uk/explore-roles/doctors/roles-doctors/surgery/general-surgery/entry-requirements-skills-and-interests.
3. US Department of Health and Human Services. US Food and Drug Administration (FDA). https://www.fda.gov.
4. Department of Health. Medicines & Healthcare Products Regulatory Agency (MHRA). http://www.mhra.gov.uk.
5. European Commission. CE Medical Devices Regulatory Framework. https://www.ema.europa.eu/en/human-regulatory/overview/medical-devices.
6. Jaiswal A, Huang KG. Energy devices in gynecological laparoscopy – archaic to modern era. *Gynecol Minim Invasive Ther.* 2017;6(4):147–151.
7. Garas G, Okabayashi K, Ashrafian H, et al. Which hemostatic device in thyroid surgery? A network meta-analysis of surgical technologies. *Thyroid.* 2013;23(9):1138–1150.
8. Obonna GC, Mishra RK. Differences between thunderbeat, LigaSure and harmonic scalpel energy system in minimally invasive surgery. *World J Lap Surg.* 2014;7(1):41–44.
9. Yildirim O, Umit T, Ebru M, et al. Ultrasonic harmonic scalpel in total thyroidectomies. *Adv Ther.* 2008;25(3):260–265.
10. Voutilainen PE, Haglund CH. Ultrasonically activated shears in thyroidectomies: a randomized trial. *Ann Surg.* 2000;231(3):322–328.
11. Timm RW, Asher RM, Tellio KR, Welling AL, Clymer JW, Amaral JF. Sealing vessels up to 7 mm in diameter solely with ultrasonic technology. *Med Devices (Auckl).* 2014;7:263–271.
12. Ethicon Endo-Surgery, Inc., Johnson & Johnson. HARMONIC HD 1000i Shears. 2017; http://www.ethicon.com/healthcare-professionals/products/advanced-energy/harmonic/harmonic-hd-1000i.
13. Arora A, Chaidas K, Garas G, et al. Outcome of TORS to tongue base and epiglottis in patients with OSA intolerant of conventional treatment. *Sleep Breath.* 2016;20(2):739–747.

14. Arora A, Garas G, Sharma S, et al. Comparing transaxillary robotic thyroidectomy with conventional surgery in a UK population: a case control study. *Int J Surg.* 2016;27:110–117.

15. Tolley N, Garas G, Palazzo F, et al. Long-term prospective evaluation comparing robotic parathyroidectomy with minimally invasive open parathyroidectomy for primary hyperparathyroidism. *Head Neck.* 2016;38(suppl 1):E300–E306.

16. Hanyong S, Wanyee L, Siyuan F, et al. A prospective randomized controlled trial: comparison of two different methods of hepatectomy. *Eur J Surg Oncol.* 2015;41(2):243–248.

17. Nawaz A, Waqar S, Khan A, Mansoor R, Butt UI, Ayyaz M. Harmonic scalpel versus electrocautery in axillary dissection in carcinoma breast. *J Coll Physicians Surg Pak.* 2015;25(12):870–873.

18. Sista F, Abruzzese V, Schietroma M, Cecilia EM, Mattei A, Amicucci G. New harmonic scalpel versus conventional hemostasis in right colon surgery: a prospective randomized controlled clinical trial. *Dig Surg.* 2013;30(4–6):355–361.

19. Kawabata R, Takiguchi S, Kimura Y, et al. A randomized phase II study of the clinical effects of ultrasonically activated coagulating shears (Harmonic scalpel) in open gastrectomy for gastric cancer. *Surg Today.* 2016;46(5):561–568.

20. Covidien Products, Medtronic, Inc. Vessel Sealing Product Portfolio. 2017; http://www.medtronic.com/covidien/en-us/products/vessel-sealing.html.

21. Chekan EG, Davison MA, Singleton DW, Mennone JZ, Hinoul P. Consistency and sealing of advanced bipolar tissue sealers. *Med Devices (Auckl).* 2015;8:193–199.

22. Amirkazem VS, Malihe K. Randomized clinical trial of Ligasure versus conventional splenectomy for injured spleen in blunt abdominal trauma. *Int J Surg.* 2017;38:48–51.

23. Hirunwiwatkul P, Tungkavivachagul S. A multicenter, randomized, controlled clinical trial of LigaSure small jaw vessel sealing system versus conventional technique in thyroidectomy. *Eur Arch Oto-Rhino-Laryngol.* 2013;270(7):2109–2114.

24. Holloran-Schwartz MB, Gavard JA, Martin JC, Blaskiewicz RJ, Yeung Jr PP. Single-use energy sources and operating room time for laparoscopic hysterectomy: a randomized controlled trial. *J Minim Invasive Gynecol.* 2016;23(1):72–77.

25. Fujita J, Takiguchi S, Nishikawa K, et al. Randomized controlled trial of the LigaSure vessel sealing system versus conventional open gastrectomy for gastric cancer. *Surg Today.* 2014;44(9):1723–1729.

26. Lamberton GR, Hsi RS, Jin DH, Lindler TU, Jellison FC, Baldwin DD. Prospective comparison of four laparoscopic vessel ligation devices. *J Endourol.* 2008;22(10):2307–2312.

27. Ioannidis JP. Perfect study, poor evidence: interpretation of biases preceding study design. *Semin Hematol.* 2008;45(3):160–166.

28. Garas G, Ibrahim A, Ashrafian H, et al. Evidence-based surgery: barriers, solutions, and the role of evidence synthesis. *World J Surg.* 2012;36(8):1723–1731.

29. Sosa JA, Bowman HM, Tielsch JM, Powe NR, Gordon TA, Udelsman R. The importance of surgeon experience for clinical and economic outcomes from thyroidectomy. *Ann Surg.* 1998;228(3):320–330.

30. Olympus Medical Systems Corp. *THUNDERBEAT Type S Next Generation of Safety and Speed*; 2017. https://www.olympus-europa.com/medical/en/medical_systems/products_services/product_details/product_details_30592.jsp.

31. Allaix ME, Arezzo A, Giraudo G, Arolfo S, Mistrangelo M, Morino M. The thunderbeat and other energy devices in laparoscopic colorectal resections: analysis of outcomes and costs. *J Laparoendosc Adv Surg Tech.* 2017;27(12):1225–1229.

32. Van Slycke S, Gillardin JP, Van Den Heede K, Minguet J, Vermeersch H, Brusselaers N. Comparison of the harmonic focus and the thunderbeat for open thyroidectomy. *Langenbeck's Arch Surg.* 2016;401(6):851–859.

33. Korolija D. The current evidence on stapled versus hand-sewn anastomoses in the digestive tract. *Minim Invasive Ther Allied Technol.* 2008;17(3):151–154.

34. Choy PY, Bissett IP, Docherty JG, Parry BR, Merrie A, Fitzgerald A. Stapled versus handsewn methods for ileocolic anastomoses. *Cochrane Database Syst Rev.* 2011;(9):CD004320.

35. Loffler T, Rossion I, Goossen K, et al. Hand suture versus stapler for closure of loop ileostomy–a systematic review and meta-analysis of randomized controlled trials. *Langenbeck's Arch Surg.* 2015;400(2):193–205.

36. Qu H, Liu Y, Bi DS. Clinical risk factors for anastomotic leakage after laparoscopic anterior resection for rectal cancer: a systematic review and meta-analysis. *Surg Endosc.* 2015;29(12):3608–3617.

37. Hiemstra E, Chmarra MK, Dankelman J, Jansen FW. Intracorporeal suturing: economy of instrument movements using a box trainer model. *J Minim Invasive Gynecol.* 2011;18(4):494–499.

38. Kayani B, Garas G, Arshad M, Athanasiou T, Darzi A, Zacharakis E. Is hand-sewn anastomosis superior to stapled anastomosis following oesophagectomy? *Int J Surg.* 2014;12(5):7–15.

39. Abellan I, Lopez V, Lujan J, et al. Stapling versus hand suture for gastroenteric anastomosis in Roux-en-Y gastric bypass: a randomized clinical trial. *Obes Surg.* 2015;25(10):1796–1801.

40. Hori S, Ochiai T, Gunji Y, Hayashi H, Suzuki T. A prospective randomized trial of hand-sutured versus mechanically stapled anastomoses for gastroduodenostomy after distal gastrectomy. *Gastric Cancer.* 2004;7(1):24–30.

41. Galetta D, Casiraghi M, Pardolesi A, Borri A, Spaggiari L. New stapling devices in robotic surgery. *J Vis Surg.* 2017;3:45.

42. Platt SR, Hawks JA, Rentschler ME. Vision and task assistance using modular wireless in vivo surgical robots. *IEEE Trans Biomed Eng.* 2009;56(6):1700–1710.

43. Roy S, Yoo A, Yadalam S, Fegelman EJ, Kalsekar I, Johnston SS. Comparison of economic and clinical outcomes between patients undergoing laparoscopic bariatric surgery with powered versus manual endoscopic surgical staplers. *J Med Econ.* 2017;20(4):423–433.

44. Citardi MJ, Yao W, Luong A. Next-generation surgical navigation systems in sinus and skull base surgery. *Otolaryngol Clin North Am.* 2017;50(3):617–632.

45. Chang CM, Jaw FS, Lo WC, Fang KM, Cheng PW. Three-dimensional analysis of the accuracy of optic and electromagnetic navigation systems using surface registration in live endoscopic sinus surgery. *Rhinology.* 2016;54(1):88–94.

46. Dalgorf DM, Sacks R, Wormald PJ, et al. Image-guided surgery influences perioperative morbidity from endoscopic sinus surgery: a systematic review and meta-analysis. *Otolaryngol Head Neck Surg.* 2013;149(1):17–29.

47. Wijsmuller AR, Romagnolo LGC, Agnus V, et al. Advances in stereotactic navigation for pelvic surgery. *Surg Endosc.* 2018;32(6):2713–2720.

48. Vavra P, Roman J, Zonca P, et al. Recent development of augmented reality in surgery: a review. *J Healthc Eng.* 2017;2017:4574172.

49. Phutane P, Buc E, Poirot K, et al. Preliminary trial of augmented reality performed on a laparoscopic left hepatectomy. *Surg Endosc.* 2018;32(1):514–515.

50. Ieiri S, Uemura M, Konishi K, et al. Augmented reality navigation system for laparoscopic splenectomy in children based on preoperative CT image using optical tracking device. *Pediatr Surg Int.* 2012;28(4):341–346.

51. Okamoto T, Onda S, Yasuda J, Yanaga K, Suzuki N, Hattori A. Navigation surgery using an augmented reality for pancreatectomy. *Dig Surg.* 2015;32(2):117–123.

52. Simpfendorfer T, Gasch C, Hatiboglu G, et al. Intraoperative computed tomography imaging for navigated laparoscopic renal surgery: first clinical experience. *J Endourol.* 2016;30(10):1105–1111.

53. Bourdel N, Collins T, Pizarro D, et al. Use of augmented reality in laparoscopic gynecology to visualize myomas. *Fertil Steril.* 2017;107(3):737–739.

54. Balog J, Sasi-Szabo L, Kinross J, et al. Intraoperative tissue identification using rapid evaporative ionization mass spectrometry. *Sci Transl Med.* 2013;5(194):194ra193.

55. Alexander J, Gildea L, Balog J, et al. A novel methodology for in vivo endoscopic phenotyping of colorectal cancer based on real-time analysis of the mucosal lipidome: a prospective observational study of the iKnife. *Surg Endosc.* 2017;31(3):1361–1370.

56. St John ER, Balog J, McKenzie JS, et al. Rapid evaporative ionisation mass spectrometry of electrosurgical vapours for the identification of breast pathology: towards an intelligent knife for breast cancer surgery. *Breast Cancer Res.* 2017;19(1):59.

57. Aziz O, Ashrafian H, Jones C, et al. Laparoscopic ultrasonography versus intra-operative cholangiogram for the detection of common bile duct stones during laparoscopic cholecystectomy: a meta-analysis of diagnostic accuracy. *Int J Surg.* 2014;12(7):712–719.

58. Chakraborty S, Zavarella S, Salas S, Schulder M. Intraoperative MRI for resection of intracranial meningiomas. *J Exp Ther Oncol.* 2017;12(2):157–162.

59. Terasawa M, Ishizawa T, Mise Y, et al. Applications of fusion-fluorescence imaging using indocyanine green in laparoscopic hepatectomy. *Surg Endosc.* 2017;31(12):5111–5118.

60. Eom BW, Kim YI, Yoon HM, et al. Current status and challenges in sentinel node navigation surgery for early gastric cancer. *Chin J Cancer Res.* 2017;29(2):93–99.

61. Mitchell CR, Herrell SD. Image-guided surgery and emerging molecular imaging: advances to complement minimally invasive surgery. *Urol Clin North Am.* 2014;41(4):567–580.

62. East JE, Vleugels JL, Roelandt P, et al. Advanced endoscopic imaging: European Society of Gastrointestinal Endoscopy (ESGE) technology review. *Endoscopy.* 2016;48(11):1029–1045.

63. Singh R, Owen V, Shonde A, Kaye P, Hawkey C, Ragunath K. White light endoscopy, narrow band imaging and chromoendoscopy with magnification in diagnosing colorectal neoplasia. *World J Gastrointest Endosc.* 2009;1(1):45–50.

64. Matsuda T, Ono A, Sekiguchi M, Fujii T, Saito Y. Advances in image enhancement in colonoscopy for detection of adenomas. *Nat Rev Gastroenterol Hepatol.* 2017;14(5):305–314.

65. Vu A, Farah CS. Narrow band imaging: clinical applications in oral and oropharyngeal cancer. *Oral Dis.* 2016;22(5):383–390.

66. Yip HC, Chiu PW. Endoscopic diagnosis and management of early squamous cell carcinoma of esophagus. *J Thorac Dis.* 2017;9(suppl 8):S689–S696.

67. Vicini C, Montevecchi F, D'Agostino G, De Vito A, Meccariello G. A novel approach emphasising intra-operative superficial margin enhancement of head-neck tumours with narrow-band imaging in transoral robotic surgery. *Acta Otorhinolaryngol Ital.* 2015;35(3):157–161.

68. Fujimoto JG, Pitris C, Boppart SA, Brezinski ME. Optical coherence tomography: an emerging technology for biomedical imaging and optical biopsy. *Neoplasia.* 2000;2(1–2):9–25.

69. Kohli DR, Schubert ML, Zfass AM, Shah TU. Performance characteristics of optical coherence tomography in assessment of Barrett's esophagus and esophageal cancer: systematic review. *Dis Esophagus.* 2017;30(11):1–8.

70. Reddy RS, Sai Praveen KN. Optical coherence tomography in oral cancer: a transpiring domain. *J Cancer Res Ther.* 2017;13(6):883–888.

71. Burns JA. Optical coherence tomography: imaging the larynx. *Curr Opin Otolaryngol Head Neck Surg.* 2012;20(6):477–481.

72. Deng F, Fang Y, Shen Z, et al. Use of confocal laser endomicroscopy with a fluorescently labeled fatty acid to diagnose colorectal neoplasms. *Oncotarget.* 2017;8(35):58934–58947.

73. Kiesslich R, Burg J, Vieth M, et al. Confocal laser endoscopy for diagnosing intraepithelial neoplasias and colorectal cancer in vivo. *Gastroenterology.* 2004;127(3):706–713.

74. Volgger V, Girschick S, Ihrler S, Englhard AS, Stepp H, Betz CS. Evaluation of confocal laser endomicroscopy as an aid to differentiate primary flat lesions of the larynx: a prospective clinical study. *Head Neck.* 2016;38(suppl 1):E1695–E1704.

75. Aeishen S, Dawood Y, Papadoukakis S, Horstmann M. [Supplementary optical techniques for the detection of nonmuscle invasive bladder cancer]. *Urologe.* 2018;57(2):139–147.

76. Inoue H, Yokoyama A, Kudo SE. [Ultrahigh magnifying endocopy: development of CM double staining for endocytoscopy and its safety]. *Nihon Rinsho.* 2010;68(7):1247–1252.

77. Flisberg K, Lindholm T. Electrical stimulation of the human recurrent laryngeal nerve during thyroid operation. *Acta Otolaryngol Suppl.* 1969;263:63–67.

78. Hu J, Fleck TR, Xu J, Hsu JV, Xu HX. Contemporary changes with the use of facial nerve monitoring in chronic ear surgery. *Otolaryngol Head Neck Surg.* 2014;151(3):473–477.

79. Silverstein H, Rosenberg S. Intraoperative facial nerve monitoring. *Otolaryngol Clin North Am.* 1991;24(3):709–725.

80. Sood AJ, Houlton JJ, Nguyen SA, Gillespie MB. Facial nerve monitoring during parotidectomy: a systematic review and meta-analysis. *Otolaryngol Head Neck Surg.* 2015;152(4):631–637.

81. Anso J, Dur C, Gavaghan K, et al. A neuromonitoring approach to facial nerve preservation during image-guided robotic cochlear implantation. *Otol Neurotol.* 2016;37(1):89–98.

82. *Medtronic Inc., APS Electrode.* 2017. http://www.medtronic.com/us–en/healthcare-professionals/products/ear-nose-throat/nerve-monitoring/nim-nerve-monitoring-systems/related-nerve-monitoring-products.html.

83. Schneider R, Machens A, Randolph GW, Kamani D, Lorenz K, Dralle H. Opportunities and challenges of intermittent and continuous intraoperative neural monitoring in thyroid surgery. *Gland Surg.* 2017;6(5):537–545.

84. Marin Arteaga A, Peloni G, Leuchter I, et al. Modification of the surgical strategy for the dissection of the recurrent laryngeal nerve using continuous intraoperative nerve monitoring. *World J Surg.* 2018;42(2):444–450.

85. Fox M, Peregrin T. 3-D printing: revolutionizing preoperative planning, resident training, and the future of surgical care. *Bull Am Coll Surg.* 2016;101(7):9–18.

86. Sarris GE, Polimenakos AC. Three-dimensional modeling in congenital and structural heart perioperative care and education: a path in evolution. *Pediatr Cardiol.* 2017;38(5):883–885.

87. Bernstein JM, Daly MJ, Chan H, et al. Accuracy and reproducibility of virtual cutting guides and 3D-navigation for osteotomies of the mandible and maxilla. *PLoS One*. 2017;12(3):e0173111.

88. Crafts TD, Ellsperman SE, Wannemuehler TJ, Bellicchi TD, Shipchandler TZ, Mantravadi AV. Three-dimensional printing and its applications in otorhinolaryngology-head and neck surgery. *Otolaryngol Head Neck Surg*. 2017;156(6):999–1010.

89. Kusaka M, Sugimoto M, Fukami N, et al. Initial experience with a tailor-made simulation and navigation program using a 3-D printer model of kidney transplantation surgery. *Transplant Proc*. 2015;47(3):596–599.

90. Jimenez Ormabera B, Diez Valle R, Zaratiegui Fernandez J, Llorente Ortega M, Unamuno Inurritegui X, Tejada Solis S. [3D printing in neurosurgery: a specific model for patients with craniosynostosis]. *Neurocirugia (Astur)*. 2017;28(6):260–265.

91. Oshiro Y, Mitani J, Okada T, Ohkohchi N. A novel three-dimensional print of liver vessels and tumors in hepatectomy. *Surg Today*. 2017;47(4):521–524.

92. Hochman JB, Rhodes C, Wong D, Kraut J, Pisa J, Unger B. Comparison of cadaveric and isomorphic three-dimensional printed models in temporal bone education. *Laryngoscope*. 2015;125(10):2353–2357.

93. O'Donoghue GM. Hearing without ears: do cochlear implants work in children? *BMJ*. 1999;318(7176):72–73.

94. Matthies C, Brill S, Varallyay C, et al. Auditory brainstem implants in neurofibromatosis type 2: Is open speech perception feasible? *J Neurosurg*. 2014;120(2):546–558.

95. Schwartz MS, Wilkinson EP. Auditory brainstem implant program development. *Laryngoscope*. 2017;127(8):1909–1915.

96. Georgalas C, Garas G, Hadjihannas E, Oostra A. Assessment of obstruction level and selection of patients for obstructive sleep apnoea surgery: an evidence-based approach. *J Laryngol Otol*. 2010;124(1):1–9.

97. Cho WSG G, Morgan A, Chaurasia M. Patient compliance to continuous positive airway pressure (CPAP) therapy for sleep apnoea: a completed audit cycle. *Ir J Med Sc*. 2013;182(suppl 12):S509–S531.

98. Garas G, Kythreotou A, Georgalas C, et al. Is transoral robotic surgery a safe and effective multilevel treatment for obstructive sleep apnoea in obese patients following failure of conventional treatment(s)? *Ann Med Surg (Lond)*. 2017;19:55–61.

99. Schwartz AR, Bennett ML, Smith PL, et al. Therapeutic electrical stimulation of the hypoglossal nerve in obstructive sleep apnea. *Arch Otolaryngol Head Neck Surg*. 2001;127(10):1216–1223.

100. Mwenge GB, Rombaux P, Dury M, Lengele B, Rodenstein D. Targeted hypoglossal neurostimulation for obstructive sleep apnoea: a 1-year pilot study. *Eur Respir J*. 2013;41(2):360–367.

101. Pengo MF, Xiao S, Ratneswaran C, et al. Randomised sham-controlled trial of transcutaneous electrical stimulation in obstructive sleep apnoea. *Thorax*. 2016;71(10):923–931.

102. Strollo Jr PJ, Soose RJ, Maurer JT, et al. Upper-airway stimulation for obstructive sleep apnea. *N Engl J Med*. 2014;370(2):139–149.

103. Kerezoudis P, McCutcheon B, Murphy ME, et al. Thirty-day postoperative morbidity and mortality after temporal lobectomy for medically refractory epilepsy. *J Neurosurg*. 2017;1–7.

104. Lozano CS, Tam J, Lozano AM. The changing landscape of surgery for Parkinson's Disease. *Mov Disord*. 2018;33(1):36–47.

105. Dalkilic EB. Neurostimulation devices used in treatment of epilepsy. *Curr Treat Options Neurol*. 2017;19(2):7.

106. Health Quality Ontario. Gastric electrical stimulation: an evidence-based analysis. *Ont Health Technol Assess Ser*. 2006;6(16):1–79.

107. Stirnimann G, Berg T, Spahr L, et al. Treatment of refractory ascites with an automated low-flow ascites pump in patients with cirrhosis. *Aliment Pharmacol Ther*. 2017;46(10):981–991.

108. Lee SH, Lee YB, Kim BH, et al. Implantable batteryless device for on-demand and pulsatile insulin administration. *Nat Commun*. 2017;8:15032.

109. Rong G, Corrie SR, Clark HA. In vivo biosensing: progress and perspectives. *ACS Sens*. 2017;2(3):327–338.

110. Litsky GS. Endoscopic surgery: the history, the pioneers. *World J Surg*. 1999;23(8):745–753.

111. Ochsner JL. Minimally invasive surgical procedures. *Ochsner J*. 2000;2(3):135–136.

112. Robinson TN, Stiegmann GV. Minimally invasive surgery. *Endoscopy*. 2004;36(1):48–51.

113. Satava RM. Surgical robotics: the early chronicles: a personal historical perspective. *Surg Laparosc Endosc Percutan Tech*. 2002;12(1):6–16.

114. Hussain A, Malik A, Halim MU, Ali AM. The use of robotics in surgery: a review. *Int J Clin Pract*. 2014;68(11):1376–1382.

115. Garas G, Tolley N. Robotics in otorhinolaryngology – head and neck surgery. *Ann R Coll Surg Engl*. 2018;100(suppl 7):34–41.

116. Shah J, Vyas A, Vyas D. The history of robotics in surgical specialties. *Am J Robot Surg*. 2014;1(1):12–20.

117. Sepehripour AH, Garas G, Athanasiou T, Casula R. Robotics in cardiac surgery. *Ann R Coll Surg Engl*. 2018;100(suppl 7):22–33.

118. Yu HY, Hevelone ND, Lipsitz SR, Kowalczyk KJ, Hu JC. Use, costs and comparative effectiveness of robotic assisted, laparoscopic and open urological surgery. *J Urol*. 2012;187(4):1392–1398.

119. Kockerling F. Robotic vs. standard laparoscopic technique - what is better? *Front Surg*. 2014;1:15.

120. Aggarwal R, Hance J, Darzi A. Robotics and surgery: a long-term relationship? *Int J Surg*. 2004;2(2):106–109.

121. Sodergren MH, Darzi A. Robotic cancer surgery. *Br J Surg*. 2013;100(1):3–4.

122. Giulianotti PC, Coratti A, Angelini M, et al. Robotics in general surgery: personal experience in a large community hospital. *Arch Surg*. 2003;138(7):777–784.

123. Liao G, Chen J, Ren C, et al. Robotic versus open gastrectomy for gastric cancer: a meta-analysis. *PLoS One*. 2013;8(12):e81946.

124. Lanfranco AR, Castellanos AE, Desai JP, Meyers WC. Robotic surgery: a current perspective. *Ann Surg*. 2004;239(1):14–21.

125. Kim VB, Chapman WH, Albrecht RJ, et al. Early experience with telemanipulative robot-assisted laparoscopic cholecystectomy using da Vinci. *Surg Laparosc Endosc Percutan Tech*. 2002;12(1):33–40.

126. Marecik SJ, Chaudhry V, Jan A, Pearl RK, Park JJ, Prasad LM. A comparison of robotic, laparoscopic, and hand-sewn intestinal sutured anastomoses performed by residents. *Am J Surg*. 2007;193(3):349–355; discussion 355.

127. Ahlering TE, Skarecky D, Lee D, Clayman RV. Successful transfer of open surgical skills to a laparoscopic environment using a robotic interface: initial experience with laparoscopic radical prostatectomy. *J Urol*. 2003;170(5):1738–1741.

128. Jackson NR, Yao L, Tufano RP, Kandil EH. Safety of robotic thyroidectomy approaches: meta-analysis and systematic review. *Head Neck*. 2014;36(1):137–143.

129. Barbosa JA, Kowal A, Onal B, et al. Comparative evaluation of the resolution of hydronephrosis in children who underwent open and robotic-assisted laparoscopic pyeloplasty. *J Pediatr Urol*. 2013;9(2):199–205.

130. Xu J, Dailey R, Eggly S, Neale A, Schwartz K. Men's perspectives on selecting their prostate cancer treatment. *J Natl Med Assoc*. 2011;103:468–478.

131. Garas G, Arora A. Robotic head and neck surgery: history, technical evolution and the future. *ORL J Otorhinolaryngol Relat Spec*. 2018;1–8.

132. Fuchs KH. Minimally invasive surgery. *Endoscopy*. 2002;34(2):154–159.

133. Look M, Chew S, Tan Y. Postoperative pain in needlescopic versus conventional laparoscopic cholecystectomy: a prospective randomised trial. *J R Coll Surg Edinb*. 2001;46:138–142.

134. Cheah WK, Lenzi JE, So JB, Kum CK, Goh PM. Randomized trial of needlescopic versus laparoscopic cholecystectomy. *Br J Surg*. 2001;88(1):45–47.

135. Antoniou SA, Koch OO, Antoniou GA, et al. Meta-analysis of randomized trials on single-incision laparoscopic versus conventional laparoscopic appendectomy. *Am J Surg*. 2014;207(4):613–622.

136. Arezzo A, Scozzari G, Famiglietti F, Passera R, Morino M. Is single-incision laparoscopic cholecystectomy safe? Results of a systematic review and meta-analysis. *Surg Endosc*. 2013;27(7):2293–2304.

137. Fan Y, Wu SD, Kong J, Su Y, Tian Y, Yu H. Feasibility and safety of single-incision laparoscopic splenectomy: a systematic review. *J Surg Res*. 2014;186(1):354–362.

138. Joseph M, Phillips MR, Farrell TM, Rupp CC. Single incision laparoscopic cholecystectomy is associated with a higher bile duct injury rate: a review and a word of caution. *Ann Surg*. 2012;256(1):1–6.

139. Garg P, Thakur JD, Singh I, Nain N, Mittal G, Gupta V. A prospective controlled trial comparing single-incision and conventional laparoscopic cholecystectomy: caution before damage control. *Surg Laparosc Endosc Percutan Tech*. 2012;22(3):220–225.

140. Milas M, Devedija S, Trkulja V. Single incision versus standard multiport laparoscopic cholecystectomy: up-dated systematic review and meta-analysis of randomized trials. *Surg*. 2014;12(5):271–289.

141. Azizi Koutenaei B, Wilson E, Monfaredi R, Peters C, Kronreif G, Cleary K. Robotic natural orifice transluminal endoscopic surgery (R-NOTES): literature review and prototype system. *Minim Invasive Ther Allied Technol*. 2015;24(1):18–23.

142. Clark MP, Qayed ES, Kooby DA, Maithel SK, Willingham FF. Natural orifice translumenal endoscopic surgery in humans: a review. *Minim Invasive Surg*. 2012;2012:189296.

143. Ko CW, Kalloo AN. Per-oral transgastric abdominal surgery. *Chin J Dig Dis*. 2006;7(2):67–70.

144. Giday SA, Kantsevoy SV, Kalloo AN. Principle and history of natural orifice translumenal endoscopic surgery (NOTES). *Minim Invasive Ther Allied Technol*. 2006;15(6):373–377.

145. Nau P, Ellison EC, Muscarella Jr P, et al. A review of 130 humans enrolled in transgastric NOTES protocols at a single institution. *Surg Endosc*. 2011;25(4):1004–1011.

146. Kozarek RA, Brayko CM, Harlan J, Sanowski RA, Cintora I, Kovac A. Endoscopic drainage of pancreatic pseudocysts. *Gastrointest Endosc*. 1985;31(5):322–327.

147. Narula VK, Happel LC, Volt K, et al. Transgastric endoscopic peritoneoscopy does not require decontamination of the stomach in humans. *Surg Endos*. 2009;23(6):1331–1336.

148. Marescaux J, Rubino F. The ZEUS robotic system: experimental and clinical applications. *Surg Clin North Am*.83(6):1305–1315.

149. Sterbis JR, Hanly EJ, Herman BC, et al. Transcontinental telesurgical nephrectomy using the da Vinci robot in a porcine model. *Urology*. 2008;71(5):971–973.

150. Nguan C, Miller B, Patel R, Luke PP, Schlachta CM. Pre-clinical remote telesurgery trial of a da Vinci telesurgery prototype. *Int J Med Robot*. 2008;4(4):304–309.

151. Kelley Jr WE. The evolution of laparoscopy and the revolution in surgery in the decade of the 1990s. *J Soc Laparoendosc Surg*. 2008;12(4):351–357.

152. Tholey G, Chanthasopeephan T, Hu T. *Measuring Grasping and Cutting Forces for Reality-Based Haptic modelling. Computer Assisted Radiology and Surgery*. London, UK: 17th International Congress and Exhibition; 2003.

153. Hu T, Castellanos AE, Tholey G. *Real-Time Haptic Feedback Laparoscopic Tool for Use in Gastro-Intestinal Surgery*. Tokyo, Japan: Fifth International Conference on Medical Image Computing and Computer Assisted Intervention; 2002.

154. Kennedy C, Desai J. *Force Feedback Using Vision*. Portugal: The 11th International Conference on Advanced Robotics; 2003.

155. Kennedy C, Hu T, Desai J. A novel approach to robotic cardiac surgery using haptics and vision. *Cardiovascular Engineering*. 2002;2(1):15–22.

156. Kennedy C, Hu T, Desai J. *Combining Haptic and Visual Servoing for Cardiothoracic Surgery*. Washington DC: IEEE International Conference on Robotics and Automation; 2002.

157. Morimoto AK, Foral RD, Kuhlman JL, et al. Force sensor for laparoscopic babcock. *Stud Health Technol Inform*. 1997;39:354–361.

158. Dario P, Ciarletta P, Menciassi A, Kim B. Modeling and experimental validation of the locomotion of endoscopic robots in the colon. *Int J Robot Res*. 2004;23:549–556.

159. Breedveld P, Van de Kouwe D, Van Gorp M. *Locomotion Through the Intestine by Means of Rolling Stents*. Salt Lake City, UT: ASME Design Engineering Technica Conference, Computers Information Engineering Conf; 2005.

160. Lehman AC, Dumpert J, Wood NA, et al. Natural orifice cholecystectomy using a miniature robot. *Surg Endosc*. 2009;23(2):260–266.

161. Lehman AC, Wood NA, Farritor S, Goede MR, Oleynikov D. Dexterous miniature robot for advanced minimally invasive surgery. *Surg Endosc*. 2011;25(1):119–123.

162. Piccigallo M, Scarfogliero U, Quaglia C, Petroni G, Valdastri P, Manciassi A. Design of a novel bimanual robotic system for single-port laparoscopy. *Mechatronics IEEE/ASME Trans*. 2010;15(6):871–877.

163. Kaur S. How medical robots are going to affect our lives. *IETE Tech Rev*. 2012;29(3):184–187.

164. Camarillo DB, Krummel TM, Salisbury Jr JK. Robotic technology in surgery: past, present, and future. *Am J Surg*. 2004;188(4A suppl):2S–15S.

165. Garas G, Patel V, Cingolani I, et al. *Process Transformation Is Required to Quantify Surgical Innovation in the Era of Data Intelligence*. London, UK: The Royal College of Surgeons of England; 2018.

166. Maier-Hein L, Vedula SS, Speidel S, et al. Surgical data science for next-generation interventions. *Nat Biomed Eng*. 2017;1:691–696.

167. Garas G, Cingolani I, Panzarasa P, Darzi A, Athanasiou T. Network analysis of surgical innovation: measuring value

and the virality of diffusion in robotic surgery. *PLoS One.* 2017;12(8):e0183332.

168. Garas G, Cingolani I, Panzarasa P, Darzi A, Athanasiou T. Beyond IDEAL: the importance of surgical innovation metrics. *Lancet.* 2019;393(10169):315.

169. *Digital Surgery™*; 2018. https://digitalsurgery.com/2018/02/12/data-driven-human-centric-surgery/.

170. Mandler AG. Touch surgery: a twenty-first century platform for surgical training. *J Digit Imaging.* 2018;31(5):585–590.

171. Nisar PJ, Scott HJ. Key attributes of a modern surgical trainer: perspectives from consultants and trainees in the United Kingdom. *J Surg Educ.* 2011;68(3):202–208.

172. Kelly BD, Curtin PD, Corcoran M. The effects of the European Working Time Directive on surgical training: the basic surgical trainee's perspective. *Ir J Med Sci.* 2011;180(2):435–437.

173. Parsons BA, Blencowe NS, Hollowood AD, Grant JR. Surgical training: the impact of changes in curriculum and experience. *J Surg Educ.* 2011;68(1):44–51.

174. Lowry J, Cripps J. Results of the online EWTD trainee survey. *Bull R Coll Surg Engl.* 2005;87(3):86–87.

175. Surgical Trainees Worried as Training Deteriorates Under European Working Time Regulations [press release]. Association of Surgeons in Training; 2009. How do you cite newspaper articles?.

176. Gladwell M. *Outliers: The Story of Success.* Boston: Little Brown and Company; 2008.

177. Chikwe J, de Souza AC, Pepper JR. No time to train the surgeons. *BMJ.* 2004;328(7437):418–419.

178. Cook DA. Web-based learning: pros, cons and controversies. *Clin Med.* 2007;7(1):37–42.

179. Larvin M. E-learning in surgical education and training. *ANZ J Surg.* 2009;79(3):133–137.

180. Fry H, Ketteridge S, Marshall S. *A Handbook for Teaching and Learning in Higher Education: Enhancing Academic Practice.* 3rd ed. New York: Routledge; 2008.

181. Vygotsky LS. *Mind in Society. The Development of Higher Psychological Processes.* Cambridge, Massachusetts: Harvard University Press; 1978.

182. Evgeniou E, Loizou P. The theoretical base of e-learning and its role in surgical education. *J Surg Edu.* 2012;69(5):665–669.

183. General Medical Council. *Good Medical Practice;* 2013.

184. Lave J, Wenger E. *Situated Learning: Legitimate Peripheral Participation.* Cambridge: Cambridge University Press; 1991.

185. Loertscher J. Cooperative learning for faculty: building communities of practice. *Biochem Mol Biol Educ.* 2011;39(5):391–392.

186. Swanwick T. *Understanding Medical Education: Evidence, Theory and Practice.* 2nd ed. Hoboken NJ: John Wiley & Sons; 2013.

187. Cook DA, Dupras DM. Teaching on the web: automated online instruction and assessment of residents in an acute care clinic. *Med Teach.* 2004;26(7):599–603.

188. Klein M. *Notes on Some Schizoid Mechanisms. Envy and Gratitude and Other Works 1946–1963.* New York: Random House; 1997:1–24.

189. Ruiz JG, Mintzer MJ, Leipzig RM. The impact of E-learning in medical education. *Acad Med J Ass Am Med Coll.* 2006;81(3):207–212.

190. Ericsson KA. Deliberate practice and the acquisition and maintenance of expert performance in medicine and related domains. *Acad Med J Ass Am Med Coll.* 2004;79(10 Suppl):S70–S81.

191. Touch surgery. https://www.touchsurgery.com/.

192. Kamin C, O'Sullivan P, Deterding R, Younger M. A comparison of critical thinking in groups of third-year medical students in text, video, and virtual PBL case modalities. *Acad Med J Ass Am Med Coll.* 2003;78(2):204–211.

193. Deering CG, Eichelberger L. Mirror, mirror on the wall: using online discussion groups to improve interpersonal skills. *Computers, informatics, nursing : CIN Plus.* 2002;20(4):150–154; quiz 155–156.

194. Walker M, Peyton JR. Teaching in theatre. In: Peyton JR, ed. *Teaching and Learning in Medical Practice.* Rickmansworth: Manticore Europe; 1998.

195. Porte MC, Xeroulis G, Reznick RK, Dubrowski A. Verbal feedback from an expert is more effective than self-accessed feedback about motion efficiency in learning new surgical skills. *Am J Surg.* 2007;193(1):105–110.

196. Office for National Statistics. https://www.ons.gov.uk/peoplepopulationandcommunity/householdcharacteristics/homeinternetandsocialmediausage. Accessed 23/10/2018.

197. Siemens G. Connectivism: a learning theory for the digital age. *ITDL.* 2004.

198. Downes S. New technology supporting informal learning. *J Emerg Technol Web Intellig.* 2010;2(1):27–33.

199. Knowles MS. *Andragogy in Action: Applying Modern Principles of Adult Learning.* Hoboken, NJ: Wiley; 1984.

200. Cheston CC, Flickinger TE, Chisolm MS. Social media use in medical education: a systematic review. *Acad Med J Ass Am Med Coll.* 2013;88(6):893–901.

201. Intercollegiate Surgical Curriculum Programme (ISCP). https://www.iscp.ac.uk/curriculum/surgical/curriculum_framework.aspx.

202. General Medical Council. *Doctors' Use of Social media;* 2013.

203. Brady RRW, Chapman SJ, Atallah S, et al. #colorectalsurgery. *Br J Surg.* 2017;104(11):1470–1476.

204. Rapp AK, Healy MG, Charlton ME, Keith JN, Rosenbaum ME, Kapadia MR. YouTube is the most frequently used educational video source for surgical preparation. *J Surg Edu.* 2016;73(6):1072–1076.

205. Al-Khatib TA. Surgical education on YouTube. *Saudi Med J.* 2014;35(3):221–223.

206. Scott DJ, Cendan JC, Pugh CM, Minter RM, Dunnington GL, Kozar RA. The changing face of surgical education: simulation as the new paradigm. *J Surg Res.* 2008;147(2):189–193.

207. Sturm LP, Windsor JA, Cosman PH, Cregan P, Hewett PJ, Maddern GJ. A systematic review of skills transfer after surgical simulation training. *Annal Surg.* 2008;248(2):166–179.

208. Tan SSY, Sarker SK. Simulation in surgery: a review. *Scottish Med J.* 2011;56(2):104–109.

209. Grober ED, Hamstra SJ, Wanzel KR, et al. The educational impact of bench model fidelity on the acquisition of technical skill: the use of clinically relevant outcome measures. *Annals Surg.* 2004;240(2):374–381.

210. Anastakis DJ, Wanzel KR, Brown MH, et al. Evaluating the effectiveness of a 2-year curriculum in a surgical skills center. *Am J Surg.* 2003;185(4):378–385.

211. Giger U, Fresard I, Hafliger A, Bergmann M, Krahenbuhl L. Laparoscopic training on Thiel human cadavers: a model to teach advanced laparoscopic procedures. *Surg Endosc.* 2008;22(4):901–906.

212. Jansen S, Cowie M, Linehan J, Hamdorf JM. Fresh frozen cadaver workshops for advanced vascular surgical training. *ANZ J Surg.* 2014;84(11):877–880.

213. Foster JD, Gash KJ, Carter FJ, et al. Development and evaluation of a cadaveric training curriculum for low rectal cancer surgery in the English LOREC National Development Programme. *Colorectal Dis.* 2014;16(9):O308–O319.

214. Arora A, Kotecha J, Acharya A, et al. Determination of biometric measures to evaluate patient suitability for transoral robotic surgery. *Head Neck*. 2015;37(9):1254–1260.

215. Gilbody J, Prasthofer A, Ho K, Costa M. The use and effectiveness of cadaveric workshops in higher surgical training: a systematic review. *Ann R Coll Surg Engl*. 2011;93(5):347–352.

216. Scott DJ, Goova MT, Tesfay ST. A cost-effective proficiency-based knot-tying and suturing curriculum for residency programs. *J Surg Res*. 2007;141(1):7–15.

217. Anastakis DJ, Regehr G, Reznick RK, et al. Assessment of technical skills transfer from the bench training model to the human model. *Am J Surg*. 1999;177(2):167–170.

218. Beard JD, Jolly BC, Newble DI, Thomas WE, Donnelly J, Southgate LJ. Assessing the technical skills of surgical trainees. *Br J Surg*. 2005;92(6):778–782.

219. Datta V, Bann S, Beard J, Mandalia M, Darzi A. Comparison of bench test evaluations of surgical skill with live operating performance assessments. *J Am Coll Surg*. 2004;199(4):603–606.

220. Beard JD. Assessment of surgical skills of trainees in the UK. *Ann R Coll Surg Engl*. 2008;90(4):282–285.

221. Jonides J, Nee DE. Brain mechanisms of proactive interference in working memory. *Neuroscience*. 2006;139(1):181–193.

222. Aggarwal R, Undre S, Moorthy K, Vincent C, Darzi A. The simulated operating theatre: comprehensive training for surgical teams. *Qual Saf Health Care*. 2004;13(suppl 1):i27–i32.

223. Sarker S, Patel B. Simulation and surgical training. *Int J Clin Pract*. 2007;61(12):2120–2125.

224. Larsen CR, Oestergaard J, Ottesen BS, Soerensen JL. The efficacy of virtual reality simulation training in laparoscopy: a systematic review of randomized trials. *Acta Obstet Gynecol Scand*. 2012;91(9):1015–1028.

225. Nagendran M, Gurusamy KS, Aggarwal R, Loizidou M, Davidson BR. Virtual reality training for surgical trainees in laparoscopic surgery. *Cochrane Database Syst Rev*. 2013;(8):Cd006575.

226. Larsen CR, Soerensen JL, Grantcharov TP, et al. Effect of virtual reality training on laparoscopic surgery: randomised controlled trial. *BMJ*. 2009;338.

227. Seymour NE, Gallagher AG, Roman SA, et al. Virtual reality training improves operating room performance: results of a randomized, double-blinded study. *Annals Surg*. 2002;236(4):458–464.

228. Grantcharov TP, Kristiansen VB, Bendix J, Bardram L, Rosenberg J, Funch-Jensen P. Randomized clinical trial of virtual reality simulation for laparoscopic skills training. *Br J Surg*. 2004;91(2):146–150.

229. Seymour NE. VR to OR: a review of the evidence that virtual reality simulation improves operating room performance. *World J Surg*. 2008;32(2):182–188.

230. Sedlack RE, Kolars JC. Validation of a computer-based colonoscopy simulator. *Gastrointest Endosc*. 2003;57(2):214–218.

231. Cisler JJ, Martin JA. Logistical considerations for endoscopy simulators. *Gastrointest Endosc Clin N Am*. 2006;16(3):565–575.

232. Lucas SM, Zeltser IS, Bensalah K, et al. Training on a virtual reality laparoscopic simulator improves performance of an unfamiliar live laparoscopic procedure. *J Urol*. 2008;180(6):2588–2591; discussion 2591.

233. Moorthy K, Munz Y, Sarker SK, Darzi A. Objective assessment of technical skills in surgery. *Br Med J*. 2003;327(7422):1032–1037.

234. Datta V, Chang A, Mackay S, Darzi A. The relationship between motion analysis and surgical technical assessments. *Am J Surg*. 2002;184(1):70–73.

235. Smith SGT, Torkington J, Brown TJ, Taffinder NJ, Darzi A. Motion analysis. *Surg Endos*. 2002;16(4):640–645.

236. Moorthy K, Munz Y, Dosis A, Bello F, Chang A, Darzi A. Bimodal assessment of laparoscopic suturing skills: construct and concurrent validity. *Surg Endosc Intervent Tech*. 2004;18(11):1608–1612.

237. Xeroulis G, Dubrowski A, Leslie K. Simulation in laparoscopic surgery: a concurrent validity study for FLS. *Surg Endosc*. 2009;23(1):161–165.

238. Corvetto MA, Fuentes C, Araneda A, et al. Validation of the imperial college surgical assessment device for spinal anesthesia. *BMC Anesthesiol*. 2017;17(1):131.

239. Hayter MA, Friedman Z, Bould MD, et al. Validation of the Imperial College Surgical Assessment Device (ICSAD) for labour epidural placement. *Can J Anaesth* 2009;56(6):419–426.

240. Modi HN, Singh H, Yang G-Z, Darzi A, Leff DR. A decade of imaging surgeons' brain function (part I): terminology, techniques, and clinical translation. *Surgery*.

241. Modi HN, Singh H, Yang GZ, Darzi A, Leff DR. A decade of imaging surgeons' brain function (part II): a systematic review of applications for technical and nontechnical skills assessment. *Surgery*. 2017;162(5):1130–1139.

242. Leff DR, Orihuela-Espina F, Atallah L, Darzi A, Yang GZ. Functional near infrared spectroscopy in novice and expert surgeons--a manifold embedding approach. *Med Image Comput Comput Assist Interv*. 2007;10(Pt 2):270–277.

243. Leff DR, Orihuela-Espina F, Atallah L, et al. Functional prefrontal reorganization accompanies learning-associated refinements in surgery: a manifold embedding approach. *Comput Aided Surg*. 2008;13(6):325–339.

244. Leff DR, Elwell CE, Orihuela-Espina F, et al. Changes in prefrontal cortical behaviour depend upon familiarity on a bimanual co-ordination task: an fNIRS study. *Neuroimage*. 2008;39(2):805–813.

245. Leff DR, Orihuela-Espina F, Leong J, Darzi A, Yang GZ. Modelling dynamic fronto-parietal behaviour during minimally invasive surgery--a Markovian trip distribution approach. *Medical image computing and computer-assisted intervention : MICCAI International Conference on Medical Image Computing and Computer-Assisted Intervention*. 11(Pt 2):595–602.

246. Shetty K, Leff DR, Orihuela-Espina F, Yang GZ, Darzi A. Persistent prefrontal engagement despite improvements in laparoscopic technical skill. *JAMA Surg*. 2016;151(7):682–684.

247. Morris MC, Frodl T, D'Souza A, Fagan AJ, Ridgway PF. Assessment of competence in surgical skills using functional magnetic resonance imaging: a feasibility study. *J Surg Edu*. 2015;72(2):198–204.

248. Duty B, Andonian S, Ma Y, et al. Correlation of laparoscopic experience with differential functional brain activation: a positron emission tomography study with oxygen 15-labeled water. *Archiv Surg*. 2012;147(7):627–632.

249. Nemani A, Intes X, De S. Surgical motor skill differentiation via functional near infrared spectroscopy. *Paper presented at: Biomedical Engineering Conference (NEBEC), 2015 41st Annual Northeast*; 17–19 April 2015.

250. Halsband U, Lange RK. Motor learning in man: a review of functional and clinical studies. *J Physiol Paris*. 2006;99(4–6):414–424.

251. Petersen SE, van Mier H, Fiez JA, Raichle ME. The effects of practice on the functional anatomy of task performance. *Proc Nat Acad Sci United States Am*. 1998;95(3):853–860.

252. Leff DR, Leong JJ, Aggarwal R, Yang GZ, Darzi A. Could variations in technical skills acquisition in surgery be explained by differences in cortical plasticity? *Annals Surg*. 2008;247(3):540–543.

253. Leff DR, Yongue G, Vlaev I, et al. 'Contemplating the next maneuver': functional neuroimaging reveals intraoperative decision-making strategies. *Annals Surg*. 2017;265(2):320–330.

254. Modi HN, Singh H, Orihuela-Espina F, et al. Temporal stress in the operating room: brain engagement promotes 'coping' and disengagement prompts 'choking'. *Annals Surg*. 2018;267(4):683–691.

255. Birkmeyer JD, Finks JF, O'Reilly A, et al. Surgical skill and complication rates after bariatric surgery. *N Engl J Med*. 2013;369(15):1434–1442.

256. Hogg ME, Zenati M, Novak S, et al. Grading of surgeon technical performance predicts postoperative pancreatic fistula for pancreaticoduodenectomy independent of patient-related variables. *Annals Surg*. 2016;264(3):482–491.

257. Tien T, Pucher PH, Sodergren MH, Sriskandarajah K, Yang G-Z, Darzi A. Eye tracking for skills assessment and training: a systematic review. *J Surg Res*. 2014;191(1):169–178.

258. Duchowski AT. Eye tracking methodology. *Theory and Practice*. 2007; 328.

259. Khan RS, Tien G, Atkins MS, Zheng B, Panton ON, Meneghetti AT. Analysis of eye gaze: do novice surgeons look at the same location as expert surgeons during a laparoscopic operation? *Surg Endosc*. 2012;26(12):3536–3540.

260. Richstone L, Schwartz MJ, Seideman C, Cadeddu J, Marshall S, Kavoussi LR. Eye metrics as an objective assessment of surgical skill. *Annals Surg*. 2010;252(1):177–182.

261. Wilson M, McGrath J, Vine S, Brewer J, Defriend D, Masters R. Psychomotor control in a virtual laparoscopic surgery training environment: gaze control parameters differentiate novices from experts. *Surg Endosc*. 2010;24(10):2458–2464.

262. Athanasopoulos LV, Athanasiou T. Are virtual clinics an applicable model for service improvement in cardiac surgery? *Eur J Cardio Thorac Surg*. 2017;51(2):201–202.

263. Yim WW, Yetisgen M, Harris WP, Kwan SW. Natural language processing in oncology: a review. *JAMA Oncol*. 2016;2(6):797–804.

264. Davenport TH, Ronanki R. Artificial intelligence for the real world. *Harv Bus Rev*. 2018;96(1–2):108–116.

265. Low SK, Zembutsu H, Nakamura Y. Breast cancer: the translation of big genomic data to cancer precision medicine. *Cancer Sci*. 2017.

Regional Surgery

18

Common Surgical Conditions of Head and Neck

CHAPTER OUTLINE

THE EAR

Embryology

During embryogenesis, the ear develops from three separate germ layers: the ectoderm, the endoderm and the mesenchyme. Beginning at approximately day 22 in utero, these primitive elements develop and grow into a complex and delicate three-part sensory organ, which provides hearing and balance to the individual, facilitates communication, spatial awareness, the ability to walk, and contributes to our unique appearance.

Anatomy

Anatomically, the ear consists of three main parts: the outer, middle and inner ear (Fig. 18.1). The outer ear includes the pinna (helix, antihelix, tragus, antitragus and ear lobe), and the external auditory canal (which has a cartilaginous outer third and is bony on the inner two thirds). The external auditory canal is lined with stratified squamous epithelium. The nerve supply to the outer ear includes the auriculotemporal nerve (upper lateral surface and anterior external auditory canal), the greater auricular nerve (lower lateral and medial surface outer ear), the lesser occipital nerve (post auricular skin), facial nerve (superior part of external auditory canal), lesser occipital nerve (posterior aspect of external auditory canal) and vagus nerve (inferior part of external auditory canal). The tympanic membrane separates the external and middle ear. It consists of an outer epithelial layer, a middle collagenous layer (which is deficient in the pars flaccida) and an inner endothelial layer. The annulus marks the junction where the tympanic membrane attaches to the external auditory canal.

The middle ear is a three-dimensional air-filled cavity within the temporal bone that lies between the tympanic membrane laterally and the stapes window medially. The roof is formed by a thin tegmen and the floor includes the jugular bulb. The middle ear is lined with epithelium and contains three articulating ossicles (malleus, incus and stapes), which lie in an angulated but continuous chain connecting the endodermal surface of the tympanic membrane and the stapes (oval) window. Tiny ligaments (annular ligaments) and muscles (tensor tympani and stapedius) also occur within the middle ear cavity; they act to dampen the domino-like motion of the ossicles and control the amount of sound energy which is presented to the delicate inner ear

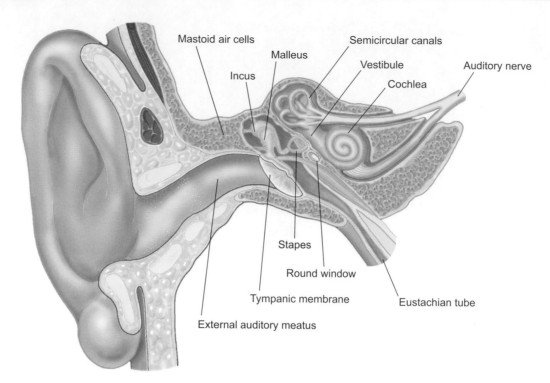

• **Fig. 18.1** Anatomy of the Ear.

components. A pressure valve known as the eustachian tube connects the middle ear cavity to the back of the nasal cavity. It opens and closes to regulate air pressure within the middle ear cavity and allow drainage of fluid as required.

The inner ear consists of a central vestibule (with appendages called the utricle and saccule), a cochlea for hearing and a semicircular canal complex for the perception of balance. The otic capsule surrounding the inner ear contains a CSF filtrate called perilymph. The inside of the bony labyrinth complex and cochlea is bathed in endolymph, which is produced by the stria vascularis. Endolymph has a finely balanced electrolyte composition to facilitate depolarization of the cochlear and vestibular nerves.

Physiology of Hearing and Balance

Each of the three parts of the ear work together to facilitate the conversion of sinusoidal sound wave energy to discrete particles of electrical activity which transmit from the cochlear and vestibular nerves to the cortex of the brain.

The outer ear effectively acts as a three-dimensional funnel, which channels sound waves towards the tympanic membrane. Once these waves of energy hit the tympanic membrane, the sound energy is converted to a mechanical vibration of the delicate three-layered tympanic membrane which oscillates through the malleus first, then the incus and finally the stapes. The movement of the ossicles is dampened by the stapedius and the annular ligaments. The tensor tympani muscle is a reflex protective muscle, which acts on the tympanic membrane to tighten it like a drum if the energy transmitted to the inner ear is too high for the delicate sensory component within.

Oscillation of the stapes against the stapes (oval) window leads to ripples of endolymph along the cochlea, causing

directional changes of tiny hair-like projections on sensory hair cells dotted along the cochlea. The change in directional configuration of the surface of these sensory cells opens and closes sodium and potassium channels, which allows action potentials to develop and depolarization of the cochlear nerve to occur. Depolarization of the cochlear nerve acts as a form of Morse code to the auditory cortex that is recognized as a perception of hearing due to neuronal plasticity in early childhood development.

Balance perception is multidimensional. It also works by the opening and closing of sodium and potassium channels within the semicircular canals: however, unlike hearing, directional movement of the head induces the movement of the fluid within the balance component of the inner ear. The vestibule, saccule and utricle govern linear acceleration, whilst the semicircular canals control perception of angular acceleration.

Clinical Examination

Thorough examination requires assessment of each of the three components of the ear. First the outer ear is inspected for asymmetry, obvious injury, wax or foreign body impaction, skin changes and obvious signs of infection such as pus. Both sides must be compared and contrasted. An auroscope allows inspection of the ear canal and the tympanic membrane. In its healthy state, the tympanic membrane is approximately 1 cm diameter, pale pink and demonstrates a cone-shaped light reflex in the anterior inferior quadrant (Fig. 18.2). The upper part of the tympanic membrane is known as the pars flaccida and the inferior part is known as the pars tensa. The lateral process and handle of the malleus are normally visible. The health of the middle ear and inner ear can be evaluated using tuning fork tests (Rinne

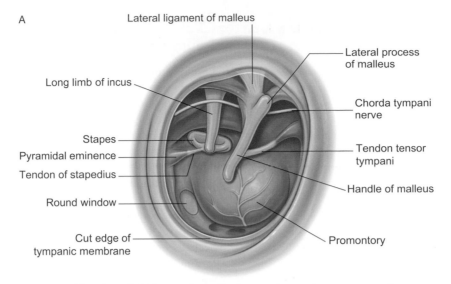

A

Lateral ligament of malleus

Lateral process of malleus

Long limb of incus

Chorda tympani nerve

Stapes

Pyramidal eminence

Tendon tensor tympani

Tendon of stapedius

Round window

Handle of malleus

Cut edge of tympanic membrane

Promontory

View into right tympanic cavity (tympanic membrane removed)

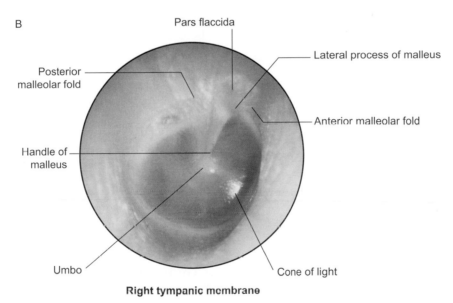

B

Pars flaccida

Lateral process of malleus

Posterior malleolar fold

Anterior malleolar fold

Handle of malleus

Umbo

Cone of light

Right tympanic membrane

• **Fig. 18.2** Healthy Tympanic Membrane. A, View into right tympanic cavity (tympanic membrane removed). B, Right tempanic membrane. (From Drake R, Wayne Vogl A, Mitchell W, eds. Gray's Atlas of Anatomy, 3rd ed. Philadelphia: Elsevier; 2021.)

and Weber test) for conductive or sensory hearing loss, audiometry for quantitative analysis of a hearing loss (Fig. 18.3) and balance tests (Romberg's, Unterberger, Hallpike) for problems with the vestibule or semicircular canals.

Surgical Disorders of the Ear

Functional Disorders of the Ear

Functional disorders of the ear include hearing loss and vertigo.

Hearing Loss

Hearing loss may be conductive (where there is a problem conducting the sound wave to the sensory part of the ear) or sensorineural (where there is a problem with the sensory cells, the nerve transmitting the electrical impulse to

the brain or the brain's ability to make sense of the message being sent to it) (Fig. 18.3).

The Weber and Rinne tests are clinical tuning fork tests, which are described in Box 18.1.

Vertigo

Vertigo is the misinterpretation of either linear or angular movement leading to dizziness or loss of balance. The Hallpike test is a diagnostic manoeuvre used to identify benign paroxysmal vertigo. The patient is lowered quickly to the supine position (face and torso facing up) with the neck extended by the clinician. The head is quickly rotated 45 degrees to the side being tested. In the presence of benign positional vertigo, the patient will report feeling dizzy, and the clinician will observe the presence of delayed nystagmus.

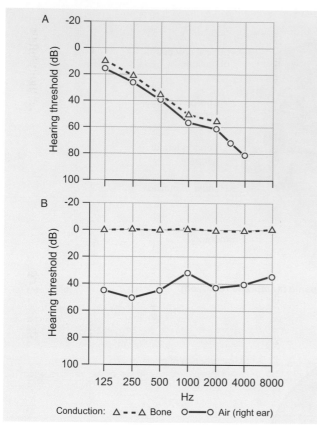

• **Fig. 18.3** An Audiogram (A) Sensorineural loss with reduced hearing levels by both air and bone conduction. (B) Conductive hearing loss with reduced hearing level by air conduction and normal bone conduction.

• BOX 18.1 Clinical Tuning Fork Tests

(Use a 512 Hz tuning fork)

Weber Test
- Base of the vibrating tuning fork is placed on the centre of the forehead.
- Ask the patient where the vibration is heard.
- If there is a sensory deficit on one side, sound will appear louder in the contralateral side.

Rinne Test
- Identifies presence of conductive hearing loss.
- Should be performed in conjunction with the Weber test.
- Base of the fork is placed against patient's mastoid process.
- When the patient no longer hears the vibration, the tuning fork is placed next to the ear on that side.
- If the sound is now heard, then the test is positive (= air conduction is better than bone conduction and there is no significant conductive hearing loss).
- In the presence of a conductive loss, sound travels better through the bone of the skull to the inner ear, leading to direct vibrations within the inner ear fluid resulting in depolarization of the hair cells. If the same tuning fork is presented to the outer ear, impediments to conduction such as wax, atretic ear canal, middle ear fluid, abnormal ossicles or cholesteatoma will prevent the full sound wave from reaching the inner ear.

Surgical Disorders of the Outer Ear

Traumatic

Foreign bodies most frequently affect the outer ear and are typically seen in early childhood. Foreign bodies must be removed by an ENT surgeon with a microscope and appropriately-sized grasping forceps or probes. Small batteries are potentially corrosive foreign bodies and when suspected must be removed immediately to prevent scarring and stenosis of the external ear canal.

Haematoma of the ear most commonly affects the outer portion or pinna. Haematoma of the outer ear must be drained under anaesthetic (local using ring block or general anaesthesia in younger patients) to prevent necrosis of the underlying cartilage and the formation of cauliflower ear deformity. Protective headwear should be worn in contact sports to prevent the occurrence of pinna haematomas.

Skin lacerations occur at the pinna or following penetrating injury to the canal. These can occur at any age. Thorough irrigation and debridement of necrotic skin may be required. Antibiotic cover should be given to prevent abscess formation and perichondritis. Repair of lacerations should be promptly performed using non-absorbable nylon sutures to the skin. This may be delayed in the case of human or animal bites.

Infectious/Inflammatory

Furuncle is a painful infection of the hair follicles. Typically, it occurs due to *Staphyloccous aureus* infection and patients will present with pain, swelling and mild hearing loss in the affected ear. Treatment requires oral antibiotics and insertion of antibiotic wicks into the ear canal.

Otitis externa is inflammation or infection of the skin of the ear canal. Patients with diabetes or dry skin who traumatize the ear canal with cotton buds or use communal swimming pools or saunas are at risk of developing this painful condition. In some cases, the infection can spread to the bone of the skull base (necrotizing otitis external (NOE)) with potential involvement of the cranial nerves, sepsis and intracranial disease. Regular aural toilet to remove debris must be performed and the use of topical antibiotics via a wick or dressing is required. If NOE is suspected, blood tests for full blood count, blood sugar level, and c-reactive protein (CRP) should be taken. Radiological assessment is with CT scan and systemic antibiotic treatment is needed.

Neoplastic

Squamous cell carcinoma (SCC) frequently occurs at the external ear. The ears are considered a high-risk site for SCC. SCC of the ear has greater metastatic potential than other sites. Cartilage invasion is a poor prognosticator. Resection with adequate margins is required and consideration should be given to performing a neck dissection with removal of dependent lymph nodes

Congenital

Congenital atresia and microtia may occur in isolation due to incomplete branchial arch development or as part of a wider syndrome. If the inner and middle ear structures are intact, hearing loss will be conductive and may be restored with bone-anchored hearing aids. Cosmesis is less important than hearing restoration; surgery to restore or reconstruct microtia or atretic ears should only be considered after the hearing has been addressed and when the child is older. Genetic conditions such as Waardenburg's, Treacher Collins and branchiootorenal syndrome should be out ruled when a patient presents with atresia or microtia.

Surgical Disorders of the Middle Ear

Traumatic

Hemotympanum is a collection of blood within the middle ear cavity. Usually associated with trauma (but also with coagulopathy), blood builds up in the cavity leading to conductive hearing loss and a dark discoloration of the tympanic membrane on auroscope examination. Patients should be evaluated for signs of head injury. Management is with analgesia and decongestants. Hearing is usually restored with resolution of the blood collection.

Ossicular discontinuity due to trauma occurs when the inner ear ossicles fall out of their normal configuration within the middle ear cavity. Ossicular discontinuity is typically associated with severe blunt force trauma and may occur in conjunction with hemotympanum. Patients presenting with a maximal conductive hearing loss should undergo CT imaging to detect the presence of temporal bone fractures. Patients may require long-term hearing aid or reconstructive surgery to restore the hearing.

Infectious/Inflammatory

Acute otitis media is an acute infection of the middle ear. It is most prevalent in children or patients with a history of congenital conditions such as cleft palate, Treacher Collins, Trisomy 21 or Apert syndrome. Middle ear effusion (or glue ear) becomes colonized by pathogens such as *Streptococcus* spp. or *Haemophilus* spp. leading to pain and conductive hearing loss. Untreated, it may lead to perforation of the tympanic membrane (Fig. 18.4), chronic suppurative otitis media or acute mastoiditis. Treatment is with broad-spectrum oral antibiotics and nasal decongestants. Patients with more than six episodes of acute otitis media in one year may require insertion of a ventilatory tube (grommet) (Fig. 18.5).

Acute coalescent mastoiditis occurs when unresolved acute middle ear infection spreads to the mastoid portion

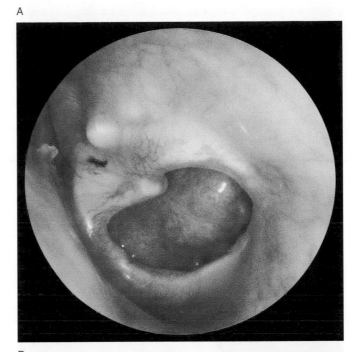

A

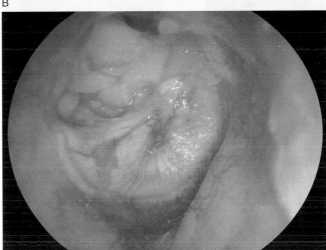

B

• **Fig. 18.4** (A) Large perforation of the tympanic membrane in the pars tensa. (B) Chronic otitis media with cholesteatoma and granulations in the attic.

of the skull to form a collection. It is a surgical emergency which, untreated, can result in meningitis, intracranial abscess formation, cranial nerve injury, deafness and death. The diagnosis is clinical. Features include aural proptosis, presence of a fluctuant red swelling behind the ear and a bulging tympanic membrane (Fig. 18.6). Emergent treatment requires grommet insertion and incision drainage of the abscess or a cortical mastoidectomy to remove the infected bone.

Neoplastic

Glomus tympanicum is the most common form of middle ear tumour. It is a benign chemodectoma or paraganglioma, which arises along the tympanic nerve in the middle ear cavity. Patients present with conductive hearing loss and a sensation of pulsatile tinnitus. Auroscope examination may reveal a red area of 'setting sun' at the tympanic membrane. CT imaging is the most sensitive diagnostic test. Larger glomus tumours may require surgical resection as destruction of the skull base can occur in rapidly growing lesions.

Cholesteatoma is a non-malignant, but locally destructive mass of squamous epithelium occurring in the middle ear. It can be classified as congenital or acquired. Acquired

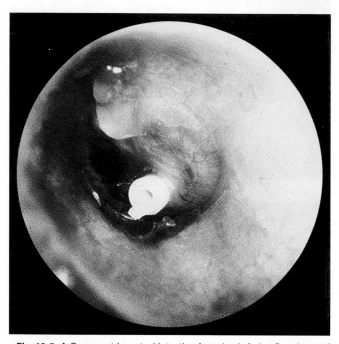

• **Fig. 18.5** A Grommet Inserted into the Anterior Inferior Quadrant of the Left Tympanic Membrane

cholesteatoma is more common and can be further divided into primary, secondary and tertiary. Local destruction can lead to ossicular erosion, intracranial empyema, labyrinthine invasion and facial nerve involvement. Treatment usually requires mastoidectomy but suction clearance may treat small easily accessible pearls of cholesteatoma where conservative management is required.

Congenital

Congenital stapes fixation is non-progressive fibrous fixation of the incus to the stapes. It is presents in childhood, and is associated with conductive hearing loss. Diagnosis is made with formal audiogram and high-resolution CT scan of the middle ear. Corrective surgery by stapedectomy/stapedotomy can be performed in older patients. Hearing aids may be used in patients who decline or are not suited for surgery.

Otosclerosis is abnormal growth of bone around the stapes that leads to progressive conductive hearing loss in young adults. Hearing loss is exacerbated in pregnancy and a link with childhood measles infection has been observed. Diagnosis is made with formal audiogram and high-resolution CT scan of the middle ear. Corrective surgery by stapedectomy/stapedotomy can be performed in appropriately selected patients.

Surgical Disorders of the Inner Ear

Traumatic

Temporal bone fractures occur due to blunt force trauma to the head. Fractures may lead to permanent

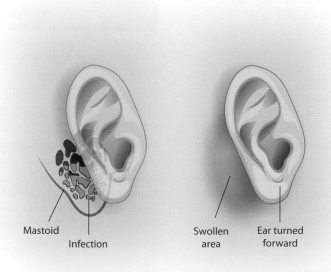

Mastoid
Infection
Swollen area
Ear turned forward

• **Fig. 18.6** Acute Coalescent Mastoiditis Featuring Aural Proptosis (From http://www.emdocs.net/acute-mastoiditis-pearls-and-pitfalls)

sensorineural hearing loss if the otic capsule around the cochlea is involved in the fracture line. Whilst hearing loss due to concussion or bruising of the inner ear may recover, hearing loss with an otic capsule involving fracture will not recover and the patient may require a hearing aid or bone anchored hearing aid. CSF otorrhea may occur and lead to meningitis

Infectious/Inflammatory

Labyrinthitis/vestibular neuronitis is inflammation of the labyrinth or nerve, which causes sudden onset severe, rotatory vertigo and vomiting due most commonly to viral infection. Treatment is predominantly symptomatic with bed rest, fluid hydration and vestibular sedatives such as betahistine.

Meniere's disease is an illness of unknown aetiology, which is characterized by rotational vertigo, tinnitus, aural fullness and fluctuating hearing loss in the low frequency ranges. Treatment options include medical management (betahistine, Stemetil, salt reduction, water restriction and diuretics) or surgery (gentamycin injection, labyrinthectomy, vestibular nerve section and endolymphatic decompression).

Neoplastic

Vestibular schwannomas are benign tumours of the vestibular nerve. They are slow growing and can exist undiagnosed for many years. The typical presentation is unilateral tinnitus with or without a hearing loss and vertigo. Later symptoms can include trigeminal neuralgia, headache or signs of increasing intracranial pressure. Management can be conservative for small tumours under 1.5 cm. For larger lesions, stereotactic radio surgery with either gamma or cyber knife will administer precise amounts of radiation to the lesion without damaging surrounding tissues. Surgical resection is generally reserved for very large tumours.

Congenital

Congenital hearing loss may arise due to maternal infection such as rubella. Absent or atretic external, middle, or inner ear components can occur when there is failure of normal branchial arch development. Neonatal hearing screening is important to evaluate the new born infant's ability to process sounds. Tympanometry, stapedius reflexes and auditory brain stem response tests are used in neonatal hearing assessment. In toddlers or older children, audiometric testing is done by means of play audiometry, distraction tests and pure tone audiometry if the child has normal or near normal cognitive ability. Hearing loss must be recognized and treated early because neuronal plasticity and the ability to collate and interpret language cease after the age of 8 in children. Treatment options to improve function may

include the use of hearing aids, bone anchored hearing aids or cochlear implants (Fig. 18.7).

THE NOSE

Function

The nose and paranasal sinuses are considered to be continuous structures of the same system with linked functions; respiration, filtration of air, humidification, olfaction and vocal resonance. It is thought that the paranasal sinuses assist in resonance and air circulation in addition to reducing the weight of the skull.

Anatomy (Fig. 18.8)

Anatomically, the nose is divided into the external nose and the nasal cavity. The paranasal sinuses are air filled extensions of the nasal cavity, which form in the facial skeleton. The upper third of the external nose is bony and the lower two-thirds consists of the upper lateral and lower lateral alar cartilages. The tip is formed from fibrous cartilage and the skin over the lower two-thirds is adherent and contains multiple sebaceous glands.

The nasal cavity is the first part of the upper respiratory tract. The nasal cavity extends from the vestibule to the nasopharynx is divided in two by the bony and cartilaginous septum, and bordered laterally by the inferior, middle and superior turbinates. The paranasal sinuses drain into the nasal cavity around the middle turbinate.

The blood supply of the nose originates from external and internal carotid artery branches including the anterior and posterior ethmoidal arteries, the sphenopalatine (maxillary artery) and superior labial arteries (facial artery). The facial and ophthalmic veins drain directly to the cavernous sinus. Sensory supply is provided by the trigeminal nerve (maxilliary division). The vidian nerve provides autonomic supply, and controls local mucosal blood flow.

The paranasal sinuses comprise of the paired maxillary, frontal, anterior ethmoidal, posterior ethmoidal and sphenoid sinuses. The anterior ethmoidal and maxillary sinuses drain into the middle meatus, and the other sinuses drain into the superior meatus and sphenoethmoidal recess.

Physiology of the Nose and Paranasal Sinuses

Numerous secretory glands and the profuse blood supply of the nasal passages allow warming and humidification of inspired air, whilst hairs at the vestibule and mucus layer remove particles of dirt so the air is cleaned prior to being transported into the lungs.

Olfaction is the sense of smell and is facilitated by the olfactory nerve cells. Olfactory nerve cells are bipolar cells which project into the superior portion of the nasal cavity via the cribriform plate. Odorant particles in a moist

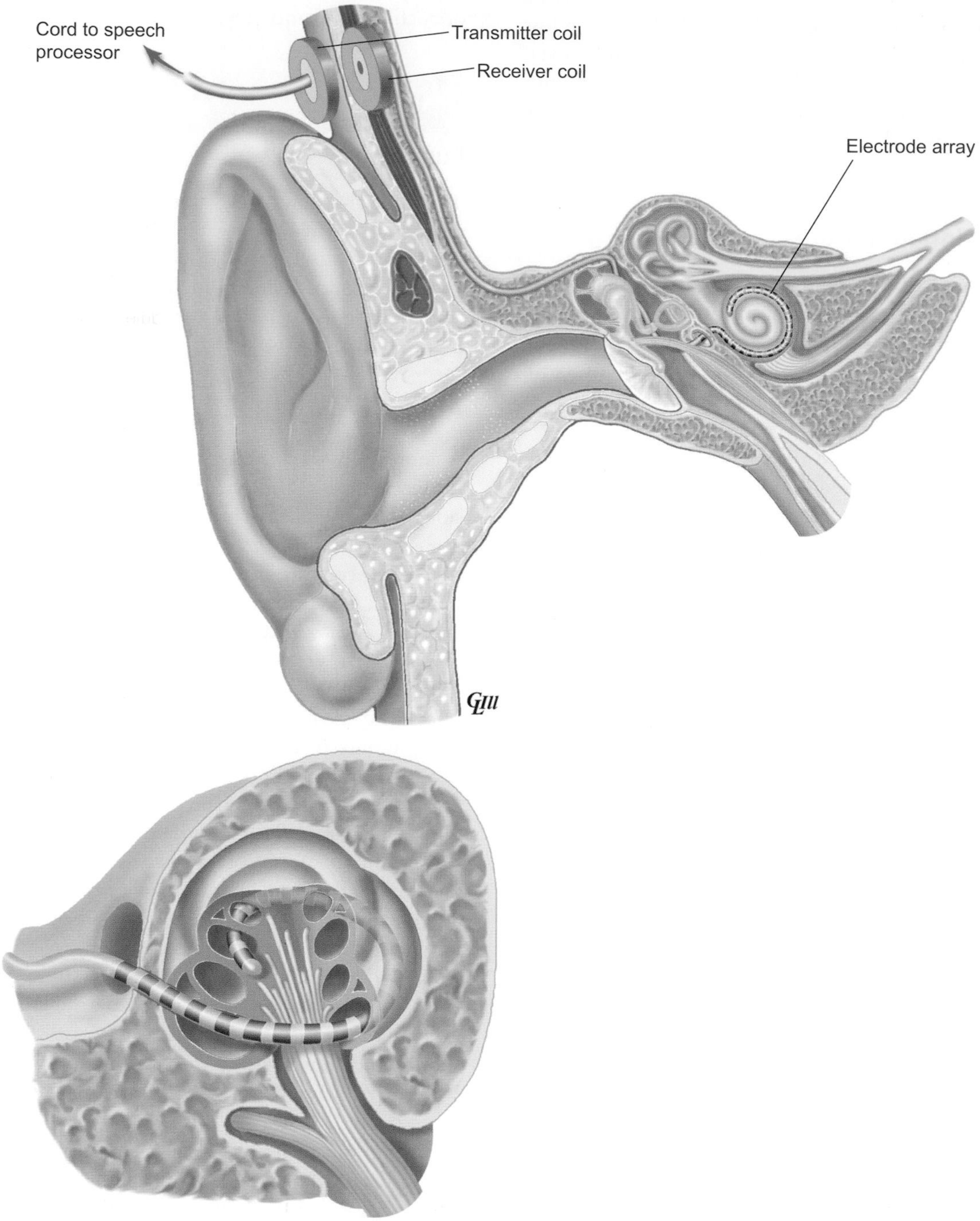

• **Fig. 18.7** Cochlear implant may be used to treat severe hearing loss in patients with sensorineural hearing loss. (Adapted from Hirsch HG. Intelligibility improvement of noisy speech for people with cochlear implants. Speech Commun. 1993; 12 (3), 261–266. Reproduced by permission of Cochlear.)

environment cause depolarization of the nerve and enable the perception of smell. Olfactory nerve cells are easily damaged by viral infection or by trauma; however, they possess a degree of plasticity not seen elsewhere in the central nervous system.

In the appreciation of flavour, a small amount of air is regurgitated across the olfactory neuroepithelial cells during deglutition. This leads to a simultaneous awareness of the taste and smell of the food being consumed.

Clinical Examination

Thorough examination requires assessment of each section of the nose and paranasal sinuses. All examination must start with inspection from the front and sides. Comparison of both sides looking for asymmetry, dorsal hump, tip depression, erythema, skin changes, obvious vesicles or discharge is made. Look for signs of obvious deformity or trauma. Gently palpate the nasal bridge and orbital margins looking

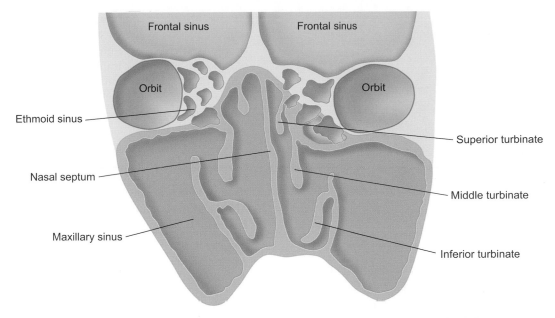

• **Fig. 18.8** Coronal Section to Show the Sinuses and Particularly the Ethmoid Air Cells

• **BOX 18.2** Flexible Fibreoptic Nasal Endoscopy

Indications include:

- Sinonasal symptoms, i.e. mucopurulent discharge, facial pain, nasal congestion, reduced sense of smell
- Evaluation of patients' response to medical treatment (e.g. polyp resolution)
- Evaluation and biopsy of nasal lesions
- Evaluation & treatment of epistaxis
- Evaluation of hyposmia or anosmia
- Foreign body removal

Relative contraindications include:

- Bleeding disorder or patients on anticoagulants
- Anxious patients or with cardiovascular disease (there is a risk of a vasovagal episode)

for asymmetry, bruising, skin lesions or obvious tumours. Displacing the tip upwards will identify collapse due to cartilage deficiency. A Thudicum or Killians speculum will allow inspection of the inside of the nasal cavity for septal deviation, nasal polyposis, tumours or foreign body.

Fibre optic nasal endoscopy under local anaesthetic should be performed to visualize the postnasal space and both Eustachian tube openings (Box 18.2). Full cranial nerve assessment and neck examination should conclude the nasal exam.

Surgical Disorders of the Nose and Paranasal Sinuses

The pathological conditions of the nose and sinuses can be broadly categorized into traumatic, infectious/inflammatory and neoplastic. Commonly encountered surgical conditions of the nose and paranasal sinuses are outlined below.

Traumatic

Foreign body in the nasal passages is a potential cause of airway obstruction or collapsed lung. Young children and psychiatric patients are prone to placing foreign bodies into the nose. Removal should be performed immediately due to the risk of airway compromise. Most can be removed without general anaesthetic.

Symptoms: Unilateral nasal blockage or malodorous rhinorrhoea.

Skin lacerations can occur as a result of human bites, isolated injury, or as a component of poly trauma. Irrigation and debridement of necrotic tissue may be required and repair is usually performed with sutures, paper stitches or glue. Antibiotic cover should be given to prevent development of cartilage infection.

Nasal fractures are very common in the emergency department setting. Deformity and nasal obstruction are the main complications but fractures may be associated with nasal septal haematoma, periorbital involvement or CSF rhinorrhoea. Manipulation is best performed immediately but, after the first few hours, swelling may prevent accurate reduction of the fracture and lead to epistaxis, therefore in settings where immediate reduction of the fracture has not been performed, manipulation is best left to 7 to 10 days post injury.

Epistaxis is a common cause for emergency department attendance. It may be spontaneous or traumatic and often occurs as sequelae of medical anticoagulation, hypertension or platelet abnormality. Initial assessment must include airway and circulation assessment and intravenous access with group and screen must be obtained. Particular attention must be paid to the platelet count and packing should be placed with extreme caution where the platelet count is low. The majority of nosebleeds occur at

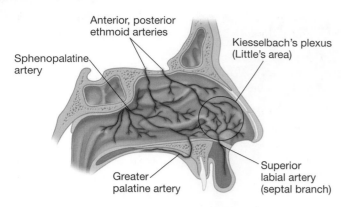

• **Fig. 18.9** Kiesselbach's Plexus (Known as 'Little's Area')

Kiesselbach's plexus at the anterior septal area known as Little's area (Fig. 18.9). Light bleeding may stop with pressure or application of silver nitrate under local anaesthetic. If conservative measures fail, anterior packing with cellulose or inflatable nasal packs may be required. For large volume bleeds, surgical ligation of the sphenopalatine, anterior ethmoidal or posterior ethmoidal arteries may be required. Patients unfit for general anaesthetic may be managed with radiologic embolization.

Orbital blow out fracture occurs where a nasal or paranasal fracture involves the floor of the orbit. Clinically, they present with cheek paraesthesia and restricted eye movements. Reduction and fixation of the fractures are required to prevent permanent visual problems.

Le Fort fractures are mid facial fractures, characterized by a free-floating palate. Typically, they occur as a result of high-speed blunt force injury as seen in road traffic injuries and they are often associated with airway compromise, neck injuries and brain injuries. Following stabilization and airway control, patients require reduction and fixation of the fractures.

Cerebrospinal (CSF) rhinorrhoea is leakage of CSF through the nose. It may be acquired or congenital and puts patients at risk of developing cerebral meningitis. Acquired CSF rhinorrhoea is the commoner of the two and is usually associated with base of skull fractures involving the paranasal sinuses. Small leaks may resolve spontaneously but larger or persistent leaks require urgent closure by either endoscopic or open surgical approach.

Infectious/Inflammatory

Vestibulitis

• This is a minor infection of the nasal vestibule, which occurs most commonly due to staphylococcal infection.
• It may lead to furunculosis, cellulitis and cavernous thrombosis.
• It must be treated promptly with topical antibiotic (Bactroban) ointment.

Rhinitis

• This is a hyper reactive nasal mucosa.
• It is broadly categorized as *allergic* or *non-allergic*.

• *Allergic rhinitis* is commoner then non-allergic rhinitis and occurs due to IgE mediated type 1 hypersensitivity reactions. It can be perennial (year-round – often due to allergies to house dust mites), or seasonal (hay-fever). It affects up to 15 % of Europeans and is characterized by prostaglandin and leukotriene release leading to vasodilatation and capillary permeability. Asthma is frequently present.
• *Non-allergic rhinitis* is hyperactive mucosa due to non-specific stimuli such as fumes or medication. The appearance of the mucosa is red and boggy compared to allergic rhinitis, which is pale and boggy.
• The diagnosis is clinical but the radio adsorbent test may be used to identify allergens and distinguish between allergic and non-allergic rhinitis.
• Treatment for both allergic and non-allergic rhinitis is with saline nasal douches and topical steroid application.

Sinusitis

• This is infection of the paranasal sinuses, which varies from a simple viral respiratory infection, to acute bacterial infection or chronic rhino sinusitis.
• Mucosal oedema, obstruction or reduced mucociliary clearance lead to stasis and bacterial or viral super infection.
• Empiric treatment for uncomplicated sinusitis is ampicillin with nasal decongestants.
• Untreated, it may progress and lead to complications including periorbital cellulitis, subperiosteal abscess, intracranial subdural abscess or meningitis.
• In cases which are refractory to treatment, CT scan can be used to identify underlying anatomical abnormality or neoplastic process.
• Sinus surgery is indicated in fungal sinusitis, sinusitis with meningitis, brain abscess, cavernous thrombosis or where an underlying neoplastic process is suspected.

Nasal Polyps

• These are pedunculated portions of nasal or paranasal mucosa, which prolapse into the nasal cavity.
• They can be simple, or neoplastic.
• Symptoms of nasal obstruction, loss of olfaction, postnasal drip, sneezing and vocal changes can occur.
• They generally occur due to untreated rhinitis but if present in children should raise the suspicion of cystic fibrosis or Kartagener's syndrome.
• A unilateral nasal polyp in a young baby could represent meningocele.
• Polyps may occur in conjunction with asthma and aspirin allergy – known as Samter's triad.
• Treatment involves endoscopic sinus surgery to restore the airway and long-term steroid nasal sprays.

Granulomatous Diseases

• They cause granuloma formation through chronic inflammation with accumulation of multinucleate giant cells and lymphocytes.

- *Wegener's disorder* is a vasculitic granulomatous disorder of unknown aetiology, which presents often with nasal congestion due to necrosis of the nasal septum. It is associated with renal and pulmonary involvement and it is diagnosed by the presence of antineutrophil cytoplasmic antibodies (ANCA). Syphilis, T-cell lymphoma and tuberculosis can lead to similar granuloma formation.

Tumours

Benign

Juvenile Nasopharyngeal Angiofibroma

- This is a benign, locally aggressive vascular tumour.
- It occurs most commonly in juvenile males.
- It presents typically with brisk unilateral haemorrhage in the setting of unilateral nasal congestion.
- CT or MRI is the diagnostic modality of choice and management includes radiotherapy, embolization or surgery.

Esthesioneuroblastoma

- This is a rare malignant tumour of neuroectodermal origin.
- It is of unknown aetiology
- It has variable prognosis.
- It is staged according to the Kadish staging system.
- Transnasal endoscopic resection may give adequate clearance but a craniofacial approach is often required in cases where the dura has been breached.

Inverting (Schneiderian Papilloma) Papillomas

- These are benign lesions arising from the mucosal surfaces of the nose or sinus, which can invert into the underlying tissues.
- They are associated with the development of squamous cell carcinoma.
- They are associated with the HPV infection.
- They have a high risk of recurrence following resection.

Malignant

Carcinoma of the Sinuses

- This is relatively uncommon.
- Adenocarcinoma and squamous cell carcinomas form the majority.
- 60–70% occur in the maxillary sinuses whilst 20–30% occur in the nasal cavity
- The risk factors are complicated and controversial. Exposure to oncogenic viruses, industrial dust and hardwood have been linked with the development of sinonasal malignancy
- The symptoms include nasal obstruction, proptosis and headaches.
- Staging of tumours requires MRI, CT or PET CT.
- Management: In maxillary sinus cancer, in stages I and II the first step is surgical excision of the cancer and/or adjuvant radiotherapy. For stages III and IV, neoadjuvant chemoradiotherapy, surgery and/or adjuvant chemoradiotherapy may be required.

Congenital

Choanal Atresia

- This is a congenital disorder which occurs as a result of failure of the bucco-nasal membrane to break down.
- It may be unilateral, bilateral, membranous or bony.
- Over 50% of babies born with choanal atresia have other abnormalities (CHARGE syndrome – coloboma, heart defects, growth retardation and ear abnormalities).
- Bilateral choanal atresia usually presents as cyanosis and an inability to feed in young babies (obligate nasal breathers for the first 3 months of life).
- Investigation should include CT and endoscopy.
- Airway management is crucial and may require intubation.
- Definitive management involves either rupture of the membrane, or drilling through the bony septum.

Cleft Palate

- This occurs as a result of failure of fusion of the nasal and palatal prominences around week 5 to week 8 of development in utero.
- Aetiology is broadly classified as genetic, intrauterine or environmental.
- The mode of inheritance is most likely to be polygenic and the risk factors for cleft development include family history; ethnicity, phenytoin, retinoid, thalidomide use; alcohol use; and folic acid deficiency.
- Management requires multiple staged surgeries as the child's facial structures grow towards adulthood.

THE LARYNX

Function

The functions of the larynx may be classified into biologic or communication. Its biologic functions include airway protection; breathing and abdominal stabilization for lifting heavy objects, and its communication function is the generation of sound waves which the phonatory system subsequently modifies to allow the production of meaningful speech.

Anatomy (Fig. 18.10)

The adult larynx is about 5 cm long and is formed by the thyroid cartilage, the cricoid cartilage and the epiglottis, with smaller paired cartilages including the arytenoids, the cuneiforms, the corniculate and the triticeal cartilages. The thyroid cartilage is the largest, butterfly shaped cartilage (forms the prominence of the Adam's apple in men). The cricoid cartilage is signet-ring shaped and sits below the thyroid cartilage.

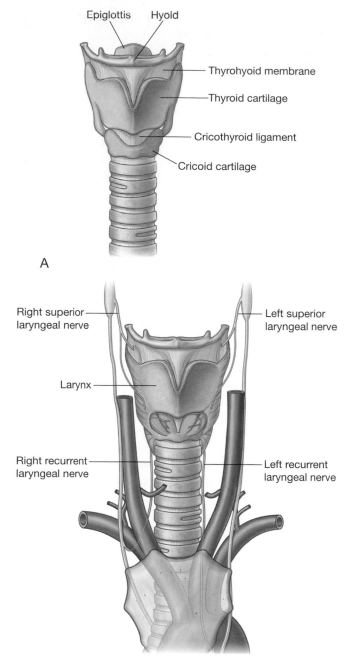

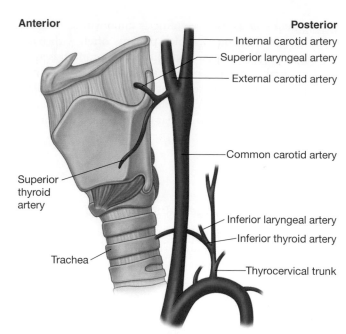

• **Fig. 18.11** Lateral View of the Larynx with Arterial Blood Supply (Adapted from Drake R, Wayne Vogl A, Mitchell W, eds. Gray's Anatomy for Students, 4th ed. Philadelphia: Elsevier; 2021.)

> **• BOX 18.3** **Recurrent Laryngeal Nerve Injury**
>
> **Symptoms**
> - Dysphagia
> - Hoarseness or aphonia
> - Dyspnoea during exercise
>
> **Causes**
> - Iatrogenic injury (i.e. thyroid/parathyroid surgery)
> - Endotracheal intubation
> - Viral infection
> - Neoplasia from neck or upper chest (i.e. thyroid or lung cancer)

• **Fig. 18.10** (A) Anterior view of the larynx. (B) Recurrent laryngeal nerve anatomy. (B, From from Drake R, Wayne Vogl A, Mitchell W., eds. Gray's Anatomy for Students, 4th ed.; 2021.)

Extrinsic and intrinsic ligaments and membranes connect the laryngeal cartilages. These ligaments allow suspension of the larynx and connect it to the adjacent structures. The vocal folds are draped over the vocal ligaments. Anatomically, the vocal fold consists of five individual layers, the deepest of which is formed by the thyroarytenoid muscle. The lamina propria, which comprises a deep (collagenous), intermediate (elastic) and superficial layer, lies beneath the mucosa and above the thyroarytenoid. The ventricular, or false vocal folds, are proximal to the true vocal folds and do not generate sound waves. The gap between the true and false cords is called the ventricle and is reduced in laryngopharyngeal reflux. The supraglottis comprises the area above the vocal folds, whilst the subglottis is the region between the inferior aspect of the vocal fold and the cricoid.

The blood supply to the larynx is provided by the superior laryngeal artery, the superior thyroid artery, and the inferior thyroid artery (Fig. 18.11). The recurrent laryngeal nerve (see Fig. 18.10B) and the superior laryngeal nerve innervate the larynx, whilst the pharyngeal nerve innervates the pharynx and soft palate. Box 18.3 describes symptoms and causes of recurrent laryngeal nerve damage.

Physiology of the Larynx

Airway protection and the prevention of food aspiration to the lungs depend on positional changes of the epiglottis and vocal folds during swallowing. The production of speech is made possible through a series of interactions between the respiratory, phonatory and articulatory systems. Voice production depends on myoelastic recoil and Bernoulli mucosal waves, where air pressure, maintained within a narrow range, pushes open the closed vocal fold, and the resulting combination of elastic recoil within the vocal folds and the Bernoulli effect sets up an acoustic pressure pulse, or sound wave, of a certain frequency. Variation in pitch and volume of voice are produced by configurational changes in the position, tension and width of the vocal folds, which are achieved by movements of the various cartilages within the laryngeal structure.

Clinical Examination

The examination of the larynx should include a thorough general inspection and neck examination for the presence of obvious lumps and bumps, scars, deformities and metastatic neck nodes. Note of the patient's body mass index should be made. Obvious hoarseness (dysphonia) or stridor (noisy breathing due to reduced airway) should be investigated with flexible nasendoscopy.

A more invasive way of assessing the vocal folds for subtle changes is *stroboscopy*, which utilizes a strobe light and a rigid scope to visualize the vocal folds and the way in which they are moving. Voice analysis software can be used to analyse different characteristics of the human voice. Direct laryngoscopy generally requires an anaesthetic and enables procurement of biopsies.

Surgical Disorders of the Larynx

Traumatic

Foreign Body Impaction in the Larynx

- This is common in children, edentulous patients, patients with neuromuscular disorders and patients with psychiatric illness.
- Common objects include fish bones and coins.
- Prompt removal is essential to prevent airway obstruction and death of the patient. Removal can be achieved with rigid bronchoscopy.

Laryngeal Fractures

- These are uncommon and typically occur following blunt trauma, seatbelt injuries or strangulation injuries.
- They can be associated with significant soft tissue oedema and pose a potential risk to the airway. Often there are intracranial or spinal injuries.
- Clinical findings include subcutaneous emphysema, haematoma of the glottis, stridor and dysphonia.
- Diagnosis usually requires a CT scan.
- Management includes bed rest, steroids and airway observation. Occasionally, tracheostomy and surgical reduction are required.

Infectious/Inflammatory

Epiglottitis

- This is caused by group B *Haemophilus* influenza infection
- It is characterized by acute swelling of the supraglottic mucosa.

- Epiglottitis is seen mainly in young children, though adults may also be affected.
- The typical history is of sudden onset of pyrexia, sore throat and dysphagia. Drooling may occur and children tend to sit in the tripod position to improve breathing.
- If epiglottitis is suspected, the patient should be immediately transferred to hospital and no attempt should be made to look in the throat or gain intravenous access. In these circumstances, total airway obstruction can occur. The airway should be stabilized under anaesthetic and, once the patient is asleep, airway control can be achieved by the insertion of a rigid bronchoscope or endotracheal tube. In certain circumstances, a tracheostomy may be performed.
- Cephalosporin antibiotics should be commenced. Siblings should be given prophylactic antibiotics. Intubated patients can usually be extubated after 48 hours.

Vocal Fold Polyps (Fig. 18.12)

- These occur as localised unilateral collections of fluid or blood, which occur on the vocal fold.
- They usually occur as a result of any combination of an initial event such as phono-trauma (vocal misuse), gastric reflux, chronic smoking and chronic laryngeal allergic reactions.
- Histologically, vocal fold polyps may contain fibrin deposits and iron laden macrophages and in some cases, they have been shown to display evidence of capillary proliferation.
- Vocal fold polyps tend to be more commonly unilateral and to occur at the middle third of the membranous part of the true vocal fold.
- Treatment requires removal of the polyp and speech therapy.

Reinke's Oedema

(Also referred to as polypoid corditis.)
- This describes a more generalized pattern of polypoid degeneration of the vocal cords.
- It is thought to occur as a separate entity from vocal fold polyps.
- Reinke's oedema is more closely associated with smoking and laryngopharyngeal reflux then with phono-trauma.
- It is characterized by the presence of diffuse swelling of the entire lamina propria or Reinke's layer and it occurs almost exclusively in smokers.
- The presence of either isolated vocal fold polyps, or Reinke's oedema, lead to an increase in the overall mass of the vocal fold with an increase in air turbulence and a lowering of the frequency of the sound produced, perceived by the listener as dysphonia or hoarseness.
- Treatment requires smoking cessation, speech therapy and surgical decompression in advanced cases.

Vocal Nodules

- These occur as symmetrical firm swellings on the vocal folds.
- They occur due to phono-trauma and are a significant cause of dysphonia.
- Treatment is with speech therapy.

Lesions of the Vocal Cords

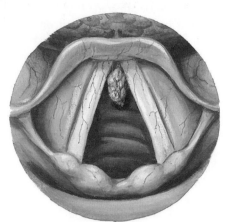

Pedunculated papilloma
at anterior commissure

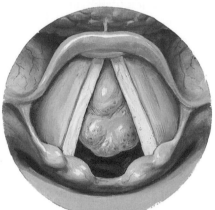

Sessile polyp

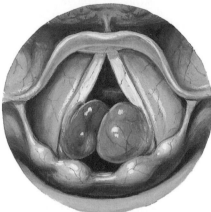

Large bilateral granulomas

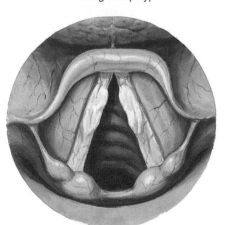

Subglottic polyp

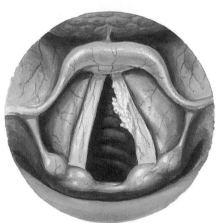

Hyperkeratosis of right cord

Bilateral leukoplakia

• **Fig. 18.12** Lesions of the Vocal Cords From top left to right: pedunculated papilloma, sessile polyp, large bilateral granulomas, subglottic polyp, hyperkeratosis at right cord, bilateral leukoplakia. (From https://www.netterimages.com/lesions-of-the-vocal-cords-labeled-runge-im-2e-otolaryngology-frank-h-netter-5614.html)

Neoplastic

Laryngeal Carcinoma

- This occurs when cells of the larynx undergo malignant transformation.
- The majority are squamous cell cancers.
- Most arise on the vocal cords.
- There is a direct causative link between smoking and alcohol consumption and the development of laryngeal cancers. Smokers are 14 times more likely, and those who consume alcohol are 7 times more likely, to develop laryngeal cancer.
- Carcinogenesis occurs in a stepwise chemically mediated process known as dysplasia. Untreated, dysplasia progresses to carcinoma in situ and invasive tumour.
- Depending on the site of the tumour within the larynx, symptoms include dysphonia, stridor, dysphagia, weight loss and metastatic disease in the neck or lungs.
- Tumours of the larynx are classified by site and by staging them according to the size of the tumour, the sites involved, the presence of neck lymph nodes and the presence of distant metastatic disease.
- Smaller non-metastatic tumours may be treated with primary radiotherapy, laser endoscopic microsurgery or partial laryngectomy, all of which are organ preserving, that is the patient will retain the speech function. Larger or metastatic tumours require multimodality treatment (often with laryngectomy followed by radiotherapy with or without chemotherapy, or with primary chemoradiotherapy).
- Tumour extent and the presence of lymph node involvement or metastatic disease determines overall survival; therefore, treatment selection requires careful preoperative assessment including triple assessment with physical examination, tissue biopsies and radiological tests such as CT, MRI and PET CT.

Congenital

Laryngomalacia

- This is the most common congenital abnormality of the larynx.
- The aetiology is unknown.
- It occurs more commonly in male babies and is a leading cause of infantile stridor.
- It is associated with gastric reflux
- It is usually self-limiting; however, it may require laser reduction of supra glottic tissues to improve the airway or tracheostomy in very extreme cases where the airway is at risk.

Laryngoceles

- These are benign but abnormal outpouchings of the larynx.
- They are typically congenital but acquired cases have been reported in glass blowers where continuous forced expiration results in increased pressure at the ventricle.

- Patients should be investigated for an underlying small carcinoma of the larynx with biopsy and CT scan should be performed for evaluation of the extent of the lesion.
- Surgical resection is usually performed via external approach.

Subglottic Stenosis

- This may occur as a congenital anomaly with incomplete canalization of the laryngotracheal tube during week 12 of foetal development, or as a result of prolonged intubation.
- Congenital subglottic stenosis can be either *membranous* or *cartilaginous*
- Surgical dilation, tracheostomy, or even laryngotracheoplasty may be required.

THE PHARYNX

Function

The pharynx connects the respiratory and gastrointestinal systems to the base of the skull. It has a dual physical role in that it acts as a passageway for air and food. It also houses lymphoid tissue in the tonsils and adenoids, which protect babies and young children from infection.

Anatomy (Fig. 18.13)

The pharynx is a conical fibromuscular cavity situated immediately behind the nasal passages and oral cavity, above the level of the oesophagus and behind the larynx. The pharynx includes the nasopharynx, oropharynx and hypopharynx. The nasopharynx connects the posterior choanae at the back of the nasal cavity, with the oropharynx. The oropharynx extends from the uvula to the base of the epiglottis (level of the hyoid bone). It houses tonsil and adenoidal tissue. The hypopharynx extends from the level of the epiglottis to the inferior edge of the cricoid. It lies between the pyriform fossae and behind the larynx. The upper middle and inferior constrictors surround the pharynx and it is elevated by stylopharyngeus, palatopharyngeus and salpingopharyngeus. Branches of the external carotid arteries supply it and innervation is derived from the glossopharyngeal and vagus nerves.

Physiology

The eustachian tube of each middle ear opens into the nasopharynx. Eustachian tube opening occurs due to pharyngeal muscle action, facilitating equalization of middle ear pressures.

The second phase of swallowing occurs in the pharynx. Chewed and moistened boluses of food are passed to the pharynx by voluntary movements of the tongue. At the pharynx, involuntary circular muscle contractions take place and the swallowing reflex is triggered to pass the bolus

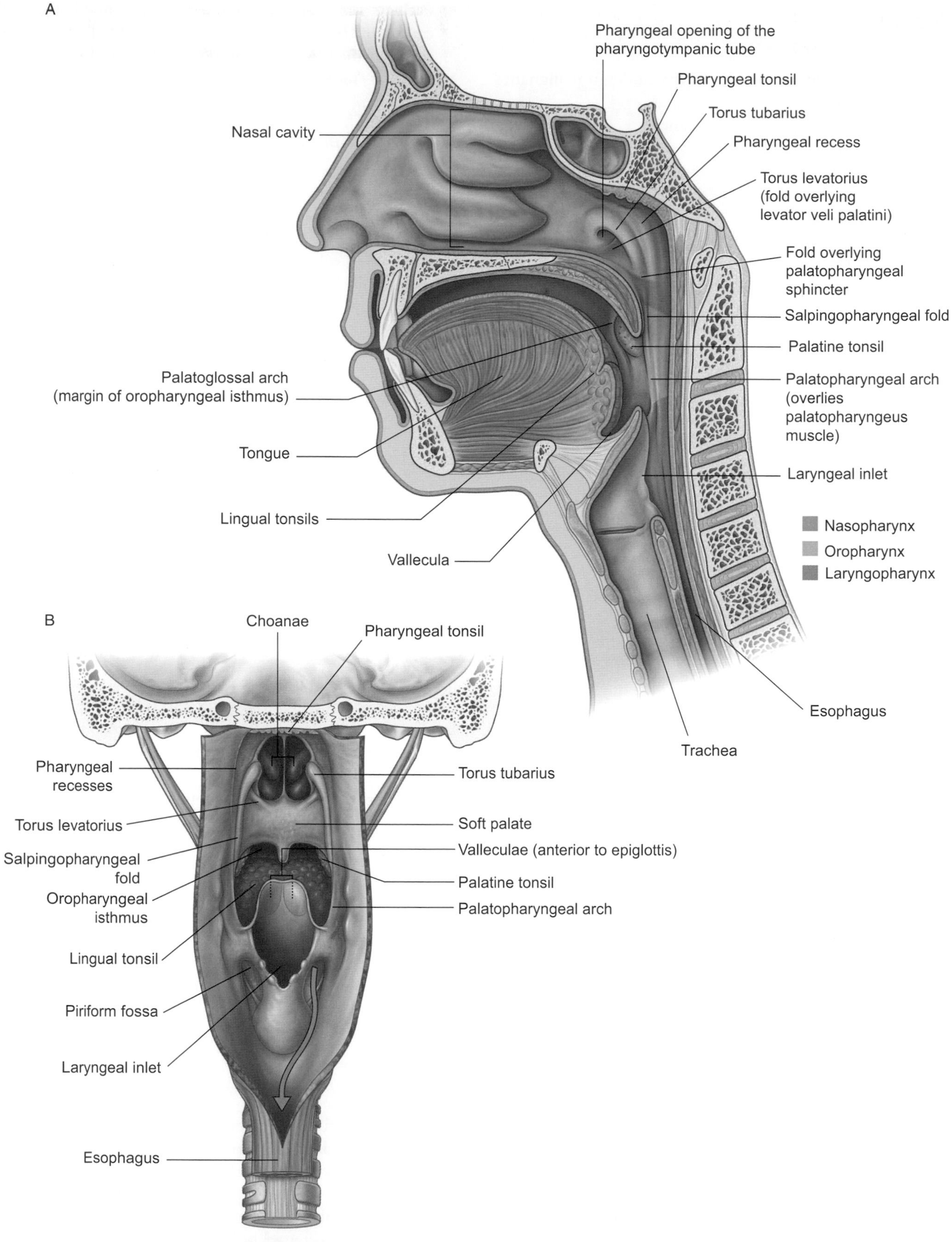

A

Nasal cavity

Pharyngeal opening of the pharyngotympanic tube

Pharyngeal tonsil

Torus tubarius

Pharyngeal recess

Torus levatorius (fold overlying levator veli palatini)

Fold overlying palatopharyngeal sphincter

Salpingopharyngeal fold

Palatine tonsil

Palatopharyngeal arch (overlies palatopharyngeus muscle)

Palatoglossal arch (margin of oropharyngeal isthmus)

Tongue

Lingual tonsils

Vallecula

Laryngeal inlet

Nasopharynx
Oropharynx
Laryngopharynx

Esophagus

Trachea

B

Choanae

Pharyngeal tonsil

Pharyngeal recesses

Torus tubarius

Torus levatorius

Soft palate

Salpingopharyngeal fold

Valleculae (anterior to epiglottis)

Oropharyngeal isthmus

Palatine tonsil

Palatopharyngeal arch

Lingual tonsil

Piriform fossa

Laryngeal inlet

Esophagus

• **Fig. 18.13** Mucosal Features of the Pharynx (A) Lateral view. (B) Posterior view with the pharyngeal wall opened. (Adapted from Drake R, Wayne Vogl A, Mitchell W, eds. Gray's Anatomy for Students, 4th ed. Philadelphia: Elsevier; 2021.)

of food into the oesophagus. In this reflex action, the epiglottis moves over the larynx to prevent food passing into the airway.

Clinical Examination

Patients should be examined sitting upright in a well-lit area with a clear view of the neck and general body habitus. A tongue depressor is placed in the midline of the dorsum of the tongue. Gentle pressure is applied so that the tonsillar pillars, tonsils, soft palate and uvula can be viewed. The posterior one-third is avoided to prevent stimulation of the gag response. Look for soft palate elevation, tonsil asymmetry and the presence of lesions around the tonsils, soft palate or posterior pharyngeal wall. The nasopharynx may be examined using a small laryngeal mirror and a headlight.

Full cranial nerve examination is performed followed by inspection and palpation of the levels of the neck to assess for tumours and lymphadenopathy. Flexible nasal endoscopy is then performed under local anaesthetic to assess for hypopharyngeal tumours, foreign bodies or lesions at the base of the tongue.

Surgical Disorders of the Pharynx

Surgical disorders of the pharynx may present with acute or chronic dysphagia (which may be for solids only, or for solids and liquids), odynophagia, weight loss, dysphonia, hyper nasal speech or regurgitation of food into the nose due to velopharyngeal incompetence.

Traumatic

Pharyngeal trauma may occur in the form of bruising or laceration. Lacerations in adults may occur due to blunt trauma or as a result of sharp foreign body ingestion. In children, pharyngeal trauma may occur as a result of non-accidental injury. Potential complications may include bleeding, retained foreign body, sepsis and CNS involvement depending on the mode of injury. Evaluation must follow ATLS assessment. Ultrasound of the neck, lateral soft tissue X-ray or CT with contrast may assist in identifying the extent of the injury.

Infectious/Inflammatory
Tonsillitis

- This is an acute infection of the parenchyma of the palatine tonsils.
- It is most commonly caused by viral infections such as adenovirus, and parainfluenza virus. Bacterial infections, such as *Streptococcus pneumoniae*, *Haemophilus influenzae* and *Moraxella catarrhalis*, account for about 20%.
- It is usually seen between the ages of 5 to 15 years old and occurs mostly in the winter and early spring.

> ● **BOX 18.4** **Centor Criteria for Diagnosis of Group A Beta-Haemolytic Streptococci**
>
> - History of fever >38°C
> - Tonsillar exudate
> - Absence of cough
> - Tender anterior cervical lymphadenopathy

- Viral tonsillitis has milder symptoms but, in bacterial tonsillitis, the sore throat will be prolonged and there may be pus on the tonsil.
- It is usually a self-limiting condition which only requires symptomatic treatment.
- Symptoms include sudden onset of sore throat and pain on swallowing which is associated with a fever of >38°C, headache, abdominal pain and vomiting. The absence of cough or coryzal symptoms makes it more likely to be a bacterial rather than viral infection.
- Clinical examination: tonsillar exudate, enlarged and erythematous tonsils. There may be an anterior cervical lymphadenopathy.
- Centor score of ≥3 (Box 18.4) in a patient older than 14 years old points to a group A beta-haemolytic streptococci. If three or four criteria are met, the positive predictive value is 40% to 60%.
- Diagnostic tests: throat culture, rapid streptococcal antigen, serological testing for streptococci, WCC and differential, vaginal/cervical/penile and rectal swabs, HIV viral load.
- Differential diagnosis includes: infectious mononucleosis, epiglottitis, peri-tonsillar abscess (Quinsy), retropharyngeal abscess, diphtheria, HIV infection.
- Treatment:
  - Analgesia: paracetamol, NSAIDs (but not aspirin in children due to risk of Reye's syndrome), over-the-counter medication to relieve sore throat
  - Penicillin-based drugs such as amoxicillin is the first-line treatment for bacterial tonsillitis. For patients who cannot complete a 10-day oral course, then a single intramuscular dose of benzathine benzylpenicillin is recommended. In allergic patients, a macrolide, a cephalosporin or clindamycin can be used.
  - The Epstein–Barr virus may also present as acute tonsillitis. Patients may have severe cervical adenopathy. The tonsils are typically enlarged and covered in greyish slough. A characteristic rash may appear if treated with ampicillin. Hepatosplenomegaly may occur, so patients should be advised to refrain from contact sports or alcohol consumption for about 6 weeks.
  - Corticosteroids are usually indicated in patients over 12 years old with almost complete inability to take any oral medication and/or signs and symptoms of airway obstruction who are already on antibiotics.
  - Tonsillectomy should be considered if the patient has experienced more than four or five episodes of bacterial tonsillitis in a year. Symptoms should be ongoing

for 2 years. Additional indication for a tonsillectomy is the presence of additional exacerbating factors, e.g. obstructive sleep apnoea, peri-tonsillar abscess, periodic fever, aphthous stomatitis, pharyngitis or adenitis syndrome. Partial tonsillectomy seems to have similar efficacy with less postoperative pain and bleeding, but more research is needed to establish who would benefit most from this procedure.

Quinsy, or Peritonsillar Abscess (Fig. 18.14)

- This occurs where pus collects between the tonsil capsule and the superior muscle constrictor of the pharynx.
- It is accompanied by trismus and the inability to swallow saliva.
- On examination, there will be unilateral swelling of the peritonsillar area with the uvula pushed to the opposite side.
- The abscess should be drained under local anaesthetic and the patient observed for complications such as septicaemia, aspiration of abscess contents leading to pneumonia, mediastinitis, involvement of the cranial nerves and erosion of the great vessels.

Retropharyngeal Abscess

- This most commonly presents in children under the age of 4.
- The onset is often after an upper respiratory tract infection, tonsillitis or dental infection. In adults, a midline prevertebral abscess is associated with tuberculosis (TB) of the spine.

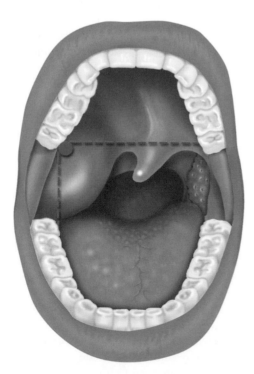

- **Fig. 18.14** Right-Sided Peritonsillar Abscess with the Point of Incision

- Management includes oxygen supplementation and airway management (which may include cricothyroidotomy or tracheostomy), intravenous rehydration, intravenous antibiotics (initial high dose ampicillin, clindamycin, cefuroxime or co-amoxiclav and then changed according to sensitivities). Surgery with drainage under general anaesthetic may be indicated.

Neoplastic

Nasopharyngeal Carcinoma (NPC)

- It accounts for less than 1% of all cancers in Europe; however, in endemic regions such as southern China, the incidence can be up to 25% of new cancer diagnoses.
- It is more prevalent in males.
- It occurs in middle age in Europe and Asia, whilst the tendency is to occur in children and adolescents in Sub-Saharan Africa.
- Nasopharyngeal carcinoma is classified into:
  - Type 1 (squamous cell carcinoma)
  - Type 2 (keratinizing undifferentiated carcinoma – most commonly associated with EBV infection) and
  - Type 3 (non-keratinizing undifferentiated carcinoma)
- Causes are multifactorial, and can be broadly classified into:
  - Infectious: the link between NPC and EBV infection is well documented
  - Environmental: tobacco, alcohol, and a diet rich in salt-cured fish and meat may increase the risk, as can exposure to hardwood dust
  - Genetic factors, i.e. having a first-degree relative
- Tumours typically arise in the fossa of Rosenmueller. Initial spread is by direct invasion and often the disease remains clinically silent until locally advanced. Metastatic neck lesions and unilateral middle ear effusion are the most common presenting symptoms, followed by epistaxis and nasal obstruction. Nasal endoscopy must be performed in any adult with unilateral middle ear effusion. Staging of tumours, requires MRI, CT or PET CT. There is no role for surgery in the initial management of NPC. Radiotherapy with or without chemotherapy is the treatment modality of choice.

Oropharyngeal Carcinoma (OPC)

- The majority oropharyngeal tumours are squamous cell carcinomas.
- OPC is more common in males than females.
- Aetiology:
  - Environmental: Risk of oral cavity squamous cell carcinoma is 4–10 times higher in alcohol consumers than others. Betel nut chewing is an important causative factor in Asian countries.
  - Infectious: Viruses such as HPV and EBV have also been linked with oropharyngeal cancer.
- Clinical examination:
  - The oral cavity and oropharynx should be examined looking for leukoplakia and erythroplakia and the neck palpated to rule out nodal metastases. Tongue mobility should be assessed.

- Investigations:
  - Biopsy of any lesion should be performed for histological diagnosis.
  - CT or MRI scan may assess deep invasion, mandible invasion and nodal status. An orthopantogram may also be helpful in assessing for mandible invasion.
- Treatment is usually multimodal. Concurrent chemoradiotherapy is often the first-line treatment with surgery reserved for salvage of radioresistant disease.

Hypopharyngeal Carcinoma

- Hypopharyngeal carcinoma of the hypopharynx includes pyriform fossa, posterior wall and post cricoid cancers.
- There is a male predominance and the peak incidence is in the sixth decade.
- Aetiological risk associations include alcohol, smoking and Plummer-Vinson syndrome (up to a 16% risk of developing post cricoid cancer).
- Tumours metastasize extensively and typically do not present till locally advanced.
- Diagnosis: Easily missed on fibre-optic nasal endoscopy, the diagnosis is often at panendoscopy or on CT or MRI imaging of the neck.
- The initial treatment is usually with concurrent chemoradiotherapy and pharyngo-laryngectomy, with free flap or gastric pull up reconstruction is usually reserved for salvage.

Congenital

Pharyngeal Pouches or Zenker's Diverticulum

- These are false herniations above the cricopharyngeus due to poor swallow coordination or increased intraluminal pressure.
- The current gold standard for diagnosis is barium swallow
- Treatment is most frequently acchieved with endoscopic stapling.

THE NECK

Function

The most important role of the neck is that it supports the weight of the head on the torso and that it protects the carotid arteries, which supply blood to the brain from the heart. The neck contains several important nerves that link the head and its vital structures to the body. The neck also houses part of the respiratory (larynx and trachea), endocrine (thyroid and parathyroid) and gastrointestinal (pharynx and salivary glands) systems. The flexibility of the neck's skeleton allows the head to turn and flex in all directions.

Anatomy

The neck contains complex neurovascular structures, muscles, ligaments and bones in layers. It contains a number of fascial layers, which divide it into compartments. These fascial layers include the investing fascia, the prevertebral fascia, pretracheal fascia and the carotid sheath (Fig. 18.15). Whilst these layers divide the neck into compartments, they also form long passages along which infection can pass – leading to significant sepsis if left unchecked, as seen with retropharyngeal and parapharyngeal abscesses.

The anterior triangle of the neck sits between the anterior border of the sternocleidomastoid muscle, the midline and the inferior border of the mandible. The prevertebral fascia forms its floor and it is further subdivided into the submental, digastric and muscular triangles. It contains the submental lymph nodes, anterior jugular vein, carotid sheath (and its contents), submandibular gland, hypoglossal nerve, lingual nerve, thyroid gland, oesophagus and larynx.

The posterior triangle of the neck sits between the posterior border of sternocleidomastoid, the anterior border of trapezius and the superior border of the clavicle. Its floor is formed by prevertebral fascia overlying the splenius capitis and scalene muscles. It contains the accessory nerve, the occipital artery, the inferior belly of omohyoid and lymph nodes.

Clinical Examination

The current best practice for describing the anatomical regions of the neck is the method developed in Memorial

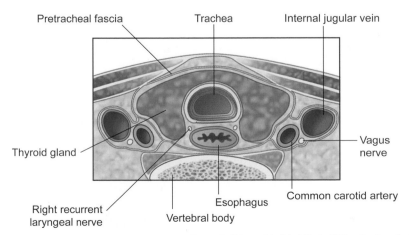

- **Fig. 18.15** Neck Transverse View (Adapted from Drake R, Wayne Vogl A, Mitchell W, eds. Gray's Anatomy for Students, 4th ed. Philadelphia Elsevier; 2021, p. 916.)

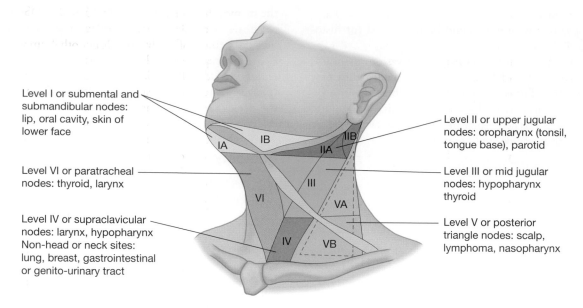

Level I or submental and submandibular nodes: lip, oral cavity, skin of lower face

Level VI or paratracheal nodes: thyroid, larynx

Level IV or supraclavicular nodes: larynx, hypopharynx Non-head or neck sites: lung, breast, gastrointestinal or genito-urinary tract

Level II or upper jugular nodes: oropharynx (tonsil, tongue base), parotid

Level III or mid jugular nodes: hypopharynx thyroid

Level V or posterior triangle nodes: scalp, lymphoma, nasopharynx

• **Fig. 18.16** Anatomical Levels of the Neck (From https://www.bmj.com/content/347/bmj.f5473)

Sloan Kettering, which divides the neck into seven anatomically distinct regions (Fig.18.16). The divisions are as follows:

Level 1: The region above the level of digastric muscle (i.e. level 1a is the submental triangle and level 1b is the submandibular triangle).

Level 2: The region between the level of the hyoid and the carotid bifurcation. Also described as the upper one-third of the internal jugular vein; it is subdivided into level 2a and 2b by the spinal accessory nerve.

Level 3: The region between the carotid bifurcation and the cricothyroid notch (or the middle third of internal jugular vein).

Level 4: The region between the cricothyroid notch and the clavicle (the lower third of the internal jugular vein).

Level 5 includes the posterior triangle as described above, whilst level 6 describes the anterior compartment around the thyroid. A further level 7 has been described as a level within the mediastinum.

Surgical Disorders of the Neck

Traumatic

Penetrating Injury

- Penetrating injury of the neck accounts for almost 10% of all trauma.
- It has a mortality of 3–6 %.
- Gunshot wounds and stabbings are on the increase and thorough investigation of all penetrating neck injuries must be performed to ensure safety of the carotid arteries and major nerves (see Ch. 36).

Infectious/Inflammatory

Lymphadenitis

- This is enlargement of the lymph nodes due to infection.

- In most cases, resolution is achieved by treatment of the underlying cause, i.e. viruses or bacteria.

Deep Neck Space Infections

- These include *parapharyngeal* and *retropharyngeal* abscesses. Deep space neck infection is potentially life-threatening because, due to the fascial layers in the neck, infection can cause local effects and can spread from one space to the next and into the mediastinum.
- Possible complications of deep neck space infection include septicaemia, aspiration pneumonia, lung abscess, mediastinitis and neural involvement of the cranial nerve and erosion of the great vessels.
- Patients with deep neck space infection present with fever, dysphagia, neck swelling and/or neck stiffness.
- CT scanning, neck ultrasound and lateral neck X-ray will assist preoperative assessment.
- Parapharyngeal abscesses typically arise following tonsillitis and dental infections.
- Potential complications include internal carotid artery rupture, internal jugular vein thrombosis and mediastinitis.
- Patients with parapharyngeal abscesses should be treated with high-dose intravenous antibiotics. Large abscess collections should be drained and patients closely monitored for complications.

Neoplastic

Metastatic Disease of Unknown Primary

- Metastatic disease of unknown primary presenting as cervical lymph node metastasis accounts for between 2 and 9% of all head and neck cancers.
- The majority of these tumours are squamous cell carcinoma.
- When the primary site is unknown, the entire pharynx and larynx is treated, to ensure all possible primary sites of the cancer are covered.

- Treatment regimens covering the entire pharynx and larynx, are a significant source of morbidity.
- Metastatic disease of unknown primary arises when an occult primary carcinoma either metastasizes early to the cervical lymphatics or develops in an anatomical site that is not easily identified with routine diagnostic tests.
- Diagnosis requires careful assessment with panendoscopy, biopsies of the tonsils and tongue base and radiological staging with CT, MRI or PET CT.
- Treatment is usually multimodal with chemoradiotherapy with or without neck dissection.

Lymphoproliferative Diseases

- These are very common.
- Lymphoma is the third most common childhood malignancy.
- Patients may present to the otolaryngologist with a neck lump and systemic symptoms of weight loss, fatigue and night sweats.
- On examination, along with cervical lymphadenopathy, patients may have diffuse adenopathy with or without hepatosplenomegaly.
- Diagnosis is made using open or core biopsy and radiological investigations including chest X-ray and CT scan of neck, thorax and abdomen.
- Treatment is with chemotherapy with or without radiotherapy.

Paragangliomas

- These are rare neoplasms which can develop at a number of sites.
- About 97% are benign and cured by surgical removal.
- The remaining 3% are malignant, and can metastasize.
- *Carotid body tumour* is the most common head and neck paraganglioma. It typically presents with a painless neck lump, but can also cause cranial nerve palsy of the glossopharyngeal, vagus, accessory and hypoglossal nerves. About 75% are sporadic; the remaining 25% are hereditary. Treatment may be conservative if slow growing, surgical if the patient is young and the lesion is growing, or radiotherapy in older patients.

Kaposi's Sarcoma (KS)

- This is caused by human herpes virus 8 (HHV8) and was originally described by Moritz Kaposi.
- It is an AIDs-defining illness, which occurs as part of a systemic disease that presents with cutaneous lesions.
- There are four subtypes:
  - Classic
  - African endemic
  - KS in iatrogenically immunosuppressed patients
  - AIDS-related KS
- Lesions may occur as plaques, nodular lesions, exophytic growths, plaques, patches, or flat macules.
- Lesions can be solitary or widespread.
- KS can involve the oral cavity, lymph nodes or internal organs.

- The mouth is the initial site in 15% of AIDS-related KS.
- Diagnosis requires tissue biopsies.
- KS is a cancer of the lymphatic endothelium which forms dense, irregular vascular channels.
- Red blood cells leak into tissues surrounding these channels, causing distinctive discoloration.
- KS is a palliative condition. Treatment is based on the type and extent of disease. Treatment modalities include: excision (for low volume localised disease), cryotherapy, chemotherapy or radiotherapy.

Congenital
Branchial Cysts

- These are congenital cystic swellings, which occur due to failure of obliteration of the pharyngeal clefts and typically present as cystic swellings anterior to the sternocleidomastoid muscle.
- There are three types of branchial cyst, and type two is the most common.
- They are more prevalent in males and typically occur on the left side.
- Histologically, the wall of a branchial cyst consists of either columnar or squamous epithelium.
- They are a potential source of deep neck space infection or malignant transformation; therefore, they should be removed.

Lymphangioma

- This is a benign hamartomatous lesion of the lymphatics, which most commonly occurs in the head and neck region.
- They have an ill-defined capsule; thus, removal may be difficult.
- Radiotherapy or cautery may also be used.

Haemangiomas

- These are benign, typically involuting tumours of vascular endothelium, of unknown aetiology, which typically occur shortly after birth and gradually involute. Port wine stains and strawberry naevus fall within the category.
- Excision may lead to profuse bleeding and most haemangiomas disappear without treatment.
- Propranolol may be used to reduce the size of haemangiomas in young children where the lesion occurs in a cosmetically sensitive area.

THE SALIVARY GLANDS

Function

The salivary glands function to produce saliva, which is essential for maintaining oral health, breaking down dietary carbohydrates and lubricating food as it passes into the gastrointestinal tract. In humans, the salivary glands are closely related to the oral cavity and pharynx, and serve the important function of secreting saliva into the mouth. They are grouped into three pairs – the parotid, submandibular and sublingual glands – and several hundred minor salivary glands. Together, they produce up to 1.5 L of saliva each day.

Anatomy (Figs 18.17 and 18.18)

The parotid gland is situated on the lateral aspect of the face in front of and below the ear. Its anatomical relations are the external auditory canal, the zygomatic arch and lower border of the angle of the mandible. Its anterior aspect lies over the masseter muscle. It is divided into a deep and a superficial part by the facial nerve, which emerges from the stylomastoid foramen

and immediately enters the gland. Here, the facial nerve divides into upper and lower divisions, which further divide to supply the muscles of facial expression. The parotid or Stensen's duct enters the oral cavity through a papilla opposite the second upper molar tooth. There are lymph nodes situated both within and around the gland.

The submandibular gland is situated under the mandible in the digastric triangle, between the anterior belly of this muscle and the stylomandibular ligament. Its posterior portion wraps around the mylohyoid muscle, and gives rise to Wharton's duct, which enters the floor of the mouth at the sublingual caruncle, beside the frenulum of the tongue. The marginal mandibular branch of the facial nerve is an important lateral relation of the gland, whilst the lingual and hypoglossal nerves lie deep to it.

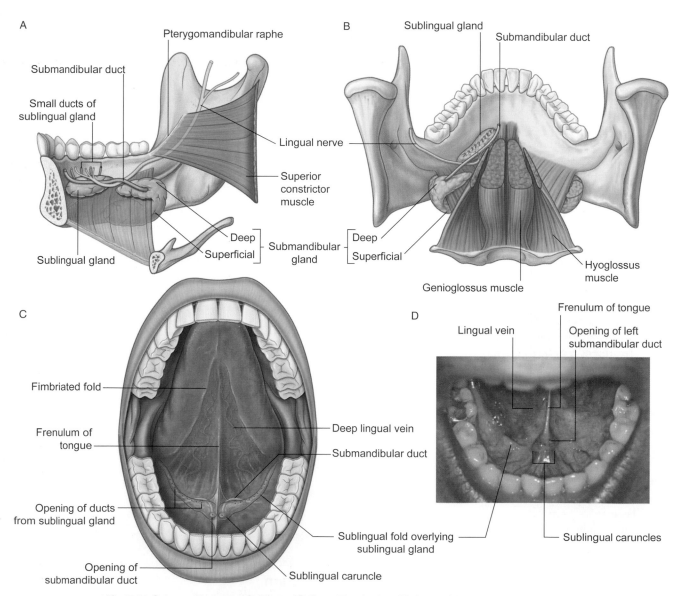

• **Fig. 18.17** Submandibular and Sublingual Salivary Glands. A and B: Internal views of the Submandibular and sublingual glands in relation to the floor of mouth muscles and the lingual nerve. C and D: Intra oral view of the sublingual caruncle overlying the sublingual glands. (Adapted from Drake R, Wayne Vogl A, Mitchell W, eds. Gray's Anatomy for Students, 4th ed. Elsevier: Philadelphia; 2021.)

The sublingual glands are found embedded in the mucous membrane of the floor of the mouth. Small excretory ducts drain these glands, some directly opening into the submandibular duct, whereas the rest drain directly into the floor of the mouth.

Physiology

Saliva production is a two-step process. Tiny acini produce isotonic primary saliva, which is secreted into terminal ends of the salivary duct system within the glands. As this primary product passes along the ductal system towards the mouth, electrolytes are reabsorbed to form a more hypotonic fluid, which is further modified by the addition of proteins from secretory granules within the acinar cells under instruction from the sympathetic nervous system. Electrolyte composition is governed by the parasympathetic nervous system.

Clinical Examination

Examination is divided into inspection and palpation. As with a neck or thyroid exam, the patient is best examined in a well-lit environment in the sitting position. Both sides should be inspected for asymmetry, overlying erythema or enlargement. Nerve involvement of the facial, lingual or hypoglossal nerve should be noted. Inspect the oral cavity for pus or stone disease at Stensen's and Warthin's ducts. Bimanual palpation is performed looking for tumours or hidden stone disease.

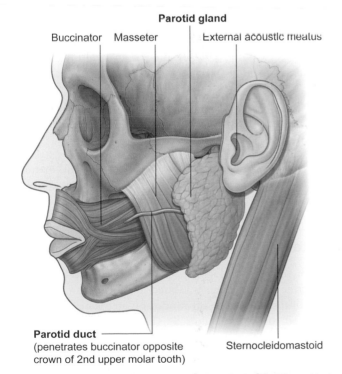

Parotid gland

Buccinator   Masseter   External acoustic meatus

Parotid duct
(penetrates buccinator opposite crown of 2nd upper molar tooth)

Sternocleidomastoid

• **Fig. 18.18** Left Parotid Gland (Adapted from Drake, R., Wayne Vogl, A., Mitchell, W., eds. Gray's Anatomy for Students, 4th ed. Philadelphia: Elsevier, 2021.)

Surgical Disorders of the Salivary Gland

Traumatic

Salivary Gland Trauma

- This is relatively uncommon but may occur as sequelae of complex facial or penetrating neck injury.
- Trauma can be categorized as acute (damage due to blunt, lacerating, avulsion or blast injuries) or chronic (damage due to irradiation, retained stones/sialolithiasis).
- Management depends on the extent of the injury, the modality of the injury, the degree of tissue contamination and the presence of associated nerve or vascular injury. Management in the acute setting requires irrigation, intravenous antibiotics and control of haemorrhage. Where nerve injury is suspected, acute salivary gland trauma requires surgical exploration.

Infectious/Inflammatory

Systemic Diseases of the Salivary Glands

- These are common.
- Non-neoplastic masses may occur in Sjogren's disease, sarcoidosis, TB, actinomycosis and cat scratch disease.
- Diagnosis requires careful history and examination, blood tests, biopsy and imaging with either MRI or CT.

Actinomycosis

- Can occur as a primary colonisation of the salivary glands, or due to spread of infection from the teeth/tonsils.
- Treatment requires incision and drainage with long-term administration of penicillin.

Sarcoidosis

- This is a chronic disease of unknown etiology, which is characterised by the presence of non caseating granulomas.
- It is a multisystem disease affecting lungs, kidneys and skin.
- Salivary gland involvement may be isolated or occur as a component of uveoparotid fever (*Heerfordt's syndrome*).

Sjögren's Syndrome

- Primary Sjrögen's disease is an autoimmune condition characterized by xerostomia and dry eyes without an associated connective tissue disorder.
- Secondary Sjögren's disease is associated with connective tissue abnormalities such as rheumatoid arthritis.
- The condition is characterized by enlargement of salivary and lacrimal glands often with recurrent sialadenitis. Schirmer's test of lacrimation and tests of salivary production and flow all help to confirm the diagnosis.
- The mainstay of treatment of Sjogren's syndrome is steroid therapy and rarely immunosuppressants. Artificial tears and saliva are used to counteract dryness of the eyes and mouth.

Sialolithiasis

- This is stone disease of the salivary glands.
- Sialolithiasis is most commonly seen in the submandibular gland due to the nature of the saliva it produces and the length and tortuosity of its duct.
- Only about 20% of calculi are found in the parotid gland.
- Patients with sialolithiasis present with a painful swelling of the gland, associated with eating.
- Stones smaller than 3 mm may pass spontaneously but with larger stones, removal with duct marsupialization, sialendoscopy or resection of the gland may be required.

Tuberculosis and Atypical Mycobacterial Infections

- These may involve the salivary glands.
- Primary tuberculosis infection of the salivary glands is rare and usually causes unilateral parotid gland involvement.
- Scrofula is the Latin word for brood sow, and it means cervical tuberculosis, which usually occurs secondary to infection in the lymph nodes.
- Extra pulmonary tuberculosis, such as scrofula, is observed most often in individuals who are immunocompromised.

Sialadenitis

- This is infection of the salivary glands, and is most commonly seen in the parotid gland.
- Patients with sialadenitis typically present with a sudden painful diffuse swelling of the involved gland.
- It occurs most often seen in elderly, debilitated and dehydrated patients.

Neoplastic

Benign Tumours of the Salivary Glands

- These are relatively common.
- Salivary gland tumours represent 3% of all neoplasms. Eighty percent are sited in the parotid gland, 10% in the submandibular gland and 10% are distributed between the sublingual and minor salivary glands.
- Benign tumours usually present as a painless enlargement in contrast to malignant tumours, which often grow quickly and are painful.
- Benign tumours include pleomorphic adenoma (Fig. 18.19), Warthin's tumour, oncocytoma and vascular tumours/malformations.

Salivary Gland Cancers

- These are more common in the submandibular and minor salivary glands.
- Fifty percent of all minor salivary gland tumours are malignant.
- Types of malignant tumour include mucoepidermoid, adenoid cystic carcinoma, acinic cell carcinoma, adenocarcinoma and squamous cell carcinoma.
- Suspicious symptoms for malignancy on presentation include pain, rapid growth, fixation and facial nerve involvement or neck metastasis.

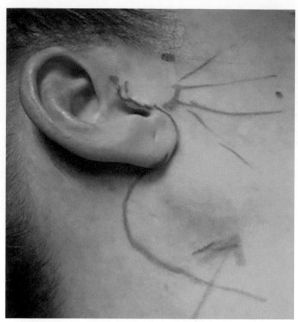

• **Fig. 18.19** Pleomorphic Adenoma of Right Parotid Gland

- Following a full history and head and neck examination, including assessment of facial nerve function, patients should have fine needle aspiration for cytology and CT or MRI scan performed.
- Optimal treatment is surgical excision with or without a neck dissection.

Congenital

Congenital Aplasia of the Salivary Glands

- This is a rare condition, which presents with dry mouth, dental cavities, pharyngitis and laryngitis.
- Though complete or partial aplasia may occur in isolation, they more typically present in conjunction with other congenital anomalies.

THYROID AND PARATHYROID GLANDS

Function

The thyroid gland governs metabolism growth and maturation of the body whilst regulating body functions through the production of hormones. The parathyroid glands regulate calcium metabolism.

Anatomy

The thyroid gland (Fig. 18.20) is a large butterfly-shaped endocrine gland, which is located in the anterior compartment of the neck. It is surrounded by pretracheal fascia and is related to the strap muscles (Fig. 18.21), the recurrent and superior laryngeal nerves, the larynx, the pharynx and the oesophagus. The small parathyroid glands are located on its posteromedial surface. Vascular supply to the thyroid and parathyroid glands is via the superior and inferior thyroid arteries and, occasionally, a thyroid inferior mesenteric artery. Joll's triangle is an anatomical triangle used to locate

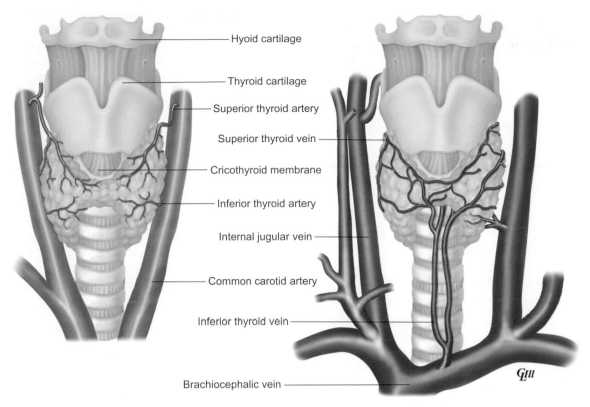

• **Fig. 18.20** The Thyroid and Its Arterial and Venous Blood Supply

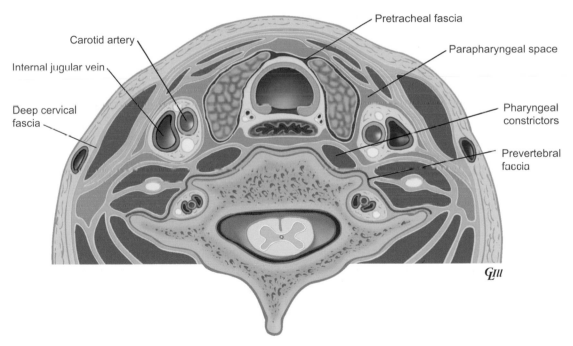

• **Fig. 18.21** Transverse View of the Neck

the superior laryngeal nerve in thyroid surgery and Beahr's triangle is an anatomical triangle to locate the recurrent laryngeal nerve.

Physiology

The functional unit of the thyroid gland is the follicular cell. Follicular cells are arranged into colloid containing spherical units known as follicles. The thyroid releases thyroid hormone at the instruction of the pituitary gland. Thyrotropin-releasing hormone secreted from the hypothalamus stimulates release of thyroid-stimulating hormone by the pituitary gland. Thyroid-stimulating hormone stimulates conversion of colloid into T3 and T4 by the thyroid gland. When blood levels of T3 and T4 increase, they exert negative feedback by suppressing the release of

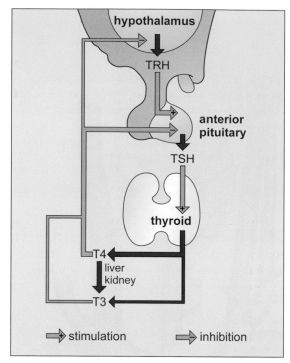

• **Fig. 18.22** The Negative Feedback Loop of Thyroxine Secretion (From Marshall J, Lapsley M, Day A, Shipman K. Clinical Chemistry, 9th ed. St. Louis: Elsevier, 2021.)

thyrotropin-releasing hormone and thyroid-stimulating hormone to maintain a steady level of T3/T4 in the blood (Fig. 18.22). T3 and T4 increase basal metabolic rate, increase heart rate and stimulate growth hormone release. Calcitonin is released by parafollicular C cells. Calcitonin aids calcium metabolism by reducing calcium resorption at the intestines, reducing phosphate loss at the kidneys and stimulating osteoblasts in the skeleton.

The parathyroid glands secrete parathyroid hormone which regulates blood calcium levels. Parathyroid hormone stimulates osteoclastic driven enzymatic degradation of bone to release calcium. Parathyroid hormone also inhibits osteoblasts, increases renal reabsorption of calcium (and magnesium) and initiates the production of 1,25-dihydroxyvitamin D, in the kidneys.

Clinical Examination

The patient should be seated in a well-lit area with the exposed neck in a neutral or slightly extended position. Note signs of cachexia and tremor. Observe the neck from the side noting any prominence beyond this normal contour of the neck. Visualisation of the thyroid gland can be optimised by observing the patient swallow a sip of water. Standing behind the patient, the thyroid is palpated bimanually. Moving laterally, palpate for discrete or multifocal masses or asymmetry. Note the presence or absence of associated lymph nodes. Ask the patient to swallow, to enhance upward movement of the gland. Repeat this with tongue protrusion. Note the site, size, consistency and shape of any masses felt. Auscultate for bruit and transilluminate if cystic

mass is identified. Pembertons test is a dynamic maneuver in which the patient is observed for signs of facial congestion following elevation of both arms above the head. In cases of very large retrosternal thyroid masses, the thoracic inlet is obstructed resulting in increased pressure within the venous system.

Surgical Disorders of the Thyroid and Parathyroid Glands

Trauma

Thyroid Gland Haematoma and Thyroid Rupture

• This may occur after severe blunt trauma.
• Both are extremely rare and can lead to airway compromise and major haemorrhage.
• In the emergent setting, where the airway is at risk, patients require urgent surgical evacuation and debridement.

Infectious/Inflammatory

Thyroiditis

• This is inflammation of the thyroid gland.
• It causes either unusually high or low levels of thyroid hormones in the blood.
• There are a number of conditions, which result in thyroiditis including De Quervain's thyroiditis, radiation induced thyroiditis, Hashimoto's thyroiditis and postpartum thyroiditis.
• Treatment requires analgesia and correction of abnormal thyroid hormone levels.

Neoplastic

Benign Thyroid Nodules

• These are very common. Clinically detectable nodules (>1 cm) are detected in about 5% of the general population, often during a routine neck examination.
• They rarely have a malignant component.
• Nodules are twice as common in females. When found in males, or in young children, thyroid nodules have an increased risk of malignancy.
• Clinically suspicious nodules, or nodules in high risk individuals, should be investigated with ultrasound and fine needle aspirate cytology (FNAC), which can give any one of four possible outcomes – benign lesion (Thy 2: 60–70%), follicular lesion (should be excised to allow further analysis), confirmed malignant cells, or non-diagnostic (Thy 1) (Box 18.5).

Thyroid Cancer

• This accounts for 1% of all cancers.
• Papillary and follicular carcinomas, which are differentiated tumours with an excellent prognosis, represent 85–90% of tumours.
• Medullary carcinoma is associated with multiple endocrine neoplasia (MEN) syndrome.
• Anaplastic is an undifferentiated form of carcinoma, which is associated with a very poor prognosis.

• BOX 18.5 FNAC Classification

- Thy 1 Non-diagnostic – cytology smears
- Thy 2 Non-neoplastic – features nodular goitre or thyroiditis
- Thy 3 Follicular lesions – unable to differentiate adenoma from carcinoma
- Thy 4 Suspicious of malignancy – approximately one-third are malignant
- Thy 5 Diagnostic for malignancy – features primary or metastatic carcinoma

---

- Risk factors include family history of thyroid carcinoma, radiation exposure, MEN syndrome, and presentation at the extremes of age (less than 16 or over 60) and male sex.
- History should include any symptoms of difficulty breathing, swallowing, hoarseness, rapid growth or pain.
- Poor prognostic factors on examination include a hard, fixed lesion, lymphadenopathy, vocal cord paralysis and size greater than 4 cm.
- The mainstay of treatment for differentiated and medullary thyroid cancer is surgery.
- Risk assessment looking at age, gender, and size of tumour in addition to the histology of the tumour will aid in the choice of treatment option.
- A partial or total thyroidectomy may be performed depending on these risk factors. Following thyroidectomy surgery, thyroid hormone is suppressed and patients can be monitored for thyroid activity with regular thyroglobulin levels. Radioiodine ablation therapy and external beam radiation are other treatment options.
- Patients at the extremes of age, male patients and tumours greater than 4 cm are associated with poorer prognosis.

Parathyroid Adenoma

- This is a benign tumour of the parathyroid gland.
- It generally causes hyperparathyroidism.
- Adenomas are often undiagnosed until found on routine blood tests that reveal high serum calcium levels.
- When symptomatic, patients may present with joint, muscle, and abdominal pain, depression, constipation fatigue and kidney stones.
- Diagnosis is with blood tests, sestamibi scan or ultrasound of the neck.
- The treatment of choice is removal of the affected gland or glands.

Parathyroid Carcinoma

- This is a rare malignancy.
- Tumours usually secrete parathyroid hormone, and patients experience severe hyperparathyroidism. Parathyroid carcinoma occurs in about 1% of patients with pre-existing parathyroid adenoma.
- Treatment requires aggressive resection of the tumour and some of the surrounding tissues. Calcimimetic drugs may be used to reduce serum calcium levels in the presence of advanced or metastatic parathyroid carcinomas.

Congenital

Congenital Hypothyroidism

- This is a congenital condition in which new born infants suffer with severe thyroid hormone deficiency.
- Causes include: aplasia of the gland, inborn error of thyroid metabolism and maternal iodine deficiency.
- Treatment is with hormone replacement.

Thyroglossal Duct Cyst

- This is a congenital abnormality, which occurs due to failure of the thyroglossal duct to close during embryogenesis.
- A remnant of thyroid tissue is often deposited along the path of the thyroid's descent and remains attached to the foramen cecum of the tongue.
- Key findings on examination are of a midline, anterior triangle neck swelling which is elevated on tongue protrusion.
- It is important to assess the neck with ultrasound examination prior to any intervention as the cyst may contain the only thyroid tissue in the neck, and removal in certain cases may result in hypothyroidism.
- Thyroglossal duct cysts should be removed because they are associated with a risk of deep neck space infection or malignant transformation in the cyst itself. Removal of a thyroglossal duct cyst is by means of *Sistrunk's procedure*. Complete removal of the cyst, its tract and the central portion of the hyoid bone are required to ensure the cyst does not recur.

GENETICALLY INHERITED CONDITIONS IN OTOLARYNGOLOGY

The otolaryngologist, and particularly the paediatric otolaryngologist, encounters a number of conditions with a strong genetic component. The key findings of some relevant conditions are outlined below.

1. **Apert syndrome** is an autosomal dominant syndrome, which is typified by craniosynostosis, syndactyly, recurrent otitis media with effusion (OME), conductive and sensorineural hearing loss. It is classified as a branchial arch syndrome and the derivatives of the first branchial arch are often affected.
2. **Congenital rubella syndrome** occurs due to intrauterine rubella infection during the first trimester. It classically causes sensorineural hearing loss, eye abnormalities and congenital heart defects such as patent ductus arteriosus.
3. **Kabuki syndrome** is a congenital disorder of suspected genetic origin (it is thought to be either autosomal dominant or x-linked recessive), which is characterized by intellectual disabilities and multiple congenital anomalies. The otolaryngologic findings include cleft or high arched palate, depressed nasal tip and prominent earlobes.

4. **Kniest dysplasia** is an autosomal dominant collagen disorder, which presents with dwarfism, clubfoot, cleft palate, laryngomalacia and myopia.
5. **Pierre Robin syndrome** is a sequence of facial abnormalities, which occurs due to deletions at chromosome 2, 11 or 17. Babies are born with micrognathia, posterior displacement of the tongue and cleft palate. Tracheotomy is often required.
6. **Stickler's syndrome** is an autosomal dominant inherited disorder of collagen 2 and 11 production. Babies' present with flattened facial features, Pierre Robin sequence, myopia, retinal detachment and arthritis.
7. **Trisomy 21** is known as Down's syndrome and it occurs because of trisomy of the 21st chromosome. This can arise because of non-disjunction at meiosis, Robertsonian translocation or mosaicism. The otolaryngology features encountered include macroglossia, low set ears, narrow external auditory canal, conductive and sensory neural hearing loss, obstructive sleep apnoea syndrome and hypothyroidism.
8. **Usher's syndrome** is a leading cause of deaf-blindness. It is characterized by hearing loss, retinitis pigmentosis and vestibular imbalance problems. Its inheritance follows an autosomal recessive pattern and there are three subtypes of which type 3 is the rarest.
9. **VACTERYL** association is a non-random association of birth defects including vertebral anomalies, anal atresia, cardiovascular anomalies, tracheoesophageal fistula, oesophageal atresia, renal/radial anomalies and limb defects.
10. **22q11 deletion syndrome** is a rare disease, which occurs due to micro deletion at chromosome 22. It presents with cardiac anomalies, abnormal facies, thymic aplasia, cleft palate and hypocalcaemia.

19

Common Surgical Conditions of Pulmonary Disease

Anatomy of the Thorax

Embryology

At 4 weeks old, the respiratory diverticulum (lung bud) appears as an outgrowth of the foregut's ventral wall. Therefore the epithelium of the internal lining of the larynx, trachea and bronchi is of endodermal origin.

The cartilaginous, muscular and connective tissue components of the trachea and lungs are derived from the mesoderm.

Initially the respiratory diverticulum communicates with the foregut and when the first expands caudally, two longitudinal ridges called the oesophagotracheal ridges develop and separate it from the foregut. These ridges later fuse to form the oesophagotracheal septum and the foregut is divided into a dorsal portion (oesophagus) and a ventral portion (trachea and lung buds).

Abnormalities in separating the oesophagus and trachea by the oesophagotracheal septum results in oesophageal atresia with or without tracheooesophageal fistulas (TEFs).

Macroscopic

Trachea

The trachea starts at the level of the lower border of the cricoid cartilage (C6) and ends at the level of the sternal angle of Louis (T4/5), just to the right of the midline. It is a cartilaginous and fibromuscular tube, which measure 10 to 12 cm in adults. The tracheal diameter varies in both men (13

to 25 mm) and women (10 to 21 mm). The tracheal wall has four layers: mucosa, submucosa, cartilage or muscle and adventitia. The posterior wall does not have cartilage and is instead supported by smooth muscle.

Bronchi

The airways consist of approximately 23 generations of branches from the trachea to the alveoli. The bronchi are composed of cartilaginous and fibromuscular elements. There are two mainstem bronchi (right and left), three lobar bronchi on the right with a total of ten segmental bronchi and two lobar bronchi on the left with a total of eight segmental bronchi.

Branches from the inferior thyroid arteries, intercostal arteries and bronchial arteries supply the trachea and bronchial tree.

The Lungs (Figs 19.1 and 19.2)

The lung includes the lung parenchyma and is mainly involved in gas exchange at the alveoli. The lung parenchyma is divided into lobes and segments. The right lung comprises ten segments: three in the right upper lobe (apical, anterior and medial), two in the right middle lobe (medial and lateral) and five in the right lower lobe (superior, medial, anterior, lateral and posterior). The left lung comprises of eight segments: four in the left upper lobe (apicoposterior, anterior, superior lingual and inferior lingula) and four in the left lower lobe (superior,

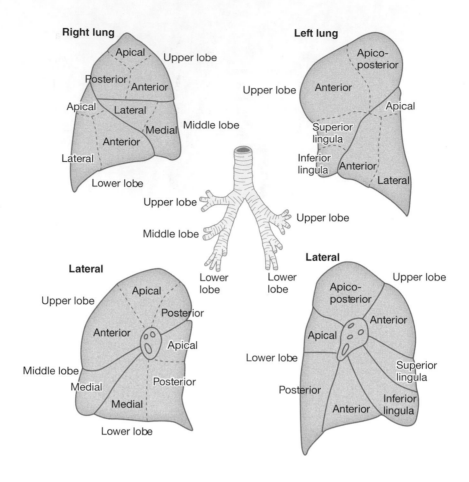

• **Fig. 19.1** Lobes and Segments of the Right and Left Lungs (From https://emedicine.medscape.com/article/1884995-overview#a)

anteromedial, lateral and posterior). Each lung is covered by the visceral pleura and this forms invaginations into both lungs, which are called fissures. There are two complete fissures in the right lung and one complete fissure in the left.

The apex of the pleura is approximately 2.5 cm above the clavicle. The pleura passes behind the sternoclavicular joint on either side to meet in the midline at the angle of Louis. The right pleural edge then passes down towards the 6th costal cartilage and then crosses the 8th rib in the midclavicular line, the 10th rib in the midaxillary line and the 12th rib at the lateral edge of the erector spinae. On the left side, the pleural edge deviates laterally at the 4th costal cartilage and follows the lateral border of the heart; the rest of the course is the same as the right side.

The main pulmonary artery originates in the right ventricle and divides into two branches; the right pulmonary artery passes posterior to the aorta and superior vena cava, emerging lateral to the atria and anterior and slightly inferior to the right mainstem bronchus. The left pulmonary artery is just anterior to the left mainstem bronchus. The

branches of the pulmonary arteries follow the branches of the bronchial tree.

The pulmonary veins originate in the alveoli and also receive drainage from the bronchial and pleural branches. There are two pulmonary veins on either side and these typically join at or near their junction with the left atrium.

The lymphatic drainage starts with the lymphatic vessels first draining into the intraparenchymal lymphatics and lymph nodes, then move to the peribronchial (hilar) lymph nodes, and subsequently move to subcarinal, tracheobronchial and paratracheal lymph nodes. The lymphatics eventually drain into the venous system via the bronchomediastinal lymphatic trunk and the thoracic duct or via the inferior deep cervical lymph nodes.

Microscopic

The trachea has multiple layers:
- Mucosa: ciliated pseudostratified columnar epithelium and mucus-secreting goblet cells. These rest on a

Pulmonary veins and arteries

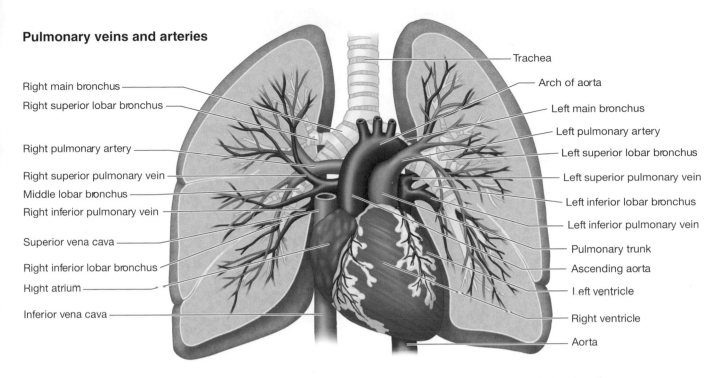

• **Fig. 19.2** Pulmonary Arteries and Veins (Reprinted with permission from Encyclopædia Britannica, © 2008 by Encyclopædia Britannica, Inc.)

basement membrane with a thin lamina propria (mainly collagenous).
- Submucosa: contains seromucous glands.
- Adventitia: cartilaginous rings that form the letter C and are open posteriorly. These are interconnected by connective tissue The open ends are connected by fibroelastic tissue and a band of smooth muscle.
The bronchus:
- Epithelium: pseudostratified columnar ciliated epithelium with numerous goblet cells. This transitions into a simple columnar epithelium and then into a cuboidal epithelium as it continues into the smaller bronchioles.
- Muscle layer: smooth muscle and elastic fibres. The cartilage support is eventually lost at the bronchial level.
The respiratory bronchiole:
- Epithelium: primarily cuboidal and may be ciliated; there are no goblet cells here. The supporting thin layer is formed by collagenous and smooth muscle. The terminal portion of the respiratory duct gives rise to alveolar sacs which are composed of multiple alveoli.
Alveoli:
- The alveolar wall is very thin (25 nm) and formed of squamous epithelium (type I cells – 98% of epithelium) covered by a thin film of surfactant fluid which is produced by type II cells. The surfactant fluid reduces the surface tension and hence keeps the alveoli open.
- The basal lamina is in contact with the capillaries from the pulmonary vascular system in order for gas exchange to occur efficiently.

Lung Cancer

Epidemiology

Lung cancer is thought to have been a rare cancer in the 19th century. Now, it is the most common cause of cancer death in the world (over 1.6 million deaths per year), more than breast, colon and prostate combined.

It is the most commonly occurring cancer in men and the third most common in women. Lung cancer deaths are expected to increase more than 1.8 times over the next 20 years.

The majority of patients with lung cancer are diagnosed with late stage disease, either locally advanced or metastatic disease. There is a growing body of evidence internationally that low dose computed tomography screening, in an at-risk population, allows the identification of early, resectable cancers and improves overall survival. International screening programs may be a game-changer in current management of the disease.

Lung cancer remains strongly associated with smoking and asbestos exposure, but is increasingly being seen in patients without these risk factors. Smoking is also often responsible for chronic obstructive pulmonary disease (COPD), but there is no direct correlation between COPD and lung cancer.

Aetiology

- **Environmental:**
  - Tobacco
There is a very clear association between lung cancer and tobacco smoking, often with a latent period of 10–30 years.

The risk factors are the number of cigarettes smoked per day, the age of onset of smoking (those who start smoking before 16 have the greatest damage to DNA), the length of time of smoking and the type of tobacco – unfiltered, high-tar and nicotine cigarettes give the highest risk. Cigar and pipe smoking are also associated with an increased risk of lung cancer, but this is of a lesser magnitude than with cigarette smoking. Passive exposure to tobacco smoke is also a risk. Following smoking cessation, the risk of developing lung cancer slowly decreases, but never reaches the level of life-long non-smokers. The risk associated with vaping is currently unknown.

- Other factors

Exposure to asbestos and certain chemicals, toxic metals and radioactive compounds and by-products (radon) also increase the risk of developing lung cancer.

- **Genetic:** Family history of lung cancer increases the risk of lung cancer.

Pathological Features

Lung cancer is generally classified as non-small-cell carcinoma (NSCLC) of epithelial origin, and small-cell lung cancer of neuroendocrine origin (Box 19.1).

NSCLC is further classified as adenocarcinoma, squamous cell carcinoma and large cell carcinoma.

Non-Small-Cell Carcinoma

According to the International Association for the Study of Lung Cancer (IASLC), NSCLC represents approximately 85% of all cases of lung cancer.

- **Adenocarcinoma**
  - Adenocarcinoma is the most common histologic subtype of lung cancer, accounting for 70–80% of all cases of NSCLC.
  - It tends to be more peripheral, arising in the small bronchial glands.
  - They have a propensity to metastasize earlier.
  - Histology reveals the presence of glands and papillary structures, round to oval nuclei with prominent nucleoli and moderate amounts of cytoplasm. Immunohistochemistry is typically positive for mucin, thyroid transcription factor 1 (TTF-1) and cytokeratin 7. TTF-1 positivity is found in 90% of primary lung adenocarcinomas, but is also found in some thyroid tumours.
  - Within adenocarcinoma, there is a widely divergent clinical, radiological, molecular and pathological spectrum of disease and there are many histological sub classifications.
  - Adenocarcinomas may progressively develop from an area of atypical adenomatous hyperplasia that may be seen as a ground glass opacity (GGO) on a CT scan. Development of solid components within the GGO suggests progression into an invasive carcinoma.

> **• BOX 19.1** **Pathological Classification of Lung Tumours**
>
> **Lung Cancer**
> - Small-cell carcinoma
> - Non-small-cell carcinoma
>   - Squamous-cell carcinoma (SCC)
>   - Adenocarcinoma
>   - Large-cell (undifferentiated) carcinoma
>
> **Neuroendocrine tumours**
> - Typical carcinoid
> - Intermediate – atypical carcinoid (= well-differentiated neuroendocrine carcinoma)
> - Malignant
>   - Large-cell neuroendocrine carcinoma
>   - Small-cell carcinoma

- **Squamous cell carcinoma**
  - Globally, squamous cell carcinoma accounts for 27–46% of NSCLC cases in men and 11–28% of cases in women.
  - It has a strong association with tobacco smoking and patients are older than in adenocarcinoma.
  - Lesions tend to be central and slow growing, with later development of metastases.
  - The growth starts as squamous metaplasia and progresses first to carcinoma in situ and then to invasive carcinoma. Although usually solitary, there may be more than one area of primary squamous carcinoma occurring both in the lung and elsewhere in the upper aero-digestive tract at the same time.
  - Histology reveals epithelial cells with a flattened appearance, intercellular bridges and individual cell keratinization. Immunohistochemistry is typically positive for p63, p40 and cytokeratin 5/6.
  - Continuing to smoke after treatment encourages further de novo development of squamous carcinoma.
- **Large-cell carcinoma**
  - These are poorly differentiated epithelial tumours which do not meet the criteria to be classified as either squamous-cell carcinoma or adenocarcinoma.
  - They represent approximately 10% of lung tumours.
  - They have no distinguishing distribution or macroscopic appearance.

Small-Cell Carcinoma

- Small-cell carcinoma (SCC) represents around 10–20% of lung tumours. Histologically, the cells are small and round.
- This is an anaplastic tumour which can occur in multiple lung sites and is highly malignant.
- Hormone production is common because its cells produce amine precursors. This causes paraneoplastic symptoms in around 15% of patients; hyponatraemia,

Cushing's syndrome and neurological syndromes such as the Eaton-Lambert myasthenic syndrome.
- The typical presentation of SCC is of a small tumour with large nodes.
- Metastases are frequently present at the time of initial diagnosis.
- SCC is generally considered inoperable because of the high incidence of disseminated disease at the time of presentation, although patients with genuinely limited disease may benefit from surgery as part of multimodality therapy.

Neuroendocrine Tumours

- There is a spectrum of neuroendocrine tumours which runs from the typical carcinoid tumour to well-differentiated neuroendocrine carcinoma (atypical carcinoid), to large-cell type neuroendocrine carcinoma and ultimately to small-cell carcinoma.
- These tumours are of increasing aggressiveness.
- Typical carcinoids are sometimes considered benign in their behaviour, although can still metastasize or recur locally after resection.

Clinical Features of Lung Cancer (Box 19.2)

- **Symptoms**
  - **General:** Weight loss, malaise and fatigue are common, especially with advanced disease.
  - **Respiratory:** Cough is the most common symptom, occurring in nearly half of patients. Sputum production is variable. Haemoptysis on at least one occasion is frequent but not usually massive. Dyspnoea can be caused by intrinsic or extrinsic airway obstruction and by pleural effusion with loss of function of part of the lung. Occasionally, pulmonary embolism (an expression of paraneoplastic syndrome, or Trousseau's syndrome) can be responsible.
  - **Other chest or local symptoms:** Non-specific chest pain, usually heaviness, is often described; specific local pain may be associated with invasion of the chest wall by tumour or involvement of the skeleton by metastases. Pain or numbness in the arm occurs from brachial plexus invasion by a superior sulcus tumour *(Pancoast tumour)*, and tumours at this site in the thoracic inlet can also invade the stellate ganglion causing a *Horner's syndrome*. Hoarseness can occur due to involvement of a recurrently laryngeal nerve by the tumour or metastatic lymph nodes. Dysphagia is the consequence of compression or invasion of the oesophagus in the same way.
- **Signs**
  - **General:** Clubbing of the fingers occurs in 30% of patients with lung cancer, and hypertrophic pulmonary osteoarthropathy in 3%, with painful swelling of the wrists and ankles. These regress rapidly with

• BOX 19.2 Symptoms and Signs of Lung Cancer

- Symptoms:
  - General: weight loss, fatigue, malaise
  - Respiratory: cough, haemoptysis, dyspnoea
  - Others: chest pain/heaviness, pain/numbness in arm, hoarseness, dysphagia
- Signs:
  - General: clubbing, hypertrophic pulmonary osteoarthropathy, raised jugular venous pressure/ distended veins in upper arms and chest in superior vena cava obstruction
  - Respiratory: localized wheeze, recurrent chest infection, inspiratory stridor, decreased air entry/bronchial breathing, dull percussion note and decreased vocal fremitus (= pleural effusion)

complete tumour resection. Distension of the jugular veins and increase in jugular venous pressure occurs with superior vena cava obstruction, and distended veins may be visible over the upper arms and chest along with swelling of the upper body from the level of the heart upwards.
- **Respiratory:** Localized wheezing can indicate a partially obstructed bronchus. Carcinoid tumours often arise within the bronchial tree and may cause recurrent chest infections. Inspiratory stridor indicates significant narrowing of the airway and mandates urgent referral to a specialist centre. An area of decreased air entry and/or bronchial breathing may occur due to an obstructed bronchus or pleural effusion. Percussion with dullness and associated decreased fremitus may indicate an effusion.
- **Signs of metastases:** Any new neurological complaint or sign such as headache, blurred vision, hallucinations, syncope, convulsions and imbalance can indicate CNS involvement. New bony or joint pain may be the sign of metastases. Enlarged scalene or supraclavicular lymph nodes may be loco-regional palpable metastases. Subcutaneous nodules may be skin metastases. Enlargement of the liver may indicate diffuse involvement. Laboratory investigations may reveal anaemia, hypercalcaemia and elevated alkaline phosphatase levels.
- **Staging of lung cancer** (Table 19.1)
  - The TNM staging of NSCLC is currently in its eighth edition as of 2017.
  - Whilst this may also be used for staging SCC, this is more commonly staged as limited or extensive disease. In limited disease, SCLC is found on only one side of the chest, involving just one part of the lung and/or lymph nodes on that side. Approximately 30% of patients diagnosed have limited stage disease. In extensive stage, disease is present in both lungs, lymph nodes on the other side of the chest or in distant organs.

TABLE 19.1 The IASLC 9th Edition of the TNM Classification for Lung Cancer.

T – Primary Tumour

TX		Primary tumour cannot be assessed, or tumour proven by the presence of malignant cells in sputum or bronchial washings but not visualized by imaging or bronchoscopy.
T0		No evidence of primary tumour
Tis		Carcinoma in situ
T1		Tumour 3 cm or less in greatest dimension, surrounded by lung or visceral pleura, without bronchoscopic evidence of invasion more proximal than the lobar bronchus (i.e. not the main bronchus)[a]
	T1mi	Minimally invasive adenocarcinoma[b]
	T1a	Tumour 1 cm or less in greatest dimension[a]
	T1b	Tumour more than 1 cm but not more than 2 cm in greatest dimension[a]
	T1c	Tumour more than 2 cm but not more than 3 cm in greatest dimension[a]
T2		Tumour more than 3 cm but not more than 5 cm; or tumour with any of the following features[c]: • Involves main bronchus regardless of distance to the carina, but without involving the carina • Invades visceral pleura • Associated with atelectasis or obstructive pneumonitis that extends to the hilar region, either involving part of the lung or the entire lung
	T2a	Tumour more than 3 cm but not more than 4 cm in greatest dimension
	T2b	Tumour more than 4 cm but not more than 5 cm in greatest dimension
T3		Tumour more than 5 cm but not more than 7 cm in greatest dimension or one that directly invades any of the following: chest wall (including superior sulcus tumours), phrenic nerve, parietal pericardium; or associated separate tumour nodule(s) in the same lobe as the primary
T4		Tumours more than 8 cm or one that invades any of the following: diaphragm, mediastinum, heart, great vessels, trachea, recurrent laryngeal nerve, oesophagus, vertebral body, carina; separate tumour nodule(s) in a different ipsilateral lobe to that of the primary

N – Regional Lymph Nodes

NX	Regional lymph nodes cannot be assessed
N0	No regional lymph node metastasis
N1	Metastasis in ipsilateral peribronchial and/or ipsilateral hilar lymph nodes and intrapulmonary nodes, including involvement by direct extension
N2	Metastasis in ipsilateral mediastinal and/or subcarinal lymph node(s)
N3	Metastasis in contralateral mediastinal, contralateral hilar, ipsilateral or contralateral scalene or supraclavicular lymph node (s)

M – Distant Metastasis

M0		No distant metastasis
M1		Distant metastasis
	M1a	Separate tumour nodule(s) in a contralateral lobe; tumour with pleural or pericardial nodules of malignant pleural or pericardial effusion[d]
	M1b	Single extrathoracic metastasis in a single organ[e]
	M1c	Multiple extrathoracic metastasis in one or several organs

Stages of Lung Cancer From the 8th Edition of TNM.

Stage	T	N	M
Occult Carcinoma	TX	N0	M0
0	Tis	N0	M0

Continued

TABLE 19.1   The IASLC 9th Edition of the TNM Classification for Lung Cancer—cont'd

Stages of Lung Cancer From the 8th Edition of TNM.

Stage	T	N	M
1A1	T1mi	N0	M0
	T1a	N0	M0
1A2	T1b	N0	M0
1A3	T1c	N0	M0
1B	T2a	N0	M0
IIA	T2b	N0	M0
IIB	T1a	N1	M0
	T1b	N1	M0
	T1c	N1	M0
	T2a	N1	M0
	T2b	N1	M0
	T3	N0	M0
IIIA	T1a	N2	M0
	T1b	N2	M0
	T1c	N2	M0
	T2a	N2	M0
	T2b	N2	M0
	T3	N1	M0
	T4	N0	M0
	T4	N1	M0
IIIB	T1a	N3	M0
	T1b	N3	M0
	T1c	N3	M0
	T2a	N3	M0
	T2b	N3	M0
	T3	N2	M0
	T4	N2	M0
IIIC	T3	N3	M0
	T4	N3	M0
IVA	Any T	Any N	M1a
	Any T	Any N	M1b
IVB	Any T	Any N	M1c

Tables courtesy of the International Association for the Study of Lung Cancer (IASLC)

[a]The uncommon superficial spreading tumour of any size with its invasive component limited to the bronchial wall, which may extend proximal to the main bronchus, is also classified as T1a

[b]Solitary adenocarcinoma (≤3 cm), with a predominantly lepidic pattern and ≤5 mm invasion in greatest dimension in any one focus

[c]T2 tumours with these features are classified T2a if 4 cm or less, or if size cannot be determined, and T2b if greater than 4 cm but not larger than 5 cm

[d]Most pleural (pericardial effusions) with lung cancer are due to tumour. In a few patients, however, multiple microscopic examinations of pleural (pericardial) fluid are negative for tumour, and the fluid is non-bloody and is not an exudate. Where these elements and clinical judgement dictate that the effusion is not related to the tumour, the effusion should be excluded as a staging descriptor

[e]This includes involvement of a single distant (non-regional node)

Evaluation of the Lung Cancer Patient

The assessment of patients prior to undergoing surgery involves the following steps, usually taken by the collective lung cancer multi-disciplinary team (MDT):

1. Diagnosis, usually obtained by CT guided biopsy, bronchoscopic biopsy or endobronchial ultrasound-guided bronchoscopic transbronchial biopsy (EBUS)
2. What is the stage of the disease?
3. What extent of resection is best to completely resect the lesion, with adequate margins (i.e. non-anatomical wedge resection, segmentectomy, lobectomy or pneumonectomy)?
4. Can the patient tolerate this planned resection?

Determination of the Stage of the Disease (Box 19.3)

- The four commonest sites of metastasis are brain, adrenal gland, liver and bone. In order to rule out the presence of distant metastasis the following investigations should be performed:
  - brain MRI (or at least a CT)
  - CT chest and upper abdomen
  - PET/CT scan (this has largely superseded bone scans). PET/CT scan has around 80–85% sensitivity and 95% specificity for the identification of lymph node disease, and identified occult metastatic disease in approximately 6% of patients.
- Other investigations which may also be of help in diagnosis and assessing the extent of the disease include:
  - *Bronchoscopy/EBUS:* to assess the airway and lymph nodes adjacent to the trachea-bronchial tree
  - *MRI* is superior to CT to determine vascular, vertebral and nerve (brachial plexus) involvement by the tumour. Whilst it is not routinely performed to assess the stage of the primary tumour (T-stage), it should be performed to assess the extent of disease in patients with superior sulcus tumours.
  - *Liver ultrasound scan* or *MRI* may provide further information regarding possible liver metastatic disease.
  - *Cervical mediastinoscopy* is performed through a small cervical incision and allows all the lymph nodes around the central airway to be identified and biopsied. Compared with EBUS, cervical mediastinoscopy allows for entire lymph glands to be removed, and is considered by many to be the gold standard for assessing mediastinal lymphadenopathy. Lymph node stations 5 and 6 are in the sub aortic and aortopulmonary regions in the left chest. They are on the lateral side of the aorta and therefore cannot be reached by mediastinoscopy. They can, however, be biopsied by an *anterior mediastinoscopy* or *video assisted thoracoscopic surgery (VATS)*.
  - If there is a pleural effusion, it is mandatory to absolutely rule out pleural involvement. If *cytological analysis of the fluid* is negative, *thoracoscopy* should be

---

• BOX 19.3 | Summary of Investigations for Staging

1. Brain MRI (or at least CT head)
2. CT chest and upper abdomen
3. PET/CT
4. Other investigations include:
   - Bronchoscopy/EBUS
   - MRI (especially in superior sulcus tumours)
   - Liver USS/MRI
   - Cervical mediastinoscopy or anterior mediastinoscopy or video-assisted thoracoscopic surgery (VATS)
   - In the presence of pleural effusion, if cytological analysis is negative, consider thoracoscopy +/− biopsy of the pleura to rule out pleural involvement

CT, Computed tomography; EBUS, endobronchial ultrasound bronchoscopy; MRI, magnetic resonance imaging; PET, positron emission tomography; USS, ultrasound scan.

---

considered to examine and, if necessary, to biopsy the pleural. Cytology has a 15–20% false-negative rate even after two to three aspirations of pleural fluid.

Determination of the Required Resection

Earlier sites of tumour progression or spread are often within the anatomical region of the lung (segment or lobe), or to the regional lymph nodes. Therefore, the standard operation for biopsy confirmed lung cancer is an *anatomical lobectomy with systematic nodal dissection (SND)*. An *anatomical segmentectomy* is often considered a reasonable alternative for small early stage lung cancers, especially if the respiratory function is significantly impaired. Lung cancer resections are considered to be incomplete without assessment of loco-regional lymph nodes and surgeons will typically remove lymphatic tissue and nodes from at least three N1 stations (within the lung of hilum) and three N2 stations (within the ipsilateral mediastinum, including the subcarinal fossa – lymph node station 7).

Pneumonectomy is far less commonly performed in the modern era, but may still be required for large central tumours. Pneumonectomy has a much greater physiological impact on the patient because of a greater loss of lung parenchyma and extensive mediastinal shift to the ipsilateral side, which may result in airway twisting or compression (post-pneumonectomy syndrome).

Pneumonectomy also has a higher incidence of bronchopleural fistula, which can be a devastating complication. In many cases where pneumonectomy was previously performed, at least one of the lobes can be preserved by performing a sleeve resection of the bronchus or carina and reimplantation of the unaffected lobe(s) (Fig. 19.3).

The extension of resection can usually be determined from the bronchoscopy and CT findings. However, in some cases it is only at the time of surgical exploration that this can be ascertained. It is therefore mandatory that the extent of resection that is physiologically tolerable by the patient be determined prior to surgery so as to allow this decision to be made safely intraoperatively.

A

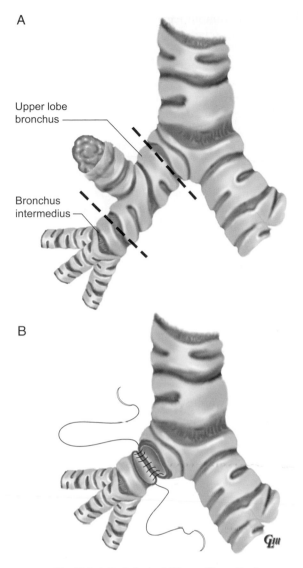

Upper lobe
bronchus

Bronchus
intermedius

B

• **Fig. 19.3** A Prototypical 'Sleeve Resection'

A non-anatomical wedge resection can sometimes be considered to completely remove a small peripheral lung tumour, although this is thought to result in a higher local disease relapse.

Preoperative Assessment of Patients with Lung Cancer

The **Thoracoscore** (Box 19.4) is a risk stratification model developed in France that gives the overall perioperative mortality risk. It probably slightly overestimates the risk of surgery but has been validated by other authors.

The assessment of any patient includes:
- general assessment of cardiovascular risk, especially as many of these patients have been smokers. This may require cardiology review, transthoracic echocardiogram or thallium scan.
- Pulmonary function assessment, which is particularly pertinent to lung surgery, and an assessment of the extent of the pulmonary resection that they will be able to tolerate without leaving them unduly dyspnoeic or oxygen

dependent. Central to these decisions are individual patient preference and the availability of other treatment options.

Most patients will tolerate lobectomy with relatively little compromise in function if they are fairly asymptomatic with normal exercise capacity. Formal lung function tests including spirometry, gas transfer, lung volumes and arterial blood gas (often taken from the ear lobe as an end capillary sample) are helpful in any patient with respiratory compromise, a history of smoking or other lung disease, or where pneumonectomy is considered a possibility. Otherwise simple spirometry may suffice.

The two strongest predictors of cardiopulmonary morbidity and mortality after pulmonary resection are the FEV_1 and the DLCO (transfer factor for carbon monoxide). Previously it was considered that we should aim to leave the patient with at least 40% predicted postoperative FEV_1 and DLCO, and this was calculated by reducing the preoperative values by a proportion consistent with the number of functional anatomical segments that are planned to be removed at surgery.

However, this may be overly conservative and deny some patients the chance of a potentially curative resection. There is, therefore, no strict cut-off with regard to lung function parameters and the final decision will need to take into consideration the patient's wishes, the magnitude of the surgery and other treatment options as well as the predicted postoperative lung function values.

A cardiopulmonary exercise test to calculate the VO_2 may provide further information when deciding if a patient can tolerate the planned resection.

A quantitative V/Q scan will allow examination of the regional perfusion (and ventilation) which may further help in the decision making, especially if pneumonectomy is anticipated.

Smoking cessation prior to surgery seems intuitively to be desirable. In fact, it takes 2 months for there to be a true benefit in terms of sputum reduction and full restitution of mucociliary function. Nonetheless, active smoking immediately prior to surgery does increase the operative risk. In a borderline patient, it can be beneficial to defer surgery for 6–8 weeks for pulmonary rehabilitation combined with smoking cessation.

Treatment of Lung Cancer

All patients with lung cancer should be discussed within a MDT setting, including representation from thoracic surgeons, respiratory physicians, clinical and medical oncologists, radiologists, histopathologists, palliative care and the clinical nurse specialist team. Other allied health professionals may help with the decision process.

Non-Small-Cell Lung Cancer

Unfortunately, most patients present with advanced disease that will not be curable with any combination of treatment modalities. In such cases, surgery may be able to assist in diagnosis or palliation to treat pleural or pericardial effusions, or airway obstruction.

However, the mainstay of their treatment will be oncological, even if it is palliative in nature. Palliative treatment is an active treatment option that seeks optimal symptom relief. The value of this treatment must not be underestimated to maintain quality of life, and every effort must be made to obtain it for all inoperable patients, especially when they become symptomatic.

Surgery should not be offered to patients with minimal chance of cure. It submits them needlessly to the risks (morbidity/mortality) of the procedure without the benefit (chance of cure).

Appropriate staging will ensure an exploratory thoracotomy ('open and shut') rate in the order of 5%. There are patients in whom only exploratory thoracotomy can assess resectability, so the rate of this procedure should not be 0%.

Surgery is still considered to be the gold standard treatment in stage 1 and 2 lung cancers, although stereotactic radiotherapy is increasingly being considered as a comparable treatment option, even though it may result in slightly higher local recurrence rate. Stereotactic radiotherapy remains a good option for patients with small tumours who do not wish (or are not fit for) surgical resection.

Stereotactic ablative techniques, usually with microwave or radiofrequency ablation, are often an alternative local treatment modality. These are often collectively referred to as RFA. These methods probably have increased rates of local recurrence as compared to surgery, and do not allow for pathological lymph node staging.

Patients with a resectable tumour and local N1 lymph node involvement are usually still considered good candidates for surgical resection, although the 5-year survival is reduced with any lymphadenopathy.

Patients with more extensive lymph node involvement (N2 disease and especially N3 disease) would normally be treated by our oncology colleagues, with a combination of chemotherapy and/or radiotherapy. Surgery may still have a role as part of multi-modality therapy especially if the disease is down-staged with regression of the lymph node disease.

Other pharmacological treatments such as tyrosine kinase inhibitors (e.g. erlotinib) can produce a profound response with regards to tumour regression when tumour gene mutations are found to be present, e.g. epidermal growth factor receptor (eGFR). The tumour response, however, is usually finite, typically 18 months.

Immunotherapy is an exciting new field of research with some very promising early results, even in extensive stage lung cancer, e.g. durvalumab, as reported by the PACIFIC study investigators.

Patients with stage IV disease because of a single, or limited, metastatic foci (e.g. brain or adrenal gland) may be considered for multi-modality therapy, including surgery.

Lung cancer involving the thoracic inlet/superior sulcus may present with neurological symptoms in the arm and hand (Pancoast syndrome). These tumours may still be resectable, but in conjunction with pre- or postoperative chemoradiotherapy.

Pancoast tumours, and indeed any lung cancer that involves the chest wall, may still be resectable en-bloc with the attached portion of the rib cage +/– diaphragm, and occasionally even a portion of the adjacent vertebra. Chest wall reconstruction may then be required with polypropylene mesh, impregnated with methyl-methacrylate cement if the defect is large, or alternatively with metal bar reconstruction.

Palliative chemotherapy has a modest effect on overall survival, but its proponents believe that it can improve quality of life significantly. This is not universally accepted. Palliative radiotherapy can obtain good relief of symptoms when there is pain from invasion into the chest wall or at the site of bone metastases. It can offer relief of superior vena cava syndrome (endovascular stenting is also a useful palliative procedure in this condition). It can also be very helpful when there is symptomatic bronchial obstruction or haemoptysis.

Small-Cell Lung Cancer

The treatment of SCC is typically combination chemoradiotherapy, including prophylactic brain irradiation. Previously, small-cell cancer was classified as only limited or extensive disease; the IASLC, however, has introduced the same lung cancer staging for SCC as in NSCLC. Patients with genuinely early stage SCC may be considered for surgery as part of multi-modality therapy.

Prognosis (Table 19.2)

According to the IASLC, the prognosis of NSCLC is relatively poor. The 5-year survival for stage one NSCLC is approximately 60%. With stage 2 disease, this falls to 30–50%. In the very highly selected stage 3 patients who are considered surgical candidates, the 5-year survival is only around 25–30%. Otherwise it is at best 10–15%, more often much less. The median survival for stage 4 disease is approximately 12 months, with 1–2% 5-year survival. Less than 20–25% of patients present with operable disease, so the overall 5-year survival for men with lung cancer in the UK is only 8%.

TABLE 19.2	5-year Survival of Non-Small-Cell and Small-Cell Lung Carcinoma.				
Stage	I	II	III	IV	Overall
NSCLC 5-yr survival	60%	30–50%	25–30% (if operable) 10–15%	1–2%	8%
SCC 5-yr survival	30%	16%	8.5%	1.9%	6%

The prognosis of SCC is far worse, with only 3–17% of patients with limited disease surviving 5 years (and only 30–40% of patients present with limited disease). For extensive stage, the median survival is 6 to 12 months with treatment and only 2–4 months without. Furthermore, the survivors present with new second aero-digestive cancers at a rate of 2–10% per patient per year. Thus, the mortality of survivors is 10 times greater than age and sex-matched cohorts.

Other Lung Tumours

- **Carcinoids**
  - They are rare malignant tumours and are, in most cases, resectable.
  - Carcinoid of the lung accounts for approximately 25–30% of all carcinoid tumours, and approximately 1% of lung tumours.
  - There are two types of lung carcinoid:
    - *Typical*, which grow slowly and rarely metastasize, and atypical which tend to grow faster and have a slightly increased risk of metastasis. Typical carcinoid has an essentially normal 5- and 10-year survival following their complete resection. The majority (70%) are central lesions. Up to 31% are asymptomatic. They can cause multiple symptoms over many years; some are due to obstruction such as wheezing, shortness of breath, cough and infection. Others are haemoptysis (frequent) or chest pain. An associated carcinoid syndrome is very rare (around 2%), as is Cushing's syndrome. Complete resection is usually considered curative. Resection should always spare as much lung parenchyma as possible. Because of their central location, these tumours often lend themselves to sleeve resections. Endoscopic resection (whatever the technique) should be reserved for frail, high-risk patients who are poor operative candidates because of the high risk of incomplete resection and recurrence. The other indication for endoscopic resection is to allow a distal pneumonitis to clear so as to permit a safe parenchyma-sparing limited resection.
    - *Atypical carcinoids* tend to be more aggressive with much more frequent lymph node metastases (30–50%). They are identified histologically by the presence of necrosis and/or 2–10 mitosis per 2 mm^2 at 10× magnification. The 5-year survival is poorer for patients with atypical carcinoids compared with carcinoid tumours without atypical features, at 40–76%. Large-cell neuroendocrine carcinomas are uncommon lesions with a poor prognosis.
- **Other rare primary pulmonary tumours**
  - Immunocompromised patients have an increased risk of presenting with solid organ lymphomas, and this includes the lungs. HIV-infected patients may also present with pulmonary Kaposi's sarcoma.
  - Hamartomas account for around three-quarters of all benign lung tumours. The definition of a hamartoma is an excessive focal overgrowth of mature normal cells and tissue in an organ, composed of identical cellular components. The majority are asymptomatic peripheral lung lesions which are discovered incidentally, and the obvious problem is distinguishing them from a small, early stage lung cancer. They often contain fat and cartilage.
  - Chondrohamartomas are purely cartilaginous, as their name indicates. Central lesions can cause symptoms of obstruction. The diagnosis of hamartoma can be made based on the radiological findings and the presence of fat and/or cartilage in a biopsy specimen. The usual indication for surgery is the uncertainty as to diagnosis. Simple excision is curative. Symptomatic lesions should be resected with as much of a parenchyma sparing technique as feasible. Asymptomatic peripheral lesions only need to be resected if large, or growing in a young, fit patient.

There is a long list of these very rare lesions which are beyond the scope of this chapter.

Metastatic Disease

Lung metastases are identified in 30–50% of all cancer patients. Whilst almost any cancer can present with secondary pulmonary deposits, the tumours that most commonly do so are colorectal, bladder, breast, prostate and sarcoma (including both osteo and soft tissue subtypes).

A limited number of lung metastases can be resected, with low morbidity and mortality, particularly in cases of colorectal cancer and sarcoma. No randomized controlled trial has been completed to prove whether patients can be cured; however, it is likely that, in selected cases, the disease progression can be delayed or a prolonged disease-free interval provided. RFA and stereotactic radiotherapy may

---

• BOX 19.5 | Indications for Chest Drain Insertion

- Pneumothorax: tension pneumothorax, persistent or recurrent pneumothorax, large spontaneous pneumothorax, pneumothorax in any ventilated patient, traumatic pneumothorax
- Pleural effusion: malignant, para-pneumonic or other non-malignant causes, e.g. heart failure
- Traumatic haemothorax
- Empyema
- Post thoracic/cardiac surgery (post drain removal surgical emphysema/pneumothorax/large fluid collection)

---

be other local treatment options, especially if the number of metastases is low.

Principles of Chest Drainage

The object of chest drainage is to obtain complete evacuation of all fluid and air from the pleural space and to allow complete re-expansion of the underlying lung (Box 19.5). If the lung cannot re-expand despite adequate drainage, then it is referred to as a trapped lung. This condition can be resolved surgically with a decortication if clinically indicated. Alternatively, an indwelling pleural catheter may allow gradual re-expansion of the lung over a longer period. If drainage cannot result in evacuation of all abnormal pleural contents, either because of loculation or coagulated blood, then surgery is usually indicated. Most cases can be managed with a thoracoscopic approach.

However, it is mandatory that all chest drains be attached to a device that allows air and fluid to escape freely from the pleural space without allowing air to enter. The traditional drainage device is the underwater seal, for example the Rocket bottle (Fig. 19.4) which is illustrated in the single-bottle drainage system seen below. Suction (typically 2 kPa) may be applied to this system if required.

The underwater seal is a cheap and safe system that works as long as the drainage bottle is well below the patient (in order to prevent negative pleural pressure from drawing the bottle fluid into the chest).

Within thoracic surgery, digital pleural drainage systems are now commonly used and in the UK they are endorsed by the National Institute of Clinical Excellence (NICE). These systems (for example, the Medela Thopaz (Fig. 19.5, as shown) provide regulated negative pressure without the need for the patient to be connected to a wall suction device.

These devices also monitor the air leak and only apply the suction required to maintain the negative pressure prescribed by the medical team. The digital display also provides real-time data of air leak and fluid drainage, as well as a 24-hour historical graph. The information displayed relating to the previous 24-hour period has been shown to allow for earlier drain removal and shorter hospital stay. This probably allows for a more accurate picture of air and fluid drainage rather than periodic observation of the bottle by different team members.

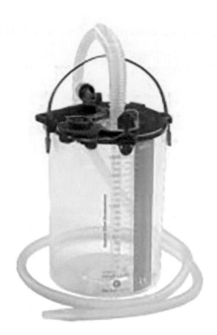

• Fig. 19.4 Rocket Medical Underwater Seal Drainage Bottle (with permission from Rocket Medical plc.)

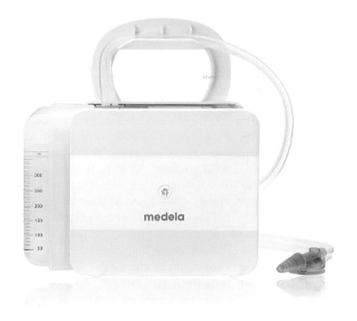

• Fig. 19.5 Medela Thopaz Digital Drainage System (with permission from Medela Healthcare)

Another system of one-way valve that is commonly used is the Heimlich valve, often integrated into a portable bag to collect drained fluid. The valve incorporates a flutter valve to allow egress of air and fluid, but prevent any return into the pleural cavity.

The standard chest drain should be place in the 4th or 5th intercostal space in the midaxillary line and directed up to the apex of the chest along the posterior chest wall. Drain insertion can be via a Seldinger or open (surgical) technique. Placing a drain can be done under ultrasound or CT guidance, and most drains placed by interventional radiologists are pigtail catheters. These can be remarkably effective, but in the author's experience, it is important to maintain their patency by irrigating them one to two times per day with 10–15 mL of sterile 0.9% saline solution.

Chest drain insertion is a well-recognized cause of morbidity and even mortality, even with smaller bore Seldinger type drains. Box 19.6 describes recognized complications of pleural drainage.

Chest Drain Insertion

All drains should be inserted by a member of staff trained and experienced in the technique of drain insertion or by members of staff supervised by others who are themselves experienced in these procedures.

Issues that need to be considered prior to drain insertion include:

- The type of drain to be used (large bore surgical drain vs Seldinger type)
- Size of drain, typically 24- or 28-F in an adult
- Whether the drain needs to be inserted immediately (elective drain insertion is often best performed in hours when higher staffing levels provide better support and monitoring)
- The most appropriate anatomical site for drain insertion
- Whether further imaging or real-time bedside USS of the chest should be obtained
- The hospital department where the drain should be inserted (ward, HDU, operating theatre)
- Who is to insert the drain and whether supervision or training is required

The 'safe triangle' should be considered in most cases as a potential site for drain insertion. This is an area beneath the axilla bounded by the mid-axillary line posteriorly, the posterior border of pectoralis major anteriorly and the horizontal level of the nipple (or 5th intercostal space) inferiorly. Seldinger type drains or pigtail catheters can be inserted at other locations, especially when guided by real time ultrasound in the case of pleural fluid. Close monitoring of the patient should be carried out during and after the procedure, and oxygen and analgesia administered as required.

Criteria for drain removal – there is much variance in local practice. Most clinicians are happy to remove the drain if there is a small air leak only (10–20 mL/min for 24 hours, as measured accurately by a digital drainage system) and <300 mL fluid output per day.

Pneumothorax

The definition of pneumothorax (PNO) is when the pleural space contains air which separates the parietal and visceral pleura, preventing the lung from occupying its normal place. Symptoms include pleuritic chest pain and dyspnoea. Physical signs may be subtle, but characteristically include reduced chest expansion on the affected side, decreased air entry and hyper-resonance to percussion.

> ● BOX **19.6** Complications of Chest Drain Insertion
>
> - Trauma to intrathoracic structures, intra-abdominal structures and lung
> - Re-expansion pulmonary oedema
> - Haemorrhage
> - Incorrect tube position
> - Blocked tube
> - Pleural drain falls out
> - Subcutaneous emphysema

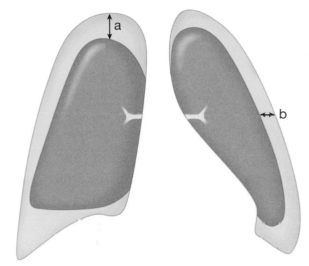

a = apex to cupola distance (American guidelines)
b = interpleural distance at the level of the hilum (British guidelines)

● **Fig. 19.6** *(a)* Distance of lung to chest wall from the apex (how size of pneumothorax used to be measured). *(b)* Distance from edge of lung to chest wall at the level of the hilum (now recommended to measure the size of pneumothorax). (Image taken from MacDuff A, Arnold A, Harvey J. on behalf of the BTS Pleural Disease Guideline Group, 2010. Management of spontaneous pneumothorax: British Thoracic Society Guideline 2010. Thorax 2010; 65 (Suppl 2): ii18-ii31.)

Current guidelines for measuring the size of pneumothorax (Fig. 19.6) is quantified on standard erect chest X-ray by measuring from the edge of the lung to the chest wall at the level of the hilum (see Fig. 19.6B). Previously this was done by measuring from the apex (see Fig. 19.6A), but this technique trended towards overestimating the volume. A 2 cm radiographic pneumothorax from the hilum approximates to a 50% pneumothorax by volume. CT scanning of the thorax is recommended for uncertain or complex cases.

Flying is contraindicated with a PNO because aeroplanes are not pressurized to sea level atmospheric pressure and so the volume of the PNO may alter, causing rapid respiratory compromise without the availability of medical intervention. Most airline companies will not allow travel with a PNO or within 4 weeks of resolution.

Spontaneous Primary Pneumothorax

- This is when a PNO occurs without an identifiable cause, although small blebs or bullae are often found, typically at the apex of the upper lobe, on CT scan or thoracoscopy.

- A *pulmonary bleb* is a small collection of sub pleural air, not greater than 2 cm in size.
- A *bulla* is usually considered to be greater than 2 cm in diameter.
  - It appears to occur most commonly in tall, thin, young, healthy individuals
  - Occurs more frequently in men than women
  - More common in smokers than in non-smokers
- The PNO can occur at any time, including at complete rest.
- Most commonly, the patient presents with onset of sudden chest pain or tightness and shortness of breath of variable severity.
- Examination shows decreased breath sounds and hyper-resonance to percussion.

Treatment

- There are three options:
  (1) Observation,
  (2) Aspiration and
  (3) Drainage.
- Treatment depends on the importance of the PNO; a <2 cm PNO will often resolve without treatment.
- Larger or increasing pneumothoraces require drainage.
- Breathlessness is an absolute indication for intervention. This should first be by needle aspiration with a wide-bore i.v. plastic cannula (with the needle removed), a three-way tap and a 50-mL syringe. Failure to aspirate the pneumothorax is an indication for insertion of an 8–14-F chest drain.
- All patients should be followed up in respiratory outpatient clinic 2–4 weeks after the initial episode.
- Hospital admission is required if there is any doubt about the PNO increasing or if the patient cannot rapidly and readily return for care if necessary, for whatever reason.
- When the episode of PNO is resolved, the risk of recurrence is around 20% following a first episode, 50% following a second episode and 80% after the third.

Surgical Treatment

- This consists of the resection of the causative bullae or bleb associated with some sort of pleurodesis procedure (a procedure which causes the visceral pleura to adhere to the parietal pleura).
- This is usually done by *pleurectomy, pleural abrasion* or *talc pleurodesis.*
- *Talc pleurodesis* is quick and easy to perform, possibly even without surgical thoracoscopy; however, some clinicians prefer not to use talc in young patients because of the theoretical risk of chest wall restriction.
- Most commonly, the surgical approach is via VATS and the risk of recurrence following surgery is 2–4%.
- Surgery is indicated after two episodes of spontaneous pneumothorax, the first episode on the contralateral side, when the current episode will not resolve despite drainage or if there is an associated haemothorax. Other

indications include bilateral pneumothorax, tension pneumothorax and those who work in high risk professions (pilots/deep sea divers).

Secondary Pneumothorax

Trauma

- If there is a lesion which causes a hole in the chest cavity, the lung may collapse.
- Usually trauma causes a hole in the lung, and air escapes into the chest cavity.
- This can be a penetrating injury into the lung or blunt trauma with a rib fracture which punctures or lacerates the lung.
- If the injury constitutes a one-way valve mechanism, a *tension pneumothorax* can ensue (see below).
- If there is a gaping hole in this chest wall, this is an *open pneumothorax*. In this case there may be respiratory failure because more ventilation occurs through the hole than through the airway.
- As clinicians, we should have a low threshold for large-bore chest drainage in any case of chest trauma.
- Another frequent cause of traumatic PNO is the various invasive diagnostic and therapeutic interventions done by doctors, including placement of central venous lines and biopsies of thoracic lesions (including lung lesions and radiofrequency ablation).

Underlying Lung Disease

- The most common cause of a secondary PNO is the rupture of an *emphysematous bulla.*
- Other causes are disease such as:
  - cystic fibrosis
  - lymphangioleiomyomatosis
  - interstitial lung disease
  - rupture of tumours or abscesses
- An uncommon cause is catamenial PNO, which is PNO that occurs at the time of menstruation due to thoracic endometrial deposits in patients with endometriosis, although the exact aetiology of this remains unclear. Many patients with catamenia PNO will have evidence of diaphragmatic ectopic endometrial tissue, with or without fenestrations.
- Any patient with either a secondary PNO >2 cm, or breathlessness should have an 8–14-F chest drain inserted immediately.
- If they are asymptomatic with a small (1–2 cm) PNO, then aspiration may be attempted. If the PNO is <1 cm in size, then they should be admitted, administered high-flow oxygen (unless suspected to have oxygen sensitivity) and observed for at least 24 hours.
- The surgical management of secondary PNO will depend on the clinical scenario and future treatment options, but may require surgery and possibly a pleurodesis procedure.

Tension Pneumothorax (Fig. 19.7)

- This occurs when pressure builds up in the pleural space, compressing the lung and collapsing it, then causing mediastinal shift to the opposite side.

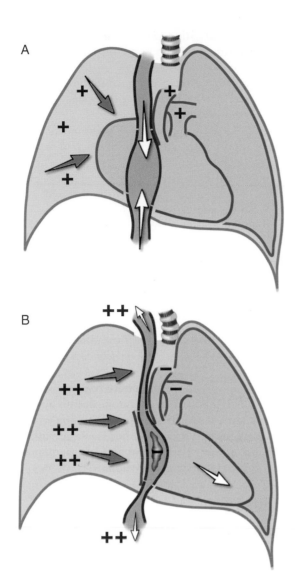

• **Fig. 19.7** In a tension pneumothorax, the mediastinum is pushed over toward the opposite side. As the pressure increases, the superior (and inferior) venae cavae are progressively kinked and pinched off where the relatively fixed and mobile parts move. As this happens, the venous return to the heart drops off and cardiac output is reduced. When this is severe enough the patient will die.

• This progressively causes reduced venous return to the heart, causing the cardiac output to drop.

Signs and Symptoms

• shortness of breath
• tachypnoea
• tracheal deviation to the opposite side
• absent breath sounds over the involved hemithorax, with hyper-resonance to percussion
• cyanosis
• tachycardia
• pulsus paradoxus

Treatment (Box 19.7)

• This is obviously a true medical emergency which requires *IMMEDIATE* action – drainage of the pleural space by

---

• BOX 19.7   Tension Pneumothorax

Tension pneumothorax: This is true life-threatening medical emergency

Signs and symptoms:

• Anxiety, agitation
• Shortness of breath
• Tachypnoea
• Pulsus paradoxus or rapid, thready pulse (↓ BP)
• Distended jugular veins
• Tracheal deviation to opposite side
• Hyperinflated hemithorax with hyper-resonance to percussion and decreased or absent breath sounds
  NB: These signs can be unreliable in a trauma patient who is bleeding

Treatment:

• DO NOT AWAIT X-RAY CONFIRMATION OF DIAGNOSIS
• Insert a first large-bore i.v. cannula in anterior chest wall in midclavicular line 1–2 rib spaces above nipple
• Repeat with one or two more cannulae, then insert definitive chest drain under aseptic technique and remove i.v. cannulae
• Obtain chest X-ray

Differential diagnosis:

The principal DD of distended jugulars and pulsus paradoxus in a trauma patient is cardiac tamponade. If insertion of cannulae does not relieve symptoms very rapidly, this diagnosis must be ruled out immediately.

Any unstable trauma or ventilated patient who has had a cannula inserted for suspected tension pneumothorax must have a chest drain inserted to prevent subsequent tension pneumothorax.

---

whatever the customary regard to aseptic technique and pain management.

• In a medical setting do NOT wait for X-ray confirmation of the diagnosis!

• First, insert one or two large-bore i.v. catheters into the chest in the midclavicular line, a little above the nipple, then insert a chest drain using controlled, aseptic technique. In the field, use literally whatever is available. Items such as ballpoint pen with the cartridge removed have saved lives in this circumstance.

Chest Trauma and Haemoptysis

Penetrating Trauma

• The most common causes of penetrating trauma are:
  • stab wounds and
  • gunshot wounds: in civilian disputes, the weapons often have low muzzle velocity, and the injury is primarily the hole made by the bullet, which can be large due to tumbling. Military weapons are now designed to be smaller calibre with high muzzle velocity to cause more indirect trauma by cavitation effects. The

injuries can thus be extensive, well beyond the hole itself.

- There are two golden rules in penetrating trauma:
  1. The intracavitary trajectory of the wounding agent is unknown, even when there is an entrance and exit wound. A bullet can ricochet off the spine, for example, and a knife blade can swing through an arc before exiting.
  2. Any wound that is below the nipple line anteriorly, and the tip of the scapula posteriorly, is a thoraco-abdominal wound until proven otherwise.
- If the heart or the great vessels are injured, the wounds are usually too rapidly fatal for the patient to reach the hospital. Therefore, the vast majority of chest wounds are managed with chest drains and do not require surgery.
- The majority of chest trauma requiring surgery involves the heart and the great vessels.
- The management of injuries to the chest should follow standard ATLS guidelines – the airway, breathing, circulation, disability and exposure approach. The lesion which represents the most immediate threat to life is managed first.
- Cardiothoracic or trauma surgical intervention may be required for the management of more extensive injuries, not resolving with simple chest drainage.

Blunt trauma

- The most common injury is a simple rib fracture caused by a fall.
- Rib fractures can occur without excessive trauma and have even been seen after vigorous coughing, but the possibility of a pathological fracture due to a neoplastic or metabolic bone disease (e.g. osteoporosis) should always be considered.
- The treatment of simple rib fractures consists of adequate pain control using oral analgesics, which must be taken as long as required. This can be for weeks.
- An initial chest X-ray should be obtained to rule out complications, but rib views are not recommended.
- Motor vehicle accidents and injuries to pedestrians are among the main causes of blunt trauma to the chest. Such patients are often multiply injured, and their management follows the same ATLS guidelines alluded to above.

Flail Chest

- Flail chest is defined radiographically as three or more consecutive ribs fractured in two or more places, so that a segment of the chest wall becomes potentially unstable.
- This can also occur with bilateral rib fractures and associated sternal fractures so that the anterior chest wall is free to move independently of the rest of the chest.
- In this condition, this segment of the chest wall will move in during inspiration and out during expiration – so called paradoxical breathing.
- This is probably a relatively uncommon phenomenon, but in severe cases, may reduce the efficiency of breathing and lead to respiratory failure.
- The mainstay of treatment is with pain control and respiratory support with either non-invasive or mechanical positive pressure ventilation.
- The published literature is conflicting, although some authors advocate rib fixation to assist with ventilatory weaning and respiratory function. There may be improvement in chronic pain if ribs are fixed.

Pulmonary Contusion

- The lung is a fragile organ and violent blows can cause contusion.
- This will cause bleeding into the lung parenchyma.
- When severe, this can spill over into the airway and the clots can obstruct the airways and hence result in respiratory failure.
- There can also be an inflammatory response with development of ARDS (adult respiratory distress syndrome). Fortunately, it is usually a limited condition with spontaneous resolution. It can also be associated with a lung laceration or injury leading to a PNO or haemopneumothorax. Care is usually simply supportive.

Haemothorax

- This is the accumulation of blood in the pleural space, whatever the cause. Treatment is usually insertion of a chest drain.
- If the drain yields more than 1500 mL initially, or more than 300–400 mL/h, immediate intervention should be considered. This may be surgery or interventional radiology to embolize a bleeding vessel.
- If the blood becomes clotted, surgery (often VATS) will be necessary to evacuate the clot.
- Haemothoraces should be evacuated to prevent the occurrence of a chronic haemothorax which will require formal decortication.

Rupture of the Diaphragm

- This is usually due to sudden blunt trauma to the abdomen or costal margin, which causes a rapid increase in intra-abdominal pressure that tears the diaphragm.
- It is more common on the left side because the liver offers protection to the right hemidiaphragm.
- It is most often seen in patients with multiple severe injuries.
- The management of these patients should follow ATLS guidelines.
- The diagnosis can be quite straightforward, based on an elevation of the involved hemidiaphragm and the obvious presence of bowel contents in the chest.

- If in doubt, a nasogastric tube should be inserted, and this will be seen to enter the abdominal cavity and then back up into the thorax.
- Lesions on the right side tend to be far subtler in their presentation and can be difficult to diagnose.
- The rupture can be initially occult and only become evident over several days as the abdominal viscera slowly migrate into the chest.
- Also, in intubated patients, positive-pressure ventilation can artificially maintain the normal position of the abdominal organs, which subsequently migrate into the chest when the physiological transdiaphragmatic pressure is restored.
- It is not uncommon for the diagnosis to be delayed months or even years, especially on the right side.
- Cross sectional imaging is likely to be helpful.
- Associated injuries are common and these include: head, CNS and limb trauma. The most common directly-related injuries are intra-abdominal and include splenic and hepatic laceration, pancreatic injury and tears of the mesentery.
- Repair is usually straightforward. In acute cases, the trans-abdominal approach may be preferred except where there is a simultaneous intrathoracic lesion which requires immediate surgical care, which is very rare. This is because of the high incidence of simultaneous intra-abdominal injury requiring surgical care. In the chronic setting, the transthoracic approach is usually preferred because, at that stage, there are often intrathoracic adhesions which are difficult to deal with through a laparotomy incision.

Haemoptysis

- This is the expectoration of blood.
- Most commonly, the cause is the rupture of a dilated bronchial artery in an area of chronic inflammation or infection (such as bronchiectasis, tuberculosis, or Aspergillus involvement of an old tuberculous cavity).
- The origin can infrequently be the pulmonary circulation, for example, after penetrating trauma to the chest or rupture of a branch of the pulmonary artery by a Swan-Ganz catheter.
- Haemoptysis can be a very limited, self-resolving event or it can be a life-threatening catastrophe. In lung cancer, there is usually just a little blood on an intermittent basis.
- The treatment of the lung cancer (including palliative radiotherapy) will usually resolve the problem.
- In the other conditions, there can be sentinel bleeds which in themselves are not serious, but that can be the precursor to a fatal bleeding episode.
- Diagnosis of the source of bleeding can be very straightforward or extremely difficult. Bronchoscopy and cross-sectional imaging may identify the source of bleeding.
  - **Treatment:**
    - Haemoptysis can lead to airway obstruction and respiratory failure.

- Treatment will depend on the underlying cause and the extent of the bleeding.
- Treatment options may include:
  - radiological embolization
  - surgical resection
  - tamponading with bronchial packing
  - double lumen intubation or bronchial blockers
  - pharmacological interventions such as tranexamic acid or correction of coagulopathy

The Pleura

Pleural Effusions

- Pleural effusions are defined as excess fluid that accumulates within the pleural cavity.
- They are common with over 50 recognized causes including: tumour, infection, pulmonary, cardiac, renal, hepatic and pancreatic disease.
- Symptoms include breathlessness and pleuritic chest pain, and symptoms associated with the underlying cause (for example, fever and productive cough in parapneumonic effusion).
- Clinical signs are tachypnoea, reduced chest expansion on the affected side, reduced air entry and stony dullness to percussion.
- Diagnostic aspiration of the pleural fluid can be useful to ascertain the cause. Pleural effusions can be classified into *transudates* or *exudates* based on the protein content of the fluid:
  - *Transudates* typically have a protein content of < 25g/L. They tend to be bilateral and causes include cardiac failure, nephrotic syndrome and hepatic failure.
  - *Exudates* have a protein content of >35 g/L, tend to be unilateral and causes include pneumonia, intrathoracic malignancy and certain inflammatory disorders.
- In cases where the protein content is inconclusive (25–35 g/L), Light's criteria can be used (Box 19.8).
- Diagnosis:
  - The diagnosis of the cause of a pleural effusion can be difficult, and surgery can play an important role.
  - *Cytology* has a false-negative rate of around 15–20% even after two or three attempts.
  - *Cultures* and blind *biopsies* can be negative in up to 50% of cases of pleural tuberculosis.
  - Biochemical fluid analysis can give indications but is often not helpful. In these cases, inspection of the pleura with appropriate biopsies is essential.

• BOX 19.8 Light's Criteria

Exudative effusions will have at least one or more of the following:
- Pleural fluid protein/serum protein ratio >0.5
- Pleural fluid lactate dehydrogenase (LDH)/serum LDH >0.6
- Pleural fluid LDH >2/3 x serum LDH upper limit of normal

- Management:
  - If a pleural effusion is symptomatic, recurrent and/or persistent and there is no satisfactory treatment of the underlying cause, then symptomatic relief can be obtained by pleurodesis or placement of an indwelling pleural catheter.
  - *Pleurodesis* is the obliteration of the pleural space by mechanical (pleurectomy of pleural abrasion) or chemical means which cause the lung to adhere to the chest wall.
  - The most effective chemical agent is *talc*. Approximately 5 g of sterile talc is either insufflated into the pleural space at the time of surgery or it is instilled into the pleural space in the form of a slurry through a drain.
  - Despite this, the effusion may return and further interventions may need to be reconsidered such as repeat drainage, repeat pleurodesis, pleural catheter or pleuro-peritoneal shunt.
  - The other commonly used agents are *tetracycline* and *bleomycin*, but they have a poorer success rate.
  - The pleurodesis induces an intense inflammatory response (which is what causes the lung to adhere to the chest wall) and it is not uncommon for the patients to have a fever and elevated white cell count and CRP levels after the procedure.
  - If the cause of an effusion is not known, then the surgery required combines a diagnostic procedure (VATS pleural examination and pleural biopsy) with a therapeutic one (pleurodesis). Some patients develop a profound inflammatory response to talc, which may be poorly tolerated, especially in frail patients such as those with end-stage malignancy.

Pleural Tumours

Primary

- Malignant pleural mesothelioma is the main primary pleural malignancy.
- It is often associated with prior asbestos exposure, with a lag time of 40 years in many cases, rarely less than 15.
- As asbestos was widely used as insulation in the building industry, the shipping industry and in brake linings with a peak in imports in the 1970s, it is expected that the current epidemic will peak in 2020.
- The patients are often in the sixth decade at the time of diagnosis.
- Histologically there are three subtypes:
  1. *epithelioid* (the purely epithelioid tend to be slightly less aggressive)
  2. *mixed*
  3. *sarcomatoid*
- The typical presentation is chest pain, shortness of breath and weight loss.
- There is blood stained pleural effusion and diffuse and bulky pleural involvement.
- The disease has a relentless course leading to death in an average of 8–10 months.

- Palliative chemotherapy can improve quality of life, and radiotherapy can alleviate pain in 50% of cases.
- The role of surgery is usually to confirm the diagnosis and to perform pleurodesis at the same time, if possible.
- Aggressive surgical resection *(extrapleural pneumonectomy followed by radiotherapy)* was shown in the *MARS feasibility study (2011)*[1] to be associated with marked increased morbidity and mortality compared with standard chemotherapy and therefore is no longer advocated routinely in the UK.
- Debulking surgery (pleurectomy and decortication) may offer valid palliation in selected cases but does not appear to increase survival.
- The *MARS 2 study*[2] is currently recruiting and randomizing patients to either chemotherapy alone or chemotherapy with extended pleurectomy decortication. It is testing the hypothesis that extended pleurectomy decortication and chemotherapy is superior (30% relative improvement) to chemotherapy alone with respect to overall survival.
- If MARS 2 shows a survival difference, it is likely that radical mesothelioma surgery may become the standard of care.

Secondary

- Pleural effusions due to secondary tumour involvement are a common problem.
- In 25–50% of cases it is the first clinical manifestation of the underlying malignancy.
- Symptoms are often a dry cough, shortness of breath and a feeling of fullness within the chest, and pain.
- Physical examination shows dullness to percussion and decreased air entry.
- The tumours commonly responsible for the condition are lung, breast, lymphoma/leukaemia, adenocarcinoma of unknown origin, genitourinary and other.
- Surgery is often required for diagnosis, as discussed previously.
- Treatment can be chemotherapy for highly chemosensitive tumours involving the pleura. In most other cases, *palliative pleurodesis* is indicated provided the lung can re-expand and occupy the entire pleural space. However, if there is a rim of tumour tissue trapping the lung and preventing its re-expansion, pleurodesis will fail.
- If the effusion is only moderately symptomatic, the conservative management should ensue.
- If the effusion is causing symptoms, then insertion of an indwelling pleural catheter will allow the effusion to be drained on an 'as needed' basis in an ambulatory setting. They are designed to minimize the risk of infecting the pleural space (their design is similar to that of a peritoneal dialysis catheter).
- The other option is for the insertion of a pleural-peritoneal shunt. This allows the fluid to drain into the peritoneal cavity, where it is reabsorbed. The success rate is around 85% and there does not seem to be a problem

with peritoneal seeding of the tumour within the lifespan of the patient.

Malignant Pericardial Effusion

- Secondary seeding of tumours in the pericardium can cause a malignant pericardial effusion.
- This can be massive and associated with cardiac tamponade.
- Clinical examination may elicit *Beck's triad* of hypotension, distended jugular veins and quiet heart sounds.
- Whilst the diagnosis is clinical, echocardiogram can be useful.
- Echocardiographic features of tamponade include pericardial effusion, a four-chamber 'floating' heart, diastolic collapse of the right ventricle, increase in interventricular respiratory dependence and IVC dilatation with loss of respiratory variation.
- Management is with needle aspiration of the pericardial fluid, radiological insertion of a pericardial drain or formal surgical intervention with a pericardial window (usually via a VATS approach).

Empyema

- An empyema is the infection of the pleural space.
- The most common cause is the infection of a para-pneumonic effusion.
- About 40% of patients with a pneumonia develop an effusion that usually resolves at the same time as the lung infection.
- Occasionally, this effusion becomes infected. The typical patient is either elderly or frail because of underlying disease.
- The typical clinical presentation is that the patient develops a pneumonia, antibiotics are prescribed and after a very brief period of improvement, the patient again becomes febrile and feels unwell. Often a new course of different antibiotics is prescribed. The patient continues to be unwell, has very poor appetite, and at this point radiology demonstrates a loculated effusion.
- Empyema can be a profoundly debilitating or fatal condition if left untreated.
- The clinical presentation can be non-specific and the laboratory findings inconclusive (indeed in chronic empyemas, the white bloods cell and CRP levels can be remarkably normal), so the early diagnosis of empyema relies heavily on a strong clinical suspicion.
- Other causes of empyema are the infection of the pleural space during or following thoracic surgery or some other intrathoracic medical intervention, primary infection of the pleural such as sometimes seen with tuberculosis, trauma, secondary to the development of a bronchopleural fistula, rupture of an abscess into the pleura, or rupture or perforation of the oesophagus.
- Microbiology: tuberculosis is an unusual cause but must be considered and ruled out in every case. In 40% of cases, the offending organism is never identified.

- This is readily understandable from the usual course of the development of the disease process as described above. A variety of Gram-positive and Gram-negative organisms and various anaerobes can cause empyema. These include *Streptococcus pneumonia*, *Streptococcus pyogenes* and *Staphylococcus aureus*.
- **Treatment of the different stages of disease:**
  - There are three stages in the disease process. They have distinct clinical features, and the treatment is different in each stage.
  - In general, pleural drainage should be achieved as early in the disease course as possible, with early VATS washout and drainage if not responding rapidly.
  - The first two stages are transient in nature, lasting only a few days for each stage. It has become more and more common to see patients only when they have reached the third stage.

(1) The Exudative or Acute Phase

This first stage is characterized by a large free-flowing effusion which is clear and exudate. At this stage, the lactate dehydrogenase (LDH) level in the fluid is moderately elevated and the pH is only slightly low. Therefore, diagnosis is not clear-cut, but this is the stage where treatment is straightforward: complete evacuation of all the pleural fluid with some sort of drain and appropriate antibiotic will resolve the infection.

(2) The Fibropurulent or Transitional Stage

This second stage of the disease is when the effusion starts to become loculated. At this stage, the loculations are very soft and friable, being entirely fibrinous. Analysis of the pleural fluid shows increasing LDH and decreasing pH levels, but these findings often remain non-specific. Ultrasound is often recommended as this is the imaging modality that best demonstrates the loculations.

However, CT has the advantage of showing the distribution of fluids throughout the entire pleural space and can aid preoperative planning. There are two treatment options for this stage:

- The first is to insert a drain in the dominant collection (or two separate drains if there are two large, non-communicating pockets of fluids). Some surgeons advocate the instillation of fibrinolytic substances (urokinase or streptokinase) into the pleural space, but there is wide debate as to their efficacy.
- The second is surgery, which at this stage will be a VATS procedure. The operation aims to remove all infected fibrinous material from within the chest.

(3) The Organizing or Chronic Phase

In this third stage of an empyema, there is fibroblast deposition and neovascularization of the fibrinous septae forming the loculations, and a smaller deposit of developing scar tissue is progressively laid down on the surface of the lung. A CT scan with i.v. contrast will show a thin layer of enhancement of the visceral and parietal pleural. At this stage, LDH levels in the pleural fluid are usually quite high and the pH is commonly <7.0.

The treatment of a chronic empyema is usually surgical removal of the cortex over the visceral pleural surface (decortication). This usually allows the lung to re-expand with immediate effect. This operation also consists of the removal of all infected material from the chest cavity. These are lengthy operations that can cause significant blood loss but they are often remarkably well tolerated even by frail patients, as they remove all infected tissue and restore function. Patients unfit for decortication can undergo a more limited drainage procedure

Chylothorax

- This is the abnormal accumulation of lymphatic fluid in the pleural cavity, commonly because of leakage from lymphatic vessels.
- The most common cause is iatrogenic – direct injury of the thoracic duct during oesophagectomy or other mediastinal surgery. The most common cause of spontaneous chylothorax is blockage or damage of the thoracic duct by tumour in the mediastinum.
- The diagnosis of chylothorax is usually very straightforward if the patient is being fed orally – the drainage from the chest drain is a characteristic milky white fluid and no laboratory confirmation is required.
- If the patient is not being fed, then the fluid appears to be serous. This is because the lymph drains the fat which is absorbed by the gut, except for medium-chain triglycerides (MCTs), which are resorbed directly into the blood stream. Laboratory analysis will show abundant lymphocytes and an elevated triglyceride level (higher than plasma levels).
- Chyle contains fat, fat soluble vitamins, high levels of protein (12–60 g/L), electrolytes, immunoglobulins and T lymphocytes. Persistent chyle leak leads to immunosuppression and sepsis can ensue. Without treatment, up to 50% of patients will die as the result of a chylothorax.
- There are currently no prospective or randomized studies in the treatment of chylothorax.
  - First-line treatment is often conservative with dietary manipulation. Conservative management aims to provide adequate fluid and electrolyte replacement, optimizing nutrition with an MCT diet (to reduce chyle volume travelling through the thoracic duct) and octreotide (a somatostatin analogue). The success rate in the literature varies from 16–75%. It is unlikely to work if the drain output is >1000 mL per day or if secondary to malignancy. If successful, then standard practice is to consolidate with ongoing MCT diet for a few weeks. The mechanism of action of octreotide is unknown, though it is known to cause splanchnic vasoconstriction reducing blood flow and triglyceride absorption. There are no prospective studies of the dose, route or duration.

- If conservative management fails (defined as 5 days of 1–1.5 L pleural fluid output in adults or 100 mL/kg per year of age in children), then surgical management should be considered. Surgery will consist either in ligation of the thoracic duct at the diaphragm (95% success rate) or in pleurodesis, usually by pleurectomy.
- Radiological intervention is an alternative to surgical treatment, with percutaneous closure of the thoracic duct by embolization or needle disruption. This procedure is complex and not available in most centres. This is worth considering but of uncertain success.

Infectious Lung Conditions Requiring Surgery

There are a variety of infectious conditions of the lung which can require surgery. These are usually complex medical problems which are beyond the scope of this chapter. This section will outline the guiding features of these conditions and very briefly summarize some of the conditions.

- **Destroyed Lung**
  - Whatever the aetiology, the lung can be destroyed by infection in part or in whole.
  - The lung can then be the source of recurrent infection with resistant organisms which put the healthy remaining lung at risk from 'spill over' contamination and infection.
  - These areas of destroyed lung can also be the source of recurrent haemoptysis.
  - Pneumonectomy for sepsis or for destroyed lung is one of the most technically challenging and dangerous operations in thoracic surgery.
- **Tuberculosis**
  - Tuberculosis is far from being eradicated; it is again increasing throughout the world and particularly in developed nations such as the UK.
  - There is a growing problem with multiresistant organisms. This increase is due to population migrations, travel and the extent of the problem in developing countries. It is also due to a large indigenous population of people below the poverty line, often drug abusers and homeless people.
  - Mycobacterium is a very slow-growing organism, and improper or inadequate treatment leads to the emergence of resistant organisms.
  - Treatment requires months of multiple-agent administration.
  - The infection is most common in precisely the populations which tend to have the poorest medical treatment and compliance with therapy.
  - Finally, tuberculosis is a very infectious disease, but most healthy people with an adequate immune system will not develop active disease.
  - The indications for surgery for tuberculosis are a localized, resectable area of active infection with a resistant organism that will not be eradicated with medical therapy or the resection of an area of past infection which has become complicated and a source of other problems such as super-infection by *Aspergillus*,

troublesome bronchiectasis or haemoptysis. When there is infection with lung destruction that merits resection, the patient should be treated medically until the sputum is completely smear negative.

- *Aspergillus*
  - There are principally two aspects of *Aspergillus* disease:
  1. The first is superinfection of a pre-existing cavity (whatever the origin). The fungus grows inside the cavity, forming a fungus ball. There is no invasive infection of the surrounding lung tissue. The principal complication of this condition is haemoptysis.
  2. Invasive aspergillosis occurs in immunocompromised patients such as those undergoing aggressive chemotherapy. Surgery is indicated for aspergilloma when there are complications or in otherwise fit patients to prevent them. Surgery for invasive aspergillosis is a more complex issue, but essentially if the disease is technically resectable and resistant to therapy, then surgery should be considered.
- **Bronchiectasis**
  - This is the abnormal and permanent dilatation of the airways.
  - It can be *cylindrical, varicose* or *saccular* (cystic).
  - The common causes are infectious – previous tuberculosis tends to involve the upper lobes, prior bacterial or viral infection in the lower lobes.
  - Other causes are ciliary dysfunction, immunoglobulin deficient states, cystic fibrosis and toxic damage to the lungs.
  - The principal consequences are chronic inflammation of the surrounding lung and the development of hypertrophied bronchial arteries (with the attendant risk of haemoptysis), increased sputum production, superinfection of the sputum by a variety of bacteria including *Pseudomonas* and airway hyperreactivity.
  - The mainstay of treatment of bronchiectasis is medical with optimal chest physiotherapy and broad-spectrum antibiotic treatment of exacerbations.
  - Surgery is reserved for the resection of localized disease when medical therapy has failed or for the management of serious complications such as haemoptysis. When the disease involves both lungs, the indications for surgery should be very restrictive.
- **Lung abscesses**
  - These are caused by infections with a bacterium which causes destruction of the underlying lung, such as *Staphylococcus aureus*, or a variety of other Gram-positive or Gram-negative organisms. This may be on a background of viral infections such as influenza.
  - The treatment of most lung abscesses is medical with antibiotics for a prolonged period (often 1–2 weeks i.v. followed by 4–8 weeks of oral therapy).
  - If larger than a few centimetres in diameter, percutaneous drainage will aid resolution.
  - The indications for surgery are:
    - the lack of response to adequate therapy after 2 weeks
    - rupture into the airway with contamination of the contralateral lung
    - rupture into the pleura causing empyema and massive haemoptysis
- The results of treatment are excellent, but this can still be a fatal condition, especially when it occurs in a debilitated host, as is often the case.
- Surgery should often be delayed, beyond the acute phase of the disease where possible.

The Mediastinum

Anatomy

Macroscopic

The mediastinum is the part of the chest between the two pleural cavities. It is commonly divided into the superior and inferior mediastinum by the transthoracic plane, an imaginary line running from the manubriosternal joint anteriorly, to the 4th thoracic intervertebral disc posteriorly (Fig. 19.8). The inferior mediastinum is further divided into the anterior, middle and posterior mediastinum. The anterior mediastinum is in front of the pericardial sac. It contains the thymus and lymph nodes. The middle mediastinum is the pericardial sac and its contents: the heart and great vessels. The posterior mediastinum is all that lies behind the pericardial sac, containing the oesophagus, posterior intercostal arteries, azygous venous system, thoracic duct and sympathetic nerve.

Pathology

- Masses arising in the mediastinum are principally tumours, cysts and vascular lesions such as aneurysms.
- The most common tumours arising in the *anterior mediastinum* are encompassed by the mnemonic four Ts:
  - Thymoma
  - Thyroid (intrathoracic goitre)
  - T-cells (lymphoma)
  - Teratoma (all the primary mediastinal germ cell tumours)

A variety of rare other tumours can arise in the anterior mediastinum, such as thymic carcinoids, thymolipomas and thymoliposarcomas.

- Ectopic parathyroid glands can be found in the thymus or within the middle mediastinum amongst the great vessels.
- In the posterior mediastinum, tumours of the oesophagus, lymphomas and neurogenic tumours are the most common neoplastic lesions.

Signs and Symptoms

- These lesions are often asymptomatic but may cause symptoms due to compression of adjacent structures.
- Thus, stridor can be heard with tracheal compression.
- Obstruction of the superior vena cava causes swelling and headaches (which worsen in the recumbent position).
- Cough and pain or discomfort often occur too.

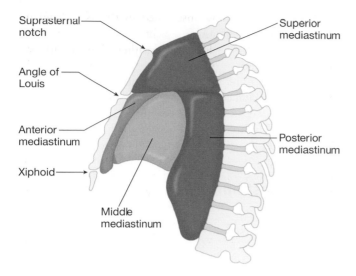

• **Fig. 19.8** The mediastinum is the part between the two pleural cavities and is divided into the superior and inferior mediastinum. The inferior mediastinum is further divided into the anterior, middle and posterior mediastinum.

Tumours

Thymomas

- Thymomas are tumours of the thymus.
- They can be well capsulated, indolent lesions or more-aggressive, invasive and/or metastatic lesions.
- Approximately 30% of patients with thymoma or thymic carcinoma have no symptoms when it is diagnosed – usually as an incidental finding of mediastinal widening on plain chest radiograph.
- Symptoms when present can include chronic cough, chest pain, muscle weakness and fatigue, shortness of breath, dyspnoea, dysphagia, anaemia and recurrent infections
- The classification of thymic cancers has been a subject of debate with many different systems suggested. To help bring some order to this issue, the World Health Organization has created a classification system for thymomas and thymic carcinoma, currently in its fourth edition as of 2015 (Table 19.3).
- One of the conceptual changes from these guidelines to previous is that all thymoma subtypes can behave in an aggressive fashion, and therefore should no longer be referred to as benign. Accordingly, their ICD-O codes now label them as malignant.
- *Thymomas* can be associated with a paraneoplastic syndrome: *myasthenia gravis (MG)* in 30–50% of cases.
  - Treatment is surgical resection for the well localized lesions.
  - Multimodality therapy including combinations of surgery, chemotherapy and radiotherapy is indicated for the invasive and/or metastatic lesions.
  - Thymomas tend to have a prolonged course even when invasive and/or metastatic.
- Thymic carcinoma is an aggressive lesion with a poor prognosis despite equally aggressive treatment.

TABLE 19.3	World Health Organization Diagnosis Criteria of Thymomas, 2015.
A	Medullary thymoma
AB	Mixed thymoma
B1	Predominantly cortical thymoma
B2	Cortical thymoma
B3	Well-differentiated thymic carcinoma
C	Thymic carcinoma

TABLE 19.4	Staging of Thymomas is Most Commonly by the Masaoka-Koga Classification.	
Stage	**Definition**	
I	Macroscopically and microscopically completely encapsulated	
IIA	Microscopic transcapsular invasion	
IIB	Macroscopic invasion into surrounding fatty tissue or grossly adherent to but not through mediastinal pleura or pericardium	
III	Macroscopic invasion into neighbouring organs (i.e. pericardium, great vessels or lung)	
IVA	Pleural or pericardial dissemination	
IVB	Lymphogenous or hematogenous metastasis	

- Increasingly thymectomy is being performed thoracoscopically or robotically rather than through a median sternotomy.
- Larger tumours or cases with invasion of surrounding structures such as pericardium are likely to require an open approach (Table 19.4)
- MG is an autoimmune disease of neuromuscular transmission.
  - Commonly it is due to the production of auto-antibodies directed against the post-synaptic acetylcholine receptor.
  - 15% of cases are associated with thymoma.
  - The principal symptom is weakness.
  - Ocular MG affects the eyelids and extrinsic muscles of the eyes.
  - Generalized MG affects all muscle groups. Bulbar MG affects the muscles of swallowing and breathing.
  - Medical treatment includes pyridostigmine (an acetylcholine esterase inhibitor), prednisolone and plasmapheresis.
  - Thymectomy is often beneficial – the earlier in the course of the disease it is performed, the better the results.
  - It can take several years for the full benefit of surgery to be reached. The results do not really depend on pathology of the thymus (normal or hypertrophied).

There is much debate on the best surgical approach and whether a simple thymectomy or an extended, radical thymectomy should be performed, and yet there is no compelling evidence of the superiority of any approach that allows complete resection of the entire thymus.

- Approximately 40% of patients will have complete remission of their MG following surgery; a further 30–40% will be improved, whereas the rest will be unchanged or worse after surgery.
- When there is a thymoma, the complete resection of the tumour principally determines the results.

Germ Cell Tumours

- Primary malignant and benign germ cell tumours can arise primarily in the thymus.
- The pathology of these lesions is identical to that of their gonadal counterparts.
- Around 15% do not have elevated tumour markers.
- With seminomas:
  - There are elevated *beta-HCG levels*, but *not* elevated alpha-fetoprotein (AFP).
  - *Elevated AFP levels* indicate mixed histology of *non-seminomatous germ cell* histology.
  - Treatment of *seminomas* is by radiotherapy, chemotherapy or both depending on the extent of the disease at the time of diagnosis.
  - Surgery is indicated in exceptional cases.
- *Non-seminomatous germ cell tumours* are treated with chemotherapy until normalization of the tumour markers.
  - If at this point there is a residual mass greater than 3 cm in diameter, this should be resected.
- The prognosis of mediastinal germ cell tumours tends to be worse than that of their gonadal counterparts, mainly because they tend to be more extensive at the time of diagnosis.

Benign Cystic Lesions

- These are predominantly bronchogenic cyst and digestive duplication cysts.
- They can arise anywhere in the middle mediastinum.
- The enteric cysts can communicate with the abdominal viscera.
- The distinction can at times be impossible to make.
- If they are symptomatic, resection is indicated.
- In young, healthy individuals, surgery is usually indicated to prevent infection, which is the principal complication of these lesions apart from compression of adjacent structure.

Surgery for Emphysema – Lung-Volume–Reduction Surgery (LVRS)

Following the results of the multi-centre trial in America (NETT study),[3] and a randomized trial in London,[4] interest in LVRS temporarily saw a resurgence in the early 2000s.

The NETT study was published in the New England Medical journal in 2003 and included 1218 patient with severe emphysema randomized to either LVRS or to best medical care. Results showed mortality rates of 0.11 deaths per person-year in both treatment groups, but improvement in exercise capacity at 24 months in 15% of the LVRS group and only 3% of the medical therapy group.

As of 2005, LVRS has been endorsed by NICE as well as the British Thoracic Society. There is now increasing interest in both surgical and bronchoscopic LVRS within the UK and the wider international community, as experienced centres report lower morality rates (typically 1–2%), and, in selected patients, the large potential improvement in lung function tests and exercise capacity as well as patient satisfaction. A multicentre randomized control trial is currently being carried out in the UK to compare surgical and bronchoscopic lung volume reduction *(CELEB trial)*.[5]

The mechanisms of action of both surgical and bronchoscopic LVRS are complex and multifactorial, but are thought to have much of their action by removing or collapsing over distended, gas-trapped, non-functional portions of the lung(s), which are taking up a large portion of the intra-thoracic volume and thereby reducing chest wall and diaphragmatic movement and function.

Patients are usually considered suitable candidates when they have marked bullous emphysema, especially if it is heterogenous and particularly when affecting the upper lobe. FEV_1 and TLCO are usually below 40%, but the surgery is particularly high risk if below 20%.

Assessment of patients should be through a COPD MDT including lung function, assessment of cardiac risk and pulmonary scintigraphy. Patient's should undergo pre-operative pulmonary rehabilitation and it is imperative that they have stopped smoking.

Surgery aims to remove between 20% and 30% of the lung using endoscopic staplers via a VATS approach. Evidence now suggests that LVRS at least can not only improve patient's symptoms but also prolong life. There remains reluctance, however, to refer patients for these treatments because of the major nature of the surgical intervention for these patients and the perceived high mortality rate, and the procedure is relatively infrequently performed in the UK, with only around 100 cases per year.

Current perioperative 30-day mortality rates are around 0–2%. Other common complications of surgery include prolonged air leak and surgical emphysema, which may be severe.

Transplantation

After many previous attempts, the first truly successful single lung transplantation was done in Toronto in 1983. The first successful bilateral transplantation was done by the same team in 1986 – and the patient was one of the longest lung transplant survivors.

Lung transplantation is usually not indicated for malignancy. Single or bilateral transplantation can be done for emphysema, intrinsic fibrosing lung disease, sarcoidosis, lymphangioleiomyomatosis and pulmonary hypertension.

Lung transplantation must always be bilateral for septic lung conditions such as cystic fibrosis and bronchiectasis.

Patients must have reached end-stage disease to justify the risks of the procedure and the obligatory immunosuppressive treatment.

The overall survival is around 50% at 5 years. Death is caused by chronic rejection, infection, lymphoproliferative disease and a variety of other causes.

Standard Thoracic Incisions

These are commonly grouped into:
- Incisions giving access to one hemithorax (or one pleural space)
- Those that lend access to both hemithoraces
- Thoracoabdominal incisions

Incisions Giving Access to One Pleural Cavity

- The most commonly used thoracotomy is the **posterolateral thoracotomy.** The patient is placed in the full lateral position and the incision swings around the tip of the scapula through the latissimus dorsi muscle onto the chest wall, which is opened in the 5th interspace (i.e. between ribs 5 and 6). Serratus anterior is usually preserved. This is the universal incision because it gives adequate access to virtually all parts of the hemithorax. Various muscle-sparing variants exist. They usually are sufficient but all do somewhat limit vision and access, and have a higher risk of postoperative seroma.
- The **anterolateral thoracotomy** is performed with the patient in a dorsal decubitus position. Therefore, it is preferred in unstable trauma patients, for example. The incision is under the breast and the pectoralis major is cut or split, the serratus anterior is split and the chest is entered in the 4th interspace. Access is somewhat more limited, especially to the hilum of the left lower lobe. True axillary mini-thoracotomies are made through the axilla into the chest via the 2nd or 3rd interspace.
- **Video assisted thoracoscopic surgery (VATS)** is a minimally invasive approach to the pleural space via one to four ports or incisions. Over the past 10 years, it has become the standard of care for early stage lung cancer. In the UK, over 50% of lung resections are conducted via this approach and this figure is likely to increase in the coming years. In malignant conditions, all the instruments should be passed through ports to avoid seeding the chest wall. Contrary to laparoscopic surgery, free passage of air into the chest is desirable to maintain the lung in a deflated condition which is essential for vision. Recovery from surgery is swifter and immediate postoperative pain is less than with thoracotomy, though the incidence of chronic pain is the same with both techniques. Hospital stays are often similar with both

techniques, so the advantages are somewhat less clear-cut than in abdominal surgery, especially since the cost of disposable instruments is high. The VIOLET study[6] in the UK is currently randomizing patients to either thoracotomy or VATS approached for lung resection and should give clarity to the benefits of a minimally invasive approach.
- **Robotic surgery** is gradually increasing in popularity, particularly for resection of thymomas and lung resections.

Incisions Giving Access to Both Pleural Cavities

- The **median sternotomy** gives good access to the anterior mediastinum, the heart and great vessels and both pleural spaces. The middle and posterior mediastinum, as well as the left lower lobe, are hard to reach.
- **The bilateral anterolateral thoracotomy with transverse sternotomy** (an incision across the sternum joining the two thoracotomies) is also known as the 'clamshell' incision. It gives fair to very good access to all parts of the thorax.
  - **Thoracoabdominal incisions:** There are a variety of thoracoabdominal incisions. The simplest is the *median sternotomy – median laparotomy.* Many other combinations joining thoracotomies with laparotomies exist.

Postoperative Care
Physiotherapy

Thoracotomy, and indeed most thoracic surgical procedures, are associated with a temporary deterioration in respiratory mechanics (partly pain related); often there is a loss of lung parenchyma. Respiratory complications are, therefore, common, outlining the need for early mobilization and respiratory physiotherapy.

Early mobilization helps overcome the dysfunction of the diaphragm, promotes lung expansion and sputum expectoration, improves ventilation-perfusion matching, is beneficial to reduce the risk of DVT and PE and promotes general well-being. Mobilization also mandates hyperpnoea, chiefly through an increase in tidal volume.

Techniques which promote deep breathing and slow, steady expiration (sometimes against moderate resistance) help mobilize secretions to a more central position where they can be removed by coughing. When the patient requires extra assistance, CPAP (continuous positive airway pressure) devices can help prevent or relieve atelectasis. If the patient is having difficulty clearing copious secretions, a mini-tracheostomy device can be inserted under local anaesthetic to aspirate them.

Enhanced Recovery Programs

Enhanced Recovery (ER) is a combination of interventions that lessen the impact of surgery on patient's recovery, helping to prevent postoperative complications and allow early discharge. Not only is this associated with improved clinical outcomes and patient satisfaction, it also helps to reduce costs associated with hospitalization.

Preoperatively the main aim is to ensure the patients are in the best possible physical condition prior to surgery. Patients are therefore encouraged to play an active role in their care and recovery with physical optimization using prescribed exercise regimes and pulmonary rehabilitation. Comorbidities such as COPD, diabetes, anaemia and malnutrition should be optimized where possible and preoperative medications should be rationalized by a pharmacist.

Perioperatively fasting should be limited and fluid management optimized to prevent dehydration. Antibiotic prophylaxis should be given prior to incision and DVT prophylaxis prescribed for all patients. VATS approaches are preferred, and invasive monitoring with urinary catheterization, arterial and central lines only used in high-risk patients.

Postoperatively aggressive pain management and anti-emetic prophylaxis is vital. Multimodal analgesia using a combination of oral analgesics, patient controlled analgesia and regional local anaesthetic blocks is recommended. Historically, epidurals have been heavily utilized; however, placement of paravertebral catheters under direct or thoracoscopic vision are being shown to be similarly effective, and can often be used in conjunction with multi-level intercostal nerve blocks, again placed under direct or thoracoscopic guidance. When possible, minimizing the number of surgical chest drains, and removing them as quickly as possible, may decrease postoperative pain.

Post-Pneumonectomy

After pneumonectomy, the space can be managed in several ways. As there is no lung, there should be no air leak, and gradual fluid accumulation will happen inevitably. Many surgeons will leave a single drain in situ, but leave it clamped, instructing the team to open the clamp for 1–2 minutes on an hourly basis in the early postoperative period. This allows for an early warning of bleeding and allows equilibration without excessive movement of the mediastinum. Usually this drain can be removed the following morning. Alternatively, the chest can be closed and some air aspirated from the empty pleural space, either by a syringe and needle or with a soft suction catheter in the pleural space which can be removed on the operating table after the anaesthetist performs a ventilatory Valsalva manoeuvre. This allows for gentle deviation of the mediastinum to the operative side. Daily chest X-rays should be obtained, and the air-fluid level in the post-pneumonectomy space would typically be seen to rise every day. A drop in this level, or sudden development of a cough with expectoration of watery red/brown fluid can be the sign of a breakdown of the bronchial stump with the development of a bronchopleural fistula. This is a medical emergency and the patient should be immediately positioned in a lateral position with the operative side down. A chest drain should be inserted to evacuate the pleural space and thus prevent contamination of the remaining lung with pleural contents. Early repair of the bronchopleural fistula is required. This bronchopleural fistula is more common after right pneumonectomy, previous radiotherapy or when the bronchial stump is not covered with muscle or other vascularized tissue.

References

1. Treasure T, Lang-Lazdunski L, Waller D, et al. Extra-pleural pneumonectomy versus no extra-pleural pneumonectomy for patients with malignant pleural mesothelioma: clinical outcomes of the Mesothelioma and Radical Surgery (MARS) randomised feasibility study. *Lancet Oncol.* 2011;12(8):763–772.

2. Warnock C, Lord K, Taylor B, et al. Patient experiences of participation in a radical thoracic surgical trial: findings from the Mesothelioma and Radical Surgery Trial 2 (MARS 2). *Trials.* 2019;20:598.

3. National Emphysema Treatment Trial Research Group. A randomized trial comparing lung-volume–reduction surgery with medical therapy for severe emphysema. *N Engl J Med.* 2003;348:2059–2073.

4. Geddes D, Goldstraw P, et al. Effect of lung-volume–reduction surgery in patients with severe emphysema. *N Engl J Med.* 2000;343:239–245.

5. Buttery S, Kemp SV, Shah PL, et al. CELEB trial: comparative effectiveness of lung volume reduction surgery for emphysema and bronchoscopic lung volume reduction with valve placement: a protocol for a randomised controlled trial. *BMJ Open.* 2018;8:e021368. https://doi.org/10.1136/bmjopen-2017-021368.

6. Lim E, Batchelor T, Shackcloth M, on behalf of The VIOLET Trialists, et al. Study protocol for VIdeo assisted thoracoscopic lobectomy versus conventional Open LobEcTomy for lung cancer, a UK multicentre randomised controlled trial with an internal pilot (the VIOLET study). *BMJ Open.* 2019;9:e029507. https://doi.org/10.1136/bmjopen-2019-029507.

20

Common Upper Gastrointestinal Surgical Conditions and their Management

CHAPTER OUTLINE

Oesophagus

Anatomy and Physiology

The oesophagus is a muscular tube that connects the pharynx to the stomach and measures 18 to 26 cm in length in an adult human. The oesophagus is predominantly lined by squamous epithelium and is guarded at both ends by sphincters. It lies anterior to the cervical vertebrae in the neck and in the posterior mediastinum in the chest and enters the abdomen through the oesophageal hiatus in the diaphragm that is located at T10 (Fig. 20.1). The last 2–3 cm of the oesophagus lie within the abdominal cavity above the gastro-oesophageal junction. The musculature of the upper two-thirds of the oesophagus is striated, which affords voluntary control, and that of the distal third consists of smooth muscle. In contrast to most of the intraperitoneal gastrointestinal tract, the oesophagus is devoid of a serosal layer – a matter of some importance to the spread of malignant disease. The oesophagus is generally divided into upper, middle and lower thirds.

The inferior thyroid artery supplies the cervical oesophagus, bronchial arteries from the descending aorta and direct aortic branches supply the thoracic oesophagus and finally the abdominal oesophagus is supplied by the ascending branches of the left gastric artery, the inferior phrenic artery and splenic artery.

The upper oesophageal sphincter is found at the pharyngo-oesophageal junction and the lower sphincter at the oesophageal opening (hiatus) in the diaphragm. Both have intrinsic and extrinsic components. The upper intrinsic sphincter has the main function of preventing access of air to the oesophagus and working in conjunction with laryngeal closure during swallowing. It relaxes on initiation of the swallowing reflex, and the superior constrictor extrinsic component contracts to expel food or liquid into the oesophagus where a wave of peristalsis carries it downwards into the stomach. The lower intrinsic sphincter (LOS) is akin to a physiological sphincter and is made up of the circular smooth muscle of the oesophagus. Its role is to prevent gastro-oesophageal regurgitation, and it is normally closed but relaxes in response to the swallowing wave. There are three major factors controlling LOS pressure: its myogenic properties, the inhibitory and the excitatory neural influences. LOS relaxation is mediated through the vagus nerve. It occurs within 2 seconds of deglutition and lasts 8 to 10 seconds. It is followed by after-contraction in the proximal part of the sphincter. Relaxation may fail in oesophageal motility disorders and low resting sphincter pressures are often seen in gastro-oesophageal reflux disease (GORD) as described later. The intrinsic sphincter is supplemented by the striated muscle of the right crus of the diaphragm, which splits to embrace the lower end of the oesophagus, but it is probably involved only in keeping the gastro-oesophageal junction closed when intra-abdominal pressure is significantly increased as in straining. Another factor which prevents reflux from the stomach is the acute angle of insertion of the oesophagus into the stomach which brings the gastric and oesophageal walls in contact when intra-abdominal pressure rises. Anatomical disorders at the diaphragmatic hiatus reduce the efficacy of the intrinsic sphincter, as is observed with hiatus hernias.

Disorders of Oesophageal Motility

Hypermotility or Acute Diffuse Oesophageal Spasm

Aetiology

- The cause of acute diffuse oesophageal spasm is not known and the condition is rare, affecting 1 in 100 000 people.
- There may well be a physiological link between this condition and achalasia.

Clinical Features

- The defining feature is intermittent, severe chest pain associated with dysphagia.
- At presentation the condition is often confused with cardiac pathology such as angina pectoris.

Investigation and Management

- A contrast study shows exaggerated oesophageal contractions which may outline the gullet as a corkscrew (Fig. 20.2A).
- Oesophagoscopy is usually normal, but manometry and the newer technique of high-resolution oesophageal manometry demonstrate exaggerated oesophageal contractions.
- Drugs that reduce smooth muscle contraction such as nitrates and calcium channel blockers occasionally provide

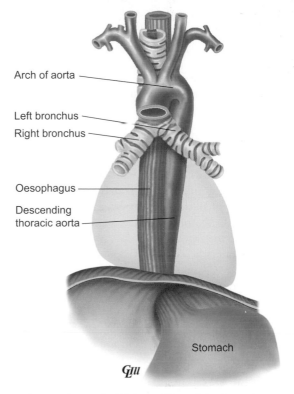

Arch of aorta

Left bronchus

Right bronchus

Oesophagus

Descending thoracic aorta

Stomach

• **Fig. 20.1** Anatomical Relationships of the Oesophagus.

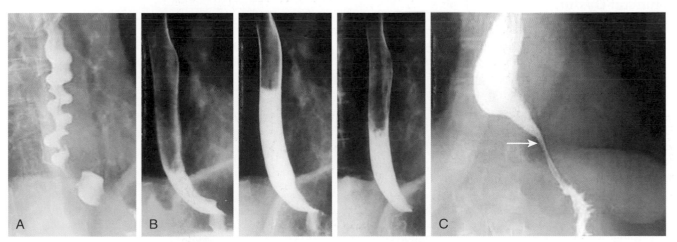

A   B   C

• **Fig. 20.2** Contrast Study Images of Oesophageal Motility Disorders. (A) Demonstrates the characteristic corkscrew appearance of the oesophagus in a patient with acute diffuse oesophageal spasm. (B) Barium contrast shows diffuse symmetrical muscular hypotonia and hypomotility with stasis of barium in the oesophagus. (C) The *arrow* demonstrates the characteristic 'rat's tail' appearance of a patient with achalasia on contrast radiography.

relief from symptoms. Balloon dilatation is also an option, but in those with severe symptoms, a long oesophageal myotomy in which all layers of muscle are divided down to mucosa are may be required for long-term symptom relief.

Nutcracker (Super-Squeeze) Oesophagus

- It is uncertain whether this condition is a distinct entity from acute diffuse oesophageal spasm.
- It is a common manometric finding in patients who present with chest pain which is of non-cardiac origin.
- The symptoms are the same as those for diffuse oesophageal spasm, as is the management.
- However, surgical treatment is rarely required.

Hypomotility
Aetiology

- The only well-recognized disorder that causes hypomotility is systemic sclerosis – a systemic condition of unknown aetiology and causes symptoms in the oesophagus, hands and skin (CREST syndrome).
- In the oesophagus, the muscle layer is replaced by fibrous tissue.
- The presence of the disease may be suspected from other features such as loss of mobility of the face and microvascular features, e.g. digital ischaemia from Raynaud's phenomenon.

Investigation and Management

- Contrast radiology shows diminished peristalsis (see Fig. 20.2B), and this can be confirmed by manometry.
- The treatment of hypomotility initially involves the treatment of associated GORD (see later).
- Smooth muscle relaxants can provide relief from pain and dysphagia.
- Second-line treatments include botulinum toxin injection and/or balloon dilatation.
- Surgery is rarely indicated.

Sphincter Dysfunction or Achalasia
Aetiology

- Achalasia is also more commonly known as cardiospasm.
- In the great majority of patients, the cause is unknown, but a similar clinical condition is found in South America as a result of infection with a protozoan organism *Trypanosoma cruzi*.
- The lower sphincter fails to relax in response to the oesophageal peristaltic wave hence food boluses are partially retained in the oesophagus.

Clinicopathological Features

- Dilatation and muscular hypertrophy occur above the lower oesophageal sphincter.
- Histological examination shows loss of ganglion cells.
- In long-standing cases, the oesophagus becomes elongated and its mucosa inflamed from stasis of food, which has been linked to increased risk of development of oesophageal cancer.

- Initially, there is not frank dysphagia but rather a slowing down of the normal rate of ingestion of food, so that at a meal the patient gets 'left behind'.
- Obvious dysphagia (Box 20.1) ultimately develops with retrosternal discomfort, regurgitation and weight loss.
- When these symptoms are reported in later life, they must be distinguished from oesophageal cancer.

Investigation

- Endoscopy is essential and, in older patients, may show a secondary cause such as infiltration of the distal oesophagus by malignant disease.
- Contrast study confirms delay at the lower sphincter and gives a characteristic 'rat's tail' appearance (see Fig. 20.2C).
- Manometry shows incomplete relaxation of the lower sphincter in response to a swallow.

Management

Medical treatment with muscle relaxants is usually unrewarding. The three effective methods for achalasia are:
- *Balloon/pneumatic dilatation*, which leads to resolution of symptoms in 80%, although it may have to be repeated and carries a small risk of oesophageal perforation.
- Longitudinal myotomy of the gastro-oesophageal junction (known to surgeons as *Heller's cardiomyotomy*) which can be done either at open operation or now, more commonly, via laparoscope or thoracoscope. Surgeons generally combine myotomy with an anti-reflux procedure because of the increased risk of GORD after the myotomy. It is reported that surgical intervention leads to symptom relief in 85% of patients.
- *Endoscopic injection of botulinum toxin* into the oesophageal wall to paralyse the lower oesophageal sphincter is effective but lasts only for a few months. Repeated injections are possible and this strategy is an effective management plan for those unsuitable for surgery.

Gastro-Oesophageal Reflux (GORD)

Features of GORD occur in association with many different oesophageal conditions, including most of the motility

---

• BOX 20.1 | History Taking in Dysphagia

- Presence of symptom when not swallowing
- Is the difficulty with solids/liquids or both?
- Exact location of symptom
- Duration and progression of symptom
- Presence of regurgitation between meals
- Presence of reflux symptoms
- Past medical history: allergic conditions (asthma, hay fever, eczema), oropharyngeal surgery/radiotherapy, stroke, connective tissue disorders
- Drug history: dopamine antagonists, anticholinergics, bisphosphonates
- Social history: smoking, alcohol

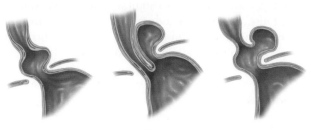

| Type 1 | Type 2 | Type 3 |

Fig. 20.3 The Anatomy of Hiatus Hernia. In type I hiatus hernia, the gastro-oesophageal junction (GOJ) moves above the diaphragm into the chest, whilst in type II, the GOJ remains in the abdomen as a separate portion of the stomach herniates into the chest. In a type III hiatus hernia, both types of hiatus hernia co-exist.

disturbances described previously. However, reflux is particularly a symptom of abnormalities at the diaphragmatic hiatus.

Pathophysiological Features

If either acid or strongly alkaline (as may occur if there are large amounts of reflux from the duodenum) secretions reach the lower oesophagus, the lower oesophageal mucosa becomes inflamed. Although in most patients this is seen at oesophagoscopy as superficial oesophagitis, two complications may result from long-term inflammation:

- Stricture – this is usually predominantly an inflammatory reaction in the mucosa and submucosa and can develop into a fibrous narrowing.
- Metaplastic change – this leads to the development of gastric-type columnar epithelium in the lower oesophagus known as *Barrett's oesophagus*, which is a premalignant lesion. It is estimated that adenocarcinoma of the lower oesophagus may develop at an estimated incidence of 0.5% per patient year with Barrett's oesophagus. Hence patients with Barrett's oesophagus must have regular surveillance of the lower oesophagus to assess for malignant transformation.

Clinical Syndromes

- There are two main causes of GORD:
  1. GORD with concomitant hiatus hernia
  2. GORD with normal anatomy
- Furthermore, there are two types of hiatus hernia:
  1. *Sliding* (type 1)
  2. *Para-oesophageal* (type 2) (Fig. 20.3)
     Occasionally, these two sub-types can both be present and are therefore referred to as *mixed* or type 3. Although only type 1 hiatal hernias are associated with GORD, both will be considered here.

GORD with Concomitant Hiatus Hernia
Sliding Hernia
Aetiology

- The proximal stomach ascends into the chest through a lax or enlarged diaphragmatic opening, taking a circumferential cuff of peritoneum with it (see Fig. 20.3).

- The normally acute gastro-oesophageal angle is reduced, so that reflux is common even though the intrinsic lower sphincter is normal.
- Risk factors for the development of hiatus hernias are:
  - obesity
  - increase in abdominal contents (pregnancy)
  - ageing
  - male gender

Clinical Features

- Generally, patients report reflux, heartburn and occasionally some lower-left chest pain shortly after eating.
- It is important, particularly with chest pain, to ensure the pain is not of cardiac origin.
- Vague indigestion is rarely caused by a sliding hernia and must be explored clinically and by investigation for an underlying cause.

Investigation

- Patients with the recent onset of symptoms, particularly if they are elderly, should be investigated for possible oesophagogastric cancer.
- Barium contrast studies can be used to establish the diagnosis of hiatus hernia but most patients are now investigated by endoscopy.
- Although it is not always easy to identify the oesophagogastric junction, this examination allows assessment of the severity of oesophagitis, and a tissue diagnosis by examination of a biopsy if relevant.
- pH monitoring and impedance studies are useful in cases of diagnostic uncertainty and as a baseline measurement before surgical treatment.

Management

The vast majority of patients can be managed by addressing risk factors and medical measures for the control of reflux, including:

- Weight loss in the obese and sleeping with the head of the bed raised to avoid nocturnal reflux.
- Alginate-containing antacids are thought to reduce free liquid in the stomach and thus reduce the volume of reflux.
- H_2-receptor antagonists (e.g. cimetidine or ranitidine) or proton pump inhibitors (e.g. omeprazole or lansoprazole). If these measures fail to control symptoms or the patient is not keen on long-term medication, then operative intervention should be considered.
- Before surgical intervention it must be absolutely clear that the symptoms of which the patient complains are the consequence of GORD, otherwise there will be minimal impact on the patients symptoms. A surgical repair is now almost always carried out at laparoscopy and is known as a *Nissen's fundoplication* (Fig. 20.4). This involves reduction of the herniated stomach below the diaphragm, removal of the circumferential peritoneal sac, re-establishment of the gastro-oesophageal angle, reduction of the intercrural

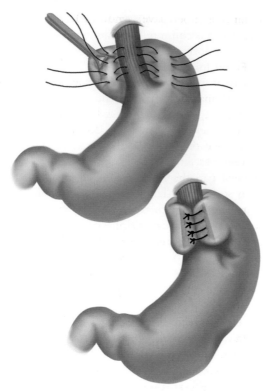

- **Fig. 20.4** A Fundoplication Operation. The gastric fundus is wrapped around the abdominal oesophagus.

space by suturing the crura together behind the oesophagus and an anti-reflux procedure (fundoplication). The fundus of the stomach is wrapped around the terminal oesophagus so that, as intra-abdominal pressure rises, the oesophagus is compressed.
- One complication of such a procedure may occasionally be the inability to belch and, in consequence, bloating – a sensation of unrelieved fullness of the stomach. In addition, some patients experience postoperative dysphagia, which is usually transient. However, the outcome is usually good, and surgery should not be withheld provided the surgeon is satisfied with the relationship between the symptoms and the hernia – particularly given evidence from oesophageal pH monitoring. The reported success rate with Nissen's fundoplication is 80–90% in patients with GORD.

Para-Oesophageal Hernia

Aetiology
- A discrete peritoneal sac occurs at the left lateral border of the oesophagus, and the fundus of the stomach rolls into this (type 2), sometimes carrying the gastro-oesophageal junction into the chest (type 3).
- More complicated examples may cause a twist of the whole stomach – a gastric volvulus, which is a surgical emergency.

Clinical Features
- These patients are usually asymptomatic, although vague upper abdominal pain may occur.

- Incarceration going on to strangulation is not common but causes acute upper abdominal pain and what appears to be vomiting but is in fact total dysphagia. This occurrence – usually in elderly frail individuals – is a surgical emergency.

Management
- Unless the patient is unfit, para-oesophageal hernias should be repaired surgically because of the risk of strangulation.
- Usually, this is done via a laparoscopic approach.

Gord with Normal Anatomy
Aetiology and clinical features
- Many patients have symptoms of GORD without any demonstrable anatomical abnormality at endoscopy or manometry.
- In some, obesity is a factor.
- Others may have hyperchlorhydria with or without a demonstrable peptic ulcer.
- In the majority, a definite cause is not identified.
- Features of heartburn and dyspepsia are universal, with regurgitation of gastric contents in some.

Investigation
- Many patients are probably treated symptomatically in general practice without investigation.
- However, those with troublesome features should have a barium swallow and/or endoscopy.
- Ambulatory monitoring of lower oesophageal pH may establish that there is persistent reflux, and oesophageal manometry identifies those with a motility disorder.

Management
- Medical management as described above is often sufficient.
- For those with oesophagitis, which is unresponsive to treatment (rare) and for patients who are not keen on long-term acid suppression therapy, an anti-reflux operation, such as Nissen's fundoplication (see Fig. 20.4), should be considered.

Oesophageal Diverticula
There are several types of oesophageal diverticula described:
- Upper oesophagus – *Zenker (pharyngeal) diverticula* are posterior outpouchings of mucosa and submucosa through the cricopharyngeal muscle that probably arise because of uncoordinated propulsion and relaxation in the pharynx.
- Mid-oesophagus – diverticula are caused by traction from mediastinal inflammatory lesions or, secondarily, by oesophageal motility disorders.
- Lower oesophagus – epiphrenic diverticula occur just above the diaphragm and usually accompany a motility disorder.

Symptoms and Signs

- A Zenker diverticulum fills with food that might be regurgitated when the patient bends or lies down. Rarely, the pouch becomes large, causing dysphagia and sometimes a palpable neck mass.
- Traction and epiphrenic diverticula are rarely symptomatic, although their underlying cause may be.

Diagnosis

- All diverticula are diagnosed by barium contrast radiography and often confirmed on upper endoscopy.

Treatment

- Specific treatment is usually not required, although surgery is occasionally necessary for large or symptomatic diverticula.
- Diverticula associated with motility disorders require treatment of the primary disorder as described previously.

Oesophageal Rupture and Mucosal Tear (Mallory–Weiss Syndrome)

Aetiology

- Vomiting is usually a coordinated event:
  - the stomach and diaphragm contract so that intragastric pressure is raised;
  - the oesophageal sphincters then relax, as does the oesophagus as a whole, and the stomach content is ejected.
- However, this orderly course may not take place if vomiting is artificially induced, or the individual is confused – usually from excessive consumption of alcohol. In such circumstances, intragastric pressure forces stomach contents into the distal oesophagus, dilating it. The oesophagus may rupture (see next section) with emptying of stomach contents into the left pleural cavity. Because the relatively elastic muscle in the oesophageal wall has a greater capacity for stretch than does the folded mucosa and submucosa, quite often only these are split to produce a longitudinal mucosal tear at the oesophagogastric junction *(Mallory–Weiss syndrome)*. These tears are usually managed conservatively once identified.

Oesophageal Rupture

Traumatic injury to the oesophagus, in response to a variety of insults is a serious event with potentially devastating consequences.

Pathophysiology

- After a perforation, negative intrathoracic pressure leads to air, food and fluids (if the stomach is full) drawn into the mediastinum and pleural cavity causing a chemical pleuromediastinitis which later causes bacterial mediastinitis, septic shock and multiorgan failure if appropriate treatment is not provided.

Aetiology

There are four categories of oesophageal rupture:
1. Iatrogenic
2. Traumatic
3. Spontaneous (Boerhaave's syndrome)
4. Tumour

Clinical Features

- The patient will have had an episode of forceful vomiting, which may be recalled.
- Vomiting may also have been induced either in a glutton or in someone who is mentally disturbed with a history of excessive eating but with the paradoxical desire not to gain weight (bulimia).
- There will be sharp left-sided pleuritic pain. This is known as Boerhaave's syndrome and named after Herman Boerhaave, the 18th century physician who first described spontaneous oesophageal rupture.
- Machler's triad: vomiting or retching (90–100%), chest pain (90%) and subcutaneous emphysema (38%) on examination. Classic triad is unusual as patients may also present with other respiratory or epigastric symptoms.

Physical Findings

- The effect of gastric content within the chest is to rapidly produce signs of severe sepsis with fever and circulatory disturbance.
- A left pleural effusion is present as usually the left posterolateral wall of the lower third of the oesophagus is perforated.
- The course is downhill with all the features of systemic inflammatory response syndrome.
- Occasionally, however, the rupture is localized and the patient is less ill with localized pleural signs and features of sepsis, which are less severe.

Management

- Detailed history of the presenting episode and past medical history to ascertain fitness for a major surgery should be taken.
- The key aspects of management are early resuscitation, early drainage, antibiotics, aggressive organ support and response to secondary sepsis.
- Parenteral or enteral (jejunostomy) nutrition is used until healing is assured, although patient mortality from oesophageal rupture remains high.
- Non-operative management is feasible in patients with small leaks when the mediastinal and pleural contamination is at a minimum. These patients need careful monitoring with nutritional support in a high-dependency setting.
- Surgical management:
  - Influencing factors include time since presentation, degree of mediastinal and pleural soiling and the general condition of the patient.
  - Primary repair: simple closure of the perforation with drainage may be successful if there is minimal contamination and patient is taken to theatre early (preferably within 24 hours). The risk of leak is high.
  - Repair and reinforcement: use of the intercostal muscle, pleura and omentum have been described as reinforcing the primary repair. The risk of a leak is still high.

TABLE 20.1	Differences between Squamous Cell Oesophageal Cancer (SCC) and Oesophageal Adenocarcinoma (AC).	
Characteristic	SCC	AC
• Location	Upper oesophagus	Lower oesophagus
• Risk Factors	Moderate	Moderate
• Alcohol	High	Not significant
• Nitrosamine	Not significant	High
• GORD	Not significant	High
• Barrett's oesophagus		
• Common Worldwide Sites	Far East	Western World

- T-tube repair: this was initially described for late presentation but it has been equally useful in unwell patients who present early. A large bore T-tube is placed in the oesophagus through the oesophageal tear – this allows a controlled fistula. Wide bore drains are placed in the mediastinum, pleural cavities and upper abdomen.
- Resection: May be used in presence of strictures but has a high morbidity in delayed reconstruction.

Cancer of the Oesophagus

Epidemiology

- There are two main types of oesophageal cancer: squamous cell carcinoma (SCC) and adenocarcinoma (AC) (usually as a result of Barrett's oesophagus).
- SCC are commoner in the Far East, especially Japan and north east China, a valley in South Africa and north east Iran.
- In the West, the adenocarcinomas are more common.
- In the UK, the oesophageal adenocarcinoma is considered a cancer of unmet need. The incidence of AC is rising in the West.
- The incidence in Europe overall is between 2 and 8 cases per 100 000 population.
- In the UK, there were around 9000 new oesophageal cancer cases in the UK every year between 2012 and 2015
- In the Far East, the incidence is in general much higher and may be between 100 and 150/100 000. Such a level warrants screening programmes within populations at high risk.
- Table 20.1 summarizes the main differences between the two types of oesophageal cancer.

Aetiology

Squamous Carcinoma

- The wide geographical variation in incidence has been attributed to social and environmental factors (see Table 20.1).
- There appears to be a strong association between cigarette and alcohol consumption and the incidence of the disease. However, diet is probably of greatest importance. Three factors are recognized:
  - high intake of nitrosamines derived from nitrates used in food preservatives
  - low intake of both vitamin A and nicotinic acid
  - iron deficiency anaemia, a known associate of hypopharyngeal cancer but probably also a factor in cancer of the body of the oesophagus. Long-standing achalasia may lead to cancer, presumably because of stasis and mucosal irritation/inflammation. The reported incidence is highly variable but may reach 2%.

Adenocarcinoma

- Cases of adenocarcinoma of the oesophagus now exceed those of squamous carcinoma in a ratio of 2:1 in the UK, whereas 30 years ago the ratio was in the reverse direction.
- Metaplastic change in the oesophageal mucosa from squamous to columnar epithelium as a result of gastro-oesophageal reflux *(Barrett's oesophagus)* predisposes to the development of adenocarcinoma.
- Endoscopic screening of all patients with significant reflux symptoms has been recommended to identify those with Barrett's oesophagus.
- The magnitude of this risk varies, with dysplastic mucosal changes, intestinal metaplasia and length of Barrett's mucosa all being factors which increase the chance of malignant change.
- Regular endoscopic surveillance with biopsy is indicated in such patients, particularly if risk factors are present, in an effort to detect early malignant change at a stage when curative treatment in the form of surgery (oesophagectomy) is possible.

Pathological Features

- Nearly all lesions are a combination of narrowing and ulceration, although the extent of each varies.
- Oesophageal adenocarcinoma can spread via multiple routes:
  - Direct invasion through the full thickness of the oesophageal wall can occur, especially as there is no serosal lining to the oesophagus, with subsequent invasion into the trachea or bronchi, the pericardium,

chest wall and diaphragm. Invasion into these adjacent structures means that the condition is incurable and life expectation is short.

- Submucosal infiltration can occur up and down the oesophagus, often causing clinicians to underestimate the extent of the disease.
- Lymph node involvement, known as lymphadenopathy, in the mediastinum and, in distal lesions, around the stomach can occur.
- Upward spread in the mediastinum may produce a sentinel node in the supraclavicular fossa known as *Virchow's nodes.*
- Haematogenous spread is unusual in the early stages, but by the time of death, up to 90% of patients may have distant metastases in the liver, lung and brain.

Clinical Features

Symptoms

- In early disease there is generally no symptoms and some patients are diagnosed whilst on endoscopic surveillance for Barrett's oesophagus.
- The lack of well-defined symptoms as the disease is developing is one reason why so few cases of oesophageal cancer are diagnosed while the condition is still in a pathologically early stage.
- There may be a feeling of something stuck in the oesophagus but this may be discounted by the patient.
- In the later stages of the disease, progressive dysphagia is common but may not be noticed until the oesophageal diameter is reduced by two-thirds.
- As a result, associated weight loss is another common feature. As dysphagia develops there is usually an associated dramatic decline in weight. More than 10–15% of the pre illness weight may be lost over 4–6 weeks.
- Acute obstruction may occasionally be precipitated in a symptomless patient by the impaction of a large (usually inadequately chewed) food bolus.
- For those patients who have developed an adenocarcinoma in an area of columnar metaplasia, a long history of heartburn suggestive of GORD may be elicited. Pain is ominous and may indicate penetration of the tumour outside the wall of the oesophagus.
- Productive cough, particularly at night, may be produced either by aspiration of retained material into the respiratory tract or by the development of a malignant oesophagotracheal fistula.
- Hoarseness may mean involvement of the recurrent laryngeal nerve and is a feature of advanced disease.
- Features of distant metastases can be the cause of presentation of a few patients.

Signs

- Clinical examination of a patient with localized oesophageal cancer usually does not reveal any abnormalities other than evidence of recent weight loss.
- A quarter of patients have palpable lymphadenopathy, which is usually in the supraclavicular region and is an indication of metastatic disease.

- Other signs of dissemination include hepatomegaly, jaundice and ascites, all of which are consistent with liver metastasis.

Investigations

1. Endoscopy

The investigation of choice to establish diagnosis is endoscopy.

This procedure is now usually done with a flexible instrument under local anaesthesia or sedation.

Endoscopy allows direct assessment of mass lesion and biopsy and/or brush cytology for pathological confirmation of the type of cancer.

There remains a risk of perforation at the time of endoscopy but this remains low (0.5% for diagnostic procedures and 5% for operative procedures).

2. Further investigation

Once the diagnosis is confirmed, further imaging studies are required to assess the stage of the disease and to determine the suitability of the patient for operative treatment.

Endoscopic Ultrasound Scanning (EUS). It is possible to obtain images from an ultrasound probe attached to an endoscope within the oesophagus, which can accurately measure the depth of penetration of the growth into the oesophageal wall and assess involvement of mediastinal and perigastric lymph nodes. This allows local staging and assessment of the tumour.

Computed Tomography (CT). CT scan of the thorax, abdomen and pelvis may also detect distant metastases but is also helpful in determining the size of the primary and whether it is attached to surrounding structures, although EUS is superior for local staging.

PET-CT Scanning. PET scanning (FDG) is increasingly used to exclude distant metastatic disease in patients being considered for radical treatment (surgical resection or chemoradiotherapy). It may identify metastases not seen on other imaging modalities such as CT.

Staging Laparoscopy and Cytology. Staging laparoscopy is carried out in selected patients with lower oesophageal and oesophagogastric junctional tumours

Screening

- The relative rarity of the condition in Western societies makes routine screening economically inappropriate and also does not fulfil Wilson's criteria.
- However, in high-risk groups, such as those with Barrett's oesophagus, it is advisable. Furthermore, in places where the incidence is high (such as China and Japan), routine flexible oesophagoscopy and/or obtaining oesophageal specimens for cytology are increasingly being recommended to detect early asymptomatic disease, thus improving long-term patient survival.

Management

Endoscopic Treatment

For very early stage oesophageal cancers (mucosal/submucosal involvement only), endoscopic therapy by *endoscopic submucosal resection (EMR)* or *radiofrequency ablation (RFA)* may be considered, particularly in patients at high risk for operative treatment. Careful and regular endoscopic follow-up is required because of the risk of local recurrence of cancer. These techniques and *photodynamic ablative therapy (PDT)* are also used for patients with high-grade dysplastic change within a Barrett's oesophagus.

Surgical Resection

- Surgical resection of oesophageal cancer is confined to patients with 'operable' disease, which is defined as locally removable cancer and no detectable distant metastatic disease, who are considered fit enough for the major operation of oesophagectomy.
- There is good evidence now that neoadjuvant chemotherapy, sometimes combined with radiotherapy, increases the frequency of complete cancer excision by downstaging the cancer and significantly improves overall survival rates and disease-free interval. Such multimodal treatment is now standard practice apart from patients with very early stage disease (T1, N0, M0).
- Surgery is precluded in those with significant co-morbidities, confirmed tracheo-oesophageal fistula or distant metastatic disease.
- During curative oesophagectomy, two basic surgical principles of resection need to be adhered to: (1) The surgeon must ensure wide resection margins and (2) radical lymph node clearance within the chest and for distal growths at the oesophagogastric junction also in the upper abdomen.
- The three main methods of access are: open operation, hybrid (thoracotomy and laparoscopic gastric mobilization) and minimally invasive.
- The conventional method of resection is by open operation which may involve opening both the abdomen and thorax known as an *Ivor-Lewis procedure* (Fig. 20.5). This approach gives better access to lymph nodes in the abdomen and chest. However, alternative surgical procedures are also available.
- In *trans-hiatal oesophagectomy* (see Fig. 20.5), the abdomen alone is opened and the oesophagus freed in the chest by blunt dissection through the diaphragmatic hiatus. The stomach (or colon) is used for surgical reconstruction by passing it through the posterior mediastinum to the neck where it is anastomosed to the upper oesophagus through a cervical incision. This procedure is used by some surgeons for patients with Barrett's oesophagus containing high-grade dysplasia. This approach may lead to limited access for thoracic lymphadenectomy.
- Left thoracoabdominal approach: this gives access to a bulky tumour and access to the gastric conduit.
- In three-stage oesophagectomy (*McKeown* procedure), the anastomosis occurs through the neck incision and is usually for more proximal oesophageal cancers
- In *minimal access oesophagectomy (MIO)*, the whole surgical procedure can now be performed by minimal access dissection within the chest (thoracoscopy) and abdomen (laparoscopy), although there is little current evidence that this method is better than open operation.
- A recently published multicentre, randomized controlled trial, involving patients from 18 to 75 years old, assigned 103 patients to hybrid-procedure and these were compared to 104 patients assigned to the open-procedure group. Hybrid minimally invasive oesophagectomy resulted in a lower incidence of intraoperative and postoperative major complications compared to open oesophagectomy, with no difference in overall and disease-free survival over 3 years.
- A single-centre randomized controlled trial conducted in the Netherlands compared open transthoracic oesophagectomy (OTE) to robotic-assisted minimally invasive oesophagectomy (RAMIE) and found that the latter resulted in a lower percentage of overall surgery-related and cardiopulmonary complications with lower postoperative pain, better shot-term quality of life and better short-term postoperative functional recovery without compromising oncological outcomes.

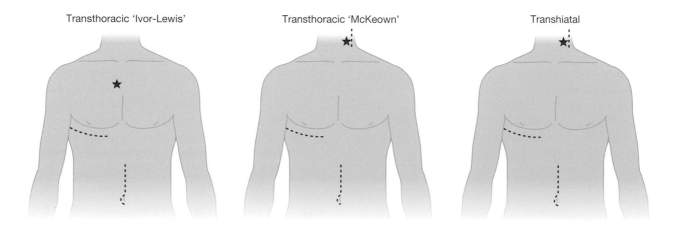

Transthoracic 'Ivor-Lewis'　　Transthoracic 'McKeown'　　Transhiatal

• **Fig. 20.5** Incisions of Open 'Ivor-Lewis', Transthoracic 'McKeown' and Transhiatal Oesophagectomies.

Other Treatments for Oesophageal Cancer

In patients unsuitable for surgical treatment, other methods can be used to treat oesophageal cancer:

Chemotherapy and/or chemoradiotherapy (e.g. with 5-fluorouracil (5-FU) and cisplatin), either alone or preferably in combination with radiotherapy, may lead to total disappearance of the local tumour in 30% of patients. Combined chemoradiotherapy (CRT) is used in some centres as primary radical treatment for squamous carcinoma of the oesophagus. Resection in these cases is reserved for local recurrent or residual cancer. In the UK, CRT is the treatment of choice for localized and proximal SCC oesophageal cancers. In the middle/lower SCC oesophageal cancers, CRT or CRT and surgery is advised.

In AC: neoadjuvant CRT improves long-term survival and in type II and III oesophagogastric junctional AC, neo- and adjuvant chemotherapy provides survival benefit.

Endoscopic insertion of self-expanding metal endoprostheses – some of which are covered with a plastic membrane through the area of tumour stricturing and may provide palliation by improving dysphagia. Covered stents can also be used to close fistulas between oesophagus and trachea.

Local endoscopic destruction of the tumour by laser or argon-beam diathermy, which can be repeated.

Prognosis

- The outcome of resection depends on the stage of the growth.
- When tumour is confined to the mucosa, a 5-year survival of 80–90% is possible, but more advanced disease means a 5-year survival of less than 5% for growths that have penetrated the full thickness of the gullet.
- Combined regimens of resection and neoadjuvant combinations of radiotherapy and/or chemotherapy are producing improved results.

Stomach

Anatomy

Macroscopic

The stomach can anatomically be divided into four principle regions: the cardia, fundus, body and pylorus as demonstrated in Fig. 20.6. The cardia is marked by the region where the oesophagus connects to the stomach and is located inferior to the diaphragm. Superior and to the left of the cardia is the fundus. Inferior to the fundus is the body of the stomach which constitutes the majority of the organ. Finally, the pylorus connects the stomach to the duodenum. Of note, the pyloric antrum provides continuity between the pylorus and body of the stomach with the distal portion of the pylorus, known as the pyloric canal, that connects to the duodenum. The smooth muscle pyloric sphincter is located at this latter point of connection and controls

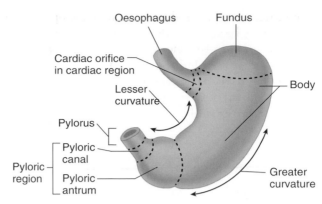

• **Fig. 20.6** Gross Anatomy of the Stomach.

stomach emptying. In the fasting state, the stomach contains large folds called *ruga*. The convex lateral surface of the stomach is called the greater curvature; the concave medial border is the lesser curvature. The stomach is held in place by the lesser omentum, which extends from the liver to the lesser curvature, and the greater omentum, which runs from the greater curvature to the posterior abdominal wall.

Microscopic

The wall of the stomach is made of the same four layers as most of the rest of the alimentary canal, but with adaptations to the mucosa and muscularis for the unique functions of this organ. In addition to circular and longitudinal smooth muscle layers, the muscularis has an inner oblique smooth muscle layer which aids mechanical digestion. The stomach mucosa's epithelial lining consists only of surface mucus cells that secrete a protective coat of alkaline mucus. There are numerous gastric pits that are the exit point of gastric glands that secretes gastric juice. Although there are differences in secretions of gastric glands depending on their location in the stomach, there are four cell types.

Parietal cells – These cells produce both hydrochloric acid (HCl) and intrinsic factor. HCl is responsible for the high acidity (pH 1.5 to 3.5) of the stomach contents and is needed to activate the protein-digesting enzyme, pepsin. Intrinsic factor is a glycoprotein necessary for the absorption of vitamin B_{12} in the small intestine.

Chief cells – These cells secrete pepsinogen, the inactive proenzyme form of pepsin.

Mucous neck cells – Secrete thin, acidic mucus that is much different from the mucus secreted by the goblet cells of the surface epithelium.

Enteroendocrine cells – These can secrete various hormones into the interstitial fluid. These include gastrin, which is released mainly by enteroendocrine G cells.

Physiology of the Stomach

The cells of the gastric glands secrete about 2500 mL of gastric juice daily. Stimulation of the parietal cells, principally by the vagus nerve, results in acid secretion. This results in the presence of the H^+/K^+ ATPase that transports the H^+ onto the luminal surface. This secretion is isotonic with other fluids and its pH is <1. The H^+ is then actively transported into the gastric lumen in exchange for K^+. Chloride ions are also actively transported into the gastric lumen. The physiological basis of stomach acid secretion has important implications for surgical pathologies affecting the stomach as discussed below.

Disorders of the Stomach and their Management

Peptic Ulcer Disease

Introduction

- For the purposes of this section, gastric and duodenal ulcers are discussed together.
- The role of surgery in the management of peptic ulcer disease is essentially limited to managing the complications that arise from this condition.
- These principally include bleeding and perforation and the approaches to each are discussed below.
- However, the surgeon does need to understand the pathophysiological mechanism causing this disease.

Epidemiology

- *Helicobacter pylori* infection was first identified as the causative factor for peptic ulcer by Barry Marshall and Robin Warren in the late 20th century and is the leading cause for the condition.
- There is a close association between peptic ulcer disease and poor socio-economic conditions, with the condition being more common in the developing world mainly as a result from the high prevalence of *H. pylori* infection.
- Other causative factors may be tobacco and alcohol consumption, which tend to be higher amongst the poor and deprived.
- In duodenal ulcer, males outnumber females by a factor of four, but gastric ulcer is equally distributed and its incidence increases with age.

Aetiology

1. The discovery of *H. pylori* as a strong associate of peptic ulceration in both the stomach and duodenum, and the additional observation that its eradication can lead to cure, has made it clear that infection with this bacterium is the cause of peptic ulceration in the majority of cases.
   - *H. pylori* is able to secrete urease creating an alkaline environment that promotes its survival. Furthermore, specific receptors (e.g. OipA) expressed by the bacteria allow it to localize to the gastric epithelium. The bacteria causes stomach mucosal inflammation, which is associated with hyperchlorhydria (increased stomach acid secretion). Inflammatory cytokines inhibit the parietal cell acid secretion. In addition, increased acid production at the pyloric antrum is associated with duodenal ulcers in 10 to 15% of the *H. pylori*

infection cases. In this case, somatostatin production is reduced and gastrin production is increased, leading to increased histamine secretion from the enterochromaffin cells, thus increasing acid production. Acidic environment at the antrum causes metaplasia of the duodenal cells, causing duodenal ulcers.
   - Moreover, there must be an idiosyncratic component to the *H. pylori*–ulcer diathesis because many people have *H. pylori* present without suffering a peptic ulcer.
2. A relationship is also apparent between acute peptic ulceration and the consumption of non-steroidal anti-inflammatory agents (NSAIDs).
   - Patients, particularly the elderly, are increasingly being prescribed these drugs, and there is therefore a rising incidence of acute ulceration with complications such as perforation and haemorrhage.
   - It is not clear whether the relationship implies a cause of peptic ulceration, but it seems more likely that NSAIDs upset the balance between mucosal regeneration and repair and therefore present a hazard for anyone who also has a peptic ulcer.
3. Other antecedents of peptic ulcer which can have a bearing on management include diet, cytomegalovirus, Crohn's disease, vasculitis and gastrinomas (e.g. Zollinger–Ellison syndrome).

Anatomical and Pathological Features

- Peptic ulcers tend to demonstrate mucosal loss accompanied by chronic inflammation with varying amounts of fibrosis.
- An ulcer penetrates to a varying depth in the gastric or duodenal wall but involvement of neighbouring organs such as the pancreas is a rare finding.
- Free perforation into the peritoneal cavity takes place when the rate of ulceration exceeds that of repair.
- In the absence of perforation, persistent inflammation promoting fibrinoid necrosis of submucosal arteries is likely to explain continued low-grade bleeding.
- Gastric ulcers can occur anywhere but are most commonly found on the lesser curvature at the junction of antral and acid-secreting mucosa.
- The long-held clinical adage that duodenal ulcers are benign and gastric ulcers malignant in a third of cases needs to be at the forefront of a surgeon's mind when dealing with this patient cohort. Whilst the immediate attention may be controlling bleeding or lavage of peritoneal contamination, the surgeon must not forget to biopsy these ulcers, in particular gastric ulcers, due to attendant risk of malignancy.

Clinical Features

Symptoms

- Both gastric and duodenal ulcers cause epigastric pain that is generally inseparable from each other, although it is often stated that patients with gastric ulcer have pain on eating and those with duodenal ulcer complain when they are hungry.

- Radiating pain to back is uncommon and should prompt the surgeon to consider other differential diagnoses such as chronic pancreatitis.
- Indigestion is often associated with the pain.
- Heartburn from acid-peptic reflux is common but needs to be differentiated from GORD as discussed previously.
- Symptomatic episodes with temporary remissions which can last weeks or months are more characteristic of duodenal than gastric ulcer.
- In both, the symptoms are relieved by antacids.
- Vomiting is a feature of gastric outflow obstruction when seen in a patient with peptic ulcer disease and suggests a chronic inflammatory process in a duodenal ulcer, although a pyloric channel gastric ulcer can also be the cause. The vomitus is usually free from bile and may contain partially digested food, recognizable as a meal taken a day or more before.
- Patients with gastric outflow obstruction often lose weight, but, unless the obstruction is complete and vomiting profuse, they do not become dehydrated in that absorption of water and electrolyte still takes place across the gastric wall.

Signs
- In uncomplicated peptic ulcer, epigastric tenderness maybe the only finding on examination.
- Rarely, gastric outlet obstruction is associated with a *succussion splash*.
- The patient displays clinical signs of dehydration (e.g. dry mucous membranes and tongue) or, more worryingly, weight loss, suggesting a more chronic process or which may be a symptom of gastro-oesophageal cancer that needs to be ruled out.

Investigations
- **Biochemical Investigations**
  - Measurement of gastric acid secretion is no longer routinely performed and only has a role in patients suspected to have Zollinger–Ellison syndrome and peptic ulcer recurrence after surgery.
  - If gastric outflow obstruction is suspected, serum concentrations of sodium, potassium and chloride and the arterial oxygen levels should be measured. These are classically associated with a hypochloremic metabolic acidosis. Attempts to correct this should be actively pursued if emergency surgery is being contemplated (e.g. haemorrhage or perforation).
  - *Helicobacter* infection – Evidence of *H. pylori* infection can be obtained by breath test following urea ingestion (containing 13 C), serum antibodies (not necessarily indicative of current infection) and faecal antigen testing.
- **Endoscopy**
  - The current initial investigation of the patient with indigestion which suggests peptic ulceration is by endoscopy, although, if this is the first episode, in young patients (<40 years) without complex features empirical treatment can be justified.

- The whole of the upper GI tract, from the oesophagus to at least the junction of the first and second parts of the duodenum is examined by direct visualization.
- All gastric ulcers are subjected to biopsy and brush cytological examination for reasons alluded to above.
- Biopsy from the antrum may be taken for urease testing – an indication of *H. pylori* infection.
- Duodenal ulcers are assessed for their depth and degree of obstruction and for any stigmata which suggest bleeding. Repeat endoscopy is essential for those with a gastric ulcer to ensure resolution and exclude a mass lesion.
- **Other Investigations**
  - Prior to the advent of flexible endoscopy, double contrast barium meal was used to confirm the diagnosis. This is now obsolete.
  - For concerning features on history, examination or in the emergency setting, cross sectional imaging in the form of contrast enhanced CT is usually performed to assess principally for malignancy or perforation.

Management
- Uncomplicated peptic ulcer is treated by:
  - Regimens to eradicate *H. pylori* if present using antibiotics such as amoxicillin and metronidazole or clarithromycin in combination with acid-reducing proton pump inhibitors (e.g. omeprazole, lansoprazole).
  - Reduction of acid secretion with H_2-receptor antagonists such as cimetidine and ranitidine; or with proton pump inhibitors, which block the hydrogen – potassium – ATP enzyme system in the gastric (parietal) cells that secrete acid.
  - After successful *H. pylori* eradication, no further treatment should be required. In patients with recurrent peptic ulcer disease in the absence of *H. pylori* infection, maintenance acid suppression therapy may be required.

The Role of Surgery
- The role of surgery in managing uncomplicated peptic ulcer disease has now been largely consigned to history. These latter procedures involved vagotomy or division of the vagus nerve. This disrupts the parasympathetic nerve supply from the stomach to the left side of the transverse colon. These surgical techniques evolved into selective vagotomy and highly selective vagotomy and could be combined with antrectomy (removal of the distal half of the stomach) to reduce the rate of recurrence. Reconstruction is performed with *gastroduodenostomy (Billroth I)* or *gastrojejunostomy (Billroth II)*, although the precise surgical nuances of these techniques are outside the scope of this chapter. The advent of pharmacological treatment and in particular, the elimination of *H. pylori*, offers patients a long-term solution without the risks of surgery.
- Complications: The role of surgery unquestionably lies in the management of complex peptic ulcer disease. Generally, the diagnosis of bleeding or perforation will

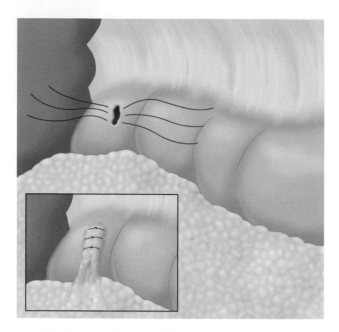

have been confirmed on endoscopy or radiology, respectively. Anatomical relationships determine that posterior duodenal wall ulcers penetrate the gastroduodenal artery that run behind the duodenal and thus bleed, whereas anterior wall duodenal ulcers penetrate the peritoneum and thus perforate into the peritoneal cavity.

a) Bleeding:
- Surgery for bleeding duodenal ulcer is generally undertaken for refractory bleeding or where satisfactory control could not be obtained at endoscopy. Following laparotomy, the anterior wall of the duodenum is opened and the base of the ulcer underrun to control bleeding from the gastroduodenal artery. Upon closure of the duodenum, it is imperative to close the duodenotomy longitudinally to avoid narrowing the duodenum.

b) Perforation:
- In the case of perforation, this surgery is now undertaken laparoscopically as long as the patient has no contraindication. The perforation is closed with a 'Graham' patch that can be formed of omentum or, rarely, falciform ligament (Fig. 20.7).

c) Gastric outflow obstruction
- As discussed above, gastric outlet obstruction suggests a more chronic process, where long-standing inflammation has caused stricturing of the duodenum.
- It is important to gain tissue samples to exclude a malignant process, which can be achieved via flexible endoscopy. Generally, a *pyloroplasty* or more commonly gastric bypass in the form of *gastroenterostomy* will alleviate the patient's symptoms. Very rarely, a partial gastrectomy may be required.

d) Gastrocolic fistula:
- In Zollinger–Ellison syndrome and, in the past, after simple gastroenterostomy, an ulcer may penetrate from stomach to colon and cause faecal contamination of the stomach and small bowel.
- The result is intractable diarrhoea. Complicated surgical revision is then required after acid secretion has been brought under control.

e) Gastroduodenal tumours:
- The majority of tumours of the stomach are adenocarcinomas and will be detailed below.
- Occasionally, gastrointestinal stromal tumours (GIST) are found in the stomach or duodenum and require surgical resection.
- Cancer arising in the duodenum is very rare and usually originates from the periampullary mucosa at the lower end of the common bile duct and necessitates pancreatic resection in the form of a *Whipple's procedure* that is discussed elsewhere in the book.

Gastric Cancer

Epidemiology

- After cancer of the colon, rectum and pancreas, carcinoma of the stomach is the most common cause of death from gastrointestinal cancer, and also the third most common cause of cancer death in men and the fourth in women.
- However, in the Western world, the incidence of this condition has diminished. Over the last decade, there has been a marked rise in the incidence of adenocarcinoma around the gastro-oesophageal junction, including the gastric cardia.
- As with oesophageal cancer, there is a worldwide variation in incidence. Gastric cancer is more common in the Far East than the West. Even in the West, racial differences occur: proximal tumours are more commonly seen in Caucasians.
- The peak age distribution is 50–70 years, but the disease can occur at any age from early adulthood; 5% of patients are less than 35 years of age.
- Gastric cancer is predominantly a male disease.

Aetiology

- The cause for gastric cancer is largely unknown. However, it is likely that factors such as prolonged *H. pylori* infection, chronic gastritis and pernicious anaemia cause gastric atrophy which causes hypochlorhydria and predisposes to gastric cancer (Box 20.2).
- Other contributory factors are similar to those seen with oesophageal cancer such as smoking and nitrate intake.
- Interestingly, previous gastric surgery, particularly in the form of partial gastrectomy, also increases the risk of gastric cancer for the reasons discussed above. In these patients, the lead time to development of cancer is up to 25 years, suggesting that these patients should have

• BOX 20.2 **Risk Factors for Developing Gastric Cancer**

- *H. pylori* infection
- Chronic gastritis
- Pernicious anaemia
- Smoking
- Nitrate intake
- Previous gastric surgery

TABLE 20.2	TMN Classification for Gastric Cancer
Stage	**Description**
Tis	In situ
T1	Limited to mucosa or submucosa
T2	Muscularis propria involved
T3	Serosal involvement
T4	Invasion outside the stomach
N0	No lymph node involvement
N1	Lymph node involved 3 cm away from tumour
N2	Regional lymph node involved
N3	Intra-abdominal distant lymph nodes involved
M0	No distant metastasis
M1	Distant metastasis

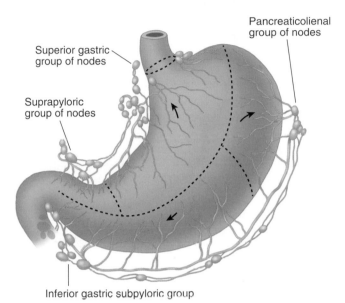

• **Fig. 20.8** The Lymphatic Drainage of the Stomach. During gastrectomy, the relevant lymph nodes must be taken along with the stomach in order to attempt to achieve a curative resection.

endoscopic surveillance of the remnant stomach. A few tumours may originate in adenomatous polyps or dysplastic mucosa.

Pathological Features

- At the time of clinical presentation, most cancers of the stomach are advanced, meaning curative surgery is not possible.
- Histologically, these tumours are *adenocarcinomas of columnar* or *cuboidal type,* although this has little relevance to treatment.
- *Adenocarcinoma* is a locally invasive tumour which directly infiltrates the full thickness of the gastric wall to involve the serosal layer and contiguous structures such as the pancreas, transverse mesocolon or left lobe of the liver.
- Peritoneal seeding *(transcoelomic spread)* may take place with either diffuse nodules and ascites or deposits on the ovaries in the female *(Krukenberg tumours)* or in the rectovesical or rectovaginal pouch *(Blumer's shelf).*
- In addition, gastric cancer is a good example of a tumour which spreads via lymphatic channels to local and regional lymph nodes and forms the surgical basis for the various forms of gastrectomy (Fig. 20.8).

- Serosal and lymphatic involvement are the most important determinants of long-term survival following surgical resection.

Staging

- Pathological staging is a very useful indicator of prognosis in patients with gastric cancer.
- A number of staging systems have been devised, the most popular of which are:
  - The Union Internationale Contre le Cancer (UICC) stage
  - The TNM system
- UICC stage I (T1, N0, M0) is often called 'early gastric cancer' and implies that the disease has not spread beyond the submucosa. At this stage, there is a high possibility of a cure. Table 20.2 illustrates the TMN staging for gastric cancer.

Clinical Features

Many patients with early stage disease have few symptoms, whilst those with late disease will usually have symptoms but be ineligible for curative treatment. As with all gastrointestinal cancer, it cannot be overemphasized that early diagnosis is the key to cure. Some early tumours are only detected by screening endoscopy. There are a series of 'red flag' symptoms that should prompt immediate investigation:

- Any feature of dyspepsia in a previously asymptomatic individual over the age of 40 should always be presumed to be caused by carcinoma of the stomach until proven otherwise.
- Dysphagia and/or early satiety – usually associated with proximal lesions.

- Significant bleeding – haematemesis and/or melaena – is not all that common, but all gastric cancers cause some oozing and this may be sufficient to produce microcytic hypochromic anaemia with the non-specific symptoms of lassitude and fatigue.
- Epigastric mass – associated with advanced disease.

Physical Findings

In patients with early stage disease there is usually no physical signs. Signs of gastric outflow obstruction discussed above may be present. The presence of metastatic spread is indicated clinically by *Virchow node* (see earlier), ascites, hepatomegaly and Bulmer's shelf.

Investigations

1. Endoscopy

In a patient suspected of having a carcinoma of the stomach, oesophagogastroscopy is the most sensitive procedure for determining the presence or absence of a gastric neoplasm. It provides information on the anatomical site and enables multiple biopsies and brush cytology to be taken. However, if the histological and cytological reports on a gastric ulcer fail to show malignant cells, this must not be taken as absolute proof that the condition is benign. A short period (6–8 weeks at the most) of appropriate treatment for peptic ulcer is given and the examination repeated. Even if there are signs of healing, this does not mean the lesion is benign, and careful examination of further biopsies from the ulcer or healed area are necessary.

2. Imaging

Double-contrast barium meal is very rarely used in the modern age. CT combined with PET scanning is very useful as it demonstrates the presence of unsuspected liver or other distant metastases and lymph node metastases. Both may also help to decide on resectability, in essence, if surgery can remove the cancer. EUS is being increasingly used to determine nodal status, depth of penetration of the primary tumour and also the extent of submucosal tumour spread. The extent of submucosal spread is particularly important for planning the extent of resection required for cancers near the pylorus and gastro-oesophageal junction.

3. Laparoscopy

This procedure has contributed considerably to identifying those cancers that are not amenable to surgical resection, i.e. irresectable. Laparoscopy is particularly adept at detecting small liver or peritoneal metastases. Laparoscopy is now usually done before a laparotomy for resection is undertaken.

Management

Surgery

- The only curative treatment for gastric cancer is surgical resection in the form of a *gastrectomy*. In the UK, only 30–40% of patients are suitable for an attempt to curative resection.
- Curative resection entails removal of the cancer with normal surrounding stomach (partial or total) and the regional lymph nodes as a single anatomical block referred to as *en-bloc*.
- The extent of resection is a subject of debate:
  - In Japan, where the best results are obtained, the stomach is removed together with the nodes within 3 cm of the tumour (N1) and the regional nodes (N2), sometimes with even more radical node resections (N3) (see Table 20.2).
  - In the West, many surgeons question the use of such radical resections because of a higher operative mortality and morbidity and because randomized controlled trials do not show a survival benefit.
- There is increasing evidence that neoadjuvant chemotherapy improves survival in patients undergoing resection for stomach cancer and standard treatment in the UK now includes pre- and postoperative chemotherapy.
- In some centres, particularly in the USA, postoperative adjuvant radiotherapy is used to reduce loco-regional recurrence.

Palliation

- Surgery may be undertaken to alleviate troublesome symptoms such as abdominal pain, dysphagia, blood loss and vomiting.
- However, because of late diagnosis and advanced disease, bypass of an obstructing lesion in the distal part of the stomach may be all that is possible.
- Laser ablation for unresectable tumours at the cardia may improve swallowing and may be performed by the use of a laser through the endoscope.
- Endoscopic insertion of a stent across the malignant stricture is increasingly used as an alternative to bypass surgery, particularly in patients with significant co-morbidities.
- A considerable proportion of patients respond to chemotherapy with carboplatin-based regimens, and this should be offered to patients with a good performance status and low co-morbidity.
- Occasionally, after chemotherapy, it is possible to resect a gastric carcinoma previously deemed unresectable on CT scanning.

Prognosis

- In the West, the majority of patients have recurrent cancer and/or metastasis within 3 years of resection but 5-year survival has been reported to be as high as 88% for early-stage disease.
- The outlook for most patients is poor and is rather worse for patients with tumours of the cardia and fundus than for those with antral lesions. Survival is very much linked to stage of cancer.

Gastrointestinal Stromal Tumours (GISTs)

Introduction

- Gastrointestinal stromal tumours (GISTs) are the most common mesenchymal neoplasms of the gastrointestinal tract.

- GISTs arise in the smooth muscle pacemaker *interstitial cell of Cajal* that are normally part of the autonomic nervous system of the intestine. They serve a pacemaker function in controlling motility.
- They are defined as tumours whose behaviour is driven by mutations in primarily the KIT gene.
- Approximately 70% of GISTs occur in the stomach and gastric GISTs have a lower malignant potential than tumours found elsewhere in the GI tract.
- All GIST tumours are now considered to have malignant potential and should be managed as such.

Epidemiology

- GISTs occur in 10–20 per one million people.
- The majority of GISTs present at ages 50–70 years
- The incidence of GIST is similar in men and women.

Pathology

- GISTs are tumours of connective tissue, i.e. sarcomas, and most GISTs are non-epithelial.
- About 70% occur in the stomach, 20% in the small intestine and less than 10% in the oesophagus.
- Small tumours are generally benign, especially when cell division rate is slow, but large tumours disseminate to the liver, omentum and peritoneal cavity.
- They rarely occur in other abdominal organs.
- Smaller tumours can usually be confined to the muscularis propria layer of the intestinal wall. Large ones grow, mainly outward, from the bowel wall until the point where they outstrip their blood supply and necrose on the inside.

Signs and Symptoms

- GISTs may present with trouble swallowing, gastrointestinal bleeding, or metastases (mainly in the liver).
- Intestinal obstruction is rare, due to the tumour's outward pattern of growth.
- Generally, patients are asymptomatic with GISTs being picked up as 'incidentalomas'.

Diagnosis

- CT scanning is often undertaken to confirm diagnosis or, conversely, is the imaging modality that initially detects the GIST.
- The definitive diagnosis is made with a biopsy, which can be obtained endoscopically, percutaneously with CT or ultrasound guidance or at the time of surgery to identify the characteristics of GISTs (spindle cells in 70–80%, epithelioid aspect in 20–30%).
- When GIST is suspected – as opposed to other causes for similar tumours – the pathologist can use immunohistochemistry (specific antibodies that stain the molecule CD117 (also known as *c-kit*)).

Management

- In localized GISTs, surgery is the primary treatment of choice.
- Lymph node metastases are rare, and routine removal of lymph nodes is typically not necessary at the time of surgery.
- Laparoscopic surgery is an excellent approach to GISTs as they tend to protrude from the organ.
- In cases of unresectable or metastatic GIST, the c-kit inhibitor *imatinib* (Glivec/Gleevec) is administered and has been shown to improve survival in these patients.

Spleen

Anatomy

The spleen lies in the left hypochondrium (Fig. 20.9A) and requires a threefold enlargement to become clinically palpable. It is predominantly supplied by the splenic artery and, if the artery is ligated during surgery, the spleen usually remains viable because of collateral blood supply via the left gastroepiploic and short gastric arteries (see Fig. 20.9B). The splenic artery usually divides before entering the substance of the spleen so that each major branch supplies a segment of the spleen. Thus the organ can be divided into transverse segments each supplied by an end artery, with relatively little blood flow between them. This anatomical knowledge is imperative in cases of splenic trauma where, depending upon the location of the injury, partial splenectomy with preservation of splenic function is possible. The spleen is drained by the splenic vein which contributes up to 40% of portal venous blood flow to the liver.

Physiology of the Spleen

The spleen consists of red pulp and white pulp. The red pulp consists of a series of sinusoids and sinuses that allow the spleen to remove aged and/or damaged red cells from the general circulation. This function of the spleen is lost after total splenectomy and abnormal erythrocytes are found in the peripheral blood including target cells and some which contain intracellular inclusions such as Howell–Jolly bodies (nuclear remnants), Heinz bodies (denatured haemoglobin) and Pappenheimer bodies (iron granules). Although the human spleen has little or no function as a red cell reservoir, it is a major storage site for iron and holds a proportion of the platelets and macrophages that are available to the circulation. The white pulp of the spleen has an important immunological function. It plays a major role in both humoral and cell-mediated immunity. Antigens are presented to dendritic cells in the germinal centres of the follicles of the white pulp to immunocompetent cells. Immunoglobulins, in particular IgM, are subsequently produced by plasma cells, resulting in hyperplastic germinal centres. The spleen is a crucial site for production of the non-specific opsonins, tuftsin and properdin which are involved in targeting

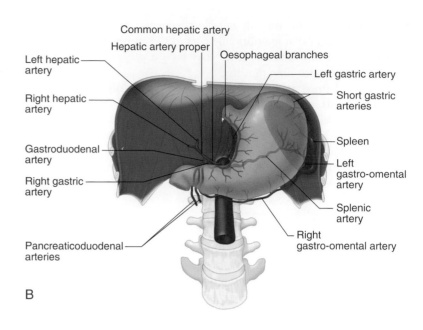

• **Fig. 20.9** (A) Position of spleen. (B) Blood supply to spleen. (Modified from Drake: *Gray's Anatomy for Students* 4e, Elsevier, 2020, Figs. 4.112 and 4.115.).

non-self–antigens for destruction. These antibodies specifically react with encapsulated bacteria, such as *Streptococcus pneumoniae*, and fungi, making them more susceptible to phagocytosis.

Disorders of the Spleen and their Management

Splenomegaly

Clinical Features

- Splenomegaly is generally painless unless the organ undergoes patchy infarction, as can occur in chronic myeloid leukaemia, vascular occlusions/crises produced by sickle cell disease or from an embolus in bacterial endocarditis.
- There may be both pleuritic and referred pain to the shoulder. Otherwise the history is that of the disease causing the splenic enlargement or hypersplenism.
- *Hypersplenism* is defined as overactivity of the spleen in one or more of its functions in relation to destruction of formed elements in the blood, with or without splenomegaly.
  - The consequences may be anaemia, leukopaenia, thrombocytopaenia or a combination of all three: pancytopaenia.

- If hypersplenism is severe and poorly responsive to non-operative treatment, splenectomy is indicated (see later).
- Other features include purpura and respiratory infections, which are the consequences of the neutropaenia. Specific symptoms related to the underlying condition may be present.

Physical Findings

These vary with the cause.
- Thrombocytopaenia is associated with purpuric skin lesions and a risk of intracranial haemorrhage.
- Leukopaenia occurs, with a variable increase in bacterial infections. There can be mild tenderness in the left upper quadrant if the spleen is enlarged secondary to an acute infection.
- A mass in the left upper quadrant of splenic origin has the following characteristics:
  - It is dull on percussion.
  - It moves downwards and medially with respiration (unlike the kidney, which moves downwards only).
  - A notch, known as the splenic notch, may be felt.
  - It cannot have its upper margin defined on palpation. In addition, care must be taken to ensure that the examining hand can get below a very large spleen; palpation is begun low down in the right iliac fossa.

Difficulty may be experienced in differentiating sple-nomegaly from the following: an enlarged left kidney, gastric or colonic tumours and masses arising from the pancreatic tail, such as a large pseudocyst.

- Ultrasonography, CT scan or magnetic resonance image (MRI) scanning shows the size of the spleen and whether it is indeed the cause of the mass. Enlargement of the spleen is termed splenomegaly. It can be classified into:
  - mild (1–3 cm below the costal margin)
  - moderate (4–8 cm below the costal margin)
  - massive splenomegaly (>8 cm). The aetiology of splenomegaly is variable and is discussed below.

Investigation of Hypersplenism

1. Blood tests

Peripheral blood films may demonstrate malarial para-sites; infectious mononucleosis gives rise to atypical lym-phocytes, and serological tests are positive (Paul–Bunnell test, Epstein–Barr virus titres).

2. Bone marrow function

A precise diagnosis is essential before proceeding to sple-nectomy because splenomegaly may, in such circumstances as infiltration of the bone marrow (malignancy, myelofibro-sis), indicate that the spleen has taken over the marrow's function in producing formed elements of the blood. Bone marrow biopsy should therefore be performed to confirm that the marrow is still active.

3. Red cell dynamics

Production can be studied by giving radiolabelled iron, and destruction by 51 Cr labelling. External scanning over the spleen demonstrates its activity in each regard. If sple-nectomy is undertaken for hypersplenism, a preoperative search by imaging, supplemented by a wide exploration at operation, must be made for accessory spleens (*splenunculi*) which could otherwise enlarge and lead to recurrence of the original condition after supposed curative surgery.

Causes of Mild Splenomegaly

- **Haemolytic anaemia**
  - Haemolytic anaemias of all types increase the work-load of the spleen in removing defective and/or dam-aged red blood cells.
  - The organ progressively enlarges and may eventually become too active in red cell destruction and exacer-bate the anaemia.
  - **a) Hereditary spherocytosis**
    - This is the commonest type of congenital hae-molytic anaemia. The critical lesion is an increase in permeability of the erythrocyte membrane to sodium. Sodium leaks into the erythrocyte, increasing its osmotic pressure. It swells, giving a typical spherical shape on a peripheral blood film and increasing osmotic fragility; periodic crises of anaemia occur, especially if the patient develops a viral illness.

- *Hereditary elliptocytosis* is a rare variant.
- Splenectomy is indicated for both spherocytosis and elliptocytosis

  b) Acquired haemolytic anaemia
- This is an autoimmune disease, which occurs either in a primary (idiopathic) form or secondary to an underlying disorder such as systemic lupus erythe-matosus or to the administration of certain drugs (e.g. penicillin).
- Splenomegaly occurs in 50% and is generally asso-ciated with mild fever and jaundice.
- The *Coombs test* is positive because the red cells are coated with immunoglobulins or comple-ment; the reaction occurs at different tempera-tures according to the presence of warm or cold antibodies.
- These haemolytic anaemias respond to splenec-tomy (which must include the removal of any accessory spleens), especially if there is a high rate of haemolysis.
- **Sickle cell disease**

  This is another common haemoglobinopathy in which normal haemoglobin A is replaced by haemoglobin S. Sickle cell disease is more likely, because of repeated minor splenic infarctions, to cause hypo- rather than hypersplenism.
- **Immune thrombocytopenic purpura (ITP)**
  - Although this disorder involves splenic destruction of platelets, the organ is rarely enlarged.
  - Splenomegaly can, however, be a feature of the sec-ondary type that develops as a consequence of lym-phoproliferative disease, infection or drugs.
  - Both types of ITP are associated with circulating anti-platelet antibodies.
  - ITP can develop acutely in children, often after a viral illness.
  - The chronic form tends to be seen in adult females.
  - In ITP, corticosteroid therapy will often (75%) improve the platelet count.
  - Splenectomy is indicated for patients who fail to respond to steroids and immunosuppressive agents (e.g. azathioprine) or who relapse when therapy is withdrawn. Steroids have a similar response rate in acquired haemolytic anaemia, but again splenectomy is indicated for treatment failures.
- **Connective tissue disorders/vasculitis**

  The above disorders, such as polyarteritis nodosa, can cause mild splenomegaly but treatment is directed at the underlying cause.
- **Infiltrative disease**

  Disorders such as amyloidosis and sarcoidosis may cause mild splenomegaly. Again, treatment is directed at the underlying disorder unless there is splenic rupture.
- **Infections**

  Mild enlargement may be seen with any acute and/or prolonged infection. Infectious causes of more serious enlargement include viruses (such as Epstein–Barr (infec-tious mononucleosis), cytomegalovirus, hepatitis and HIV), bactcrial (infective endocarditis), tuberculosis, brucellosis and syphilis. Splenomegaly during the course of an acute infectious illness is treated with the appropriate antimicrobial agents.

- **Splenic abscess**

This is an uncommon lesion usually associated with severe systemic infection and a high mortality rate. Sources of metastatic abscess of the spleen are typhoid and paratyphoid fever, osteomyelitis, otitis media and puerperal sepsis. Splenic abscesses are drained as part of the overall management of severe septic states. The drainage may be performed percutaneously under ultrasonic or CT guidance.

- **Splenic cyst**

This is a rare condition. Cysts can be either congenital in origin (dermoid and mesenchymal inclusion cysts) or parasitic from echinococcal (hydatid) infestation. Occasionally, a traumatic pseudocyst results from liquefaction of a previous splenic haematoma. Splenic cysts need to be distinguished from pancreatic pseudocysts formed in the lesser sac following severe acute pancreatitis and from neoplastic cysts arising from the pancreatic tail. Partial and/or total splenectomy may indicated recurrent cysts, failure of drainage or symptoms.

Causes of Moderate Splenomegaly

- **Portal hypertension**

Whatever the underlying cause, the spleen enlarges but seldom to a great extent. Features of liver disease and of hypersplenism may be present. Splenic vein thrombosis without occlusion of the portal vein may produce segmental or left-sided portal hypertension (sinistral) with splenomegaly and oesophageal varices, for which splenectomy alone is curative.

- **Lymphoma and leukaemia**

The spleen is very frequently enlarged in patients with tumours of the lymphoid system, e.g. lymphoma, Hodgkin's disease and other, rarer disorders which are more difficult to classify. The role of operative treatment in these disorders is establishment of the diagnosis by lymph node biopsy and, very occasionally, to remove a massive spleen that is causing symptoms or hypersplenism.

- **Thalassaemia**

Thalassaemia, common in those from the Mediterranean littoral and sub-Saharan Africa, is the result of a defect in haemoglobin peptide synthesis which is transmitted as a dominant trait. The disease is a group of related disorders – alpha and beta – depending on which haemoglobin peptide chain has reduced synthesis. Heterozygotes have a mild form of anaemia, whereas homozygotes have severe chronic anaemia and retardation of growth (thalassaemia major). The characteristic malar hypertrophy is due to overactive haematopoiesis in the upper jaw. Splenectomy is sometimes indicated for symptoms.

- **Storage diseases**

Porphyria is a hereditary error of catabolism of haemoglobin resulting in porphyrinuria, abdominal crises precipitated by barbiturates, anaemia, photosensitivity and neurological or mental symptoms in advanced stages. Splenomegaly is often present. In *Gaucher's disease*, the spleen actively stores the abnormal lipoid glucocerebroside, leading to enormous enlargement of the spleen. There is associated anaemia, brown discoloration of the skin of the hands and face and conjunctival thickening (pinguecula) and if symptoms are present, splenectomy is indicated.

Causes of Massive Splenomegaly

- **Chronic myeloid leukaemia (CML)**

CML is a cancer of the white blood cells characterized by the increased and unregulated growth of myeloid cells in the bone marrow and the accumulation of these cells in the blood. It is a type of myeloproliferative neoplasm associated with a characteristic chromosomal translocation called the Philadelphia chromosome. The spleen can become massively enlarged and lead to symptoms from its size necessitating splenectomy.

- **Myelofibrosis**

Many types of myeloproliferative disease are characterized by splenomegaly, including myeloid and lymphocytic leukaemia, polycythaemia rubra vera and myelofibrosis (also called myelosclerosis).

In myelofibrosis, extramedullary haematopoiesis develops in the liver and spleen as a result of obliteration of the bone marrow by fibrous tissue. Massive splenomegaly and secondary hypersplenism may result. The huge spleen causes dragging abdominal discomfort, which may be exacerbated by the pain of recurrent splenic infarcts. Hypersplenism predisposes to fatigue and dyspnoea (because of anaemia), spontaneous bleeding (thrombocytopaenia) and opportunist infection (neutropaenia).

- **Primary lymphoma of spleen**
  - hairy cell disease
  - tropical diseases

Diseases such as malaria, kala-azar (leishmaniasis) and schistosomiasis can lead to massive splenomegaly, which is then susceptible to minor trauma. The massive enlargements seen particularly in the tropics may require splenectomy because of pain and/or secondary hypersplenism.

Traumatic Splenic Injury

Aetiology

- In blunt abdominal trauma, the spleen is the most vulnerable organ despite its relatively protected site under the rib cage.
- The mechanism is usually a direct blow or fall such as road traffic accidents or sports injuries.
- Rupture is often associated with fractures of the overlying ribs.
- Other injuries – particularly to the head – may also occur and appear to dominate the damage profile.

- In most patients, the spleen is healthy and of normal size, but if there is splenomegaly, relatively minor trauma can cause bleeding (e.g. infectious mononucleosis and malaria).
- Spontaneous rupture can occasionally occur, although, in such circumstances, very minor trauma may have been forgotten.
- The spleen can also be damaged inadvertently during the course of an abdominal operation which involves procedures in the left upper quadrant, when a relatively minor capsular tear may cause persistent bleeding.

Pathological Features

- Elaborate classification of the extent and nature of splenic rupture has been devised and can assist the surgeon in deciding whether to attempt splenic conservation.
- The important practical distinction is between *immediate* and *delayed* rupture.
  - *Immediate rupture:* the capsule and, to a greater or lesser extent, the underlying organ are torn and bruised, bleeding is extensive and the clinical presentation is prompt. The most extreme example is when the spleen is completely avulsed from its artery or vein.
  - *Delayed rupture*: the capsule remains initially intact or, on occasion, the leak of blood is local and only into the left upper quadrant. Presentation may then be delayed for hours, days or even weeks.

Clinical Features

History

- An obvious injury to the left chest wall or the abdomen may have been sustained.
- Conscious patients complain of abdominal pain that is generalized but usually most severe in the left upper quadrant. Pain may also be felt in the tip of the left shoulder because irritation of the undersurface of the diaphragm stimulates the phrenic nerve (C4 dermatome: *Kehr's sign*).
- An unconscious patient cannot report these symptoms, and there is danger that the abdominal condition may be overlooked unless very careful attention is paid to the clinical findings.
- Head injuries do not cause circulatory collapse. To ensure correct patient management, Advanced Trauma & Life Support (ATLS) guidelines and protocols should be followed.

Physical Findings

- Hypovolaemia: in frank rupture there is considerable rapid blood loss into the peritoneal cavity, and pallor, low blood pressure, rapid pulse and restlessness develop.
- There may be external bruising and tenderness over the upper left abdomen and lower left ribs – the latter suggesting fracture.

- Typically, there is abdominal tenderness, guarding and rigidity.
- Occasionally a splenic mass is felt if there is pre-existing splenomegaly or a large subcapsular haematoma.
- *Delayed rupture* has an insidious presentation with anaemia, vague left upper quadrant and left shoulder pain and mild tenderness in the left upper quadrant. The signs may become acute if free rupture eventually takes place.

Investigation

- *Chest X-ray* taken as part of the ATLS guidelines often shows fractured ribs, and the left hemidiaphragm may be elevated by the underlying haematoma.
- *Abdominal X-ray* is *not* usually indicated, but if done may show splenomegaly or a subdiaphragmatic soft tissue mass.
- Few tests are required when frank rupture of the spleen causes a haemoperitoneum.
- In other patients, imaging may be required to confirm the diagnosis of rupture or a subcapsular haematoma.
- As a general rule in a **haemodynamically stable** patient radiological imaging can be utilized to confirm the diagnosis BUT in **haemodynamically unstable** patients, prompt surgery with splenectomy can be life-saving.
- *Focused Ultrasound Scan in Trauma (FAST scan)* and *CT* may demonstrate the rupture of the splenic capsule and show free blood in the peritoneal cavity. A subcapsular haematoma can be demonstrated.
- In a haemodynamically stable patient, the progress or resolution of a haematoma may be assessed by repeated scanning.

Management

- Until recently, any but the most trivial splenic injury was regarded as an indication for splenectomy.
- Nowadays, because of better recognition of the risk of postsplenectomy sepsis, an attempt is made to preserve splenic tissue.
- Splenic salvage is particularly desirable in children, who are at greater risk.
- However, the prime goal is to save the patient's life, and attempts at splenic preservation should not be continued if there is continuous bleeding.
- Management may follow three main courses:
  - Non-operative – splenic injury is suspected, but there are few clinical signs, and imaging shows a limited haematoma; the patient is admitted for a few days for observation and repeat imaging to show either no enlargement or resolution.
  - Initial non-operative followed by operation – indicated by increasing physical findings and/or haemodynamic instability which imply continued bleeding.
  - Emergency operation – a patient in hypovolaemic shock is, if possible, resuscitated immediately and then proceeds to laparotomy; sometimes it may be necessary to operate in the presence of hypotension in order to control bleeding.

Splenectomy

Operation

The spleen can be safely removed via a left subcostal or midline laparotomy, but extension into the chest is occasionally needed if the organ is massive. Laparoscopic splenectomy is widely used for small or moderate-sized spleens, notably for ITP in the elective setting. A preoperative ultrasound scan should be made for (pigment) gallstones in patients with haemolytic anaemia and, if found, cholecystectomy considered at the same time as splenectomy. Accessory spleens, which can cause recurrence of haemolytic and thrombocytopenic disorders, should be removed if found in such patients. If the organ is large and adherent, it may be advisable to expose and ligate the splenic artery at an early stage. Adhesions to the diaphragm and mesocolon need to be divided before the peritoneal attachments of the spleen are incised and the organ is mobilized into the wound. Care must be taken when dividing the short gastric vessels not to injure the stomach and, when the splenic vessels are ligated, to avoid injury to the tail of the pancreas.

In the emergency setting at operation, a rapid search is made for other sites of bleeding, notably from the liver and tears in the mesentery. Unless the organ is extensively shattered or bleeding is uncontrollable, an attempt is made to preserve it. Simple manoeuvres may suffice, such as topical haemostatic agents (e.g. oxidized regenerated cellulose: Surgicel) applied with gentle pressure over a swab. Alternatively, the organ is mobilized and accurate suture is performed with or without ligation of the splenic artery to reduce blood flow. Enclosing the spleen in a bag of absorbable mesh may also control bleeding. Finally, segmental resection may be feasible, especially with modern haemostatic technologies such as ultrasonic dissection and topical haemostatic agents being available. If splenectomy proves unavoidable, some surgeons leave splenic tissue behind within an omental pocket, but the function of such autotransplants is doubtful. Operation is also indicated for a delayed rupture that presents with late haemoperitoneum or (rarely) drainage for an infected splenic haematoma.

Complications of Splenectomy

1. Bleeding

This may result from persistent oozing in the splenic bed and is the commonest cause of subphrenic haematoma and abscess. These complications are more frequent in patients with preoperative thrombocytopaenia.

2. Thrombocytosis

This is the rule after splenectomy, but venous thromboembolism is not especially common; antiplatelet agents or subcutaneous heparin may be given if the platelet count rises above 1000×10^9/L.

3. Overwhelming postsplenectomy infection (OPSI)

OPSI is the most serious late complication of splenectomy. Thus immunization is required not only when splenectomy is planned but also in operations on adjacent organs in which the spleen may form part of the dissection – e.g. total gastrectomy and operations on the distal pancreas. As discussed above, the functional role of the spleen is protection from infection, particularly against encapsulated organisms such as pneumococci and meningococci. The commonest form of OPSI is therefore pneumococcal or meningococcal septicaemia. In addition, infections with *Haemophilus influenzae* are an important risk. Postsplenectomy sepsis often starts insidiously but can rapidly develop into a fulminant infection. There is fever, vomiting, dehydration and circulatory collapse often without specific features that alert the clinician to the diagnosis. In this setting, intravenous administration of fluids and antibiotics should be started on an empirical basis without waiting for the results of culture and organism sensitivities. The mortality rate is at least 50%, which emphasises the need for prophylaxis.

Prophylaxis

The occurrence of OPSI could be much reduced if vigorous preventative measures were used in those at risk. Although the condition was originally thought to be limited to infants and children, it is now known to occur at all ages, which justifies universal prophylaxis after splenectomy. There is no absolute agreement on regimens, but guidelines advised vaccinations against *S. pneumoniae* (pneumococcus – repeated every 5 years), *Neisseria meningitidis* and *H. influenzae*. In addition, patients should receive yearly influenza vaccination, take penicillin V lifelong, or erythromycin in cases of penicillin allergy, and wear a Medicare bracelet to alert healthcare professionals that the patient is asplenic. The lifetime risk of developing OPSI is estimated at 2–4% and is higher in children than in adults; the risk is also greater if the spleen is removed because of a haematological disease (thalassaemia, lymphoma) rather than for trauma.

21

Common Colorectal Surgical Conditions

CHAPTER OUTLINE

Anatomy

Large Bowel

Embryology

The midgut, in the 5-week-old embryo, is attached to the dorsal abdominal wall by a short mesentery. In adulthood, the midgut begins just distal to the bile duct entrance to the duodenum and ends at the junction of the proximal two-thirds of the transverse colon with the distal third.

The hindgut gives rise to the distal third of the transverse colon, all the way to the upper part of the anal canal. It also gives rise to the internal lining of the bladder and urethra.

The distal part of the anal canal is derived from the ectoderm.

Their blood supply reflects their embryological origin with the superior mesenteric artery supplying the midgut, the inferior mesenteric artery supplying the hindgut and the inferior rectal arteries (which are branches of the internal pudendal arteries) supplying the caudal part of the anal canal.

Macroscopic

The large bowel measures approximately 150 cm and extends from the ileo-caecal valve to the junction of the rectum and anal canal. Its diameter is approximately 6 cm.

The caecum, which typically starts in the right iliac fossa, extends upwards to become the ascending colon, then turns to the left at the hepatic flexure, to pass across the abdomen as a long (~50 cm) dependent loop, called the transverse colon and at the splenic flexure, turns down to become the descending colon, to reach the brim of the pelvis. Below this point, the bowel becomes the sigmoid colon and projects into the pelvis before it ends retroperitoneally as the rectum.

The appendix is a blind-ending tube varying from 2 to 20 cm in length and arises from the posteromedial aspect of the caecal wall, whose anatomical position in the pelvis may vary considerably:

- Behind the caecum (retrocaecal) ~65%
- Projects downwards into the pelvis (pelvic) ~31%
- Immediately below the caecum (subcaecal) ~2%
- In front of the terminal ileum (pre-ileal) ~1%
- Behind the ileum (post-ileal) ~0.4%

The appendix, transverse colon and sigmoid colon all have mesenteries. The rest of the colon does not.

The rectum is the last 15 cm of the gastrointestinal tract and lies anterior to the sacrum and coccyx.

The distal 3–4 cm is called the anal canal. This is derived from a fusion of the embryological hindgut and the proctodeum, therefore is made up of both visceral and somatic structures.

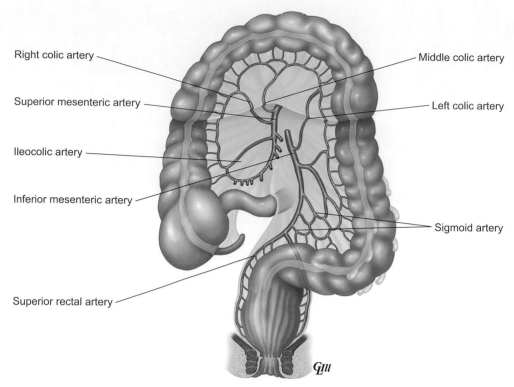

Right colic artery

Superior mesenteric artery

Ileocolic artery

Inferior mesenteric artery

Superior rectal artery

Middle colic artery

Left colic artery

Sigmoid artery

Gʲ

• **Fig. 21.1** Arterial Blood Supply to Colon

Microscopic

The wall of the colon is comprised of four layers:

1. Mucosa: this is the inner lining and is comprised of a layer of simple columnar epithelium, areolar connective tissue and a thin layer of smooth muscle (muscularis mucosae). The epithelium mostly contains absorptive and goblet cells that are for water absorption and mucus secretion, respectively.
2. Submucosa: this consists of areolar connective tissue that binds the mucosa to the muscularis. It contains blood and lymphatic vessels for absorbing nutrients. It also contains the submucosal plexus or plexus of Meissner, which is a network of neurons forming part of the enteric nervous system.
3. Muscularis: this is comprised of smooth muscle that is found in two sheets – an inner sheet of circular fibres and an outer sheet of longitudinal fibres. Portions of the longitudinal muscle are thickened, forming three bands called the taeniae coli which run along most of its length. When these bands contract, they gather the colon into a series of pouches called haustra. Between the layers of the smooth muscle lies a second plexus of the enteric nervous system, the myenteric plexus or plexus of Auerbach.
4. Serosa: this is part of the visceral peritoneum. Small pouches of the visceral peritoneum filled with fat are attached to the taeniae coli and are called epiploic appendages.

Blood Supply

Arterial

The superior mesenteric artery originates from the T12/L1 level of the aorta and supplies the colon up to two-thirds of the transverse colon via the ileocolic, right colic and middle colic arteries (Fig. 21.1).

The inferior mesenteric artery originates from L3 level of the aorta and its branches are: left colic artery (descending colon), sigmoid artery (sigmoid colon), superior rectal artery (rectum and upper part of the anal canal).

The marginal artery of Drummond is an arterial anastomosis which is formed from both the mesenteric arteries and runs along the mesenteric border of the colon. This ensures that, in case the inferior mesenteric artery is ligated, the descending and sigmoid colon receive sufficient arterial blood supply.

The inferior rectal arteries, which are branches of the internal pudendal arteries, supply the distal part of the anal canal.

Venous

Venous drainage from the colon passes in the inferior and superior mesenteric veins and, once these join the splenic vein, they form the hepatic portal vein behind the neck of the pancreas. The portal vein then passes in the free edge of the lesser omentum and then divides into right and left branches before reaching the liver.

Lymphatic

The midgut lymphatic drainage is to the nodes in the mesentery and preaortic nodes around the origin of the superior mesenteric artery. It then passes into the cisterna chyli and the thoracic duct.

The hindgut lymphatic drainage is to the nodes of the posterior abdominal wall and the sigmoid mesentery and preaortic nodes around the origin of the inferior mesenteric artery which then passes to the cisterna chyli and thoracic duct.

Physiology

Functions of the large intestine include haustral churning and peristalsis of the contents along the colon towards the rectum and the defaecation and absorption of some water, ions and vitamins. The bacteria present in the large intestine also produce some B vitamins and vitamin K.

Sodium and Water Absorption

Normally, about 1.5 L of water, 200 mmol of sodium and 100 mmol of chloride pass through the large intestine per day. From the 1.5 L entering the large intestine, approximately 95% of the sodium and water in it is reabsorbed as it moves through the colon.

Sodium is usually transported from the lumen into plasma by two energy-dependent mechanisms:
- sodium–potassium exchange in the cell membrane
- sodium–proton exchange at the luminal surface

Chloride absorption is down an electrical gradient and by exchange for bicarbonate.

Water moves from the lumen into the cell because the latter is at a higher osmotic pressure, due to the active transport of solutes, especially sodium, chloride and short chain fatty acids.

Bacterial Metabolism and Fermentation

The colon contains 99% of the organisms in the gastrointestinal tract, and more than 400 different types have been identified. Bacteria make up approximately 80% of the weight of normal faeces.

Bacteria in the colon are important because:
- They cause fermentation (anaerobic release of energy) by breaking down the carbohydrates to produce short-chain fatty acids (SCFAs).
- They are the source of potentially lethal complications if the mucosal barrier is damaged.

The colonic bacteria to produce SCFAs break down dietary fibre, which is non-starch polysaccharides such as cellulose and other plant components, like dextrin, inulin, beta-glucans and oligosaccharides. By increasing dietary fibre intake, the colonic motility is increased, partly because of the water-absorbing properties of fibre, and because of the increased bacterial activity and fermentation. SCFAs are absorbed and form part of the body's energy cycle. A by-product of these chemical reactions is gas (flatus), a mixture of carbon dioxide, hydrogen and methane with varying amounts of other gases, such as hydrogen sulphide, depending on the substrate.

• BOX 21.1   Causes of Constipation

- Inadequate dietary fibre
- Neoplasms of the colon, rectum and anus
- Benign lesions of the anus
- Endocrine disease, e.g. myxoedema
- Drugs, e.g. codeine phosphate
- Hirschsprung's disease
- Slow-transit constipation
- Psychological and behavioural abnormalities
- Neurological causes: cerebral, e.g. stroke; spinal, e.g. multiple sclerosis, paraplegia, neoplasm

---

Storage and Evacuation of Faeces

When the faeces enter the rectum, the resulting distention of the rectal wall stimulates stretch receptors which initiate a defaecation reflex that empties the rectum. The receptors send sensory signals to the sacral spinal cord and then motor impulses travel along parasympathetic nerves back to the descending, sigmoid colon and rectum. The muscles contract and increase the pressure within the rectum and, along with the voluntary contraction of the abdominal muscles and diaphragm, open the internal sphincter. The external anal sphincter is comprised of skeletal muscle and has voluntary control.

Factors controlling colonic motility are:
- Fibre content of the diet
- Amount of fluid in the colon
- Laxative use
- Hormones, e.g. cholecystokinin
- Psychological factors
- Food in the stomach, which can initiate a reflex colonic contraction (gastrocolic reflex)
- Circadian rhythm (resting tone is considerably reduced at night)

BENIGN COLORECTAL DISEASE

Functional Bowel Disorders

Functional Constipation

This is defined as either excessive straining at stool or the passage of two or fewer stools in a week (the Rome IV criteria[1] for functional bowel disorders).

In 2014/15, 66,287 people in the UK were admitted to hospital with constipation as the main condition. The total cost to hospitals for treating unplanned admissions due to constipation was £145 million in that same year. The prescription cost of laxatives to the NHS is £101 million. The common causes of constipation are summarized in Box 21.1.

The aetiology of functional constipation is considered to be either due to a slow gut transit ('colonic inertia'), rectal evacuatory dysfunction or a combination of both. The commonest cause of a slow transit gut is due to medication

---

• BOX 21.2 Causes of Faecal Incontinence

- Trauma (obstetric, surgical, accidental)
- Colorectal disease (haemorrhoids, rectal prolapse, IBD, tumours)
- Congenital (spinal bifida, operations for imperforate anus, Hirschsprung's disease)
- Neurological (cerebral, spinal, peripheral)
- Miscellaneous (behavioural, impaction, encopresis)

• BOX 21.3 Treatment Summary of IBS

- Lifestyle modification
  - Reduce caffeine and sorbitol in patients with IBS-D
  - Increase soluble fibre intake, although that may exacerbate bloating
- Pharmacological treatment
  - Loperamide/Laxatives (IBS-D/IBS-C)
  - Tricyclic antidepressants (peripheral and central actions)
  - Amitriptyline
  - Probiotics
  - Linaclotide/Prucalopride (IBS-C)
  - Plecanatide (US approved)
- Psychological treatment
  - Cognitive behavioural therapy
  - Hypnotherapy
- Surgery
  - Try and Avoid!

---

like opiates, anticholinergics, antihypertensives, iron tablets, antacids and non-steroidal anti-inflammatories. Other causes include neurological disease (multiple sclerosis, Parkinson's disease and diabetic autonomic neuropathy), endocrine (hypothyroidism) or electrolyte disturbances (hypercalcaemia, hypokalaemia).

Investigations after a full clinical history and examination of the patient such as a simple blood test could detect the hormonal or electrolyte disturbances described above. Luminal examinations are for patients with short history or alarm symptoms to exclude colorectal cancer. Colonic transit studies can be used as a fairly simple investigation for slow colonic transit. One way is by ingesting a capsule of markers and then take a plain abdominal film on day 5. Patients who have expelled at least 80% of the markers have a normal colonic transit.

Another investigation to evaluate the anatomical and physiological disturbances of rectal evacuation in these patients is a defecating proctography. This is using either plain X-ray or MRI to assess defecation in a patient after inserting barium or magnetic resonance gel per rectum. Another method is the balloon expulsion test, which also assesses for pelvic floor dysfunction, rectocele, rectal prolapse and other disturbances of rectal evacuation. Anorectal manometry in patients with chronic constipation can exclude Hirschsprung's disease, which usually presents shortly after birth and, very occasionally, first presents in adults.

Slow transit constipation does not respond to laxatives or dietary fibre. Biofeedback therapy may help but patients may need surgical treatment. This means having a total colectomy and ileorectal anastomosis.

Faecal Incontinence

This is a socially disabling condition with an incidence of 1–2% and is defined by the Rome IV criteria as the 'uncontrolled passage of solid or liquid stool which occurs at least two times in a four-week period'. It affects more women than men and its peak incidence occurs in the elderly.

The major aetiological factors are listed in Box 21.2. The commonest cause in women is due to obstetric trauma.

It is important to take an accurate history of the frequency and severity of the incontinence and include past history of anal surgery and careful obstetric history in females. It is useful to quantify the degree of incontinence using a scoring system, e.g. the Cleveland Clinic scoring system.

Specific investigations after full examination include three-dimensional manometry to examine resting and squeeze pressures, anorectal ultrasound and anal mucosal electrosensitivity and rectal compliance measurements.

Treatment in patients with troublesome faecal soiling, with an identified sphincter defect due to obstetric injury or trauma by manometry or ultrasound, is more likely to be surgical (direct sphincter repair, sphincter augmentation procedures). Conservative treatment is usually more appropriate for patients with neurological causes. Sacral nerve stimulation has shown promising results in patients with intact anal sphincters and some preservation of pudendal nerve function. Other procedures like anal plug and stoma formation have their own value and the latter is performed if all else fails.

Irritable Bowel Syndrome (IBS)

This is a functional bowel disorder, which is characterized by chronic abdominal pain, discomfort, bloating and alteration of bowel habit. Rome IV criteria for diagnosing IBS include recurrent abdominal pain at least 1 day per week in the last 3 months with symptom onset at least 6 months before diagnosis with two or more of the following criteria: related to defecation, associated with a change in frequency of stool, and associated with a change in stool consistency/appearance.

There are three main subtypes: IBS-C (predominant constipation), IBS-D (predominant diarrhoea) and IBS-M (mixed bowel habits). If they do not fit into any of these categories, then they are considered to have IBS unclassified. They can also be grouped into sporadic or post-infectious/inflammatory bowel disease-associated types.

It is important to note that IBS diagnosis is made after exclusion of organic disease, so the presence of alarm symptoms (i.e. symptom onset after 50 years old, rectal bleeding, weight loss or abdominal mass) should prompt luminal investigations. It is important to consider coeliac disease as the differential.

Treatment includes lifestyle modification, pharmacological, psychological and surgical treatment (Box 21.3).

Solitary Rectal Ulcer Syndrome (SRUS)

This is an uncommon but benign disease which is defined by a combination of clinical and histological findings. It affects men and women equally, who often complain of rectal bleeding, mucus discharge, prolonged excessive straining, perineal and abdominal pain, tenesmus, constipation and rectal prolapse. Histological findings described include obliteration of the lamina propria by fibrosis and smooth muscle fibres extending through the muscularis mucosa to the lumen. Collagen deposition in the lamina propria and abnormal smooth muscle fibre extensions are helpful to distinguish it from other conditions.

Ulcers are only found in 40% of the patients and 20% have a solitary ulcer.

Aetiology is less clear and it may be caused by paradoxical contraction of the anal sphincter muscle during defaecation, direct digital trauma and perhaps primary neuromuscular pathology.

Treatment includes dietary changes, bulking agent and biofeedback defaecation retraining. Surgical intervention is rarely indicated for patients who have a concomitant prolapse or patients who are still symptomatic despite conservative management. Surgical resection without biofeedback does not seem to be effective. Rectopexy has a failure rate of up to 50% but stapled transanal rectal resection in solitary rectal ulcer which is associated with prolapse showed promising results with 80% of patients showing good results.

Chronic Rectal Pain Syndrome

The term 'chronic proctalgia' in the Rome III classification was used to describe the levator ani syndrome, unspecified anorectal pain and proctalgia fugax. This umbrella term was eliminated from the updated Rome IV criteria and the separate types are kept individually.

Rectal Prolapse (see Ch. 22)

Diverticular Disease

Diverticular disease can be either acquired or congenital.

In the more common acquired type, the diverticula are serosa-covered outpouchings of mucosa alone through gaps in the muscularis propria which transmit the blood vessels. In the far less common congenital diverticular disease, the diverticula contain all layers of the normal colon.

The diverticula are usually in the left side of the colon, especially the sigmoid, but quite frequently involve the entire colon. The rectum with a complete layer of longitudinal muscle rarely develops diverticula.

Epidemiology and Aetiology

Acquired diverticular disease is rare under the age of 35, after which there is a progressive increase in incidence, so that 50% of those in their eighth or ninth decade are affected, though not necessarily symptomatic. The condition is common in Western countries but rare in China, India and Africa.

TABLE 21.1	Hinchey Classification	
Class	**Pathology**
I	Mesenteric/Pericolic abscess
II	Pelvic abscess
III	Purulent peritonitis
IV	Faecal peritonitis

The aetiology is not well understood but it has been long thought that a low-fibre diet with high intraluminal pressures caused the outpouching of the mucosa alongside blood vessels. Although there is an epidemiological link between low-fibre diet and diverticular disease, there is no evidence in recommending high-fibre diet as treatment.

Smoking or use of non-steroidal anti-inflammatory drugs (NSAIDs) have also been associated with a higher incidence of diverticular disease.

Pathological Features

Diverticula have a narrow neck and faeces can accumulate in them causing any of the following:
- Persistent inflammation in a segment of bowel wall
- Local inflammation of the affected diverticulum, leading to perforation

Perforation may in turn be:
- Local into pericolic tissues
- Into the peritoneal cavity causing generalized peritonitis
- Into an adjacent organ causing a fistula (e.g. uterus, vagina)

Clinical Features

Symptoms

These are frequently absent and the diagnosis is made following a colonoscopy or barium enema or CT pneumocolon done for other reasons, chiefly to exclude a large-bowel carcinoma. There may be mild left lower abdominal pain, which accompanies a long-standing irregularity of bowel habit with episodic slight diarrhoea or more usually constipation with the passage of small quantities of hard faecal pellets.

Classification of diverticular disease is challenging yet necessary to avoid unnecessary operations in patients with good prognosis. The Hinchey classification is the most well-known and it is used for findings in surgery for perforated diverticulitis (Table 21.1).

Signs

In uncomplicated disease, signs are absent or minimal. There is occasionally tenderness over the descending colon, and this portion of the bowel may be palpable. Signs of focal or generalized peritonitis are present in case of perforation.

Investigations

In the case of asymptomatic diverticulosis found in investigations for another disorder, then no further investigations are needed.

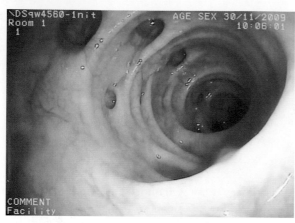

• **Fig. 21.2** Diverticula in Colonoscopy

In symptomatic patients who have suspected diverticular disease, patients often have to undergo luminal investigations to rule out bowel cancer (Fig. 21.2). In the case of the emergency presentation of patients with complications, CT scan is the investigation of choice and any endoscopic investigations should be deferred.

Management

In symptomatic but uncomplicated diverticular disease, patients are advised on increasing dietary fibre intake, weight loss and exercise, as well as management of their constipation with bulk-forming laxatives if diet alone is not enough. Although there is little evidence that high fibre diet will improve their symptoms, it may well prevent from development of further diverticula. In addition to this, patients are advised to avoid non-steroidal anti-inflammatory drugs (NSAIDs) which have been linked to diverticular disease.

Elective surgery of the affected colonic segment in patients with intractable symptoms may only be performed in exceptional cases.

Inflammation/Abscess

Involvement of a segment of bowel wall may cause severe abdominal pain, pyrexia and tenderness over the affected segment. Inflammation may progress to perforation or pericolic abscess. Investigation with a CT scan or ultrasound may help with the diagnosis. Management of these patients depends on the local centre and patient's clinical picture. Antibiotics should be initiated to patients unwell enough to attend hospital.

Management options for patients with complicated or uncomplicated diverticulitis who do not respond to conservative management include radiological (CT/ultrasound) drainage of abscess, laparoscopic lavage (although a recent meta-analysis[2] found a higher incidence of pelvic abscesses compared to surgery), emergency surgery (resection with either primary anastomosis +/- stoma, Hartmann's procedure, defunctioning stoma).

Diverticular Bleeding

Large-volume rectal haemorrhage, which is thought to be due to erosion of a vessel in the neck of a diverticulum, is a well-recognized complication. This is usually painless and the colour of the blood depends on the site of origin, i.e. bright red with clots from the left side and dark red from the right side.

Most cases of bleeding are managed non-operatively but ongoing bleeding warrants further investigation. An important differential is vascular malformations causing the bleeding. Selective angiography of the large-bowel arteries is usually required, after which embolization or surgical resection is performed.

Fistulation

The clinical features depend on the organs involved. The commonest sites of fistulation are into the bladder or vagina and they are characterized by the passage of gas and faecal material into urine or vagina respectively. Fit patients with colovesical fistula should undergo surgery with resection of the affected colonic segment.

Rectal Bleeding

Rectal bleeding is a very common symptom in adults of all ages. One-year prevalence of rectal bleeding is 10% in the UK. The majority of patients with rectal bleeding have a benign anal cause for this, e.g. haemorrhoids or anal fissure. However, rectal bleeding can be a sign of colorectal cancer (CRC) or inflammatory bowel disease. Causes of rectal bleeding are summarized in Box 21.4.

In the emergency setting, if the patient presents with acute large-volume rectal bleeding, it may be appropriate to first exclude an upper GI bleed, before proceeding to a colonoscopy and/or mesenteric angiography. Usually, the source of rectal bleeding in the older patient is due to diverticular disease or arteriovenous malformation. However, sometimes no cause is identified for massive haemorrhage and therefore a subtotal colectomy has to be performed.

In the elective setting, a patient with rectal bleeding should have routine blood tests including full blood count and, in the younger population with suspected inflammatory bowel disease, a faecal calprotectin is also useful. If there is any suspicion for malignance, the patient should be urgently referred for further investigations.

INFLAMMATORY BOWEL DISEASE

Ulcerative Colitis

Epidemiology and Aetiology

This condition is common in Scandinavia, the UK and North America. There is a higher incidence in rural dwellers. Current smoking may protect against ulcerative colitis, whereas it increases the risk of Crohn's disease. Females are more commonly affected than males, and the condition is prevalent in late adolescence and early adult life.

The cause is not known but the following may be involved.

Genetics

There is a higher familial incidence of ulcerative colitis than would be expected by chance. However, no clear genetic pattern of expression has been identified.

- Haemorrhoids
- Anal fissure
- Diverticular disease
- Colorectal or anal cancer
- Colorectal polyps
- Arteriovenous malformations
- Ischaemia
- Trauma
- Colitis
- Solitary rectal ulcer
- Other anal conditions
  - Fistula
  - Squamous carcinoma
  - Sexually transmitted diseases

- Crypt abscess formation
- Goblet cell depletion
- Destruction of surface epithelium (ulceration)
- Mucosal oedema
- Dysplasia

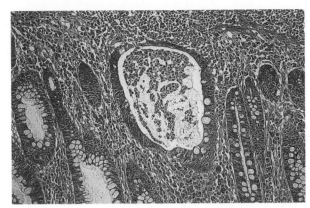

• **Fig. 21.3** Histological Appearance of a Crypt Abscess in Ulcerative Colitis

Transmissible Agents

The histological and clinical features of the disease have some things in common with those that occur in acute bacterial infections of the colon, but, in spite of intensive microbial investigation, a specific organism has not been identified.

Diet

The prevalence of the disease in countries in which the diet is low in fibre and contains additives suggests that the use of highly milled flour and certain additives (e.g. carrageen) may be factors. A small number of patients with ulcerative colitis are made symptomatically worse by taking milk protein, which is the consequence of mucosal hypolactasia.

Psychodynamics

Introversion and depression are commonly seen, and the symptoms are often made worse by psychological stress. However, it is probable that these matters are secondary rather than causative.

Immunology

The failure to find any infective agent has led to the suggestion that the destructive inflammation of the colonic mucosa is autoimmune, similar to that found in, for example, thyroiditis. However, markers of autoimmune disease such as antinuclear factor are no more common in these patients than in the normal population.

Pathological Features

The major feature is inflammation of the mucosa with increased vascularity and haemorrhage. In spite of the name of the disease, macroscopic ulceration is not common except in very severe and advanced disease. The changes are usually most marked in the rectum (proctitis) and spread for a varying degree proximally into the colon. Rarely, the entire large bowel is involved but the disease does not extend proximal to the ileocaecal valve although a 'backwash ileitis' may affect the terminal ileum. Box 21.5 lists the histological features; the most diagnostic of these is the

crypt abscess (Fig. 21.3). Dysplastic change is thought to be a marker for the risk of malignant change (see later).

Symptoms

The most characteristic symptom is bloody diarrhoea with associated social embarrassment and discomfort. There are periods of remission followed by acute relapse. Disease confined to the rectum is usually mild and without systemic effects. More extensive colonic involvement leads to ill health, weight loss, symptoms of anaemia and complaints of abdominal pain.

Signs

In mild disease, physical signs are few or absent. Those with a more severe or extensive condition look ill, show signs of weight loss, anaemia and dehydration. Abdominal examination may show colonic distension and tenderness.

Complications

Fulminant colitis

The severity of colitis can be assessed using the Truelove and Witts' criteria (Table 21.2). Severe attacks require admission to hospital for intensive medical management and often require urgent colectomy.

Toxic Megacolon (Acute Dilatation)

The medical management of severe colitis is complex and beyond the scope of this book. Severe inflammation

TABLE 21.2	Truelove and Witts' Classification of Severity of Ulcerative Colitis			
Activity	Mild	Moderate	Severe	
Number of bloody stool per day (n)	<4	4–6	>6	
Temperature (°C)	Afebrile	Intermediate	>37.8	
Heart rate (beats per minute)	Normal	Intermediate	>90	
Haemoglobin (g/dL)	>11	10.5–11	<10.5	
Erythrocyte sedimentation rate (mm/h)	<20	20–30	>30	

NOTE: six or more bowel motions per day associated with at least one other 'severe' criterion is indicative of a severe attack
From Truelove SC, Witts LJ. Cortisone in ulcerative colitis: final report on a therapeutic trial. Br Med J. 1955; 2 (4947): 1041–1048.

may cause the colon (particularly the transverse part) to dilate.

There is severe acute systemic disturbance with:

- toxaemia
- anaemia from bleeding
- acute loss of water and electrolyte
- progressive abdominal distension

The last of these may lead to perforation of the colon with general peritonitis, which carries a high mortality and gives the complication its sinister reputation.

Treatment is with water and electrolyte replacement and intensive medical treatment (see below). High-dose hydrocortisone (400 mg/day) is started and antibiotics may also be given. Close monitoring of both the systemic condition (such as 12-hourly blood analysis including inflammatory markers such as C-reactive protein and white cell count) and the degree of colonic dilatation (by serial plain X-ray and measurement of the diameter of the caecum or ascending colon) is required to detect deterioration or the likelihood of perforation. Blood transfusion is required if haemoglobin is less than 10 g/dL. Parenteral nutrition is often required. The patient should be assessed jointly by an experienced physician and surgeon on a 12-hourly basis during the acute phase of colitis. Failure to respond to intensive medical therapy after 48–72 hours, or deterioration in the patient's condition during this period, is an indication for intravenous cyclosporine therapy or operation. Surgery involves urgent removal of the colon – usually leaving the rectum intact – and a diverting ileostomy may be required. Once the patient has recovered, further surgery may be considered as discussed below.

Massive Haemorrhage

This is rare and usually responds to transfusion and intensive treatment of the disease.

Carcinoma

Adenocarcinoma develops as a result of dysplastic change in long-standing colitis. The risk is very small in those who have had the disease for less than 10 years. Thereafter, it increases in those who have total colitis, so that by 20 years it approaches 20%. The hazard is much less in patients with limited disease. The presence of a cancer is an absolute indication for surgery.

Complications Other Than in the Gastrointestinal Tract

Systemic complications (Box 21.6) are uncommon and are usually an indication of the severity of the colitis. If this is successfully treated, such complications usually resolve. An exception is urinary calculus after removal of the colon and ileostomy. It is thought that this is partly the result of increased water loss via the ileostomy which leads to a more concentrated urine. However, disorders of oxalate metabolism may also be involved.

Investigation

All patients suspected of having ulcerative colitis should have a sigmoidoscopy and biopsy of the rectal mucosa. Stool cultures are carried out to exclude an infective cause. Except in the mildest cases, in which the proximal limit of the disease can be seen at sigmoidoscopy, a barium enema (Fig. 21.4), or more commonly a colonoscopy, is used to determine the extent. The latter, accompanied by multiple biopsies, is the most precise method and may also reveal an unsuspected carcinoma. Colonoscopy may be delayed until after treatment in patients with severe attacks because of the risk of perforation. CT or MRI scanning may be useful to define the extent of disease and identify complications such as perforation.

Management

Medical

Most patients have minimal disease which can be adequately managed by a combination of 5-aminosalicylic acid (5-ASA) or prednisolone suppositories. Oral sulfasalazine or other 5-aminosalicylic acid based drugs such as mesalazine (fewer side-effects) are effective in more extensive disease. Beclometasone dipropionate or prednisolone can be added

- Skin disorders, e.g. erythema nodosum, pyoderma gangrenosum
- Eye disorders, e.g. iritis, episcleritis
- Arthritis, e.g. ankylosing spondylitis, peripheral rheumatoid-type arthritis
- Liver disorders, e.g. chronic liver disease, sclerosing cholangitis
- Renal disorders, e.g. ureteric calculi following ileostomy, secondary amyloidosis, glomerulonephritis

- Severe exacerbations of colitis (more than 8 × bowel movements per day, pyrexia, tachycardia, low albumin, low haemoglobin, high platelet count or C reactive protein)
- Severe exacerbations of non-gastrointestinal manifestations
- Toxic colon/acute dilatation
- Chronic colitis refractory to medical treatment
- Development of premalignant changes (dysplasia) in colon/rectum
- Development of carcinoma of colon/rectum

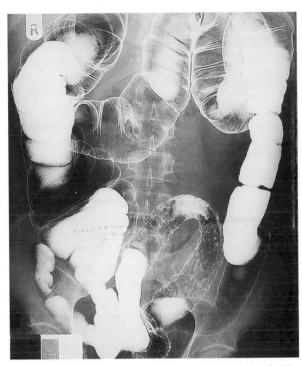

• **Fig. 21.4** Barium Enema in a Patient with Ulcerative Colitis

to induce remission. More extensive disease with incapacitating symptoms may require admission to hospital for systemic steroids, immunosuppression (e.g. oral tacrolimus, mercaptopurine or azathioprine). If the patient suffers from moderate to severe ulcerative colitis which does not respond to conventional therapy, then additions of infliximab, adalimumab, vedolizumab and golimumab can be discussed. The choice is made on a patient-to-patient basis after discussion with the patient.

Surgical

Apart from special circumstances when a temporary diversion of the faecal stream by ileostomy alone is done, the objective of surgery is to remove all, or nearly all, diseased large bowel. The indications for surgery are given in Box 21.7.

When there is time, electrolyte balance, toxaemia and anaemia are corrected preoperatively. Mechanical preparation of the bowel is contraindicated because of the risk of perforation. Perioperative antibiotic prophylaxis is essential.

If either a temporary or a permanent stoma is contemplated (which is common – see later), a specialist in stoma care as well as the surgeon should discuss the matter with the patient. The patient should be given information about all available treatment by a specialist, what they can expect in the short and long term after surgery and they should also be given the opportunity to discuss information on diet, sexual function, effects on lifestyle, psychological well-being, and stoma care.

Operative Procedures

- Proctocolectomy with permanent ileostomy

This is the standard procedure in elective or semi-elective cases (Fig. 21.5): all diseased or potentially diseased bowel is removed and the patient is rapidly restored to full health. However, the permanent stoma requires an appliance to be worn and can have its own complications (Box 21.8), although these can usually be avoided. In urgent cases, a total colectomy with ileostomy is performed, but the rectum is left in situ.

Patients usually adapt well to the alteration of body image inevitably produced, but their occasional difficulty in doing so and a natural distaste for a stoma in both themselves and their surgeons has led to the development of other techniques.

- Ileorectal anastomosis after colectomy

In some patients, the rectal disease may not be severe or may resolve after colectomy and temporary diverting ileostomy; ileorectal anastomosis (Fig. 21.6) may then produce a good functional result. However, there is risk of subsequent carcinoma in the rectum, and inflammation may recur. Lifelong surveillance is necessary.

- Continent ileostomy

The objective is to improve the cosmetic appearance of the stoma by avoiding a spout and to do away with the need for an appliance to be worn continuously.

The technique is to fold the distal ileum on itself to form a pouch with a valve at its end (Fig. 21.7). The pouch is emptied at the patient's convenience with a tube. The procedure is complex and has had a high incidence of complications and failure of continence.

- Ileal pouch and ileo-anal anastomosis

The technique is to form a similar pouch but to anastomose it to the anal verge after all large-bowel mucosa has

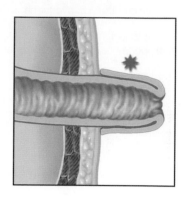

• **Fig. 21.5** Operation of Proctocolectomy and Ileostomy

• BOX 21.8	Complications Related to Ileostomy

- Para-ileostomy hernia
- Protrusion/prolapse of ileostomy
- Renal calculi
- Electrolyte imbalance
- Para-stomal dermatitis
- Psychological/sexual problems

been removed (Fig. 21.8). Patients usually defecate normally (although usually fairly frequently) and, in some cases, they need to empty the pouch by use of a per-anal tube. The operation is technically complex with a significant complication rate, but is a major advance over proctocolectomy and permanent ileostomy.

Crohn's Disease of the Colon

This condition characteristically affects the small intestine (for more detailed treatment, see Ch. 22) but may involve the large bowel either in isolation (20% of cases) or in combination with small-intestinal disease (50% of cases).

Clinical Features

Symptoms

The diarrhoea and other complaints are often indistinguishable from those of ulcerative colitis, and the systemic upset is the same. However, there may be associated complaints of perianal problems such as fissure and fistula (Ch. 22).

Patients with ileocolic Crohn's disease usually have less diarrhoea and more abdominal pain.

Clinical Findings

The abdominal findings may be non-specific, although a mass in the right iliac fossa or an abdominal wall abscess/fistula are very suggestive. There is a high incidence of anal lesions such as:

- fistula
- perianal abscess
- chronic fissure
- anal ulceration
- oedematous skin tags

Investigation

Sigmoidoscopy or colonoscopy may not distinguish the disease from ulcerative colitis. Characteristic histopathological features may be found on biopsy including transmural inflammation, crypt abscesses and granuloma formation.

Barium enema (Fig. 21.9) shows segmental and discontinuous involvement of the large bowel and the presence of fissures and fistulae in the bowel wall. Strictures are not uncommon. CT and/or MRI scanning may give additional information about the extent of disease (especially the presence of small bowel disease, which may also be demonstrated on barium follow-through examinations) and complications such as localized perforation or internal fistula. They may also be useful in the assessment of perianal disease.

Management

The medical treatment is similar to that for ulcerative colitis (see above). In the acute setting, a corticosteroid

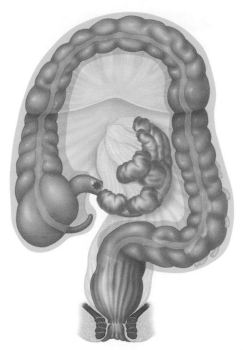
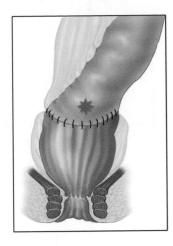

• **Fig. 21.6** Colectomy and Ileorectal Anastomosis

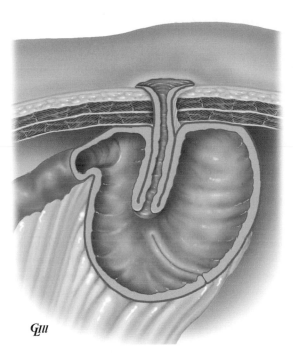

• **Fig. 21.7** The Continent Ileostomy

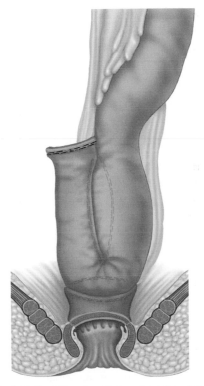

• **Fig. 21.8** Ileal Pouch with Ileo-Anal Anastomosis

as monotherapy or addition of azathioprine may help in inducing a remission. Biological therapy with infliximab or adalimumab can also be added. Colectomy may be required for severe or intractable disease.

Ischaemic Colitis

This condition is uncommon in those under the age of 50. The frequent occurrence at the splenic flexure, where the arterial anastomotic loops are least well developed, suggests that the cause is reduced arterial input, perhaps from the development of degenerative arterial disease.

Clinical Features
Symptoms
Symptoms are:
- acute left-sided abdominal pain
- dark red rectal bleeding

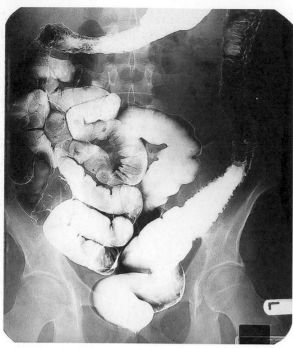

Fig. 21.9 Barium Enema in a Patient with Crohn's Disease of the Large Bowel Note deep ulcers and sparing of rectum.

Clinical Findings

Clinical findings are:
- fever
- hypotension
- abdominal tenderness

Investigation and Management

A plain abdominal X-ray may show a distended splenic flexure in which oedematous mucosa may be detected. This finding is confirmed by CT scanning or barium enema where the thumbprinting of the mucosa is apparent. In some cases, the diagnosis may be confirmed by colonoscopic biopsy, but the risk of perforation is increased.

Spontaneous resolution is the rule. Occasionally, progression leads to gangrene, for which emergency surgery is required. Intermediate between these is ischaemia that leads to late stricture, for which surgery is needed.

Infective Diseases

There is a wide variety of organisms capable of causing colitis (Box 21.9). They are of surgical importance only because of the need to detect treatable infective agents in patients who may at first sight seem to have ulcerative colitis or Crohn's disease.

Radiation Colitis and Proctitis

Radiation therapy is an important part of treatment of patients with gastrointestinal and pelvic malignancies. However, one of its main adverse outcomes is radiation colitis/proctitis.

• BOX 21.9 Infective Causes of Colitis/Proctitis

Bacterial
- *Salmonella*
- *Shigella*
- *Mycobacterium tuberculosis*
- *Staphylococcus*
- *Gonococcus*
- *Campylobacter*
- *Clostridium difficile*

Viral
- *Enteroviruses*
- *Cytomegaloviruses*
- *Herpes*

Spirochaetal
- *Treponema pallidum*

Chlamydial
- *Lymphogranuloma pallidum*

Protozoal
- *Entamoeba histolytica*

Metazoal
- *Schistosoma mansoni*
- *Mycotic*
- *Histoplasma capsulatum*

Pathological Features

Histological changes in radiation-related intestinal damage include:
- Transient mucosal atrophy
- Submucosal oedema
- Inflammation and infiltration of the lamina propria with polymorphonuclear leucocytes and plasma cells
- Obliterative endarteritis of the small vessels of the bowel wall in chronic radiation injury

Aetiology

Radiation injuries to the bowel wall are due to damage to the lipid layer of the cell membrane, proteins and cellular DNA. The effects are maximal in cells with a high mitotic rate.

Patient-related risk factors associated with an increased risk of radiation-induced colitis are listed in Box 21.10.

Clinical Features

The commonest symptoms are colicky abdominal pain, tenesmus, nausea and vomiting, anorexia, diarrhoea, per rectal bleeding and fever. Rarely, they present with massive lower GI bleeding or bowel perforation.

Almost all patients who receive more than 1.5 Gy per day develop acute radiation enteritis either while undergoing therapy or shortly after treatment is completed.

Radiation proctitis is seen in patients with prostate, cervical and anal cancers.

Chronic radiation colitis may present months or years after completion of radiation therapy or can continue from the acute phase. Most patients develop symptoms at a median 8 to 12 months after completion of radiotherapy.

Investigations

Blood tests may show evidence of chronic anaemia and malnutrition due to chronic blood loss and malnutrition. In the case of perforation or bowel obstruction, the inflammatory markers may also be high.

CT is the best study to reveal bowel obstruction (partial or complete) secondary to radiation colitis. Endoscopy is generally avoided in the acute phases of radiation enteritis because of the risk of perforation. However, it may still be necessary for establishing the diagnosis or treating the haemorrhage. In this case, colonoscopy should be performed with caution and little bowel insufflation.

Findings include a friable intestinal and rectal mucosa with areas of superficial ulceration.

In chronic radiation colitis, the mucosa appears thin, friable and pale with prominent submucosal telangiectasias. There is also fibrous induration and ulceration. The cardinal sign in chronic radiation damage is the presence of small-vessel vasculopathy.

In acute colitis, biopsies show mucosal inflammation with necrosis and ulceration, crypt atrophy and crypt abscesses.

Management

Prevention involves trying to minimize the dose of radiation to the bowel while maximizing the dose to the tumour itself. Amifostine administered intravenously has shown promise in preventing symptoms of acute proctitis and decreasing the severity of chronic proctitis symptoms.

Treatment of radiation proctitis includes medical management (sucralfate enemas, 4 weeks of metronidazole, SCFAs, vitamin A, tropical formalin, hyperbaric oxygen), endoscopic (dilatation for strictures, thermoelectric cauterization, cryotherapy, argon plasma coagulation, radiofrequency ablation) and surgical therapies (diversion stoma, resection surgery).

NEOPLASIA

Benign Neoplasms

Adenomas

Aetiology and Epidemiology

Benign large-bowel neoplasms are associated with a number of different conditions, many of which have a genetic

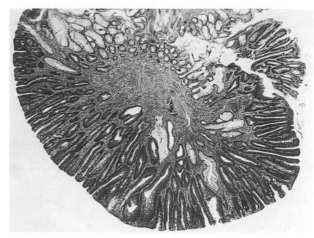

• **Fig. 21.10** Histological Appearance of a Tubular Adenoma of the Colon

component (see, for example, familial adenomatous polyposis, later). The lifetime incidence in the Western world's population is 20–25%, but elsewhere the condition is much less common. Adenomas are linked to a low-fibre, high red meat, high-fat diet. The majority of colonic cancers arise from pre-existing adenomatous polyps.

Pathological Features

The most common and important neoplasm is an adenoma which arises from the glandular or epithelial cells. The tumour is most often a polyp with a stalk, but flat (sessile) lesions also occur. The histological appearance is a basis for classification into tubular, villous or tubulovillous (Fig. 21.10). Tubular polyps tend to be pedunculated and spherical; the other two types are more often multi-fronded and sessile.

They may be single or multiple, and, in some hereditary syndromes, many hundreds or thousands are present. The important clinicopathological correlate of an adenoma is that it is a premalignant lesion and exposure of its surface over the years to the faecal stream may initiate the development of an adenocarcinoma. This polyp–cancer sequence is most likely in lesions over 1 cm in diameter. Not all polyps are adenomas. The other causes of protrusions of mucosa that are anatomically polyps are given in Box 21.11.

Clinical Features and Diagnosis

Most adenomas are both asymptomatic and devoid of signs. Unless there is a family history or there are so many lesions that bleeding is obvious, the diagnosis is made either as the result of a screening programme (see later) or on incidental examination of the large bowel by colonoscopy or CT colonoscopy (virtual colonoscopy, CT colonography) for unexplained iron deficiency anaemia or other symptoms.

A rare clinical syndrome is when a villous adenoma in the rectum is sufficiently large that large quantities of potassium-rich mucus are lost from it and the patient becomes hypokalaemic.

• BOX 21.11 Classification of Colorectal Polyps

Neoplastic
- Adenoma
  - Tubular
  - Tubulovillous
  - Villous

Non-neoplastic
- Hamartoma
  - Juvenile
  - Peutz–Jeghers
- Inflammatory
  - Lymphoid
  - Inflamed oedematous mucosa
- Miscellaneous
  - Metaplastic
  - Connective tissue polyps

Management

The finding of an adenomatous polyp, particularly if it is larger than 1 cm, requires the following action:
- Complete examination of the large bowel by colonoscopy to exclude or identify other similar neoplasms
- Removal of all lesions, which can usually be achieved endoscopically
- Regular lifelong surveillance for recurrence and/or the development of large-bowel cancer in selected cases (Fig. 21.11)

Familial Adenomatous Polyposis (FAP)

This is an autosomal dominant condition with a high degree of penetrance.

Pathological Features

Multiple adenomatous polyps develop in the colon and also sometimes in the small bowel, especially the duodenum. The colonic polyps usually start between the ages of 13 and 30 years, although sometimes this does not take place until the fourth decade. Progression through the polyp–cancer sequence is inevitable. Not infrequently, there are other manifestations outside of the colon, including desmoid tumours, congenital hypertrophy of the retinal pigment epithelium (CHRPE), fibromas, osteomas or sebaceous cysts. The latter three conditions linked with FAP are known as Gardner's syndrome.

Clinical Features

The condition is initially asymptomatic, although a family history may be present. Blood from the rectum is the most common symptom, and there may be other less specific complaints such as tenesmus and diarrhoea.

Diagnosis and Management

The diagnosis is made by endoscopy. Wireless capsule endoscopy of the small bowel should be done to exclude small-bowel polyps. Siblings should be examined. Total colectomy is essential because of the universal progression to cancer. An ileo-anal pouch reconstruction is usually possible.

Malignant Neoplasms

Epidemiology and Aetiology

Malignant tumours of the large bowel are common and are the third commonest cause of cancer death in the UK at 18,000 per year. The highest incidence of adenocarcinoma, which accounts for 98% of the tumours, occurs in New Zealand, Australia, Western Europe and North America. The lowest is in Asia, Africa and South America, although Argentina is an exception. The disease can develop at any age from the second decade, but the peak incidence is in the sixth and subsequent decades. The important aetiological factors are described below.
- *Dietary factors*

  Bile salt conversion: There is indirect evidence that a diet rich in animal fat is a major risk factor. It is suggested that such a diet, common in the Western world, produces an environment within the gut which favours bacteria that convert bile salts to carcinogens, and work on experimental animals supports this hypothesis.

  Low intake of fibre has also been claimed to predispose to neoplasia because it slows transit and thus increases the time of exposure of the mucosa to carcinogens.
- *Adenomatous polyps*

  The polyp–cancer sequence is considered above. It probably accounts for the development of the great majority of large bowel cancers, a matter which emphasizes the importance of screening (see later).
- *Genetic factors*

  Familial adenomatous polyposis (FAP) as an inevitable cause of cancer is described above. There is a two- to three-fold increased risk to a first-degree relative of a patient with adenocarcinoma. Hereditary non-polyposis colon cancer (HNPCC, also known as Lynch syndrome) is an autosomal dominant condition, which has a high risk of colon cancer and other cancers including endometrium, ovary, stomach, small intestine, hepatobiliary tract, upper urinary tract, brain and skin. The increased risk is due to inherited mutations that impair DNA mismatch repair with resultant micro-satellite instability. MLH1, MSH2 and MSH6 gene mutations account for almost all cases. HNPCC leads to between 2% and 7% of colorectal cancers.
- *Inflammatory bowel disease*

  Long-standing and total ulcerative colitis as a cause is described above. Crohn's disease is also associated with a fourfold increase in the risk of colorectal carcinoma.

Pathological Features

Distribution

The anatomical distribution of colonic carcinoma is as follows:
- Rectum 37%
- Sigmoid 27%
- Caecum 14%
- Ascending colon 7%
- Descending colon 5%
- Transverse colon 4%
- Hepatic flexure 3%
- Splenic flexure 3%

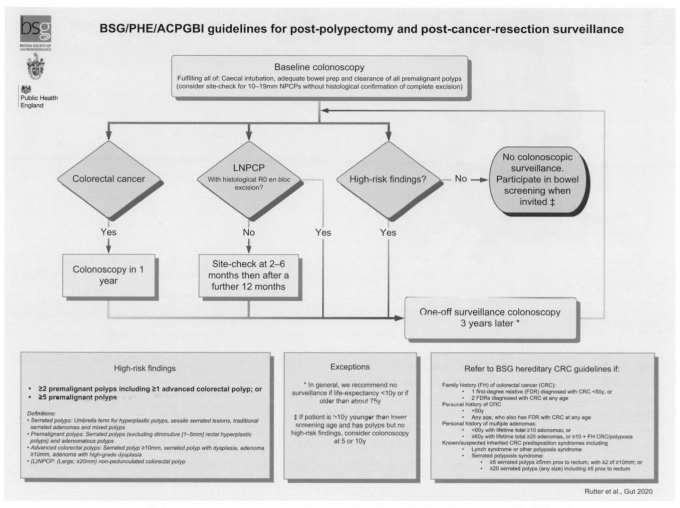

• Fig. 21.11 Colonoscopic Follow-Up of Colonic Adenomas (From Rutter MD, East J, Rees CJ, et al. British Society of Gastroenterology/Association of Coloproctology of Great Britain and Ireland/Public Health England post-polypectomy and post-colorectal cancer resection surveillance guidelines. Gut. 2020; 69, 201–223.)

Synchronous Lesions

Up to 3% of patients have one or more synchronous cancers, and 75% have at least one benign adenoma.

Macroscopic Classification

Tumours are classified as follows:

- polypoidal
- ulcerating
- annular
- semi-annular
- mucinous

Spread

Direct extension in the transverse axis of the bowel wall eventually causes complete encirclement. Tumour cells which arise in the mucosa penetrate the submucosa and muscle to reach the serosal surface of the bowel, or, where the bowel is extraperitoneal, as in the rectum, they spread into the fascia and the structures contained in it such as the sacral plexus (posteriorly), the ureters (laterally), and the bladder in the male or the uterus and cervix in the female (anteriorly).

Lymphatic permeation and embolization carry tumour cells initially to local (paracolic) nodes and from there to

nodes which lie on the course of the blood supply to the bowel. In consequence, spread is largely upwards towards the aorta and the portal vein.

Haematogenous: Malignant cells can often be seen within the lumen of capillaries and small veins in sections taken from colorectal tumours. They are probably the source of emboli which enter the tributaries of the portal vein and so reach the liver, which may be involved at the time of treatment in up to 40% of cases. Spread beyond the liver to lung, kidney and bone is uncommon at diagnosis.

Transcoelomic implantation follows penetration to the serosal surface and causes ascites. Cells may also be implanted on the ovaries

Direct implantation: Exfoliated cells remain viable within the lumen of the bowel and may be implanted if the mucosa is breached – as at the site of an anastomosis or in a haemorrhoidectomy wound if that procedure is carried out in a patient with an unsuspected proximal carcinoma.

Staging

The conventional method of staging is by the Dukes classification (Fig. 21.12):

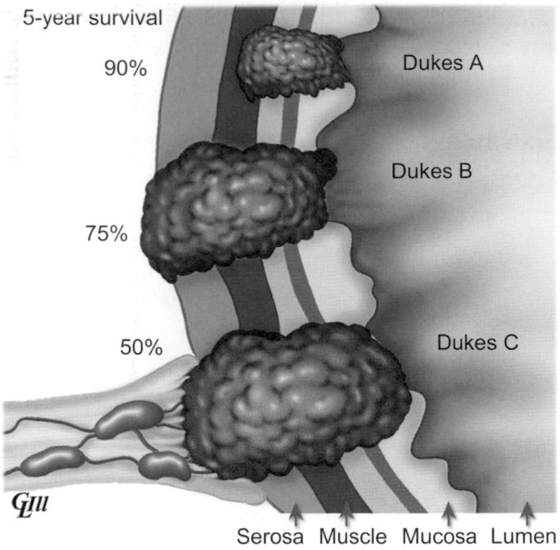

• **Fig. 21.12** Dukes Staging of Colonic Carcinoma

• Stage A – the neoplastic cells are confined to the mucosa. The 5-year survival is 90%.
• Stage B – the tumour has extended through all muscle layers and possibly reached the serosa; metastases to lymph nodes are absent. The 5-year survival is 75%.
• Stage C – lymph node metastasis has occurred. The 5-year survival is 50%. Stage C cases are often divided into C1 (local lymph node involvement only) and C2 (more proximal nodes involved). C2 carries a worse prognosis than C1.
• Stage D – this was not part of the original classification but is often used to describe a patient with disseminated metastatic disease. The 5-year survival is 6%.

The TNM (Table 21.3) system is also widely used.

Screening for Colorectal Cancer

The good results obtained in Dukes stage A cancer and the known polyp–cancer sequence encouraged the idea that attempts should be made to detect asymptomatic polyps and early cancers. A nationwide screening programme is available offering testing for faecal occult blood every 2 years from the age of 60 to 70 years. If blood is detected, individuals are invited to undergo colonoscopy. This test has shown significant limitations; for example, a sensitivity of only 50%, being less sensitive in detecting cancer in women and also in patients with rectal or right-sided cancer. Finally, uptake is only 50%.

Another screening test introduced in England to improve early detection is a flexible sigmoidoscopy to both women and men at the age of 55. This resulted in a reduction in disease incidence. Again, with limitations due to the practicality issues it poses in delivering such a service, yet another stool test called faecal immunochemical testing (FIT) was being introduced in 2018 in England. There are significant advantages as it is easier to use and can be measured more reliably by a machine than by human eye, it is more sensitive in detecting blood in stool, has an increased sensitivity

TABLE 21.3	TNM Staging in Colorectal Cancer
TNM Staging	
T (Primary tumour)	
Tx	Primary tumour cannot be assessed
T0	No evidence of primary tumour
Tis	Carcinoma in situ
T1	Tumour invades mucosa and submucosa
T2	Tumour invades muscularis propria
T3	Tumour invades through muscularis propria into subserosa or into non-peritonealized pericolic or perirectal tissues
T4	Tumour perforates the visceral peritoneum or directly invades other organs or structures
N (Regional lymph nodes)	
Nx	Regional lymph nodes cannot be assessed
N0	No regional lymph node metastasis
N1	Metastasis in 1–3 pericolic or perirectal lymph nodes
N2	Metastasis in 4 or more pericolic or perirectal lymph nodes
M (Distant metastasis)	
M0	No distant metastasis
M1	Distant metastasis

in detecting cancers and has a higher compliance to the faecal occult blood test.

Regular screening should reduce deaths from colorectal cancer by 16%. High-risk groups (strong family history, e.g. HNPCC, those with previous adenomatous polyps, etc.) should already be included in a more intensive screening programme, and start testing at an earlier age.

Clinical Features

Symptoms

Common symptoms include change in bowel habit, rectal bleeding, mucus discharge per rectum, abdominal pain, malaise, weight loss and tenesmus.

A distinction can be drawn between the presentation of tumours in the right side, the left side and the rectum.

Right-sided tumours have non-specific complaints such as malaise, weight loss, vague abdominal pain and, occasionally, a self-detected mass in the abdomen. A frequent reason for the patient seeking medical advice is the development of symptoms of iron deficiency anaemia: any patient who does so and in whom the cause is not obvious should undergo urgent full investigation of the large bowel and upper GI tract, usually done by combined upper GI endoscopy and colonoscopy. The liquid nature of the contents of the right side make presentation with intestinal obstruction rare.

Left-sided tumours are more likely to present with obstructive symptoms, because the stool is semi-solid or completely solid and the calibre of the bowel is less. There is colicky abdominal pain and a change in bowel habit which may include either constipation or diarrhoea, or alternation between the two. A distal tumour may lead to the passage of mucus which is confused with a loose motion. Visible blood in the stool is rare (10%). Acute intestinal obstruction may supervene.

Rectal tumours are more likely to be associated with rectal bleeding, usually on defecation, and mucous discharge is common as is tenesmus.

A growth that has spread locally may cause:
- faecal incontinence from invasion of the anal sphincters
- back pain because of involvement of the sacral plexus
- urinary infection, a rectovesical fistula or renal failure through infiltration of the ureters

Physical Findings
These are often absent. A mass may be palpable in the abdomen or on rectal examination. In advanced disease, weight loss may be obvious, there may be evidence of spread (ascites and hepatomegaly) and signs of bowel obstruction may be present.

Investigation

Sigmoidoscopy
All patients with symptoms that suggest a large-bowel carcinoma must have a digital rectal examination and colonoscopy. Any mucosal abnormality is biopsied. However, sigmoidoscopy can only see, at best, as far as the mid-sigmoid colon (about 25 cm) using the rigid instrument, or to the splenic flexure with a flexible sigmoidoscope. Full visualization of the large bowel requires colonoscopy, barium enema or CT colonoscopy (virtual colonoscopy).

Colonoscopy
Direct visualization of the entire colon is the investigation of choice, but the procedure is expensive in time and resources and can be technically difficult. It carries a small risk of perforation (1 in 500–1000 procedures). Even if a distal colonic or rectal cancer is found, it is important to examine the proximal colon to exclude synchronous tumours or polyps.

Barium Enema
Barium enema was the traditional method of investigating the colon. Lesions appear as an 'apple-core' stricture, although false negatives can be up to 7%. Identified lesions require follow-up colonoscopy for biopsy or treatment (Fig. 21.13). This modality is largely defunct given other techniques would offer the same or better image quality.

CT Pneumocolon (Virtual Pneumocolon)
After bowel preparation, air is insufflated into the rectum and colon. Prone and supine scans are acquired and mucosal lesions readily identified. In the case of a probable cancer being seen, the scan may also be used to exclude metastatic disease. The scan also picks up incidental extra-colonic abnormalities.

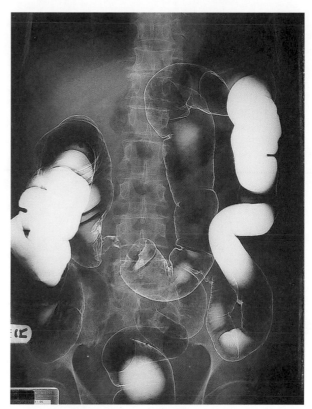

• **Fig. 21.13** Barium Enema Demonstrating an 'Apple-Core' Lesion

Biomarkers
Tumour Markers
- Carcinoembryonic antigen (CEA) is currently used in practice to monitor CRC recurrence and as a prognostic factor. Its overall sensitivity for detecting primary CRC is 37%. Due to its low sensitivity and specificity, it is not used as a diagnostic marker but instead it is currently the most useful marker in early detection of liver metastasis in patients diagnosed with colorectal cancer.
- Examples of tissue biomarkers:
  - Microsatellite instability (MSI): these are short sequences of 1–6 base pairs in the genome and have a high risk of mutations which are corrected by the MMR systems. Localized CRC with MSI have a better prognosis than the ones with microsatellite stability.
  - KRAS: mutations to this gene cause an activation of the eGFR pathway. Mutations to this gene confer resistance to anti-eGFR antibodies, cetuximab and panitumumab. It is therefore an important predictive factor to response to treatment with eGFR inhibitors.
  - BRAF: This gene is frequently mutated in CRC. BRAF V600E mutation in the presence of microsatellite stable (MSS) form, is associated with poor prognosis.

A preoperative CT scan is required to assess the local extent of the tumour and also exclude or define metastatic disease. In some cases, PET scanning may be used to better assess metastatic disease. MRI scanning is the best modality to assess the local extent of rectal cancers.

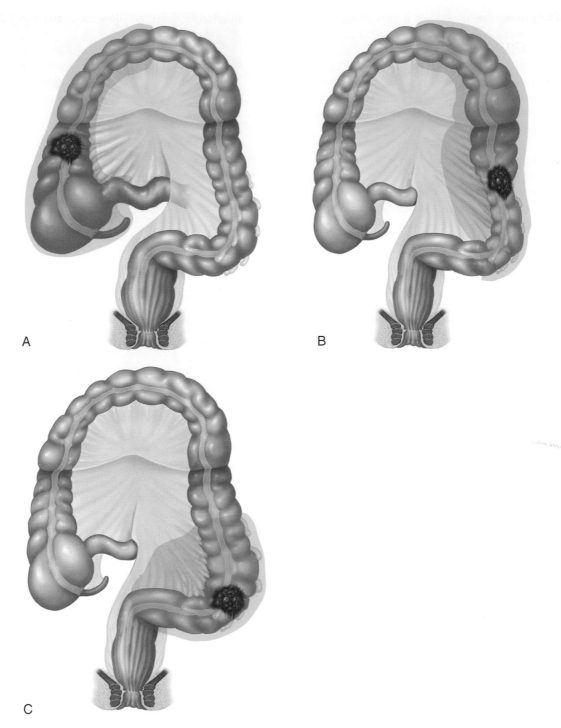

• **Fig. 21.14** (A) Right hemicolectomy, (B) left hemicolectomy and (C) sigmoid colectomy

Management

The management of colorectal cancer has become a truly multispecialty program in which the surgeon plays a vital role. Patients are discussed at a multidisciplinary meeting (MDT) and a treatment plan agreed. Laparoscopic or laparoscopic-assisted operations are being increasingly performed for patients with colorectal cancer. These usually result in less postoperative pain, smaller scars and a more rapid recovery compared with traditional open operations. There is good evidence that, performed in

well-trained hands, laparoscopic colorectal resection does not compromise tumour clearance or lymph node harvest.

Colon Carcinoma

The treatment of Dukes A to C disease is primarily by surgical removal, and this is accompanied in B and C tumours by adjuvant therapy. Right-sided tumours are removed by a right hemicolectomy and those on the left by a resection tailored to the segment of bowel involved (Fig. 21.14). The

- Bowel preparation by oral laxative or whole gut irrigation
  - not used by all surgeons
- Antibiotic chemoprophylaxis
- Thromboembolism prophylaxis
- Correct anaemia
- Correct electrolyte deficiencies

- Haemorrhage
- Ureteric damage
  - Urinary leakage
  - Ureteric stricture
- Damage to bladder function
  - Acute retention
  - Urinary incontinence
- Impaired sexual function – erectile dysfunction, retrograde ejaculation – nerve injury
- Damage to duodenum (right hemicolectomy)
- Damage to spleen (left hemicolectomy)
- Anastomotic complications
  - Stricture
  - Leakage
- Complications of stoma
  - Parastomal hernia
  - Prolapse
  - Electrolyte imbalance
  - Ischaemia
  - Stenosis
- Diarrhoea/constipation

preoperative preparation and the common complications of surgery are given in Boxes 21.12 and 21.13.

Rectal Carcinoma

Patients with early rectal cancer (T1 tumours <3 cm in diameter) and who are suitable for local resection with transanal endoscopic microsurgery (TEMS) should be discussed in a unit which has an early rectal cancer MDT.

Patients with rectal cancer, particularly the more locally advanced tumours that extend close to the proposed surgical resection margin, are usually treated preoperatively with chemoradiotherapy – a combination of radiotherapy with concomitant chemotherapy (either intravenous fluorouracil or oral capecitabine, the latter sometimes combined with irinotecan). Such treatment shrinks most tumours and reduces the risk of 'margin positive' resections and consequently also local pelvic recurrence.

A tumour in the mid- or upper rectum is removed by resecting the distal colon and involved rectum and restoring continuity by joining the large bowel to the stump of rectum – this is called an anterior resection (Fig. 21.15A). The anastomosis may be done with either sutures or staples, and the latter are particularly useful when the rectal stump is short and access difficult. The patient may have a proximal

defunctioning stoma to allow the anastomosis to heal, especially in low rectal anastomoses. Decisions are tailored to each individual patient's comorbidities, age, potential bowel function and preferences. A low rectal tumour may require the removal of the whole rectum and adjacent sphincters – this is called an abdominoperineal excision and end colostomy (see Fig. 21.15B). Abdominoperineal excisions can be extra-levator or intersphincteric. The advocated advantages of the extra-levator are to improve cancer clearance and reduce local recurrence.

The operations can be open, laparoscopic, robotic or transanal. The CLASICC[3], COLOR II[4] and COREAN[5] trials compared open versus laparoscopic operations for rectal cancer and found the laparoscopic oncological outcome results to be as good as for open procedures. However, laparoscopic procedures for low rectal tumours can be technically challenging and results from ACOSOG Z6051[6] and ALaCaRT[7] trials showed an involved circumferential margin rate of 11.3% versus 9% in open operations. The trans anal total mesorectal excision (TaTME), which allows the surgeon to start the operation transanally and can first assess whether distal transection can be performed with clear margins and the feasibility of performing a sphincter-preserving procedure, has been advocated as a way to avoid the increased rates of involved circumferential margins. TaTME is also credited with lower operative times, although that would mean a two-team approach. The St Gallen consensus,[8] from 37 colorectal surgeons from 20 countries and 5 continents published in March 2018, suggested that the TaTME may be technically easier than the abdominal TME in patients with a narrow pelvis, obese patients and patients with bulky mid/distal rectal tumours. Reports of higher than expected local recurrence by the Norwegian Colorectal Cancer Group has brought TaTME under scrutiny and further studies looking at its safety profile. The literature is still divided on the potential benefits of this approach and more research is being undertaken currently.

Robotic surgery has also been proposed to deal with the limitations of conventional laparoscopy. It has a high cost and longer operatives compared to laparoscopy; however, its conversion rates compared to laparoscopic procedures are significantly reduced. Other advantages include a clear view of planes via a three-dimensional view with a high definition camera controlled by the surgeon, intuitive instrument handling and endowrist instruments. The ROLARR[9] trial, which randomized 471 patients to robotic assisted or to conventional laparoscopic surgery for high anterior resection or low anterior resection or APE, showed that robotic surgery had a conversion rate of 8.1% and the laparoscopic group had a 12.2% conversion rate ($P = 0.16$). It did not show a significant difference in postoperative or intraoperative complications, 30-day mortality, sexual dysfunction and bladder dysfunction. It did, however, show a difference in patients with difficult pelvic anatomy, such as in obese males.

Ultimately, the choice of surgery will be decided on patient factors, surgeon preference and expertise as well as the facilities and equipment available at each hospital.

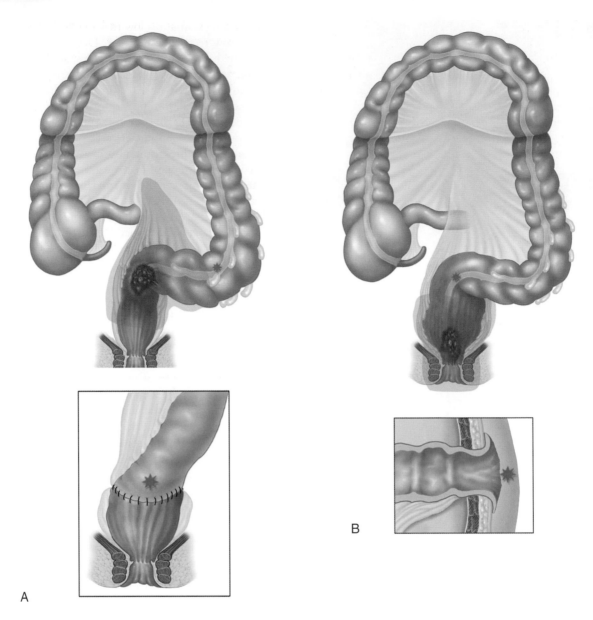

• **Fig. 21.15** Rectal Carcinoma Surgery (A) Anterior resection of rectum. Shaded area resected. (B) Abdominoperineal excision of rectum and anus. Shaded area is resected.

Neoadjuvant Therapy

In rectal cancers, the addition of pre-operative (chemo) radiotherapy (CRT) is to reduce the incidence of local recurrence and facilitate clear circumferential margins (CRM).

Radiation

Radiotherapy is used for some rectal cancers before surgery (see earlier). It can also be used to treat early rectal cancer – either alone or after local excision, locally advanced colon cancer after margin-positive resection or for palliation of metastatic disease.

Chemotherapy

Patients with lymph node metastases confirmed after colonic resection for adenocarcinoma are offered adjuvant chemotherapy with FOLFOX (a combination of folinic acid (leucovorin), 5-fluorouracil and oxaliplatin) or CAPEOX (oxaliplatin and capecitabine) or single agent capecitabine.

In patients with stage I (Dukes A) colorectal cancer, adjuvant chemotherapy is not recommended. In stage II, patients with a high risk should be considered for adjuvant chemotherapy and, if they have a low risk, should be considered for clinical trials if available. In patients with stage III, adjuvant chemotherapy is recommended to those who are fit. In stage IV with both operable and inoperable metastasis, chemotherapy is recommended. Cetuximab (a monoclonal epidermal growth factor inhibitor) is now also recommended in addition to these regimens for patients with metastatic disease confined to the liver.

Hepatic Metastases

Liver metastases, when the only site of secondary or recurrent cancer, are increasingly being treated by liver resection (see Ch. 23) or other ablative techniques such as radiofrequency ablation (RFA), microwave treatment or cryotherapy. These alternative technologies are usually given using image guidance – ultrasound or CT scanning – either percutaneously using specially designed probes or at open operation when they may be combined with hepatic resection. In all cases, patients are also treated with chemotherapy before and/or after resection or ablation using the agents described above for palliative treatment of metastatic disease. Prolonged survival is increasingly seen, even in the presence of liver secondaries, as a result of such multi-modality treatment.

Further Reading

Association of Coloproctology of Great Britain and Ireland (ACPGBI). *The Case for Colorectal Cancer Screening*; 2013.

NICE guidelines. *Management of Crohn's Disease*; Published 3 May 2019 (www.nice.org.uk/guidance/ng129).

NICE guidelines. *Management of Ulcerative Colitis*; Published 3 May 2019. NICE guideline [NG130].

Phillips RKS. *Colorectal Surgery: A Companion to Specialist Surgical Practice*. 4th ed. Edinburgh: Elsevier Saunders; 2009.

References

1. Lacey BE, Mearin F, Chang L, et al. Bowel disorders. *Gastroenterology*. 2016;150:1393–1407.
2. Ceresoli M, Coccolini F, Montori G, Catena F, Sartelli M and Ansaloni L. Laparoscopic lavage versus resection in perforated diverticulitis with purulent peritonitis: a meta-analysis of randomized controlled trials. *World J Emerg Surg*. 2016;11(1):42.
3. Jayne DG, Guillou PJ, Thorpe H, et al. Randomized trial of laparoscopic-assisted resection of colorectal carcinoma: 3-year results of the UK MRC CLASICC Trial Group. *J Clin Oncol*. 2007;25(21):3061–3068.
4. van der Pas MH, Haglind E, Cuesta MA, Fürst A, Lacy AM, Hop WC, et al. Laparoscopic versus open surgery for rectal cancer (COLOR II): short-term outcomes of a randomised, phase 3 trial. *Lancet Oncol*. 2013;14(3):210–218.
5. Kang SB, Park JW, Jeong SY, Nam BH, Choi HS, Kim DW, et al. Open versus laparoscopic surgery for mid or low rectal cancer after neoadjuvant chemoradiotherapy (COREAN trial): short-term outcomes of an open-label randomised controlled trial. *Lancet Oncol*. 2010;11(7):637–645.
6. Fleshman J, Branda M, Sargent DJ, Boller AM, George V, Abbas M, et al. Effect of laparoscopic-assisted resection vs open resection of stage II or III rectal cancer on pathologic outcomes: the ACOSOG Z6051 randomized clinical trial. *JAMA*. 2015;314(13):1346–1355.
7. Stevenson AR, Solomon MJ, Lumley JW, Hewett P, et al. Effect of laparoscopic-assisted resection vs open resection on pathological outcomes in rectal cancer: the ALaCaRT randomized clinical trial. *JAMA*. 2015;314(13):1356–1363.
8. Adamina M, Buchs NC, Penna M, Hompes R, St. Gallen Colorectal Consensus Expert Group. St Gallen consensus on safe implementation of transanal total mesorectal excision. *Surg Endosc*. 2018;32:1091–1103.
9. Jayne D, Pigazzi A, Marshall H, et al. Effect of robotic-assisted vs conventional laparoscopic surgery on risk of conversion to open laparotomy among patients undergoing resection for rectal cancer: the ROLARR randomized clinical trial. *JAMA*. 2017;318(16):1569–1580.

22

Common Anal Conditions

Anatomy

Embryology

The hindgut gives rise to the distal third of the transverse colon, the descending colon, the sigmoid, the rectum and the upper part of the anal canal. The distal part of the anal canal is derived from the ectoderm. The junction between the endodermal and ectodermal regions of the anal canal is delineated by the pectinate or dentate line. Failure of the separating membrane between the endoderm and ectoderm results in *imperforate anus*. At this point, the epithelium changes from columnar to stratified squamous epithelium. It also means that the distal aspect of the anal canal is supplied by the inferior rectal arteries (derived from the internal pudendal arteries) and the caudal part is supplied by the superior rectal artery, a continuation of the inferior mesenteric artery.

Macroscopically

- The anal canal measures approximately 4 cm long and is directed downwards and backwards from the rectum to end at the anal orifice.
- The anal canal walls form a powerful sphincter mechanism and is comprised of:
  - The internal anal sphincter: involuntary muscle, which extends caudally with the circular muscle of the rectum.
  - The external anal sphincter: voluntary muscle, which surrounds the internal sphincter and extends downwards and medially to occupy a position which is below and lateral to the lower end of the anal sphincter. At the upper end, the external sphincter merges with the levator ani fibres (Fig. 22.1A). The *anorectal ring* is where the deep part of the external anal sphincter fuses with the internal

sphincter and levator ani, marking the end of the anal canal and the beginning of the rectum. The anorectal ring lies about 2.5 cm from the anal margin.
- Relations:
  - Posteriorly: anococcygeal body and coccyx
  - Laterally: ischiorectal fossa
  - Anteriorly: perineal body, penis (males)/vagina (females)
- Arterial supply: superior rectal artery (derived from the inferior mesenteric artery) and corresponding superior rectal vein which drains into the inferior mesenteric vein and portal vein, for the caudal part. Inferior rectal vessels derived from the internal pudendal and ultimately the internal iliac artery and vein for the distal part of the anal canal. The two venous systems communicate and therefore form one of the porto-systemic anastomoses.
- Lymphatic system: above the dentate line, the lymphatic vessels drain along the superior rectal vessels to the lumbar nodes, whereas the lymphatics below the dentate line drain to the inguinal nodes.
- Nerve supply: to the upper canal this is via the autonomic plexuses, whilst the lower part is innervated by the somatic inferior rectal nerve, a terminal branch of the pudendal nerve.

Microscopically (see Fig. 22.1B):

- The upper part of the canal (proximal to the dentate line) is lined with columnar epithelium and presents vertical columns of mucosa *(the columns of Morgagni)* connected at the distal ends by valve-like folds called the *'valves of Ball'*.
- The distal part of the canal is lined by squamous epithelium.

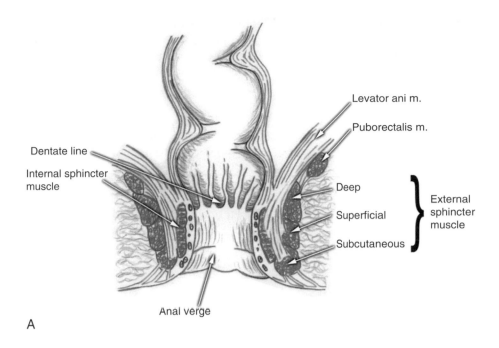

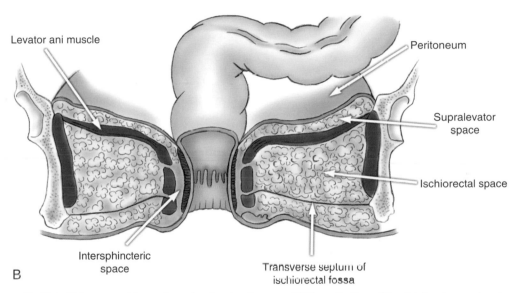

• **Fig. 22.1** (A) Anatomy of the anal canal and perianal spaces. (B) The epithelium of the distal rectum and anal canal. (Image reproduced with permission from Medscape Drugs & Diseases (https://emedicine.medscape .com/), Fistula-in-Ano, 2020, available at: https://emedicine.medscape.com/article/190234-overview.)

- Table 22.1 summarizes the differences of the anal canal above and below the dentate line.

Haemorrhoids

The anal canal mucosa contains vascular structures that are part of the normal continence mechanism and are referred to as the anal cushions.[1] When the anal cushions become enlarged and/or symptomatic, they are then considered to be pathological and are referred to as haemorrhoids. The prevalence of haemorrhoids is equal between male and female populations and they are reported to occur mostly between the fourth and sixth decades of life.[2]

Classification

The classification of Goligher (Fig. 22.2) is the most widely used categorization and it is based on the degree of prolapse[3]; however, it should be appreciated that there is a degree of inter-observer variation when this score is used. Furthermore, haemorrhoids may appear more prominent when the patient is placed in the lithotomy position under general anaesthesia and thus inter-observer variation may also confound the accuracy of this classification.

1. Grade I – do not prolapse below the dentate line
2. Grade II – prolapse out the anal canal with defecation or straining and spontaneous reduction

3. Grade III – prolapse out the anal canal with defecation or straining with manual reduction required
4. Grade IV – irreducible

Aetiology

The pathogenesis of symptomatic haemorrhoids is most likely due to weakening of the anchoring connective tissue that fixes the anal cushions above the dentate line, which then leads to

prolapse. Factors that increase intra-abdominal pressure, such as straining, constipation, pregnancy and prolonged sitting, aggravate the symptoms.[4–6] It should be appreciated that the exact aetiology of haemorrhoid formation remains unknown.

Symptoms

Patients may present with:
• painless per rectal bleeding,
• prolapse,
• mucus discharge and
• pruritus.
    Haemorrhoids can also become painful if they become strangulated or thrombosed.

Diagnosis

• The diagnosis is based on the history and physical examination, including rigid sigmoidoscopy and proctoscopy.
• Anal inspection may not reveal the presence of haemorrhoids unless they are prolapsed. It should be remembered that the prevalence of haemorrhoids is sufficiently high that they should not be assumed to be the cause of rectal bleeding.
• Endoscopic assessment of the lower gastrointestinal tract is mandatory in all but the youngest or frailest of patients, with the patient's age and other symptoms used to decide between the use of flexible sigmoidoscopy or full colonoscopy.

Management

• All patients should be advised to adopt a high-fibre diet, to avoid straining during defaecation or spending a protracted amount of time on the toilet.[7–9]

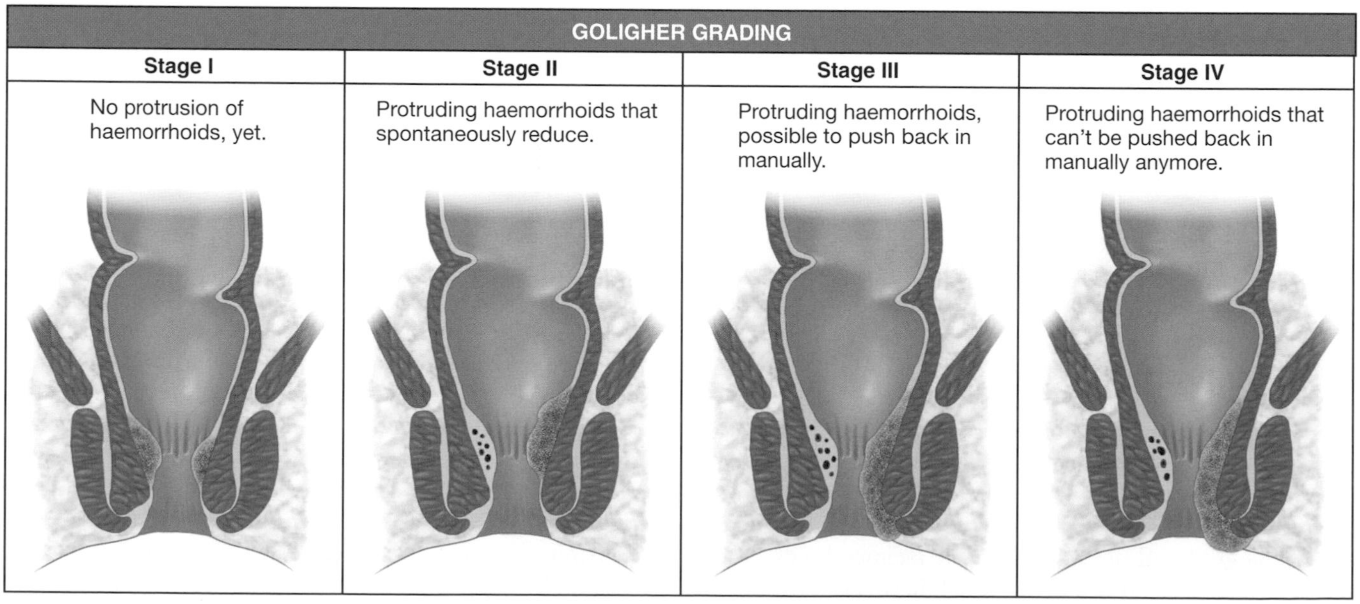

TABLE 22.1	Summary of Differences of Anal Canal Below and Above the Dentate Line.	
Above the Dentate Line	**Below the Dentate Line**
Columnar epithelium	Squamous cell epithelium
Autonomic sensory nerve supply Therefore banding or injections here are not painful	Somatic innervation
Sensitive to stretch	Sensitive to pain/touch and temperature
Hindgut arterial supply (superior rectal artery from IMA)	From inferior rectal artery (from internal pudendal artery which is a branch of the internal iliac artery)
Venous drainage to IMV and portal venous system	Venous drainage into internal pudendal vein
Lymphatic drainage follows the arterial supply to inferior mesenteric nodes	Lymphatic drainage to inguinal nodes

IMA, Inferior mesenteric artery; IMV, inferior mesenteric vein.

GOLIGHER GRADING			
Stage I	**Stage II**	**Stage III**	**Stage IV**
No protrusion of haemorrhoids, yet.	Protruding haemorrhoids that spontaneously reduce.	Protruding haemorrhoids, possible to push back in manually.	Protruding haemorrhoids that can't be pushed back in manually anymore.

• **Fig. 22.2** Goligher Grading of Internal Haemorrhoids (From https://www.slideserve.com/benjamin/gol igher-grading)

- Patients who remain symptomatic after dietary modifications and changes to their defecatory dynamics are candidates for 'office-based' procedures.
- The most widely used are:
  - rubber band ligation
  - sclerotherapy
  - infrared coagulation
- The aims of these office-based procedures are to decrease the blood flow to the haemorrhoids, reduce redundant tissue and increase haemorrhoidal fixation to the rectal wall.[10]

Rubber band ligation (RBL) (Fig. 22.3) is the most popular of the office-based procedures in the UK.[11] RBL involves placement of an elastic band to the base of the haemorrhoid to strangulate it. This results in ischaemia and necrosis of the haemorrhoid with scarring that facilitates mucosal fixation to the rectal wall. The most frequent complications are perianal pain due to misplacement of the band near or below the dentate line or bleeding. Bleeding presents 7–10 days after the procedure and is believed to be due to the resulting ulcer. RBL is the first-line procedure for second degree haemorrhoids, and a good first-line treatment for third-degree haemorrhoids.[12–14] A recent randomized study compared RBL to the haemorrhoidal artery ligation procedure (HAL). Although RBL was demonstrated to have a higher recurrence rate for second- and third-degree haemorrhoids (up to 49%), it was reported to be superior to HAL as RBL is less painful, does not require general anaesthesia and is easily repeated in the office setting.[15]

Sclerotherapy involves injection of a sclerosing agent into the apex of the haemorrhoid which results in fibrosis. It is an effective treatment for second-degree haemorrhoids but has limited efficacy for third-degree haemorrhoids.[10,11] Sclerotherapy is safer for patients with coagulation disorders, such as thrombocytopaenia or patients who receive antiplatelet or anticoagulation treatment when compared to RBL.[16] In recent years, the popularity of this technique has waned in the UK as it is not thought to offer significant benefit over improvements in diet and defecatory dynamics.

Infrared coagulation cauterizes the haemorrhoid by contact application of infrared waves. This results in sclerosis and fibrosis of the haemorrhoid. It can be used for first- and second-degree haemorrhoids with similar results to RBL but it is infrequently used in the UK.[17,18]

Surgical Treatment

For patients who report that office procedures have failed, those who cannot tolerate these procedures and those with fourth-degree haemorrhoids, surgical treatments can be considered.

Conventional haemorrhoidectomy involves excision of the haemorrhoidal tissue, the anoderm and the associated perianal skin. It is more effective for grade III haemorrhoids when compared to office procedures, but it is more painful and is associated with higher complication rates.[14] Different approaches for haemorrhoidectomy (open or closed), and using a variety of surgical devices (e.g. scissors, diathermy, laser, LigaSure or Harmonic scalpel) have been described.

Despite conventional surgical teaching there is no proven superiority for the closed technique versus the open technique when comparing recurrence and pain at defecation, with the possible exception of healing time.[19] LigaSure and harmonic scalpel haemorrhoidectomy are faster to perform and associated with less postoperative pain compared to conventional haemorrhoidectomy techniques, which may be due to decreased thermal injury.[20] There are some published data supporting open haemorrhoidectomy as the best

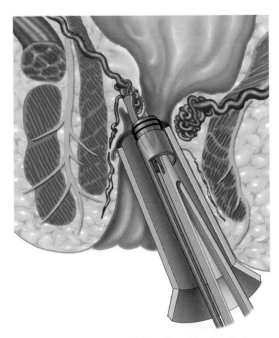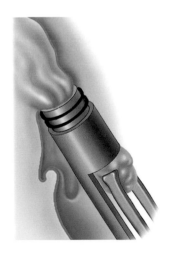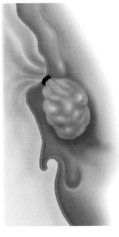

• **Fig. 22.3** Rubber band ligation for haemorrhoids. (From https://abdominalkey.com/ligasure/)

approach for refractory and fourth-degree haemorrhoids because of its low recurrence rate.[21]

Stapled haemorrhoidopexy uses a circular stapler that resects a ring of rectal mucosa above the haemorrhoids. This results in cephalad relocation of the haemorrhoids and interruption of their blood supply. It is highly effective for prolapsing internal haemorrhoids but not for haemorrhoids with external components.[22] It is reported to be less painful than conventional haemorrhoidectomy if the staple line is correctly placed, and also to have a lower postoperative complication rate.[23] Higher long-term recurrence rates have been documented when compared to conventional haemorrdoidectomy.[21,24] Furthermore, several unique complications (e.g. rectovaginal fistula, staple line bleeding and stricture at the staple line) have been described in the literature and, for the reasons outlined previously, this technique has fallen out of favour in the UK.[25]

Haemorrhoidal artery ligation is performed with the use of a Doppler probe that helps locate the haemorrhoidal artery branches. Ligation of the arterial branches above the dentate line reduces the blood flow to the haemorrhoids. For prolapsing haemorrhoids, mucosal plication is performed as well (haemorrhoidopexy). Haemorrhoidal artery ligation has less postoperative pain than haemorrhoidectomy. It is recommended for grade II and III haemorrhoids but not for fourth-degree as recurrence rates are high. The low cost, low complication rate, shorter operating time and decreased postoperative pain associated with this procedure suggest this method is a safe, quick and easy initial surgical option that patients should be offered.[26-29]

Management of Thrombosed Haemorrhoids

A thrombosed external haemorrhoid appears as a tender blue lump that is easily recognized on the anal verge. Excision of the thrombus along with the overlying skin is advised if the onset of symptoms is less than 48–72 hours. Excision of the thrombus allows rapid pain relief, lower incidence of recurrence and longer remission intervals. If the patient presents later than 72 hours, the clot will already be resolving and there is no need for surgical intervention. After 72 hours, the majority of patients report significant improvement in their pain and can be treated conservatively with dietary modifications, mild laxatives, oral and topical analgesics and sitz baths as necessary.[30-32] Ultimately, the haemorrhoid will fibrose to become an external skin tag.

Anorectal Abscess

Aetiology

- With the exception of simple skin infections, the most common theory explaining the development of true anorectal abscesses is sepsis arising from the blockage of an anal crypt gland, i.e. *cryptoglandular theory*.[33]
- Anorectal abscesses are more frequent in men than women.

- They typically occur between the second and the fourth decades of life.[34]
- This infection develops in the intersphincteric space and spreads vertical (upwards or downwards), horizontally or even circumferentially. It can then present as *perianal*, *ischiorectal* and, less often, as *supralevator* or *horseshoe* abscesses.
- New theories suggest Crohn's disease-associated fistulae result from an epithelial barrier defect whose repair is diminished.[35]

Symptoms

- A patient with a perianal or ischiorectal abscess will present with:
  - severe pain,
  - induration or erythema of the perianal skin, and
  - fever.
- An ischiorectal abscesses may take longer to become visible externally on the perianal skin.
- A patient with a supralevator abscess may present with signs of sepsis and report only vague discomfort in the rectum with no external manifestation.
- Similarly, patients with intersphincteric abscesses may present with very severe pain and no obvious abnormalities around the perianal skin.

Surgical Treatment

- Incision and drainage through the perianal skin is the definitive treatment of an anorectal abscess:
  - Digitation of the abscess cavity should be performed to break down loculations.
  - Identifying an internal opening in the acute phase and attempting to formally treat an underlying fistula risks injury to the sphincter or creation of new tracts and is not routinely recommended.[36,37]
  - Furthermore, only 15–30% of abscesses fail to heal and are found to be associated with a fistula, raising the possibility that some underlying fistulae might spontaneously heal.
- The management of high pelvic abscesses differs to that of other anal abscesses and it is crucial to establish if the abscess is above or below the levator ani, which can be determined by the use of short inversion recovery pelvic MRI.
- If the abscess originates from an upward extension of an intersphincteric abscess, and thus is cranial to the levator ani, then it should be internally drained via incision of the rectal wall to prevent the development of an incurable high fistula.[38]

Fistula in Ano

Aetiology

- Fistula in ano is an epithelialized tract that connects the perianal skin to the anal canal.

- It most frequently occurs as a result of the chronic phase of an anorectal infection.
- Other causes include Crohn's disease, chlamydia infection, HIV infection, anorectal cancer, anal fissure, radiation proctitis and iatrogenic causes, e.g. obstetric injuries.[33]
- 15–30% of patients with anal abscess will develop a fistula in ano during the 12 months after abscess drainage as a result of epithelialization of the abscess drainage tract.[36,39,40]

Symptoms

A patient with a fistula in ano may present with:
- chronic purulent discharge,
- pruritus and
- mild pain.

Classification

Fistulae are classified into four main groups by their relation to the anal sphincter muscles as reported by Parks (Fig. 22.4).[38]

1. **Intersphincteric** in which the fistula tracks along the intersphincteric plane only; it is the commonest configuration (45%).
2. **Transsphincteric** in which the track passes from the intersphincteric plane through the external sphincter into the ischiorectal fossa (30%).
3. **Suprasphincteric** in which the track passes in the intersphincteric plane over the top of the puborectalis, then downwards again to the ischiorectal fossa (20%).
4. **Extrasphincteric** in which the track passes from the rectum or more proximal colon, through the levator muscles,

the ischiorectal fat and then anal skin. It is outside the external sphincter complex altogether. Extrasphincteric fistulae are typically not cryptoglandular in origin and should raise suspicion of another underlying abdominal pathology, e.g. diverticular disease or Crohn's disease (5%).

Fistula in ano can also be classified by complexity.[41,42]

Complex fistulae:
- These include high transsphincteric fistulae that involve ≥30% of the external sphincter, suprasphincteric, extrasphincteric, horseshoe fistulae and fistulae associated with Crohn's disease, radiation, malignancy, pre-existing faecal incontinence and chronic diarrhoea.
- In women, fistulae involving the anterior sphincter complex may also be considered complex.

Simple fistulae:
- These include superficial, intersphincteric and low transsphincteric primary fistulae that involve <30% of the external sphincter.

Clinical Features and Investigation

- The diagnosis of a fistula is based on patient's history and physical examination.
- The history may reveal associated intestinal pathology, previous anal surgery or obstetric trauma.
- Inspection reveals a perianal skin lesion with intermittent or constant purulent discharge and perhaps a surgical scar.
- Palpation of the skin may reveal induration due to an underlying track that can be followed toward the anal margin.

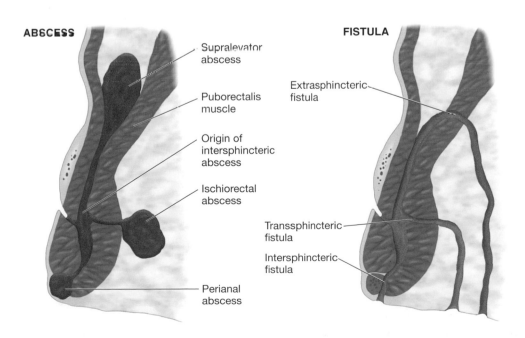

• **Fig. 22.4** Parks Classification of Fistulae

- In most cases, digital rectal examination (DRE) will allow the identification of the internal opening, an assessment of the presence or absence of secondary tracks and will allow assessment of sphincter function and length.[43]
- Surgical decisions should be made in the office as relaxation of the anal canal and levator ani under general anaesthesia complicates assessment, particularly of the amount and quality of sphincter that would remain if fistulotomy is performed.
- *Simple fistulae* do not require cross sectional imaging prior to surgery, whereas patients with *complex fistulae*, especially those in the setting of Crohn's disease, and recurrent fistulae may benefit from preoperative imaging. *MRI* and *endoanal ultrasound* are most commonly used, with MRI considered superior due to its resolution and lack of inter-operator variability.[44]
- An examination under anaesthesia may be useful to clarify fistula anatomy that was unclear in the office. Gentle probing of the external opening will confirm the presence of a tract; this should be performed very carefully in order to avoid creating false tracts.[45] *Goodsall's rule* (Fig. 22.5) suggests that an anterior fistula enters the anal canal in a radial fashion and posterior fistulae are often configured in a curved fashion from an internal opening in the posterior midline at the 6 o'clock position.[46] It is important to emphasise that Goodsall's rule is helpful but is *not* always accurate. Dilute hydrogen peroxide or dilute povidone iodine infused via a small catheter into the external opening of the fistula while examining the anal canal with a proctoscope can help identify internal openings.[47]

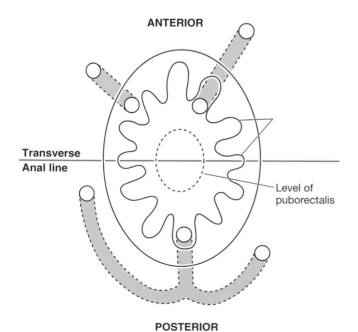

ANTERIOR

Transverse
Anal line

Level of
puborectalis

POSTERIOR

• **Fig. 22.5** Goodsall's Rule

Surgical Treatment

- The key to successful treatment of a fistula in ano is to drain the infection, eradicate the primary track and avoid recurrence while preserving continence.
- The optimal surgical approach depends on the aetiology of the fistula, the anatomy of the fistula, sphincter function and structure.

(a) Fistulotomy: Simple fistulae in ano in the setting of normal anal sphincter function may be treated with fistulotomy with an efficacy of 90% and with minimal risk of faecal incontinence.[48,49] Risk factors for postoperative incontinence are preoperative incontinence, female sex, recurrent or complex disease with previous surgery. In an otherwise healthy man with no previous anal surgery, one-third of the anal sphincter can be safely divided.[50,51] The amount of healthy sphincter that is divided is much less important than the amount of sphincter that remains, with 2 cm of normal muscle being adequate to maintain normal continence. The fistula tract should be laid open rather than excised as fistulectomy results in delayed healing, larger wounds and higher rates of incontinence.[43] Marsupialization of the wound edges post fistulotomy improves healing and reduces bleeding.[52,53]

Other procedures are available if fistulotomy is deemed inappropriate.

(b) Seton: *A draining seton* should be placed initially to eradicate sepsis and let secondary tracts heal with a second sphincter-sparing procedure 6 or more weeks later. A draining seton can be used as a therapeutic option in its own right and may permit slow division of the enclosed muscle, despite being loose.[43] A *cutting seton* is a tight suture or an elastic vessel loop that is placed through the fistula tract and tightened every 2 weeks in the office. It slowly cuts through the tract causing scarring, although the extent of sphincter division or resulting deformity can lead to incontinence.[54] A cutting seton is now thought to be no safer than primary fistulotomy; however, if this technique is used, it is imperative to cut the anoderm before the tight seton is placed for patient comfort.

(c) Endoanal advancement flap involves curettage of the fistula tract, suture closure of the internal opening with mobilization of a segment of proximal healthy anorectal mucosa, submucosa and muscle to cover the site of the fistula. This procedure is most effective for patients who have redundant rectal mucosa as this minimizes the tension placed on the flap. Success rates of 70% have been reported and it can be used for complex transsphincteric and suprasphincteric fistulae. Contraindications are active proctitis due to Crohn's disease, undrained sepsis, persisting secondary tracks, malignant or radiation-related fistula and severe perianal scarring because of previous surgery.[55,56]

(d) Ligation of the intersphincteric fistula tract (LIFT) is a sphincter-sparing procedure that involves a radial incision over the intersphincteric space and blunt dissection of the intersphincteric component of the fistula to fully mobilize this section. The portion of the fistula exposed in the intersphincteric space is then suture ligated flush with both the internal and external sphincters, followed by transection of the fistula between these sutures and loose approximation of the skin. It is a safe approach for simple and complex transsphincteric fistulae with good success rates but is contraindicated when intersphincteric sepsis is present.[57,58]

(e) Fistula plug is a collagen matrix that is placed through the fistula and sutured in place causing the internal opening to be closed. Early data suggested excellent success rates but more recent results have been considerably less promising. Reasons for early failure are untreated underlying sepsis or plug dislodgement.[59]

(f) Fibrin glue is a sphincter-sparing method that may treat simple and complex anal fistulae after track debridement. It seals the fistula tract and is thought to initiate collagen formation. Recurrence rates have been documented from 0% to 100% in the longer term. Fibrin glue is simple to use, has a minimal morbidity and theoretically is still attractive as a first-line treatment in complex fistulae, although it has fallen out of favour in the UK given the above results.[60]

The treatment of Crohn's fistulae in ano is mainly medical. Surgery is reserved to control anal sepsis with placement of a draining seton. Anti-TNF agent therapy is the first-line treatment after sepsis control.

Prognostic factors for healing include absence of proctitis, smoking cessation, short duration of disease and simple fistula anatomy. Severe perianal Crohn's disease may require diverting stoma or proctectomy to control symptoms.[61]

(g) Others: Laser application, video-assisted fistula treatment (VAAFT) and **over-the-scope clip (OTSC)** are new techniques to treat fistulae in ano but further studies are needed to evaluate their results.[37]

Anal Fissure

- Anal fissure is a longitudinal tear/split in the anal canal, that is almost always distal to the dentate line.
- It has equal distribution between men and women and occurs mostly between the second and fourth decades of life.
- Most fissures are located in the posterior midline, but in 12.6% of women and 7.8% of men, it can also occur in the anterior midline.[62]

Aetiology

- The pathogenesis of anal fissures is uncertain but it has been hypothesized this process begins with defecation associated trauma, followed by ischaemia and elevated anal pressure.
- In the posterior midline, where most fissures occur, the blood flow is lower than the other quadrants of the anal canal.[63,64]
- The perfusion of the anoderm is strongly influenced by the anal resting pressure as the higher the resting pressure,

the poorer the blood flow, resulting in relative anoderm ischaemia.
- When a fissure occurs, it begins a cycle of pain that results in increased anal sphincter tone, increased pressure within the anal canal and more anoderm ischaemia.[65–70]
- Anal fissures that are not in the anterior or posterior midline occur more rarely. When non-midline fissures are identified, multiple fissures are present or painless fissures are noted, an underlying disease should be considered such as Crohn's disease, tuberculosis, syphilis, HIV, leukaemia or anal cancer.

Classification

- An *acute fissure* looks like a simple tear of the anoderm.
- If the fissure fails to heal within 8 weeks, it is characterized as *chronic* and it is often much deeper than an acute fissure with associated oedema and fibrosis.
  - Fibres of the internal anal sphincter may be visible at the fissure base.
  - Features that accompany the chronic fissure are a 'sentinel pile' (skin tag) at the distal margin or hypertrophied anal papillae in the anal canal proximal to the fissure.

Symptoms

- Patients with anal fissure usually present with:
  - pain during or immediately after defecation; it is described as sharp, tearing, 'like passing knives' or 'shards of glass'
  - the pain is associated with fresh rectal bleeding that is usually limited to the toilet paper.

Diagnosis

- Gentle traction of the buttocks will demonstrate the fissure.
- If the diagnosis is not apparent, then an examination under anaesthetic is advised in order to exclude occult anorectal sepsis or an alternative anorectal pathology, e.g. cancer.[71]

Management

- Treatment focuses on breaking the cycle of pain, anal spasm and ischaemia. Initial measures aim to relax the anal sphincter, manage the associated pain with dietary modifications and use laxatives to soften the stool in order to minimize trauma to the anal canal.
- Warm sitz baths may ease pain but they do little to treat the underlying pathology for patients with chronic fissures.[72–74]
- Acute anal fissures may resolve within a few days with the use of simple measures, including the use of dietary fibre supplements.[75]
- Topical therapies:

- These include *nitroglycerin* ointment and ointments containing *calcium channel blockers* (e.g. nifedipine and diltiazem) that aim to reduce anal resting tone through relaxation of the internal anal sphincter, which in turn improves anoderm blood flow.
- These agents have success rates of approximately 60%.[71]
- Up to 30% of patients report headaches with the use of nitroglycerin in a dose dependent manner.[76]
- Diltiazem is rarely associated with headache and should be considered first-line treatment as it is better tolerated, although it can cause pruritus ani.[77,78]
- *Botulinum toxin* can be used either as the primary treatment for anal fissure or following failure of topical therapies.
  - Botulinum toxin binds to presynaptic nerve terminals preventing acetylcholine release and thereby prevents neural transmission and reduces anal resting pressure.
  - This effect lasts for 2–3 months until acetylcholine reaccumulates in the nerve terminals.[79]
  - There is no clear evidence regarding the optimal dose or injection site of botulinum toxin.[80]
  - Botulinum toxin has similar results to topical therapies when used as a first-line therapy for chronic anal fissures,[81,82] with modest improvement in healing rates when used as second-line therapy.
  - However, sequential combination therapy utilizing topical therapies and botulinum toxin will allow sphincterotomy to be avoided for up to 90% of patients.[83]

Surgical Treatment

Persistent symptomatic anal fissures that fail to heal with non-operative management require surgical treatment.

Lateral Sphincterotomy

- This is superior to topical therapies and botulinum toxin, with healing rates of 88 to 100% reported after sphincterotomy, although incontinence will occur in approximately 4% of patients with normal preoperative sphincter function.[84,85]
- Division of the internal sphincter should be tailored and be made the same length as the fissure (Fig. 22.6).
- There are no significant differences in outcome measures when comparing the *open* (sphincterotomy under direct vision though radial anoderm incision) or *closed* (sphincterotomy via a stab incision) techniques, with similar rates of persistent symptoms, recurrence and the need for reoperation.[86,87]
- Those with obstetric injuries, patients with significant previous anorectal operations or a documented anal sphincter injury should not be considered for sphincterotomy.

Anocutaneous flap is an alternative surgical approach for those with normal or low anal resting pressures. These patients represent a subset of the anal fissure cohort and the

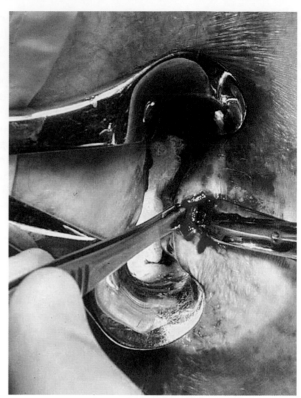

• **Fig. 22.6** Open Lateral Sphincterotomy

aetiology of fissures in the setting of normal or low anal tone is poorly understood. Fissure healing rates of 81–100% and minor faecal incontinence of 0–6% have been reported.[71,88] The anoderm flap can be constructed in a number of ways depending on surgeon preference.[89,90] Redundant rectal mucosa should not be used as a flap due to associated mucus secretion.

Fissurectomy

- This includes excision of the fibrotic edge of the fissure, curettage of the base, and excision of the sentinel pile and/or anal papilla if present.
- Healing of medically refractory anal fissure is improved if combined with botulinum toxin[91] and can be considered as a first-line surgical treatment due to low incontinence rates when compared to sphincterotomy.[92]

Anal Dilatation

- This is significantly associated with incontinence and heals fewer fissures than sphincterotomy, therefore it is not indicated for the treatment of anal fissure.[71]

Rectal Prolapse

Rectal prolapse or procidentia is the protrusion of the rectum through the anus. This can be either mucosal or full-thickness. On inspection, it classically appears as concentric rings of rectal mucosa, although eccentric prolapse can occur that may make the diagnosis more difficult in the early stages.

Mucosa Prolapse

Usually occurs in combination with obstructive defecation syndrome and solitary rectal ulcer syndrome. Symptoms include passage of mucus or blood per rectum, constipation and straining to open bowels.

Treatment is started with bulking laxatives and increased fibre intake. If this is not effective, procedures like suction banding or sclerotherapy, surgical excision or plication and radiofrequency ablation of the prolapse can be considered.

Full-Thickness Prolapse

This is circumferential protrusion of all of the rectal wall layers through the anus. Conservative treatment described above may be beneficial to some extent, but the definitive treatment is likely to be surgical. Surgical repair methods are summarized in Table 22.2.

Epidemiology

- The prevalence of external rectal prolapse is less than 0.5%
- It occurs more frequently in women with a peak incidence in the seventh decade.
- Many women with rectal prolapse also suffer from generalized pelvic floor weakness, and almost one-third have a concomitant uterine/vaginal prolapse, enterocele, rectocele or cystocele.[93]

Aetiology

- There is a hypothesis that rectal prolapse progresses from intussusception, to external mucosal prolapse, then to full thickness rectal prolapse.[94,95]
- The underlying cause of rectal prolapse remains unclear, although there are some known risk factors (Box 22.1).

Diagnosis

- The diagnosis of full rectal prolapse is based on history and physical examination.
- Symptoms:
  - the main complaint will be a lump extruding from the anus
  - constipation

BOX 22.1 Risk Factors for Rectal Prolapse

- Abnormally deep pouch of Douglas
- Lax pelvic floor muscles
- Weak internal and external anal sphincters
- Lax lateral ligaments of the rectum
- A redundant sigmoid colon
- Connective tissue disorders: Ehlers-Danlos, Marfan syndromes[96]
- Psychiatric disorders[97]
- Obesity
- Multiparity
- Instrumental delivery

TABLE 22.2 Surgical Options for Repair of Full-Rectal Thickness Prolapse.

Approach	• Transabdominal (Open/Laparoscopic/Robotic)				Perineal	
Patient group	Fit patients				Frail, elderly patients	
Other factors to consider	Gender, sexual activity, presence of genital prolapse, preoperative constipation, evacuatory difficulties, faecal incontinence, history of pelvic floor injury					
Type of operation	Suture	Resection	Anterior/ Posterior mesh rectopexy	Ventral mesh rectopexy	Delorme's	Altmeier's
Advantages	Low recurrence rate	Low recurrence Decreased constipation	Low recurrence rate	Spares autonomic nerves Low recurrence rate	Low morbidity Low mortality Minimal impact on continence	Low mortality rates With pelvic floor repair
Disadvantages/risks	Autonomic denervation Functional constipation	Risk of anastomotic leak	High morbidity Mesh infection/ invasion	Technically challenging Mesh infection/ invasion Rectal stricture Rectovaginal fistula	High recurrence rate (5–26%)	Pelvic sepsis Recurrence rate 10–16%

- faecal incontinence
- obstructed defecation
- mucus drainage and/or per rectal bleeding
- The patient's urological and gynaecological symptoms should be assessed as they may also require surgical correction.
- A prolapse is easier identified with the patient in the squatting position or sitting on a commode. If the prolapse is not reproducible in clinic, the patient should be encouraged to document it with a photo.[98]
- DRE may detect a patulous anus or reduced sphincter tone, and careful examination of perineum may revel concomitant pelvic floor pathology, e.g. rectocele, cystocele or uterine prolapse.
- On occasion, patients may present with an incarcerated rectal prolapse that requires reduction by a doctor or, more rarely, a gangrenous prolapse that requires amputation (see Altemeier's procedure later).

Diagnostic Tests

- Although the diagnosis is mainly clinical, other tests may be required including colonoscopy, contrast enema, defecography, MRI proctogram, transit studies, electromyography and anal manometry.[99]
- The primary role of colonoscopy is to rule out an additional colonic pathology. A mass or polyp can on occasion be the lead point for a rectal prolapse.
- Associated findings at colonoscopy are a solitary rectal ulcer in 10–15% of patients that may initially be confused with malignancy, or erythema of the prolapsing rectal mucosa.
- Contrast enema is used to assess sigmoid colon redundancy as prolapse repair may have to be combined with a sigmoid resection to minimize recurrence or concomitant constipation.
- Colonic transit studies are only ordered for patients who suffer with severe constipation.
- Patients with constipation are poor candidates for posterior rectopexy, division of the lateral ligaments during rectal mobilization or levatorplasty, as these procedures are thought to exacerbate constipation.[100]
- Patients with slow transit constipation may require subtotal colectomy, ileo-rectal anastomosis and rectopexy, although this is only justified in a very small proportion of patients.
- Conventional defecography or MRI proctography are performed in cases where rectal prolapse is not reproducible in clinic.
- An MRI proctogram may also reveal anatomical defects and other associated pelvic organ prolapse that may alter surgical planning.[101]
- Anorectal manometry and electromyography are recommended by some authors as these tests may reveal low resting sphincter pressure and predict poor postoperative continence but these tests do not alter surgical management.[98,102]

Medical Management

- Medical management is only appropriate for the smallest of prolapses and is otherwise only offered to patients who are unfit for surgery under spinal anaesthesia or for those who refuse a surgical repair.
- Patients are advised to have adequate fluid and fibre intake.
- Enemas and suppositories can minimize straining in the setting of severe constipation, which may decrease episodes of prolapse.[103]
- Table sugar or salt have been described to reduce oedema of incarcerated rectal prolapses when applied topically and may facilitate reduction.[104]

Surgical Treatment (see Table 22.2)

- Surgery is the definitive treatment for rectal prolapse.
- A range of surgical interventions have been described that are broadly divided into *transabdominal* or *perineal* approaches.
- As a general principle, procedures that require pelvic dissection should be avoided in young men due to the risk of associated sexual dysfunction.
- The surgical approach should be individualized based on each patient's symptoms, bowel habit, anatomy, comorbidities, age and sexual activity.
- Perineal procedures are mostly performed for elderly and frail patient as they are felt to be less invasive and carry less morbidity risks.[105] However, there are studies suggesting that the morbidity and mortality of the perineal approaches have been underestimated.[106]

Perineal Approaches

Perineal rectosigmoidectomy (Altemeier's procedure) involves full-thickness disconnection of the prolapsed rectal wall from the everted anus while preserving the anal transition zone, delivery of the redundant rectum and sigmoid through the anus, excision of the redundant bowel, followed by a hand-sewn coloanal anastomosis. It is extremely difficult to perform this procedure if the prolapse is short (<5 cm). This procedure has historically been combined with levatorplasty, a procedure to tighten the pelvic floor muscles, in an attempt to improve continence, although there is very little evidence to support that strategy.

Delorme's procedure is appropriate for patients with a short (<5 cm), full-thickness rectal prolapse. The rectal mucosa is stripped from the prolapsed rectum, the rectal wall is plicated, then the redundant mucosa is excised and a mucosal–anoderm anastomosis is constructed to restore epithelial continuity.

Transabdominal Approaches

Transabdominal rectopexy aims to anchor the rectum to the sacrum without resection. That can be accomplished by using a fixation material (e.g. mesh, suture, tack). If a mesh is used, it can be placed anterior, posterior, completely or partially encircling the rectum. The rectum can be fully mobilized with or without division of the lateral ligaments prior to fixation. The procedure can be performed either open, laparoscopically or robotically.

Transabdominal resection rectopexy removes the redundant sigmoid colon via an abdominal approach. This procedure is popular in the USA and should not be combined with a mesh rectopexy due to the risk of mesh infection. The extent of the bowel resection may vary from a sigmoidectomy to subtotal colectomy, after which suture rectopexy is undertaken to minimize tension on the anastomosis.

Ventral mesh rectopexy (VMR) is very popular in Europe since it was first introduced in 1996; however, the technique was originally described in the USA during the 1960s but was technically difficult to perform prior to the advent of laparoscopy. This procedure involves dissection of the rectum from the vagina (or prostate) down to the perineal body and minimal posterior rectal dissection. After rectal mobilization, a synthetic or biologic mesh is anchored on the anterior wall of the rectum and then secured to the sacral promontory to suspend the rectum. This procedure is reported to have a low recurrence rate of 4% and a postoperative constipation rate of 23%. Mesh-related complications have been documented in up to 5% of patients over a 10-year follow-up period.[107,108] Recently there have been major concerns in the media regarding pelvic mesh-related complications and, as such, the popularity of procedures using mesh seems to be waning. Relative contraindications for VMR include obesity, previous pelvic radiotherapy, high-grade endometriosis and diverticulitis. Absolute contraindications include pregnancy, hostile abdomen or pelvis, severe proctitis or anismus resistant to biofeedback. VMR can be challenging technically and high profile cases of significant complications have been reported. Therefore, VMR should only be performed by experienced surgeons after discussion at a pelvic floor MDT with specific clinical governance arrangements made at each institution to collect appropriate outcome data.[109]

- Studies comparing recurrence after these different surgical approaches have failed to demonstrate superiority of one technique over another.
- There are no significant differences regarding recurrence or postoperative incontinence when comparing Altemeier's and Delorme's procedures.
- Similarly, there are no differences in recurrence when comparing abdominal and perineal approaches.
- Resection rectopexy has, however, been demonstrated to be associated with lower rates of postoperative constipation.
- Division of the lateral ligaments during rectal mobilization has been thought to be associated with constipation and decreased recurrence rates, although the evidence supporting these associations is poor.
- The laparoscopic approach is generally thought to be preferable as it is associated with fewer complications and a more rapid recovery; however, there may be higher recurrence rates with this approach due to fewer adhesions or improperly placed sutures.[103,110]

- It is worth highlighting that patients with multivisceral prolapse require a multidisciplinary approach and management.[111]
- Finally, male patients should be offered the perineal approaches described above in order to avoid erectile dysfunction as a complication of rectal mobilization during abdominal approaches.[112]

Anal Warts (Condyloma Acuminata)

Aetiology

- An anal wart is the clinical result of an infection of the perianal skin with human papillomavirus (HPV).
- There are over 40 HPV subtypes that infect the human anogenital tract but HPV types 6 and 11 are most commonly detected in anogenital warts.[113]
- HPV is the most common sexually transmitted disease, with most sexually active women (>50%) being infected by one or more genital HPV types.[114] The infection is transmitted through contact with infected skin, mucosa or fluid and it is hypothesized that anal intercourse is not necessarily required for anal infection to occur.[115,116]
- Increased sexual exposure, HIV infection[117] and smoking[118] are risk factors for HPV infection.

Pathogenesis

- HPV are small double-stranded DNA viruses that integrate into the DNA of epithelial cells.
- HPV has an incubation period of 3 weeks to a few months.[119]
- Epithelial cells surrounding visible lesions may be infected as well in a latent manner for several months and are responsible for relapsing infections.

Diagnosis

- Diagnosis is based on history and clinical examination. Patients usually complain of a lump in the area, bleeding, pruritus and discomfort.
- The warts can be single or multiple, pinkish-white, cauliflower-shaped or pinhead-sized lesions.
- Anal warts may also develop in the anal canal distal to the dentate line. These appear as small flat-topped to globoid-shaped papules.
- Examination should be thorough in order to exclude associated genital lesions.
- Proctoscopy is necessary to exclude anal canal lesion.
- Malignant degeneration is rare but more likely to occur in immunosuppressed, HIV-positive patients[120] and disease above the dentate line.[121]

Management

- Treatment options are directed by location, number, size of lesions, patient preference and physician experience.

- **Podophyllotoxin** 0.15% cream or 0.5% solution is applied twice a day for 3 consecutive days followed by a gap of 4 days. The treatment duration is 4 weeks. Podophyllotoxin inhibits mitotic division and acts as a cytotoxic agent. Side effects are burning, pain, erosion, itching and inflammation. Erosions are shallow and heal within a few days. Reduction in the number of the warts can be accomplished in up to 70% of cases; however, relapse may occur in up to 55% of patients.[122]
- **Imiquimod** 5% cream is a local immunomodulator and has the potential to eradicate HPV from mucocutaneous surfaces. The cream has to be applied overnight three times a week and should be washed off carefully in the morning with soap and water. Side-effects include erythema, erosion, excoriation, itching and burning. Side effects may be controlled by lowering the frequency of applications to twice or even once a week. The treatment can be continued until wart clearance or for a maximum of 16 weeks.[123] A meta-analysis comparing cure rates for imiquimod and podophyllotoxin did not show statistically significant differences, although imiquimod had less serious side-effects.[124] The release of the patient's own skin-derived interferons and other cytokines, as well as the induction of apoptosis in HPV-infected keratinocytes, which both seem to be the most important effects of topically applied imiquimod, open a new era of topical warts treatment.
- **Cryotherapy** acts through necrosis and thrombosis of the dermal microvasculature. It has the advantage of being simple, easy to repeat and inexpensive. It can be effective in up to 88% of cases and is associated with a recurrence rate of 39%.[125]
- **Trichloroacetic acid** is a caustic agent that is applied directly to anal warts. It is suitable for small lesions and requires weekly treatments for up to 4 weeks. It can cause deep ulceration, pain and scaring. It has good response rates of up to 81% but recurrence rates of 36% have been reported.[126]

Surgical Treatment

- A variety of surgical options are available including electrocautery, electrofulguration, scissors excision, curettage, laser and, more recently, argon therapy.[127]
- *Electrocautery* or *scissor excision* can achieve clearance rates of 90–100% with recurrence rates of 19–29%.
  - Excision of larger lesions can lead to anal stenosis.
- *Electrofulguration* may be more appropriate for larger lesions, while curettage is only effective for small numbers of lesions.
- *Laser* ablation vaporizes intracellular water and destroys target lesions and argon lasers produce thermal coagulation allowing superficial tissue destruction.
- *Electrosurgery*, *laser* and *argon* surgery can potentially transmit viral particles, detected in the smoke. Consequently, if electrocautery is used, it is best to excise the lesions with scissors and use cautery to achieve haemostasis as this minimizes aerosolization of the HPV vaccine. Surgical masks and the use of a smoke evacuator are also recommended.
- Treatment can be performed in an outpatient setting using local anaesthesia for small lesions, whereas broad-based lesions will require regional or general anaesthesia.
- Tissue for histopathology should be obtained in order to exclude anal intraepithelial neoplasia or squamous cell carcinoma in high-risk patients, e.g. HIV-positive and transplant patients with impaired immune system.

Pruritus Ani

- Pruritus ani (PA) is described as itching or burning affecting the perianal skin.
- It may be present for a short period or progress to be a chronic problem.
- It is more common in male populations between the fourth and sixth decades of life.[128]

Classification

- PA is classified as *primary (idiopathic)* when the cause is unknown and *secondary* when a causal link has been identified.
- *Idiopathic PA* accounts for the majority of cases, estimated to be responsible for between 50–90% of patients, although some authors suggest a cause can be identified in up to 75% of cases.[129]

Aetiology

- Fifty percent of patients with PA suffer from loose stools or incomplete evacuation. These conditions lead to occult faecal contamination and soiling of the perianal skin.[130]
- Additionally, the anal sphincters of individuals with PA may relax more easily to rectal distension, which contributes to soiling.[131,132]
- Coffee, tea, cola, alcohol, milk products, chocolate, spices, grapes and tomatoes may contribute to faecal soiling by causing loose stools, increased defecatory frequency or reduction of anal sphincter tone.
- Smoking can be responsible for loose stool.[133]
- Drugs as colchicine, quinidine, peppermint oil and topical steroid creams or benzocaine found in haemorrhoidal creams all can cause itching.[134]
- Anorectal diseases associated with PA include haemorrhoids, abscesses, fissures, fistulae and skin tags.[128]
- Anal surgery may change the morphology of the anal canal and lead to soiling and itching.
- Dermatological diseases as psoriasis, Lichen sclerosus, atopic dermatitis, contact dermatitis, hidradenitis suppurativa, Bowen's disease and Paget's disease can present with anal itching.[135]
- Furthermore, perianal skin infections like *Candida*, sexually transmitted diseases (e.g. anal warts, herpes,

syphilis, gonorrhoea), streptococcal and staphylococcal infections, erythrasma due to *Corynebacterium minutissimum* and parasites have also been described as causes of PA.[136]

- Obesity along with excessive sweating and poor anal hygiene leads to itching. On the other hand, excessive anal hygiene measures can have the same outcome and wet wipes exacerbate the matter further.[137,138]
- Systemic diseases have also been associated with PA including iron deficiency anaemia, diabetes mellitus, hyperbilirubinemia, lymphoma, leukaemia, renal failure and thyroid disorders.[129]
- Finally, PA may be the manifestation of anxiety and depression, but psychogenic pruritus should be a diagnosis of exclusion only.[139]
- It should not be forgotten that the disease itself can also cause great distress.

Diagnosis

- A diagnosis is based on history and physical examination.
- The history of the patient should include the duration of the symptoms, co-existing skin conditions, medical history, current medications, alcohol intake, bowel habit, dietary habits, sexual history, psychiatric background and personal hygiene practice.
- Examination should not be limited only to the perineum especially if there is suspicion of a dermatological disease.
- DRE and proctoscopy complete the clinical examination.[140]
- The perianal skin may look completely normal or be erythematous or lichenified with erosions and ulcerations.[141]

Investigations

- If the patient complains of systematic symptoms, then laboratory tests should be ordered, including a full blood count, liver, thyroid and kidney function tests, blood glucose and tissue transglutaminase to detect coeliac disease.
- Serology for syphilis is advised if the suspicion is raised.
- Swabs can identify bacterial or sexual transmitted infections
- Skin scrapings help diagnose fungal infections.
- If contact dermatitis is suspected, a patch test may be necessary.
- Biopsy is only required if neoplasia is suspected.
- Colonoscopy will also exclude a colonic pathology in patients with altered bowel habit.

Treatment

- Where an underlying cause is identified the appropriate management plan should be instituted.
- On the other hand, patients with idiopathic PA may improve with dietary modifications, bowel-habit modifications and use of a mild steroid cream such as hydrocortisone 1% for 2 weeks along with barrier creams.

- Topical steroids will alleviate the symptoms but are not used long-term as they are associated with skin atrophy and a deterioration in symptoms.[142]
- Patients should be advised to wash after using the toilet but without soap and instead use soap-free cleanser and dry the area with a soft cloth or hairdryer.
- Loose natural fabric undergarments should be used to minimize perspiration.
- If the patient complains of excessive sweat, baby powder and a dry cotton tissue on the anal verge can improve symptoms.
- If the itching is the predominant symptom at night, an antihistamine can be prescribed.
- For patients with refractory symptoms, capcaicin[143] and intradermal 1% methylene blue injection[144] have been described but more studies are needed to prove their efficacy.

Faecal Incontinence

- Faecal incontinence (FI) is the involuntary loss of solid or liquid faeces from the anus.
- The prevalence is age-related
- FI is more frequent in individuals with inflammatory bowel disease, coeliac disease, irritable bowel syndrome and diabetes.[145]
- Faecal incontinence is associated with female gender, pregnancy, parity and instrumental vaginal delivery.[146]

Aetiology

- Continence and defecation are multifactorial processes depending on functional anal and pelvic floor muscles, rectal capacity, compliance, sensation and stool consistency.
- Compromise or alteration of any of the above factors may lead to FI.
- Common causes of incontinence are obstetric trauma and injury of the sphincters due to anal surgery (e.g. fistulotomy).
- FI can be associated with rectal prolapse and rectocele.
- Radiation proctitis and inflammatory bowel disease can also result in FI.
- Peripheral neuropathy (e.g. pudendal nerve injury) or systemic neuropathy due to diabetes has been reported as cause of incontinence too.
- Individuals with dementia, stroke, brain tumours, multiple sclerosis, spinal cord injury, spina bifida or central nervous system disorders are at greater risk of FI.
- Less frequently, FI may be due to sphincter degeneration secondary to scleroderma or idiopathic degeneration.
- Patients with diarrhoea either due to irritable bowel syndrome or after colonic resection are at high risk of FI.
- It should be remembered that FI can be a manifestation of behavioural disorders.[147,148]

Classification

- FI can be classified as *urge, passive, post defecatory* or *mixed.*
- Patients with *urge FI* experience a strong and urgent desire to defecate, but are often unable to defer defecation until they can reach the toilet.
- Patients with *passive incontinence* are not aware of the need to defecate and may be unaware of incontinence until it is visually apparent.
- Patients with *urge incontinence* have reduced anal squeeze pressures and frequently have external sphincter defects.
- In contrast, patients with *passive incontinence* have lower anal resting pressures and are more likely to have internal anal sphincter defects, with or without concomitant defects in the external sphincter.
- *Nocturnal incontinence* is a frequently reported symptom but is particularly prevalent for patients with diabetes or scleroderma related FI.[149,150]
- FI scoring symptoms have been developed to quantify severity and response to treatment; however, outwith specialist pelvic floor clinics, they are predominantly used as research tools.[151]

Assessment

- Assessment focuses on the clinical history and physical examination.
- The history should explore bowel and dietary habits, surgical and obstetric history, medical and neurological conditions.
- Co-existence of urinary incontinence suggests the possibility of an underlying neuropathy.
- Clinical examination includes inspection of the perineum and DRE. DRE will exclude the presence of a low rectal carcinoma/polyp, faecal impaction, allows assessment of the anal resting and squeeze pressures and identification of sphincter defects.

Management

- Initial management starts with dietary modification to improve diarrhoea or constipation accordingly.
- Food and stool charts are advised.
- Scheduled toileting with the use of enemas or suppositories is recommended along with skin care.[152]
- If diarrhoea persists, antidiarrhoeal drugs such as loperamide hydrochloride should be the first choice. It can be used long term in doses from 0.5 mg to 16 mg per day as required.
- Alternatively, for people who cannot tolerate loperamide, codeine phosphate can be offered.[148]
- Patients who do not respond to these measures should be referred for biofeedback/pelvic floor muscle training.
- The purpose of this therapy is to improve anorectal sensation, coordination, strength of the pelvic floor and endurance of the external sphincter. Although these therapies are widely employed, much larger prospective studies are needed to confirm their utility.[153]

Investigations

- If conservative measures fail to improve FI, anorectal physiologic assessment is undertaken to identify the functional or anatomic problems underlying symptoms of FI.
- Anal manometry is utilized to assess sphincter function by recording the anal resting and squeeze pressures and the presence or absence of the rectoanal inhibitory reflex.
- Endoanal ultrasound complements anal manometry by assessing the structural integrity of the anal sphincters and demonstrating anatomical defects.
- Rectal balloon expulsion and rectal sensory volumes demonstrate pelvic floor coordination and rectal afferent sensation respectively, with rectal barostat used selectively to assess rectal compliance.
- Electromyography or pudendal nerve motor terminal latencies can be used to investigate pudendal neuropathy; however, this is infrequently undertaken and the latter investigation is considered obsolete.
- MRI proctography or defecography may be used prior to surgery for patients suspected to have a rectocele, intussusception and perineal descent.[154]
- Finally, colonoscopy should be performed if colorectal polyps, inflammatory bowel disease or cancer is suspected.[155]

Surgical Treatment

Patients with acute traumatic anal sphincter injuries (e.g. obstetric injuries) or faecal incontinence due to rectal prolapse should be treated with surgery without offering conservative management.[156,157]

Overlapping anal sphincter repair is appropriate for patients with >90-degree defects in the external anal sphincter in the presence of good quality sphincter function; however, patients with defects approaching 180 degrees are not suitable for this procedure. Patients should be warned that the efficacy of the procedure deteriorates with time but that it can be repeated with similar results to the index procedure.[148]

Injection of bulking agents improves symptoms for up to 50% of patients but improvements can be short lived and further studies are needed.[156]

Artificial neosphincters and **sphincter augmentation procedures** (e.g. transposition of the gracilis muscle) are associated with significant complication rates (such as infection, erosions, device malfunction, migration) and should only be performed in specialized centres. These procedures should be reserved for patients with severe incontinence, with sphincter defects >180 degrees, failed repairs and anal sphincter aetiologies of FI.[148]

Sacral nerve stimulation should be considered the first-line surgical option for patients with and without sphincter defects. It shows very encouraging results, although high-quality studies are still required to prove its long-term efficiency.[158]

Percutaneous tibial nerve stimulation has been also been proposed as a treatment for FI. Although initial results were promising, more recent data suggest less encouraging outcome measures.[159]

Malone antegrade colonic enema (MACE) or **end stoma** formation are additional options for paediatric and adult patients who have failed other management strategies, respectively.[160]

Although there is a plethora of non-surgical and surgical options reported in the literature, there is no consensus upon the optimal sequence of treatments and for many patients, a combination of therapies or treatments might be necessary to improve FI symptoms.[161]

References

1. Thomson WH. The nature of haemorrhoids. *Br J Surg*. 1975;62(7):542–552.
2. Johanson JF, Sonnenberg A. The prevalence of hemorrhoids and chronic constipation. An epidemiologic study. *Gastroenterology*. 1990;98(2):380–386.
3. Goligher JC, Duthie HL, Nixon HH. *Surgery of the Anus, Rectum and Colon*. Vol 5. London: Bailliere Tindall; 1984:98–149.
4. Loder PB, Kamm MA, Nicholls RJ, Phillips RK. Haemorrhoids: pathology, pathophysiology and aetiology. *Br J Surg*. 1994;81(7):946–954.
5. Haas PA, Fox TAJ, Haas GP. The pathogenesis of hemorrhoids. *Dis Colon Rectum*. 1984;27(7):442–450.
6. Foxx-Orenstein AE, Umar SB, Crowell MD. Common anorectal disorders. *Gastroenterol Hepatol*. 2014;10(5):294–301.
7. Alonso-Coello P, Mills E, Heels-Ansdell D, et al. Fiber for the treatment of hemorrhoids complications: a systematic review and meta-analysis. *Am J Gastroenterol*. 2006;101(1):181–188.
8. Johannsson HO, Graf W, Pahlman L. Bowel habits in hemorrhoid patients and normal subjects. *Am J Gastroenterol*. 2005;100(2):401–406.
9. Garg P, Singh P. Adequate dietary fiber supplement and TONE can help avoid surgery in most patients with advanced hemorrhoids. *Minerva Gastroenterol Dietol*. 2017;63(2):92–96.
10. Cocorullo G, Tutino R, Falco N, et al. The non-surgical management for hemorrhoidal disease. A systematic review. *G Chir*. 2017;38(1):5–14.
11. Davis BR, Lee-Kong SA, Migaly J, Feingold DL, Steele SR. The American society of colon and rectal surgeons clinical practice guidelines for the management of hemorrhoids. *Dis Colon Rectum*. 2018;61(3):284–292.
12. Shanmugam V, Thaha MA, Rabindranath KS, Campbell KL, Steele RJC, Loudon MA. Rubber band ligation versus excisional haemorrhoidectomy for haemorrhoids. *Cochrane Database Syst Rev*. 2005;2005(3):CD005034.
13. Brown SR, Watson A. Comments to "Rubber band ligation versus excisional haemorrhoidectomy for haemorrhoids". *Tech Coloproctol*. 2016;20(9):659–661.
14. MacRae HM, McLeod RS. Comparison of hemorrhoidal treatment modalities. A meta-analysis. *Dis Colon Rectum*. 1995;38(7):687–694.
15. Brown S, Tiernan J, Biggs K, et al. The HubBLe Trial: haemorrhoidal artery ligation (HAL) versus rubber band ligation (RBL) for symptomatic second- and third-degree haemorrhoids: a multicentre randomised controlled trial and health-economic evaluation. *Health Technol Assess*. 2016;20(88):1–150.
16. Yano T, Nogaki T, Asano M, Tanaka S, Kawakami K, Matsuda Y. Outcomes of case-matched injection sclerotherapy with a new agent for hemorrhoids in patients treated with or without blood thinners. *Surg Today*. 2013;43(8):854–858.
17. Marques CFS, Nahas SC, Nahas CSR, Sobrado CWJ, Habr-Gama A, Kiss DR. Early results of the treatment of internal hemorrhoid disease by infrared coagulation and elastic banding: a prospective randomized cross-over trial. *Tech Coloproctol*. 2006;10(4):312–317.
18. Poen AC, Felt-Bersma RJ, Cuesta MA, Deville W, Meuwissen SG. A randomized controlled trial of rubber band ligation versus infra-red coagulation in the treatment of internal haemorrhoids. *Eur J Gastroenterol Hepatol*. 2000;12(5):535–539.
19. Bhatti MI, Sajid MS, Baig MK. Milligan-Morgan (open) versus Ferguson haemorrhoidectomy (closed): a systematic review and meta-analysis of published randomized, controlled trials. *World J Surg*. 2016;40(6):1509–1519.
20. Nienhuijs S, de Hingh I. Conventional versus LigaSure hemorrhoidectomy for patients with symptomatic hemorrhoids. *Cochrane Database Syst Rev*. 2009;2009(1):CD006761.
21. Simillis C, Thoukididou SN, Slesser AAP, Rasheed S, Tan E, Tekkis PP. Systematic review and network meta-analysis comparing clinical outcomes and effectiveness of surgical treatments for haemorrhoids. *Br J Surg*. 2015;102(13):1603–1618.
22. Tjandra JJ, Chan MKY. Systematic review on the procedure for prolapse and hemorrhoids (stapled hemorrhoidopexy). *Dis Colon Rectum*. 2007;50(6):878–892.
23. Nisar PJ, Acheson AG, Neal KR, Scholefield JH. Stapled hemorrhoidopexy compared with conventional hemorrhoidectomy: systematic review of randomized, controlled trials. *Dis Colon Rectum*. 2004;47(11):1837–1845.
24. Jayaraman S, Colquhoun PHD, Malthaner RA. Stapled hemorrhoidopexy is associated with a higher long-term recurrence rate of internal hemorrhoids compared with conventional excisional hemorrhoid surgery. *Dis Colon Rectum*. 2007;50(9):1297–1305.
25. Porrett LJ, Porrett JK, Ho Y-H. Documented complications of staple hemorrhoidopexy: a systematic review. *Int Surg*. 2015;100(1):44–57.
26. Giordano P, Overton J, Madeddu F, Zaman S, Gravante G. Transanal hemorrhoidal dearterialization: a systematic review. *Dis Colon Rectum*. 2009;52(9):1665–1671.
27. Lehur PA, Didnee AS, Faucheron J-L, et al. Cost-effectiveness of new surgical treatments for hemorrhoidal disease: a multicentre randomized controlled trial comparing transanal Doppler-guided hemorrhoidal artery ligation with mucopexy and circular stapled hemorrhoidopexy. *Ann Surg*. 2016;264(5):710–716.
28. Pucher PH, Sodergren MH, Lord AC, Darzi A, Ziprin P. Clinical outcome following Doppler-guided haemorrhoidal artery ligation: a systematic review. *Colorectal Dis*. 2013;15(6):e284–e294.
29. Ratto C, Parello A, Veronese E, et al. Doppler-guided transanal haemorrhoidal dearterialization for haemorrhoids: results from a multicentre trial. *Colorectal Dis*. 2015;17(1):O10–O19.
30. Greenspon J, Williams SB, Young HA, Orkin BA. Thrombosed external hemorrhoids: outcome after conservative or surgical management. *Dis Colon Rectum*. 2004;47(9):1493–1498.

31. Jongen J, Bach S, Stubinger SH, Bock J-U. Excision of thrombosed external hemorrhoid under local anesthesia: a retrospective evaluation of 340 patients. *Dis Colon Rectum*. 2003;46(9):1226–1231.

32. Chan KKW, Arthur JDR. External haemorrhoidal thrombosis: evidence for current management. *Tech Coloproctol*. 2013;17(1):21–25.

33. Parks AG. Pathogenesis and treatment of fistula-in-ano. *Br Med J*. 1961;1(5224):463–469.

34. Sainio P. Fistula-in-ano in a defined population. Incidence and epidemiological aspects. *Ann Chir Gynaecol*. 1984;73(4):219–224.

35. Dignass AU. Mechanisms and modulation of intestinal epithelial repair. *Inflamm Bowel Dis*. 2001;7(1):68–77.

36. Sahnan K, Askari A, Adegbola SO, et al. Natural history of anorectal sepsis. *Br J Surg*. 2017;104(13):1857–1865.

37. Ommer A, Herold A, Berg E, et al. German S3 guidelines: anal abscess and fistula (second revised version). *Langenbeck's Arch Surg*. 2017;402(2):191–201.

38. Parks AG, Gordon PH, Hardcastle JD. A classification of fistula-in-ano. *Br J Surg*. 1976;63(1):1–12.

39. Vasilevsky CA, Gordon PH. The incidence of recurrent abscesses or fistula-in-ano following anorectal suppuration. *Dis Colon Rectum*. 1984;27(2):126–130.

40. Henrichsen S, Christiansen J. Incidence of fistula-in-ano complicating anorectal sepsis: a prospective study. *Br J Surg*. 1986;73(5):371–372.

41. Fazio VW. Complex anal fistulae. *Gastroenterol Clin North Am*. 1987;16(1):93–114.

42. Sangwan YP, Rosen L, Riether RD, Stasik JJ, Sheets JA, Khubchandani IT. Is simple fistula-in-ano simple? *Dis. Colon Rectum*. 1994;37(9):885–889.

43. Williams JG, Farrands PA, Williams AB, et al. The treatment of anal fistula: ACPGBI position statement. *Colorectal Dis*. 2007;9(suppl 4):18–50.

44. Wise PE, Schwartz DA. The evaluation and treatment of Crohn perianal fistulae: EUA, EUS, MRI, and other imaging modalities. *Gastroenterol Clin North Am*. 2012;41(2):379–391.

45. Gonzalez-Ruiz C, Kaiser AM, Vukasin P, Beart RWJ, Ortega AE. Intraoperative physical diagnosis in the management of anal fistula. *Am Surg*. 2006;72(1):11–15.

46. Cirocco WC, Reilly JC. Challenging the predictive accuracy of Goodsall's rule for anal fistulas. *Dis Colon Rectum*. 1992;35(6):537–542.

47. Gunawardhana PA, Deen KI. Comparison of hydrogen peroxide instillation with Goodsall's rule for fistula-in-ano. *ANZ J Surg*. 2001;71(8):472–474.

48. Owen HA, Buchanan GN, Schizas A, Emmanuel A, Cohen R, Williams AB. Quality of life following fistulotomy – short term follow-up. *Colorectal Dis*. 2017;19(6):563–569.

49. Vogel JD, Johnson EK, Morris AM, et al. Clinical practice guideline for the management of anorectal abscess, fistula-in-ano, and rectovaginal fistula. *Dis Colon Rectum*. 2016;59(12):1117–1133.

50. Cavanaugh M, Hyman N, Osler T. Fecal incontinence severity index after fistulotomy: a predictor of quality of life. *Dis Colon Rectum*. 2002;45(3):349–353.

51. Garcia-Aguilar J, Belmonte C, Wong WD, Goldberg SM, Madoff RD. Anal fistula surgery. Factors associated with recurrence and incontinence. *Dis Colon Rectum*. 1996;39(7):723–729.

52. Ho YH, Tan M, Leong AF, Seow-Choen F. Marsupialization of fistulotomy wounds improves healing: a randomized controlled trial. *Br J Surg*. 1998;85(1):105–107.

53. Pescatori M, Ayabaca SM, Cafaro D, Iannello A, Magrini S. Marsupialization of fistulotomy and fistulectomy wounds improves healing and decreases bleeding: a randomized controlled trial. *Colorectal Dis*. 2006;8(1):11–14.

54. Ritchie RD, Sackier JM, Hodde JP. Incontinence rates after cutting seton treatment for anal fistula. *Colorectal Dis*. 2009;11(6):564–571.

55. Jones IT, Fazio VW, Jagelman DG. The use of transanal rectal advancement flaps in the management of fistulas involving the anorectum. *Dis Colon Rectum*. 1987;30(12):919–923.

56. Ozuner G, Hull TL, Cartmill J, Fazio VW. Long-term analysis of the use of transanal rectal advancement flaps for complicated anorectal/vaginal fistulas. *Dis Colon Rectum*. 1996;39(1):10–14.

57. Alasari S, Kim NK. Overview of anal fistula and systematic review of ligation of the intersphincteric fistula tract (LIFT). *Tech Coloproctol*. 2014;18(1):13–22.

58. Hong KD, Kang S, Kalaskar S, Wexner SD. Ligation of intersphincteric fistula tract (LIFT) to treat anal fistula: systematic review and meta-analysis. *Tech Coloproctol*. 2014;18(8):685–691.

59. El-Gazzaz G, Zutshi M, Hull T. A retrospective review of chronic anal fistulae treated by anal fistulae plug. *Colorectal Dis*. 2010;12(5):442–447.

60. Hammond TM, Grahn MF, Lunniss PJ. Fibrin glue in the management of anal fistulae. *Colorectal Dis*. 2004;6(5):308–319.

61. Lee MJ, Heywood N, Sagar PM, Brown SR, Fearnhead NS. Association of coloproctology of Great Britain and Ireland consensus exercise on surgical management of fistulating perianal Crohn's disease. *Colorectal Dis*. 2017;19(5):418–429.

62. Hananel N, Gordon PH. Re-examination of clinical manifestations and response to therapy of fissure-in-ano. *Dis Colon Rectum*. 1997;40(2):229–233.

63. Klosterhalfen B, Vogel P, Rixen H, Mittermayer C. Topography of the inferior rectal artery: a possible cause of chronic, primary anal fissure. *Dis Colon Rectum*. 1989;32(1):43–52.

64. Schouten WR, Briel JW, Auwerda JJ, De Graaf EJ. Ischaemic nature of anal fissure. *Br J Surg*. 1996;83(1):63–65.

65. Schouten WR, Briel JW, Auwerda JJ. Relationship between anal pressure and anodermal blood flow. The vascular pathogenesis of anal fissures. *Dis Colon Rectum*. 1994;37(7):664–669.

66. Hancock BD. The internal sphincter and anal fissure. *Br J Surg*. 1977;64(2):92–95.

67. Farouk R, Duthie GS, MacGregor AB, Bartolo DC. Sustained internal sphincter hypertonia in patients with chronic anal fissure. *Dis Colon Rectum*. 1994;37(5):424–429.

68. Keck JO, Staniunas RJ, Coller JA, Barrett RC, Oster ME. Computer-generated profiles of the anal canal in patients with anal fissure. *Dis Colon Rectum*. 1995;38(1):72–79.

69. Lin JK. Anal manometric studies in hemorrhoids and anal fissures. *Dis Colon Rectum*. 1989;32(10):839–842.

70. Gibbons CP, Read NW. Anal hypertonia in fissures: cause or effect? *Br J Surg*. 1986;73(6):443–445.

71. Cross KLR, Massey EJD, Fowler AL, Monson JRT. The management of anal fissure: ACPGBI position statement. *Colorectal Dis*. 2008;10(suppl 3):1–7.

72. Dodi G, Bogoni F, Infantino A, Pianon P, Mortellaro LM, Lise M. Hot or cold in anal pain? A study of the changes in internal anal sphincter pressure profiles. *Dis Colon Rectum*. 1986;29(4):248–251.

73. Jiang JK, Chiu JH, Lin JK. Local thermal stimulation relaxes hypertonic anal sphincter: evidence of somatoanal reflex. *Dis Colon Rectum*. 1999;42(9):1152–1159.

74. Gupta P. Randomized, controlled study comparing sitz-bath and no-sitz-bath treatments in patients with acute anal fissures. *ANZ J Surg.* 2006;76(8):718–721.

75. Jensen SL. Treatment of first episodes of acute anal fissure: prospective randomised study of lignocaine ointment versus hydrocortisone ointment or warm sitz baths plus bran. *Br Med J.* 1986;292(6529):1167–1169.

76. Bailey HR, Beck DE, Billingham RP, et al. A study to determine the nitroglycerin ointment dose and dosing interval that best promote the healing of chronic anal fissures. *Dis Colon Rectum.* 2002;45(9):1192–1199.

77. Sajid MS, Whitehouse PA, Sains P, Baig MK. Systematic review of the use of topical diltiazem compared with glyceryltrinitrate for the nonoperative management of chronic anal fissure. *Colorectal Dis.* 2013;15(1):19–26.

78. Kocher HM, Steward M, Leather AJM, Cullen PT. Randomized clinical trial assessing the side-effects of glyceryl trinitrate and diltiazem hydrochloride in the treatment of chronic anal fissure. *Br J Surg.* 2002;89(4):413–417.

79. Jones OM, Brading AF, Mortensen NJM. Mechanism of action of botulinum toxin on the internal anal sphincter. *Br J Surg.* 2004;91(2):224–228.

80. Lin JX, Krishna S, Su'a B, Hill AG. Optimal dosing of botulinum toxin for treatment of chronic anal fissure: a systematic review and meta-analysis. *Dis Colon Rectum.* 2016;59(9):886–894.

81. Samim M, Twigt B, Stoker L, Pronk A. Topical diltiazem cream versus botulinum toxin A for the treatment of chronic anal fissure: a double-blind randomized clinical trial. *Ann Surg.* 2012;255(1):18–22.

82. Sajid MS, Vijaynagar B, Desai M, Cheek E, Baig MK. Botulinum toxin vs glyceryltrinitrate for the medical management of chronic anal fissure: a meta-analysis. *Colorectal Dis.* 2008;10(6):541–546.

83. Lindsey I, Jones OM, Cunningham C, George BD, Mortensen NJM. Botulinum toxin as second-line therapy for chronic anal fissure failing 0.2 percent glyceryl trinitrate. *Dis Colon Rectum.* 2003;46(3):361–366.

84. Garg P, Garg M, Menon GR. Long-term continence disturbance after lateral internal sphincterotomy for chronic anal fissure: a systematic review and meta-analysis. *Colorectal Dis.* 2013;15(3):e104–e117.

85. Nelson RL, Manuel D, Gumienny C, et al. A systematic review and meta-analysis of the treatment of anal fissure. *Tech Coloproctol.* 2017;21(8):605–625.

86. Wiley M, Day P, Rieger N, Stephens J, Moore J. Open vs. closed lateral internal sphincterotomy for idiopathic fissure-in-ano: a prospective, randomized, controlled trial. *Dis Colon Rectum.* 2004;47(6):847–852.

87. Garcia-Aguilar J, Belmonte C, Wong WD, Lowry AC, Madoff RD. Open vs. closed sphincterotomy for chronic anal fissure: long-term results. *Dis Colon Rectum.* 1996;39(4):440–443.

88. Sahebally SM, Walsh SR, Mahmood W, Aherne TM, Joyce MR. Anal advancement flap versus lateral internal sphincterotomy for chronic anal fissure – a systematic review and meta-analysis. *Int J Surg.* 2018;49:16–21.

89. Singh M, Sharma A, Gardiner A, Duthie GS. Early results of a rotational flap to treat chronic anal fissures. *Int J Colorectal Dis.* 2005;20(4):339–342.

90. Magdy A, El Nakeeb A, Fouda EY, Youssef M, Farid M. Comparative study of conventional lateral internal sphincterotomy, V-Y anoplasty, and tailored lateral internal sphincterotomy with V-Y anoplasty in the treatment of chronic anal fissure. *J Gastrointest Surg.* 2012;16(10):1955–1962.

91. Lindsey I, Cunningham C, Jones OM, Francis C, Mortensen NJM. Fissurectomy-botulinum toxin: a novel sphincter-sparing procedure for medically resistant chronic anal fissure. *Dis Colon Rectum.* 2004;47(11):1947–1952.

92. Sileri P, Stolfi VM, Franceschilli L, et al. Conservative and surgical treatment of chronic anal fissure: prospective longer term results. *J Gastrointest Surg.* 2010;14(5):773–780.

93. Nygaard I, Barber MD, Burgio KL, et al. Prevalence of symptomatic pelvic floor disorders in US women. *J Am Med Assoc.* 2008;300(11):1311–1316.

94. Wijffels NA, Collinson R, Cunningham C, Lindsey I. What is the natural history of internal rectal prolapse? *Colorectal Dis.* 2010;12(8):822–830.

95. Hotouras A, Murphy J, Boyle DJ, Allison M, Williams NS, Chan CL. Assessment of female patients with rectal intussusception and prolapse: is this a progressive spectrum of disease? *Dis Colon Rectum.* 2013;56(6):780–785.

96. Carley ME, Schaffer J. Urinary incontinence and pelvic organ prolapse in women with Marfan or Ehlers Danlos syndrome. *Am J Obstet Gynecol.* 2000;182(5):1021–1023.

97. Marceau C, Parc Y, Debroux E, Tiret E, Parc R. Complete rectal prolapse in young patients: psychiatric disease a risk factor of poor outcome. *Colorectal Dis.* 2005;7(4):360–365.

98. Bordeianou L, Hicks CW, Kaiser AM, Alavi K, Sudan R, Wise PE. Rectal prolapse: an overview of clinical features, diagnosis, and patient-specific management strategies. *J Gastrointest Surg.* 2014;18(5):1059–1069.

99. Patcharatrakul T, Rao SSC. Update on the pathophysiology and management of anorectal disorders. *Gut Liver.* 2018;12(4):375–384.

100. Bordeianou L, Paquette I, Johnson E, et al. Clinical practice guidelines for the treatment of rectal prolapse. *Dis Colon Rectum.* 2017;60(11):1121–1131.

101. Kaufman HS, Buller JL, Thompson JR, et al. Dynamic pelvic magnetic resonance imaging and cystocolpoproctography alter surgical management of pelvic floor disorders. *Dis Colon Rectum.* 2001;44(11):1574–1575.

102. Glasgow SC, Birnbaum EH, Kodner IJ, Fleshman JW, Dietz DW. Preoperative anal manometry predicts continence after perineal proctectomy for rectal prolapse. *Dis Colon Rectum.* 2006;49(7):1052–1058.

103. Tou S, Brown SR, Nelson RL. Surgery for complete (full-thickness) rectal prolapse in adults. *Cochrane Database Syst Rev.* 2015;2015(11):CD001758.

104. Myers JO, Rothenberger DA. Sugar in the reduction of incarcerated prolapsed bowel. Report of two cases. *Dis Colon Rectum.* 1991;34(5):416–418.

105. Brown AJ, Anderson JH, McKee RF, Finlay IG. Strategy for selection of type of operation for rectal prolapse based on clinical criteria. *Dis Colon Rectum.* 2004;47(1):103–107.

106. Fang SH, Cromwell JW, Wilkins KB, et al. Is the abdominal repair of rectal prolapse safer than perineal repair in the highest risk patients? An NSQIP analysis. *Dis Colon Rectum.* 2012;55(11):1167–1172.

107. Consten ECJ, van Iersel JJ, Verheijen PM, Broeders IAMJ, Wolthuis AM, D'Hoore A. Long-term outcome after laparoscopic ventral mesh rectopexy: an observational study of 919 consecutive patients. *Ann Surg.* 2015;262(5):742–748.

108. Samaranayake CB, Luo C, Plank AW, Merrie AEH, Plank LD, Bissett IP. Systematic review on ventral rectopexy for rectal

prolapse and intussusception. *Colorectal Dis.* 2010;12(6):504–512.

109. Mercer-Jones MA, Brown SR, Knowles CH, Williams AB. Position statement by the pelvic floor society on behalf of the Association of Coloproctology of Great Britain and Ireland on the use of mesh in ventral mesh rectopexy. *Colorectal Dis.* 2020 Oct;22(10):1429–1435.

110. Senapati A, Gray RG, Middleton LJ, et al. PROSPER: a randomised comparison of surgical treatments for rectal prolapse. *Colorectal Dis.* 2013;15(7):858–868.

111. Kapoor DS, Sultan AH, Thakar R, Abulafi MA, Swift RI, Ness W. Management of complex pelvic floor disorders in a multidisciplinary pelvic floor clinic. *Colorectal Dis.* 2008;10(2):118–123.

112. Phillips, R. Colorectal Surgery: A Companion to Specialist Surgical Practice. 4th ed. Saunders Elsevier, 2009.

113. Gross G, Ikenberg H, Gissmann L, Hagedorn M. Papillomavirus infection of the anogenital region: correlation between histology, clinical picture, and virus type. Proposal of a new nomenclature. *J Invest Dermatol.* 1985;85(2):147–152.

114. Baseman JG, Koutsky LA. The epidemiology of human papillomavirus infections. *J Clin Virol.* 2005;32(suppl 1):S16–S24.

115. Nyitray AG. The epidemiology of anal human papillomavirus infection among women and men having sex with women. *Sex Health.* 2012;9(6):538–546.

116. Sonnex C, Scholefield JH, Kocjan G, et al. Anal human papillomavirus infection in heterosexuals with genital warts: prevalence and relation with sexual behaviour. *BMJ.* 1991;303(6812):1243.

117. Abbasakoor F, Boulos PB. Anal intraepithelial neoplasia. *Br J Surg.* 2005;92(3):277–290.

118. Kaderli R, Schnuriger B, Brugger LE. The impact of smoking on HPV infection and the development of anogenital warts. *Int J Colorectal Dis.* 2014;29(8):899–908.

119. Oriel JD. Natural history of genital warts. *Br J Vener Dis.* 1971;47(1):1–13.

120. Frisch M, Biggar RJ, Goedert JJ. Human papillomavirus-associated cancers in patients with human immunodeficiency virus infection and acquired immunodeficiency syndrome. *J Natl Cancer Inst.* 2000;92(18):1500–1510.

121. Metcalf AM, Dean T. Risk of dysplasia in anal condyloma. *Surgery.* 1995;118(4):724–726.

122. Lacey CJN, Goodall RL, Tennvall GR, et al. Randomised controlled trial and economic evaluation of podophyllotoxin solution, podophyllotoxin cream, and podophyllin in the treatment of genital warts. *Sex Transm Infect.* 2003;79(4):270–275.

123. Schofer H. Evaluation of imiquimod for the therapy of external genital and anal warts in comparison with destructive therapies. *Br J Dermatol.* 2007;157(suppl 2):52–55.

124. Yan J, Chen S-L, Wang H-N, Wu T-X. Meta-analysis of 5% imiquimod and 0.5% podophyllotoxin in the treatment of condylomata acuminata. *Dermatology.* 2006;213(3):218–223.

125. Abdullah AN, Walzman M, Wade A. Treatment of external genital warts comparing cryotherapy (liquid nitrogen) and trichloroacetic acid. *Sex Transm Dis.* 1993;20(6):344–345.

126. von Krogh G, Lacey CJ, Gross G, Barrasso R, Schneider A. European course on HPV associated pathology: guidelines for primary care physicians for the diagnosis and management of anogenital warts. *Sex Transm Infect.* 2000;76(3):162–168.

127. Lacey CJN, Woodhall SC, Wikstrom A, Ross J. 2012 European guideline for the management of anogenital warts. *J Eur Acad Dermatol Venereol.* 2013;27(3):e263–e270.

128. Daniel GL, Longo WE, Vernava 3rd AM. Pruritus ani. Causes and concerns. *Dis Colon Rectum.* 1994;37(7):670–674.

129. Nasseri YY, Osborne MC. Pruritus ani: diagnosis and treatment. *Gastroenterol Clin North Am.* 2013;42(4):801–813.

130. Smith LE, Henrichs D, McCullah RD. Prospective studies on the etiology and treatment of pruritus ani. *Dis Colon Rectum.* 1982;25(4):358–363.

131. Eyers AA, Thomson JP. Pruritus ani: is anal sphincter dysfunction important in aetiology? *Br Med J.* 1979;2(6204):1549–1551.

132. Farouk R, Duthie GS, Pryde A, Bartolo DC. Abnormal transient internal sphincter relaxation in idiopathic pruritus ani: physiological evidence from ambulatory monitoring. *Br J Surg.* 1994;81(4):603–606.

133. Muller-Lissner SA, Kaatz V, Brandt W, Keller J, Layer P. The perceived effect of various foods and beverages on stool consistency. *Eur J Gastroenterol Hepatol.* 2005;17(1):109–112.

134. Siddiqi S, Vijay V, Ward M, Mahendran R, Warren S. Pruritus ani. *Ann R Coll Surg Engl.* 2008;90(6):457–463.

135. Zuccati G, Lotti T, Mastrolorenzo A, Rapaccini A, Tiradritti L. Pruritus ani. *Dermatol Ther.* 2005;18(4):355–362.

136. Bowyer A, McColl I. A study of 200 patients with pruritus ani. *Proc R Soc Med.* 1970;63(suppl 1):96–98.

137. Aucoin EJ. Pruritus ani. *Postgrad Med.* 1987;82(7):76–80.

138. Jones DJ. ABC of colorectal diseases. Pruritus ani. *BMJ.* 1992;305(6853):575–577.

139. Caccavale S, Bove D, Bove RM, Montagna MLA. Skin and brain: itch and psychiatric disorders. *G Ital Dermatol Venereol.* 2016;151(5):525–529.

140. MacLean J, Russell D. Pruritus ani. *Aust Fam Phys.* 2010;39(6):366–370.

141. Ansari P. Pruritus ani. *Clin Colon Rectal Surg.* 2016;29(1):38–42.

142. Al-Ghnaniem R, Short K, Pullen A, Fuller LC, Rennie JA, Leather AJM. 1% hydrocortisone ointment is an effective treatment of pruritus ani: a pilot randomized controlled crossover trial. *Int J Colorectal Dis.* 2007;22(12):1463.

143. Gooding SMD, Canter PH, Coelho HF, Boddy K, Ernst E. Systematic review of topical capsaicin in the treatment of pruritus. *Int J Dermatol.* 2010;49(8):858–865.

144. Samalavicius NE, Poskus T, Gupta RK, Lunevicius R. Long-term results of single intradermal 1 % methylene blue injection for intractable idiopathic pruritus ani: a prospective study. *Tech Coloproctol.* 2012;16(4):295–299.

145. Menees SB, Almario CV, Spiegel BMR, Chey WD. Prevalence of and factors associated with fecal incontinence: results from a population-based survey. *Gastroenterology.* 2018;154(6):1672. e3–1681.e3.

146. MacLennan AH, Taylor AW, Wilson DH, Wilson D. The prevalence of pelvic floor disorders and their relationship to gender, age, parity and mode of delivery. *BJOG.* 2000;107(12):1460–1470.

147. Wald A, Bharucha AE, Cosman BC, Whitehead WE. ACG clinical guideline: management of benign anorectal disorders. *Am J Gastroenterol.* 2014;109(8):1141–1157;(Quiz) 1058.

148. Norton C, Thomas L, Hill J. Management of faecal incontinence in adults: summary of NICE guidance. *BMJ.* 2007;334(7608):1370–1371.

149. Engel AF, Kamm MA, Bartram CI, Nicholls RJ. Relationship of symptoms in faecal incontinence to specific sphincter abnormalities. *Int J Colorectal Dis.* 1995;10(3):152–155.

150. Bharucha AE, Wald AM. Anorectal disorders. *Am J Gastroenterol.* 2010;105(4):786–794.

151. Jorge JM, Wexner SD. Etiology and management of fecal incontinence. *Dis Colon Rectum.* 1993;36(1):77–97.

152. Bochenska K, Boller A-M. Fecal incontinence: epidemiology, impact, and treatment. *Clin Colon Rectal Surg.* 2016;29(3):264–270.

153. Norton C, Cody JD. Biofeedback and/or sphincter exercises for the treatment of faecal incontinence in adults. *Cochrane Database Syst Rev.* 2012;2012(7):CD002111.

154. Bharucha AE. Update of tests of colon and rectal structure and function. *J Clin Gastroenterol.* 2006;40(2):96–103.

155. Paquette IM, Varma MG, Kaiser AM, Steele SR, Rafferty JF. The American Society of colon and rectal surgeons' clinical practice guideline for the treatment of fecal incontinence. *Dis Colon Rectum.* 2015;58(7):623–636.

156. Maeda Y, Laurberg S, Norton C. Perianal injectable bulking agents as treatment for faecal incontinence in adults. *Cochrane Database Syst Rev.* 2013;2013(2):CD007959.

157. Norton C, Whitehead WE, Bliss DZ, Harari D, Lang J. Management of fecal incontinence in adults. *Neurourol Urodyn.* 2010;29(1):199–206.

158. Falletto E, Brown S, Gagliardi G. Sacral nerve stimulation for faecal incontinence and constipation in adults. *Tech Coloproctol.* 2018;22(2):125–127.

159. Simillis C, Lal N, Qiu S, et al. Sacral nerve stimulation versus percutaneous tibial nerve stimulation for faecal incontinence: a systematic review and meta-analysis. *Int J Colorectal Dis.* 2018;33(5):645–648.

160. Alavi K, Chan S, Wise P, Kaiser AM, Sudan R, Bordeianou L. Fecal incontinence: etiology, diagnosis, and management. *J Gastrointest Surg.* 2015;19(10):1910–1921.

161. Brown SR, Wadhawan H, Nelson RL. Surgery for faecal incontinence in adults. *Cochrane Database Syst Rev.* 2013;2013(7):CD001757.

23

Surgical Pathology of the Liver, Pancreas and Biliary Tract

CHAPTER OUTLINE

THE LIVER

Liver and Biliary Embryology and Anatomy

The primordial liver and biliary system appears at week 3 in the embryo as an anterior thickening and outgrowth from the endodermal epithelium of the foregut (future duodenum). This hepatic diverticulum or bud penetrates the septum transversum, where it enlarges and divides into two parts. The larger portion forms the hepatic parenchyma, biliary apparatus and hepatic sinusoid network and the smaller portion expands to form the gallbladder and its stalk and the cystic duct. Haematopoiesis begins during week 6 and the liver becomes a bright red colour.

Clinical Anatomy

The liver lies below the right diaphragm. The liver is adherent to the under-surface of the diaphragm where the peritoneal covering of the liver reflects to form the coronary and triangular ligaments (Fig. 23.1).

Ventrally, the covering reflects to form the falciform ligament in which runs the ligamentum teres, the obliterated fetal umbilical vein. This latter vein carries oxygenated blood from the placenta to the fetus. The vein runs along the under-surface of the liver to drain into the ductus venosus, between the caudate lobe and the left lateral section, to reach the inferior vena cava. Following birth, the umbilical vein fibroses and forms the round ligament lying in the falciform ligament. In the adult, the fibrosed ductus venosus is seen as the Arantius' ligament and in patients with chronic liver disease, the umbilical vein can recanalize and gives rise to the clinical finding of caput medusae on the abdominal wall.

The liver has a unique dual blood supply (Fig. 23.2). Blood flow to the liver is derived from both the portal vein (80%) and the hepatic artery (20%). The portal vein carries blood returning from the gastrointestinal tract and forms behind the head of the pancreas as a continuation of the superior mesenteric vein and confluence with the splenic vein. It then passes in the free edge of the lesser omentum to the liver hilum where it divides into a left and right branch. Arterial anatomy to the liver can be

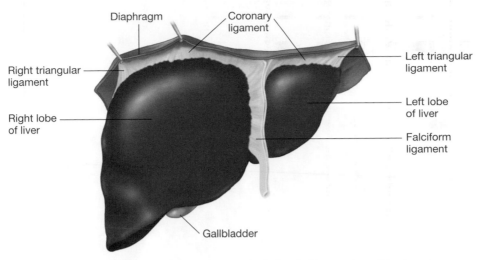

• **Fig. 23.1** The Gross Anatomy of the Liver Including its Ligamentous Attachments

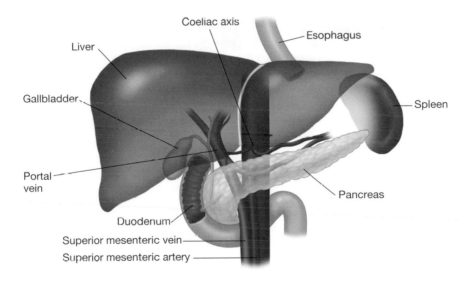

• **Fig. 23.2** The Blood Supply to the Liver The portal vein supplies 80% of the liver blood and lies posteriorly in the free edge of the lesser omentum. It is formed by the union of the SMV and splenic vein behind the neck of the pancreas. The hepatic artery supplies the remaining blood to the liver and is a branch of the coeliac axis of the aorta. The bile duct is the most lateral structure in the porta hepatis with the hepatic artery lying medial to it. SMV, Superior mesenteric vein.

highly variable. The hepatic artery usually arises from the coeliac artery on the ventral surface of the aorta and passes to the right along the superior border of the pancreas to ascend in the free edge of the lesser omentum to the liver hilum, where it divides into left and right branches. However, the hepatic artery can arise solely from the coeliac trunck, superior mesenteric artery or, indeed, the aorta. The bile duct also lies in the free edge of the lesser omentum. The triad of the bile duct, the portal vein branches and the arterial branches are enclosed in a fibrous (Glisson's) sheath, which is a continuation of Glisson's capsule that covers the liver.

Venous drainage of the liver is through three central hepatic veins (right, middle and left), which have a very short extrahepatic length before reaching the inferior vena cava (IVC) just below the diaphragm (Fig. 23.3). There are a variable number of short veins draining directly into the retrohepatic IVC that often require division during major hepatectomy. The caudate lobe of the liver (or segment 1, see below) has specialized venous drainage, and drains separately and directly into the IVC. This specialized drainage of the caudate lobe is life-saving in diseases such as Budd–Chiari syndrome. In this rare disease, there is thrombosis of all the main hepatic veins but the caudate lobe remains functional because of its direct drainage into the IVC (essentially bypassing the hepatic veins) and can hypertrophy to completely envelope the IVC while the remaining liver undergoes necrosis.

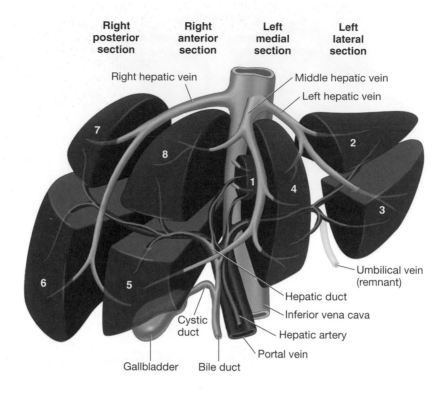

Right posterior section | Right anterior section | Left medial section | Left lateral section

Right hepatic vein   Middle hepatic vein
Left hepatic vein

Umbilical vein (remnant)
Hepatic duct
Inferior vena cava
Cystic duct   Hepatic artery
Portal vein
Gallbladder   Bile duct

• **Fig. 23.3** The liver is divided into eight separate and distinct segments as per Couninad's classification. Each segment has its own arterial and portal blood supply and its own biliary drainage. Segments 2, 3 and 4 make up the left liver and segments 5–8 the right liver. Segment 1 or the caudate lobe is a specialized lobe of the liver (see text).

Sectional/Segmental Liver Anatomy

In simple terms, the anatomy of the liver is based upon the divisions of the hepatic artery and bile ducts and, on this basis, the liver is divided into two hemilivers, each supplied by a branch of the hepatic artery (see Fig. 23.3) and the plane of separation between the right and left hemilivers lies along a virtual line (Cantlie's line) drawn between the tip of the gallbladder fossa and the IVC. The right and left hemilivers can be further subdivided into sections based upon the divisions of the hepatic artery and biliary system. Hence, the left hemiliver can be divided into a medial and lateral section and the right liver into anterior and posterior sections. In the right liver, the medial and lateral sections are separated in the plane of the right hepatic vein and, in the left liver, the medial and lateral sections are separated by the plane of the left hepatic vein. The arterial divisions further divide the liver into eight functional units called segments, named after the French surgeon Claude Couinaud who originally described them. In this nomenclature, segments 2–4 comprise the left hemiliver and 5–8 the right liver (see Fig. 23.3). These distinct anatomical segments allow for resection of separate segments of the liver. Hence, based upon the above terminology, it is possible to perform a left lateral sectionectomy, right posterior sectionectomy, left hepatectomy or segment 2 resection as

long as these important anatomical principles are borne in mind. Non-anatomical resections of the liver are ones that are performed across boundaries without specific regard for the segmental anatomy. As described above, segment 1 is also referred to as the caudate lobe and has a distinct blood supply and biliary drainage compared to the rest of the liver and this is of paramount importance when surgical management of biliary tract cancers or cholangiocarcinoma is being considered (see later).

Biliary System

The bile canaliculi around the hepatocytes unite to form intralobular bile ductules, then interlobular ducts eventually converge to form the right and left hepatic ducts (see Fig. 23.3). The bile ducts are lined by specialized epithelial cells known as cholangiocytes. The union of the left and right hepatic ducts forms the common hepatic duct and, from the insertion point of the cystic duct, the common bile duct lying in the free edge of the lesser omentum. The biliary anatomy can be highly variable and the conventional anatomy described above is present in only 57% of the population (Fig. 23.4). The common bile duct terminates at the ampulla of Vater where it is joined by the terminal end of the pancreatic duct (see Fig 23.2). The

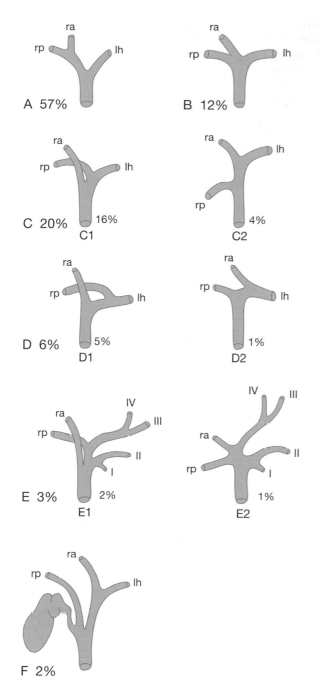

Parenchymal

Hepatocytes	Metabolism of protein, steroids, bile secretion, sugar storage, xenobiotic metabolism
Cholangiocytes	Cytokine secretion and regulation of inflammation
Sinusoidal endothelial cells	Filtration and transport of nutrients from the blood, modulating vascular tone and antigen presentation
Hepatic stellate cells	Fat-storing cells, vitamin A storage and growth factors

Non-parenchymal

Kupffer cells	Phagocytosis and cytokine production
T- and B-lymphocytes	Regulation of inflammation

Gallbladder

The gallbladder is a pear-shaped structure whose size varies depending upon fasting state. The gallbladder sits on the underside of the liver in the gallbladder fossa and thus between segments 4 and 5. Gallbladder and biliary anatomy is relevant for cholecystectomy (see below). Importantly, Calot's triangle should not be confused with the hepato-cystic triangle (see Fig. 23.13). The gallbladder is described as having a fundus, body and neck and derives blood from the cystic artery, which is usually a branch of the right hepatic artery.

Hepatobiliary Physiology

The liver is a complex and highly specialized organ with diverse functions and as such has multiple cell types within it. These are broadly divided into parenchymal and non-parenchymal cells (Box 23.1). These are briefly discussed below.

Hepatocytes

Hepatocytes play a dominant role in metabolism and storage of dietary molecules. Carbohydrates are stored as glycogen and released in response to changes in blood sugar concentration to meet bodily requirements. Fats are metabolized – to ketone bodies – for energy transfer and release. Some special products, such as cholesterol, are synthesized. Fat-soluble vitamins (A, D and K) are principally or exclusively stored in the liver. The liver is the only source of albumin and alpha-globulin. Many other specialized proteins, such as clotting factors, are synthesized in the liver. Operations on patients with liver disease and defective protein synthesis require management of deficiency states. The liver detoxifies a variety of endogenous and exogenous substances (chiefly drugs) mainly by conjugating them into less active forms.

• **Fig. 23.4** Variations in Biliary Anatomy Only in 57% of the population does normal biliary anatomy occur (A) where the right posterior (rp) duct joins the right anterior (ra) duct to form the right hepatic duct which then joins the left hepatic (lh) duct. Many variations can exist as illustrated above. Important clinical variations include C2 where the (rp) duct inserts into the common bile duct and can be mistaken for the cystic duct at the time of cholecystectomy.

exit of the ampulla of Vater is guarded by a circular muscle known as the sphincter of Oddi. Importantly, the biliary system is supplied only with arterial blood derived from the hepatic artery and hence problems with hepatic arterial blood flow to the liver preferentially lead to bile duct damage such as that seen after thrombosis of the hepatic artery which can lead to bile duct necrosis or biloma/biliary abscess formation.

The production, storage and release of bile into the duodenum is a fundamental function of the liver. Bilirubin is a breakdown product of the cleavage of haem from red blood cells by the reticuloendothelial system. On release into the circulation, it is unconjugated (fat-soluble) and transported in the plasma bound to albumin. On extraction from the plasma by the hepatocyte, it is conjugated with glucuronide by the enzyme glucuronyl transferase to become water-soluble and is excreted continuously in the bile. Bacterial deconjugation in the colon produces stercobilin, which colours the faeces brown. If there is infection in the biliary tree, deconjugation may take place within it, and the bilirubin may aggregate to form stones (see 'Oriental cholangiohepatitis'). Although bile is secreted continuously by the liver cells, one of its main functions is assisting in digestion. Under physiological circumstances, bile is intermittently released into the duodenum. Between meals, the gallbladder acts as a reservoir in which bile is concentrated from 5 to 20 times by removal of sodium and water. Release of bile into the duodenum begins shortly after the ingestion of food – in response to stimulation of the vagus. The main flow, which is accompanied by gallbladder contraction and relaxation of the sphincter of Oddi, takes place as the result of the secretion of cholecystokinin from the duodenal wall in response to the presence of fat in the lumen. Contraction of the gallbladder in this manner against an obstructing stone causes pain (biliary colic). In addition to concentrating bile, mucin is secreted from the gallbladder mucosa and this is believed to have a role in preventing stone formation.

Non-Parenchymal Cells

Reticuloendothelial Function

Sixty-five percent of the reticuloendothelial system is located within the liver, giving it an integral immunological role. Kupffer cells within the liver sinusoids are responsible for filtering and destroying bacteria and their products that arrive in the liver through the diet and are absorbed from the gut. This has important implications for the surgeon as often, during liver surgery, the liver vascular inflow is temporarily clamped, known as Pringle manoeuvre, to lessen blood loss. However, the build-up of these toxins during clamping causes a phenomenon known as ischaemia-reperfusion injury after release.

Jaundice

Jaundice or icterus is the clinical manifestation of an increased concentration of bilirubin in serum, the normal upper limit of which is 17 μmol/L. When hepatic uptake and excretion are decreased, the excess bilirubin in plasma spills over into the interstitial space so that the tissues become stained yellow. Bilirubin has a high affinity for the protein elastin and therefore, because the sclera of the eye contains the highest abundance of this protein in the body, it is the eyes that appear most

---

• **BOX 23.2** **Classification of Jaundice**

Type of Bilirubin	Causes Raised
Medical	
Prehepatic/haemolytic Unconjugated	Haemolysis Antibodies Drugs Thalassemia
Hepatic/Hepatocellular Unconjugated and conjugated	Hepatitis Gilbert's syndrome Drugs
Surgical	
Post-hepatic/Obstructive Conjugated	Gallstones Biliary Pancreatic tumours

---

prominently yellow. A symptom that often accompanies jaundice is itching or pruritus and is probably caused by the excessive build-up of bile salts in the tissues. Clinically, it is important to distinguish between jaundice that occurs because of increased bilirubin production (termed medical jaundice) or jaundice that has developed because of an obstruction to excretion of bile (termed surgical jaundice) (Box 23.2). Defining jaundice as medical or surgical ensures that the appropriate medical teams manage the patient.

Prehepatic

This phenomenon occurs because of the increased and/or excessive breakdown of red cells – haemolysis. The rate of production of bilirubin is sufficiently fast to saturate the conjugation mechanisms within the liver. The bilirubin in plasma is unconjugated and therefore is not excreted by the kidney, resulting in acholuric jaundice.

Hepatic

Hepatic jaundice generally occurs when there is damage to the liver parenchyma, meaning either uptake, conjugation or secretion of bilirubin are impaired. Importantly, diseases affecting the cholangiocytes that line the bile canaliculi can also occur in hepatic jaundice. Hepatic/intrahepatic cholestasis occurs when there is a failure to excrete conjugated bilirubin into the canaliculi within the liver, and it is a common occurrence in patients with hepatocellular jaundice. Jaundice may be caused by:
- Defective uptake occurs with mild intermittent jaundice in otherwise healthy individuals (Gilbert's syndrome).
- Congenital absence of glucuronyl transferase is associated with severe jaundice and early death (Crigler–Najjar syndrome).

- Congenital impairment of excretion of conjugated bilirubin into the bile is known as Dubin–Johnson–Rotor syndrome.

All the above conditions are rare, apart from Gilbert's syndrome.

The common causes of hepatocellular jaundice are:
- viral diseases of the liver cell – hepatitis A, B, C, D and E
- other hepatic infections
- alcoholic liver disease
- hepatotoxic drugs, such as the phenothiazines

Post-Hepatic

Post-hepatic jaundice is also termed obstructive or 'surgical' jaundice, which implies that the cause is a mechanical obstruction in the extrahepatic biliary tree (extrahepatic cholestasis). The term identifies those patients whose jaundice may be capable of relief by some form of mechanical intervention – either by surgery, endoscopy or interventional radiology. In these patients, the relatively intact hepatocyte conjugates bilirubin, which is then released back into the plasma and excreted by the kidney so that the urine is dark and the stools pale. The same phenomenon occurs in patients with intrahepatic cholestasis caused by canalicular obstruction within the liver. Causes of extrahepatic cholestasis include:
- obstruction in the lumen of the biliary tree – gallstones
- obstruction in the wall of the ducts – biliary atresia; bile duct carcinoma (cholangiocarcinoma); postoperative stricture
- extrinsic compression – pancreatitis; pancreatic tumour; secondary deposits in the hilar lymph nodes of the liver

Investigations
Biochemical

It is highly informative to measure liver functions tests (LFTs) in a patient with jaundice. Generally, these are made up of three serum measurements: bilirubin, alkaline phosphatase and the transferases (Box 23.3):
- **Bilirubin:** A raised level of plasma bilirubin indicates disruption of its normal passage from blood, through the hepatocyte and down the biliary collecting system into

the duodenum. Serial measurements are helpful in following the course of hepatic or biliary disease.
- **Alkaline phosphatase (ALP):** This substance is secreted predominantly from the cells of the biliary collecting system, which proliferate in the presence of obstruction. A raised serum level in the presence of jaundice is therefore a good indicator of cholestasis – either extrahepatic or intrahepatic. Another serum enzyme called gamma-glutamyl transferase (gGT) can also be used in conjunction with ALP.
- **Transferases:** These enzymes are constituents of the hepatocyte. If their serum levels are raised, the implication is that there is hepatocellular damage. Usually this is primary, within the hepatocyte, but, in long-standing extrahepatic obstruction, secondary interference with hepatocellular function may take place. The commonly measured transferases are alanine aminotransferase (ALT) and aspartate aminotransferase (AST).

Other measurements that may be of value in jaundice are:
- **Albumin concentration:** This gives a guide to the synthetic capacity of the liver and the nutritional state of the patient.
- **Clotting factors:** These are synthesized in the liver. The most easily assessed is prothrombin. Vitamin K is a cofactor in its synthesis. Because the vitamin is fat soluble and is therefore not well absorbed from the intestine in the absence of bile, its limited hepatic stores soon become exhausted. The hypoprothrombinaemia of jaundice responds to the administration of parenteral vitamin K provided that hepatocyte function is preserved, as is nearly always the case when the jaundice is caused by obstruction. Measurement of the prothrombin time is therefore an essential preliminary before operation in a jaundiced patient.
- **Alpha-fetoprotein (AFP):** See hepatocellular carcinoma, later.
- **Hepatitis virus markers**

Imaging
- **Ultrasound**

Ultrasound is a very useful investigation to differentiate between medical and surgical jaundice and is also noninvasive. Ultrasound scanning reliably detects dilated biliary system and, when this feature is found, the presence of surgical jaundice is suggested. In addition, cysts, abscesses and tumours can be delineated, and guided fine-needle aspiration and biopsy are possible but should be carefully used as aspiration of tumour can cause seeding.
- **CT scanning**

CT scan provides much more precise and detailed anatomy of the liver with less operator variability but at the expense of a radiation dose. The image is enhanced with oral contrast medium to delineate the bowel and with an intravenous contrast agent to show vascular structures. CT scans are also used to stage patients with suspected and/or proven cancer prior to consideration of liver surgery.

• BOX 23.3 LFT Findings During Different Causes of Jaundice

Prehepatic – Normal AST/ALT and ALP with abnormal haematological tests depending on cause (e.g. Thalassemia screen)

Hepatic – AST/ALT very high and ALP 2–3 times increased compared to normal

Post-hepatic – AST/ALT increased and ALP 10–12 times increased

ALP, Alkaline phosphatase; ALT, alanine transaminase; AST, aspartate transaminase; LFT, liver function tests.

- **Magnetic resonance cholangiopancreatography (MRCP) and magnetic resonance imaging with contrast**

  MRCP now provides good images of the biliary and pancreatic ductal system and this non-invasive method has replaced diagnostic endoscopic retrograde cholangiopancreatography (ERCP) and percutaneous transhepatic cholangiography (PTC) as the preferred choice for imaging the biliary system. MRCP are performed without the need for contrast but do not provide a therapeutic option.

  When mass lesions within the liver are included within the differential diagnosis, MRI liver with contrast is a valuable investigation and, in many instances, superior to CT scanning (Fig. 23.5). Contrast agents such as Primovist are used and distribute to the vascular and extravascular spaces during the arterial, portal venous and late dynamic phases, and then progressively into the hepatocytes and bile ducts during the hepatobiliary phase.

- **Cholecystography/cholangiography**

  PTC is achieved by introducing a fine needle through the substance of the liver into a bile duct. Success rates are reduced if the biliary system is not dilated. PTC is of particular value in determining the anatomical level and the nature of obstructing hilar lesions. Furthermore, ERCP is usually not able to relieve obstruction at the hilum and thus most such patients require PTC (see Fig. 23.5).

  ERCP similarly delineates the biliary tract but also can show the pancreatic ductal system. At both ERCP and PTC,

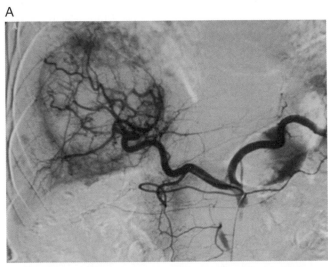

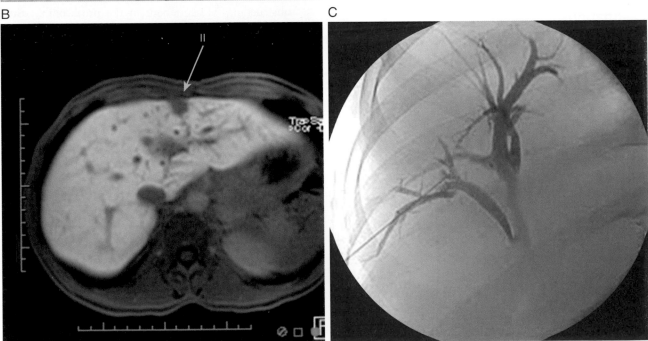

• **Fig. 23.5** (A) Illustrates a coeliac artery angiogram showing a large tumour blush in the right liver. (B) MRI liver demonstrating a metastasis within the left liver from a colorectal primary. (C) A percutaenous transhepatic cholangiogram (PTC). A Chiba wire has been used to puncture the biliary system within the right liver and contrast is injected to obtain a cholangiogram.

bile may be aspirated for microbiological examination and cells may also be obtained for cytological assessment. Both procedures are usually now performed only for therapy, such as the placement of biliary stents to relieve obstruction or the removal of biliary stones by endoscopic sphincterotomy or dilatation of the sphincter of Oddi.

- **Arteriography**

  Selective coeliac and superior mesenteric angiograms can show the abnormal circulation of a tumour (tumour blush – see Fig. 23.5). The late-phase images of an angiogram demonstrate the portal vein, and therefore neoplastic involvement of both arterial and venous vessels can be assessed. However, vascular reconstruction using CT or MRI images is comparable to direct angiography. Invasive angiography is now usually performed only as a precursor to embolization as shown in Fig. 23.5, where angiography is needed to embolize a ruptured hepatocellular carcinoma.

- **Laparoscopy**

  Laparoscopy permits direct visualization of the liver and may be combined with laparoscopic ultrasound to provide both accurate staging and biopsy of diseased liver tissue. Because of the accuracy of modern staging imaging, many surgeons do not use laparoscopy prior to resection. If laparoscopy is used, it is normally performed immediately before planned laparotomy for liver resection. Some evidence suggests that the use of laparoscopy in patients with pathologies such as hilar cholangiocarcinoma may detect small volume peritoneal metastasis not visible on radiological imaging.

- **Biopsy**

  Percutaneous liver biopsy is an invasive procedure which is used in the diagnosis of diffuse liver disease or for confirmation of metastatic malignancy. Accuracy is increased when insertion of the needle for biopsy or liver cytology is guided by ultrasound, CT or at laparoscopy. However, if pathology is confidently identified by a liver radiologist, then biopsy is not required prior to definitive management.

General Management

Preparation for Liver Surgery

Major liver resections may require specialized support for abnormalities in the clotting system and for postoperative nutrition by either the enteral or parenteral route. For these reasons this type of surgery is usually carried out by specialized centres.

The Jaundiced Patient

- **Clotting**

  The most likely problem is vitamin K deficiency, which can be corrected by parenteral administration of the synthetic derivatives menadione or phytomenadione (K1). The synthesis of prothrombin, set in motion by restoring supplies of vitamin K, takes some hours, so the prothrombin time must, except in dire emergencies, be rechecked before operation is undertaken. In emergency cases, fresh frozen plasma may be used to correct clotting.

- **Antibiotic prophylaxis**

  Sepsis from organisms that originate in the GI tract is a major cause of death in the surgical management of jaundice, partly because of interference with hepatic reticuloendothelial function. Prophylactic antibiotics against enteric organisms, such as cefuroxime or ciprofloxacin, are used routinely at the time of surgery or invasive procedures such as PTC and ERCP.

- **Preliminary biliary decompression**

  In a patient who will subsequently require an operation, liver function may be improved by biliary decompression which is done by one of the following methods:

- passing a catheter percutaneously into the liver substance and then into a bile duct at PTC (see Fig. 23.5)
- ERCP with or without dilatation of an obstructing lesion and insertion of biliary stent (plastic or expanding metal). Generally, plastic stents are used in benign conditions and metal expanding stents in malignant disease

Hepatorenal Syndrome

This condition is probably one variant of the systemic inflammatory response syndrome (SIRS) in which renal and hepatic failure develop in response to severe injury or sepsis, especially if there is dysregulation of the immune system. A patient with jaundice is particularly liable to develop acute kidney injury, and measures to prevent this include:

- adequate preoperative hydration
- avoidance of nephrotoxic medication
- avoidance of intraoperative hypotension
- maintenance of high urine flow by the use of an osmotic diuretic (mannitol) which opposes the action of increased secretion of antidiuretic hormone on the distal tubule after operation; and also by administration of a low dose of inotrope which increases renal plasma flow and glomerular filtration rate

Benign Conditions of the Liver

Congenital Diseases

Biliary Atresia

Aetiology and Pathological Features

- The commonest cause of prolonged neonatal jaundice is extrahepatic biliary atresia. The cause is not known.
- There may be single or multiple points of obstruction, and the proximal biliary ducts may dilate considerably.

Clinical Features

Mild jaundice is not uncommon in the neonatal period. However, persistence and progression beyond 2 weeks is abnormal and then the distinction has to be made between obstruction and hepatitis. This can usually be achieved by the biochemical profile and ultrasound scanning as discussed above.

Management

There are two management options:

- For the majority of infants, hepatic portoenterostomy or Kasai operation should be attempted within 60 days of birth at a specialist centre. Delay beyond this time is associated with the rapid development of intrahepatic fibrosis and a reduced survival.
- When evidence of deteriorating liver function is apparent, liver transplantation should be considered.

Prognosis

- If not relieved, liver failure ultimately ensues with death in the first year of life; only a few infants surviving beyond 6 months.

Congenital Cystic Liver Disease

- Cysts may be solitary or multiple (Fig. 23.6).
- Multiple cysts are frequently associated with polycystic disease of the kidney and may be linked to a defective polycystin protein.

Clinical Features

- The cysts are often small, asymptomatic and found only incidentally either at laparotomy or during investigation of other symptoms.
- Large cysts may present with pain in the right upper abdomen, which may radiate to the right shoulder and is believed to be caused by stretching of the liver capsule *(Glisson's capsule).*

Management

- In a few instances, percutaneous aspiration under image control is used but refilling of the cyst after needle aspiration is common as most cysts are connected to the biliary system.
- In symptomatic and/or large cysts, surgical decompression by fenestration or 'de-roofing' is required which, in the modern era, can be achieved via the laparoscopic approach.
- Rarely, in cases of multiple cysts located in the right or left liver, liver resection may be indicated.
- In patients showing multiple bilateral cysts (e.g. polycystic liver disease) with compromise of the quality of life and/or reduced functioning liver parenchyma, liver transplantation should be considered.
- In cases of polycystic liver and kidney disease associated with renal failure, combined liver and renal transplantation is the treatment of choice.

Choledochal Cyst

- This term is used to describe dilatation of all or part of the extrahepatic biliary tree, with or without associated cystic change of the intrahepatic bile ducts (see Fig. 23.6).
- Choledochal cysts are classified as follows:
  - **Type I**: *cystic* (**Ia**), *segmental* (**Ib**), or *fusiform* (**Ic**) dilatation of the extrahepatic bile duct
  - **Type II**: the cyst forms a diverticulum from the extrahepatic bile duct

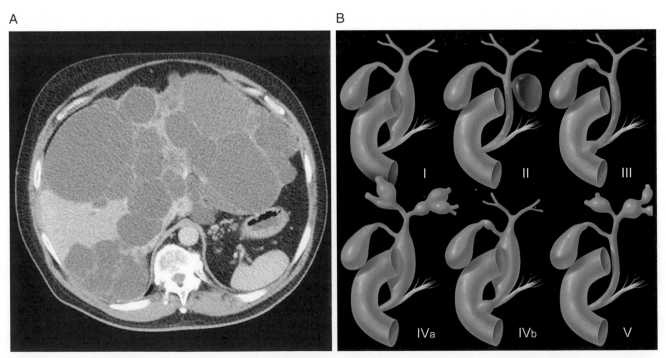

A   B

• **Fig. 23.6** (A) Demonstrates an axial CT scan with multiple cysts in the liver – the characteristic feature of polycystic liver disease. (B) The Todani classification of choledochal cyst. Type I–IV require resection of the bile and Roux-en-Y hepaticojejunostomy and type V requires liver transplantation if widespread or liver resection if localized to one liver lobe. (B, from Kamaya, A., Diagnostic Ultrasound for Sonographers, Elsevier 2019, Chapter 42.)

- **Type III**: cystic dilatation (*choledochocele*) of the distal common bile duct lying mostly within the duodenal wall
- **Type IV**: type I associated with intrahepatic bile duct cysts.
  - **Types I** and **IV** are usually associated with an anomalous biliary–pancreatic ductal junction which allows pancreatic juice to flow retrogradely into the biliary tree.
  - These types of choledochal cyst in particular are associated with an increased risk of cholangiocarcinoma development.
  - Patients may present with upper abdominal pain and raised liver enzymes and amylase.
  - Others are found incidentally on ultrasound scanning.
  - Surgical excision of the cyst with Roux-en-Y hepaticojejunostomy (see below) is recommended to reduce the risk of cholangiocarcinoma.
- **Type V (Caroli's disease):**
  - This is a rare congenital but non-familial disorder with saccular dilatation of the intrahepatic ducts.
  - The cause is not known.
  - The syndrome is usually diffuse but is occasionally confined to one liver segment or lobe.
  - Clinical features are of recurrent upper abdominal pain and cholangitis in childhood or early adult life.
  - Cholangitis is treated with systemic antibiotics. Localized disease to the liver is managed with liver resection.
  - Chronic cholangitis may lead to *secondary biliary cirrhosis* – a phenomenon where repeated infections in the bile duct causes chronic inflammation and, eventually, strictures in the smaller bile ducts leading to liver failure.
  - Bile duct carcinoma is described in some cases. Liver transplantation should be considered in patients presenting with a secondary biliary cirrhosis.

Liver Trauma

- The liver can be injured either by blunt or penetrating injury to the abdomen or chest.
- The commonest causes are road traffic accident, falls and non-accidental injury.
- In all cases, the attending medical team should retain a high index of suspicion for other injuries.
- Most liver injuries in the UK arise from blunt rather than penetrating trauma and this is in contrast to countries where gun crime is common.

Clinical Features

- In blunt trauma, the liver is the second most common site of injury within the abdomen, after the spleen.
- Liver trauma complicates about 15–20% of blunt injuries to the abdomen and of these, about half will have splenic trauma.
- The mechanism of the injury, a sudden compression of the liver between the ribs and the spine, disrupts the hepatic substance and results in a diversity of injury from contusions, subcapsular (contained beneath an intact Glissonian capsule) haematomas or lacerations (Box 23.4).
- The surgical right side of the liver is far more likely to be injured and most blunt injuries involve segments 4, 6, 7 and 8.
- Associated gallbladder injury or portal triad injury is uncommon and occurs in about 5% of blunt injuries to the liver but is more common in penetrating injuries.
- Massive haemorrhage, bile leaks and fistulae are not uncommon in portal triad injury and early mortality or long-term complications are more likely to occur.

• BOX 23.4	Classification of Liver Trauma (American Association of Surgery for Trauma)	
Grade		**Injury Description**
I.	Hematoma	Subcapsular, nonexpanding, <10 cm surface area
	Laceration	Capsular tear, nonbleeding, <1 cm parenchymal bleeding
II.	Hematoma	Subcapsular, nonexpanding, 10 to 50% surface area; Intraparenchymal nonexpanding <10 cm in diameter
	Laceration	Capsular tear, active bleeding; 1–3 cm parenchymal depth <10 cm in length
III.	Hematoma	Subcapsular, >50% surface area or expanding; Ruptured subcapsular hematoma with active bleeding; Intraparenchymal hematoma >10 cm or expanding
	Laceration	>3 cm parenchymal depth
IV.	Hematoma	Ruptured intraparenchymal hematoma with active bleeding
	Laceration	Parenchymal disruption involving 25% to 75% of hepatic lobe
V.	Laceration	Parenchymal disruption involving >75% of hepatic lobe
	Vascular	Juxtahepatic venous injury (i.e. retrohepatic vena cava)
VI.	Vascular	Vascular avulsion

- The risk of mortality from blunt abdominal trauma rises with the severity of the liver injury and with an increase in the number of other organs involved.
- Small injuries may not manifest any clinical signs.
- Larger injuries may show signs of loss of circulating volume but it is possible that even an extensive injury may be undetected clinically unless a complication results later.

Management

- All patients should be managed in accordance with Advanced Trauma Life Support (ATLS) guidelines and in line with the grade of liver injury (see Box 23.4).
- In general, a patient who is haemodynamically stable should undergo cross sectional imaging alongside resuscitation.
- The sensitivity and specificity of CT imaging has been demonstrated to be high and CT can be used to classify the severity of injury (see earlier), but is not necessarily a guide to management.
- In *unstable* patients, the surgeon should consider operative intervention in conjunction with other specialists, depending upon injuries.
- However, surgeons have moved increasingly to a non-operative strategy in the management of both blunt and penetrating liver trauma.
- Most cases of *grade I–III* are likely to be haemodynamically stable and can be managed by a trauma service without a specialized liver unit.
  - The survival should approach 100% in this setting.
  - The more severe injuries should be transferred to the care of a specialist unit, depending of course on the stability of the patient and other concomitant injuries that might take precedence.
  - Even some high-grade injuries in stable patients can be managed non-operatively but complications such as re-bleeding, biloma, abscess, compartment syndrome or other event requiring intervention occur in about 15%.
  - While re-bleeding tends to occur in the early days after injury, infective or biliary complications may not manifest themselves for weeks or months after injury.
- Injury *grade IV or V* and requirement for blood transfusion is predictive for a complication in the non-operatively managed patient.
- In the *unstable* patient or where laparotomy is performed for other reasons, the initial management of liver trauma, especially by a non- specialist, is simply to control the damage by perihepatic packing using gauze rolls in anticipation of resuscitation and radiological re-evaluation of the liver with possible arterial embolization if required.
- The involvement of more than one hepatic vein or a portal triad injury increases the probability that operative management will be required.

- Immediate vascular or biliary reconstructions are really only for the specialist unit and bile injuries should be controlled by peritoneal drainage and, if possible, bile duct intubation.
- Massive haemorrhage from a portal vein injury might be controlled by ligation but the resulting liver and bowel ischaemia leads to a very high mortality. Arterial ligation in the presence of intact portal venous inflow is unlikely to cause mortality.

Liver Infections

Pyogenic Liver Abscess

Aetiology

- This condition is uncommon in the UK and usually affects the elderly or debilitated.
- In 25–50% of cases the primary site of infection remains unknown.
- Biliary infection (cholangitis) is the commonest source with the other main cause being bacterial seeding via the portal vein (portal pyaemia) from an intra-abdominal site – an abscess related to appendicitis, pancreatitis, diverticular disease or perforation of the GI tract.
- Pyogenic liver disease needs to be distinguished from amoebic abscess (see later).

Pathological Features

- About half of all liver abscesses are multiple.
- Solitary abscesses are usually found in the right lobe of the liver, directly under the diaphragm. Common organisms are: *Streptococcus milleri*, *Escherichia coli*, *Streptococcus enterococcus*, *Staphylococcus aureus* and anaerobes such as *Bacteroides* spp, (Box 23.5).

Clinical Features

Presenting symptoms are variable but there is often fever, malaise, anorexia and upper abdominal pain. Jaundice is rare.

• BOX 23.5 Aetiology of Pyogenic Liver Abscesses		
Hepatobiliary	Benign	Cholecystitis, biliary-enteric anastomosis, endoscopic biliary procedures, percutaneous biopsy
Portal	Malignant Benign	Diverticulitis, pelvic sepsis, perforation
Arterial	Malignant	Gastric, colonic cancer
Traumatic		Endocarditis, ENT
Cryptogenic		or dental infection
Direct spread of adjacent infection		chemoembolization or trauma

Investigation

- Bloods:
  - There may be a neutrophil leucocytosis, secondary anaemia and hypoalbuminaemia.
- Cross-sectional imaging such as CT and MRI are the best methods with which to establish the diagnosis and, with prophylactic antibiotics, may be used to guide aspiration to obtain pus for microbiological analysis, often combined with percutaneous drain insertion.

Management

- All patients are treated with systemic antibiotics which, in multiple abscesses, may be the only form of treatment feasible.
- Those large enough to be readily detected on imaging rarely respond to antibiotics alone and require drainage.
- The morbidity and mortality are high if abscesses are multiple or inadequately drained; in such cases, either multiple drains should be placed percutaneously or a surgical procedure will be required.

Hydatid Disease

- This is a liver disease that is caused by the parasite *Echinococcus granulosus* and may present with hepatomegaly, which, if the cyst is active or infected, is associated with tenderness.
- Ultrasound and CT (Fig. 23.7) will show whether a cyst is single or multiple.
- Calcified cysts are usually dead and therefore do not require treatment.
- Obstructive jaundice or cholangitis by daughter cysts obstructing the common bile duct is managed initially by endoscopic biliary stenting.
- Large, superficially placed and symptomatic cysts may require surgical evacuation with special precautions (covering the surgical field with betadine or ceramide gauze) being taken to kill the brood capsules before the contents are released whilst the patient is taking albendazole prior to and after surgery.

Amoebic Liver Abscess

- Amoebic liver infection and abscess is a complication of *Entamoeba histolytica* colitis.
- The amoebae enter the portal circulation through an ulcer in the colonic mucosa.

Pathological Features

The amoebae establish a colony which first leads to hepatitis and then to liver necrosis and abscess formation. Extension of the focus may lead to pleural effusion, bronchopleural fistula and lung abscess. Rupture into the peritoneal cavity may also occur.

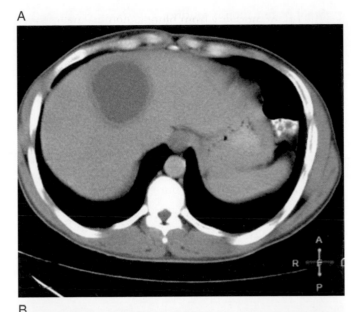

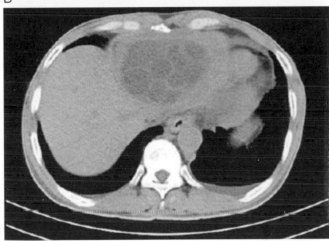

• **Fig. 23.7** (A) CT scan demonstrating a hydatid cyst in the left liver. Daughter cysts can be seen within the main cyst. (B) An axial CT image that shows an amoebic abscess within the liver.

Clinical Features

History

- There may or may not have been a background of colitis.
- There is progressive painful right upper-quadrant pain with sweating, rigors and a swinging pyrexia.
- Involvement of diaphragm and lung may lead to respiratory symptoms.
- Shoulder pain is not uncommon.

Physical Findings

- Right upper-quadrant tenderness, hepatomegaly and jaundice are common findings.

Investigation

- **Ultrasound or CT** delineates the abscess (see Fig. 23.7) and may be used for image-guided aspiration to obtain a specimen for microscopy and bacteriological culture when secondary contamination is suspected.

- Stool examination is routine.
- **Serology:** The amoebic fluorescent antibody titre is raised in 90% of patients.

Management

- Metronidazole is specific for amoebic infection, although resistance is increasing.
- If the patient's condition does not rapidly improve, antibiotics effective against enteric organisms should be prescribed because of the frequency of secondary infection.
- Abscesses may need to be aspirated percutaneously under ultrasound/CT guidance, but only occasionally is open operation required.

LIVER TUMOURS

Benign Liver Tumours

- Benign liver tumours are commonly detected as incidentalomas and are usually asymptomatic.
- However, larger lesions might cause abdominal pain or present because of biliary obstruction. Table 23.1 describes the main features of the common benign liver tumours on imaging.

Haemangioma

- The most common benign tumour is *cavernous haemangioma.*
  - These are composed of thin-walled dilated vessels.
- Haemangiomas are often found as incidental lesions on cross sectional imaging
- There is a female preponderance (5:1).
- Small haemangiomas are asymptomatic but compression of adjacent structures may cause discomfort.
- Indeed, compression of hepatic venous outflow can be a cause of *Budd–Chiari syndrome.*
- In large or giant haemangioma, rupture or a consumptive coagulopathy (*Kasabach–Merritt syndrome*) may occur.
- Imaging by ultrasound shows acoustic enhancement behind the lesion due to improved transmission through the blood within.

- Triple-phase CT has a high sensitivity and specificity for haemangioma and characteristically shows hypoattenuation in the unenhanced phase, intense enhancement in the arterial phase and pooling of contrast in the venous phase.
- MRI has a higher degree of sensitivity and specificity for haemangioma.
  - T1-weighted images show hypoattenuation, whereas T2-weighted images are very bright.
  - Use of contrast agents shows peripheral nodular enhancement with centripetal filling.
- The specificity of imaging does not reach 100% and confusion with other hypervascular lesions such as hepatoma, focal nodular hyperplasia and hypervascular adenomas and metastases is possible.
- When confirmed, small haemangiomas require no surgical intervention or radiological follow-up.
- Where these lesions cause symptoms or show rapid increase, surgical intervention in the form of liver resection should be considered.

Focal Nodular Hyperplasia (FNH)

- This is a benign tumour nearly always in women in the third or fourth decade.
- FNH is composed of all the normal elements of liver tissue but they are present in a disorganized way.
- Large malformed blood vessels sit in a fibrous stroma forming a well-defined mass surrounded by normal liver.
- FNH is usually solitary and asymptomatic.
- Diagnosis is usually incidental on scanning and confirmed either by CT or MRI to demonstrate the central scar which is present in 80% of FNH. However, diagnostic overlap can occur with well-differentiated hepatocellular carcinoma (HCC) or fibrolamellar HCC. A sulphur colloid scan may help and, if confirmed by an expert hepatobiliary radiologist, FNH does not require biopsy and may be safely left alone if asymptomatic.

Adenoma

- Hepatic adenomas are composed of normal liver tissues. They may comprise biliary elements and these are common, usually <1 cm, and are called biliary hamartomas.

TABLE 23.1 **The Common Features of Benign Tumours on Imaging.**

	Haemangioma	FNH	Adenoma
USS	Hyperechoic and well-defined lesion	Hypoechoic and well-defined lesion	Hypoechoic and usually well-defined lesion
CT	Low density with peripheral enhancement over 5–10 minutes	Hypo/isodense with a central scar	Well-defined hypodense lesion with transient enhancement
MRI	Round lobulated mass with high intensity on T2 weighted images	High T2 weighted signal with central scar	Isointense T1 signal

CT, Computed tomography; FNH, focal nodular hyperplasia; MRI, magnetic resonance imaging; USS, ultrasound scan.

- Adenomas composed of hepatocytes are rare but more common in females.
- There is a strong association with oestrogen exposure through contraceptive pill use, which raises the incidence.
- Hepatic adenoma can complicate pregnancy and is also linked to glycogen storage disease and diabetes. Indeed, the oral contraceptive pill can sometimes cause reduction in the size of the adenoma.
- Large adenomas can cause discomfort or rupture and haemorrhage. Malignant transformation is recorded but very uncommon in small lesions <5 cm.
- Distinguishing benign adenoma from malignant lesions is very difficult and no single test is specific.
  - A smooth border, intralesional fat or bleeding, and a pseudocapsule suggest, but are not diagnostic of, adenoma.
- In some cases, excision or needle biopsy may be considered.
- Alternatively, if the clinical history and imaging do not suggest malignancy, the background liver is normal and the AFP is not elevated, these patients can be observed with imaging and AFP monitoring and cessation of oral contraceptives.
- Larger tumours should be considered for resection not only because of the risk of malignant transformation but also because of the hazard of rupture.

Malignant Tumours

Hepatocellular Carcinoma

- HCC is one of the most common tumours worldwide with a reported incidence of 6.2/100 000 in 2011 but this is increasing due to the rise in the prevalence of viral hepatitis, mostly hepatitis C.
- HCC demonstrates high prevalence in North America and Western Europe and secondly in sub-Saharan Africa, Central/Southeast Asia.
- Viral hepatitis increases the risk of developing HCC by about 100-fold over the non-infected person.
- Hepatitis B virus immunization has been shown to reduce the incidence of HCC in Taiwan.
- However, all causes of cirrhosis, including alcoholic liver disease, non-alcoholic fatty liver disease, metabolic diseases and cryptogenic causes, can lead to HCC.
- Indeed, HCC occurs very infrequently in a normal liver and most HCC (80%) occur in the cirrhotic liver. This is because dysregulated attempts at liver regeneration in a cirrhotic liver leads to the development of HCC.

Clinical Features

- The patient with HCC is typically in the fifth or sixth decade with a strong male preponderance.
- The presentation can be very varied and vague especially if superimposed upon the general malaise of chronic liver disease.

- Patients at risk because of known cirrhosis or viral hepatitis may be under regular follow-up within a liver clinic and HCC diagnosed by routine investigations (AFP or scanning).
- Pain, weight loss, jaundice and ascites signify advanced disease.
- Physical examination might reveal hepatomegaly and the signs of chronic liver disease.
- Features of metastatic disease such as pleural effusion, bone pain, pulmonary embolism or neurological symptoms may be present and indicate disseminated disease.

Diagnosis

- Imaging initially is likely to consist of ultrasound scan and about 75% of HCC are multifocal.
- CT is likely to be more reproducible and precise, whereas MRI is more likely to show up smaller lesions not demonstrated on CT and also tumour thrombus in the portal vein, a feature of HCC.
- Generally, HCC classically demonstrate arterial enhancement and 'washout' in the venous phase (Fig. 23.8).
- AFP is also elevated in about 80% of cases and the presence of an enlarging mass >2 cm with radiological characteristics of HCC on two modalities or an enlarging mass >2 cm on one imaging modality but with AFP elevation <500 ng/mL is sufficient to be certain of the diagnosis.
- Confirmation by percutaneous needle biopsy needs to be carefully considered as there is a risk of tumour seeding into the abdomen and along the needle track and is generally not recommended. In patients where the diagnosis is uncertain, surveillance imaging at a short interval usually resolves diagnostic dilemma.
- As discussed above predisposing factors for HCC are:
  - chronic viral hepatitis (hepatitis B or C infection)
  - alcoholic liver disease/non-alcoholic fatty liver disease
  - aflatoxin exposure from *Aspergillus flavus*
  - hereditary haemochromatosis and Wilson's disease
  - alpha-1 antitrypsin deficiency
  - glycogen storage disease
  - HIV infection

Management

- The initial principles of management of HCC are to manage the sequelae of liver cirrhosis such as varices, jaundice, coagulopathy and malnutrition.
- The only curative modalities for HCC are liver resection or liver transplantation.
- Liver resection has the significant advantage of removing the HCC completely; however, only 20% of HCC occur in a normal liver and therefore only these patients would qualify for resection. Importantly, liver resection in a cirrhotic liver yields universally poor results as the liver is unable to regenerate because of the previous damage to the liver parenchyma. In these patients, careful work-up and selection for transplantation based on the Milan criteria can give good patient survival (Box 23.6).

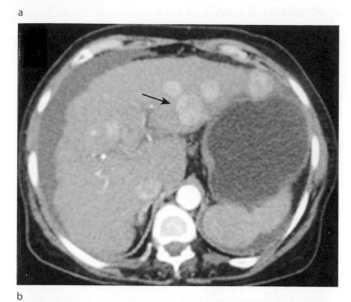

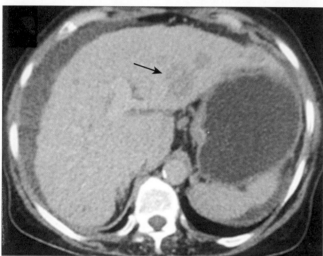

• **Fig. 23.8** Axial CT Scans (A) Demonstrates arterially enhancing lesions within a cirrhotic liver that show complete washout during the porto-venous phase (B) and is consistent with multifocal HCC. Also note the finding of ascites around the liver which is common in patients with cirrhosis.

• **BOX 23.6 Milan Criteria for Liver Transplantation for HCC**

Single HCC ≤5 cm *score 1*
Up to 3 tumours ≤3 cm *score 1*
No extrahepatic involvement *score 1*
No major vessel involvement *score 1*

- Other treatments include:
  - *Transcatheter arterial chemoembolization (TACE)* through the hepatic artery based on the same principle to deliver targeted drug, usually doxorubicin, to the tumours. The drug is usually bound to lipiodol which binds to the tumour hepatocytes thus keeping the drug within the tumours. TACE leads to a modest

TABLE 23.2	Management of HCC.
Treatment Modality	**Status of HCC**
Liver Resection	Well preserved liver function with limited HCC (usually in one liver lobe)
Liver Transplantation	Cirrhotic liver with HCC within Milan criteria
Radiofrequency Ablation (RFA)	Small HCCs (≤2 cm) in a cirrhotic liver where the patient may not be fit for transplantation or be outside Milan criteria
Transcatheter Arterial Chemoembolization (TACE)	Large HCC (approx. 5 cm) in a cirrhotic liver
Sorafenib	Metastatic disease

benefit over supportive care alone and is generally recommended for HCC of approximately 5 cm.
- Local tumour ablation by direct alcohol injection or thermoablation using RFA or microwave, cryotherapy and, more recently, yttrium-90 labelled glass microsphere embolization for tumours of approximately 2 cm.
- Systemic therapies for metastatic disease or multifocal disease include various cytotoxic regimens, sometimes in combination with immunomodulatory agents such as interferon-alpha, have been studied but as yet the only agent to show statistically significant benefit in phase III studies is the multi-targeted tyrosine kinase inhibitor sorafenib. Current management paradigms for HCC are summarized in Table 23.2.

Fibrolamellar HCC

- This variant of HCC has its own characteristics and natural history that distinguishes it from the common form of HCC discussed above.
- Fibrolamellar HCC occurs in a much younger population (second or third decade) and usually on the background of a normal liver and has a female preponderance.
- The clinical presentation may be with pain, mass or cachexia.
- The LFTs are usually abnormal but the AFP is not elevated and patients do not usually have hepatitis or cirrhosis.
- Prognosis is reported to be better than HCC and liver resection is indicated if the disease can be resected.
- Diagnosis can be made confidently on CT scan but diagnostic confusion between fibrolamellar HCC and FNH can occur as fibrolamellar HCC can have a central scar in some cases.
- In cases of diagnostic uncertainty, liver resection may be performed, if safe, for both oncological and diagnostic reasons.

Intrahepatic Cholangiocarcinoma

Aetiology and Pathological Features

- Cholangiocarcinoma may be either *intra-* or *extrahepatic.*
- Although the tumours are usually sporadic, some diseases can predispose to developing cholangiocarcinoma such as:
  - primary sclerosing cholangitis,
  - exposure to thorotrast (although this is now historic) and
  - infection with liver fluke.
- *Extrahepatic* cholangiocarcinoma is strongly associated with smoking and the tumour causes a fibrous stricturing of the bile ducts. The presentation is almost always with features of painless biliary obstruction (see later).
- Viral hepatitis, HIV infection and fatty liver disease are linked to increased risk of *intrahepatic* cholangiocarcinoma.

Clinical Features

- The symptoms of intrahepatic cholangiocarcinoma may be vague with:
  - upper abdominal discomfort,
  - malaise or
  - a right upper quadrant mass.
- Pain, weight loss, jaundice or ascites are features of disseminated disease.

Investigations

- The tumour marker CA19.9 is sometimes elevated and can be used to monitor the disease burden.
- A combination of ultrasonography and CT or MRI may provide the diagnosis and location but distinguishing intrahepatic cholangiocarcinoma from HCC on cross-sectional imaging may be difficult and often not possible.
- However, intrahepatic cholangiocarcinoma, unlike HCC, occurs in a normal liver and therefore this can sometimes aid in making the diagnosis.
- In cases of irresectable tumour or in patients unsuitable for radical surgical treatment, the diagnosis may be confirmed by needle biopsy.
- The needle is directed into the tumour under ultrasound or CT scan guidance.

Management

- Liver resection is the optimal treatment as these tumours are poorly responsive to chemotherapy and resection ensures complete removal of the tumour.
- Transplantation is proposed as an alternative treatment in some patients but, outside of highly specialized centres, is not standard treatment.

Metastatic Cancer to the Liver

Epidemiology

- Metastatic disease to the liver commonly arises from primary cancers in the colon, pancreas, stomach, oesophagus, breast, lung and small intestine.
- In Western countries, a solid mass in the liver is much more likely to be metastatic disease than a primary liver cancer.

Clinical Features

- Liver metastases do not usually cause symptoms and are normally found as incidental findings in the investigation of other tumour-related symptoms.
- Liver metastasis detected during the staging process of known primary cancers are termed *synchronous* metastasis and those found at least 6 months after a primary tumour has been resected are termed *metachronous* metastasis.

Investigation

- The detection of metastatic disease involves the use of the extracorporeal imaging modalities of CT/MRI and CT-PET scanning.
- CT-PET is an excellent modality for the detection of extrahepatic metastases.
- MRI is specific for intrahepatic metastatic disease and is used for surgical planning.
- The majority of livers with metastatic disease will have multiple lesions and only about 10% are solitary metastases.
- Bilobar disease is not uncommon but, as discussed later, in the modern surgical era these lesions can be successfully resected.

Management

- The presence of liver metastases is a poor prognostic feature and, untreated, these patients are unlikely to survive more than a few months.
- Liver resection can be considered if all disease can be removed (or ablated) whilst leaving adequate functioning liver tissue.
- Liver surgery is usually performed in the absence of extrahepatic metastatic disease.
- However, in patients with limited and operable lung metastasis, liver and lung surgery can be considered to resect all disease.
- In most patients, liver surgery is performed after resection of the colorectal adenocarcinoma.
- In general, when planning liver surgery there are three important prerequisites:
  1. There must be portal and arterial inflow to the future liver remnant.
  2. There must be venous outflow for the future liver.
  3. There must be at least 30% normal liver volume in the future liver remnant.

- The treatment of metastatic colorectal cancer has improved vastly in the past decade and is now commonly treated by surgery in the form of liver resection.
- Data accumulated from many large prospective and retrospective cohort studies all suggest that long-term cure following the surgical removal of liver-only metastases in patients with otherwise curable colorectal cancer is possible in about 50–60% of cases.
- Other forms of treatment, such as chemotherapy, embolization and radiation, may reduce disease burden but, in many patients (80%), the disease will recur.
- However, only approximately 25–30% of liver metastases from colorectal cancer are resectable at presentation. Here the use of systemic chemotherapy to downsize bulky disease increases the resectable population and adjuvant chemotherapy following complete resection of liver metastases appears to reduce the risk of relapse in the liver and has been shown to improve long-term survival.
- Previously, a wide margin of tumour clearance (>1 cm) was thought to be necessary for adequate resection; however, now histologically clear margin in the resected specimen yields equivalent results. Importantly, positive margins at resection lead to a high local recurrence rate.
- Newer surgical techniques have evolved that allow even more radical liver surgery to be performed. These include *preoperative portal vein embolization*, *staged* or *two-stage hepatectomy* and *ALPPS procedure* (Fig. 23.9).

- Prognostic factors that predicate a poor prognosis following liver resection of metastases from colorectal cancer are:
  - a short disease-free interval
  - multiple large metastases
  - bilaterality
  - positive margins following resection
  - extrahepatic disease
  - poor response to systemic chemotherapy
  - very high preoperative carcinoembryonic antigen (CEA)
  - synchronous presentation
- Other tumour types where liver resection for metastases has an important role are *neuroendocrine* tumours of the GI tract. The presence of liver metastases often gives rise to physical symptoms or functional syndromes from hormone production. Complete surgical removal or debulking of metastatic disease in selected cases can be a most useful treatment.

Complications of Surgery

- Liver surgery for metastatic disease is not without complication.
- *Major complications* such as bile leak, abscess and haemorrhage occur with a frequency of about 2–5% and postoperative liver failure in about 2–3% of resections.
- Preoperative chemotherapy has a significant damaging effect on the liver, causing steatosis and fibrosis, and increases the risk of complications and, in some patients,

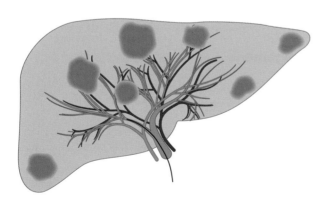 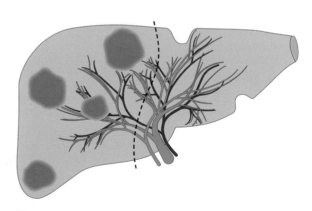

A   B

• **Fig. 23.9** The management of bilobar liver metastasis in the modern era has evolved considerably and now many of these patients are considered for liver resection where previously they would have been deemed non-resectable. In the case of solitary metastasis, the surgical planning is relatively straightforward and may involve segmentectomy, sectionectomy or hemihepatectomy. In the above example, the liver has extensive bilobar metastasis and clearly resecting all lesions in a single operation would mean leaving inadequate future liver volume, meaning patient mortality. Two alternative approaches are available to the surgeon. Firstly, a two-stage hepatectomy could be performed – at the first operation, all the metastasis in the left liver are resected. After an adequate break (usually 6–8 weeks) liver regeneration would be complete and a second operation is performed to carry out a right hepatectomy (dotted line) leaving a full left liver. In cases where rapid liver regeneration is required, the ALPPS procedure (Associating Liver Partitioning with Portal Vein Ligation for staged hepatectomy) can be utilized. Here, at the first operation, the liver is divided (dotted line) and the metastasis in the left liver cleared. The portal vein to the right liver is also divided but the hepatic artery is left alone. After a short interval (7 days), the left liver rapidly grows meaning that the right liver can be removed.

the effect of chemotherapy on the liver can be so severe (chemotherapy associated liver injury) that liver resection is not possible as the risk of failed liver regeneration in the future liver remnant is prohibitively high.

GALLSTONES (CHOLELITHIASIS)

Epidemiology

- Gallstones are very common with a reported prevalence of 10–15% in the general population.
- Gallstones can affect patients of all ages and both sexes, although they are 2–4 times more common in women (Box 23.7).
- Cholesterol is the principal constituent of the great majority of gallstones, either as pure cholesterol stones (20%) or as mixed gallstones combined with deconjugated bile pigment, especially bilirubin (75%). Stones composed of pigment alone account for the remaining 5%.

Aetiology

- The development of gallstones is multifactorial and is dependent upon the type of stone.
- Although cholesterol is insoluble in water, in bile it is normally solubilized by micelles. If the concentration of cholesterol in bile is high, the capacity of this mechanism may be exceeded, leading to a state of cholesterol supersaturation.
- Cholesterol supersaturation can occur when plasma oestrogen levels are increased (e.g. pregnancy and in women taking oral contraceptives) and when there is depletion of the bile acid pool (e.g. in resection or disease of the terminal ileum that interrupts the enterohepatic circulation).
- Gallstones formation is also encouraged when there is biliary stasis, as is observed in the fasting state because of lack of food stimulus to gallbladder emptying.
- In addition, total parenteral nutrition and truncal vagotomy also encourage biliary stasis.
- Bilirubin is kept in solution in bile by conjugation with glucuronide. Pigment stones are encountered when there

---

• BOX 23.7 Risk Factors for Gallstone Formation

Obesity
Rapid weight loss
Childbearing
Multiparity
Female gender
First-degree relatives
Drugs: ceftriaxone, postmenopausal oestrogens
Total parenteral nutrition
Ethnicity: highest in Native American (Pima Indian)
Ileal disease, resection or bypass
Age

---

is increased breakdown of red blood cells, as seen in haemolytic disorders such as spherocytosis, sickle cell disease and malaria, or when there is failure of conjugation, as described in hepatocyte insufficiency in the formation of glucuronide, or excess glucuronidase

Clinical Features

Asymptomatic Stones

- Gallstones anywhere in the biliary tree can remain asymptomatic and therefore undetected for many years.
- Ultrasound scanning done on patients with vague abdominal symptoms has resulted in more frequent discovery of such incidental gallstones.
- In the absence of symptoms, it is currently not recommended to offer patients surgical intervention.
- Only about a third of patients will become symptomatic, with an annual incidence of symptom development of approximately 1%. Therefore, for most patients, cholecystectomy is not advised.
- Operation may be considered in the following cases:
  - There is a non-functioning gallbladder or a poorly functioning gallbladder (gallbladder dyskinesia) which is thought to render an attack of acute cholecystitis more likely. Non functioning gallbladder are confirmed using hepatobiliary iminodiacetic acid (HIDA) scans and cholecystectomy can be offered to such patients even in the absence of gallstones.
- In diabetics, because this condition carries a greater risk of complications following the development of such features as biliary colic or cholecystitis; elective operations for silent stones may pre-empt this risk.
- A cholecystenteric fistula has been identified.

Symptomatic Stones

Stones become clinically evident by the complications they cause, which are classified according to their anatomical site (Fig. 23.10).

Stones in the Gallbladder

Biliary Colic

Clinical Features

- Gallstone impaction at Hartmann's pouch or the cystic duct can cause pain.
- Although often referred to as *colic*, the pain is usually constant in the epigastrium and right upper quadrant and may radiate through to the back in the region of the inferior angle of the scapula.
- Attacks last for a few minutes to half an hour and may be exacerbated by ingestion of fatty food that stimulates the release of *cholecystokinin (CCK)* and consequent gallbladder contraction.
- Vomiting is common because of vagal stimulation.

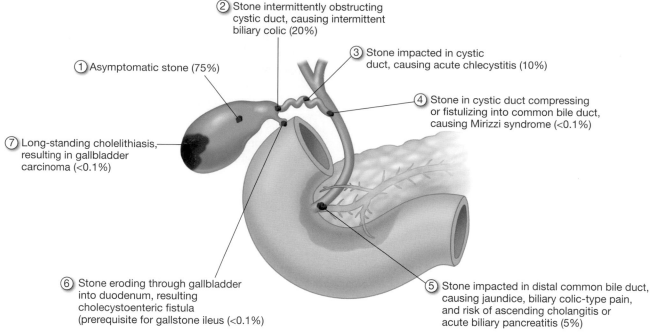

② Stone intermittently obstructing cystic duct, causing intermittent biliary colic (20%)

① Asymptomatic stone (75%)

③ Stone impacted in cystic duct, causing acute chlecystitis (10%)

④ Stone in cystic duct compressing or fistulizing into common bile duct, causing Mirizzi syndrome (<0.1%)

⑦ Long-standing cholelithiasis, resulting in gallbladder carcinoma (<0.1%)

⑥ Stone eroding through gallbladder into duodenum, resulting cholecystoenteric fistula (prerequisite for gallstone ileus (<0.1%)

⑤ Stone impacted in distal common bile duct, causing jaundice, biliary colic-type pain, and risk of ascending cholangitis or acute biliary pancreatitis (5%)

• **Fig. 23.10** Complications Arising from Gallstones (1) Most gallstones are asymptomatic. Stones within the gallbladder may cause biliary colic (2), acute cholecystitis (3) or, rarely, Mirizzi syndrome (4). Impaction of gallstones on the common bile duct and pancreatic duct causes obstructive jaundice and pancreatitis (5). Large gallstones can erode into the duodenum (choleduodenal fistula) and cause small bowel obstruction (6). Finally, long-standing gallstones predispose to gallbladder cancer (7).

- Importantly, fever is absent.
- The pain spontaneously settles when the stone either becomes disimpacted or, less commonly, is passed into the common bile duct. Recurrent attacks are common and often of variable duration and severity. There are usually no findings on physical examination.

Investigation

- The white cell count, serum amylase and C-reactive protein are usually normal.
- There may be mild elevation of ALP and/or AST/ALT.
- Ultrasound abdomen reliably detects 98% of gallbladder stones (Fig. 23.11) but is less reliable in identifying those that are within the bile ducts (termed *choledocholithiasis*).
- In addition, ultrasound can also provide information about:
  - the thickness of the gallbladder wall, an increase above normal being indicative of past or present inflammation,
  - the diameter of the common bile duct and
  - the architecture of the liver and pancreas and any other mass lesions.

Management

- The initial administration of a parenteral analgesic such as morphine or pethidine relieves the acute exacerbations of pain and, over a few hours, the condition nearly always resolves.
- If the diagnosis is confirmed by imaging, subsequent cholecystectomy is usually indicated (see later). In the

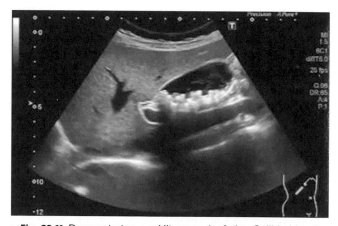

• **Fig. 23.11** Demonstrates an Ultrasound of the Gallbladder The gallbladder contains multiple gallstones, confirmed by the characteristic acoustic shadow. This arises because gallstones reflect ultrasonic waves, creating a shadow on the scan behind them.

modern era, this is completed by the minimal access approach such as laparoscopy but robotic cholecystectomy is being increasingly used in specialized centres.

Acute Cholecystitis

- When a gallstone impacts at the outlet of the gallbladder, water continues to be absorbed through the gallbladder wall, and the concentrated bile can initiate a *chemical cholecystitis.*
- Secondary bacterial infection causes *acute cholecystitis.*

Clinical Features

- The symptoms are similar to those of biliary colic, but the pain is generally more severe and persistent.
- Nausea and vomiting are common and fever is usually present (an important distinguishing feature from biliary colic).
- Tenderness and guarding are often present in the right upper quadrant. In less severe instances, laying the hand lightly on the upper right abdomen and asking the patient to take a deep breath causes a catch in breath because of pain when the inflamed gallbladder impacts on the examining hand – *Murphy's sign.*
- Hyperaesthesia of skin over the right ribs 9–11 posteriorly *(Boas' sign)* may also be present.
- If inflammation spreads beyond the gallbladder, a mass, composed of the enlarged gallbladder and adherent omentum and bowel, may be palpated under the right costal margin and may also be consistent with a gallbladder empyema.

Investigation

- There is leucocytosis with a prominent neutrophilia and the bilirubin concentration and liver enzymes may be mildly raised, either as a result of partial obstruction of the common hepatic duct by a stone lodged in Hartmann's pouch or because of local inflammation.
- In patients with long-standing repeated symptoms, the possibility of *Mirizzi syndrome* should be entertained (see Fig. 23.10).
- The serum amylase concentration may be moderately elevated but not to the levels seen in acute pancreatitis.
- Ultrasound shows the enlarged gallbladder with gallstone(s), a thickened wall and a surrounding rim of pericholecystic fluid from local oedema – the hallmark of acute cholecystitis.
- Further radiological investigations are not usually required.

Management

- Initial treatment is non-operative, with pain relief and systemic broad-spectrum antibiotics.
- Intravenous fluids may be required.
- Most attacks resolve, and definitive treatment by cholecystectomy is performed during the index hospital admission if possible (see Cholecystectomy, later).
- The worldwide literature now supports no increased risk of open conversion or bile duct injury in performing laparoscopic cholecystectomy in the emergency setting. Thus, interval surgery (4–6 weeks) is now less common.
- In a few patients, the initial attack does not resolve with antibiotic treatment because of a perforation of the gallbladder or the formation of an empyema.
- If progression is thought to be taking place despite antibiotic treatment, as judged by failure of symptoms to resolve and the persistence of local signs, the gallbladder should be drained percutaneously by ultrasound-guided cholecystostomy with a view to delayed cholecystectomy.

Free Perforation

- This is caused by a progressive rise in tension in the gallbladder; the blood supply of the wall is reduced, and gangrene occurs, usually at the fundus.
- Abdominal pain becomes increasingly severe and more generalized.
- Perforation may lead to diffuse peritonitis or a pericholecystic abscess which demands urgent exploration, peritoneal lavage and a cholecystectomy.
- In cases of severe inflammation, it may be necessary to perform a subtotal cholecystectomy to mitigate the risk of bile duct injury.

Mucocele

- A stone may impact in the neck of the gallbladder without causing inflammation either from the concentrated bile or from secondary infection.
- The result is a mucocele – a distended gallbladder full of clear mucus.
- Cholecystectomy is indicated and often the diagnosis is made at surgery.

Common Bile Duct Stones (Choledocholithiasis)

Obstructive Jaundice

- Impaction of a stone in the common bile duct, usually at the duodenal papilla, causes obstructive jaundice, giving a clinical picture consistent with surgical jaundice as described earlier.
- There is usually accompanying abdominal pain that often distinguishes choledocholithiasis from malignant aetiologies that are typically painless (see below).
- Clinical examination usually yields little by way of findings.

Investigation

- Ultrasound is usually the initial investigation and demonstrates dilatation of the intra- and extrahepatic bile ducts and may even identify ductal stones.
- T2-weighted MRCP (Fig. 23.12) or ERCP confirms the diagnosis and with ERCP allowing definitive management.

Management

- There is a choice for management of bile duct stones depending upon surgical expertise and patient choice/fitness.
- The choice lies between endoscopic (ERCP) extraction of common bile duct gallstones followed by cholecystectomy if appropriate or laparoscopic/open cholecystectomy with on-table bile duct exploration.
- ERCP with sphincterotomy of the lower bile duct sphincter of Oddi (or balloon sphincter dilatation) and extraction of the ductal stone(s) is commonly used.

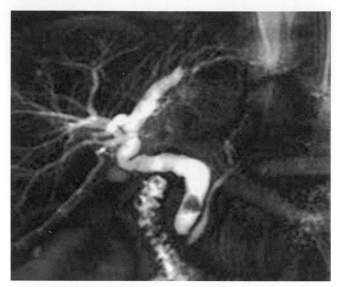

• **Fig. 23.12** MRCP Demonstrating a Common Bile Duct Stone MRCP are performed with T2 weighting where fluid appear bright (white) and fat containing structures black (dark). In the fasting state, the sphincter of Oddi is closed and the bile in the biliary system appears as a standing column of fluid – with any lesions appearing as filling defects. Note fluid in the duodenum. Importantly, MRCP is performed without contrast.

- Alternatively, during surgery for laparoscopic/open cholecystectomy with on-table bile duct exploration, bile duct clearance can be achieved using either a transcystic (via the cystic duct) or choledochotomy (incision into the common bile duct) technique and bile duct closure is performed without the need of T-tube insertion.

Acute Cholangitis

Aetiology and Pathological Features

- Organisms enter the biliary tree either from the gastrointestinal tract via the duodenal papilla or by excretion in the bile after reaching the liver via the bloodstream (a phenomenon known as *cholovenous reflux*).
- In the bile, they multiply in the presence of obstruction to cause inflammation.
- Ductal stones are the primary cause in the Western world. In the East, parasitic infections with liver flukes *(Clonorchis sinensis)* and ascariasis are associated with secondary bacterial cholangitis. The causative organism is usually a Gram-negative enteric bacterium, typically *Escherichia coli*. Infected bile in the biliary tree is potentially fatal because it may lead to septicaemia and hepatorenal failure.
- Long-term sequelae of repeated attacks of cholangitis include liver abscesses, secondary biliary cirrhosis (see earlier) with subsequent liver failure and portal hypertension.

Clinical Features

- A past history of biliary disease may be obtained.
- Presentation is with abdominal pain, high fever with rigors and jaundice (referred to as *Charcot's triad*).

- In addition, elderly patients are often confused and hypotensive *(Reynold's pentad)*.
- The gallbladder is impalpable. Cholangitis indicates ascending biliary infection.

Investigation

- The white cell count will usually reveal neutrophilia, whilst liver function tests will show cholestasis.
- There is a positive blood culture in 40% of patients.
- Ultrasound or CT scanning may show gallbladder stones, a dilated duct and sometimes a ductal stone.

Management

- Resuscitation with intravenous fluids and parenteral broad-spectrum antibiotics (including anaerobic cover) is mandatory.
- A prompt response will result in relief of symptoms, resolution of fever and rapid reduction in jaundice.
- Failure to achieve this indicates the need for bile duct drainage by urgent ERCP or PTC. If possible, stones should be extracted, but effective biliary drainage is the first essential requirement.
- Definitive treatment of cholelithiasis, as described earlier, can be deferred until the acute episode has settled.

Stones in the Small Intestine

Gallstone Ileus

Aetiology

- A gallbladder which contains gallstones, particularly large stones, may erode into adjacent small bowel, usually the duodenum.
- Stones can then be shed through this cholecystenteric fistula into the gut.
- A large stone that has a diameter greater than the narrowest part of the small bowel (terminal ileum) may impact to produce small-bowel obstruction.

Clinical Features

- This pathology usually presents in elderly patients and gives very few symptoms initially.
- Vague attacks of colic may have occurred as the stone passes down the gut. Eventually, the history is of small-bowel obstruction with clinical findings of abdominal distension and possible abdominal tenderness.

Investigation

- In addition to the characteristic features of small-bowel obstruction on a plain radiograph or CT scanning, it may be possible to see:
  - air in the biliary tract (aerobilia) – also observed after any instrumentation of the biliary tract (e.g. ERCP)
  - a calcified gallstone in the right lower quadrant

Management

- The condition can be found at operation for small-bowel obstruction without preoperative diagnosis.
- The gallstone can be milked retrogradely and extracted via a small enterotomy. This can also be performed laparoscopically. The small bowel proximal to the obstruction is carefully examined to exclude other stones.
- Treatment of the choledochofistula should be deferred and may not be required.

Acalculous Cholecystitis

Aetiology and Pathological Features

- Acute cholecystitis may develop in the absence of gallstones. This primary (or acalculous) cholecystitis usually afflicts very ill, often diabetic, patients in an intensive care unit.
- The condition is a severe form of acute cholecystitis that often progresses to gangrene and perforation.
- The mortality may approach 15%.

Clinical Features

- The coexistence of other serious illnesses in a patient who may be unconscious often masks the diagnosis.
- It is important to retain a high index of suspicion in order to make this diagnosis in this cohort of patients.

Investigation

- Diagnostic features on ultrasound or CT scanning are those of gallbladder dilatation with oedema in the gallbladder wall.
- In many cases, ultrasound at the bedside can clinch the diagnosis

Management

- Percutaneous cholecystostomy under ultrasound guidance with gallbladder drainage and parenteral antibiotics may suffice unless perforation has occurred, in which case urgent cholecystectomy is required.

Sphincter of Oddi Dysfunction

Aetiology and Pathological Features

- Two mechanisms are involved in the development of sphincter of Oddi dysfunction.
  1. There may be stenosis, or narrowing of the sphincter of Oddi or
  2. alteration in the function of the sphincter of Oddi.
- Individuals with stenosis of the sphincter of Oddi may have had recurrent passage of gallstones through the ampulla of Vater, trauma from ERCP, biliary surgery or infections of the common bile duct.
- In contrast, dyskinesia of the sphincter of Oddi is a functional disorder due to spasms.

Clinical Features

- In many patients, sphincter of Oddi dysfunction only becomes apparent after cholecystectomy and is classed as a post-cholecystectomy syndrome.
- Both stenosis and dyskinesia can obstruct flow through the sphincter of Oddi and can, therefore, cause retention of bile in the biliary tree and pancreatic juice in the pancreatic duct.
- Patients with sphincter of Oddi dysfunction present with abdominal pain resembling that of gallstones.
- Among other characteristics, the pain is typically in the upper part of the abdomen or in the right upper quadrant of the abdomen.
- In some patients, the cause of abdominal pain may indeed be sphincter of Oddi dysfunction and gallstones are an incidental finding.

Investigation

- Sphincter of Oddi dysfunction is best diagnosed using manometry at the time of ERCP to measure the pressures within surrounding ducts to determine whether or not the muscle is functioning normally.

Management

- Medication to prevent spasms such as injection of Botulinum toxin into the muscle gives variable relief.
- The alternative is sphincterotomy (procedure to cut the muscle) at ERCP or surgery.

Gallbladder Tumours

Benign

Adenoma

- This is an uncommon tumour and often described as a gallbladder polyp which predisposes to gallbladder carcinoma.
- It is usually an incidental finding on ultrasound scanning.
- Adenomas less than 1 cm in diameter can be observed, but larger ones or ones that demonstrate rapid increase in size should be removed by cholecystectomy as there is a risk of underlying malignancy.

Three other conditions can mimic the appearance of an adenoma on ultrasound:

- **Cholesterolosis,** in which plaques of cholesterol are laid down in the gallbladder mucosa and cause a thickened irregular mucosal appearance which is sometimes known as *strawberry gallbladder*. Cholecystectomy is indicated in patients with symptoms provided these are clearly related to the biliary tree.
- **Soft adherent non-calcified stones** that may be difficult to distinguish from adenomas on scanning and may not give the characteristic acoustic shadow.

- **Adenomyoma** is a localized collection of cystic spaces in the gallbladder wall; it is a benign condition and, in its generalized form, is known as adenomyomatosis.

Malignant

Epidemiology, Aetiology and Clinical Presentation

Cancer of the gallbladder is rare and is most commonly adenocarcinomas.

- The peak incidence is in the 60–80-year age range.
- There is a wide geographic variation of incidence. The highest incidence is among women in India, South America and the Far East.
- The vast majority of gallbladder adenocarcinoma is associated with gallstones.
- Other risk factors include:
  - previous cholecystitis
  - a family history of gallbladder cancer or gallstones
  - a porcelain gallbladder (calcification of the gallbladder wall)
  - smoking
  - obesity
  - the presence of a gallbladder adenoma
- The presentation might be with vague symptoms of malaise, upper abdominal discomfort and nausea.
- Pain, jaundice or a palpable right upper quadrant mass imply advanced disease. Careful examination of routine cholecystectomy specimens where gallbladder cancer was not suspected preoperatively suggests an incidence of 1%.

Pathological Features

- Gallbladder cancers tend to invade locally into the adjacent liver.
- They have a dismal prognosis because the great majority have invaded the liver beyond resectability at the time of presentation.
- The overall 5-year survival is 2–5%.
- The only tumours with a favourable prognosis are those early cancers found during pathological examination of a gallbladder removed for biliary symptoms.

Surgical Management

- The standard operation for gallbladder carcinoma is the 'en bloc' cholecystectomy, which means cholecystectomy with resection of liver segments V–IV.
- In some cases, lymphadenectomy of the hepatoduodenal ligament extended to the hepatic artery is performed.
- Patients having a diagnosis of an incidental carcinoma found on histopathology after routine cholecystectomy should be considered for radical surgery depending on the stage and site of the tumour (Table 23.3).
- Many early cancers are cured by cholecystectomy alone. Importantly, if the cystic duct margin is found to be involved with carcinoma the patient requires hepaticojejunostomy (see Fig 23.19).

TABLE 23.3 **Management of Gallbladder Cancer.**

Extent of Cancer	Management
Cancer involving mucosa only	Simple cholecystectomy
Cancer extending to muscle only	Simple cholecystectomy
Cancer breaching muscle or involving serosa	Radical cholecystectomy
Cancer involving cystic duct	Radical cholecystectomy, portal lymphadenectomy and hepaticojejunostomy

Cholecystectomy

- Cholecystectomy is a commonly performed operation and, in the modern era, is routinely performed by the laparoscopic route.
- There is also a newer development of performing cholecystectomy via robotic surgery and, in circumstances when these approaches are not possible or fail, surgery is completed by the open approach.
- As discussed earlier, cholecystectomy is the optimal management for many gallbladder pathologies including those related to gallstones or, indeed, malignancy.
- Regardless of the surgical approach, key anatomical landmarks are used to ensure cholecystectomy is carried out safely.
- Generally, at laparoscopy, the fundus of the gallbladder is grasped and displaced in the cephalad direction. Depending upon the level of inflammation, there may be omentum or other abdominal viscera adherent to the gallbladder – these are safely dissected free of the gallbladder. The goal of the operation is to safely dissect the *hepatocystic triangle* (Fig. 23.13) and create a safe posterior window behind the gallbladder, termed the *critical view of safety* as described by Strasberg.
- This dissection ensures that only the cystic duct and artery are divided during cholecystectomy and all other hepatic structures remain in-situ. Note there is no corresponding cystic vein.
- Importantly, the hepatocystic triangle is a distinct anatomical triangle from *Calot's triangle,* although they are often used interchangeably.
- If, during surgery, there is any doubt about biliary anatomy, the surgeon should perform an intraoperative cholangiogram to clarify biliary anatomy prior to division of any structures (see Fig. 23.13). Some surgeons perform intraoperative cholangiogram routinely, whilst others perform it on a selected basis.
- Despite these standardized surgical steps, common bile duct injury is reported in 0.05–0.3% cases.

A

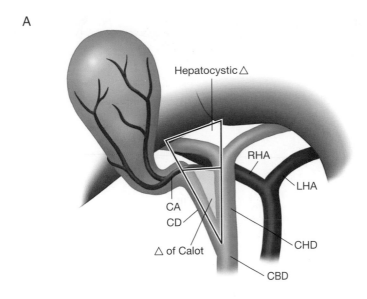

B

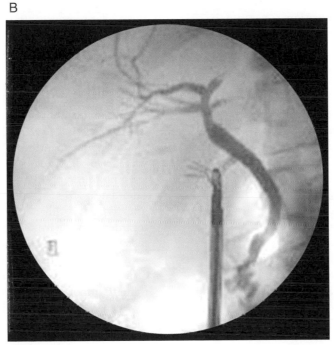

• **Fig. 23.13** (A) Demonstrates both the hepatocystic and Calot's triangle. The *hepatocystic triangle* is bounded by the cystic duct *(CD)*, inferior border of the liver and common hepatic duct *(CHD)*. It contains the cystic artery *(CA)*, a branch of the right hepatic artery *(RHA)*. *Calot's triangle* is bounded by the cystic artery, cystic duct and common hepatic duct. (B) An intraoperative cholangiogram performed via the cystic duct (transcystic approach) that confirms biliary anatomy and demonstrates distal flow into the duodenum. This test can also be used to investigate for common bile duct stones at the time of surgery, as well as confirming biliary anatomy. *LHA*, left hepatic artery.

Cholangiocarcinoma

- Cancers of the bile ducts are not common, comprising about 2% of all GI tract malignancy with an incidence of 1/100 000 and are predominantly adenocarcinomas.
- Cholangiocarcinomas may arise anywhere in the biliary system and, for surgical purposes, are divided into *intrahepatic* (see previously), *hilar* (occurring at the liver hilum) or *extrahepatic*.

- *Extrahepatic* cholangiocarcinoma occurs at the terminal end of the bile duct. The tumours show a sub-mucosal growth pattern and microscopic examination shows the cancer spreading 10–20 mm either side of the visible disease, which poses a particular problem for cholangiocarcinoma at the liver hilum as these tumours can require extended liver resections that are incompatible with patient surgery or the tumour extends so far into the liver that resection is not possible.

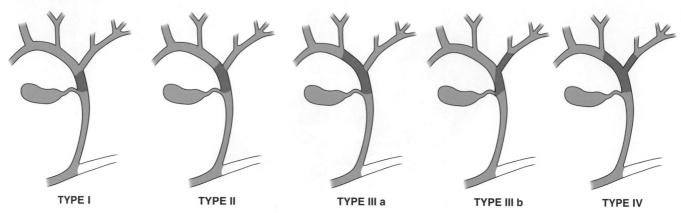

TYPE I   TYPE II   TYPE III a   TYPE III b   TYPE IV

• **Fig. 23.14** Bismuth-Corlette classifies hilar tumours into 4 groups. *Type I* involves the common hepatic duct distal to the biliary confluence. *Type II* involves the biliary confluence, whilst *type IIIa* involves the biliary confluence and right hepatic duct and *type IIIb* involves the biliary confluence and left hepatic duct. *Type IV* extends to the bifurcation of the left and right hepatic ducts or multifocal.

- Lymphatic and/or neurovascular invasion are common and the presence of nodal disease is a strong predictor of poor patient outcome.
- Only about 20% of patients are candidates for surgical resection.
- The proximity of the bile duct to other structures in the hepatic ligament such as the portal vein and hepatic artery means that invasion of these vital structures can occur early, and often the local extent of disease prevents curative surgery or distant metastatic disease is already evident.
- All cholangiocarcinomas are poorly sensitive to chemotherapy and the only curative modality is radical surgical resection.
- These are aggressive cancers and prognosis is poor except for cancers detected and operated for early-stage disease.
- *Hilar/extrahepatic cholangiocarcinoma*:
  - The presentation is usually (>90%) with painless jaundice as the tumour obstructs the bile duct.
  - The patient initially undergoes evaluation of the site of obstruction by non-invasive investigations such as CT and MRI. Distal bile duct cholangiocarcinomas may show as a mass in the periampullary region or, more classically, '*double duct*' sign (dilatation of the bile and pancreatic duct), whilst a hilar cholangiocarcinoma may produce a mass in the liver hilum.
  - Distal cholangiocarcinomas are managed in the same way as cancer of the head of pancreas (see later).
  - Hilar cholangiocarcinomas, or, as they are sometimes called, *Klatskin tumours* after the surgeon who originally described them, involve the upper end of the bile duct at the biliary confluence.
  - Choledochal cysts, primary sclerosing cholangitis and infestation with parasites such as *Clonorchis sinensis* and *Opisthorchis viverrin* are recognized predisposing conditions.
  - Other risk factors are smoking and oriental cholangiohepatitis. The Bismuth-Corlette classification divides these hilar tumours into four groups according to site (Fig 23.14).
- Involvement of the local vessels, the portal vein and hepatic artery are particularly important in the surgical evaluation of hilar cholangiocarcinoma. This can usually be satisfactorily achieved by CT angiography or MR angiography.
- The use of PET scan in the staging of hilar cholangiocarcinoma identifies a further 20% of patients who have disease not identified on conventional imaging, meaning that these patients are not surgical candidates.
- The type IV hilar cholangiocarcinoma is often regarded as being irresectable. Surgery usually involves resection of the extrahepatic biliary system combined with partial hepatectomy and the same prerequisites of liver surgery described earlier apply here too. It is thought important to resect the caudate lobe (segment 1) when dealing with a hilar cholangiocarcinoma as the caudate lobe bile ducts drain into both the left and right biliary systems, as discussed above.
- Preoperative cytological or histological confirmation is difficult to obtain and the decision to treat surgically is based on the clinical history and imaging findings.
- Inoperable patients are treated by relief of the jaundice by biliary stenting. Biliary stents can be deployed either at ERCP or by PTC. A plastic stent might last 3–4 months before becoming occluded by biliary debris. Metallic expanding biliary stents, although more costly, have prolonged patency.
- Palliative therapies such as chemotherapy, radiotherapy or photodynamic therapy are usually contingent upon obtaining histological or cytological proof of malignancy.
- Liver transplant has occasionally been employed in hilar cholangiocarcinoma, but its use is currently very limited to highly specialized centres.

PANCREAS

Anatomy and Physiology

Embryology

Pancreatic development begins as ventral and dorsal buds of the foregut, each with its own drainage duct. As the foregut rotates and develops, the two buds fuse to partially surround the superior mesenteric vessels. The larger dorsal pancreas forms the body, tail and upper part of the head, and the ventral pancreas forms the rest of the head and the uncinate process. Fusion of the duct systems results in the duct of the ventral bud becoming the main duct (of Wirsung) that drains into the duodenum through a shared opening with the common bile duct at the ampulla of Vater (see Fig. 23.2). The duct of the dorsal bud persists as the smaller accessory duct of Santorini, which drains into the duodenum through the minor papilla.

Anatomy

The pancreas lies across the posterior abdominal wall at the level of L1. The head is surrounded by the concavity of the duodenum. The uncinate process and lower part of the head pass posteriorly and to the left of the superior mesenteric vessels (see Fig. 23.2). The body of the pancreas forms the main bulk of the gland and extends across the midline, ending in a tail lying close to the splenic hilum. The main pancreatic duct leads from the tail to the head of the organ, gradually increasing in size as it drains ductules from the pancreatic substance. It usually joins the common bile duct to open into the second part of the duodenum through a common channel and single orifice. This opening is visible from the luminal surface of the duodenum as a small nipple – the major papilla – and is an essential landmark during ERCP.

Developmental Anomalies of the Pancreas

Pancreas divisum is a relatively common (5%) anatomical variation in which most of the pancreas drains into the duodenum through the duct of Santorini and the minor papilla.

Annular pancreas is a rare cause of extrinsic compression of the second part of the duodenum from failure of the two developing pancreatic buds to fuse. Both pancreas divisum and annular pancreas may be associated with drainage abnormalities and rare causes of pancreatitis.

Accessory budding of the primitive duodenum results in nodules of pancreatic tissue in abnormal positions such as the stomach, duodenal wall, jejunum or in a Meckel's diverticulum known as *heterotropic pancreas*. Heterotopic nodules are present in 20% of the population.

Physiology

The human pancreas is both an endocrine and an exocrine organ. The majority of the gland consists of acinar cells which synthesize the exocrine pancreatic enzymes and drain into the intraglandular ductules which are tributaries of the main pancreatic duct. The principal hormones that control release of exocrine secretions are secretin and cholecystokinin (CCK), which are produced from the APUD group of cells in the duodenum and upper jejunum. Secretin is released into the bloodstream when acidic gastric contents enter the first part of the duodenum. It stimulates secretion of a watery, alkaline pancreatic juice rich in electrolytes. CCK is released when fatty acids and amino acids enter the duodenum; it stimulates contraction of the gallbladder and relaxation of the distal bile/pancreatic duct sphincter of Oddi, as well as secretion of a pancreatic juice rich in enzymes. These enzymes are involved in the breakdown of carbohydrates, fats and proteins, the most important of which are amylase, lipase, colipase, phospholipase and a family of proteases: trypsinogen, chymotrypsinogen and elastase. The proteases are secreted in inactive forms (pro-enzymes: zymogens) that are subsequently activated in the lumen of the duodenum by enterokinase, which is probably secreted from the same source as secretin and CCK.

The endocrine portion of the human pancreas is arranged as islands of endocrine tissue (the islets of Langerhans) within the exocrine gland. The islets have a rich vascular supply, and the endocrine cells secrete hormones directly into the portal blood. These include alpha cells (secreting glucagon), beta cells (secreting insulin) and delta cells (secreting somatostatin).

Measurement of Function

A large number of physiological tests have been devised to measure both the exocrine and endocrine functions of the pancreas. Only tests utilized in routine clinical practice are discussed here.

Secretin Pancreatic Function Test

- The secretin pancreatic function test measures the ability of the pancreas to respond to the hormone secretin.
- The small intestine produces secretin in the presence of partially digested food.
- Normally, secretin stimulates the pancreas to secrete a fluid with a high concentration of bicarbonate. This fluid neutralizes stomach acid and is necessary to allow a number of enzymes to function in the breakdown and absorption of food. Patients with chronic pancreatitis, for instance, will have abnormal pancreatic function.
- In this test, a fine tube is placed in the duodenum and secretin is inserted. with aspiration of the duodenal contents. for approximately 1 hour. These are subsequently analyzed.

Faecal Elastase Test

- The faecal elastase test measures elastase-1, an enzyme found in fluids produced by the pancreas, using an enzyme-linked immunosorbent assay (ELISA).

- Elastase digests and degrades various kinds of proteins.
- For this test, a patient's stool sample is analyzed for the presence of elastase. Levels of faecal elastase lower than 200 μg/g of stool indicate an exocrine insufficiency.

Imaging

Endoscopic Ultrasonography (EUS)

- Endoscopic ultrasound (EUS – an ultrasound probe attached to the end of a flexible endoscope) is increasingly used to assess and evaluate pancreatic disease.
- The body of the gland is well visualized because of its close proximity to the posterior aspect of the stomach, and the head is within the duodenal loop and also easily seen.
- Vascular invasion may be assessed and guided needle biopsies taken through the endoscope.
- Cyst fluid may be aspirated for cytology, amylase and CEA concentrations, which can be used to discriminate between the inflammatory and neoplastic cystic disease (see later).
- EUS is also good at detecting very small gallbladder or bile duct stones (microlithiasis) not seen on other imaging.

ERCP

- ERCP involves passage of a flexible, side-viewing endoscope into the duodenum and cannulation of the major duodenal papilla. Contrast medium is injected to outline the pancreatic duct *(pancreatography)* and the bile ducts *(cholangiography).*
- The procedure is described as retrograde because the contrast medium flows in the opposite direction to normal biliary and pancreatic juices. The technique produces good images of the pancreatic duct and is useful in the diagnosis of pancreatic duct strictures and their cause, for the identification of bile duct and pancreatic duct stones and for defining congenital abnormalities and leaks from the biliary or pancreatic ductal systems.
- Transient asymptomatic hyperamylasaemia after ERCP is common (>75% of patients).
- Complications of diagnostic ERCP occur in 2–3% of patients and include acute pancreatitis, cholangitis, bleeding and, rarely, perforation.
- The advent of MRCP for diagnosis of biliary and pancreatic abnormalities has meant ERCP is almost exclusively reserved for therapeutic purposes.
- As discussed above, ERCP can be used for extraction of common bile duct stones, sphincterotomy and/or balloon dilatation of biliary strictures. Plastic or expanding metal tubes (stents) can be placed through strictures of the bile and pancreatic ducts to relieve obstruction and brushings taken from strictures for cytology.

Pancreatitis

Classification

- Pancreatitis is the most important benign condition of the pancreas and is defined as inflammation of the pancreas associated with autodigestion.
- The incidence of acute pancreatitis is reported to range between 5–80/100 000 with the highest incidence reported in the United States and Finland.
- It is important to distinguish between:
  - *acute,*
  - *chronic* and
  - *acute-on-chronic* pancreatitis.
- In acute pancreatitis, endocrine and exocrine function, as well as the morphology of the gland, return to normal after resolution of the attack unless complications ensue.
- In chronic pancreatitis, there are permanent structural changes that can lead to a small, fibrotic gland with either exocrine or endocrine functional impairment or both.
- Recurrent attacks of acute pancreatitis may lead to the changes of chronic pancreatitis and, importantly, acute pancreatitis can occur in the background of chronic pancreatitis.

Acute Pancreatitis

Acute pancreatitis exhibits a broad spectrum of clinical severity, ranging from mild and self-limiting (in most cases), to a rapidly fatal disorder associated with multi-organ failure and death. Classification of acute pancreatitis is shown in Box 23.8.

Aetiology

A number of conditions are known to predispose to pancreatitis (Table 23.4).

- The most common cause of pancreatitis (60–70%) are gallstone disease and alcohol consumption.
- The mechanism by which these aetiological factors trigger pancreatitis is not clear and may differ between patients.

• BOX 23.8 Revised Atlanta Classification of Acute Pancreatitis

A. Mild acute pancreatitis
  (i) no organ failure
  (ii) no local or systemic complications
B. Moderately severe acute pancreatitis
  (i) organ failure that resolves within 48 hrs (transient organ failure) and/or
  (ii) local or systemic complications without persistent organ failure
C. Severe acute pancreatitis: persistent organ failure (>48 hrs)
  (i) single organ failure
  (ii) multiple organ failure

TABLE 23.4	Causes of Acute Pancreatitis.			
Toxic-metabolic	**Idiopathic**	**Genetic**	**Autoimmune**	**Obstructive**

Alcohol
Smoking
Hypercalcemia
Hyperparathyroidism
Medication
Toxins
	Early onset
	Late onset
	Tropical
		CFTR mutations
		SPINK1 mutations
		Alpha-1-antitrypsin
		  deficiency
			Isolated
			Associated with other
			  autoimmune diseases
				Pancreatic divisum
				Sphincter of Oddi disorders
				Duct obstruction (gallstones
				  and tumour)
				Choledochal cysts
				Inflammatory bowel disease

- Intraglandular activation of pancreatic juice, obstruction to drainage of secretions, metabolic intralobular changes and ischaemia have all been suggested as putative mechanisms.

Gallstones

- The mechanisms by which gallstones cause acute pancreatitis are not fully understood. However, it is known that patients with multiple small stones in the gallbladder are more likely to develop pancreatitis than those with large or solitary stones.
- It has therefore been postulated that acute pancreatitis may follow passage of a stone through the major papilla.
- Less commonly, a stone may be identified impacted in the papilla during an attack. In either circumstance, reflux of bile or duodenal contents along the pancreatic duct may follow with intraductal activation of pro-enzymes by enterokinase or possibly infected bile. Autodigestion of the pancreas (particularly by trypsin and phospholipase A) then occurs. Once enzymes are activated, cell membranes are digested, and oedema, proteolysis, vascular damage and necrosis – hallmarks of acute inflammation – may follow.
- Gallstones rarely lead to chronic pancreatitis but are often associated with recurrent attacks of acute pancreatic inflammation unless they are surgically removed by cholecystectomy (see later).

Alcohol

- Alcohol alone can damage the pancreas, and excessive alcohol consumption can precipitate an acute episode of pancreatitis.
- Recurrent episodes of acute pancreatitis may occur in heavy consumers of alcohol, and may lead to chronic pancreatitis (see later). The precise mechanism of action is not known.

Pathological Features

- The mildest form of pancreatitis is characterized by interstitial oedema with inflammatory exudate. In more severe forms, there is glandular necrosis, termed necrotizing pancreatitis, which results from microcirculatory stasis within the gland leading to infarction.
- Surrounding peripancreatic tissues may also develop necrotic changes.

- Secondary infection may also supervene leading to infected necrosis by translocation of bacteria from adjacent colon.
- This is usually bacterial infection but occasionally fungal infections can supervene.

Clinical Features

- The symptoms vary with the severity of the attack of pancreatitis and may evolve with time.
- The principal symptom is abdominal pain, usually localized to the epigastrium or upper abdomen, that radiates to the back in the upper lumbar region or between the scapulae, which is relieved by leaning forward. Pain ranges from mild discomfort to an excruciating level in severe cases.
- Rarely, acute pancreatitis can occur in the absence of pain.
- Nausea and repeated vomiting from Vagus nerve stimulation are present in most instances.
- General findings may be of an acutely ill patient with signs of circulatory insufficiency.
- In the abdomen, the degree of tenderness, guarding and rigidity found depends on the amount and nature of the inflammatory process.
- Rarely, body wall ecchymoses occur, around the umbilicus (Cullen's sign) or in the flanks (Grey Turner's sign). Both are a consequence of haemorrhagic fluid tracking from the retro-peritoneum. The remaining clinical features depend on the local and systemic complications that occur.

Diagnosis

- The clinical manifestations of acute pancreatitis are so varied that the condition must be considered in the differential diagnosis of all instances of abdominal pain until the serum amylase concentration has been demonstrated to be within the normal range (see below).
- Hyperamylasaemia can occur in other pathologies such as biliary and bowel obstruction and, if the patients presents days after the onset of abdominal pain, the amylase may be normal despite pancreatitis having occurred.

Investigation

Serum Amylase Concentration

- Elevation of the serum amylase level occurs in a number of acute abdominal emergencies, such as acute cholecystitis, bowel ischaemia and perforated peptic ulcer, but a concentration in excess of 1000 IU/L (or >four times the upper limit of normal) is highly suggestive of acute pancreatitis.
- Very rarely, other causes of hyperamylasaemia (such as *macro-amylasaemia* – a benign condition associated with amylase molecules of abnormally large molecular weight which are not adequately cleared by the renal tubules) may confuse the diagnosis.

Serum Lipase Concentration

- Elevated serum lipase levels are also seen in acute pancreatitis (two to five times normal values), the level rising within 4 hours of the attack and remaining elevated for 4–7 days.
- The elevation of serum lipase lasts longer than amylase and this test is therefore particularly useful in patients with delayed presentation of abdominal pain.

Liver Function Tests

- Significant elevation of the LFTs, especially the ALP, at presentation is highly suggestive of gallstone aetiology.
- Jaundice raises the possibility of a persisting, obstructing common duct stone, and should raise concern about possible concurrent acute cholangitis, both of which require urgent treatment to prevent mortality.

Imaging

- In patients with acute abdomen, an erect chest X-ray is performed to assess for gastrointestinal perforation even if the serum amylase is elevated.
- In unwell patients with a normal erect chest X-ray, CT scan can be performed to aid in diagnosis. CT abdomen may be useful in clinching the diagnosis by demonstrating an oedematous pancreas with inflammatory changes in the surrounding tissues (Fig. 23.15) and identifying the underlying cause, particularly gallbladder stones, although these are better seen on ultrasound.
- Contrast enhanced CT scanning is also used at a later stage (usually after 72 hours) to assess the extent of pancreatic necrosis and the development of other complications (see later). It is indicated in patients with persisting organ failure, signs of sepsis or clinical deterioration – typically occurring 6–10 days after onset of acute pancreatitis.

Prognosis

- The severity of an attack of acute pancreatitis can be assessed in a number of ways including *Glasgow* and *Ranson* scoring systems. In modern hepatopancreatobiliary practice, the role for scoring systems has declined as the regular

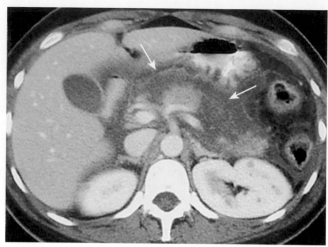

• **Fig. 23.15** Axial CT Abdomen Demonstrating Features of Acute Pancreatitis There is peripancreatic oedema *(white arrows)* and very little enhancement of the pancreas, suggesting necrosis.

review and examination of patients provides a much better assessment of the patients' clinical cause and potential to develop complications. Some important points aside from this include:

- **CRP >350** on admission and **high BMI** are predictive of complications during an episode of acute pancreatitis
- More recently, the APACHE II score has been applied and gives a semi-continuous assessment of severity of pancreatitis, as it does of any acute surgical illness. However, this tool is not practical as it requires the entry of multiple criteria and is not specific for acute pancreatitis.

Mortality Rates

- The overall mortality from acute pancreatitis is 5–10%.
- Most patients (70%) have a mild attack, as defined by the Revised Atlanta criteria, and a low mortality (0–2%). A severe attack of acute pancreatitis carries a higher mortality (20–30%). Death occurs for three principal reasons:
  - early – from multisystem organ failure in fulminant attacks
  - from co-morbid conditions – mainly cardiorespiratory diseases, particularly in the aged
  - late – from local complications, mainly infected necrosis but, more rarely, colonic necrosis or haemorrhage from eroded retroperitoneal vessels

Management

- Management is, in general, supportive, with management of complications if and when they develop.
- *Mild pancreatitis* usually resolves with parenteral fluid replacement, bowel rest (nothing by mouth and nasogastric intubation and drainage because of ileus and abdominal distension) and analgesia. Opiate analgesia is often necessary, but morphine is avoided because it is associated with contraction of the sphincter of Oddi.

- A *severe* episode requires more intensive support, ideally in a high-dependency or intensive care unit.
  - Treatment includes intravenous replacement of large amounts of fluid lost into the retroperitoneum, respiratory support, which may include endotracheal ventilation, the treatment of renal failure and often antibiotics – either prophylactic or as a result of bacterial culture. These measures are instituted alongside invasive monitoring of the patient (arterial line, central venous catheter and urinary catheterization).
  - Paralytic ileus may be prolonged and intravenous nutrition is then necessary.
  - Fluid balance requires careful monitoring: normal saline, plasma substitutes (colloids) and blood may all be required.
  - Urgent ERCP with sphincterotomy and gallstone extraction is indicated in severe gallstone-related pancreatitis, particularly if there is concern about an associated acute cholangitis.
  - In many patients, nutrition can be adequately achieved by nasojejunal tube enteral feeding until oral intake is resumed.

Complications

The more severe the attack of acute pancreatitis the more likely it is that complications will develop (Table 23.5).

Systemic

Systemic complications usually occur soon after the onset of the acute attack (within 0–7 days), although they can take place after this time. They include:

- haemodynamic instability because of hypovolaemia from massive exudation of fluid into the retroperitoneal tissues and the release of inflammatory cytokines;

cardiac function may also be directly depressed; hypoxia is common and of multifactorial origin – abdominal distension, cytokine release and bacterial translocation from the gut; Adult Respiratory Distress Syndrome may develop

- hypocalcaemia – thought to be the result of calcium deposition in areas of fat necrosis
- hyperglycaemia – from disturbances of insulin metabolism
- acute coagulopathies including disseminated intravascular coagulation

Local

- Local complications usually occur more than a week after onset of pancreatitis.
- Pancreatic and peripancreatic inflammation may lead to tissue necrosis and collections of inflammatory fluid.
- Secondary infection of these may follow, probably by bacterial translocation from the gut, and lead on to infected collections, abscess, bacteraemia and a secondary systemic inflammatory response.
- Biliary obstruction may be caused by inflammation or fluid collections around the head of the gland.
- Inflammation may also cause portal or, more commonly, splenic vein thrombosis.
- CT changes in the early stages of the disease (multiple fluid collections, extensive pancreatic necrosis as indicated by non-enhancement of necrotic areas on contrast enhancement) may also give an early indication of local complications.

Necrosis and Infection

- Necrotic areas within the pancreas gland or surrounding tissues may, if they remain sterile, resolve over time.
- However, when these areas are infected and there is a systemic response, they should usually be removed.
- This can, in many cases, by achieved by percutaneous drainage, sometimes with multiple drains.
- If, however, this fails to improve the patient, surgical debridement in the form of necrosectomy can be considered. This has usually been achieved by either using minimal access surgery such as video-assisted surgery or with laparotomy. At surgery, there is full exploration of the pancreas, lesser sac and surrounding areas of fat necrosis. Necrotic tissue is debrided and large-bore drains left close to the areas of necrosis/pancreatic remnant. Postoperative retroperitoneal irrigation through the surgically placed drains is then often undertaken.

Acute Fluid Collections/Pseudocysts

Acute fluid collections are relatively common, and many will resolve spontaneously. They may mature into pseudocysts after 4–6 weeks as a wall of granulation and fibrosis is formed (Fig 23.16).

- They start either as 'sympathetic' inflammatory collections (usually in the lesser sac of the peritoneum) or as

TABLE 23.5	Complications of Acute Pancreatitis.
Pancreatic	Phlegmon
	Pseudocyst
	Abscess
	Ascites
	Fat necrosis
Hepatobiliary	Jaundice
	Bile duct obstruction
	Portal vein/splenic vein thrombosis
Intestinal	Paralytic ileus
	Gastrointestinal haemorrhage
Systemic	Malnutrition
Metabolic	Hypocalcaemia
	Hyperglycaemia
Haematological	Disseminated intravascular coagulation
Renal	Acute renal failure
Cardiac	Hypovolemic shock
Respiratory	Hypoxia
	Adult respiratory distress syndrome

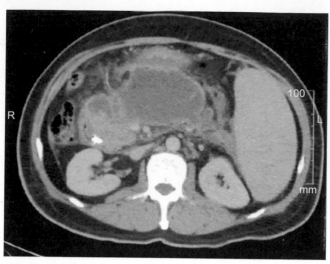

• **Fig. 23.16** Axial CT of a Patient 8 Weeks After an Acute Episode of Pancreatitis There is a mature pseudocyst that demonstrates an enhancing wall. This would ideally be treated with endoscopic cyst-gastrostomy.

the consequence of rupture of the pancreatic duct or one of its tributaries.

• When a peripancreatic fluid collection is of the first kind, it usually resolves spontaneously.

• Pseudocysts larger than 6 cm diameter that persist for longer than 6 weeks are more often in communication with the pancreatic duct and require drainage. In the modern era, this can be achieved without the need for surgery by using EUS to perform cyst gastrostomy. In rare cases when this fails, surgery can be considered, either as laparoscopic or open, to perform cyst jejunostomy.

Chronic Pancreatitis

Aetiology and Pathological Features

Alcohol excess is the usual cause of chronic pancreatitis, accounting for 80% of cases in the developed world. Pancreatitis can also occur in other conditions where free drainage of the pancreatic duct is impeded such as pancreas divisum, papillary or pancreatic tumours, biliary stents and traumatic duct stricture. Hereditary/familial pancreatitis is also an important cause of chronic pancreatitis and, in tropical countries, nutritional causes are responsible for many cases. Table 23.6 illustrates the major causes of chronic pancreatitis.

As with acute pancreatitis, the precise underlying mechanisms leading to the development of chronic pancreatitis are not fully understood. Heavy consumption of alcohol is a common association and it is in such circumstances that the morphological changes within the pancreas become evident. The earliest change appears to be deposition of plugs of protein within the smaller pancreatic ducts. The lumen becomes obstructed, and dilatation follows. Atrophy of the acini then occurs. There may be an accompanying inflammatory infiltrate, but this is variable. Fibrosis takes place around the affected ducts. Eventually only a few acinar and islet cells remain, with widely dilated pancreatic ducts.

TABLE 23.6	Causes of Chronic Pancreatitis.
Common	**Frequency (%)**
Alcohol	65–80
Idiopathic	15–30
Uncommon	
Autoimmune	3–5
Obstructive	3–5
Rare	
Hereditary	<1
Hypertriglyceridemia	<1
Hyperparathyroidism	<1

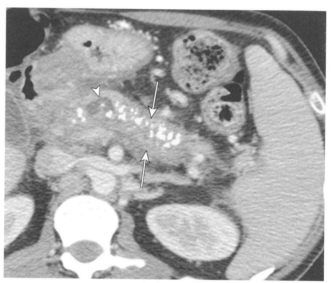

• **Fig. 23.17** CT Scan Demonstrating Typical Features of Chronic Pancreatitis There is extensive calcification throughout the pancreas that is atrophic (solid white arrows). There is also pancreatic duct dilatation (triangular white arrow) as a result of stricturing in the duct. Note also splenomegaly, a likely result of portal hypertension and likely secondary to alcoholic liver disease.

Intraluminal calcification of the protein plugs also occurs, so that pancreatic ductal stones form. Other changes seen in chronic pancreatitis include ductal strictures and dilatation, intrapancreatic cysts and chronic pseudocysts.

Chronic pancreatitis is not reversible, but it is possible that progress can be arrested if the causative factor, such as alcohol, is withdrawn. Fig. 23.17 demonstrates a CT of a patient with chronic pancreatitis with typical findings of the disease.

Clinical Features

History

The predominant symptom is chronic abdominal pain, mainly in the epigastrium or upper abdomen. It may radiate to the back, can be continuous, severe and relentless. An alternative course is chronic pain with acute exacerbations that resemble acute pancreatitis. These bouts of pain may become resistant to even opiate analgesia and mean the patient has multiple recurrent hospital admissions. In many patients this can lead to opiate addiction. Chronic pain may be accompanied by severe weight loss caused by anorexia and fat malabsorption. Depression is also a common symptom.

Steatorrhoea occurs when the secretion of pancreatic lipase is reduced by 90% and is present in about half the patients. The development of diabetes is more common. Both occur more often when the pancreas is calcified. A relatively short clinical presentation suggestive of chronic pancreatic inflammation should always raise the suspicion of cancer of the gland (see below). Furthermore, chronic pancreatitis carries an increased risk for the development of pancreatic cancer. Less commonly, chronic pancreatitis causes obstructive jaundice and occasionally cholangitis. Obstruction and/or thrombosis of the splenic vein can lead to segmental portal hypertension (sinistral hypertension) with gastric varices and upper gastrointestinal bleeding.

Evidence of malnourishment on clinical examination may be obvious. Other signs may be few, but some patients show the characteristic features of alcoholic liver disease.

Investigation

Endocrine Function
In patients with long-standing symptoms, diabetes may be present and, if there is clinical suspicion of this, then a glucose tolerance test should be performed.

Exocrine Function
Tests have been outlined above but are not often used for diagnostic purposes.

Concentration of Serum Amylase
In the diagnosis of chronic disease this is not of value, although the level may be increased during an acute episode of pain.

Imaging

Plain X-ray can show a characteristic transverse outline of the calcified gland, although this investigation is not indicated for investigation of chronic pancreatitis.

Ultrasound and CT can demonstrate both a reduction and an increase in the size of the gland, duct dilatation or the presence of calcification. They may also demonstrate intra-pancreatic cysts or chronic pseudocysts.

ERCP and MRCP are also useful to confirm the anatomical abnormality – a dilated and/or strictured main (chain of lakes), blunted side branches and sometimes associated stones. ERCP is usually only now performed when endoscopic therapy is planned: for example, stone removal, ductal dilatation or stenting.

It is often difficult to distinguish between chronic pancreatitis and carcinoma, especially as cancer may develop on a background of chronic pancreatitis. Pancreatic imaging combined with EUS and targeted needle biopsy may be helpful. However, it must be remembered that a needle biopsy which shows chronic pancreatitis does not exclude

carcinoma, as secondary inflammation is often found adjacent to a carcinoma. In some cases, particularly if obstructive jaundice has developed, resection of a pancreatic mass is recommended without a definite pathological diagnosis of malignancy, the final diagnosis only being made on histopathology.

Management

Measures for Control
In alcohol-induced chronic pancreatitis, complete cessation of alcohol is needed but rarely achieved. Control of pain may require long-term use of opiates that may lead to addiction. In some cases, EUS and coeliac plexus block may help reduce abdominal pain.

Steatorrhoea is treated with pancreatic supplements, usually combined with stomach acid suppression therapy. Diabetes mellitus may be unstable and difficult to control. The insulin requirement is often greater than in idiopathic diabetes, perhaps because pancreatic glucagon is lacking.

Surgical Intervention
The indications for surgical intervention in chronic pancreatitis are:

- correctable anatomical complications which are considered to be associated with either pain or recurrent exacerbations of pancreatitis – e.g. an obstructed pancreatic duct. In these scenario, the Partington-Rochelle procedure may be considered (Fig. 23.18)
- obstructive jaundice secondary to an inflammatory biliary stricture can be managed with hepaticojejunostomy
- rarely, intractable pain with a diffusely damaged gland can be managed with total pancreatectomy
- the development of a possible malignant mass (see later)
  Operation involves either drainage of cysts (similar to acute pancreatitis) or drainage of obstructed pancreatic duct, or partial or complete pancreatic resection for intractable pain or a suspicious mass. If total pancreatectomy is performed, islet cell transplantation can be considered in an attempt to prevent the development of brittle diabetes mellitus. Hypoglycaemia is a not uncommon cause of death after total pancreatectomy. Surgical management for chronic pain is controversial. Good results are only obtained if other factors, such as alcohol and smoking, are controlled and patients are well motivated and carefully selected.

Complications

Pancreatic Pseudocyst
This is the commonest complication found, especially if careful cross-sectional imaging is performed, and they usually arise from within pancreatic tissue. Small cysts do not usually require drainage. Larger ones can give rise to localized pain, nausea and vomiting or even biliary obstruction. A smooth, tender mass is occasionally palpable in the epigastrium, but a cyst can be easily identified on ultrasound or CT scan. Surgical intervention is now rarely used as endoscopic cyst-gastrostomy can successfully manage almost all cysts.

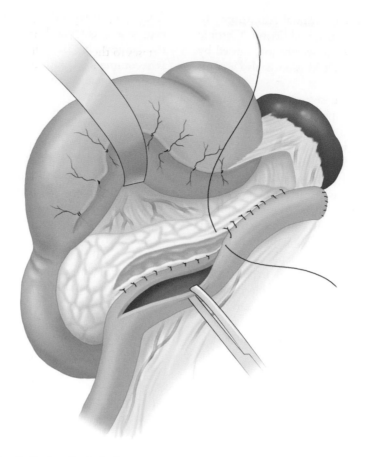

• **Fig. 23.18** The Partington-Rochelle Procedure This surgical procedure is used to relieve a pancreatic duct obstruction and/or remove pancreatic ductal stones. After opening the pancreatic duct, a Roux loop is fashioned and a longitudinal pancreatico-jejunostomy is fashioned.

Pancreatic Ascites

Alcoholic pancreatitis with a communication between the pancreatic duct and the peritoneal cavity is the usual cause of this rare complication. The amylase content of the ascitic fluid is very high. Treatment is by temporary endoscopic insertion of a stent into the pancreatic duct, operative drainage of the duct fistula into a jejunal loop or resection of the portion of the gland that contains the fistula.

Pancreatic Carcinoma

Cancer of the exocrine pancreas (pancreatic adenocarcinoma (PDAC)) is an aggressive disease with a poor prognosis. At diagnosis many patients have advanced/metastatic disease and are not candidates for surgical resection. Unfortunately, even in those patients where surgery is undertaken, the long-term survival is modest at best with little improvement in the last two decades.

Epidemiology

Pancreatic cancer has now overtaken gastric cancer to become the fourth leading cause of death from malignant disease in Western society. In the UK, this amounts to some 5000 deaths a year and is continuing to increase steadily. Across western Europe, the disease causes some 30 000 deaths a year. The peak incidence occurs between the ages of 50 and 70 years, although it occasionally occurs in those as young as 30. Pancreatic cancer is a disease of the developed world.

Aetiology

The risk factors for PDAC are shown in Box 23.9. However, their exact contribution is unclear. All studies show the disease to be commoner in men than in women, although there is evidence of a rising incidence in women in some countries. There is an established link between pancreatic cancer and cigarette smoking, perhaps through nitrosamine inhalation. Other factors include employment in chemical industries and obesity. The role of alcohol consumption is also unclear, although chronic pancreatitis has been linked to the development of pancreatic cancer. A causal relationship with diabetes mellitus has been confused by the fact that up to 15% of patients with pancreatic cancer develop diabetes in the period before presentation, although new onset diabetes in later age should prompt investigations to exclude pancreatic cancer. A family history of pancreatic cancer (first-degree relative) and a number of identified cancer genetic risk factors (e.g. BRCA 1 or 2, familial adenomatous polyposis (FAP) and hereditary nonpolyposis colorectal cancer (HNPCC)) all increase the risk of pancreatic cancer.

Low increase (<5-fold increase in risk)	Alcohol High BMI BRCA1 gene carrier Type 2 diabetes mellitus Familial adenomatous polyposis Smoking First-degree relative with PDAC Hereditary non-polyposis colorectal cancer
Moderate increase (5–10-fold increase in risk)	BRCA2 gene carrier Chronic pancreatitis Cystic fibrosis Two first-degree relatives with PDAC
High increase (>10-fold increase in risk)	Hereditary pancreatitis Peutz-Jeghers syndrome Family history of PDAC in at least 3 first- or second-degree relatives

Pathological Features

All but 5% of cancers are adenocarcinomas which originate from the pancreatic ducts; the remainder are of acinar origin and thought to be less aggressive. Seventy percent of PDAC occur in the pancreatic head. Only 1% have a cystic component (cystadenocarcinomas). Spread of the growth is by four typical routes:

- Direct invasion of neighbouring tissues including perineural spread – typically this will involve the duodenum but importantly means the tumour remains resectable. Cancers arising in the pancreatic head invade and obstruct the lower end of the common bile duct to produce extrahepatic obstructive jaundice (see surgical jaundice earlier). The development of obstruction causes the biliary tract to dilate and, in many circumstances, the pancreatic duct also dilates. The gallbladder in these patients is usually not diseased and also distension becoming clinically palpable – this is the basis of Courvoisier's sign – in that if the gallbladder is palpable in the presence of jaundice, the cause cannot be gallstones because stones cause inflammation and fibrosis, causing gallbladder contraction. Furthermore, in 15–20% of those with a carcinoma in the pancreatic head, direct invasion of the duodenum can result in gastric outflow obstruction and vomiting. Local infiltration of retroperitoneal tissues – the coeliac plexus, splenic and portal veins – may be responsible for some symptoms and may also determine irresectability.
- Lymph node involvement – only lymph node involvement outside the normal resectional field would deem the tumour non-operable. The nodes adjacent to the gland, the pre-aortic coeliac glands and the nodes at the porta hepatis are all frequently involved.

- Vascular – the tumour drains into the portal vein, and liver metastases are most common. Blood-borne metastases to the liver and lungs – non-operable.
- Within the peritoneal cavity – transcoelomic spread – again non-operable.

Clinical Features

History

The typical presenting history is of a middle-aged patient with painless obstructive jaundice and pruritus which may have similar features to hilar cholangiocarcinoma (see earlier). There may be associated weight loss and epigastric pain which radiates through to the back and can sometimes be alleviated by sitting crouched forward in a similar manner to that described in acute pancreatitis. If duodenal invasion has occurred, vomiting is present and can be indicative of an advanced tumour. A carcinoma of the body or tail almost always presents late because of the insidious progression of the tumour before symptoms occur. However, in retrospect, there is often a non-specific prodromal phase of vague symptoms of malaise, weight loss and epigastric pain radiating to the back. The major clinical diagnostic problem is that early symptoms mimic other commoner disorders such as peptic ulcer, oesophagitis with heartburn, angina and biliary colic. PDAC of the pancreatic tail similarly gives very little in the way of symptoms.

Physical Findings

Examination may reveal only jaundice. There may be scratch marks over the trunk and limbs as a consequence of bile salt-induced pruritus. Other possible findings include a palpable enlarged gallbladder (Courvoisier's law – see above) and a palpable mass in the epigastrium which characteristically transmits aortic pulsation. In advanced disease, abdominal distension, ascites and/or a palpable, hard, left supraclavicular lymph node may be found (Virchow's gland).

Investigation

Biochemical

Liver function demonstrates an obstructive picture. Both carbohydrate antigen 19-9 (CA 19-9) and CEA may be elevated in PDAC. CA 19-9 is usually elevated in patients with pancreatic cancer but is also raised in obstructive jaundice of any cause and is therefore unreliable in patients with unrelieved jaundice. Although these markers are not specific enough to be diagnostic, they often support a clinical diagnosis, particularly if there is a progressive rise on repeated estimations. In the presence of jaundice, prothrombin time/INR is prolonged.

Imaging

Ultrasound may show a normal common bile duct or demonstrate a dilated intra- and extrahepatic biliary tree (in the presence of jaundice), a mass in the head of the pancreas and possible liver metastases. A CT scan is invaluable in demonstrating the relationship of the tumour to the superior mesenteric vessels and portal vein, which is essential in determining if the tumour is resectable. It may also demonstrate the presence of a 'double duct' sign which is pathogenomic of PDAC. In addition, it may show lymphatic and hepatic metastases. Endoscopy can demonstrate a malignant mass infiltrating the medial wall of the second part of the duodenum from which a biopsy may be obtained. Endoscopic ultrasound is becoming increasingly useful in the detection, evaluation and local staging of small pancreatic lesions, including endocrine tumours, by assessing vascular invasion of the superior mesenteric vessels or portal vein. PET scanning may be used in patients being considered for surgical resection to exclude metastatic disease not seen on other staging investigations. Laparoscopy is also often used to exclude small peritoneal or liver metastases before an attempt at resection, although it is not mandatory.

Management

Surgical Resection

Surgery offers the only realistic option of long-term cure from PDAC. However, only 20% of patients with PDAC are resectable at the time of presentation. The tumour is most commonly found in the pancreatic head. The most common operation performed is a pylorus preserving pancreatoduodenectomy as opposed to the traditional Whipple's procedure. The pancreatic head, lower common bile duct (and gallbladder), duodenum (apart from the proximal section of the first part of duodenum), a short length of proximal jejunum and the surrounding tissues including lymph nodes are resected. The remaining common bile (or hepatic) duct, the body and tail of the pancreas and the remaining duodenum are then anastomosed separately to the jejunum (Fig 23.19). This is a major procedure but, in expert hands, the hospital mortality is less than 5%. Tumours found at operation to be irresectable are palliatively treated by biliary and, usually, also duodenal bypass.

Alleviation of Obstructive Jaundice

Endoscopic, percutaneous radiological or surgical methods can be used to achieve this. There is now a move within the field of pancreatic surgery to operate on patients with resectable disease without the need to relieve jaundice prior to surgery. At present, although this is being carried out, it should be considered non-standard until further results are available.

Endoscopic stenting at ERCP – The major papilla is cannulated via the endoscope and a plastic or expanding metal stent placed through the obstructing tumour. Bile and pancreatic juice can be collected or ductal brushings or biopsy taken for cytological or histopathological analysis. The mortality is 1–2%, associated with introducing infection (cholangitis) into an obstructed biliary system – prophylactic antibiotic cover is required. In some patients (maybe 10%), ERCP stenting is unsuccessful. A percutaneous cholangiogram (PTC) can be performed and a plastic or metal stent inserted along the track into the biliary tree and through the bile duct stricture.

Palliative surgical decompression – This can be undertaken by direct anastomosis of a loop of isolated jejunum to the dilated hepatic duct (hepaticojejunostomy). Both can be

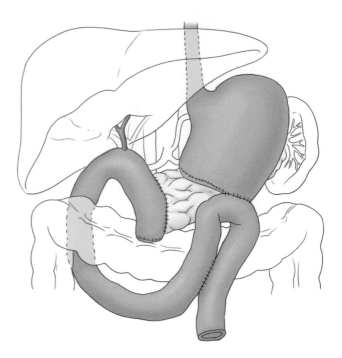

• **Fig. 23.19** Demonstrates the Typical Postoperative Reconstruction Following Pylorus Preserving Pancreaticoduodenectomy The remaining small bowel (jejunum) is moved into the supracolic compartment and a pancreatico-jejunostomy and hepaticojejunostomy are fashioned. The operation is finished with a gastrojejunostomy that is at least 70 cm beyond the hepaticojejunostomy to prevent biliary reflux of gastric contents.

combined with a gastroenterostomy to manage duodenal obstruction – currently the most frequent indication for operative palliation, although increasingly being replaced by endoscopic duodenal stenting.

Pain Relief

Many patients with pancreatic cancer require strong analgesic (usually opioid) use to deal with intractable pain caused by invasion of the coeliac plexus. Relief may be achieved by a coeliac plexus nerve block with alcohol or radiofrequency ablation (RFA), either at the time of operation or under radiological control.

Treatment of Exocrine and Endocrine Pancreatic Insufficiency

The clinical features of this condition are malabsorption with weight loss and steatorrhoea. Pancreatic enzyme supplements are prescribed, and the patient is advised to take as much with each meal as is necessary to control the loose motions. Diabetes secondary to pancreatic cancer occasionally requires insulin for control. Dietary carbohydrate restriction, sometimes supplemented by oral hypoglycaemic agents, is usually adequate.

Chemotherapy and Radiotherapy

In patients with advanced/metastatic disease, chemotherapy regimens that have shown some response (10–30%) are based on combination therapy using 5-fluorouracil (5-FU),

TABLE 23.7	Biochemical and Morphological Characteristics of Pancreatic Cysts.			
	Pseudocyst	**SCN**	**MCN**	**IPMN**
Location	All pancreas	All pancreas	Tail	Head
Cytology	Pigmented histiocytes	Bland PAS+	Mucinous	Mucinous
Viscosity	Low	Low	Increased	High
Cystic Amylase	High	Low	Low	High
Cystic CEA	<200 ng/mL	<0.5 ng/mL	>200 ng/mL	>200 ng/mL
K-Ras mutations	Negative	Negative	Positive	Positive

CEA, Carcinoembryonic antigen; MCN, mucinous cystic neoplasm; IPMN, intraductal papillary mucinous neoplasm; SCN, serous cystic neoplasm.

although this is not curative. Single agent gemcitabine is also widely used, sometimes combined with capecitabine (an oral form of 5-FU). Adjuvant chemotherapy following surgical resection provides a survival advantage of up to 10% at 3 years as reported by the ESPAC-1 trial. In addition, external beam radiotherapy and, more recently, cyber-knife radiotherapy are used for localized but irresectable cancers, often combined with palliative chemotherapy.

Prognosis

PDAC carries a poor prognosis and most patients are dead within 2 years of diagnosis – more than half within 6 months. Even for those patients fortunate to present with a surgically resectable lesion, the 5-year survival after successful removal is less than 20%. Early involvement of palliative care services is important for most patients.

Pancreatic Cysts

Pancreatic cysts are fluid collections in or around the pancreas gland. They can be divided into inflammatory and non-inflammatory types. They are usually found as incidentalomas during investigation of upper abdominal pain or as part of investigations for jaundice or acute pancreatitis. Investigations of pancreatic cysts are performed using a combination of ultrasound, CT, MRI and, occasionally, PET scanning. Cyst appearance and size, calcification on CT, the presence of pancreatic ductal dilatation and evidence of malignant change (wall thickening, positivity on PET scanning, evidence of metastatic spread) may establish a provisional diagnosis and guide management. Where there is diagnostic uncertainty EUS may be helpful, especially when combined with cyst aspiration for fluid analysis (cytology, amylase and CEA levels). A high amylase suggests intraductal papillary mucinous neoplasm (IPMN) (or a pseudocyst) and a high CEA is indicative of a mucinous cystadenoma/cystadenocarcinoma. A summary of the biochemical and morphological characteristics of pancreatic cysts is given in Table 23.7.

Inflammatory cysts follow an attack of acute pancreatitis. They do not have an epithelial lining and are surrounded by granulation tissue and termed pancreatic pseudocysts. They may cause abdominal pain or occasionally obstruct the bile duct (jaundice) or duodenum (vomiting). Pseudocysts may resolve over the course of a few weeks. However, if they are connected to the pancreatic ductal system, they will persist and often require drainage into the stomach that is usually performed by an endoscopic method, although surgery may be required if this fails. Pseudocysts will have a high fluid amylase level if aspirated and confirms the diagnosis.

Non-inflammatory cysts are neoplastic lesions that may be benign, premalignant or malignant. They are often asymptomatic or may cause mild abdominal pain, or occasionally jaundice or even acute pancreatitis. The difficulties in management are, firstly, identifying the type of cystic lesion and, secondly, advising on whether the patient should undergo pancreatic resection.

Serous cystadenomas consist of multiple small cysts and may have central calcification on imaging. They are benign and usually asymptomatic. Occasionally, when large they are resected because of abdominal pain.

Mucinous cystadenomas have larger cysts and sometimes peripheral calcification. They are potentially malignant and can develop into an adenocarcinoma. For this reason, resection is normally recommended for any cyst greater than 3 cm in diameter, provided the patient is fit enough for operation.

Intraductal papillary mucinous neoplasm (IPMN) is a condition associated with dilatation of the pancreatic ducts with excess mucin production. Mucous secretions may be seen at the pancreatic ductal orifice at endoscopy. IPMN is divided into main duct and side branch types, although there is overlap. Cystic components are often seen. There is a high risk of malignant change (adenocarcinoma) particularly in the main duct type. Resection of the involved pancreas is normally advised.

Solid pseudopapillary tumours of the pancreas are rare neoplasms occurring mainly in young Asian and black women. They may be large and are potentially malignant. Resection is recommended, with a good prognosis after complete excision.

24

Small-Bowel Disease and Intestinal Obstruction

Introduction

Small-bowel pathology requiring surgical assessment and treatment is associated with mechanical (such as obstruction), infective and bleeding pathology. Whilst the gastroenterology team plays a greater role in the pathology of the small bowel, the management of small-bowel conditions often involves teams of physicians, surgeons and radiologists working together. A multidisciplinary approach to care is often recommended for many small-bowel conditions.

Anatomy

For an average adult, the length of small bowel is 6 meters (22 feet). The length of small bowel may vary greatly, with taller people generally having a longer small intestine. Whilst the duodenum is technically part of the small bowel, many consider it separately. The small bowel proper commences at the duodeno-jejunal flexure located to the left of the second lumbar vertebra in the root of the transverse mesocolon. At this location, a developed fold of the peritoneum can be found called the ligament of Treitz. The mesenteric root runs obliquely downwards and to the right for 12 to 15 cm to lie over the right sacroiliac joint. The proximal half of the small bowel is referred to as the jejunum, whilst the distal half is the ileum. There is no abrupt distinction between the two but a gradual transition from one to the other. The jejunum is approximately 2.5 meters in length, has a different pattern of vascular arcades, less fat in the mesentery and wider diameter than the ileum. The jejunum is the midsection of the small intestine and connects the duodenum to the ileum. The ileum is the final section of the small intestine. The arterial supply to the jejunum and ileum is from the superior mesenteric artery (SMA), a branch of the aorta that leaves at the level of L1 inferior to the coeliac trunk. The SMA moves between layers of the mesentery and splits into 20 branches. The branches form loops (arcades) where straight arteries, called vasa recta, arise. The venous drainage is via the superior mesenteric vein (SMV). The SMV combines with the splenic vein at the neck of the pancreas, forming the hepatic portal vein. Lymphatic drainage is into the superior mesenteric nodes. The prominent muscular folds (valvulae conniventes) of the small bowel can be visualized on a plain abdominal radiograph. Intestinal mucosal cell turnover is rapid with a lifecycle of a few days. There is a constant flow of digestion and recycling of cell tissue. The entire intestinal tract contains lymphoid tissue, and, specifically, the submucosa of the distal ileum contains well-defined collections of lymphoid tissue, called Peyer's patches. Whilst the exact function is unknown, it is believed they mount an immune response to intraluminal antigens from gut bacteria.

Vitellointestinal Abnormalities

In human embryology, the vitelline duct (vitellointestinal duct) is a narrow tube joining the yolk sac to the mid gut of a developing fetus. It typically appears in the fourth week. Generally, the duct obliterates in the fifth to sixth week of egg fertilization. However, the vitellointestinal duct may persist and present clinically in several forms:

1. Vitellointestinal fistula: an open communication between the ileum and umbilicus
2. Meckel's diverticulum, which is a free diverticulum in the terminal ileum

3. A fibrous strand connected to the umbilicus, attached at the antimesenteric border of the ileum or at the apex of a Meckel's diverticulum. The clinical significance is that it may cause an obstruction or strangulation.

Physiology

Motility

There are two main movements of the small bowel:
1. Peristalsis – this is a coordinated, wave-like contraction of the muscle of the small intestine over several centimetres which propels food contents forward.
2. Segmental movements – these are typically over a short distance and mix the bowel contents together.

It is the interaction between liquid and air that causes bowel sounds. Peristalsis causes a loud gurgle (borborygmus) and lasts over several seconds. Segmental movements produce faint 'clicks' which last over a shorter period of time and auscultate anywhere across the abdominal wall. When auscultating the abdominal wall, one should remain anywhere across the abdomen in a fixed position and listen for a full minute to conclude bowel sounds are absent. An increase in activity of the small intestine, for example due to an obstruction or diarrhoea, may cause both types of bowel sounds to become louder and more frequent.

Secretion and Digestion

Secretion and digestion both commence in the mouth and stomach and continue throughout the length of the small bowel. These processes are completed in the small bowel where nutrients and minerals are absorbed. The small intestine secretes the succus entericus, also called intestinal juice, which has an electrolyte concentration approximately the same as that of the extracellular fluid. When nutrients are found in the small intestine, a hormone called cholecystokinin causes bile from the gallbladder and pancreatic enzymes to be released into the small intestine. Many of the digestive enzymes released from the pancreas and liver enter the small intestine through the pancreatic duct. The overall flow of liquid though the small intestine in 24 hours is large, but the alimentary tract normally contains at any one moment only about 1 L of secretion. Diversion of intestinal content because of obstruction, fistula or diarrhoea, rapidly causes extracellular fluid volume depletion.

Absorption

The small intestine is the principle site for water and electrolyte absorption. Proteins are broken down into peptides and amino acids prior to absorption. The jejunum absorbs glucose, simple peptides and amino acids. Fat is emulsified by bile salts and degraded to fatty acids and monoglycerides. These form micelles which are aggregates of bile salts, fatty acids, cholesterol and monoglycerides that are absorbed at the mucosal surface. Complex molecules such as bile salts are absorbed in the terminal ileum and transported by the portal circulation to the liver for resecretion into bile. This enterohepatic circulation is a mechanism for preservation of molecules which require complex synthesis. Resection or pathology of the terminal ileum interrupts the enterohepatic circulation and reduces the absorption of complex molecules, such as the B_{12} and intrinsic factor complex, which may cause macrocytic anaemia. Furthermore, resection of significant length of small bowel may lead to 'short bowel syndrome' where the remaining length of the small intestine is not enough to allow adequate nutrient and electrolyte absorption.

Adaptability

The principle goals in surgical resection is to preserve as much bowel as possible to preserve healthy bowel function. However, the bowel can undergo extensive resection without obvious effects. For survival, a total length of at least 30 cm has been suggested. In cases of very short lengths of functioning small bowel, parenteral nutrition is needed for survival. Surgical procedures exist for attempting to increase the length of the available small intestine. Another option is small-bowel transplantation.

Fistula

A fistula is an abnormal connection between two epithelialized surfaces. It is possible to have a fistula between the small bowel and the skin, called an enterocutaneous fistula (ECF). This may occur due to disease processes (such as Crohn's disease) or a complication of surgery (such as enterotomy or an anastomotic leak). It is possible to have an ECF arising from the duodenum, jejunum or ileum. A proximal fistula involving the duodenum or jejunum produces large fluid losses (>1 L/day) and can lead to significant volume deficiency within a few days. The skin around the fistula can also be digested due to the enzymes in the fluid. In contrast, a distal ileum fistula has a lower fistula output (approximately 500 mL/day) and is easier to manage. Successful treatment of fistulas requires several methods including eradicating sepsis, protecting the adjacent skin, controlling fistula output and maintaining nutrition. Fistulas may eventually spontaneously resolve or may require surgical closure.

Microbiology

Most organisms ingested are destroyed by both acid and pepsin found in the stomach, and relatively sterile conditions are found in a healthy small bowel. However, large inoculum (such as gastroenteritis) or bacteria resistant to digestion (e.g. *Mycobacterium tuberculosis*) may survive. Organisms remain within the small bowel due to the protective action of the mucosal barrier; however, in cases of

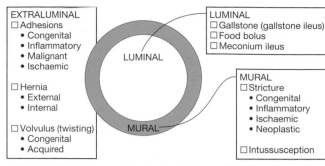

• **Fig. 24.1** The Causes of Mechanical Obstruction Classified in Their Relation to the Bowel Wall

bowel ischaemia or bowel obstruction, there is a breakdown of this protection. Once organisms enter the interstitial space of the gut wall, it is possible to enter the portal circulation. Bacterial endotoxins entering the circulation can lead to systemic inflammatory response syndrome (SIRS), sepsis and multi-organ failure.

Intestinal Obstruction

There are several classification systems for bowel obstruction, and this is required as different types of bowel obstruction have varying aetiology, present with varying symptoms and require different treatment. The distinction between mechanical obstruction and paralytic ileus is important. Mechanical obstruction is caused by a blockage and further passage of small-bowel contents is prevented, but the bowel itself is normal and active. In paralytic ileus, the bowel is inactive.

Mechanical Obstruction

There are further classification systems for mechanical obstruction. Clinically, bowel obstruction may be acute, subacute and chronic. The causes of bowel obstruction may be classified into the position in relation to the bowel wall – i.e. luminal, mural or extramural (Fig. 24.1).

The obstruction can be an 'open loop' where the bowel content can escape proximally because there is no obstruction proximally, or 'closed loop' in which the bowel segment is obstructed proximally and distally. In large-bowel obstruction, there is a risk of a closed loop obstruction because a competent ileocaecal valve may prevent regurgitation of bowel contents from the caecum to the terminal ileum. Eventually, the blood supply may become compromised; the venous drainage is the first to be affected and, later, arterial obstruction can lead to haemorrhagic infarction.

Pathophysiology

If there is a bowel obstruction, intestinal contractions are increased and become more frequent. As the bowel diameter increases, contractions may eventually fail. As the

bowel wall becomes oedematous, there is a reduced reabsorption of secretions which causes extracellular volume deficiency. As the bowel distends, the intramural vessels become stretched and may compromise the blood supply, which can lead to ischaemia, infarction and perforation. In cases of strangulation, the bowel becomes ischaemic resulting in SIRS and lactic acidosis. If the strangulated loop does not resolve, it will infarct, usually within 4 hours, and perforate, causing bacterial peritonitis which may be fatal. If there is gross distension of the abdomen due to dilated loops, diaphragmatic movement is limited and respiratory function is impaired. Vomiting may result in inhalation and may lead to airway compromise and aspiration pneumonia.

Clinical Findings

Symptoms

There are four main symptoms of small-bowel obstruction, summarized in Box 24.1.

Abdominal pain may be the first symptom and it is a central colicky abdominal pain, which appears in waves with pain free intervals of several minutes. If the bowel becomes ischaemic or perforated, the pain becomes constant and more severe.

Vomiting, initially containing food debris and dark green fluid (bile) but, if the bowel obstruction is long-standing and is from mid-jejunum and distally, then the fluid may resemble faeculent material and change to a dark brown colour with offensive smell.

Distension is usually evident and is a common symptom of small-bowel obstruction. Distension is more marked when the site of the small-bowel obstruction is more distal.

Constipation can be partial or complete. In complete obstruction, there is no passage of flatus or faeces from the rectum. In large-bowel obstruction, complete obstruction occurs earlier than in small-bowel obstruction. It is possible to have an incomplete obstruction due to a progressive tumour. This may present as a change in bowel habit with a reduction in the size and frequency of stool, as well as the presence of blood or mucus.

Physical Findings

General

Dehydration occurs due to vomiting, decreased fluid absorption and fluid loss in the bowel, including loss of water and electrolytes. Dehydration may be associated with tachycardia, loss of skin turgor and increased capillary refill time. Temperature changes may occur with a raised temperature in cases of bowel ischaemia.

Abdominal Examination

The abdominal examination findings can be summarized in Fig. 24.2.

Inspection

Distension, the more distal the obstruction in the small bowel the greater the distension.

Scars across the abdomen which may suggest adhesional small-bowel obstruction.

Peristalsis may be visible in thin patients.

Palpation may identify:
- an abdominal or pelvic mass
- irreducible mass in a hernia orifice suggestive of a strangulated hernia
- tenderness and guarding may suggest small-bowel strangulation and ischaemia

Percussion may produce a tympanic note due to gas filled loops of bowel, although in slowly developing distal small-bowel obstruction, fluid may predominate.

Auscultation may reveal increased frequency bowel sounds that are high pitched and tinkling. Loud peristaltic noises may coincide with an attack of colic. Bowel sounds may be absent in advanced conditions or in cases of peritonitis due to bowel perforation.

A rectal or vaginal examination may reveal a pelvic mass or an empty collapsed rectum.

Investigations

Imaging

A plain abdominal radiograph is taken supine. Four questions to be asked are:
1. Is this an obstruction?
2. If obstruction is present, is it in the small or large bowel?
3. Is it possible to identify the level of obstruction in the small or large bowel?
4. Can specific causes of obstruction be identified?

Small-bowel obstruction on a radiograph is shown as distended small-bowel loops, containing gas and fluid, with fluid levels in the erect position. The levels are frequently arranged in a step ladder pattern (Fig. 24.3). In the jejunum, the valvulae conniventes may be visible. Adjacent loops may be separated by a variable distance giving an indication of the amount of oedematous fluid in the bowel wall. There is not normally gas in the large bowel. Large-bowel obstruction causes accumulation of gas, which outlines its wall proximally and which is maximal in the caecum, with no small bowel dilation in cases of a competent ileocaecal valve.

The gas patterns on a radiograph may help to identify the location of the obstruction with bowel dilatation proximal to a transition point at the site of the obstruction and collapsed bowel distal to the transition point. Gastrografin (a hyperosmolar water-soluble contrast

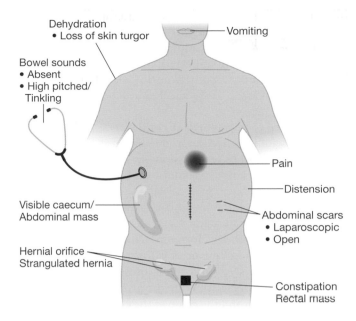

• **Fig. 24.2** Possible Examination Findings in Bowel Obstruction

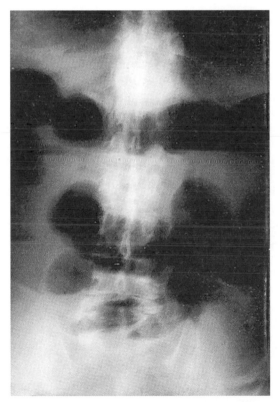

• **Fig. 24.3** Small-Bowel Obstruction – Erect X-Ray

medium) swallow and follow-through can be used to identify the site of the small bowel obstruction. Another advantage of gastrografin is its potential therapeutic role, especially in cases of adhesional small bowel obstruction. The use of gastrografin in adhesive small bowel obstruction has been shown to be safe and may reduce the need for surgery if conservative treatment fails. Several X-rays are taken over some hours to show the transit of contrast through the bowel. If there is contrast entry in the large bowel after 1–2 hours, complete small bowel obstruction may be excluded. In suspected large-bowel obstruction, a retrograde contrast study from the rectum may be performed to review a truly mechanical obstruction from pseudo-obstruction.

Computed tomography (CT) of the abdomen and pelvis is a very useful investigation in the diagnosis of small-bowel obstruction. It is preferably done with intravenous contrast, but there is a risk of contrast nephrotoxicity, especially in patients with acute prerenal failure due to small-bowel obstruction. The intravenous contrast allows better delineation of the bowel anatomy and demonstrates the blood supply to the bowel, which is important if suspecting bowel strangulation and ischaemia. A CT scan can correctly confirm the diagnosis of mechanical small-bowel obstruction versus ileus. Also, a CT scan can identify the site of the small-bowel obstruction and the cause of the obstruction, allowing the surgeon to plan the surgery appropriately. In cases of neoplastic disease, a CT scan can identify the primary tumour and examine for metastatic or peritoneal disease.

Blood Tests

Blood tests are useful in small-bowel obstruction. A raised white cell count may indicate infection, inflammation or bowel ischaemia. Small-bowel obstruction is associated with water and electrolyte disturbances. Small-bowel obstruction may lead to prerenal failure with rise in urea and creatinine. Raised lactate levels may suggest dehydration which should improve with fluid resuscitation, or intestinal ischaemia which requires immediate surgery. In upper abdominal obstruction, the serum amylase may also increase, although the rise may not be more than four times the upper limit of normal as in acute pancreatitis.

Management

The management is classified into non-operative (conservative) and operative. The indications for non-operative management are:

1. Previous abdominal surgery and high risk of adhesional small-bowel obstruction.
2. No evidence of threat to the viability of the bowel either through strangulation or perforation (suggested through signs of shock, hypovolemia, systematic inflammatory response and peritoneal irritation).
3. The obstruction is incomplete and features suggest non-progression, e.g. Crohn's disease in the small bowel.

Non-operative management includes:

- insertion of a nasogastric tube for proximal decompression with continuous free drainage and aspiration at regular intervals
- antiemetic medications
- suitable analgesia, using the WHO analgesia ladder, starting with paracetamol and moving towards opiates

- intravenous antibiotics if patient is at risk of aspiration pneumonia
- water and electrolyte replacement through intravenous replacement. The electrolytes for patients with bowel obstruction should be checked daily and corrected appropriately
- a catheter should be placed to accurately record urine output and to calculate fluid balance and to guide intravenous fluid replacement
- repeated (4–6-hourly) evaluation of the clinical state – abdominal girth, development of tenderness, changes in bowel sounds and in cardiovascular status
- in individual circumstances, repeated plain X-rays or contrast studies and haematological and biochemical reassessment of the features of strangulation

A limit of 5 days or less is usually placed on non-operative management, although this may be extended in patients with a history of multiple previous operations or significant co-morbidities. During the period of non-operative management, the nutritional state of the patient should be assessed and total parenteral nutrition should be considered in prolonged periods of small-bowel obstruction.

Operative Management

The indications are:

- established or suspected small-bowel strangulation, including those with irreducible external hernia
- worsening abdominal pain
- rising inflammatory markers
- failure of resolution after a period of non-operative management
- a cause (e.g. carcinoma) requiring surgical removal

Operative management is preceded by a brief period of application of the measures outlined under non-operative management – gastric suction, fluid resuscitation, water and electrolyte replacement. The only indication for urgent operation is when strangulation or other causes of non-viability of the bowel are likely. At operation, the obstruction is relieved and, if possible, the underlying cause removed. If the underlying cause cannot be removed (e.g. irresectable cancer), then it is bypassed, or the bowel is exteriorized as a stoma proximal to the obstruction if there is adequate length of bowel from the duodenum to the ileostomy. Dead or damaged intestine must be excised, and, if the remaining intestine is healthy, then perform an anastomosis or, if there are concerns about the state of the remaining bowel, then perform an ileostomy.

Causes of Mechanical Bowel Obstruction

The commonest classification of mechanical small-bowel obstruction is: intraluminal, mural and extramural. The commonest causes of small-bowel obstruction are:

1. *Adhesions* – usually postoperative
2. *Hernias* – either external or internal

Intraluminal

Gallstone 'Ileus'

It is possible that, in cases of large gallstones, they may erode through into the adjacent duodenum. There may be an initial presentation of acute cholecystitis or recurrent chronic cholecystitis. It is possible that inflammation of the gallbladder and surrounding structures can lead to adhesion formation. The pressure effect and inflammation may lead to erosion of the gallbladder wall and a fistula from the gallbladder to adjacent structures, normally the duodenum. On entering the duodenum, the gallstone may then transit distally until it causes a mechanical impaction in a narrow lumen in the gastrointestinal tract. Less than 1% of causes of intestinal obstruction are due to gallstone 'ileus'. In the developed world, this condition is rare as most people have early management of gallstones. There is a higher frequency in the elderly and those with many medical co-morbidities.

Clinical Features

Many signs and symptoms of gallstone ileus are non-specific. The presentation of gallstone ileus normally has a history of prior biliary symptoms. The initial presentation may be one of intermittent obstruction. Symptoms are variable and can involve nausea, vomiting, central abdominal pain and distension. If the gallstone is causing obstruction in the proximal small bowel, the vomit is normally of gastric contents and bile, whilst a distal obstruction can lead to a more faeculent vomit.

Investigations

A plain abdominal radiograph is useful in the diagnosis. It may be possible to see air in the biliary tree (pneumobilia), partial or complete intestinal obstruction, aberrant gallstones and a change in the position of the gallstone on serial films. An ultrasound can assess for other gallstones and assess the biliary tree. A magnetic resonance cholangiopancreatography (MRCP) may be useful in certain cases where diagnosis is uncertain. A CT scan of the abdomen and pelvis, as discussed previously, provides significant information such as the exact site of obstruction by the gallstone, cholecystoduodenal fistula, signs of perforation such as free air or free fluid, the blood supply to the small bowel and other significant pathologies, such as incidental finding of neoplasm.

Management

Gallstones are removed at laparotomy through an enterotomy proximal to the point of impaction. All the proximal small bowel is checked for the presence of additional stones. If the bowel looks healthy after the stone is removed, then the enterotomy is closed. If the bowel looks unhealthy, then small-bowel resection is performed with anastomosis or defunctioning ileostomy if the patient is critically unwell. Although not essential, a further procedure may be performed to deal with the disease in the biliary tree. In most patients, there is no requirement for cholecystectomy.

Food Bolus

The common causes of food bolus are:
- poor chewing of food in an edentulous patient
- a previous gastric resection which has destroyed the pylorus
- high consumption of indigestible fibre (e.g. orange pith)
- occasionally, partial obstruction for some other reason with impaction of partially digested food at the site of narrowing

Management

Operation is indicated if the symptoms persist. The bolus can often be milked distally into the large intestine, and it is rarely necessary to open the bowel and risk contamination of the peritoneal cavity. If that is not possible, then perform enterotomy for removal of the food bolus. Foreign bodies may be able to pass through the gastrointestinal tract. This depends on the size, shape, and material of the foreign body. Some foreign bodies may need to be removed urgently, such as batteries and large sharp objects.

Meconium 'Ileus'

This is discussed in Chapter 9.

Mural

Neonatal Obstructions and Intussusception

These are discussed in Chapter 9.

Inflammatory

Crohn's disease, tuberculosis and, in the large bowel, diverticulitis may all produce obstruction by inflammation or fibrous strictures or adherence to bowel loops in the inflamed area. Diverticulosis of the large bowel causes small-bowel obstruction by forming adhesions between the inflamed colon and the small bowel. Patients with autoimmune diseases and vasculitis may have episodes of small-bowel obstruction with abdominal distension and significant abdominal pain, which most times resolves with non-operative management. Also, ingestion of NSAIDs may be associated with intestinal stricture and bleeding.

Neoplastic

Colorectal carcinoma is a common cause of large-bowel obstruction (see Ch. 13). Small-bowel neoplasms occasionally also cause obstruction (see later).

Extramural

Adhesions

Worldwide, adhesions are second only to strangulated external hernia as the commonest cause of small-bowel obstruction. In developed countries, where hernias are usually treated early, they are the leading cause.

Aetiology

A minority of adhesions are attributable to developmental disturbances (congenital adhesions). However, the vast majority are scars on the peritoneum caused by previous inflammation. The peritoneal mesothelial cells have a potent fibrinolytic mechanism based on the tissue conversion of plasminogen to plasmin. In consequence, any fibrin produced by inflammation in the peritoneal cavity is usually broken down before it can become 'organized' into fibrous tissue. If fibrinolysis fails, usually due to peritoneal inflammation, then the usual process of wound healing takes place and fibrous tissue is deposited. The small bowel, rather than moving freely within the peritoneal cavity, becomes attached to itself or to an adjacent fixed point and can therefore kink or twist (Fig. 24.4).

Adhesions may be a simple isolated band that can trap the bowel and narrow it, or they may be complex and dense involving the whole peritoneal cavity. The time course of adhesion formation is comparable to that of the inflammation/ischaemia which are the underlying causes. Acute processes can produce adhesions in a matter of days – although this does not necessarily mean that obstruction follows, and an adhesion can lie dormant for months or years. Therefore, post-surgical adhesional obstruction may manifest either within a few days of an operation – when it may be difficult to distinguish from a persistent paralytic ileus – or years or decades after the operation.

Apart from the causes shown in Table 24.1, it has often been postulated by exasperated surgeons, re-operating for the umpteenth time on a patient with adhesive obstruction, that there are patients who are 'adhesion formers', although at present there is no convincing evidence of this.

Clinical Features

It is unknown whether or not adhesions cause pain other than that associated with intestinal obstruction. Chronic or recurrent pain is often ascribed to their presence, particularly pelvic pain in women. Although there is no strong evidence to support this association, pelvic adhesions are the commonest cause of secondary female infertility.

Management

A non-operative management is tried initially, including: nasogastric tube, nil by mouth, intravenous fluid resuscitation, urinary catheter, management of fluid and electrolyte disturbances. If the adhesional obstruction is prolonged, then consider intravenous total parenteral nutrition. Also, consider gastrograffin swallow and follow through. If the adhesional obstruction persists or the patient develops symptoms or signs of bowel ischaemia/strangulation/perforation (worsening abdominal pain, pyrexia, tachycardia, tachypnoea, peritonism, raised inflammatory markers) then proceed with an operation. Surgery includes adhesiolysis to resolve the small-bowel obstruction, and small-bowel resection if part of the small bowel is not viable. Adhesiolysis should be performed carefully to avoid serosal tears and enterotomies.

External Hernia

This is discussed in Chapter 30.

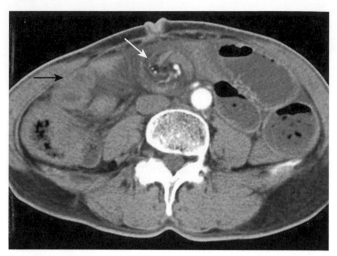

• **Fig. 24.4** Small-Bowel Volvulus on CT with Evidence of the 'Whirlpool Sign' (From Liu, W., et al.: Multisection spiral CT in the diagnosis of adhesive small bowel obstruction: the value of CT signs in strangulation. Clinical Radiology, 76:1:75.35-75.311, 2021, Fig. 2A, p. 75.e9)

TABLE 24.1	**Adhesions**	
Classification	**Underlying cause**	**Examples**
Congenital	Abnormality or arrest of development	Duodenal obstruction
	Ischaemia	Persistent vitellointestinal duct with volvulus
Acquired	Trauma	Post-surgical obstruction
Cell damage	Irradiation	Pelvic radiotherapy for gynaecological cancer
Intraperitoneal inflammation	Inhibition of fibrinolysis	Peritonitis
		Focal inflamed areas, e.g. diverticulitis of the colon
		Peritoneal dialysis in renal failure
Ischaemia	Inhibition of fibrinolysis	Partially devascularized bowel
		Surgical procedures
Peritoneal loss	Lack of local fibrinolysis	Wide surgical excision
Intraperitoneal foreign materials	Foreign body inflammation	Surgical materials: implants, sutures
Abnormality of fibrous tissue	Unknown	Colectomy for polyposis coli
		Stromal fibrous response to malignant disease

Internal Hernia

This is an uncommon cause of small-bowel obstruction but may be increasing in frequency. This takes place into a recess of a peritoneal fold formed either during development (e.g. around the junction of the duodenum and jejunum at the ligament of Treitz) or as a consequence of operation (e.g. lateral to a colostomy or ileostomy). They are increasingly seen after laparoscopic gastric bypass for obesity, when small bowel may herniate between the jejunal and transverse colon mesenteries (*Peterson's space*). Transmesenteric hernia is the most common type, especially after the creation of a Roux-en-Y anastomosis, e.g. gastric bypass, liver transplantation.

Clinical Features and Management

Features are of intestinal obstruction without obvious cause. The clinical trap is that a loop of bowel may be strangulated but is not in contact with the anterior parietal peritoneum and therefore does not produce symptoms and signs of peritoneal irritation. In consequence, disastrous delay may occur. A CT scan is a useful investigation to help in the diagnosis of an internal hernia. Internal hernias may initially be reducible spontaneously and cause intermittent symptoms which are clinically silent for a long time. Occasionally, an internal hernia may be found incidentally at surgery for an unrelated cause.

Volvulus

This is caused by a twist of the bowel around the mesenteric axis. A closed loop may result in obstruction and ischaemia of the involved loop. It is less common in the small bowel than large bowel.

Small Bowel

The usually highly mobile small bowel may be tethered by adhesions, often to the abdominal wall or adjacent viscera, causing rotation of the bowel around this. If rotation is greater than 180 degrees, strangulation may occur.

Large Bowel

The rotation occurs at two main sites:
- caecum – when there is a persistent mesentery
- sigmoid colon – when the existing mesentery is usually more extensive than normal; this is the commoner cause of large-bowel volvulus
  Caecal volvulus can occur in adults of 30 years of age or more, and sigmoid volvulus is more common in older people.

Clinical Features and Management

Small Bowel

The symptoms and signs are similar to that of acute small-bowel obstruction with localized abdominal pain if strangulation has developed. In cases of involvement of a considerable length of small bowel, if strangulation occurs, there may be associated marked circulatory disturbance (shock). A CT scan of the abdomen and pelvis should be able to demonstrate small-bowel volvulus. During surgery, the volvulus is untwisted, the cause relieved and any bowel with ischaemia or doubtful viability is resected.

Large Bowel

Caecal volvulus presents with features of small-bowel obstruction and sigmoid volvulus presents with features of large-bowel obstruction, occasionally with a background of repeated episodes. In caecal volvulus, although obvious intestinal obstruction is present, the clinical and radiological features may be confusing. CT scan of the abdomen and pelvis is useful to delineate the anatomy and provide the diagnosis of caecal volvulus. Sigmoid volvulus is, in theory, easier to diagnose. The patient is elderly. The features are those of large-bowel obstruction, perhaps with previous episodes. The presentation may be acute with signs of circulatory insufficiency because of ischaemia or infarction. A grossly distended, drum-like abdomen is characteristic. A plain supine abdominal X-ray may be diagnostic with a 'coffee bean' sign. CT scanning is usually diagnostic of both caecal and sigmoid volvulus.

In caecal volvulus, there is only a limited place for non-operative management because this is a closed-loop obstruction. Particularly if signs of peritoneal irritation are present, operation is immediately undertaken, the ileum and right colon resected and the bowel reconstructed by ileotransverse anastomosis. In sigmoid volvulus unlike caecal volvulus, non-operative treatment is the initial choice. A rigid sigmoidoscope is introduced under visualization, a wide-bore flatus tube is passed along it and the sigmoid loop decompressed by careful negotiation of the obstructed loop. Alternatively, a flexible sigmoidoscope is introduced under visualization, the bowel is untwisted and is assessed for any ischaemic changes, the colon proximal to the volvulus is decompressed and a wide-bore flatus tube is left in situ. If there is any failure of decompression or concerns over ischaemia, an urgent operation is required, and the affected colonic segment is resected either with or without primary anastomosis. After decompression has been achieved, a decision on surgical excision of the mobile sigmoid colon can be taken at a later date. The decision on surgery is based on the number of episodes of sigmoid volvulus and the patient's fitness for surgery and co-morbidities.

Tuberculosis

Aetiology

Tuberculosis enters the intestine via the lymphoid follicles found in the mucosa of the ileum. The source is either ingested or acquired from a focus of infection already present, such as swallowed sputum associated with an open pulmonary lesion. Both human and bovine strains of *Mycobacterium tuberculosis* can be the cause, but the latter is more uncommon in the UK. In immunodeficiency states (for example AIDS), unusual strains of mycobacteria such as *M. avium intracellulare* may be identified. Although tuberculosis affecting the small intestine is uncommon in developed countries, it remains a feature of communities with poor nutrition and hygiene, where there may be a continuous focus of tubercular infection.

Pathological Features

Typically, tuberculosis inflammation affects the wall of the ileum and is associated with:

- ulceration
- lymph node enlargement and subsequent caseation and calcification
- bowel stricture formation

In addition, tuberculosis may involve the peritoneum to produce tuberculous peritonitis characterized by the presence of miliary nodules and the development of ascites.

Clinical Features

The patient may be suffering with weight loss, low-grade pyrexia, anaemia, diarrhoea, ascites and vague abdominal pain. Ulceration of the intestine may cause frank rectal bleeding. The formation of an inflammatory mass or the development of a stricture may cause acute intestinal obstruction. A mass in the right iliac fossa has to be distinguished from one caused by Crohn's disease, which it resembles closely.

Investigation

CT or MRI scan of the abdomen may identify thickened small-bowel loops, intestinal obstruction, lymph node enlargement, abscess formation or ascites. A barium follow-through can outline the small bowel and demonstrate areas of inflammation and strictures. The radiological appearances may be difficult to distinguish from those of Crohn's disease. Half of patients with tuberculous ileitis also have a radiologically identified pulmonary lesion.

Management

As with all other manifestations of tuberculosis, the primary treatment is with antituberculous medications, although this is becoming increasingly problematic with the development of resistant strains. The surgeon may be required to establish the diagnosis by laparoscopy or laparotomy if necessary, or to manage complications such as bleeding and obstruction if they fail to respond to medical treatment.

Radiotherapy Effects

Tissues that divide rapidly, such as the mucosa of the small and – to a lesser extent – the large bowel, are sensitive to irradiation. Abdominal or pelvic radiotherapy for the treatment of cancer results in damage to the intestinal mucosa and to the small blood vessels of the bowel wall. This was especially common with high radiotherapy doses used in the past for gynaecological malignancies. Currently, lower radiotherapy doses and improved radiotherapeutic techniques have decreased the risk of intestinal injury due to radiotherapy.

Clinical Pathological Features

The major pathological changes related to irradiation are mucosal atrophy and intramural fibrosis. Other clinical features include strictures causing low-grade intestinal obstruction and ulceration with bleeding. Patients may present with gastrointestinal bleeding, bowel obstruction, bowel perforation, fistula formation and intra-abdominal or pelvic collections.

Management

Surgical excision of the affected small-bowel loops damaged by radiotherapy may be required. It is important not to resect a significant amount of small bowel leading to short bowel syndrome, especially since the remaining bowel may also be affected by irradiation. Also, healthy unirradiated bowel should be used for reconstruction of the intestinal continuity, otherwise healing with stricture formation or anastomotic breakdown may occur.

Diverticula of the Small Bowel

Meckel's Diverticulum
Anatomy and Epidemiology

A remnant of the vitellointestinal duct may persist in the form of a Meckel's diverticulum. The presentation of a Meckel's diverticulum follows the 'law of 2s': the prevalence is 2% of the population, it is found at a distance of 2 feet (60 cm) from the ileocaecal valve, it is 2 inches (5 cm) long, and it is twice as common in males than females (Fig. 24.5).

Clinical Presentation

Meckel's diverticulum may have various clinical presentations:

- acute diverticulitis which may mimic appendicitis
- worsening diverticulitis which may lead to perforation with peritonitis
- retained foreign body (e.g. fishbone) within the diverticulum which may cause perforation
- persistent vitello-umbilical fistula
- bowel obstruction if the diverticulum or an associated band is attached to the umbilicus resulting in small-bowel volvulus or internal hernia
- bowel obstruction due to ileo-ileal intussusception
- pain or bleeding from a peptic ulcer secondary to the presence of ectopic parietal cells within the

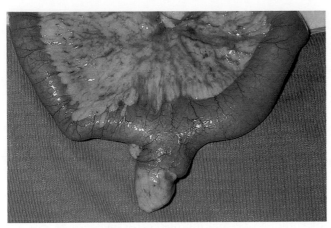

• **Fig. 24.5** Meckel's Diverticulum

diverticulum. The peptic ulcer occurs on the mesenteric border of the ileum, and the presentation is of pain and distal small-bowel bleeding which can be very heavy. It commonly affects children or young adults and may be diagnosed with gastrointestinal angiography or radionuclide scanning with Technetium TC-99M sodium pertechnetate which detects the presence of the ectopic gastric mucosa.

Management

Symptomatic Meckel's diverticulum is treated according to the complications it may cause, but commonly it is resected. If it is discovered incidentally during abdominal surgery, it may be left, or can be resected especially in children.

Jejunal Diverticula

Jejunal diverticula are multiple herniated areas through the mesenteric aspect of the jejunum, usually bulging to one side. They are uncommon and of unknown aetiology and may be congenital. The clinical presentation may include:
- diverticulitis, which may lead to bowel perforation
- macrocytic anaemia thought to be the consequence of infection with small-bowel bacterial overgrowth
- enterolith formation with small-bowel obstruction

Management

If asymptomatic, no treatment required. Antibiotics can be used for diverticulitis and bacterial overgrowth. Resection of the affected intestinal segment may be needed for perforation or bowel obstruction, or recurrent diverticulitis not responding to antibiotics.

Small-Bowel Tumours

Epidemiology and Aetiology

Primary tumours of the small bowel are rare and account for only 5% of gastrointestinal neoplasms. Unfortunately, small-bowel neoplasms are often discovered when they have metastasized to distant sites or at surgery when indicated

for other diagnosis or intestinal obstruction. Small-bowel cancers are made up of adenocarcinomas (30–40%), carcinoid tumours (35–42%), lymphomas (15–20%), sarcomas (10–15%), and gastrointestinal stromal tumours (GISTs; 7–15%). Predisposing factors include inherited conditions, immunocompromise (particularly Kaposi sarcoma, adenocarcinoma and lymphoma), and Crohn's disease.

Inherited Conditions

The inherited conditions associated with small-bowel tumours include:
- Familial adenomatous polyposis (FAP), although most of the neoplasms arise in the duodenum
- Peutz–Jeghers syndrome, where intestinal polyps are identified mainly in the jejunum and marginal pigmentation around the buccal and anal mucosa. A common presentation is with intussusception.
- Gardner's syndrome, which is a rare disorder with small-bowel adenomas, neoplasms and desmoid tumours and with skeletal abnormalities.

Immunocompromise

Causes of immunocompromise predisposing to small-bowel tumours include:
- Coeliac disease in which there is gluten-sensitive enteropathy with a wide variety of other manifestations of atopy and there is an increased incidence of small-bowel neoplasms.
- Acquired immunodeficiency, such as in AIDS, which makes the patient liable to Kaposi sarcoma and lymphoma.
- Immunosuppression, such as in transplant patients, which is associated with small-bowel lymphomas.

Crohn's Disease

Crohn's disease is associated with an increased incidence of small-bowel adenocarcinoma.

Pathological Features
Benign Tumours

- Adenomas may present anywhere in the small bowel, but they are commoner in the duodenum, particularly in association with FAP.
- Lipomas are commoner in the large than in the small bowel and may cause intussusception.
- Neurofibromas can occur in isolation or as part of the general picture of neurofibromatosis, causing bleeding or obstruction.

Malignant Tumours

- Adenocarcinomas may affect any part of the small bowel, but they are commoner in the duodenum.
- Gastrointestinal stromal tumours (GIST) are intra- or extraluminal, may give rise to bleeding or obstruction

and may metastasize, particularly if they are large and have a high mitotic rate.

- Lymphomas may be small-bowel primary or part of a systemic disorder.
- Secondary or metastatic small-bowel tumours are rare but may occur with lung cancer, breast cancer, or melanoma.

Management

Tumours are usually identified and staged by CT scanning. Biopsy may be possible in proximal lesions by endoscopy. Surgical resection of the involved segment of small bowel is indicated in bowel cancer such as in adenocarcinoma and GIST. Curative surgery depends on the extent to which the surgeon can remove the entire cancer during the operation. Emergency surgery may also be needed for relief of bowel obstruction, with resection or bypass if the obstructing tumour itself cannot be removed safely. Adjuvant chemotherapy is often given after resection of adenocarcinoma and imatinib after resection of high-risk GIST. Several chemotherapy medications may have some efficacy in the treatment of small-bowel cancer; however, given how rare small-bowel cancer is, very few clinical trials have been completed showing the benefits of chemotherapy in its the treatment. For benign tumours, resection is only indicated if they are causing significant symptoms, such as obstruction or bleeding, or there is concern about possible malignant tumour formation. Lymphoma is usually treated by cytotoxic chemotherapy, although perforation or obstruction may necessitate emergency resection.

25

Common Endocrine Surgical Conditions

CHAPTER OUTLINE

Introduction

The endocrine system is distributed throughout the body and results in medical conditions in widespread locations that do not follow the anatomical demarcation of much of modern medical practice.

Conditions can be benign or malignant, and can be associated with endocrine dysfunction of hyper- or hypofunction. Some conditions are genetically linked and a fundamental knowledge of anatomy, embryology, physiology, pathology and the associations of surgical conditions is essential to manage patients.

Multidisciplinary team working is essential and involves endocrinology, endocrine surgery and anatomically based surgical specialties: e.g. thoracic, hepatobiliary, skull base, neurology, ear, nose and throat (ENT) and colorectal to name only a few, radiology and interventional radiology, nuclear medicine, radiotherapy, oncology and genetics.

THYROID

Embryology

- The thyroid is derived from a midline epithelial proliferation in the floor of the pharynx. The primitive thyroid descends from the back of the tongue in the midline to its resting place in front of the trachea. The descent can leave a remnant tract with thyroid tissue present at any point, the *thyroglossal tract*. The tract usually disappears but can persist; its origin leaves a trace at the back of the tongue represented by the *foramen caecum*.
- Thyroid tissue can persist or present anywhere along the tract:
  1. *Lingual thyroid* is tissue at the back of the tongue — as additional thyroid tissue or, rarely, the sole thyroid tissue present.

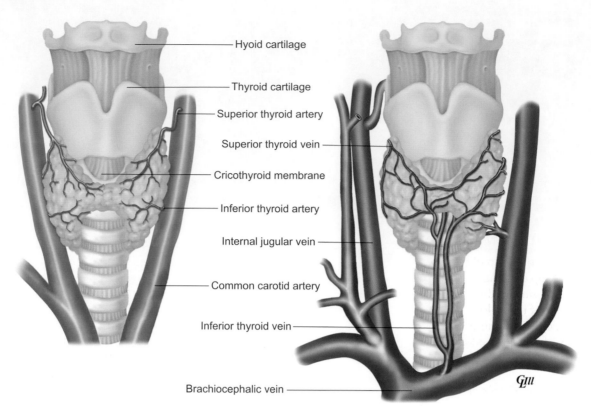

Hyoid cartilage

Thyroid cartilage

Superior thyroid artery

Superior thyroid vein

Cricothyroid membrane

Inferior thyroid artery

Internal jugular vein

Common carotid artery

Inferior thyroid vein

Brachiocephalic vein

• **Fig. 25.1** The Arterial and Venous Blood Supply of the Thyroid

2. *Thyroglossal cyst* presents in the region of the hyoid bone where the tract is adherent to the hyoid bone. The attachments to the tongue are responsible for movement on protrusion of the tongue.
3. Pyramidal lobe is a variable extension of tissue from the thyroid isthmus upward toward the hyoid.

Anatomy

• Pretracheal fascia envelops the thyroid and binds it to the trachea and is responsible for the movement of the thyroid on swallowing. The fascia fuses anteriorly with fascia that envelops the strap muscles that cover the thyroid anteriorly, principally sternothyroid and sternohyoid muscles.
• The thyroid has a rich blood supply with feeding vessels forming an anastomotic network throughout the thyroid.
• There are two main arteries (Fig. 25.1):
  1. The inferior thyroid artery which arises from the subclavian artery via the thyrocervical trunk and reaches the thyroid by passing deep to the carotid sheath and is typically found in the mid thyroid region. Terminal vessels feed the thyroid and are also the commonest supply to the parathyroid glands.
  2. The superior thyroid artery is a branch of the external carotid artery. It feeds the thyroid at its superior pole.

• There are three named veins (see Fig. 25.1):
  1. Middle thyroid veins are delicate and drain direct to the jugular. They need control and division in the early stages of thyroidectomy to enable mobilization of the thyroid.
  2. The superior and inferior thyroid poles have venous drainage with the same named veins. These veins drain to the jugular and the brachiocephalic veins.
• The *recurrent laryngeal nerve (RLN)* supplies motor and sensation to the larynx and, particularly, the muscles that control the vocal cords. Identification and preservation is crucial in thyroid surgery to prevent voice change. The RLN has a variable position but classically runs near the trachea-oesophageal groove and crosses behind, through and, rarely, in front of, the branches of the inferior thyroid artery (ITA).
• The *external branch* of the *superior laryngeal nerve* is variably found at the superior thyroid pole with the superior thyroid vessels but can be more cranial in position. Care is needed in individually controlling the superior pole vessels at surgery to avoid injury. The nerve supplies the cricothyroid muscle and its function is important in voice quality and projection such as singing.
• Upper and lower parathyroid glands are present on each side near the thyroid, although can be ectopic in location. Parathyroid glands should be preserved during thyroid surgery, where possible. Transplantation of excised or ischaemic glands to the sternocleidomastoid muscle can help preserve parathyroid function. One fully

functional parathyroid is required to avoid postoperative hypocalcaemia due to parathyroid dysfunction, which can be temporary or permanent.
- The first lymph nodes draining the thyroid are found in the fatty tissue surrounding the thyroid; the central neck compartment or level 6 is bounded laterally by the carotid sheath, superiorly by the cranial aspect of the thyroid cartilage and inferiorly by the sternal notch.
- Lateral lymph node compartment involves the carotid sheath and lateral tissue bounded by the medial border of trapezius muscle, clavicle and mastoid process – otherwise classified as levels 2, 3,4 and 5.

Microscopic

- The thyroid is made up of tightly packed follicles. A follicle is made up of a single layer of cuboidal cells forming a sphere and surrounding a lumen containing colloid. Enlargement of the colloid centre and coalescence of follicles, associated with fibrosis and scarring, occurs in the formation of a multi nodular goitre. Thyroid follicular cells and follicles are key in the production of *thyroid hormone*.
- *Parafollicular* or *C cells* are of neural crest origin and found between the follicles. They secrete *calcitonin*. Embryologically, C cells originate as the ultimobranchial body from the fourth pharyngeal pouch and descend with the upper parathyroid and infiltrate into the thyroid.

Physiology

- *Thyroid stimulating hormone* (TSH) is secreted by the anterior pituitary and stimulates the thyroid to produce thyroid hormones (T4 and T3).
- There is negative feedback between TSH and thyroid hormones. TSH is regulated by thyrotropin releasing hormone (TRH) from the hypothalamus.
- Thyroid hormones increase metabolic rate and sensitize tissues to the sympathetic nervous system.
- Calcitonin is involved with calcium metabolism but has little physiologic role in humans and does not require replacement following thyroidectomy. Its main use in clinical practice is as tumour marker in medullary thyroid cancer.

Thyroid Hormone

- Large amounts of iodine (I⁻) are required to make thyroid hormone which is actively transported into thyroid follicular cells.
- TSH binds to the TSH receptor of the thyroid. This triggers the process within the follicular cells whereby iodine is captured and added to tyrosine residues, most importantly within the protein *thyroglobulin* (TG).
- *Thyroid peroxidase* (TPO) catalyses the processes of thyroid hormone production.

- TG is a protein containing tyrosine residues produced within the thyroid follicular cells and is subsequently secreted into the follicular cell lumen.
- Mono- (MIT) and diiodotyrosine (DIT) residues within TG crosslink to form the hormones T3 and T4 under the influence of TPO.
- There is a large reservoir of thyroid hormone combined with thyroglobulin within the follicular cell lumen ready for release under TSH control. TG is recycled, and thyroid hormone is released into the circulation.

Diseases Influencing the Thyroid

- *Chronic iodine deficiency* causes thyroid hypertrophy and goitre formation
- *Pituitary adenoma with TSH production* (rare) causes thyrotoxicosis
- *Struma ovarii (ovarian dermoid tumour)* is an unusual cause of thyrotoxicosis
- *Autoimmune antibodies:* Anti-thyroperoxidase (TPO Ab) and antithyroglobulin (TG Ab) antibodies can cause thyroid atrophy and hypothyroidism, whilst TSH receptor stimulating antibody (TSHR Ab) results in thyrotoxicosis.
- *Genetic defects* e.g. mutation of *PDS* gene affects thyroid iodide transport in Pendred syndrome (association of goitre and deafness)
- *Goitrogens* are substances which interfere with pathways of thyroid hormone production.

Evaluation of Thyroid Disease

Introduction

- Patients can present with thyroid enlargement *(goitre)*, or with a clinical state of altered thyroid hormones. These conditions can coexist.
- A presenting thyroid nodule can be solitary or part of a multinodular process.
- A goitre can grow anteriorly, posteriorly, inferiorly or superiorly or have a combination of growth features.
- The growth pattern can influence symptoms, as can the disease process affecting the thyroid, e.g. firmness of thyroid tissue in thyroiditis, meaning that apparent goitre size may not correlate with symptoms.
- There may be associated conditions such as eye disease.

History
Neck Symptoms

- Dysphagia – compression of the oesophagus – sensation lump on swallowing
- Dyspnoea – compression or deviation of the trachea:
  - minimal – cough at night
  - moderate – SOB exacerbated on activity
  - severe – stridor
- Voice change – due to mass effect or involvement of RLN in cancer
- Other lumps – lymph node, thyroglossal cyst

Functional State

- Euthyroid – normal thyroid function
- Hyperthyroid – increased thyroid hormones (T4/3)
- Hypothyroid – reduced T4/3
- Thyroid hormones:
  1. Affect metabolism and
  2. Sensitize the sympathetic nervous system.
     - Apathetic thyrotoxicosis can occur in elderly patients when features of sympathetic reactivity are absent, and patients can present with depression, weight loss and slow atrial fibrillation.

Associated Features

- Family history – genetic causes
- Drugs – amiodarone, antithyroid drugs, lithium
- History of radiation exposure – geographic or medical treatment
- Contrast containing radiology
- Age
- Pregnancy

Examination

- Thyroid – movement upwards on swallowing is the clinical feature that differentiates a lump of thyroid origin from other neck lumps.
- Thyroglossal cyst – moves upwards on protrusion of the tongue.
- When examining a lump consider the following:
  - Site, size, shape, surface, surrounds, lymph nodes.

When a thyroid lump is suspected it is important to consider whether a lump is solitary or part of a multi-nodular process.

- Is there evidence of retrosternal extent? Is it possible to get below the nodule (either initially or on swallowing)?
- Is the trachea central or deviated?
- Is there evidence of lymph node involvement?

The systemic features of hypo- and hyperthyroidism are shown in Tables 25.1 and 25.2, respectively.

Investigation of Thyroid Disease

- Triple assessment in most situations, although cytology is not always necessary.
  - Thyroid function
  - Imaging
  - Cytology

Tests of Thyroid Function

- The diagnosis of thyroid disease and monitoring of thyroid treatment is simplified with the use of assays for TSH and free T4 and free T3.
- Free levels of T3 and T4 are not affected by changes in protein levels as occur in some medical conditions and pregnancy, and which affected results of earlier assays of total T4 and T3.
- A normal TSH suggests a euthyroid state.

TABLE 25.1 **Symptoms and Signs of Hypothyroidism.**

Symptoms of Hypothyroidism	Signs of Hypothyroidism
Fatigue	Hypersomnolence
Poor appetite, weight gain	Slow relaxing tendon reflexes
Memory impairment	Nerve entrapments – carpal tunnel syndrome
Intolerance of cold environment	Cool, dry and thickened skin
Depression, psychosis, coma	Peripheral and periorbital oedema
Dry skin and course dry hair	Hoarse voice
Muscle aches	Bradycardia
Menstrual disturbance	Cardiomegaly
Heart failure	

TABLE 25.2 **Symptoms and Signs of Thyroid Hyperactivity.**

Symptoms of Thyroid Hyperactivity	Signs of Thyroid Hyperactivity
Subjective – nervousness, irritability, behavioural change	Anxiety
Weight loss, in spite of a good appetite	Excessive purposeless movements
Diarrhoea	Diffuse fine tremor, best elicited in the outstretched fingers
Muscle weakness	Signs of recent weight loss – loose skin, little subcutaneous fat
Tremor	Warm and often moist peripheries with vasodilatation
Intolerance of a hot environment, preference for cold	Sinus tachycardia and systolic hypertension
Loss of libido and, in women, oligomenorrhoea	Atrial fibrillation and cardiac failure, especially in the older patient
Eye complaints (Table 25.3)	Eye signs (see Table 25.3)
	Pretibial myxedema – infiltration of the shin, present only in those with eye signs
	Proximal myopathy, particularly in the upper limbs

TABLE 25.3	Eye Features in Hyperthyroidism.	
Symptoms	**Signs**	
Poor sight for both near and distant objects	Ophthalmoplegia	
Double vision	Conjunctival oedema (chemosis)	
Grittiness in the eye	Exophthalmos	
Exophthalmos	Lid retraction	
	Lid lag	

TABLE 25.4	Classification of Thyroid USS and the Positive Predictive Value (PPV) of Malignancy.	
	Result	**PPV Malignancy**
U1	Normal thyroid	<1%
U2	Benign	<2%
U3	Indeterminate	10–15%
U4	Suspicious	30–40%
U5	Malignant	60–70%

- Free T4 and T3 can be mildly reduced in acute and chronic illness of non-thyroid origin, although the TSH remains normal.
- An elevated TSH and low T4 establishes a diagnosis of *hypothyroidism*. It should be noted that the TSH may rise before thyroid hormones reduce and suggests impending hypothyroidism.
- A suppressed TSH and elevated T4 or T3 establishes a diagnosis of *hyperthyroidism*.
- A suppressed TSH with normal T4/3 suggests subclinical or impending hyperthyroidism.
- *Thyroid antibodies*
  - Raised titres of *antithyroglobulin* (TG) antibodies (Ab) and *anti-thyroid peroxidase* (TPO) antibodies (Ab) are present in up to 30% of women over the age of 45.
  - In *Hashimoto's thyroiditis* and *Graves' disease,* they are present in up to 97%. They can be measured when there is clinical evidence of hypothyroidism to clarify cause and before considering a thyroid lobectomy to consider future risks of hypothyroidism with reduced thyroid tissue post-surgery.
  - *TSH Receptor Ab* is characteristic of *Graves' disease.* It is present in 90% of patients with very high specificity.

Imaging

1. **Ultrasound** (Table 25.4)
   - Key routine investigation of palpable and non-palpable thyroid nodules, remaining thyroid tissue and lymph nodes.
   - Nodules are stratified using ultrasound criteria for risk of malignancy.
   - Nodules that are classified benign (U2) do not require fine-needle aspiration (FNA).
   - Nodules with risk factors (U3–5) are targeted with ultrasound-guided FNA for cytological clarification.
2. **CT or MRI**
   - Used for anatomical clarification of retrosternal extent, tracheal narrowing and, in malignancy, to assess local invasion of local structures and lymph node extent.
3. **Radiographs**
   - Chest X-ray and neck X-ray may detect a goitre during evaluation of non-thyroid disease. Thoracic inlet X-ray was used to assess potential tracheal narrowing but is no longer routinely used.

4. **PET CT**
   - Increasingly, thyroid nodules are being detected during evaluation of other cancers and referred for evaluation.

Cytology

1. **Fine-needle aspiration cytology (FNAC)** (Table 25.5)
   - FNAC is a routine assessment of any thyroid nodule that is classified as U3–5 and where there is clinical concern despite a reassuring USS.
   - It can also be used for aspiration of symptomatic thyroid cysts.
   - Ultrasound guidance ensures accurate targeting. Gold standard assessment includes the presence of a cytology technician to provide an assessment of adequacy of specimen for analysis.
   - This enables repeat needle passes if required and reduces acellular yields. A preliminary cytological assessment is possible when a cytologist is present. Results are classified as Thy 1–5.
   - Subsequent management of patients depends upon the clinical context, size and symptoms of goitre and not simply the cytology result.
   - Cytology results should be reviewed in multidisciplinary meetings (MDMs) and results subjected to regular audit to ensure standardization.
2. **Core biopsy**
   - Performed in more complex situations when a larger tissue specimen is required.
   - The needle is larger and takes a core of tissue.
   - Histological examination is performed.
   - Used in large masses when FNAC has been non-diagnostic, or when histological tissue is required as in lymphoma to direct non-surgical treatment.

Radioisotope Scans

- I^{123} and Tc^{99m} scanning – used to differentiate causes of *hyperthyroidism.*
  - *Solitary toxic nodule:* hot nodule increased uptake with suppression of remaining tissue
  - *Toxic multinodular goitre (MNG):* diffuse patchy increased uptake
  - *Graves' disease*: diffuse symmetrical increased uptake
  - *Subacute thyroiditis:* absent uptake. Hyperthyroidism is due to release of preformed thyroid hormone from damage to follicles

TABLE 25.5	Classification of Thyroid FNAC, PPV of Malignancy and Management.		
		PPV Malignancy on Histology	**Management of Cytology**
Thy 1/Thy 1c	Acellular/simply cyst	~15%	Repeat FNA
Thy 2/Thy 2c	Benign/colloid cyst	<10%	Reassure
Thy 3	Indeterminate		
	Thy 3a atypical	10–30%	Repeat FNA/TL
	Thy 3f follicular lesion	30–35%	TL
Thy 4	Suspicious for malignancy	55–70%	TL/TT
Thy 5	Malignant	100%	TL/TT

FNAC, Fine-needle aspiration cytology; PPV, positive predictive value; TL, thyroid lobectomy; TT, total thyroidectomy.

- Isotope scanning can be used to assess presence of ectopic thyroid tissue – lingual thyroid, mediastinal thyroid or unusual sites of thyrotoxicosis, e.g. struma ovarii.
- The role of isotope scans to determine hot and cold nodules for assessment of cancer risk has largely been replaced by USS and FNA.

Surgical Thyroid Conditions

1. **The solitary thyroid nodule**
   - Thyroid nodules can present with a clinical lump or be detected as incidental findings on ultrasound or other imaging modalities such as MRI or PET scans.
   - Nodules are commoner in women.
   - At the age of 30 years, around 20–30% of women will have some form of thyroid nodule on an ultrasound scan and this percentage increases with age.
   - The majority of nodules are benign and the majority of patients are euthyroid.
   - It is important to evaluate nodules for cancer risk and thyroid status.
   - Risk factors:
     - Family history of malignancy
     - History of radiation exposure – particularly in childhood
   - Clinical features:
     - Clinical assessment of the thyroid does not differ from basic principles.
     - The nodule under assessment may be solitary in nature or part of a multi nodular process.
     - This may be clinically evident or based on imaging.
   - **Investigations**
     - Thyroid status
     - TSH, free T4/T3
     - Thyroid antibodies
     - Imaging and FNA – ultrasound is the key investigation
     - Nodules are characterized and stratified for risk of malignancy
     - Lymph node size and morphology is assessed

- Reporting is based on the BTA (British Thyroid Association) criteria (see Table 25.4)
- Ultrasound-directed FNA performed of thyroid nodules at increased risk of malignancy (U3–5) and any lymph nodes considered suspicious
- **Management**
  - *Benign nodules (U2 or Thy 2)* are managed according to symptoms and patient preference.
    - Smaller and asymptomatic nodules are treated conservatively.
    - Larger nodules causing compressive symptoms or cosmetic effects can be treated with thyroid lobectomy.
  - *Indeterminate nodules (Thy 3 and 4)*
    - These are treated with thyroid lobectomy to establish a histological diagnosis.
    - Any nodules subsequently shown to be malignant are typically treated with a 'completion' thyroid lobectomy of the contralateral side.
  - *Malignant nodules (Thy 5)* undergo definitive surgical treatment (see section on thyroid cancer).

2. **Non-toxic goitre**
   - A (nodular) goitre may develop from a chronic, low grade and intermittent stimulation of the thyroid.
   - Initial diffuse thyroid hyperplasia progresses through areas of focal hyperplasia, combined with necrosis, haemorrhage and scarring to the development of nodules.
   - A relative rise in TSH is thought to drive the process. Several causes are recognized which produce a relative deficiency in iodine for hormone production.
   - Frequently the cause in a given patient is unknown:
     a. Iodine deficiency – dietary deficiency still occurs in certain geographic areas e.g. Central Africa, Central Asia. Iodination of salt has reduced the incidence in many countries.
     b. Physiological demand – usually diffuse hyperplasia transiently during puberty and pregnancy
     c. Goitrogens – dietary, e.g. found in cassava and cabbage (especially when combined with iodine deficiency), medication, e.g. amiodarone, lithium

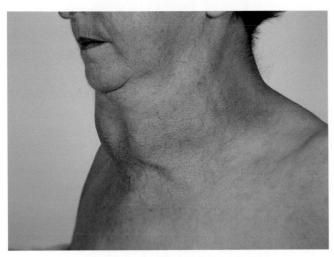

• **Fig. 25.2** Large, Diffuse, Nodular Goitre

d. Defects in thyroid hormone synthesis pathway – defects in many steps of the pathway have been identified, e.g. impaired transport of iodine (Pendred syndrome – goitre associated with deafness)

e. Thyroiditis, e.g. Hashimoto's thyroiditis – common cause of hypothyroidism, may cause a goitre

f. Benign and malignant neoplasm

3. Multinodular goitre

- Present as a painless goitre with evidence of more than one nodule clinically or on imaging.
- More common in women than men with a 5:1 ratio.
- The natural history of an MNG is enlargement over time.
- Some appear to grow fairly quickly, whereas others appear static for many years.
- Patients are usually euthyroid, although, in some elderly patients, autonomous function of nodules develops causing hyperthyroidism.
- Symptoms relate to size and compression of local structures such as trachea, oesophagus.
- Goitres that grow posterior or retrosternal can have significant size without marked visible appearance on inspection of the neck.

Examination

- The texture of an MNG is variable – can be soft or firm.
- Discrete nodules may be palpable or the goitre may be diffusely enlarged with the impression of vague nodularity (Fig. 25.2).
- The trachea may be deviated if there is asymmetric growth of the thyroid.
- Compression within the chest or thoracic inlet can cause engorgement of neck veins; elevation of the arms may induce venous compression causing redness of the face and neck – *Pemberton's sign.*
- Regional lymph nodes should be assessed as the nature of individual nodules needs to be evaluated on an individual basis to exclude malignancy.
- Thyroid status should be assessed.

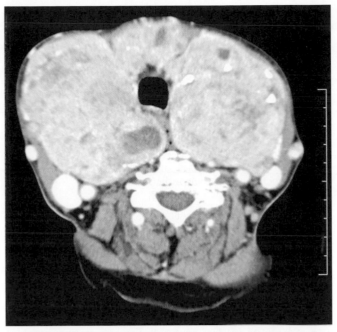

• **Fig. 25.3** Axial CT (Portal Venous Phase) of a Multi-Nodular Goitre (From https://radiopaedia.org/articles/multinodular-goitre; Case courtesy of Dr Varun Babu. Radiopaedia.org, rID: 18398)

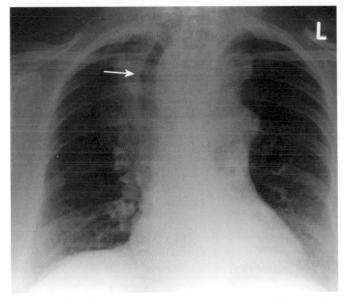

• **Fig. 25.4** Chest Radiograph Showing Tracheal Deviation to the Right from an MNG

Investigation

- It is important to exclude malignancy and assess size of thyroid and evidence of local compression in an MNG:
  - Thyroid function tests confirm a euthyroid state in most patients. Elderly patients can have biochemical hyperthyroidism without clinical features.
  - Ultrasound scan – evaluates number and malignancy risk for individual nodules, size of thyroid, and lymph nodes. USS-guided FNA of suspicious nodules should be performed.
  - CT scan – to assess trachea compression and posterior/retrosternal extent when suspected clinically or on USS (Figs 25.3 and 25.4).

TABLE 25.6	Causes of Thyrotoxicosis.	
Thyrotoxicosis (overproduction)	Graves' disease	70%
	Toxic MNG	20%
	Toxic nodule	5%
	Iodine induced	<1%
	TSH-secreting pituitary adenoma	<1%
	Neonatal thyrotoxicosis	<1%
Associated with thyroid destruction	Subacute thyroiditis	3%
	Silent thyroiditis	3%
	Amiodarone-induced (type 2)	<1%
Non-thyroidal origin	Factitious	All very rare
	Struma ovarii	
	Metastatic thyroid cancer	

Management

- **Indications for surgery:**
  - Suspicious nodule on FNA
  - Compressive symptoms or evidence tracheal narrowing
  - Significant size or growth of thyroid on surveillance
  - Retrosternal goitre
  - Cosmetic appearance
  - Hyperthyroid state
  - Patient preference
- **Surgical treatment:**
  - Total thyroidectomy is preferred for an MNG.
  - Subtotal operations aim to leave adequate thyroid function and avoid thyroxine treatment; however, leaving significant thyroid tissue frequently leads to regrowth of goitre and the subsequent need for re-operative surgery with increased risk of injury to RLN and parathyroid glands.
  - Large retrosternal component may need sternotomy to enable resection, although the majority can be removed via a neck approach.

Thyrotoxicosis

Thyrotoxicosis is the clinical syndrome that results from exposure to elevated circulating levels of thyroid hormones. Hyperthyroidism refers to thyrotoxicosis due to overproduction of thyroid hormones by follicular cells. *Graves' disease* is the commonest cause. Less frequently, thyroid destruction results in the release of stored hormone in the absence of hyperthyroidism, e.g. subacute thyroiditis. The following three conditions that affect the thyroid account for 95% of the causes of thyrotoxicosis. All causes are listed in Table 25.6.

- Graves' disease (70%)
- Toxic multinodular goitre (20%)
- Toxic solitary adenoma (5%)

Presentation

The clinical features of thyrotoxicosis (Table 25.7) depend upon the severity and duration of disease, age of patient

TABLE 25.7	Systemic Features of Thyrotoxicosis.
System	**Effects**
General	Weight loss, anxiety, irritability, heat intolerance, fatigue, insomnia, thinning hair
Skin	Warm moist palms, hyperhidrosis, itching, exacerbation of eczema
Eye	Lid lag and retraction
Central nervous system	Irritability, worsening psychiatric conditions, stupor, coma
Cardiovascular system	Tachycardia, cardiomegaly, heart failure, rhythm disturbance
Respiratory	Dyspnoea
Bone	Reduced bone mineral density
Reproduction	Gynaecomastia, infertility, light or absent menstrual periods
Metabolic	Hypercalcaemia, hyperglycaemia
Gastrointestinal	Diarrhoea, hyperdefecation
Neuromuscular	Tremor, proximal myopathy, paralysis

and specific cause, which may include extra thyroidal manifestations.

1. **Graves' disease**
   - Graves' disease (GD) is an autoimmune condition that occurs in all age groups, with peak incidence in women aged 20–40 years.
   - It affects 2% of women with a female to male ratio of 10:1.
   - It is named after the Irish physician Robert Graves.
   - In mainland Europe it is known as the Maladie de Basedow.
   - Aetiology
     - Stimulatory antibodies to the TSH receptor (TRAb) are present in the sera of 90% of patients and cause the unregulated overproduction of thyroid hormone.
     - Genetic and environmental factors are involved in the production of antibodies, although the precise mechanism has not been elucidated.
     - Antibodies to TG and TPO are also frequently present.
     - Some antibodies have a destructive effect and the balance of antibodies may explain the variable clinical course in response to treatment in patients.
     - Inflammatory cells infiltrate the thyroid with the production of cytokines.
     - There is associated hyperplasia and hypertrophy of thyroid follicles, causing goitre formation.
     - Extra thyroidal manifestations are associated with GD (Table 25.8).
     - Other autoimmune conditions are associated with GD (Box 25.1).

TABLE 25.8	Extrathyroidal Manifestations of Graves' Disease.	
Ophthalmopathy	Grittiness and periorbital oedema	
	Proptosis	
	Extra-ocular muscle involvement	
	Corneal involvement	
	Optic nerve compression	
Dermopathy	Pretibial myxedema	
Acropachy	Clubbing	
Lymphoid Hyperplasia		

> **• BOX 25.1 Autoimmune Disorders Associated with Graves' Disease**
>
> Addison's syndrome
> Chronic lymphocytic thyroiditis
> Immune-mediated thyrombocytopenia
> Myasthenia gravis
> Pernicious anaemia
> Rheumatoid arthritis
> Systemic lupus erythematosus
> Vitiligo

- The cause of ophthalmopathy
  - Eyelid retraction and lid lag can occur in all causes of thyrotoxicosis due to sensitization of the sympathetic nervous system by excess thyroid hormone.
  - Sympathetic fibres run with the third cranial nerve and innervate levator palpebrae superioris muscle.
  - Specific GD ophthalmopathy is thought to be due to an immune response to retroorbital antigens similar to the thyroid, or cross reactivity of thyroid receptor Ab to TSH receptors present on fibroblasts and adipocytes within the retroocular tissues.
  - Resulting inflammation, oedema and fibrosis affects the retroorbital tissue and ocular muscles.
  - Ophthalmopathy can be unilateral and is more common in smokers.
- Clinical features
  - The presence of thyrotoxicosis, diffuse goitre with a bruit and specific eye signs makes the diagnosis clinically evident. However, only 50% of patients have a clinically apparent goitre, while 30% have clinically evident GD ophthalmopathy.
  - The natural course of GD is variable:
    - Approximately half of patients will show remission with medical treatment,
    - However, up to half of the patients able to stop medical treatment will subsequently relapse and require further medical treatment and subsequent definitive treatment in the form of radioiodine ablation or surgical excision.
    - Half of patients will not achieve remission with medical treatment and are offered definitive treatment.
- Investigation
  - Blood tests confirm hyperthyroidism (suppressed TSH and raised T4/T3)
  - Anti TPO and TG are present in 90%, though non-diagnostic
  - TRAb are elevated in >90% of patients – sensitivity and specificity for GD are in upper 90%
  - Thyroid nodules can be present in GD and a thyroid USS is indicated in their presence.
  - Isotope scan (Tc^{99}) shows diffuse increased thyroid uptake.

2. **Toxic multinodular goitre and toxic nodule**
   - A longstanding MNG can develop autonomous functioning nodules leading to hyperthyroidism. It is the commonest cause of thyrotoxicosis in those aged over 60 years.
   - Presentation may be precipitated by iodine loading that occurs with contrast containing radiology investigations.
   - Hyperthyroidism due to a solitary thyroid nodule occurs in 5% of cases of hyperthyroidism.
   - The function of the remaining thyroid tissue is suppressed.
   - Investigation
     - Blood tests: A suppressed TSH in the presence of normal T4/3 suggests developing autonomy.
     - Imaging: In both presentations, it should be remembered to assess the thyroid as per non-hyperthyroid patients, with USS evaluation of thyroid nodules. The thyrotoxic state may not be clinically evident at presentation.
     - Thyroid scintigraphy: demonstrates a hot nodule with suppression of the remainder of the thyroid in a toxic nodule; and patchy increased uptake throughout the thyroid in a toxic MNG.
   - **Management of thyrotoxicosis**
     - A precise diagnosis is important in discussion and treatment planning with patients.
     - The aim of initial treatment is to render the patient euthyroid by controlling the production of thyroid hormone.
     - The half-life of thyroxine is 7 days, meaning thyroid control can take several weeks to be achieved.
   - Management of patients with Graves' disease
     - *Medical*: Patients with GD are typically treated with antithyroid drugs for 6 to 18 months to assess for remission. Those not undergoing remission, or who subsequently relapse, are offered definitive treatment.
     - *Definitive treatment*: removal of intrinsic thyroid hormone production with radioiodine ablation or total thyroidectomy.
     - Following definitive treatment, patients are warned they will require life-long thyroid hormone replacement.

- *Radioiodine ablation* suitable in:
  - small goitres, majority of patients
  - absent/mild ophthalmopathy
- Contraindicated in:
  - pregnancy,
  - planning pregnancy within 6 months,
  - breastfeeding,
  - severe ophthalmopathy,
  - close contacts with children post treatment.
- Surgery is treatment choice in:
  - large and symptomatic goitres
  - FNA suspicious malignancy
  - severe ophthalmopathy
  - children
  - patient preference
- Management of toxic MNG and nodule
  - Remission does not occur in toxic MNG or toxic nodule.
  - Medical: antithyroid drugs are used to control the thyroid function, followed by definitive treatment.
  - Surgery: total thyroidectomy for MNG; lobectomy for toxic nodule.
  - Radioiodine: leaves the goitre in place but destroys function. In a toxic nodule, the suppressed thyroid tissue outside the nodule does not take up the radioiodine and maintains function post therapy; however, the treated nodule remains.

Antithyroid Drugs

- Two thionamide antithyroid medications are used in the UK:
  - *Carbimazole* and
  - *Propylthiouracil* (PTU)
- These drugs interfere with the action of TPO enzyme, blocking thyroid hormone production.
- PTU is preferred in the first trimester of pregnancy as it is less likely to cross the placenta due to protein binding.

Titration regime – Carbimazole (or PTU) dosage is reduced over many months as monitored thyroid hormone levels come under control and treatment potentially stopped when TSH is normal or rising while on a low dose.

Block and replace – High-dose carbimazole maintained and thyroxine added when thyroid hormone levels fall. Treatment is maintained for approximately 6–12 months, then stopped to see if remission has occurred.

Major side effects are rare but include agranulocytosis, aplastic anaemia, hepatitis and vasculitis (with PTU) and require medication to be stopped.

Patients should be warned to seek medical advice should they develop a fever, sore throat or mouth ulceration during treatment.

β-Blockers e.g. propranolol – can be used to control sympathetic symptoms during early antithyroid treatment before thyroid control achieved.

Thyroid Cancer

- There has been an increased incidence throughout the world, largely due to the detection of small incidental cancers picked up on ultrasound scan.
- In 2015, there were 3528 new cases of thyroid cancer in the UK.
- Thyroid cancer is quite rare and makes less than 1% of the total cancer cases in the UK.
- Clinically insignificant, microscopic occult thyroid cancers are detected in 5–10% of autopsies.
- Types of thyroid cancer:
  - Differentiated thyroid cancer (DTC): papillary and follicular thyroid cancer (PTC, FTC)
  - Medullary thyroid cancer
  - Hurthle cell thyroid cancer
  - Anaplastic thyroid cancer
  - Small cell lymphoma of the thyroid (rare)
- **Differentiated thyroid cancer (DTC)** arises from the thyroid follicular cells and accounts for 95% of thyroid cancers.
  - **Predisposing factors**
    - Radiation exposure in childhood; medical treatment involving radiotherapy or living in areas exposed to nuclear fallout, e.g. Chernobyl.
    - *Genetic*
    - DTC 5–15% may be genetically linked
      - Syndromic familial adenomatous polyposis (FAP) associated with PTC
      - PTEN/Cowden syndrome associated with follicular adenoma and FTC
      - Non-syndromic familial non-medullary thyroid cancer
      - Medullary thyroid carcinoma (MTC) 25%, may be genetically linked; multiple endocrine neoplasia type 2 (MEN2), familial medullary thyroid cancer (FMTC)
  - **Pathological classification of thyroid cancer**
    - Papillary (~80%)
    - Follicular (~15%)
    - Poorly differentiated and anaplastic
    - Medullary
    - Lymphoma
    - Secondary tumours (metastases)[*]
  - Presentation
    - Clinical presentation with a neck (thyroid or lymph node) lump for evaluation. The majority of patients do not have symptoms that will differentiate a benign from malignant lump.
    - Features which are statistically associated with an increased risk for cancer are:
      - Age <20 or >60 years old
      - Hoarse voice – suspicious for involvement of *recurrent laryngeal nerve*
      - Airway symptoms – stridor

---

[*]DTC comprises PTC and FTC.

- Rapid growth
- Firm lump with fixation
- Enlarged cervical lymph nodes
- History of neck irradiation
- Family history of thyroid cancer
- Unexpected/incidental histological finding in a thyroid excised for benign reasons

Differentiated Thyroid Cancer (DTC)

Papillary Thyroid Cancer

- PTC is the commonest thyroid cancer
- Mean age of presentation is 35–45 years old
- Seventy percent occur in women
- Typically spreads via lymph nodes
- Thirty to fifty percent of tumours are multifocal
- Overall 10-year survival is 98%
- Investigations
  - A preoperative diagnosis can be made for classical PTC on FNA (Thy 5) due to distinctive cytological features
  - Patients are typically euthyroid
  - Ultrasound confirms suspicious features of nodule (U3–5) and FNA confirms diagnosis (Thy 5) or is suspicious (Thy 3/4)
  - Cytology: nuclear inclusions and grooves, papillary formations, absence of colloid
  - Histology: growth pattern is typically finger-like papillary structures with nuclear characteristics similar to cytology. Psammoma bodies present in 50%

Follicular Thyroid Cancer

- FTC has an older mean age at presentation than PTC at 40–60 years. FTC is also commoner in women (75%). FTC spreads via haematogenous route with lymph node involvement in less than 10%.
- Investigation:
  - Ultrasound show a suspicious nodule and FNA is reported as indeterminate follicular lesion (Thy 3F).
  - A definitive cytological diagnosis is not possible in local disease because differentiation between a benign follicular adenoma and a follicular cancer requires histological detail of capsular and vascular invasion. Consequently, these lesions have similar FNA appearances and are classified as Thy 3F.
  - Definitive diagnosis is made following diagnostic thyroid lobectomy for histological assessment.
  - Lesions are classified as:
    a. *Minimally invasive FTC* – capsular invasion alone without vascular invasion or with limited vascular invasion
    b. *Widely invasive FTC* – wide invasion of thyroid tissue and extra thyroidal tissue

Staging of DTC

- DTC differs from other thyroid cancers and most other tumours in its good prognosis. Disease recurrence rates are 10–30%. A small number of patients have aggressive disease that is resistant to standard treatment and are incurable.

- Consequently, the TNM staging has been adapted.
- In patients under the age of 45 years, only stages 1 and 2 are recognized. Patients with metastatic lung or bone disease are classified as stage 2 in this age group in recognition of the excellent prognosis for most patients with treatment.
- Patients aged 45 years and older are, however, classified into stages 1–4.

Management of DTC

There remains ongoing debate regarding the extent of thyroid surgery, lymph node dissection and postoperative radioiodine treatment for DTC. The principles of management of DTC are:

a. **Surgery**
  - For tumours less than 1 cm size, with no adverse features and clinical and radiological absence of lymph node disease, a thyroid lobectomy may be considered as sole treatment.
  - For patients with larger tumours and lymph node involvement, a total thyroidectomy and level 6 lymph node dissection is usually performed.
  - The main principle behind performing a total thyroidectomy is to facilitate radioiodine ablation postoperatively because the presence of normal thyroid tissue in the neck concentrates the radioiodine and makes treatment and scanning less effective and would require larger radioactivity doses.
  - When there is evidence of wider lymph node disease, a level 2–5 lymph node dissection may be required. Lymph nodes are less responsive to radioiodine treatment and are excised when involved.

b. **Radioiodine**
  - Approximately 4–6 weeks post total thyroidectomy, radioiodine ablation is performed using I^{131}.
  - DTC behaves like normal thyroid tissue and concentrates iodine.
  - Radioiodine ablation destroys microscopic residual thyroid cells and enables scanning to assess for the presence of wider disease.
  - To maximize I^{131} uptake in thyroid cells, TSH stimulation is required. This is achieved through either thyroid hormone withdrawal to increase endogenous TSH or administration of recombinant TSH to raise the TSH.
  - The objective of radioiodine treatment is to render the thyroglobulin undetectable, which is used as a surrogate for absence of thyroid tissue and hence thyroid cancer.

Surveillance

- Long-term TSH suppression is usually performed with thyroxine treatment. This reduces the potential stimulation that TSH has on any residual thyroid cancer cells.

- Thyroglobulin blood test monitoring is performed. A rise suggests recurrent disease.
- Thyroglobulin antibody is measured as it interferes with the assay leading to potentially falsely reassuring TG results.
- Periodic ultrasound is performed to assess for lymph nodes and ensure thyroid bed is clear.

Anaplastic Thyroid Cancer

- This is a rare but aggressive tumour with poor prognosis that occurs in patients over the age of 60.
- It typically presents as a rapidly growing neck mass.
- Anaplastic cancer may occur due to de-differentiation of an unrecognized DTC.
  - **Presentation**
    - Rapidly growing mass
    - Stridor
    - Fixed hard mass on examination
    - Evidence of vocal cord palsy
  - **Investigations**
    - USS-guided FNA/core biopsy distinguishes this from lymphoma, which may present in a similar manner.
    - Evidence of local structure invasion in neck and metastatic and mediastinal disease on CT is common.
  - **Treatment**
    - Surgical excision is performed when feasible but is rarely possible.
    - Frequently treatment is supportive.
    - Radioiodine is ineffective as de-differentiation means the tumour does not concentrate iodine.
    - Radiotherapy may be used.
    - Survival is frequently only several months.

Medullary Thyroid Cancer (MTC)

- Accounts for 5–10% thyroid cancers.
- It is a neuroendocrine tumour that derives from the C-cells (also known as parafollicular cells) within the thyroid.
- C-cells derive embryologically from the ultimobranchial body which are of neural crest origin.
- C-cells secrete calcitonin and are used as a tumour marker.
- MTC has a high frequency of involvement of cervical lymph nodes.
- Seventy-five percent are sporadic with a mean age 40–60 years.
  - Eighty percent are solitary
- Twenty-five percent are familial with a mean age 35 years.
  - Ninety percent are bilateral and multifocal, associated with diffuse C-cell hyperplasia, which precedes the development of cancer.

- Many are associated with other endocrine conditions: *phaeochromocytoma* and *primary hyperparathyroidism* in *multiple endocrine neoplasia (MEN) 2*.
- *MEN2A* and *2B* and *FMTC* are due to germline RET proto-oncogene mutations.
  - RET is located on chromosome 10.
  - Inheritance is autosomal dominant.
  - Risk of development of MTC increases with age in patients with MEN2, and penetrance varies with the specific codon mutation.
- **Presentation**
  - Neck or lymph node mass.
  - Phaeochromocytoma – subsequent neck exam or calcitonin screening identifies MTC.
  - Following screening of an affected family member.
  - Prophylactic surgery is offered to known family members with RET. This is performed in childhood to reduce risks of malignancy – by 5 years of age in MEN2A and earlier for MEN2B in known families.
- **Investigation**
  - Ultrasound demonstrates a suspicious thyroid nodule and lymph nodes.
  - FNA confirms the diagnosis on thyroid and or lymph node.
  - Blood calcitonin is raised.
  - Further imaging with CT and PET may be considered depending on size of tumour and level of calcitonin to assess for local and metastatic disease.
  - Any new patient with MTC should have screening tests such as plasma metanephrines and 24-hour urine metanephrines/catecholamines to exclude phaeochromocytoma before proceeding to neck surgery.
  - Genetic screening in MTC patients for familial causes and assessment of future risk of other endocrine conditions is also performed.
  - Family screening is offered when an inherited cause is identified.
- **Treatment**
  - Treatment is surgical and offers the only chance of cure in localized neck disease. Lymph nodes are frequently involved but may be very small and difficult to identify on imaging.
  - Meticulous total thyroidectomy (Box 25.2) and level 6 lymph node dissection (Box 25.3) is performed as a minimum procedure with a low threshold for bilateral level 2–5 lymph node dissection depending on clinical context. Postoperative undetectable calcitonin is the aim of surgery but may not be achieved. Prognosis depends on stage of disease but is less than DTC.

Lymphoma

- Lymphoma accounts for a small number of thyroid malignancies (3–4%). Frequently, it occurs on a background of Hashimoto's thyroiditis.

- **Thyroid lobectomy:** is removal of an entire thyroid lobe – typically includes isthmus and pyramidal tract tissue.
- **Thyroid isthmectomy:** is removal of the isthmus of the thyroid
- **Total thyroidectomy:** is removal of all thyroid tissue
- **Subtotal thyroidectomy:** surgeon leaves tissue on one side or both sides of neck with a volume large enough to avoid thyroxine treatment. Reduced risk to recurrent laryngeal nerve (RLN) and parathyroids. This is still performed in countries when thyroxine medication is not widely available but is otherwise rarely performed today. Judging quantity of thyroid tissue to maintain euthyroid state is not straightforward. Patients risk recurrent goitre in years ahead and potential re-operative surgery which increases risk of injury to RLN and parathyroids due to scar tissue. This procedure is contraindicated in the presence of malignancy.

- **Central lymph node clearance (or level 6)** – perithyroidal lymph nodes in the fatty tissue near the thyroid. The anatomical boundaries are the sternal notch inferiorly, carotid sheath laterally and the thyroid cartilage superiorly. These lymph nodes are excised in many thyroid cancer operations.
- **Lateral lymph node clearance (levels 2,3,4,5)** – lymph nodes up and down the carotid sheath and laterally placed to the medial aspect trapezius muscle. These nodes are cleared in advanced cancers.

- Diffuse B-cell lymphoma and marginal zone B-cell are the commonest types to involve the thyroid.
- It occurs more frequently in women and a mean age is >60 years.
- Lymphoma presents with rapidly enlarging mass and airway compromise and is frequently an urgent admission.
- Distinguishing the condition from anaplastic cancer is important as treatment differs and prognosis improved in lymphoma.
  - **Investigation**
    - Diagnosis may be suspected on FNA.
    - Histology is required for lymphoma typing to guide treatment so a core biopsy is the procedure of choice. Occasionally, an open surgical biopsy is required.
    - Staging is done with CT and PET scans.
  - **Management**
    - Initial treatment with high dose steroids results in a dramatic improvement in tumour size and symptoms in the acute phase.
    - Ongoing management is by haemo-oncology.
    - Treatment options include chemotherapy and radiotherapy.

Parathyroid Transplantation

- Patients require one fully functional parathyroid gland to maintain normal calcium homeostasis.
- Ischaemic or accidentally-removed parathyroid glands during thyroid surgery can be transplanted to a muscle pocket in the sternocleidomastoid muscle to increase likelihood of long-term normocalcaemia.
- Transplant function typically becomes evident 3–4 weeks post-surgery. Parathyroid glands that are left in situ can also recover post-surgery.
- Monitoring of PTH and calcium is required.

Surgical Management of Thyroid Patient

- Preoperative
  - Investigations that are specific to thyroid surgery include:
    1) *Blood tests:*
        a) Full blood count – Agranulocytosis can occur with antithyroid drugs
        b) Thyroid function tests – to ensure euthyroid state in those with thyroid dysfunction
        c) Albumin corrected calcium – parathyroid conditions can co-exist with thyroid disease and can be dealt with at the same time provided this has been considered
    2) *Direct laryngoscopy* – to inspection vocal cords and to assess function prior to surgery.
- Informed consent should cover:
  - **Thyroxine replacement** for life in those undergoing a total thyroidectomy and increased risk of requiring thyroxine following thyroid lobectomy in those with positive autoantibodies
  - **Temporary and permanent requirement for calcium supplementation** in total thyroidectomy – relative risk is increased in cancer operations and GD due to associated lymph node excision in cancer and 'hungry bones' in GD.
  - Calcium (ionized or albumin corrected) and PTH levels are checked post-surgery. An initial low PTH suggests calcium levels may fall in the postoperative period even though initial calcium levels seem satisfactory (Box 25.4).

Management of Complications:

- **Hypocalcaemia:**
  - Patients are usually started on regular oral calcium supplements following total thyroidectomy, e.g. 1.5 g calcium carbonate two to three times daily.
  - Oral calcium supplements are rapidly absorbed and should be given while waiting for blood results in symptomatic patients.
  - Cholecalciferol (vitamin D_3) or one-alphacalcidol (1-hydroxycholecalciferol) are vitamin D supplements/analogues that have a powerful effect in raising calcium levels. One-alphacalcidol is added when

• **BOX 25.4** Symptoms and Signs of Hypocalcaemia

Symptoms of hypocalcaemia

- Pins and needles sensation or numbness in the fingers/feet and perioral area
- Carpopedal spasm (in cases of very low calcium)

Signs of hypocalcaemia

- Chvostek's sign – twitching of the facial muscles on tapping over the facial nerve in the pre-auricular area
- Trousseau's sign – carpopedal spasm on insufflation of a blood pressure cuff above the systolic pressure for 3 minutes

- Sit the patient up
- Administer oxygen
- Call for senior surgical and anaesthetic help
- Alert theatres and organize transfer of patient if stable
- If patient requires intubation on the ward and if this cannot be achieved, the wound may need opening:
  - Rapidly clean skin with chlorhexidine/alcohol-based prep.
  - Open wound: for skin use clip removers or stitch cutter if subcuticular sutures or glue used.
- Platysma stitches will need to be cut to fully open the skin flap.
- Sternohyoid muscle sutures closing the strap muscles over the trachea may also be cut to release clot from deeper in the neck.
  - Further neck exploration is performed by senior surgeon in theatre.

calcium is less than 2 mmol/L or symptoms persist despite regular oral calcium supplements. The dosage is adjusted according to response of blood calcium level.

- Intravenous calcium gluconate raises calcium rapidly and is prescribed in symptomatic patients when calcium is less than 1.9 mmol/L or when carpopedal spasm is present. Repeated administration may be necessary. Oral supplements should also be commenced with one-alphacalcidol and calcium as intravenous calcium raising effects will be temporary.

- **Voice change:**
  - Injury to the recurrent laryngeal nerve can result in a hoarse or weak voice, whilst injury to the external branch of the superior laryngeal nerve results in an underpowered projection of voice and inability to hit higher notes when singing.
  - A temporary praxia is reported in 3–10% but recovers after 3–4 months in the majority. Incidence of permanent palsy should be not more than 1–2%.
  - Bilateral RLN injury is rare. It can result in adduction of the vocal cords with resultant stridor and airway obstruction that requires tracheostomy.

- **Bleeding/haematoma:**
  - Incidence is rare (1–2%) and is highest in the first few hours following surgery and then risk declines during the 12 hours post-surgery.
  - Mass effect in a constricted space can occur but, importantly, blood is an irritant and causes secondary laryngeal oedema which contributes to airway obstruction.
  - The combined effects can necessitate urgent intubation and surgery to evacuate the clot and arrest the bleeding.
  - In a small number of cases when the anaesthetist has difficulty in intubation, the wound may need to be opened on the ward to evacuate clot and facilitate views of the airway.
  - Thyroid patients require close observation following surgery for the development of neck haematoma,

which can develop rapidly, or more gradually over an hour or two. Early senior review is required if there is concern and most crisis situations can be avoided with early recognition.

- Postoperative haematoma formation can pose a threat to the airway and is an emergency (Box 25.5).

- **Thyroid storm:**
  - This is a rare but potentially life-threatening situation caused by an acute exacerbation of thyrotoxicosis with marked hypermetabolism and adrenergic response.
  - Adequate preoperative thyroid function control in thyrotoxic surgical patients makes this very unlikely following surgery.
  - It can occur in thyrotoxic patients following parturition or with a severe illness, e.g. uncontrolled diabetes or severe infection. Patients are managed in an intensive care environment.
  - Features include: hyperpyrexia, tachycardia, atrial fibrillation, heart failure, agitation, confusion, shock and coma.
  - Management focuses on reducing thyroid hormone secretion with antithyroid drugs, providing supportive treatment (e.g. external cooling, β-blockers, steroids, i.v. fluids) and treating underlying causes, e.g. diabetes and infection.

Thyroiditis

Thyroiditis describes a mixed group of disorders that result in inflammation of the thyroid (Table 25.9).

- **Infective thyroiditis**

TABLE 25.9	Classification of Thyroiditis.

Infections
- Bacterial, fungal, parasitic

Subacute thyroiditis
Autoimmune thyroiditis
Hashimoto's thyroiditis
Lymphocytic thyroiditis
Postpartum thyroiditis
Thyroiditis associated with other disorders
GD
Focal thyroiditis in PTC
Radiation thyroiditis
Miscellaneous
Sarcoidosis
Drug associated (amiodarone, lithium)
Amyloidosis
Riedel's thyroiditis

- A rare condition that presents with pain and tenderness over the thyroid and an elevated temperature. Gram-positive streptococcal and staphylococcal bacteria are the commonest agents that spread to the thyroid via the blood.
- Investigation and management:
  - WCC and inflammatory markers may be raised
  - Ultrasound with guided-FNA for microbiology culture
  - Blood cultures
  - Antibiotic therapy is usually curative. Thyroid lobectomy may be required in recurrent cases
- **Subacute thyroiditis (De Quervain's thyroiditis)**
- A painful thyroid inflammation causing thyrotoxicosis from the release of stored thyroid hormone. On examination, the thyroid is firm, moderately enlarged and tender.
- The thyrotoxicosis is self-limiting and resolves over 2 to 3 months.
- It is commoner in women.
- The trigger is thought to be a viral infection and some patients have symptoms of a sore throat and muscle aches.
- Sweats and weight loss can result from thyrotoxicosis.
- Investigations and management:
  - Thyroid antibodies are raised
  - ESR and CRP are raised
  - TSH is suppressed, T4 and T3 are raised or high normal
  - Isotope scan shows absent uptake in the thyroid
- Treatment is directed at symptom control with anti-inflammatory medications and patient reassurance.
  - β-Blockers for thyrotoxic-related symptoms may be necessary.
  - Corticosteroids are used in cases with severe local inflammatory neck symptoms.
  - Transient hypothyroidism may occur in the recovery phase.

- **Hashimoto's thyroiditis**
- This is an autoimmune thyroiditis with associated lymphocytic infiltration of the thyroid. The precise nature and aetiology have not been fully elucidated. Thyroid antibodies (TPO and TG) are usually demonstrable.
- Clinical presentation is variable and ranges from asymptomatic to pressure symptoms with neck discomfort and a sensation of a neck lump out of proportion to goitre size.
- Most patients are euthyroid, although hypothyroidism is a common finding, may develop over time and requires monitoring.
- Rarely, patients can present with thyrotoxicosis (hashitoxicosis).
- On examination, an atrophic, firm, slightly nodular thyroid is a common finding.
- Treatment is with thyroxine replacement when TSH rises. Symptom control with anti-inflammatory agents may be needed.
- Surgery does not have a major role but may be considered for patients with intractable neck symptoms.
- **Riedel's thyroiditis**
- Very rare chronic inflammatory condition with dense fibrous tissue replacing thyroid tissue and invading local surrounding structures. It can be part of a systemic disorder of multifocal fibrosclerosis which features retroperitoneal and mediastinal fibrosis, and sclerosis cholangitis.
- Clinical findings are of a rock hard, painless goitre, with associated hoarse voice secondary to RLN involvement. Tracheal and oesophageal compression can occur.
- Differentiation from cancer is important.
- Core biopsy or open biopsy may be required due to the extensive fibrosis.
- Surgical decompression or tracheostomy may be required. Total thyroidectomy is rarely possible. Corticosteroids may benefit and tamoxifen is also used for progressive fibrosis.
- Thyroxine is required when TSH starts to rise.

PARATHYROID

Embryology and Anatomy

There are usually four parathyroid glands, upper and lower on each side of the neck. Macroscopically, they are yellow brown in colour. Normal glands weigh <60 μg each and are approximately the size of a small grain of rice or lentil.

Superior parathyroids derive from the fourth pharyngeal pouch and descend with the ultimobranchial body to the mid portion of the thyroid. They are classically described as being located within a 1 cm radius of the junction of the ITA and RLN, although this is variable

Inferior parathyroids derive from the third pharyngeal pouch and descend with the thymus to the lower pole of thyroid and below in the thyrothymic tract.

Embryological descent can be arrested or continue anywhere along the pathway of descent, resulting in ectopic parathyroid locations within the neck, carotid sheath, thyroid or mediastinum.

Cadaveric studies have shown the presence of a true supernumerary parathyroid in less than 5% of cases and additional microscopic 'rests' of parathyroid tissue in the thyrothymic tract in around 7%. These additional rests of tissue are important in secondary hyperparathyroidism (HPT) and MEN1 as potential sites of parathyroid tissue growth.

The terminal branches of the ITA are the usual blood supply to the parathyroid glands, although supply can be taken from nearby vessels in ectopic locations.

Histology

Parathyroid glands have a delicate capsule surrounding small epithelial cells which are arranged in acini. There is intervening stromal fat between cells. The amount of fat increases with age.

There are two types of secretory cells, as follows.

Chief Cells

These cells secrete PTH. They are small cells with eosinophilic staining and prominent nucleus.

Oxyphil Cells

These are acidophilic staining cells with uncertain function. Less numerous but larger than chief cells, they contain many mitochondria. Numbers increase with age and may form nodules within the parathyroid gland.

Physiology

Ninety-nine percent of calcium is stored in the skeleton. Calcium in the blood exists as albumen bound (50%) and ionized. Ionized calcium is involved in many physiologic functions including muscle contraction, nerve transmission and blood coagulation.

Calcium levels are tightly controlled with normal range albumen corrected levels 2.2–2.55 mmol/L.

Control of calcium levels involves PTH, vitamin D and calcitonin, although the presence of calcitonin is not essential for life. Regulation of calcium metabolism involves the GI tract, kidneys and skeleton.

Parathyroid Hormone

PTH is an 84-amino acid (aa) peptide produced as pre pro form which is cleaved to make active PTH. The first 34 aa are required for activation of PTH receptors. The half-life of PTH is 2–4 minutes. Parathyroid cells detect small changes in calcium levels via the calcium sensing receptor (CaSR).

In normal physiology, there is an inverse relationship between calcium levels and PTH secretion:

With a raised calcium, PTH is low, whilst with a low calcium, PTH is raised in an attempt to normalize calcium levels.

PTH raises calcium via three mechanisms:
- Actions on bone – increased osteoclast activity and osteoblasts
- Actions on kidney – increased active renal tubular absorption of calcium ions in DCT (up to 99% with normal renal function) and inhibiting phosphate reabsorption in the PCT
- Promotes absorption calcium from small intestine (particularly the duodenum and jejunum) by stimulating renal production of active vitamin D (1,25 DHCC)

Vitamin D

Only a small number of foods naturally contain vitamin D, including fatty fish and egg yolks, whilst cereals and milk are fortified with vitamins. The major source of vitamin D is via the action of UV light on the skin from the precursor 7 dehydrocholesterol. Vitamin D is concentrated in the liver where it is hydroxylated to 25 hydroxycholecalciferol (DHC). Further hydroxylation in the kidney stimulated by PTH produces 1,25 dihydroxycholecalciferol (DHCC) and 24 DHCC (less active form) (Fig. 25.5 (metabolism vitamin D)).

Calcitonin

Secreted by the C-cells of the thyroid. calcitonin inhibits osteoclast bone resorption and renal resorption of calcium and phosphate. Raised calcitonin in advanced MTC and

---

Differential Diagnosis of Hypercalcaemia

Primary HPT and cancer are the most frequent causes of hypercalcaemia.
- Endocrine
  - Primary HPT
  - Tertiary HPT
  - Thyrotoxicosis
  - Phaeochromocytoma
- Malignancy
  - Secondary spread – bronchus, breast, thyroid, prostate, kidney
  - Rare tumours, e.g. bronchus secreting PTH related peptide
  - Multiple myeloma
  - Lymphoma
- Infection
  - TB
- Other
  - Sarcoid
  - Familial hypocalciuric hypercalcemia (FHH)
- Drugs
  - Vitamin D/calcium tablets
  - Lithium
  - Thiazide diuretic

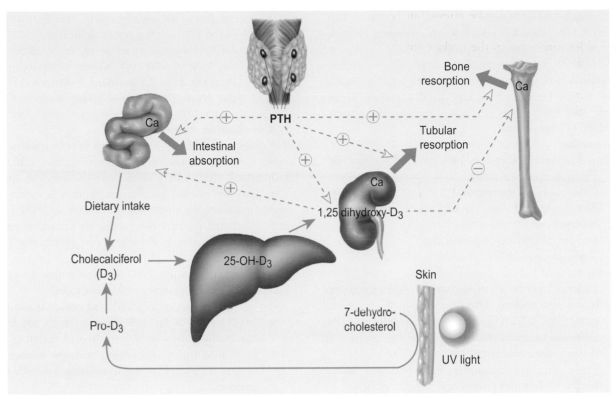

• **Fig. 25.5** Metabolism of vitamin D.

total thyroidectomy result in no clinically significant alteration of calcium or phosphate homeostasis. Calcitonin is
used as a tumour marker in MTC.

Hyperparathyroidism

Primary

- Autonomous PTH production from parathyroid
  gland(s).
- There is loss of negative feedback and loss of the normal
  relationship of PTH and calcium.
- Calcium is raised and PTH is inappropriately high.
- In normocalcaemic HPT, there is a high normal calcium
  with a high normal (inappropriate) PTH.

Secondary

- Renal failure induces low calcium and raised phosphate,
  which cause a secondary rise in PTH, as an initial appropriate response.
- Raised PTH can become uncontrolled and have detrimental effects.
- Medical treatment may control the PTH rise but, in a
  small number of dialysis patients, this may require surgical control.
- Vitamin D deficiency through lack of sunlight, intake or
  GI malabsorption can also cause secondary rise in PTH.
- Calcium is low in renal failure and PTH is very high.

Tertiary

- Autonomous uncontrolled PTH production that occurs
  following the correction of a secondary cause, e.g. renal
  transplant.
- Calcium becomes raised and PTH remains high.

Primary Hyperparathyroidism (PHPT)

- PHPT occurs in all ages but is commoner in women and
  incidence increases with age, with a peak incidence over
  60 years age.
- **Aetiology and genetics**
  - A solitary parathyroid adenoma is the commonest
    cause.
  - Intraoperative PTH testing has enabled surgeons to
    assess functionality of enlarged glands.
  - Traditionally, it was thought 15% of patients had
    multi-gland hyperplasia. This figure has been reduced
    to 5–10% with the advent of functional testing.
  - Solitary adenoma/hyperplasia 90–95%.
  - Double adenoma 2–3%.
  - Multi-gland hyperplasia 5–10%.
  - Parathyroid carcinoma 1%.
  - The molecular and genetic events leading to parathy-
    roid adenoma formation are complex and still being
    elucidated. Most parathyroid adenomas are thought
    to be monoclonal, whereas diffuse hyperplasia is
    polyclonal.

- Genes identified include:
  - *PRAD1* (Parathyroid adenoma oncogene 1)
  - *MEN1* gene (encodes menin)
  - *HRPT2* (encodes parafibromin)
- Parathyroid carcinoma is rare – neck irradiation may be a risk factor. Hereditary predisposition is very rare and includes hyperparathyroidism-jaw tumour (HPT-JT) syndrome.
- **Presentation**
  - Raised serum calcium may be identified because of:
    - Evaluation of symptoms
    - Classical HPT symptoms
    - Blood testing in renal stone, pancreatitis, osteoporosis
    - Incidental finding on blood test
    - Screening in MEN1
  - Symptoms of PHPT
    - Patients may be asymptomatic with an incidental blood test finding. Direct questioning may reveal symptoms which may be attributable to HPT; however, many of these symptoms are common in the population at large.
    - Symptoms are classically described as 'Stones, bones, abdominal groans and psychic moans'.
    - Fatigue, lack of general well-being, lack of concentration, emotional lability, depression and aches in the joints are common symptoms.
    - Abdominal pain with constipation or renal stones and, rarely, pancreatitis can occur.
    - Extreme hypercalcaemia can cause confusion, coma and cardiac arrest.
- **Examination**
  - There are no specific examination findings.
  - Neck examination rarely reveals a palpable parathyroid.
  - A palpable lump is most likely a coincidental thyroid pathology but requires evaluation with USS.
- **Diagnosis and investigation**
  - The following are required to ensure a biochemical diagnosis:
    - (a) Blood tests
      - Ionized calcium or albumin adjusted calcium are raised.
      - The presence of an inappropriate high PTH excludes non-parathyroid causes.
      - Replete vitamin D (low levels can cause a secondary rise in PTH).
      - Normal renal function.
    - (b) Urine tests
      - Raised calcium excretion is common.
      - An adequate calcium excretion in urine on 24-hour collection is used to exclude FHH which does not benefit from surgery.
      - FHH is caused by inactivating mutations to the CaSR resulting in raised calcium and raised PTH with very low urinary calcium excretion. Genetic testing is performed when calcium/creatinine ratio <0.02.
  - Assessment of organs affected in PHPT:
    - (a) Renal USS – renal tract calcification
    - (b) DEXA bone scan to assess bone mineral density (BMD) – WHO criteria for osteoporosis are BMD that lies 2.5 standard deviations (SD) below the average value of a young woman (T score <–2.5SD)
- **Localization studies:**
  The diagnosis of PHPT is based on a firm biochemical diagnosis. Once a decision has been made to proceed to surgery, localization studies help determine the surgical approach. The rationale behind localization studies is based on the high frequency of single gland disease in PHPT which makes targeted parathyroidectomy an attractive option to limit neck dissection. In the absence of parathyroid localization, a bilateral neck exploration (BNE) to inspect all four glands is usually undertaken. An experienced surgeon will identify the culprit glands in >95% of cases.
    - (a) ^{99m}Tc sestamibi (MIBI) radionuclide scanning
    - MIBI uptake is dependent on the mitochondria present in the pathological parathyroid. MIBI is sequestered into the mitochondria and low mitochondrial counts may explain negative images in 30–40% of patients.
    - MIBI can be used in isolation or combined with a technetium isotope scan of the thyroid in which the thyroid images are subtracted from the MIBI images.
    - Combination of MIBI with single-photon emission CT (SPECT) may enhance anatomical detail.
    - (b) Neck ultrasound scan
    - Enlarged parathyroid glands may be visible on USS but is operator dependent.
    - Imaging in re-operative cases for persistent and recurrent disease
    - Recurrent and persistent disease cases can be complex and it is important to reconfirm the biochemical diagnosis. Imaging to focus surgery and reduce surgical risks of injury to the RLN and remaining normal parathyroids is important.
  Additional options include:
    - (c) PET
    - (d) 4D CT
    - (e) MRI
    - (f) Neck venous sampling
  - Peripheral samples are compared to neck samples from specific veins to identify a gradient of PTH and localize hyperfunctioning parathyroid tissue in re-operative cases.
- *Indications for surgery include:*
  - Symptoms suggestive of PHPT
  - Age <50 years irrespective of symptoms
  - Calcium >2.75 mmol/L
  - Evidence of osteoporosis
  - Renal tract calcification
  - High urine calcium excretion (>10 mmol/24)
  - Reduced creatine clearance (>30%)
  - Patient choice

- *Management of hypercalcaemia*
  - The majority of patients with hypercalcaemia related to PHPT are satisfactorily managed on an outpatient basis with advice to stay well hydrated.
  - Symptomatic patients with calcium >3.5 mmol/L may require hospital admission for i.v. fluids for rehydration.
  - Bisphosphonate administration is rarely required in cases where calcium does not fall with fluid administration.
  - Cinacalcet is a calcimimetic drug that enhances sensitivity of the calcium sensing receptor (CaSR) resulting in a decrease in PTH secretion. Its main therapeutic use is in complex dialysis patients with SHPT. It is used in complex cases of PHPT with severe hypercalcaemia.
  - The definitive treatment of PHPT is surgical and is offered to patients fit for surgery.
- **Surgery in PHPT**
  - The aim of parathyroidectomy is to remove hyper-functioning parathyroid tissue.
  - Patients should be warned of the small (1–2%) risk of persistent HPT in the event of multi-gland or ectopically placed parathyroid tissue.
  - Risks to the RLN are similar to those in thyroid surgery (1%).
  - Risks of hypoparathyroidism and hypocalcaemia are very low in first-time surgery. Risks are increased in re-operative cases where the neck is scarred and parathyroid tissue has already been excised.
  - Bleeding can rarely occur following parathyroid surgery with risks of airway compromise and management as in thyroid surgery.
  - Surgical strategies are:
    - Targeted surgery on an image-detected lesion
    - Unilateral exploration to identify pathologic and normal parathyroid on one side
    - BNE with inspection of four parathyroid glands and excision of pathologic gland(s)
    - *Subtotal parathyroidectomy* is the identification of all four parathyroids with the preservation of a well-vascularized remnant of parathyroid tissue the size of a normal parathyroid and excision of remaining tissue and thymus. This is reserved for patients with four-gland disease, e.g. MEN1.
  - Intraoperative PTH monitoring (IOPTH) can be used to confirm adequate excision of overactive parathyroid tissue during surgery and reduce the risk of operative failure in patients with multi-gland disease.
    - IOPTH provides results within 15 minutes that can guide surgery in the operating room.
    - Blood is taken post anaesthetic intubation and immediately pre-excision of pathologic parathyroid tissue.
    - The highest of these results sets the maximum result from which a drop of a minimum 50% is expected following successful excision.
    - Blood is drawn 5- and 10-minutes post parathyroid excision. Failure to achieve a fall in PTH suggests hyper-functioning parathyroid tissue remains and further neck exploration is required.
- Postoperatively
  - Day surgery is suitable in selected patients.
  - Symptoms of hypocalcaemia can occur due to a true hypocalcaemia from parathyroid dysfunction, 'hungry bones', or as a short term readjustment phenomena to the relative drop of calcium into the normal range.
  - PTH and calcium levels are checked postoperatively.
  - Calcium may be orally administered for several days postoperatively. In patients undergoing subtotal parathyroidectomy or re-operative surgery, calcium and Vitamin D supplementation may be required as in total thyroidectomy.

Parathyroid Carcinoma

- It is rare and affects <1% of patients with PHPT.
- It affects the sexes equally.
- Prior neck irradiation is a risk factor.
- It occurs in 15% of patients with HPT-JT syndrome.
- It is more likely to be associated with severe manifestations of HPT, although carcinoma may be an unexpected intraoperative finding due to evidence of local invasion of surrounding structures.
- Very high preoperative calcium and PTH and a palpable neck lump give rise to preoperative suspicion, although the majority of lesions in this context will be benign.
- **Investigation**
  - When suspected clinically, CT of neck and chest is useful to assess for local structure invasion and chest metastases.
- **Treatment**
  - Surgery involves excision of the parathyroid with the thyroid lobe and surrounding (level 6) lymph node.

Secondary Hyperparathyroidism (SHPT)

- *Aetiology*
  - Most important cause is chronic renal failure with dialysis
  - Chronic malabsorption of calcium
  - Vitamin D deficiency
  - Long-term lithium therapy
  - Hypermagnesaemia

Chronic Renal Failure

- Renal failure and reduced GFR/dialysis results in a strong drive to parathyroid hyper-function secondary to:
  - Retention of fixed acid and acidosis
  - Reduced filtered phosphate with resulting hyperphosphataemia
    - Raised phosphate stimulates PTH secretion
    - Calcium-phosphate binding lowers serum calcium
  - Reduced one-alpha hydroxylase activity

- Low vitamin D with reduced absorption of calcium from GI tract

Signs and Symptoms of SHPT

- Pruritus (>50% on haemodialysis)
- Vascular calcification:
  - Reduced arterial vessel compliance leads to hypertension and cardiac complications
- Soft tissue calcification
  - Eye, lung, heart, joints
- Skin calcification
  - Calciphylaxis is due to small vessel and skin calcification causing skin necrosis on hands and lower limbs
- Bone
  - Osteoporosis and fracture resulting from high bone turnover
  - Adynamic bone disease from low bone turnover
  - Osteitis fibrosa cystica (rare)
- Medical treatment aims to reduce PTH by reducing the stimulating effects:
  - Reduce phosphate
    - reduce intake with low protein diet
    - phosphate binding agents
    - dialysis
  - Treat vitamin D deficiency
    - calcitriol and alphacalcidol
  - Calcimimetic agents
    - cinacalcet
- Surgery
- Medical treatment controls PTH levels in the majority of patients but when PTH levels are uncontrolled (>800) or when there are complications of SHPT, surgery may be required. Surgical options are aimed at reducing PTH while maintaining some PTH for bone metabolism in both the short- and longer-term, as the underlying cause persists unless renal transplantation occurs. Risks of recurrent hyperparathyroidism are increased with lesser forms of parathyroid surgery.:
  - Subtotal parathyroidectomy with cervical thymectomy
  - Total parathyroidectomy with or without parathyroid transplantation to muscle in the forearm.

ADRENAL GLANDS

Embryology and Anatomy

The adrenal glands are retroperitoneal organs located at the superior medial aspect of the upper pole of each kidney. Each gland is approximately 5 cm in length, 3 cm wide and has a 1-cm thickness and is made up of an outer cortex and inner medulla. The right adrenal is triangular in shape, whilst the left adrenal is crescent shaped.

From the fifth week of gestation, mesothelial cell proliferations develop between the urogenital ridge and root of the dorsal mesogastrium, forming the primitive adrenal cortex. Ectodermal chromaffin-staining neural crest cells, which are part of the sympathetic nervous system, invade the medial aspect of the developing cortex forming the medulla. Chromaffin cells are widespread in the fetus but subsequently regress, except in the medulla. Persistence of these cells can be responsible for the presence of ectopic adrenal tissue in the adult in the presence of elevated ACTH levels. After birth, the fetal cortex regresses, with the outer layer persisting as the reticularis. The adult structure of the cortex arises around puberty.

The cortex is divided into three distinct zones with predominant secretion:

- outer glomerulosa mineralocorticoid, largely independent of ACTH
- middle fasciculata glucocorticoid, ACTH-dependent
- inner reticularis androgens

There are three adrenal arteries arising from aorta, renal and phrenic arteries.

The main venous drainage is via a solitary adrenal vein which drains directly to the IVC on the right and renal vein on the left.

Physiology

Cortex

- The adrenal cortex is a component of the hypothalamic-pituitary-adrenal (HPA) axis, which regulates the production of glucocorticoids by the adrenal.
- The common precursor of steroid hormones is cholesterol.
- Cholesterol is converted by CYP11A1 to pregnenolone (a C-21 steroid), which is the precursor for all steroid hormones.
- See Fig. 25.6 (Major Steroid Pathways).
- Hormone products are classified into five groups based on the receptor to which they bind:
  1. *Glucocorticoids* i.e. cortisol
  2. *Mineralocorticoid* i.e. aldosterone
  3. *Androgens* i.e. testosterone
  4. *Oestrogens*
  5. *Progesterones*
- HPA axis:
  - Glucocorticoids are secreted with diurnal variation.
  - There is an early morning peak at around 6 AM and late evening/overnight trough.
  - Stress causes an increase in glucocorticoid level of 5–10-fold.
- Actions of glucocorticoids:
  - Glucocorticoid receptors (GR) are present in all cells and regulate genes involved in metabolism and immune response.
  - Glucocorticoids are important in body fluid homeostasis and fetal development (e.g. surfactant production).
  - There are many different actions throughout the body:
    - Anti-inflammatory effects: up-regulation of anti-inflammatory proteins and down regulation of pro-inflammatory proteins.

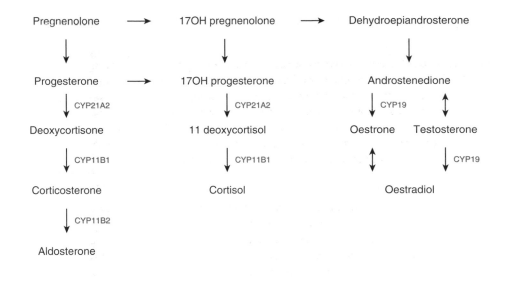

• **Fig. 25.6** Metabolism of vitamin D.

• Metabolic effects: stimulates gluconeogenesis in the liver, proteolysis and lipolysis for gluconeogenesis. Insulin resistance and hyperinsulinaemia.
• Side effects of excess glucocorticoids are seen in Cushing's syndrome (see later).
• Evaluation of an adrenal lesion
  • Presentation
    • Symptoms of hyper-function
    • Incidental finding on CT or other imaging (MRI, USS)
    • Follow-up of a malignancy
  • In patients without a known history of a malignancy, the vast majority of adrenal lesions are benign, and, in patients with a history of malignancy, metastasis is present in nearly 50%.
  • Dedicated **Adrenal CT** is performed for characterization. Both pre- and post-contrast characteristics are assessed. CT features require expert assessment in an MDM.
    • Features of a benign lesion include:
      • **Non-contrast images:** Well circumscribed homogeneous lesion with Hounsfield units (HU) <10 suggests a lipid rich adenoma. When HU >10, contrast images with washout calculation may help characterize the lesion as benign.
      • **Contrast images:** early scan at 80 seconds and a delayed attenuation scan after 10 minutes demonstrating contrast washout >50% suggests a lipid poor adenoma.
  • Features of malignancy include:
  • Irregular margin

• Heterogeneous enhancement
• HU >30 on non-contrast scan or low washout values
  • **MRI:** chemical shift images can be used to assess the nature of adrenal lesions.
  • **18F FDG PET scan:** combined with CT increases the sensitivity, specificity and PPV of malignancy and is used in selected cases and, particularly, oncology patients.
• Hormonal Assessment (see individual sections later)
  • Screen for Conn's syndrome
  • Screen for Cushing's syndrome
  • Screen for phaeochromocytoma
  • Urinary steroid profile may be indicated if malignancy considered
• Non-functioning lesions with benign features do not require treatment. Follow up imaging to ensure no growth or change at 6 months may be indicated.
• Functioning tumours are recommended for surgical excision.
  • Patients with Cushing's syndrome and pheochromocytoma will typically require treatment of these conditions before undertaking interventions for other conditions.

Adrenal Cortex

Cushing's

Harvey Cushing defined pituitary driven glucocorticoid excess in 1932. Today, glucocorticoid excess is known as Cushing's syndrome, while the pituitary cause is known as Cushing's disease. Cushing's syndrome is a rare disorder, and is classified as either *ACTH dependent* (80%) or *ACTH independent disease* (20%). Pituitary tumours and ACTH independent disease are more common in women aged 20–40, whereas ectopic ACTH occurs in a slightly older age group (30–50 years) and is more common in men.

- **Causes of Cushing's syndrome**
  (1) ACTH dependent
  - Pituitary (70%)
  - Ectopic ACTH (10%)
  - Lung (Small cell lung constitute majority ~50%), carcinoid, MTC, pancreas, thymus, phaeochromocytoma
  (2) ACTH independent
  - Adrenal adenoma (10%)
  - Adrenocortical cancer (10%)
  - Bilateral macronodular hyperplasia (rare)
  - Medication – excess steroid intake (rare)
- **Diagnosis**
  - Clinical suspicion is required to make an early diagnosis.
  - Onset of signs can be insidious and close contacts to patients and patients themselves may not notice changes for many months or even years in rare instances.
  - Symptoms and signs include:
    - Central obesity
    - Moon/round face
    - Buffalo hump
    - Thin skin and easy bruising
    - Poor wound healing
    - Muscle wasting and proximal weakness
    - Purple striae
    - Hirsutism
    - Depression
    - Menstrual irregularity
    - Hypertension
    - Osteoporosis – inhibition osteoblasts and bone formation, reduced GI absorption of calcium
    - Diabetes/impaired glucose tolerance
- **Screening tests**
  - 24-hour collection for urinary free cortisol is elevated.
  - Overnight low dose dexamethasone suppression test (ODS) does not suppress cortisol.
  - There is loss of diurnal rhythm of cortisol secretion and basal cortisol (plasma or salivary) may be raised
  - ACTH is raised in pituitary Cushing's syndrome and undetectable in ACTH independent causes.
- **Localizing tests**
  1. ACTH dependent:
     - Pituitary source of ACTH tends to have a more indolent course than causes of ectopic ACTH, which can be rapidly progressive in nature.
     - Sources of ectopic ACTH may be due to very small tumours which can be difficult to localize.
     - **High dose dexamethasone suppression testing** – there is partial sensitivity to feedback in pituitary disease and this has been used to distinguish pituitary from an ectopic ACTH cause.

- **MRI** pre- and post-gadolinium enhancement for pituitary adenomas.
- **Bilateral inferior petrosal sinus sampling** pre- and post-CRH stimulation confirms a pituitary source.
- **Chest/abdominal CT** for sources of ectopic ACTH.

Octreotide scanning may be helpful in identifying small lung carcinoids not visualized on other techniques as these tumours may express somatostatin receptors.

  2. ACTH independent:
     - CT pre- and post-contrast identifies an adrenal cause and imaging characteristics are used to asses benign and potentially malignant adrenal disease.
     - MRI also used to identify and characterize adrenal tumours.

Treatment

Medical
- Surgery is the treatment modality of choice. Patients with extreme hypercortisolism may benefit from a period of medical control pre-surgery and it is also used in patients with recurrent disease or who not suitable for surgery.
- Ketoconazole (blocks adrenal steroid synthesis)
- Metyrapone (11-beta-hydroxylase inhibitor)
- Mitotane is an inhibitor of cortical function and is cytotoxic to the cortex inducing permanent atrophy. It is used in adrenocortical cancer.

Pituitary Adenoma
- Trans-sphenoidal excision is successful in 80%.
- For persistent/recurrent disease, treatment options include re-operative pituitary surgery, radiotherapy, stereotactic radiosurgery and bilateral laparoscopic adrenalectomy.

Ectopic ACTH
- Treatment is directed at the underlying cause when identified. Medical management of the glucocorticoid excess may adequately control disease; however, patients with persistent glucocorticoid excess may be offered bilateral laparoscopic adrenalectomy.

ACTH-Independent Disease
- Imaging distinguishes unilateral from bilateral disease.
- *Benign adenoma* – surgery is curative. Options are laparoscopic adrenalectomy either via a transabdominal or retroperitoneal approach. Large tumours may require an open approach. Intraoperative and postoperative steroid replacement is required as the contralateral adrenal gland will be atrophied and non-functional. Functional recovery of the contralateral gland can take place over many months but many patients require steroid replacement for life.
- HPA axis testing is required by assessing an adequate cortisol response to synthetic ACTH before steroid replacement can be stopped.

Subclinical Cushing's Syndrome
- Adrenal nodules without overt steroid excess but that do not suppress cortisol adequately on low-dose

dexamethasone suppression are considered to have sub-clinical Cushing's syndrome or to have low grade 'autonomous cortisol secretion'.
- Hypertension, type 2 diabetes, obesity and osteoporosis are found with increased frequency, and many of these patients are elderly.
- Adrenalectomy aims to improve hypertension and glucose tolerance.
- Steroid replacement over many months is required until HPA axis testing shows recovery of the contralateral adrenal gland.
- Decisions regarding medical or surgical treatment in this group of patients requires multidisciplinary discussion.

Adrenocortical Cancer (ACC)

- ACC is a rare tumour affecting 1–2 per million population annually.
- There is a bimodal distribution with peak incidence in children under 5 years of age and in adults aged 30–40 years.
- Families with Li-Fraumeni syndrome have an increased risk.
- Approximately 70% of tumours secrete excess hormones, Cushing's syndrome being the commonest clinical presentation. Evidence of virilization is a feature that raises suspicion of malignancy.
- Investigation
  (1) **Hormonal evaluation:**
  - Basal cortisol, ACTH, 24-hour urine for urine free cortisol, ODS
  - Renin, aldosterone, potassium
  - Plasma and urinary steroid profiles are particularly helpful in characterizing ACC
  - Plasma metanephrines
  (2) **Radiological:**
  - Abdominal and chest CT.
  - Adrenal features are frequently of large (>6 cm) heterogenous tumours, high HU on non-contrast CT, irregular margins and evidence of local invasion to surrounding structures and tumour thrombosis extending along major veins such as left renal vein and IVC.
  - There may be evidence of lung or liver metastases.
  - It is important to exclude phaeochromocytoma as radiological features can be similar. Preoperative biopsy is contraindicated in adrenal tumours due to the risk of needle tract seeding with tumour.
- **Management**
  - Treatment is aimed at complete surgical excision with open surgery.
  - Mitotane is used as adjuvant treatment either alone or with combination chemotherapy.
  - Five-year survival is approximately 60% after successful surgery but only 20–35% overall.

Hyperaldosteronism

- **Aetiology**
  (1) Primary hyperaldosteronism (PHA)
  - Unilateral adenoma (60–70%)

  - Bilateral hyperplasia (30%)
  - Glucocorticoid remedial (1–3%)
  - ACC (<1%)
  (2) Secondary hyperaldosteronism
  - Reduced renal blood flow causing raised renin, e.g. renal artery stenosis, heart failure

Primary hyperaldosteronism
Jerome Conn first described primary hyperaldosteronism (PHA) in 1955. PHA is a common cause of secondary hypertension and, overall, is responsible for 5–13% of cases of hypertension and around 20% of cases of resistant hypertension. Hyperaldosteronism has been shown to be associated with increased cardiac mortality independent of the hypertension it causes.

Sixty-six percent of cases are due to unilateral disease, although there is a spectrum from pure unilateral adenoma to bilateral hyperplasia. One-third of cases are due to bilateral disease and are treated medically.

Physiology

- Renin is secreted by the afferent arteriole of the renal glomeruli in response to reduced perfusion pressure and sympathetic stimulation.
- Renin converts the liver-produced angiotensinogen to angiotensin I, which in turn is converted into the active angiotensin II by ACE in the lungs.
- Angiotensin II stimulates aldosterone production; causes arteriolar constriction increasing BP; enhances NaCl resorption by the PCT; and stimulates ADH secretion
- Aldosterone is produced by the glomerulosa cells of the adrenal cortex; it causes reduced sodium chloride excretion by stimulating Na absorption with loss of potassium in the distal convoluted tubule (DCT) and collecting duct, resulting in increased extracellular fluid (ECF).
- PHA causes sodium and fluid retention and potassium loss leading to hypertension and hypokalaemia.

Diagnosis

(1) *Aldosterone renin ratio (ARR)* is the best initial test. Ratio >20–40ng/dL suggests *Conn's syndrome.*
  - It is important to also have a raised aldosterone (>15ng/dL) and low plasma renin activity (PRA) to avoid spurious elevated ratios.
  - Mineralocorticoid antagonist medications need to be stopped pre-testing.
(2) Salt loading/saline suppression testing for suppressibility of renin and aldosterone is used as a confirmatory test
(3) CT and venous sampling:
  - Once a diagnosis is confirmed, it is important to lateralize the secretion if surgery is considered.
  - A typical Conn's adenoma is up to 2.5 cm in size with benign features on CT. However, the presence of an adenoma does not equate to function.

- Larger lesions with indeterminate CT features (HU >30) raises the possibility of an aldosterone producing ACC.
- Due to concerns that CT may misidentify the secretory side in around a third of patients, *venous sampling (VS)* has become the gold standard for localization. In VS, the aldosterone level of both sides is compared. The right adrenal vein is short with an acute angle to the IVC and is more difficult to cannulate than the left adrenal vein. Cortisol levels are checked as a control to ensure the adrenal vein was appropriately cannulated.

Treatment

- Unilateral PHA is treated with laparoscopic adrenalectomy.
- Bilateral disease is treated medically with mineralocorticoid antagonist drugs.

Phaeochromocytoma and Paraganglioma

- Neuroendocrine tumours of the adrenal medulla are phaeochromocytomas and extra adrenal chromaffin tissue of the sympathetic ganglia are paragangliomas.
- Approximately 80% originate in the adrenal.
- They are rare tumours with an incidence of 1–2 per million population and are a rare cause of secondary hypertension.
- They produce excess catecholamines in an episodic manner.
- The majority are sporadic and non-malignant, although 25–30% are familial, with at least 10 predisposing genetic mutations now identified.
- Malignancy is more common in extra adrenal sites. Genetic screening is considered in patients presenting at a young age (<40 years).
- Cesar Roux first described the successful excision of a pheochromocytoma in 1926 in Lausanne.
- Associated syndromes include:
  - MEN2A and B
  - Von Hippel-Lindau (VHL)
  - Succinate dehydrogenase (SDH)
    - SDHB – extra adrenal paraganglioma with 40–80% malignant
    - SDHD – head and neck paraganglioma, usually benign
  - Neurofibromatosis type 1
- **Physiology**
  - Catecholamines are derived from tyrosine which is converted to DOPA, dopamine and norepinephrine within sympathetic nervous system tissue and the adrenal medulla.
  - The conversion of norepinephrine to epinephrine requires the enzyme phenylethanolamine-N-methyltransferase (PNMT) which is only found in the adrenal medulla and organ of Zuckerkandl.

- Consequently, adrenal phaeochromocytomas can secrete epinephrine and norepinephrine, whilst paragangliomas outside the organ of Zuckerkandl secrete norepinephrine.
- Catecholamines are metabolized in the liver and kidney by monoamine oxidase (MAO) and catechol-O-methyltransferase (COMT) into breakdown products that include VMA, metanephrines and normetanephrines.
- Epinephrine and norepinephrine act via alpha receptors causing arterial vasoconstriction; beta 1 receptors of the heart causing positive inotropic and chronotropic effects; and beta 2 receptors in a wide range of non-cardiac tissue causing smooth muscle relaxation.
- Epinephrine and norepinephrine stimulate glycogenolysis and oppose the action of insulin. Following excision of a pheochromocytoma, patients require monitoring of blood glucose for hypoglycaemia.
- **Clinical features**
  - Phaeochromocytoma may be detected due to:
    - Incidental lesion on imaging
    - Symptom evaluation
    - Surveillance in known genetic predisposition, e.g. MEN2
- **Symptoms**
  - Secretion of excess catecholamines is episodic and symptoms are variable and may be related to the anatomical location of the tumour.
  - Severe headache, difficult to control hypertension, anxiety, fear and sweating are classical features.
  - Life-threatening crises can occur with heart failure, myocardial infarction and CVA.
  - Release of catecholamines may be triggered by activity, e.g. induction of anaesthesia, adrenal biopsy (which is contraindicated for most adrenal conditions).
  - Micturition may cause symptoms in a bladder-located paraganglioma.
- **Investigations**
  - Measurement of plasma metanephrines is the most accurate single test and can be measured at clinic visit (requires patients to lie down for 20 minutes).
  - 24-hour urine collection for metanephrines has replaced measurement of catecholamines and VMA.
  - CT and MRI to localize the site.
  - I[123] MIBG is taken up by most pheochromocytoma tissue and useful for location of extra adrenal sites and metastases.
  - PET scan in malignancy for metastatic lesions.
- **Preoperative preparation**
  - Safe preparation for surgery is essential to minimize risks of extreme intraoperative blood pressure changes such as severe hypertension during tumour mobilization, and hypotension following tumour removal.
  - Patients are alpha blocked for 4–6 weeks preoperatively. Once fully alpha blocked, beta effects may supervene and β-blockers may be added if there is excessive tachycardia.

- During the period of alpha blockade, vasoconstriction is reduced and the vascular volume is gradually improved.
- In the UK, phenoxybenzamine (a non-competitive α-blocker) or doxazosin (a competitive blocker) are used. Dose is gradually titrated until postural hypotension is achieved. Nasal congestion is a regular symptom.
- **Surgery**
  - Laparoscopic adrenalectomy or open adrenalectomy for larger and malignant lesions.
  - Phaeochromocytomas have an indeterminate malignancy potential with apparent benign lesions presenting with metastases many years following apparently successful surgery. Consequently, patients require long-term monitoring of metanephrines following surgery. Diagnosis of malignancy requires evidence of local organ invasion at the time of surgery or metastases outside the usual sites of the sympathetic nervous system.
- **Malignancy**
  - Therapeutic MIBG is an option for lesions that take up MIBG.
  - Debulking surgery has a role in selected malignant cases.
  - Combination chemotherapy has reported response rates of around 50–60%.

Neuroblastoma

- Third commonest childhood malignancy after leukaemia and cerebral cancer.
- It accounts for 6–10% of childhood cancer but 15% of childhood cancer mortality.
- Ninety percent occur in children under 5 years age.
- It is rare in adults.
- The tumours arise from neural crest elements of sympathetic neural tissue and can present anywhere along the sympathetic nervous system.
- The adrenal is the commonest site.
- The vast majority are sporadic.
- Rare familial associations are associated with the ALK gene mutations. There is also an association with NF type 1 and Beckwith–Wiedemann syndrome.

Clinical Features

- Symptoms are often vague and may relate to site of disease.
- In adrenal disease, patients may present with malaise, weight loss, constipation and an abdominal mass.
- Fifty to sixty percent of neuroblastoma patients have metastatic spread at diagnosis and this may precipitate presentation (skull, orbit and liver are common sites).
- Investigation
  - Plasma and urine metanephrines are usually elevated
  - MIBG uptake
  - CT

Treatment

- Requires treatment in a specialist centre with a multidisciplinary team working.
- Disease is classified into low-, intermediate- and high-risk.
- Treatment options include surgery, chemotherapy, radiotherapy, bone marrow stem cell transplantation, isotretinoin and immunotherapy.
- Cure rates for low and intermediate disease are 70–90% and around 30% in high-risk disease.

Gastroenteropancreatic Neuroendocrine Tumours (GEP-NET)

- Cells that can develop neuroendocrine tumours (NET) are found in endocrine organs (e.g. MTC), nervous tissue (e.g. paragangliomas) and diffuse cells such as enterochromaffin (Kulchitsky) cells and enterochromaffin-like (ECL) cells in the GI tract and lungs.
- The cells that lead to NETs are a heterogeneous group that have similar features of secretary granules and produce a variety of vasoactive polypeptides and amines, e.g. serotonin and histamine.
- GEP-NET are a group that includes bronchial and intestinal NET (formerly carcinoid tumours) and pancreatic endocrine tumours. They can be classified as originating from:
  - *Foregut* – lung, bronchus, thymus, pancreas, stomach, duodenum. A variety of vasoactive amines may be produced including histamine and ACTH. Typically, there is low serotonin release
  - *Midgut* – second/third part of duodenum to distal two-thirds of transverse colon. High serotonin and tachykinin release
  - *Hindgut* – low serotonin release
- Biochemical markers:
  - Chromogranin A – present in secretory granules of chromaffin cells. Frequently elevated in NET and used to monitor disease response/progression.
  - 5HIAA – serotonin metabolite measured in urine, with 75% sensitivity and near 100% specificity for midgut NET.
- Imaging:
  - CT and MRI – useful to assess for liver metastases and mesenteric desmoplastic reaction
  - Somatostatin receptor scintigraphy (SRS) – NET frequently have somatostatin receptors
  - PET – gallium 68 dotatoc (somatostatin analogue with activity assessed by PET)
  - Endoscopic USS and endoscopy
  - Angiography with stimulation – for assessing gastrinoma and insulinoma
- Classification:
  - Grade (G) assesses the biological aggressiveness of tumours based on an assessment of rate of proliferation.

- WHO grading criteria for NET based on:
  - mitotic count (per 10 hpf)
  - Ki-67 index (%)
- G1 and G2 tumours show <20 mitoses and <20% Ki-67, while G3 have >20 mitoses and >20% Ki-67 and behave as neuroendocrine carcinomas (NEC).
- Further classification can be used based on differentiation. G1 and G2 are typically well- and intermediate-differentiated, whilst G3 are poorly-differentiated.
- TNM staging varies based on anatomical location of primary tumour.
- Treatment principles
  - Complete surgical excision, including lymph nodes where possible
  - Tumour debulking with excision primary tumour as palliation in metastatic disease may aid symptom control and render adjuvant treatments more effective. This may involve surgical excision or embolization of liver metastases
  - PRRT (peptide receptor radionuclide therapy)
  - Chemotherapy

Pancreatic Endocrine Tumours

- **Anatomical considerations**

The pancreas has exocrine and endocrine function. The endocrine component are the islets of Langerhans, which make up only a small amount of pancreas mass (2–3%). Four cell types exist, as can be seen in the following table:

		Location	Hormone	Tumour
A	10%	Body and tail	Glucagon	Glucagonoma
B	70%	Throughout the pancreas	Insulin	Insulinoma
D	5%	Throughout the pancreas	Somatostatin	Somatostatinoma
PP	15%	Uncinate process	Pancreatic Polypeptide	PPoma

- **Clinical features**
  - Pancreatic NET can be functional and associated with a recognized clinical syndrome, whilst others may be non-functional (includes PPoma).
  - Symptoms may also be based on tumour size and metastases.
  - Non-functioning pancreatic NET are twice as common as insulinomas.
  - Ninety percent pancreatic NET are malignant with insulinomas being the exception.

Insulinoma
Epidemiology

- Despite being the commonest islet cell tumour, insulinomas are rare.

- The incidence is 1–4 per million. They are more common in women (3:2 female:male ratio).
- Ninety percent are solitary and 10% multiple.
- Less than 10% are malignant and about 8% are associated with MEN1.

Symptoms

- These tumours secrete excess insulin resulting in episodes of hypoglycaemia. Features of which are:
  1. Autonomic – e.g. sweating, anxiety, hunger, palpitations
  2. Neuroglycopenic – e.g. confusion, tiredness, inability to concentrate, difficulty in communication, speaking and thinking, mood change, e.g. aggression and anger, seizures, loss of consciousness

Diagnosis

- This is based on '*Whipple's triad*'
  1. Symptoms of hypoglycaemia
  2. Confirmed low blood glucose (<2.5 mmol/L) associated with symptoms
  3. Correction with administration and normalization of blood glucose.
- The diagnosis is confirmed with a supervised fast over 72 hours. Symptoms terminate the fast.
- Blood is drawn for glucose, insulin, C peptide, proinsulin and sulphonylurea.
- The majority of patients will develop symptoms before the end of the 72-hour period.
- Insulin is produced as a preprohormone by the beta cells of the pancreatic islet which is rapidly converted to the pro insulin.
- Insulin is made up of A and B chains (51 aa) that are cross-linked with disulphide bridges. An additional 31 aa make up the C peptide which is cleaved from the A and B chains in proinsulin to liberate insulin. A small amount of proinsulin circulates.
- The half-life of insulin is 3–5 minutes. C peptide and proinsulin are not present in medically administered insulin. The presence of C peptide, proinsulin and absence of sulphonylurea excludes medication administration as the cause of the hypoglycaemia.
- **Localization**
  - 80% of insulinomas are <2 cm in size, intrapancreatic and can be found throughout the pancreas.
  - Imaging options:
    1. contrast CT
    2. endoscopic USS
    3. selective arterial calcium injection with hepatic vein sampling can be used in complex cases
    4. intraoperative USS

Management

- Medical
  Diazoxide inhibits the release of insulin and controls blood sugar levels in the preoperative period.
- Surgical

- Surgery is the only curative treatment.
- Surgical enucleation is the treatment of choice for sporadic solitary tumours via laparoscopic or open surgery.
- Distal subtotal pancreatectomy with enucleation of head tumours is considered in MEN1 patients with increased risk of multiple tumours and recurrence.

Malignancy

- This can be an indolent disease.
- Palliative resection may alleviate symptoms.
- Diazoxide for symptom control.
- Chemotherapy e.g. streptozotocin, 5FU and doxorubicin.
- Treatment of liver metastasis may include:
  - Hepatic metastasectomy, embolization or radio frequency ablation.

Nesidioblastosis and NIPHS

Nesidioblastosis is a term that describes excessive function of islet beta cells with histologic features of beta cell hyperplasia and budding from pancreatic duct epithelium. It was previously used to describe features seen in a mixed group of causes of rare congenital hyperinsulinism affecting infants. Similar histological features have recently been described in adults with post prandial hypoglycaemia or that have undergone bariatric surgery (particularly gastric bypass procedures) and develop episodes of hyperinsulinaemic hypoglycaemia many months following surgery, referred to as noninsulinoma pancreatogenous syndrome (NIPHS). These patients have a negative 72-hour fast. Some patients may benefit from partial pancreatectomy.

Glucagonoma

This is a very rare tumour of the A (alpha) cells secreting glucagon. Incidence is 1 in 20 million.

Most lesions are solitary, slow growing, large and 70% are malignant. Metastases to lung and liver are commonly present at presentation. Tumours are located in the body and tail of the pancreas.

Glucagon is secreted in response to low glucose levels, stress, exercise and surgery. Glucagon stimulates liver glucose production (glycogenolysis and gluconeogenesis) and is very catabolic.

Clinical Features

Distinctive skin rash of migratory necrolytic erythema affects 75% of patients and can affect any part of the body, especially friction areas. There is necrosis of the epidermis and healing while new rash forms elsewhere. The rash is very pruritic. Diabetes and marked weight loss also occur.

Diagnosis

- Raised plasma glucagon levels confirms the diagnosis.
- CT detects most lesions.

Treatment

- Surgical excision offers the only chance of cure.
- Patients require preoperative preparation to reverse catabolic effects and control hyperglycaemia.
- DVT prophylaxis is particularly important.
- Octreotide may help with symptom control and rash.
- Chemotherapy in malignancy.
- Surgical debulking and embolization of liver metastases has a role in selected malignant cases.

Gastrinoma

This is the second commonest islet cell tumour, with an incidence of around 2 per million population. Gastrinomas are small neuroendocrine tumours (NETs), and can occur outside the pancreas. The majority are found in the **Gastrinoma Triangle,** bounded by the junction of the cystic duct and CBD, junction of the second and third part of duodenum and junction of neck and body of pancreas. More than 50% are malignant, with early metastasis to peripancreatic lymph node and liver in 70%.

- 75% Sporadic – likely solitary
- 25% MEN1 – multiple

The production of excess gastrin (produced by G-cells in gastric antrum in individuals without disease) leads to parietal cell hyperplasia in the gastric body and release of histamine from ECL-like cells, resulting in excess HCl production. This may present as simple peptic ulcer disease (PUD) initially but ulcers may be multiple, and follow a complicated course with features of Zollinger–Ellison syndrome (ZES).

Clinical Features

- Epigastric pain is a common complaint
- Severe reflux oesophagitis
- Diarrhoea or steatorrhoea (excess HCl inactivates pancreatic enzymes)
- Dehydration and weight loss
- Complications of PUD – bleeding and perforation
  - Ulcer recurrence or failure to heal
- Associated hyperparathyroidism raises the possibility of MEN (hypercalcaemia is also a secretagogue for gastrin)

Investigation

- The criteria for diagnosis are:
  - Elevated fasting serum gastrin.
  - Increased gastric acid secretion (and excludes achlorhydria of atrophic gastritis). Provocation testing with secretin causes a rise in gastrin in gastrinoma but not other causes of hypergastrinaemia and can be used in cases of diagnostic dilemma.
- Other causes of raised gastrin levels should be excluded:
  - Proton pump inhibitor medication
  - Renal failure
  - Atrophic gastritis with/without pernicious anaemia
  - G-cell hyperplasia

- Pyloric stenosis
- Localization
  - SRS identifies >90% primary tumours larger than 2 cm but only 30% <1 cm
  - Selective arterial stimulation (SASI) using secretin or calcium gluconate as secretagogue can localize small gastrinomas
  - CT is useful to identify liver metastases
  - Intraoperative ultrasound is helpful to confirm pancreas lesions and intraoperative duodenoscopy for small duodenal wall lesions

Management

- All gastrinomas should be treated as malignant. Local lymph node involvement is common (>60%) and liver metastasis occur in 10% of duodenal and 60% of pancreatic lesions.
- Medical:
  - Proton pump inhibitors control acid production in preparation for surgery or palliation.
- Surgery:
  - Is indicated unless there are widespread irresectable liver metastases. The extent of surgery depends on the location of the primary tumour (duodenal vs. pancreatic) and the presence of MEN1. Options include pancreaticoduodenectomy, pylorus preserving pancreaticoduodenectomy and pancreas preserving total duodenectomy.
  - Chemotherapy and somatostatin analogue therapy (Octreotide) are options in metastatic disease

VIPoma

- Very rare islet cell tumour producing VIP. Greater than 50% are malignant. Extrapancreatic lesions are rarely found in paediatric patients as ganglioneuromas or ganglioneuroblastomas.

Clinical Features

- Are due to the actions of VIP on the GI tract
- Verner-Morrison syndrome
  - secretory watery diahorrhoea (>3 L/day), hypokalaemia and acidosis, achlorhydria.

Diagnosis

- Clinical suspicion is raised with persistent diarrhoea despite fasting and with exclusion of other causes of diarrhoea.
- Raised levels of plasma VIP.
- Imaging e.g. CT.
- SRS scintigraphy.
- Treatment is surgical excision where possible. Surgical debulking may help symptom control in malignancy and treatments aimed at liver metastasis as described previously.
- Octreotide inhibits VIP release and helps control symptoms.

Intestinal NET

- Foregut
  - Generally detected on endoscopy
  - Oesophagus – very rare and frequently malignant
  - Stomach –
- type 1 is associated atrophic body gastritis and hypergastrinaemia
- type 2 is associated with MEN1
- type 3 is sporadic with no associated background disease
  - Small (1–2 cm) type 1 and 2 lesions have low malignant potential and may be suitable for endoscopic removal and surveillance. Sporadic type 3 are more frequently malignant and are generally treated with surgical resection and local lymph node resection.
- **Duodenum**
  Only 2% NET are primary duodenal lesions. Gastrinomas, somatostatinomas, benign ganglioneuromas and very rare malignant lesions occur. Small lesions detected at endoscopy may be suitable for endoscopic removal.
- Midgut
  - These are rare tumours. Patients tend to present with a long history of vague and non-specific abdominal symptoms including pain; or tumours are detected at laparotomy.
  - Local lymph node involvements and wider metastases are common at presentation.
  - Midgut NET secrete serotonin which causes a desmoplastic reaction within the mesentery causing fibrosis and contraction. Bowel obstruction and vascular occlusion causing ischaemia may occur, resulting in an emergency presentation with an acute abdomen.
  - Appendix NET are identified in 1 in 200 appendicectomies. Ninety percent are found at the tip of the appendix and do not require further treatment once removed. Larger lesions (>2 cm) and those at the base of the appendix are more likely to have lymph node involvement and are usually treated with a right hemicolectomy.
- Hindgut
  - Colorectal NETs from the transverse colon to anus.
  - The majority are found in the rectum (85%).
  - Ninety-five percent are G1 with about 2% NEC, and 93% have local disease at presentation, with the remainder having wider metastatic disease.
  - Local resection with endoscopic procedures is possible for many patients. Colorectal resection, such as left hemicolectomy, may be required.
- Carcinoid syndrome
  - Occurs in 5–10% of patients with NET. Vasoactive substances, e.g. serotonin and kallikrein (converted to bradykinin), that reach the systemic circulation are responsible for carcinoid syndrome.
  - In patients with G1, NET occurs in the presence of substantial liver metastases or cirrhosis whereby the vasoactive substances in portal circulation bypass liver degradation.

- NET from outside the GI tract may also produce carcinoid syndrome. The majority of cases are due to midgut NET.
- Features:
  - Skin flushing
  - Telangiectasia
  - Abdominal pain
  - Diarrhoea
  - Bronchospasm
  - Secondary restrictive cardiomyopathy
- Diagnosis:
  - High levels of 5-HIAA are found in urine.
  - Elevated chromogranin A
  - CT demonstrates liver metastases
- Treatment
  - Somatostatin analogues control symptoms and are the mainstay of treatment.
  - Treatment of underlying condition as per principles of treatment. Complete surgical excision is rare and treatment is frequently aimed at liver metastases.
  - Preoperative preparation with octreotide is important to prevent a carcinoid crisis should surgical intervention be considered.
  - Long-term survival with octreotide treatment is possible in many patients as this is often an indolent disease.

Multiple Endocrine Neoplasia

MEN1

Autosomal inherited condition whereby mutations affecting gene for 'menin' (chromosome 11) causes MEN1. The associated conditions are:
- Primary HPT
- Pituitary adenomas, e.g. prolactin, growth hormone, TSH
- Pancreatic endocrine tumours, e.g. insulinoma, PPoma, gastrinoma
- Thymic and bronchial NET

Hyperplasia affecting all parathyroid glands occurs and is a common presenting feature. Non-functioning pancreatic NET are common, and pancreatic NET are typically multiple throughout the gland. Residual parathyroid and pancreatic tissue post-surgery is prone to develop further disease. Surgery is therefore a compromise between radical surgery to reduce recurrence and prolong the disease-free period, and morbidity from the extent of surgery in young people. Surgery for conditions in MEN1 is discussed in relevant sections.

A small number of patients with similar clinical presentation to MEN1 do not have proven genetic mutations of menin and mutations in CDKN1B (chromosome 12) have been identified in <4% (MEN4). Both menin and CDKN1B act to control expression of p27 which is involved in controlling cell growth (inhibits cyclin E and CDK2). Mutations result in reduced expression of p27 and uncontrolled cell growth.

MEN2

Autosomal mutation of RET protooncogene located on chromosome 10 cause MEN2. Traditionally known as MEN2A (exon 10 mutations) and MEN2B (exon 16 mutations), they are also known as MEN2 and MEN3. Associated conditions for MEN2A are:
- MTC
- Phaeochromocytoma
- Primary HPT

It is important to exclude pheochromocytoma in any new patient with a diagnosis of MTC before undertaking surgery and consider MEN2 as a diagnosis. Families with known MEN2 undergo screening to identify gene carriers and offer prophylactic thyroid surgery before the advent of MTC and annual surveillance for the early detection of phaeochromocytoma. Thyroidectomy is typically offered at 5 years of age in MEN2A and before 12 months in MEN2B.

MEN2B is a more aggressive form of MEN2, with MTC presenting at an earlier age and with some additional clinical features:
- Marfanoid habitus
- Multiple mucosal neuromas – 'bumpy' lips and tongue
- FMTC is due to mutations in RET but in whom other features on MEN2 are absent

Anterior Pituitary Tumours

Anatomy

The pituitary is a pea-sized gland that sits in the sella turcica of the sphenoid bone beneath the diaphragma sellae. Above lie the optic nerves and chiasm. Dura mater separates the pituitary from the cavernous sinus. Within the walls of the cavernous sinus are the cranial nerves III–V. The posterior pituitary derives from neuroectoderm and is an extension neurological tissue of the hypothalamus through which it connects via the pituitary stalk. The anterior pituitary forms as a bud from the roof of the primitive mouth as Rathke's pouch and is part of the endocrine system.

Pituitary tumours account for approximately 10% of intracranial neoplasms with around 1000 new cases diagnosed in the UK per year. The vast majority of pituitary tumours are benign but they can cause morbidity due to local extent, e.g. chiasmal compression causing visual field defects (CNII), and rarely parasellar extension causing raised intracranial pressure and wider cranial nerve defects (CN III–V). Around 75% cause hormonal excess, most commonly prolactin, growth hormone or ACTH. Functioning tumours are rarely associated with MEN1.

Classification

(A) Non-functioning
(B) Functioning

- Prolactin (PRL)
- Growth hormone (GH)
- ACTH
- TSH – rare
- FSH – very rare
- LH – very rare

Tumours less than 1 cm in size are micro adenoma and those >1 cm are macro adenomas.

Clinical Presentation

- Endocrinological syndrome, e.g. Cushing's syndrome, acromegaly
- Neurological deficit
  - bi-temporal hemianopia – optic chasm (CN II) compression
- Seizures
- Raised intracranial pressure (rare)
  - headache, vomiting, ocular palsy, papilloedema, altered consciousness
- Hypopituitarism
  - compression of normal pituitary causing loss of hormone production

Assessment

- Hormonal
  - Will be influenced by clinical presentation:
  - GH (can be raised or normal in acromegaly)
  - Insulin-like growth factor 1 (IGF 1) is simulated by GH and is the screening test of choice for GH abnormalities as levels do not vary as much as GH
  - Glucose tolerance test demonstrates failure to suppress GH in acromegaly
  - PRL
  - FSH, LH
  - ACTH/cortisol and thyroid function assessment are discussed in relevant sections

Imaging

- MRI with gadolinium is the investigation of choice for pituitary.
- CT can be helpful for preoperative surgical planning for anatomical detail.
- CT angiogram for detailed vascular anatomy.
- Visual field assessment:
  - Confrontation visual field assessment
  - Static, e.g. Humphrey Perimetry
  - Kinetic, e.g. Goldman Perimetry

Management

Patients require close management by endocrinology and discussion in pituitary MDMs to determine appropriate management. Functioning tumours, tumours that enlarge during a period of monitoring, those with neurological deterioration and non-responsiveness to medical treatment are considered for surgery. Surgical outcome depends on tumour size and functional status.

Conservative/monitoring of small incidental and non-functional tumours with serial imaging for enlargement may be appropriate.

Medical

- Prolactinoma – bromocriptine and cabergoline (dopamine receptor agonists) are effective and first-line treatment for the majority of prolactinomas.
- Acromegaly – GH receptor antagonist, e.g. pegvisomant and somatostatin analogues, have a role alongside surgery, which is usually first choice treatment.
  - Cushing's disease (CD) – ketoconazole and metyrapone are discussed in the section on adrenals and are an adjunct to pituitary surgery.

Surgery

- Transsphenoidal
  - Microscopic technique
  - Endoscopic technique

Access can be via a sublabial incision and tunnel to the nasal passage or via a direct transnasal route. Complete gross tumour resection is reported in around 68%, with remission of hormone excess in around 70–80% using endoscopic surgery. CD tends to be due to micro adenomas and remission rates of 86% are reported in this group using either surgical technique.

Radiotherapy and stereotactic radiosurgery can be used in complex and recurrent tumours

- Complications of pituitary surgery include:
  - Persistent disease
  - CSF leak
  - Diabetes insipidus
  - Hypopituitarism
  - Syndrome of inappropriate antidiuretic hormone secretion (SIADH)
  - Infection
  - Cranial nerve defects (III–VI)
  - Vascular injury (CVA)
  - Visual field defects

Prolactinoma

Prolactinoma is the commonest functioning pituitary tumour. Micro-prolactinomas may be present in up to 10% of postmortems.

Symptoms

- Excess prolactin:
  - Amenorrhoea
  - Galactorrhea
  - Reduced libido and sterility
  - Hypogonadism
  - Gynecomastia
  - Impotence
  - Reduced facial and body hair
- Mass effect

First-line treatment with dopamine agonists are effective at controlling prolactin levels and reducing tumour size in around 80%. Nausea, vomiting and hypotension are side-effects. Surgery may be offered to those intolerant or non-responding to medication.

Growth Hormone Excess

Gigantism occurs when GH secreting adenoma presents in prepuberty before fusion of bony epiphyses. Affected individuals are very tall. Early recognition and treatment by paediatric endocrinologists and surgery make this rare today.

Acromegaly

GH excess after puberty and fusion of epiphyses results in acromegaly. Unlike gigantism, it may present in an insidious manner and it may take several years before diagnosis. It is a very rare condition with a prevalence of 40 per million.

Clinical Features

- Coarse facial appearance and overgrowth of the hands and feet.
- Glucose intolerance.
- Osteoporosis.
- Hypertension.

Cushing's Disease

See 'Adrenal' section

Complications of Management of Pituitary Disorders

- **Nelson's Syndrome**
  - Can follow bilateral adrenalectomy for pituitary Cushing's disease.
  - It presents with skin hyperpigmentation due to high ACTH which closely resembles melanocyte stimulating hormone, and a rapidly expanding pituitary tumour due to loss of negative feedback on the pituitary. Prophylactic radiotherapy in patients not undergoing pituitary surgery has reduced the incidence.
- **Diabetes Insipidus**
  - Reduced antidiuretic hormone (secreted from posterior pituitary) can follow pituitary surgery. DI may be last <72 hours or be of longer duration. Polyuria with the production of large quantities of dilute urine (low osmolality) results in thirst, dehydration and raised plasma sodium and osmolarity. Treatment is with an ADH analogue desmopressin (DDAVP).

26

Common Breast Surgical Conditions

Breast surgery is a rapidly advancing area within general surgery. Success in treating breast cancer has enabled a focus on aesthetic excellence in addition to optimal cancer outcomes. This has led to the development of innovative advancements in reconstructive surgery, and constant evaluation and investigation into breast and axillary conserving treatment. This chapter introduces the concept of managing benign and malignant breast disease and covers common benign and malignant pathologies.

Clinical Anatomy

The female breast overlies the second to sixth rib. It is made up of approximately 20 lobules of glandular tissue, which are surrounded by fat (Fig. 26.1). The lobules are separated by the ligaments of Cooper which are fibrous septa running from the subcutaneous tissue to the fascia of the chest wall. Each lobule drains via a duct to the nipple. The nipple is surrounded by the pigmented areola. The male breast is rudimentary and is composed of small ducts supported by fibrous tissue and fat.

The breast receives its blood supply via three sources: the axillary artery (via its lateral thoracic and acromiothoracic branches), the internal thoracic artery (via its perforating branches) and from the intercostal arteries via their lateral perforating branches (small source of blood supply to the breast). The venous drainage follows the corresponding arteries.

The lymph drainage follows the pathway of its blood supply; 75% of the total lymphatic drainage travels along the tributaries of the axillary vessels to the axillary lymph nodes. The rest travels along the internal thoracic vessel tributaries, along the internal thoracic chain. There is tendency for the lateral part of the breast to drain towards the axilla and the medial part to the internal thoracic chain. The axillary lymph nodes also drain the lymphatics of the pectoral region, upper abdominal wall and the upper limb. The lymph nodes in the axilla are arranged in five groups:
- Anterior: deep to pectoralis major along the lower border of pectoralis minor
- Posterior: along the subscapular vessels
- Lateral: along the axillary vein
- Central: in the axillary fat
- Apical: through which all the other axillary nodes drain

Referral

Patients are referred to breast surgeons through a number of pathways:
1. Screening (if an abnormality is identified on their screening mammogram)

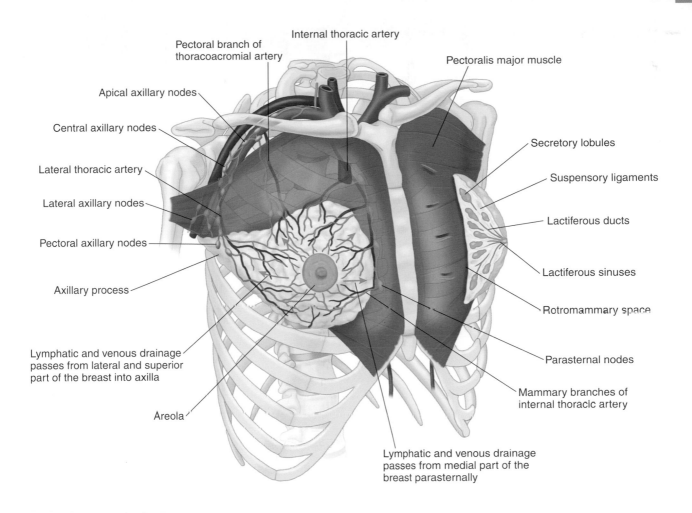

• **Fig. 26.1** Right Breast Anatomy (Redrawn from Drake: Gray's Anatomy for Students, 4th edition, Elsevier, 2020, Fig. 3.16, p. 141.)

• **BOX 26.1** **'One-Stop-Clinic' Referrals Through Primary Care**

National Institute for Health and Care Excellence (NICE) guidance (NG12) has the following recommendations:
Refer people using a suspected cancer pathway referral (for an appointment within 2 weeks) for breast cancer if they are:
- aged 30 and over and have an unexplained breast lump with or without pain or
- aged 50 and over with any of the following symptoms in one nipple only:
  • discharge
  • retraction
  • other changes of concern
Consider a suspected cancer pathway referral (for an appointment within 2 weeks) for breast cancer in people:
  • with skin changes that suggest breast cancer or
  • aged 30 and over with an unexplained lump in the axilla
Consider *non-urgent referral* in people aged under 30 with an unexplained breast lump with or without pain.

---

2. Through primary care to a *'one-stop-clinic'* (with new breast symptoms; Box 26.1)
3. The emergency department (with a breast abscess or an implant problem)

• **BOX 26.2** **Principles of a One-Stop-Clinic**

1. Single route into the system
2. Straight to test approach
3. Timely decision-making
4. Appropriate follow-up

The One-Stop-Clinic

The one-stop-clinic was initially designed to streamline the diagnostic pathway for patients with suspected breast cancer by providing access to a specialist clinic within 2 weeks of referral (Box 26.2). It was later extended to include *any* symptomatic breast patient whether breast cancer was suspected or not. The idea was to provide rapid access to diagnostic services for women with breast pathology where consultation, imaging and tissue biopsy were performed within the same hospital visit.

During the clinic, patients are seen by a consultant breast surgeon, registrar or clinical nurse specialist, a focused history is received and examination performed

• BOX 26.3 Elements of a Focused Breast History

Focused Breast History

1. Lumps (generic lump history plus associated symptoms below)
2. Nipple changes (new inversion, rash, eczema, itch, discharge)
3. Nipple discharge (colour, multi/single duct, spontaneous or only on expressing, volume, frequency, uni- or bilateral)
4. Skin changes (dimpling, tethering, colour)
5. Lymph nodes (axilla, supraclavicular fossa)
6. Pain (breast pain cyclical/non-cyclical, bony pain)
7. Breast cancer risk factors (see Box 26.4)

• BOX 26.4 Risk Factors for Breast Cancer

Breast Cancer Risk

- Age
  Odds of developing breast cancer in the next 10 years:
  1 in 1 732 aged 20
  1 in 69 aged >40
  1 in 26 aged >70
- Female gender
  100 times the risk than men
- Genetic mutations
  See Box 26.5
- Personal history of breast cancer
  2–5 times the risk
- Personal history of a high-risk breast lesion (atypical ductal hyperplasia, atypical lobular hyperplasia)
  Up to 5 times the risk
- Oestrogen exposure
  Use of oral contraceptive pill (14% per 10 years use)
  Hormone replacement therapy
  Early menarche (risk increases by a factor of 1.05 per year earlier)
  Late menopause
  Nulliparity or aged over 30 at first pregnancy
  Post-menopausal obesity
- Alcohol

(Boxes 26.3, 26.4 and 26.5). Ultrasound-scan and mammogram are available, in addition to core biopsy, fine-needle aspiration (FNA) and punch biopsy where indicated. A grading system based on clinical suspicion of cancer is allocated at each stage of the pathway to enable an informed discussion with the patient and arrangement of appropriate follow-up and support (Box 26.6).

A considerable proportion of one-stop clinics involve the diagnosis and management of benign breast disease. One in ten women presenting to a clinic will be diagnosed with a breast malignancy. A variety of breast pathology is seen in the one-stop-clinic including:

- benign lumps
- nipple discharge
- nipple inversion

• BOX 26.5 BRCA1 and BRCA2 Genetic Mutations and Breast Cancer Risk

Genetics
Most well-known are the BRCA1 and BRCA2 mutations (5–10% of all breast cancers)
Cancer risk by age 70 is:

Breast	60% for BRCA1 carriers
	55% for BRCA2 carriers
Ovarian	59% for BRCA 1 carriers
	16.5% for BRCA2 carriers
Median age at breast cancer diagnosis	
	42 years for BRCA 1
	45 years for BRCA 2

High-risk women in this category are referred for discussion of risk-reduction strategies which can include risk-reducing mastectomy.

From Mavaddat et al. EMBRACE Study *J. Nat. Cancer Inst. 2013;* 105: 812–22

- mastalgia (breast pain)

• BOX 26.6 Clinical Grading System

Clinical Grading Systems

A letter is allocated to identify which modality has been used to identify the risk.

P	physical examination
U	ultrasound
M	mammography

A number is then allocated to indicate suspicion of cancer

1	normal breast tissue
2	likely benign breast pathology
3	indeterminate lesion
4	likely cancer
5	highly likely to be cancer

Histological analysis on core biopsy will confirm or refute the clinical diagnosis. It is important that the clinical examination and the histology are concordant: if not, further assessment is required. The biopsy result is also categorized 1–5, with 5 sub-categorized into B5a and B5b (pre-malignant & invasive, respectively).

Examples

1. A 79-year-old lady presenting with a tethered hard lump, with ultrasound and mammographic evidence suspicious of a cancer would be categorized as:
   P5, U5, M5   A biopsy would be taken
2. A 45-year-old lady with a breast lump consistent with a small cyst on clinical examination, ultrasound scan and mammogram would be categorized as:
   P2, U2, M2   No biopsy is required

- gynaecomastia
- breast cancer
- congenital breast disease (less commonly)

BENIGN BREAST DISEASE (B1 AND B2)

Congenital Breast Disease

There is a vast range of congenital disorders of the breast, including but not limited to:
- Hypermastia (the presence of accessory mammary glands), which occurs in 2–6% of women
- Symmastia (webbing across the midline between breasts)
- Amastia (congenital absence of the breast and nipple)
- Amazia (absent breast with nipple present)
- Polythelia (supernumerary nipples)
- Hyperadenia (presence of mammary tissue without a nipple)

Poland syndrome, named after British surgeon Alfred Poland, is a rare (1 in 20 000) congenital disorder in which there is absence of pectoralis major on one side of the body (usually the right), and is associated with cutaneous syndactyly (webbed fingers) on the ipsilateral side. It is associated with many other clinical features including breast hypoplasia (underdevelopment) and chest wall deformity.

Cysts

- Breast cysts are a benign pathology that form during involution of breast lobules.
- In fibrocystic disease, the overgrowth of glandular and connective tissue tends to block ducts, causing lobules to widen and fill with fluid.
- They are more common in peri-menopausal women; however, they can occur at any age.
- They often present as a smooth, mobile lump, which may fluctuate in size through the menstrual cycle.

Diagnosis and Treatment

- Cysts are easily identified on ultrasound scan.
- Women over the age of 40 should also be offered a mammogram.
- No treatment is required; however, larger cysts are often aspirated for symptomatic relief.
- In the case of a bloody aspirate, cyst fluid is sent for cytology.
- Occasionally, a residual mass is present after aspiration, in which case triple assessment should be conducted.
- Cysts may contain a solid intra-cystic focus or 'debris', in which case they are occasionally biopsied to exclude intra-cystic carcinoma.

Fibroadenoma

- Fibroadenoma is the most common benign breast lesion in younger women.
- Originating from breast lobules, these slow growing oestrogen-dependent lesions are comprised of stromal and epithelial cells.
- Fibroadenomas develop at menarche (at the same time as the physiological hyperplasia of lobular breast tissue), hence they are commonly found in younger women (although can be found at any age).

Clinical Features

- Most commonly between 1 cm and 3 cm in diameter, fibroadenomas usually present as a freely mobile, rubbery, smooth, painless lump in the breast, although not uncommonly women describe tenderness and even pain.
- They can be multiple and bilateral.
- These lesions do not have malignant potential; however, women not infrequently request surgical excision due to discomfort or anxiety.

Diagnosis

- Diagnosis is made on clinical examination, imaging and, in certain cases, core biopsy.
- Typically, women in their early 20s are diagnosed on clinical examination and focused ultrasound scan. Women aged over 26 are subject to core biopsy for histological analysis.
- Women aged 40 and over also have a mammogram. Core biopsy may be performed on women aged under 26 if any atypical findings are present, the lesion is large (>3 cm) or has grown rapidly in size.
- The differential diagnosis in this scenario is *phyllodes tumour*.

Treatment

- The natural history of fibroadenoma is such that 20% resolve with no treatment, 40% remain the same and 20% enlarge in size.
- Depending on the size and location of the lesion and the patient's symptoms, no treatment may be necessary, and they can be reassured and discharged with advice to monitor the lesion and re-present should anything change.
- For symptomatic, rapidly growing, or large (>3 cm in diameter) lesions, surgical excision should be considered to exclude phyllodes and to address sampling error.
- Surgical excision remains the mainstay of treatment. The lesion is enucleated or 'shelled' from the breast with its characteristic capsule intact.
- The morbidity from surgical excision includes scarring, asymmetry, numbness, infection and further surgery if, on histological analysis, a malignant phyllodes tumour is found.

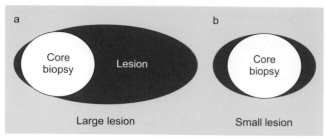

• **Fig. 26.2** Sampling Error Core biopsy of a smaller sized lesion (b) is more proportionally representative of the lesion than a core biopsy of a large lesion (a).

- With larger lesions, the diagnostic uncertainty from a core biopsy increases. This is due to 'sampling error' (Fig. 26.2) in which, with a larger lesion (A), the tissue taken from a standard size core biopsy represents a smaller proportion of the total lesion compared with a core biopsy of a smaller lesion (B). Hence, there is more chance of 'missing' malignant cells.
- The morbidity from surgical excision has led to development of minimally invasive treatments such as high-intensity focused ultrasound (HIFU), vacuum-assisted excision, and cryo-ablation.
- These novel treatments are intended to improve cosmetic outcome, preserve the breast parenchyma and avoid scarring; however, presently these are not common treatments in everyday practice.

Multiple Fibroadenomas

- Women with multiple fibroadenomas present a challenge for both treatment and surveillance. Evidently, surgical excision of multiple lesions can result in poor cosmetic outcome and unacceptable morbidity.
- This subset of patients may prove an ideal group for minimally invasive techniques.
- Monitoring multiple lesions with traditional hand-held ultrasound is challenging. Automated breast volume scans (ABVS) can offer an alternative to traditional ultrasound.
- ABVS can produce a 3D reconstruction of lesions enabling more accurate analysis and allowing more sensitive monitoring than traditional hand-held ultrasound.

Mastalgia

- Mastalgia (breast pain) represents 60% of all breast referrals.
- It affects women of all ages.
- Two-thirds of pre-menopausal women will experience breast pain.
- In 50% of women, mastalgia will affect their quality of life.

• **BOX 26.7** **Extra-Mammary Causes of Mastalgia**

Extra-mammary causes of mastalgia
- Referred pain from cervical spine pathology
- Musculoskeletal pain
- Costochondritis (Tietze's syndrome)
- Shingles
- Lung disease

- Mastalgia can be categorized into two groups: 'cyclical' and 'non-cyclical' and the distinction helps to identify the likely cause.

Cyclical Mastalgia

- This is where breast pain is related to the menstrual cycle.
- The exact aetiology remains unclear; however, it is thought to relate to fluctuations in hormone levels making breast tissue more sensitive, leading to pain.
- Most cases of cyclical pain resolve without treatment and resolves at menopause; however, women who take HRT may remain symptomatic.
- The type of symptoms described include heaviness, stabbing, pricking, burning or tightness in the breast and/or nipple areolar complex. It can be unilateral or bilateral and may radiate into the axilla or scapula.

Non-Cyclical Mastalgia

- Where breast pain is not related to menstrual cycle, it is referred to as 'non-cyclical'.
- This type of pain can affect pre- and post-menopausal women and can sometimes be linked to benign breast disease, for example, fibrocystic disease.
- Extra-mammary (outside of the breast) causes may also be responsible for the perceived pain in the breast and need consideration (Box 26.7)
- Non-cyclical breast pain can be unilateral or bilateral, constant or intermittent. Symptoms are described as for cyclical pain, the difference being the pattern.
- Approximately 50% will resolve spontaneously.

Diagnosis

- In the majority of cases, no underlying cause will be identified.
- The focus is to exclude breast pathology or identify an extra-mammary cause.
- Women with breast pain and a normal clinical examination can be reassured and discharged with advice on lifestyle changes that may alleviate their symptoms (see treatment section).
- Women over 40 with unilateral mastalgia require a mammogram.
- If abnormality is found on clinical examination or mammography, then investigation should ensue along the appropriate pathway.

Treatment

- Reassurance that breast pain is not related to an underlying malignancy is the most effective treatment for mastalgia and is effective in 70% of women (non-randomized studies).
- Simple lifestyle changes (weight management, exercise, smoking cessation, wearing a well-fitting bra) and dietary modification (reducing caffeine, alcohol, tobacco, dietary fat and chocolate) can offer some relief. Topical non-steroidal anti-inflammatory drugs (NSAIDs) are successful for the majority of women. Topical NSAID use has been demonstrated to clinically reduce breast pain in 90% of women and is reported to be superior to evening primrose oil and placebo. Whilst there is no clinical evidence base for the use of evening primrose oil in the management of mastalgia, it is commonly used and some patients may derive benefit.
- A minority of women will have severe, ongoing, life-restricting breast pain, refractory to simple interventions. Medical management includes, but is not restricted to, synthetic steroids (danazol, gestrinone), taxifen (unlicensed for breast pain), and non-steroidal selective oestrogen receptor modulators (toremifene and afimoxifene). The use of bromocriptine is no longer recommended due to its unacceptable side-effect profile (nausea, postural hypotension, dizziness and constipation).

Mastitis and Breast Abscess

Mastitis is a painful inflammatory condition of the breast and is a common cause for morbidity in women in the puerperal period. It classically presents as a red, hot, tender breast (part or whole). Systemic symptoms may also be present including fever and malaise. Although most cases of mastitis resolve with simple treatments, complications can be severe and include sepsis, abscess, chronic or recurrent infection, fistulae and scarring. Mastitis itself is not a diagnosis and must be categorized into either *lactational (puerperal)* or *non-lactational mastitis* since the management is tailored to the type of mastitis.

Lactational Mastitis

- Lactational mastitis affects 0.4–11% of post-partum women and is a cause for morbidity and difficulties breastfeeding.
- The primary cause is milk stasis, leading to an inflammatory response, which may lead to infection.
- The most common organism isolated from nipple swabs or breast milk culture is *Staphylococcus aureus.*

Treatment

- The mainstay of treatment and prevention of further episodes is based upon efficient milk clearance (continuing to feed from the affected breast/using a mechanical breast pump/hand expressing).
- Women are encouraged to nurse from the affected breast even with an infective aetiology.
- Paracetamol is the analgesia of choice in lactating women; however, if NSAIDs are required, ibuprofen is preferred.
- It is difficult to differentiate clinically between infection or inflammation, so, in general, if symptoms have not settled within 12–24 hours with effective milk removal, an infective cause should be considered.
- In suspected infective cases, antibiotics should be commenced as soon as possible and continued for 10 days to reduce the risk of abscess formation.
- If infection is suspected, nipple swabs and breast milk culture may help to identify the causative organism.
- Penicillin is ordinarily the first-line treatment (clindamycin if penicillin allergic) but local protocols should be adhered to.

Non-Lactational Mastitis

- Non-lactational mastitis is associated with infection, the most common organisms responsible being *Staphylococcus aureus*, Enterococci, and anaerobic bacteria (such as *Bacteroides* spp. and anaerobic *Streptococci*).
- Non-lactational mastitis often starts within a defined region of the breast, which can indicate the aetiology of the mastitis.

Peri-Ductal Mastitis

- Retro-areolar mastitis is often associated with peri-ductal mastitis.
- Peri-ductal mastitis is an inflammatory condition of the mammary ducts due to bacterial infection.
- It usually, but not exclusively, occurs in younger women who smoke.
- It typically presents as a red, hot, tender, central breast.
- It can present with a retro-areolar lump, purulent nipple discharge (green and offensive, occasionally bloody) or nipple inversion.
- It can be bilateral or unilateral.
- Complications include abscess and fistula formation. If an abscess is identified, aspiration under ultrasound guidance is the recommended treatment, and, in the case of suspected malignancy, triple assessment must be performed.

Treatment

- The mainstay of treatment is broad-spectrum antibiotics (with anaerobic cover in smokers) and simple analgesia.
- Smoking cessation is recommended to reduce recurrence.
- Ultrasound-guided aspiration is the treatment of choice if there is evidence of fluid collections or abscess.
- In severe refractory cases, surgical treatment may be necessary including abscess drainage and laying open of fistulae in the acute setting, and excision of chronic abscess cavities or fistulous tracts in chronic disease.
- Operating within a chronically inflamed/infected field increases the risk of postoperative infection,

multiple operations, scarring and recurrence, highlighting the importance of preventative measures as the first-line approach.

Peripheral Mastitis

- Peripheral mastitis is less common, and is associated with diabetes mellitus, trauma or treatment with corticosteroid.
- A rare cause of peripheral mastitis is idiopathic granulomatous mastitis (IGM).

Idiopathic Granulomatous Mastitis (IGM)

- IGM is a benign, non-caseating, chronic, granulomatous disease, the aetiology of which remains unclear.
- It presents with symptoms ranging from recurrent mastitis to chronic abscess with fistulation.
- It is often refractory to antibiotic treatment.
- Surgery should be avoided for this condition; it rarely expedites resolution, has high rates of complications and can lead to breast deformity.
- More recently, steroid and immunosuppressive agents such as methotrexate have been trialled with a reported high rate of resolution.
- IGM can mimic signs of breast cancer (distortion and ulceration) so thorough investigation and surveillance is required.
- Prior to initiating treatment, it is imperative that the lesion is subject to core biopsy to differentiate it from a malignancy, other granulomatous conditions (*Mycobacterium tuberculosis*), systemic pathology (e.g. sarcoidosis) or a foreign body reaction.

Breast Abscess

- Breast abscess is a surgical emergency and should be referred to the general surgical team for diagnosis and management.
- It may be clinically detectable as a tender, firm or fluctuant lump with red, hot, overlying skin.
- Not all cases are palpable, but should be suspected in cases of mastitis which have not responded to antibiotics.
- Breast abscess can cause sepsis.

Diagnosis

- Diagnosis is based on clinical history, examination, and ultrasound-guided aspiration.
- All cases of presumed breast sepsis should be confirmed by a breast surgeon, to exclude cancerous mastitis.
- Additionally, review in the breast unit will enable image-guided aspiration of any abscess, a procedure that often needs to be repeated to ensure complete resolution.

Treatment

- Historically, all breast abscesses were drained surgically; however, this procedure is associated with poor aesthetic results and higher morbidity than needle aspiration.
- There have been reports of successful management of breast abscess using vacuum-assisted drainage.
- This technique could be advantageous over needle aspiration as the wider bore needle and ability to perform lavage may negate the need for repeated aspiration.
- It may also provide an alternative to surgery where repeated needle aspiration has failed.

Protocol-Guided Management of Mastitis

As lactational mastitis is a common presentation to accident and emergency departments, evidence-driven management schemes have resulted in clarification of admission criteria, correct antibiotic use and early access to a Breast Unit for confirming diagnosis and image-guided aspiration, repeated in a few days if needed. This approach saves precious resources, minimizes hospital stay and minimizes disruption to the mother and baby. One such algorithm of management implemented by the authors' team across three large London hospitals demonstrated a substantial reduction in hospital admission rates; ensuring that only unwell patients with systemic signs of sepsis were admitted. Moreover, compliance with appropriate antibiotic therapy improved, fewer patients were subjected to incision-drainage and a higher proportion received needle-guided aspiration and follow-up in a specialist breast unit (Fig. 26.3).

Nipple Discharge

- Nipple discharge is a common complaint seen in the breast clinic.
- It represents a wide spectrum of benign and malignant pathologies and can be a variation of normal for some women.
- Causes include:
  - natural changes of the breast (duct ectasia, post lactation – for up to three years post-partum)
  - infection or inflammation (periductal mastitis, abscess)
  - endocrine disorders (prolactinoma)
  - medication (combined oral contraceptive pill)
  - injury or trauma to the breast
  - intra ductal papilloma
  - ductal carcinoma-in-situ (DCIS)
  - Paget's disease of the nipple
  - breast cancer
- It is important to elicit whether the discharge is:
  - unilateral or bilateral
  - from single or multiple ducts
  - bloody or offensive smelling
  - spontaneous or requires pressure on the breast to express
  - large volume or frequent (to ascertain the impact on quality of life)

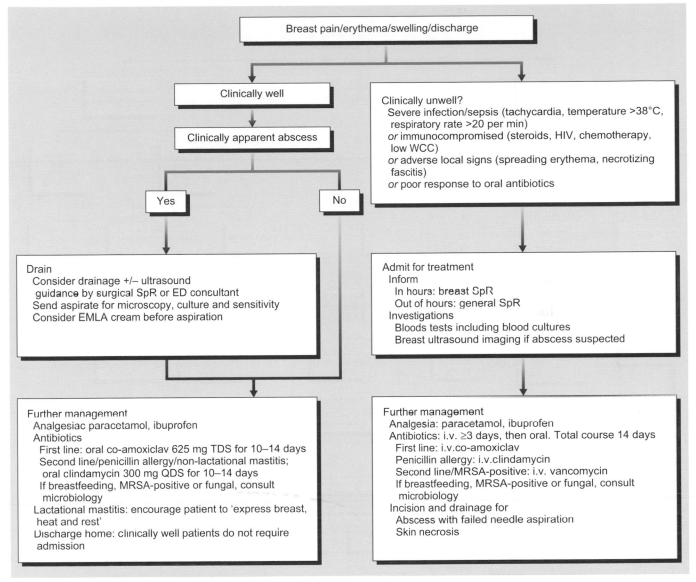

• **Fig. 26.3** Breast Abscess and Mastitis Pathway *BD,* Twice daily; *ED,* emergency department; *HIV,* human immunodeficiency virus; *MRSA,* methicillin-resistant *Staphylococcus aureus; QDS,* four times a day; *SpR,* specialist registrar; *TDS,* three times a day; *WCC,* white cell count. (From Patani, et al. Best practice care pathway for improving management of mastitis and breast abscess. Br. J. Surg. 2018; 105 (12): 1615–1622.)

- associated with any other changes in the breast (lump, skin dimpling, erythema, eczematous nipple changes)
- Unilateral, spontaneous, persistent and/or bloody nipple discharge in women over 50 or any nipple discharge in men requires a 2-week-wait referral to exclude a malignancy.
- A pathway for patients presenting with nipple discharge provides a structure within which to investigate, monitor and treat patients. A suggested approach is demonstrated in Fig. 26.4.

Duct Ectasia

- Duct ectasia is a benign condition which normally occurs in older, parous women.

- It is a result of lactiferous ducts becoming shorter and wider as part of normal breast involution.
- Inspissated luminal secretions collect within the duct and can present as a retro-areolar lump, nipple discharge (can be watery, thick, or bloody), nipple retraction/inversion, infection or non-cyclical breast pain.
- It is also a cause of asymptomatic calcification on screening mammogram.

Diagnosis and Treatment

- Once diagnosed, duct ectasia does not mandate further treatment.
- Antibiotics in the presence of infection, analgesia if required, and smoking cessation are the mainstay of treatment.

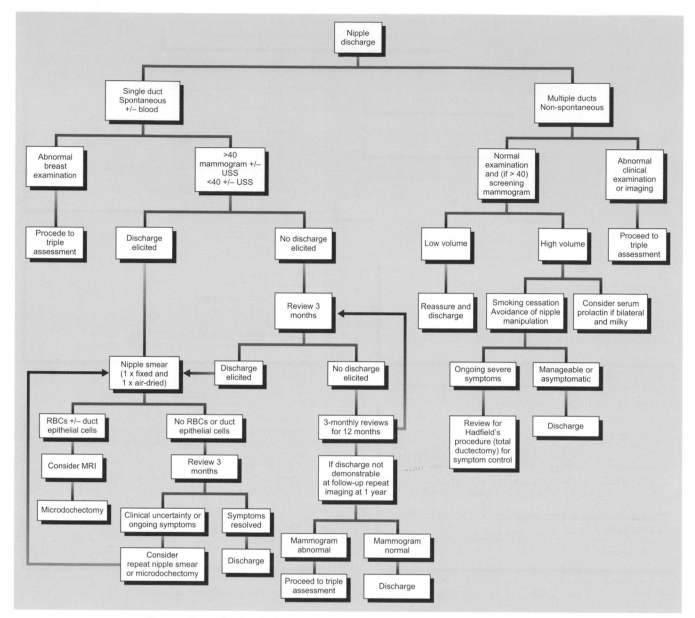

• **Fig. 26.4** Example of a nipple discharge algorithm. RBC, red blood cells; USS, ultrasound

• A supportive well-fitting bra, warm compresses and breast pads for nipple discharge can help manage symptoms.
• Women who experience troublesome nipple discharge may go on to have microdochectomy (excision of one duct) or total duct excision.

Intra-Ductal Papilloma

• Intra-ductal papillomata are benign warty growths within the lactiferous ducts.
• They can be solitary or multiple, central (close to the nipple) or peripheral. Intra-ductal papilloma can be a cause of spontaneous, single duct, bloody nipple discharge. They can also present as a palpable lump. Triple assessment is mandated to differentiate from a malignancy.
• The significance of intra-ductal papilloma depends on whether atypical cells are detected on histology. Due

to the heterogeneous nature of papillomata, in order to assess for atypia, the entire lesion must be examined.
• For this reason, all papillomata were traditionally subject to surgical excision biopsy.
• The upgrade rate to a malignant diagnosis was around 3–12% if atypical cells were absent on initial histology, which increased to around 33–36% if present. The risk of upgrade was higher in patients over 50 years old, larger lesions (>1 cm) and peripheral lesions (>3 cm from the nipple).
• The majority of surgical excision specimens for papilloma generated benign histology (70–90%); therefore, these patients were being subjected to 'unnecessary' operations with the associated risks.
• Even in cases of an 'upgrade' to malignant pathology, patients would still require further, definitive surgery.

- With the advent of vacuum-assisted biopsy performed under local anaesthetic in the outpatient unit, surgical excision biopsy can normally now be avoided.
- Women with multiple papillomata or atypia are at higher risk of developing a malignancy in the future, and therefore require surveillance.
- This varies between institutions, as there is no nationally agreed protocol.

Gynaecomastia

- Gynaecomastia is enlargement of the male breast due to glandular hypertrophy.
- It is usually bilateral and is physiological in up to 90% of cases, i.e. neonates, puberty, obesity and ageing.
- *Pseudo gynaecomastia* is caused by lipid deposition, in the absence of glandular hypertrophy.
- It is caused by an increased oestrogen:testosterone effect, for which there are many causes.
- Only 1% of cases will result in a malignant diagnosis; however, male breast cancer is more often diagnosed at a later stage than female cancers.
- The management is similar.
- An irregular firm lump, ulceration, nipple abnormality or lymphadenopathy raises the suspicion of cancer.
- Breast tissue has receptors for androgens, oestrogens and progesterone. Put simply, oestrogen and progesterone stimulate breast development, and androgens inhibit oestrogens. An imbalance can be caused by increased oestrogen levels or sensitivity or decreased testosterone levels or sensitivity.
- *Neonatal gynaecomastia* results from transfer of maternal hormones and can persist for months. *Pubertal gynaeco mastia* occurs in up to 60% of boys and is a result of a threefold surge in oestrogen that peaks before the 30-fold surge in testosterone. Free testosterone decreases with age and obesity becomes more common, giving rise to gynaecomastia in older men (55–60% of men over 50 years old).
- Disease can result in gynaecomastia via multiple mechanisms:
  - a low testosterone state (e.g. Klinefelter's syndrome, Kalman's syndrome, infection, trauma, infiltration)
  - a high androgen and high oestrogen state (Leydig tumour)
  - high oestrogen state (Sertoli cell tumour, starvation and refeeding)
  - multifactorial mechanisms (cirrhosis, renal failure)
- Medications are a common cause of gynaecomastia and include inhibition of testosterone synthesis (metronidazole and spironalactone), inhibition of testosterone action (finasteride, cimetidine), high androgen levels resulting in high oestrogen levels (anabolic steroids), high oestrogen levels/sensitivity (phenytoin, digoxin) and multiple mechanisms (amiodarone, ACE inhibitors).

Diagnosis

- A focused history should be sought including age of onset, duration of symptoms, red flags for malignancy, family history, illegal drug use, history of mumps/testicular pathology and medications.
- Clinical examination should include the axilla and external genitalia.
- Stigmata of feminization, renal or liver disease may give a clue as to the aetiology.
- Blood tests should include full blood count (FBC), renal, liver and thyroid function, luteinising hormone (LH) and follicle stimulating hormone (FSH), prolactin, alpha fetoprotein(AFP), beta human chorionic gonadotropin (BHCG) and testosterone levels.
- Abnormalities may warrant onward referral to an appropriate physician. In physiological gynaecomastia, no imaging is required.
- Ultrasound and mammogram may be indicated if the aetiology is uncertain. If malignancy is suspected, triple assessment is mandated.

Treatment

- Surgical treatment is rarely required for gynaecomastia and is associated with variable cosmetic outcome.
- It is reserved for severe symptomatic cases and, at the time of writing, is not routinely funded on the NHS.
- Open surgery in the form of a limited excision of breast tissue through a peri-areolar incision is one approach.
- Some breast tissue is left behind in order to reduce the risk of a 'saucer' deformity.
- In cases where a large amount of breast tissue is present, a reduction mammoplasty approach with skin reducing incision may give a better result.
- Thick skin flaps are important in order to improve cosmesis.
- Liposuction can be used as a less invasive option compared to open surgery and is becoming increasingly popular in an attempt to improve aesthetic outcome.
- Gynaecomastia can recur if the stimulus is still present postoperatively. Treating the underlying cause or removing the stimulus where possible can help to reduce gynaecomastia.

B3 LESIONS

- Indeterminate lesions are graded B3 (Box 26.8) for one of three reasons:
  1. The lesion is known to be heterogenous and there is a chance the biopsy is not representative of the entire lesion (sampling error).
  2. The lesion is known to be associated with in situ or invasive cancer.
  3. The lesion is known to be associated with both in situ and invasive cancer.

- Papillomata (with or without atypia)
- Radial scar (with or without atypia)
- Mucocoele-like lesions
- Cellular fibroepithelial lesion
- Flat epithelial atypia (FEA)
- Atypical intra-ductal epithelial proliferation (AIDEP)
- Non-pleomorphic lobular neoplasia (LN)
- Spindle cell lesions

- The incidence of B3 lesions has increased with the introduction of breast screening and the increased sensitivity of mammograms with digital technology. The increasing use of core biopsy as vacuum-assisted biopsy may also play a role in the increasing diagnosis of these lesions.
- The significance of B3 lesions is the associated risk of 'upgrade', meaning on further sampling/surgical excision, the diagnosis is altered to an in situ or invasive ductal carcinoma.
- Depending on the lesion type, number, size and presence or absence of atypia, the upgrade rate ranges from <2% to 40%.
- Investigating and managing B3 lesions is where the challenge lies.
- Traditionally, the majority of lesions were subject to surgical excision. A great deal of surgical excision specimens were benign; thus, the patient arguably received an unnecessary operation.
- Core biopsy is often not sufficient to represent the entire lesion.
- Vacuum-assisted biopsy is a middle ground, which can provide a greater volume of excision without the morbidity from open surgery.

DUCTAL CARCINOMA-IN-SITU

DCIS is an intra-ductal cancer that has not invaded the basement membrane. It is characterized by epithelial hyperplasia with atypia. DCIS represents 25% of new breast cancers. DCIS represents a heterogenous spectrum of disease that does not behave in a uniform manor. Some, but not all, will progress to an invasive ductal carcinoma. It is estimated that, without treatment, 20–30% of DCIS will progress to invasive cancer. Age remains the biggest risk factor for DCIS, with women age 70–84 having double the risk of women aged 40–49.

DCIS is categorized according to features that may predict how it is likely to behave:
- progress to invasive cancer
- recur
- recur as an invasive cancer

The grading system is based on the cell nuclei and split into low (grade 1), intermediate (grade 2) and high (grade 3), grade 3 being the most rapidly growing, and hence most aggressive. Size matters with DCIS, and larger lesions convey a higher chance of recurrence. The presence of comedo necrosis (dead cells in the centre of the ducts) also conveys higher risk disease. ER and HER-2 receptor status also help identify risk, with higher grade lesions being less likely to be ER positive and more likely to be HER-2 positive. Histologically, 1 mm of micro-invasion is 'permissible' for the lesion to still be termed DCIS; anything greater than 1 mm is termed invasive cancer.

Diagnosis

Screening has changed the way DCIS is presented and the type of DCIS we see. Historically, DCIS would present with symptomatic disease, i.e. a lump, bloody nipple discharge or Paget's disease of the nipple. Women now mostly present with asymptomatic screen-detected DCIS. Typically, screen-detected disease is of a lower grade and size. It usually presents as micro-calcification on mammogram. Not all calcification seen on mammography is cancer, but different patterns give clues as to the diagnosis. Multiple clusters of fine calcifications are typically seen in low-grade disease, whereas continuous, branching coarse calcifications are often seen in high-grade DCIS. Biopsy is required to determine the presence of DCIS.

Treatment

All patients with DCIS will be discussed at the breast cancer multi-disciplinary team meeting (MDM). Breast conserving surgery (BCS) or mastectomy will be recommended depending on, amongst other factors, the size of the lesion. In the case of BCS, a wire is sited under image-guidance, with the tip indicating the centre of the lesion, to guide the excision. Based on current consensus guidelines, a margin of 2 mm of healthy breast tissue is recommended for complete excision of DCIS. Further surgery to re-excise margins, or mastectomy in some cases, may be recommended if the margins are involved. NICE guidelines recommend sentinel lymph node biopsy (SLNB) when performing a mastectomy for DCIS due to the risk of detecting an occult invasive cancer (19.2–29.2%, mean 23.6%). In certain high-risk cases, adjuvant radiotherapy or endocrine therapy may be recommended at the post-operative MDT. Radiotherapy has been shown to reduce local recurrence by half but has not been shown to offer a survival advantage.

The natural history of DCIS is still not fully understood. Historic data describes a different end of the spectrum of disease than we are facing. Current research is striving to identify predictive factors for recurrence and progression to invasive cancer in order to detect high-risk lesions to target with endocrine therapy and radiotherapy. Surgery for DCIS improves survival for both intermediate and high-grade DCIS but not for low-grade disease. LORIS is a prospective randomized controlled trial comparing surgery with active monitoring (mammogram annually for 10 years) for women with low risk DCIS, with the aim of establishing whether some women may safely avoid surgery.

Follow-up

Follow-up arrangements can vary between patients. Annual mammogram for 5 years is the minimum recommended.

MALIGNANT BREAST DISEASE

Breast cancer accounts for 25% of female cancers worldwide and is the leading cause of cancer death for women. As the most common cancer in the UK, breast cancer accounts for 15% of all new cancer diagnoses. Specifically, there are 54 900 new cases per year. For women, the lifetime risk of developing a breast cancer is 1 is 8, and for men, 1 in 870. Over the past decade, the incidence of breast cancer has risen by 6% for females and has remained stable in men. White women are more commonly affected than Asian or Black women. Breast cancer is less common in women living in the most deprived areas. The majority of cases are sporadic; a minority are due to known genetic mutation. There are modifiable risks; however, more research is necessary to understand fully the difference between causation and association.

Pathology

The most common types of invasive breast cancer are ductal (80%) and lobular (15%) cancer. Other types including inflammatory, Paget's, papillary and medullary comprise the remaining 5%. The culmination of different elements of the histology report not only indicate prognosis, but also guide treatment.

Grade

The histological grade of the tumour is strongly related to prognosis. It comprises three elements: (1) nuclear atypia and pleomorphism, (2) tubule/acinar/glandular formation and (3) mitotic count. Scores from the three domains are combined to give an overall grade on a scale of 1–3. Grade 1 represents well-differentiated, slow-growing tumours conveying the best prognosis to grade 3, which are the most aggressive.

Tumour Size

Estimating tumour size on clinical examination is well-recognized to be inaccurate. Imaging improves the accuracy somewhat; however, the gold standard is to measure the tumour size in three dimensions at histological analysis of the surgical specimen. A small tumour (<15 mm) is a positive prognostic indicator and conveys less risk of lymph node involvement. Small, node negative tumours exceed 90% survival at 10 years. This said, with our ever-increasing knowledge of breast cancer, more emphasis is now placed on tumour biology for how a cancer is likely to behave or respond to treatment.

Lymphovascular Invasion

The presence of lymphovascular invasion is a poor prognostic indicator, inferring higher risk of local recurrence and worse survival. It is of particular interest in node negative breast cancers, as its presence is associated with inferior outcomes.

Biomarkers

Oestrogen and Progesterone Receptor

Hormone receptor status is important to ensure woman receive appropriate adjuvant treatment. Oestrogen (ER) and progesterone (PgR) receptor status is routinely reported in all breast cancer specimens. Eighty percent of UK breast cancers are ER positive. Women with ER positive cancer are offered tamoxifen (if pre-menopausal), or an aromatase inhibitor (if post-menopausal) or a combination of the two over time. Hormone receptor status can be accurately reported on a core biopsy enabling the identification of suitable patients for neoadjuvant hormone treatment or chemotherapy. ER and PgR status are given a score out of 8 (Allred score) which is based on the frequency and intensity of receptors within the specimens. A score of 0 or 2 defines an ER/PgR negative cancer.

Human Epidermal Growth Factor-2 Receptor

Human epidermal growth factor-2 (HER-2) status is overexpressed in 14% of breast cancers. HER-2 positive cancer traditionally had a poorer prognosis. The introduction of anti-HER-2 therapies (trastuzumab (Herceptin) and pertuzumab) has improved survival of women with HER-2 positive cancers. HER-2 is also scored based on frequency and intensity of immunohistology staining. A score of 0/1+ is negative, 2+ is equivocal and 3+ is positive. A HER-2 result of 2+ requires further testing by dual in-situ hybridization (D-ISH) or fluorescence in-situ hybridization (F-ISH) to further classify the HER-2 amplification to ascertain the likely benefit from anti–HER-2 therapy.

Breast Cancer Subtypes

A shift of focus has been observed for predicting the recurrence of breast cancer from using traditional clinic-pathological data to using intrinsic subtypes. This information is used in conjunction with genomic information to ascertain which group of patients are most likely to benefit from adjuvant chemotherapy in order to improve patient selection. This is not only to ensure women who will benefit most receive the right treatment, but also to avoid overuse in women that would see very little benefit.

Luminal A and B

Luminal A and B cancers are both ER positive. Luminal A are always HER-2 negative. Luminal B can be HER-2 positive or negative. The Ki67 score differentiates between luminal A and B subtypes. Ki67 is a protein encoded by the MK167 gene. It is present in all active phases of the

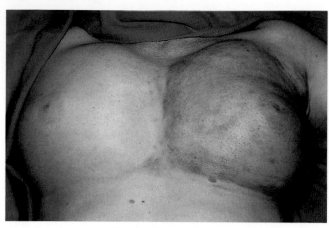

• **Fig. 26.5** Peau d'Orange

cell cycle but absent in quiescent cells, hence it is a marker of cellular proliferation. A Ki67 score of <14% represents low cellular proliferation, luminal A. A Ki67 score of >14% represents luminal B cancers. Luminal A cancers have a low-risk of recurrence, as opposed to luminal B which have a high-risk of recurrence on multi-gene expression assay.

Her-2 Enriched (Non-Luminal)

In this cancer subgroup, HER-2 is overexpressed; however, the ER status is negative. This subtype of cancer gains the most benefit from neoadjuvant chemotherapy.

Triple Negative Breast Cancers (TNBC)/Basal

Triple negative breast cancers represent a heterogenous category of breast cancer, which are ER, PgR, HER-2 negative (sometimes very low expression of ER). TNBC is associated with a higher grade, more aggressive tumour. The aggressive nature of TNBC plus fewer targets for treatment (ER and HER-2 negative) results in worse outcomes. TNBC respond less favourably to standard anthracycline-based chemotherapy but may benefit from a taxane-based regime. The addition of platinum-based chemotherapy in the neoadjuvant setting has shown promising results; however, further work is required to identify which patients within this subgroup will benefit from this therapy.

Diagnosis

The gold standard for breast cancer diagnosis is triple assessment, including clinical examination, imaging and tissue diagnosis. Most early cancers are diagnosed via the screening programme as they are largely asymptomatic. Symptomatic patients present through one-stop-clinics with a variety of symptoms, classically a breast lump.

Clinical Examination

The observable stigmata of breast cancer include skin dimpling (peau d'orange, Fig. 26.5) or tethering, breast distortion, nipple retraction or eczema and skin-colour change (redness associated with inflammatory cancers). Breast cancers may occasionally present as ulcerating or fungating lesions. Palpation may reveal a firm, irregular lump, which may be adherent to the overlying skin or underlying chest wall. There may by lymphadenopathy in the axilla or supra clavicular fossa.

Imaging

Mammography

Mammography in addition to ultrasound scan is routine for breast cancer diagnosis in women aged 40 or older. Women who are aged less than 40 years but have ultrasound evidence of a suspicious lesion or a biopsy-proven malignancy will also undergo mammography. Mammogram is more sensitive for ductal cancers and in less dense breast tissue; hence, young women with dense (less atrophic) breasts and those with lobular cancers may require MRI to assist in diagnosis.

Abnormal findings on mammography include masses, distortions, calcifications and asymmetries. Malignant lesions are typically irregular masses, with indistinct margins and a density the same or greater than the normal breast tissue. Benign features include oval or round lesions with distinct borders of variable density.

Ultrasound

Ultrasound is superior to mammography at differentiating between solid and cystic lesions. It is the first-choice imaging modality for tumour localization for both core biopsy and guide wires (sited preoperatively to guide surgical excision). Features consistent with malignancy on ultrasound include spiculation, microlobulation, lesions deeper than they are tall, hypoechoic lesions and thick hyperechoic halos. Benign lesions are typically compressible, well-circumscribed and hyperechoic.

All women with a suspected cancer on breast imaging will go on to have an ultrasound of the ipsilateral axilla and core biopsy/FNA of any abnormal lymphadenopathy.

Histological Diagnosis

Core biopsy is usually the first-line invasive diagnostic investigation for a suspected breast malignancy. The report will give details as to the type of cancer (ductal, lobular or other), grade (1–3), the hormone receptor status (oestrogen and progesterone receptor positive or negative) and the HER-2 receptor status (positive or negative). Sometimes further stains are required to clarify the tumour type, such as E-cadherin to differentiate between lobular and ductal phenotypes. The histological data from core biopsy not only provides a definitive diagnosis in most cases, but it also helps guide treatment. Furthermore, detailed information becomes available on analysis of the surgical specimen where the entire extent of the tumour is examined.

Staging

The clinical stage of breast cancer is determined by clinical examination and radiological findings. Nuclear medicine bone scans and CT thorax abdomen and pelvis is indicated to identify potential distant disease in patients with large cancers, positive lymph nodes and those who will undergo chemotherapy.

Pathological staging can only be achieved following analysis of the surgical specimen and may be different to clinical staging, especially if the patient has undergone neoadjuvant treatment with the intention of shrinking the tumour. Pathological staging gives more detailed information about the size and characteristics of the tumour and provides additional information such as excision margins, lymphovascular invasion and peri-neural invasion.

TABLE 26.1	Predicted 10-Year Survival According to the Nottingham Prognostic Index.		
NPI	**Score**	**Cancer-specific 10-year survival**	**All-cause 10-year survival**
I (Excellent)	≤2.4	96%	88%
II (Good)	>2.4 but ≤3.4	93%	86%
III (Moderate)	>3.4 but ≤5.4	78%	74%
IV (Poor)	>5.4	44%	42%

From Fong, Y. et al. The Nottingham Prognostic Index: five- and ten-year data for all-cause survival within a screened population. Ann. R. Coll. Surg. Engl. 2015; 97 (2). 137–139.

Prognostic Tests

The *Nottingham Prognostic Index* was introduced into clinical practice over 30 years ago to predict survival. It combines lymph node stage, histological grade and tumour size to give a numerical result, which can be used to subdivide women into 4 groups according to the predicted 10-year survival (Table 26.1).

$$NPI = \text{Lymph node stage } (1-3) + \text{Histological Grade} (1-3) + \{\text{Tumour size} \times 0.2^*\}$$

*The correction factor of 0.2 is representative of tumour size being of less prognostic value than lymph node stage and histological grade.

The use of the NPI has declined since the introduction of web-based prognostic indicators (e.g. Predict) which encompass additional prognostic factors. Predict (developed in the UK; available at: https://breast.predict.nhs.uk) has the additional benefit of representing survival prospects at 5 and 10 years without treatment, and the likely benefit from adjuvant systemic treatment (see Figs 26.6 and 26.7 for examples of using Predict).

Treatment

Treatment for breast cancer is multi-faceted and may include surgery and radiotherapy for loco-regional control, and chemotherapy, endocrine and biologic therapies for systemic control.

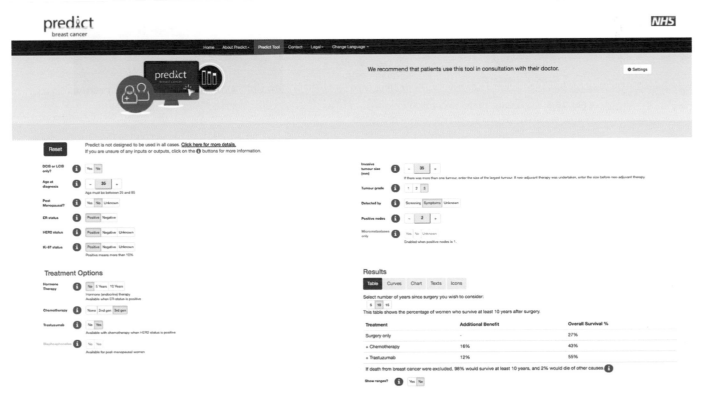

• **Fig. 26.6** Example of a High-Risk Cancer from Predict (https://breast.predict.nhs.uk, Public Health England)

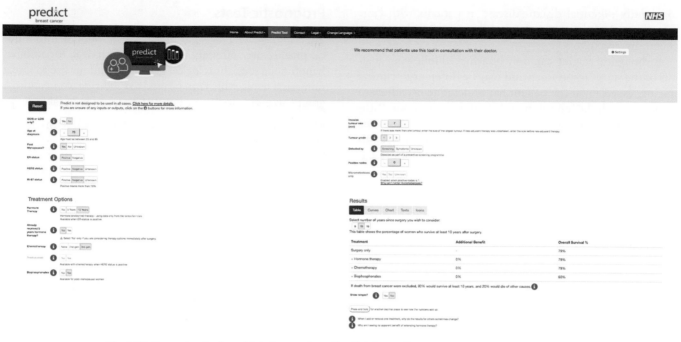

• **Fig. 26.7** Example of a Low-Risk Cancer from Predict (https://breast.predict.nhs.uk, Public Health England)

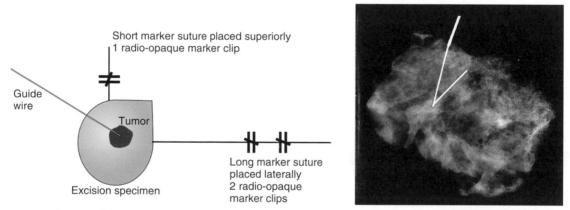

Short marker suture placed superiorly
1 radio-opaque marker clip

Guide wire

Tumor

Excision specimen

Long marker suture placed laterally
2 radio-opaque marker clips

• **Fig. 26.8** Schematic of the orientation for a wide local excision specimen (left) and intra-operative X-ray of an orientated specimen with the wire in situ (right).

Surgery

Surgery to the Breast

The two main options are breast conserving surgery (BCS) and mastectomy. BCS is usually coupled with radiotherapy; mastectomy may be performed in isolation, or with the addition of radiotherapy if the patient is found to be heavily node positive (> four nodes) or have a tumour of certain size (>50 mm). The primary focus of surgery is to provide loco-regional control. Aesthetic outcome is important and has been demonstrated to have psychosocial and quality of life implications. With excellent survival statistics for most breast cancers, the importance of aesthetic outcome for psychosocial wellbeing is brought to the fore.

Breast Conserving Surgery

BCS aims to remove the tumour plus a margin of healthy breast tissue while conserving the breast. In occult tumours, image-guided wires are sited preoperatively with their tip inside the tumour to direct surgical excision. Once excised, the specimen (with wire in situ if one is used) is orientated using sutures and radio-opaque markers clips (Fig. 26.8) and specimen radiology is performed perioperatively (usually in theatre using a specimen X-ray system). If the tumour appears close to an excision margin, further tissue can be excised prior to closure. The remaining breast tissue can be mobilized in order to close the defect. Alternative localisation techniques including radioactive and magnetic seeds are in development and are anticipated to become more common in the near future.

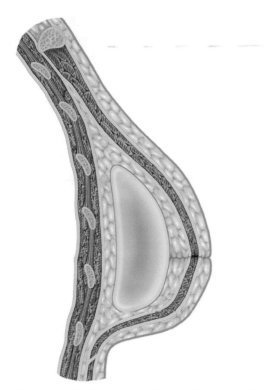

• **Fig. 26.9** Schematic of a Sub-Pectoral Implant Reconstruction

The postoperative surgical histopathology will give detailed information on margin clearance and, if required, further surgery to excise close or involved margins will follow. Women may require mastectomy following BCS if satisfactory margin clearance cannot be achieved. Women who have BCS will also require radiotherapy to the breast. Previous radiotherapy (i.e. mantle radiotherapy for Hodgkin's lymphoma) to this area may negate further radiotherapy, in which case BCS may not be appropriate and mastectomy would be the treatment of choice.

Mastectomy

Mastectomy is indicated for (but not limited to) women with unfavourable tumour to breast size ratio, multifocal or inflammatory cancers and women in whom radiotherapy is contraindicated (see above). Some women opt for a simple mastectomy with no reconstruction. Options for reconstruction can be subdivided into:

1. delayed versus immediate
2. implant versus autologous
3. nipple sparing versus nipple sacrificing

Each has its own benefit and risk and is a shared decision between surgeon and patient.

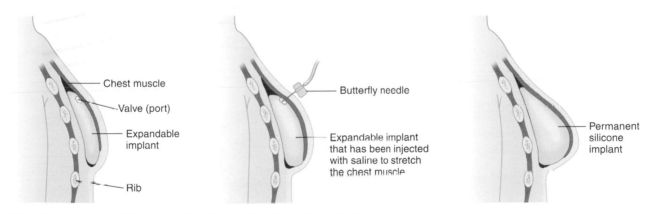

Traditional two-stage expander-implant breast reconstruction without mesh

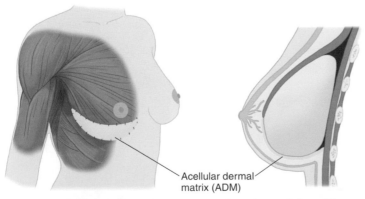

Single-stage submuscular implant reconstruction with mesh (matrix)

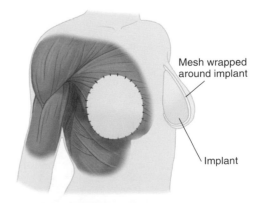

Single-stage subcutaneous implant-based reconstruction with mesh

• **Fig. 26.10** Schematic of Implant-Based Breast Reconstruction (From Potter, et al., Does the addition of mesh improve outcomes in implant based breast reconstruction after mastectomy for breast cancer. BMJ 2018;362:k2607.)

Immediate versus Delayed

Immediate reconstruction can either be implant-based or using autologous tissue. With implant-based immediate reconstruction, the skin envelope is preserved, and the implant is traditionally sited underneath pectoralis major (Fig. 26.9). Often an acellular dermal matrix (ADM) is used in order to provide extra coverage between the implant and the skin in the area with no muscle coverage, and it better supports the lower pole. Pre-pectoral implant reconstruction where ADM envelopes the implant, which is sited superficial to pectoralis major, is currently being trialled but has not yet been widely adopted (Fig. 26.10). This has potential advantages of less postoperative pain (muscle mobilization is avoided), and a more natural breast movement as it is not confined by pectoralis major.

Delayed reconstruction can also be autologous or implant-based. In the case of implant-based reconstruction, an expander implant is required to stretch the skin and muscular envelope to the required size before a permanent implant can be sited. The expander is sited in a partially collapsed state with an access port fixed under the skin. Postoperatively, once the tissues have had time to heal, sterile saline is injected into the expander port at regular intervals in clinic until the desired size is achieved. The expander implant then can be exchanged for a permanent one.

Implant versus Autologous

Both methods carry their own advantages and disadvantages. Implant reconstruction is generally a faster operation with less immediate surgical risk and possibly more freedom with regard to size (as it does not depend upon amount of 'spare tissue' the patient has). There is a greater risk of infection as essentially a foreign body remains in situ, and implants have a finite life span, so require replacement. Capsular formation, implant rupture and migration may also result in further surgical intervention.

Autologous reconstruction uses the patients' own tissue to recreate a breast. Flaps can be pedicled (where the blood supply to the flap remains in situ i.e. latissimus dorsi muscle reconstruction; Fig. 26.11), or free flaps (where the blood supply to the flap is disconnected and re-anastomosed to a local vessel i.e. deep inferior epigastric perforator (DIEP) reconstruction; Fig. 26.12). Autologous reconstruction requires the patient to have enough 'spare' tissue for reconstruction so is not suitable for all. It requires a much longer operation with a higher immediate surgical risk; however, the tissue is the patients' own, so it not only has advantages regarding rejection and infection, it also feels more natural to the patient (it is warm and moves more naturally) and can yield improved symmetry owing to a more natural ptosis (droop). Another advantage of autologous reconstruction is that it is more often definitive surgery (i.e. there is no need for implant exchanges, etc).

In certain cases, an implant can be used in conjunction with an autologous flap where additional volume or soft tissue coverage is desired or required.

Nipple Sparing versus Nipple Sacrificing

Nipple-sparing mastectomy has been demonstrated to be oncologically safe in selected patients and can provide

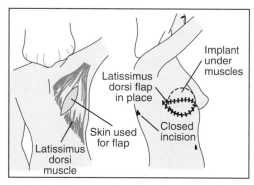

• **Fig. 26.11** Latissimus Dorsi Flap (From Elsevier's 2021 publication ICD-10-CM/PCS Coding: Theory and Practice ISBN 978-0-323-76414-8)

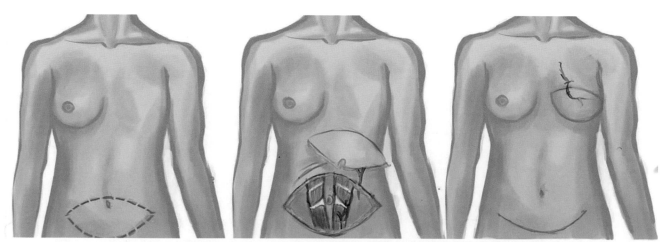

• **Fig. 26.12** Deep Inferior Epigastric Perforator (DIEP) Free Flap (From Adrian, C.: Breast Cancer and Gynecologic Cancer Rehabilitation, Elsevier, 2021)

superior cosmetic outcome. Evidence of nipple involvement, Paget's disease or bloody nipple discharge are contraindications to nipple-sparing techniques. A tumour to nipple distance of >2 cm is deemed oncologically safe in the absence of the above features. The risk of sparing the nipple is anchored around potential disruption to the blood supply causing necrosis and, in extremis, nipple loss. In cases of nipple-sacrificing procedures, nipple reconstruction can be performed using local (skin from the breast, i.e. a CV flap) or distant tissue (nipple share from the contralateral nipple, labial tissue transfer). The areolar pigment can be recreated using tattoo. Some women opt to use a prosthetic nipple,

which adheres to the skin, whereas others are comfortable with no nipple.

Surgery to the Axilla

Surgical management of the axilla is a current hot topic and a perpetual 'moving target 'in breast cancer surgery. The focus of axillary surgery is to provide information to guide adjuvant treatments and to provide local control. On the one hand, axillary recurrence is very unpleasant for patients and includes painful plexopathies, but on the other, morbidity from axillary surgery is not insignificant and can include lymphedema of the arm (~5% SLNB vs. ~30% ALND), which can be detrimental to quality of life. The mainstay of surgery to the axilla for breast cancer involves sentinel lymph node biopsy (SLNB) and axillary lymph node dissection (ALND). A simplified surgical approach to the axilla is represented in Fig. 26.13.

Sentinel Lymph Node Biopsy

SLNB is indicated for patients with a clinically negative axilla. It employs a dual technique to identify the first draining lymph nodes from the breast for a targeted excision (Fig. 26.14). An injection of radioactive isotope to the ipsilateral breast is performed the day before surgery and blue dye is injected into the breast preoperatively. The lymphatic drainage is traced intra-operatively using both a gamma probe (audible beeps to indicate a high count e.g. nodes with the most radiation) and blue dye (visibly blue lymph nodes) in order to excise the sentinel nodes (maximum of four). SLNB is accurate with a false negative rate of under <5%.

If, following SLNB, the nodes are negative, contain isolated tumour cells, or micrometastasis, no further surgery is recommended. If there is large volume nodal metastasis or macrometastasis within the node, ALND is recommended. In the case of low volume nodal involvement, ALND or radiotherapy can be offered.

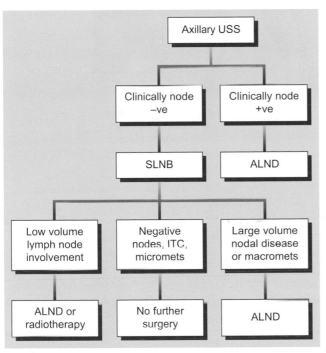

• **Fig. 26.13** Simplified Approach to the Axilla ALND, Axillary lymph node dissection; ITC, isolated tumour cells; SLNB, sentinel lymph node biopsy; USS, ultrasound.

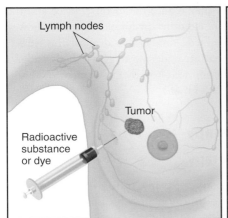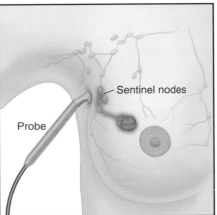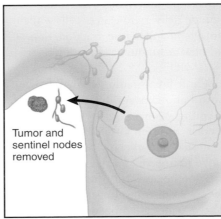

• **Fig. 26.14** Sentinel Lymph Node Biopsy. © 2010 Terese Winslow LLC, U.S. Govt. has certain rights.

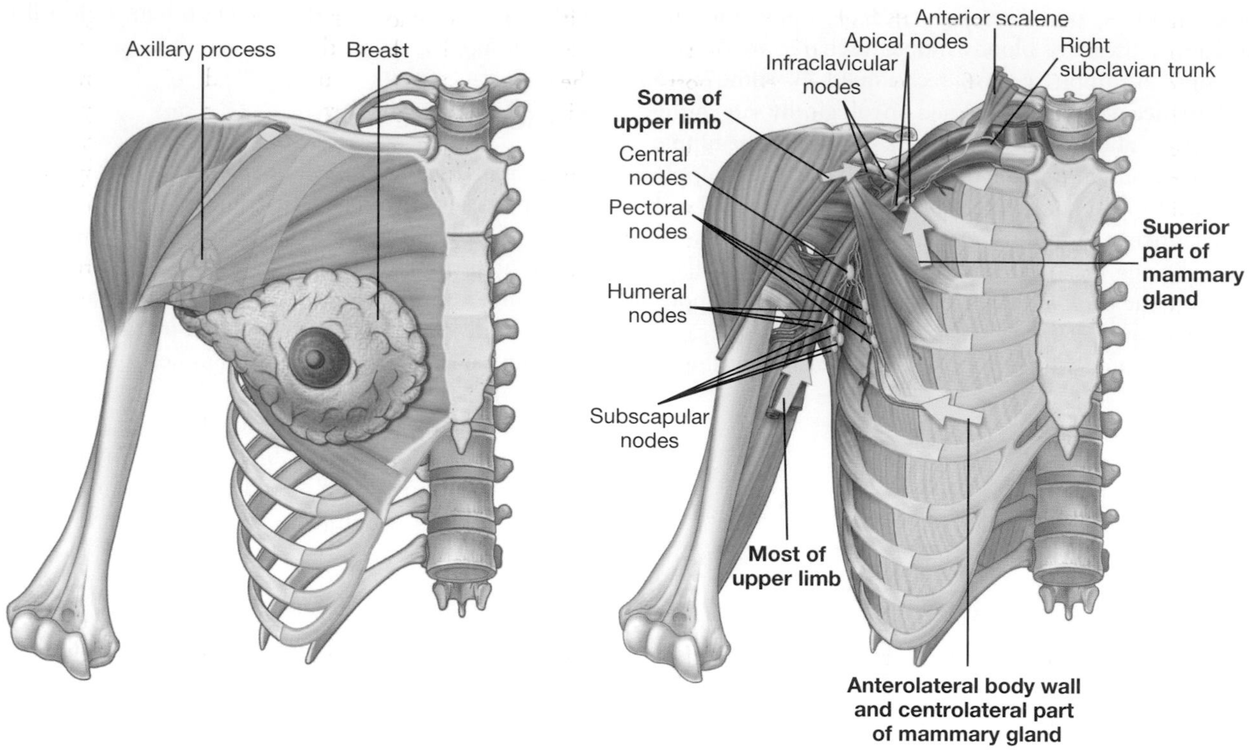

• **Fig. 26.15** Anatomy of the Axilla (From Drake/*Basic Anatomy* 2e, Elsevier, 2018, Figures 7.43 and 7.44)

Axillary Lymph Node Dissection

ALND is performed in the clinically node positive (ultrasound and core biopsy) axilla. It is a more extensive operation and aims to remove all nodes in level I and II (Fig. 26.15) plus any palpable abnormal nodes from level III. Care must be taken to avoid the large axillary vein at the apex of the axilla, the thoracodorsal pedicle (to latissimus dorsi), long thoracic nerve (to serratus anterior) and the intercostobrachial nerve (sensation to the upper inner arm).

Radiotherapy

The aim of radiotherapy is to fatally target cancer cells while preserving underlying structures. Three ways to enable accurate delivery to cancer cells while minimizing collateral damage include dose fractionation, CT-guided planning and new techniques such as intensity-modulated radiotherapy (IMRT).

Whole breast radiotherapy following BCS provides local control and conveys breast cancer specific survival benefit. In young women, with close resection margins, lymphovascular invasion or involved regional lymph nodes, an additional radiotherapy boost to the tumour bed has been shown to improve local control.

Radiotherapy is also recommended in some women following mastectomy. In general, women with more than four positive axillary lymph nodes or involved surgical margins are offered radiotherapy. The radiotherapy field can also be extended to include supra- and infra-clavicular, internal mammary and axillary nodes in certain clinical situations.

Side-effects of radiotherapy may include skin damage (blistering, burns, ulceration), breast oedema, pain, tiredness and fatigue. Longer-term damage to underlying structures including the heart and lungs, fibrosis of the breast (leading to shrinkage and asymmetry) and telangiectasia may occur. Rare consequences include secondary tumours such as angiosarcoma.

Radiotherapy can be administered to breast reconstruction, although may affect the aesthetic result. Neoadjuvant radiotherapy in DIEP reconstruction is currently being investigated (PRADA). Intra-operative radiotherapy is currently a topic of expert debate. It is thought that intra-operative radiotherapy to the breast cavity may reduce the inconvenience and travel demands of adjuvant radiotherapy for older patients; however, the additional anaesthetic time is not ideal for this subset of patients. Current trials are underway to assess whether adjuvant radiotherapy can be omitted altogether in women with low risk of recurrence (PRIMETIME).

Systemic Therapy

Endocrine Therapy

The role of endocrine therapy is to reduce the growth stimulating effect of hormones on breast cancer cells. Premenopausal women are offered tamoxifen for 5 years. Ovarian suppression and an aromatase inhibitor should be considered for young women with high-risk disease. In post-menopausal women, letrozole or anastrozole should be offered for 5 years. Tamoxifen may still be used in post-menopausal women if aromatase inhibitor cannot be tolerated. Women with high-risk disease, who reach menopause after 5 years of tamoxifen, can be considered for an aromatase inhibitor. The risk of recurrence from breast cancer remains present for at least 15 years after the initial diagnosis. Extended course endocrine therapy has a role in pre-menopausal women (further 5 years of tamoxifen) and post-menopausal (further 5 years of aromatase inhibitor).

Post-menopausal women with ER-positive tumours may be appropriate for neoadjuvant aromatase inhibitors to enable breast conservation.

Chemotherapy

Chemotherapy is a systemic therapy used in women with high risk of cancer recurrence. Adjuvant chemotherapy in addition to locoregional treatment for breast cancer has led to a 25% per year reduction in breast cancer recurrence and a 14% reduction in mortality.

Traditionally, chemotherapy was reserved for patients with large tumours of a high grade with involved lymph nodes. However, recent evidence has suggested that some women with node negative disease benefit from chemotherapy and conversely some with node positive disease do not. More emphasis is now being placed on tumour biology and genomic profiling to ascertain *how much* benefit will be gained in proportion to *adverse effects* of systemic treatment enabling more informed decision-making processes. This may identify subsets of patients in whom chemotherapy (with its associated morbidity) can be avoided, and also may highlight additional subsets of patients who may gain additional benefit.

Genomic Assays

Genomic assays are being used within breast cancer to further classify risk of recurrence and identify those who will gain most benefit from systemic therapy; therefore, it is not just an indicator of prognosis but a predictive indicator too. The most widely used genomic assay in the UK is the Oncotype Dx, which looks at the activity of 21 genes and delivers a score between 0–100. A score <18 conveys a low risk of recurrence, between 18 up to and including 30 is an intermediate risk and greater than or equal to 31 represents a high risk of recurrence. This information in conjunction with clinic-pathological and biological information is being used to inform discussions with patients regarding the use of adjuvant chemotherapy in ER positive, HER-2 negative, node negative cancers. The recently published Trial Assigning Individualized Options for Treatment (Rx) or TAILORx study used the Oncotype Dx to stratify women with node negative, hormone receptor positive, HER-2 negative cancers into low (0–10), intermediate (>10 <25) and high risk (>25) groups in order to ascertain non-inferiority of endocrine treatment alone versus endocrine plus chemotherapy for women with intermediate-risk disease. The low-risk group was treated with adjuvant endocrine therapy alone, the high-risk group was treated with chemotherapy and endocrine therapy, and the intermediate-risk group was randomized to receive endocrine plus chemotherapy or endocrine therapy alone. The results demonstrated non-inferiority of endocrine therapy alone versus chemotherapy and endocrine therapy for women at intermediate risk of recurrence. The caveat to these results is that subgroup analysis of pre-menopausal women and women under 50 at the upper end of the intermediate risk group revealed that chemotherapy might offer some benefit.

Chemotherapy Agents

Anthracyclines have largely replaced the traditional cyclophosphamide/methotrexate/fluorouracil (CMF) chemotherapy. Adriamycin (doxorubicin) and epirubicin are the most common anthracyclines in use. The addition of a taxane to adjuvant anthracycline regimes has been shown to be beneficial in some cases. The most common taxanes in use are paclitaxel (Taxol) and docetaxel (Taxotere). The addition of carboplatin to neoadjuvant chemotherapy is beneficial in some cases (e.g. TNBC).

Neoadjuvant Chemotherapy

With the recognition of breast cancer as a systemic disease and the improved outcomes observed from the addition of systemic therapy to loco-regional treatment, the concept of neoadjuvant chemotherapy was borne. Despite no appreciable advantages in survival, two important benefits from neoadjuvant chemotherapy exist:

1. Prognostic information regarding tumour response to therapy
2. Downsizing of the tumour to enable breast conservation in 25% of patients initially planned for mastectomy

Neoadjuvant chemotherapy is not a guarantee for breast conservation, even if the tumour demonstrates a response. Tumours regress in different patterns, some shrink concentrically enabling BCS, some shrink concentrically but not enough to enable BCS, and some will fragment so that, although the volume of tumour is less, the diameter is not reduced, thereby inhibiting BCS. Tumour subtype affects the response rate of neoadjuvant therapy with the most benefit observed in the HER-2 positive ER/PgR negative tumours, followed by triple negative cancers.

Clinical versus Pathological Response

A complete clinical response (CCR) is where the tumour in no longer detectable on imaging or clinical examination. It is vital to site a marker clip within the tumour prior to neoadjuvant treatment to enable the localization of the tumour site for excision in the case of CCR.

CCR differs from a complete pathological response (Path CR) which can only be determined on histological analysis of the surgical specimen. Some tumours may not be visible on imaging or detectable clinically, but invasive cancer may still be present in the surgical specimen, hence, a complete clinical response but not a complete pathological response. This has implications on planning further adjuvant treatment.

Biological Therapy

Trastuzumab

Trastuzumab (Herceptin) is a monoclonal antibody targeted toward the HER-2 receptor which is overexpressed in 15–20% of breast cancers. HER-2 positive breast cancers have a worse prognosis. The HER-2 receptor plays an important role in tumour growth. Addition of Herceptin to adjuvant chemotherapy has demonstrated a survival benefit in women with HER-2 positive breast cancer, including those with metastatic disease.

Pertuzumab

Pertuzumab is a monoclonal antibody directed to the HER-2 receptor. It can be given in the neoadjuvant setting to women with early or locally advanced HER-2 positive breast cancer with a high risk of recurrence. It is given alongside Herceptin and chemotherapy. Pertuzumab can also be used for secondary breast cancer when Herceptin and chemotherapy has not previously been given for metastatic disease.

Surveillance

Surveillance and follow-up can vary between institutions. The guidance set out by NICE recommends annual mammography until eligibility for the NHS Breast Screening Programme (NHSBSP). If the patient is already eligible for the NHSBSP, 5 years of annual mammography is recommended before enrolling back into the NHSBSP.

Education is provided so women remain 'breast aware' and are advised to re-engage with the breast service should they have any concerns. Some hospitals will review their patients clinically for 5 years after treatment, some longer. Other institutions have an open access follow-up facility where no routine follow-up is offered following the completion of the primary treatment; however, open access to the breast care team enables them to seek advice and/or clinical review should any issues arise. The Open Access Follow-up (OAFU) programme can offer access to doctors, nurses, psychologists, complimentary therapists, lymph oedema teams and patient support groups, amongst other services.

SURVIVORSHIP

The progress in our understanding, diagnosis and management of cancer has inevitably resulted in more people living with, and beyond, treatment. This has prompted a shift of focus towards the after effects of treatments, not just on measuring the ability to 'cure'. More energy has been placed into understanding how people normalize their experiences and move on with their lives, while maintaining vigilance regarding red flags for recurrence. Each patient has an individual experience and hence, unique needs following treatment completion. Some will experience physical side-effects, some psychological. Sequelae may present immediately and some may be delayed. Personality type, family support, friendship dynamics, and individual beliefs and coping strategies all interplay and contribute to how an individual adjusts to their new normal, as a cancer survivor. Nurse specialists offer a wealth of knowledge in this area and maintain contemporary knowledge of services available to people living beyond cancer ranging from complementary therapies to financial advisory services.

Further Reading

Breast Cancer Care. Available at: www.breastcancercare.org. Accessed August 2018.

Cancer Net. https://www.cancer.net/cancer-types/breast-cancer/risk-factors-and-prevention. Accessed August 2018.

Cancer Research UK. Available at: https://www.cancerresearchuk.org/about-cancer/breast-cancer. Accessed August 2018.

Duffy SW, Dibden A, Michalopoulos D, et al. Screen detection of ductal carcinoma in situ and subsequent incidence of invasive interval breast cancers: a retrospective population-based study. *Lancet Oncol.* 2016;17(1):109–114. https://doi.org/10.1016/S1470-2045(15)00446-5.

Early Breast Cancer Trialists' Collaborative Group (EBCTCG). Tamoxifen for early breast cancer: an overview of the randomised trials. Early Breast Cancer Trialists' Collaborative Group. *Lancet.* 1998;351(9114):1451–1467.

Giuliano AE, Hunt KK, Ballman KV, et al. Sentinel lymph node dissection with and without axillary dissection in women with invasive breast cancer and sentinel node metastasis: a randomized clinical trial. *J Am Med Assoc.* 2011;305(6):569–575.

Kirwan, C. C., Coles, C. E., Bliss, J., & PRIMETIME Protocol Working Group. (2016). It's PRIMETIME. Postoperative avoidance of radiotherapy: biomarker selection of women at very low risk of local recurrence. *R Coll Radiol, 28*(9), 594–596.

LORIS. Available at: http://www.associationofbreastsurgery.org.uk/research/current-trials/loris. Accessed August 2018.

Macmillan Routes from Diagnosis. The most detailed map of cancer survivorship yet. Available at: https://www.macmillan.org.uk/_images/Routesfromdiagnosisreport_tcm9-265651.pdf. Accessed August 2018.

Mavaddat N, Peock S, Frost D, et al. Cancer risks for BRCA1 and BRCA2 mutation carriers: results from prospective analysis of EMBRACE. *J Natl Cancer Inst.* 2013;105:812–822.

NICE Guidelines for Early and Locally Advanced Breast Cancer. Available at: https://pathways.nice.org.uk/pathways/early-and-locally-advanced-breast-cancer. Accessed August 2018.

Pinder SE, Shaaban A, Deb R, Desai A, et al. NHS Breast Screening multidisciplinary working group guidelines for the diagnosis and management of breast lesions of uncertain malignant potential on core biopsy (B3 lesions). *Clin Radiol.* 2018;73:682–692.

POSNOC. Available at: http://www.posnoc.co.uk. Accessed August 2018.

Public Health England. *NHS Breast Screening Programme. Clinical Guidance for Breast Cancer Screening Assessment.* 4th ed. 2016.

Sim YT, Litherland J, Lindsay E, et al. Upgrade of ductal carcinoma in situ on core biopsies to invasive disease at final surgery: a retrospective review across the Scottish Breast Screening Programme. *Clin Radiol.* 2015;70(5):502–506.

Sparano JA, Gray RJ, Makower DF, et al. Adjuvant chemotherapy guided by a 21-gene expression assay in breast cancer. *N Eng J Med.* 2018;379(2):111–121.

TAILORX. Available at: https://www.cancer.gov/types/breast/research/tailorx. Accessed August 2018.

Virnig BA, Tuttle TM, Shamliyan T, Kane RL. Ductal carcinoma in situ of the breast: a systematic review of incidence, treatment, and outcomes. *J Natl Cancer Inst.* 2010;102(3):170–178.

27

Common Vascular Conditions

CHAPTER OUTLINE

VASCULAR SURGERY

Introduction

Vascular disease affects the circulatory system, which consists of arteries, veins and lymphatics. Vascular pathologies affect blood flow and lymphatic drainage. Flow obstruction can lead to incomplete drainage or end-organ impairment and poor tissue perfusion. Abnormalities of the endothelial wall and vascular tissue can also lead to life-threatening conditions that require expedited treatment. Vascular reconstruction involves the art of plumbing, which can be broken down into three components: the inflow, the outflow and the conduit (the pipe) as well as the main pump, the heart. Without these, any vascular treatment is doomed to failure.

Arterial Physiology

Arterial disease exerts major haemodynamic effects upon the circulation, which in turn manifest as clinical symptoms and signs of the disease. Haemodynamics pervade most aspects of vascular surgery; hence, in order to understand these processes, it is necessary to have a basic grasp of normal arterial physiology.

Normal Arterial Physiology

Blood vessels represent a highly complex and dynamic network. The vessel wall serves as an insulator preventing dissipation of energy and also provides capacitance, maintaining the ability to store energy during the systolic phase of the cardiac cycle which is later released in the diastolic phase. This results in a more continuous flow of energy throughout the cardiac cycle.

Blood flow is governed by the following parameters:
- Blood pressure, velocity and blood viscosity
- The anatomy of the arterial tree
- The mechanical characteristics of the arterial wall
- The properties of the vascular endothelium

Blood Pressure

Conventionally, blood pressure (P) is measured in millimetres of mercury (mmHg). It is dependent upon:
- The force of cardiac contraction
- Circulatory volume
- Tone – the pressure exerted by the muscular effect of the arterioles

Resistance to Flow

The energy provided by the heart is transformed into heat. The viscosity of blood itself limits flow – it is three to four times more viscous than water and uses up energy. The configuration of the arterial tree, with multiple branches and bends, leads to inertial losses.

The diameter of peripheral vessels has the greatest effect on peripheral resistance and (given normal blood viscosity), at flow rates found within the human circulation, resistance increases markedly when vessel diameter falls below approximately 3 mm. Resistance in the human circulation is therefore from the:
- Microcirculation – small arteries, arterioles and capillaries (70%)
- Venous circulation (10%)
- Large and medium-sized arteries (20%)

Patients with significantly diseased large arteries, therefore, are often less affected than those with predominantly microvascular changes, such as those with diabetes.

Patterns of Arterial Flow

Three main forms are recognized:
- **Laminar** – when the motion of the blood can be described by a series of concentric rings parallel to the wall of the vessel; the flow velocity is greatest in the centre and least at the vessel wall
- **Turbulent** – a disorderly flow pattern where velocity varies randomly across the diameter of the vessel
- **Disturbed** – midway between laminar and turbulent where, at certain points in the circulation, there is transient disruption of laminar flow which is re-established further downstream.

In healthy individuals, the only part of the human circulation in which there is turbulent flow is the ascending aorta, although disturbed flow may occur at arterial branch origins. In the presence of atherosclerosis, turbulent flow is common.

Boundary Effects

The boundary layer is the blood flowing adjacent to the vessel wall. At branch points and where the lumen suddenly changes size, the layer may slow down, change or even reverse its direction, which is called boundary layer separation (BLS). BLS leads to complex local flow patterns at arterial bifurcations, anastomoses and sites of arterial disease. Atherosclerotic plaques have been observed to occur particularly at points where BLS leads to reversed or stagnant flow, e.g. at the carotid bifurcation (Fig. 27.1). The reasons for this are unknown but may relate to mechanical changes in frictional forces (shear stress) between blood and vessel wall or to prolonged contact between the blood and endothelium at these points.

Pulsatile Nature of Flow

Blood flow in vivo is pulsatile. The haemodynamic principles outlined above are useful but depend upon steady laminar flow within a straight, frictionless tube. In consequence, they do not provide a precise description of the events that occur in the human circulation. Therefore, instead of

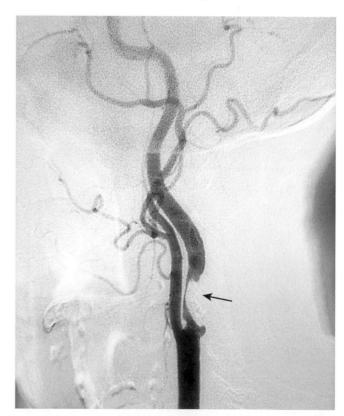

• **Fig. 27.1** Intra-arterial digital subtraction angiogram showing a 90% stenosis of the internal carotid artery (arrow). Note how the vessels proximal and distal to the lesion appear almost normal. This is one of the few areas of the body where arterial disease is often localized and thus amenable to endarterectomy.

using the term vascular resistance, *'vascular impedance'* better describes the opposition of the circulation to pulsatile flow and includes the effects of viscosity, bends, branches, changes in diameter, arterial elasticity (compliance) and wave reflections. In order that blood should flow, mean arterial pressure (MAP) must fall, although in health the gradient in MAP between the heart and the ankle is only of the order of 10 mmHg. Therefore, as the pressure wave moves distally, MAP and diastolic pressure fall. However, due to reflected waves from the distal circulation, systolic pressure actually increases and pulse pressure widens. For these reasons, in healthy individuals, the systolic ankle:brachial pressure index (ABPI) is normally slightly greater than 1 and does not fall on exercise. Very high ABPI measurements are abnormal as seen in diabetics due to vessel calcification and subsequent incompressibility. An accepted normal range for an accurately performed resting ABPI is 0.9–1.2 (ankle systolic pressure of 108–144 mmHg in a patient with a systolic pressure of 120 mmHg).

Phases of Arterial Flow

Arterial flow is normally triphasic, consisting of:
- An initial large forward flow caused by ventricular contraction
- A short period of reverse flow in early diastole
- A third phase of forward flow in late diastole

The duration of the reverse flow phase depends upon peripheral resistance: when increased (vasoconstriction on exposure to cold), the reverse flow period is extended; when decreased (exercise, exposure to heat) the opposite is the case.

Structure of the Arterial Tree

Arterial Wall Compliance

Blood flow is affected by the arterial wall itself and depends on the relative amounts of collagen, elastin and smooth muscle. The compliance (elasticity) of the artery allows blood energy to be stored during systole and to be returned to the blood in diastole. As the distance from the heart increases, the elastin:collagen ratio decreases so that the more distal arteries do not store as much energy in this way and act more as passive conduits.

Law of Laplace

This law describes the relationship between surface tension (*T*), radius (*r*) and intraluminal pressure (*P*):

$$T = Pr$$

Thus, the greater the diameter, the greater the tension in the vessel wall for a given blood pressure. This relationship also explains why blood pressure increases arterial wall stress and why hypertension is such a strong risk factor for aneurysmal dilatation, rupture and dissection (see later).

Abnormal Arterial Physiology

As can be seen, the haemodynamic forces in healthy individuals are complex, and become more so with the onset of disease.

Arterial Narrowing (Stenosis)

This is the commonest arterial lesion. Blood flow and blood pressure reduce at approximately the same magnitude of narrowing. Because flow along the length of the artery at a localized stenosis must remain constant, velocity increases. Thus, potential energy (pressure) is converted into kinetic energy and back to potential energy, costing energy as heat. If the stenosis is short, smooth, tapering and low grade, laminar flow is preserved and little energy is lost. By contrast, if it is long, irregular, abrupt and high grade, turbulence is produced and energy is dissipated.

Critical Arterial Stenosis

This is somewhat arbitrarily defined as a stenosis which produces a reduction in flow (and usually pressure) and is normally associated with a 50% reduction in diameter ($\approx$ 75% reduction in cross-sectional area – area = Πr^2). The greater the velocity of the blood, which flows into the stenosis, the greater the energy losses and so the greater the fall in pressure across the stenosis. Flow through stenosis can be augmented by exercise or any other factor that results in peripheral vasodilatation and so reduces the vascular resistance of the distal circulation. Therefore, a stenosis may not be haemodynamically and symptomatically significant (critical) at rest but becomes so at high flow rates. This is the basis for exercise or 'stress' testing – and is commonly seen in stenosed large vessels such as iliac arteries.

Atherosclerotic stenoses are frequently multiple. Viscous energy losses are proportional to the length of the stenosis, so one 4-cm stenosis is equivalent to two 2-cm stenoses of the same calibre. This is not true for inertial energy losses, as the two 2-cm stenoses cause more turbulence than a single 4-cm stenosis. Thus, a series of separately non-critical stenoses may act as one critical stenosis to reduce flow and pressure. When two lesions are of equal severity, both should be corrected; where they are not, the narrower one should be dealt with first.

Arterial stenosis leads to loss of energy and loss of pressure. At first, only peak systolic pressure (PSP) is affected, MAP being preserved. Reduction in PSP is thus the most sensitive measure of stenosis. Stenosis also leads to changes in the normal triphasic waveform, with damping of the PSP, loss of the normal forward flow in late diastole (biphasic pattern) and then loss of normal reverse flow in early diastole (monophasic pattern). Such changes can be used to assess arterial disease by non-invasive means such as hand-held Doppler ultrasound.

Collateral Circulation

The increase in size of vessels that run parallel to a site of obstruction is a vital compensatory mechanism that affects the clinical manifestations of arterial disease and potential treatment options. Through mechanisms that are not well understood, but which almost certainly involve a response by the endothelium to shear stress, increased flow through an artery leads to hypertrophy and dilatation. This enlargement of existing vessels provides an alternative pathway for blood flow. Effective collateral circulation is dependent upon the normal anatomy of the area involved. Disease of the superficial femoral artery with collateral flow through the profunda femoris system is perhaps the most common example of effective collateral circulation.

Collateral dilatation takes time, so that gradual development of a stenosis has a better outcome than sudden narrowing or occlusion. The formation of a collateral circulation can be augmented through exercise because the reduction in peripheral resistance on walking increases flow through the alternative pathway. A number of growth factors (such as vascular endothelial growth factor, nitric oxide) are secreted secondary to the induced ischaemia following exercise that contributes to the formation of new collaterals. However, no matter how well a collateral circulation develops, the vessels are of lower overall diameter than that which they replace, the peripheral resistance is greater and so the blood supply to the organ or limb is poorer.

Normal Arterial Anatomy

Arterial Wall Structure

Arteries are normally distensible, compliant and have three layers:
- **Intima** – a single-cell endothelial layer which rests on a basement membrane
- **Media** – separated from the intima by the internal elastic lamina, composed mostly of smooth muscle cells but also, in large vessels, containing numerous elastin fibres
- **Adventitia** – a meshwork of connective tissue which contains the vasa vasorum that provide blood to the media; between the media and adventitia is the external elastic lamina

Arterial Endothelium

The endothelium is not merely an inert lining (Box 27.1). The biology of the endothelial cell is complex and still imperfectly understood. Any disease process that leads to endothelial dysfunction has major effects upon arterial autoregulation, blood coagulation and fibrinolysis.

Effects of Ischaemia–Reperfusion Injury

Ischaemic Injury

All tissues rely on the circulation to deliver oxygen and nutrients and to remove the waste products of metabolism. Any pathological process that reduces the blood supply leads to the replacement of aerobic by anaerobic metabolism and the build-up of the potentially harmful products of metabolism, particularly carbon dioxide and lactic acid, with the accumulation of hydrogen ions. Through mechanisms that are poorly understood, tissues can adapt to a degree of ischaemia, especially if it develops gradually rather than acutely. However, after a certain point, irreversible

---

• BOX 27.1   Properties of the Normal Endothelium and Arterial Wall

Endothelium
- Controls microvascular permeability
- Non-thrombogenic, pro-fibrinolytic surface through production of prostacyclin, heparins and activation of fibrinolytic cascade
- Modulation of the inflammatory response through cytokine and adhesion molecule release or expression
- Modulation and initiation of thrombus formation through platelet and coagulation cascade activation
- Production of vasoactive substances such as nitric oxide, angiotensin-converting enzyme (ACE) and endothelin

Arterial wall
- Storage of blood energy
- Autoregulation – contraction and relaxation in response to myogenic and metabolic factors
- Lipid metabolism
- Production of connective tissue
- Arterial repair through migration and proliferation of smooth muscle cells

---

ischaemic injury and loss of function occurs, even if normal arterial flow is eventually restored. Tissues differ widely in their tolerance of ischaemia: irreversible damage to neurons occurs after only a few minutes, but skin may survive for up to 24 hours. This variability in tissue tolerance affects the clinical manifestations of arterial disease in different parts of the body as well as the urgency and success of surgical intervention.

Reperfusion Injury (RI)

When tissues are rendered ischaemic, the endothelium lining within the affected vascular bed is activated. Instead of providing a smooth, non-adherent surface, activated endothelial cells release pro-coagulant substances, express adhesion molecules that attract and bind leucocytes and release cytokines. Cytokines act upon the white cells to produce more cytokines and oxygen-derived free radicals. When the tissue is re-perfused, the activated endothelium produces an inflammatory response leading to tissue damage. In addition, some activated leucocytes and their products escape into the general circulation and can contribute to organ failure, such as renal failure, myocardial insult and adult respiratory distress syndrome.

Clinical Complications

Compartment Syndrome

Compartment syndrome occurs when the musculature within a fixed fascial compartment swells due to insult. When severely ischaemic tissues are re-perfused, the microcirculation is very permeable, and plasma leaks through the damaged capillary endothelium into the interstitial space. Ischaemic cells also swell because of membrane injury. Whilst arterial inflow continues, the microcirculation and then venous outflow is compromised leading to malperfusion and congestion. The overall result is marked tissue swelling and oedema, leading to a vicious circle of increasing pressure and poor tissue oxygenation. Clinically, the affected limb appears enlarged, with pain on palpation and plantar or dorsiflexion of the distal aspect, especially upon passive movement. Raised plasma levels of creatine kinase (CK) and myoglobinuria are characteristic but late features of compartment syndrome. Fasciotomy is therefore often necessary at the same time as revascularization. Abdominal compartment syndrome may also occur, often leading to renal failure and respiratory compromise. Treatment involves decompression of the affected compartment.

General Metabolic Effects
Ischaemic tissues essentially act in isolation until revascularized. On reperfusion, the re-instated blood flow washes out all the anaerobic and tissue damage metabolites leading to a sudden surge of toxins in the greater circulation. This often leads to arrhythmias and haemodynamic instability. Cardiac arrest even several hours later is not uncommon.

Myoglobinuria
Irreversible damage to muscle cells causes release of myoglobin into the circulation on reperfusion. Renal tubular injury and renal failure may follow. Management comprises adequate hydration and sometimes forced alkaline diuresis; however, this often leads to fluid overload and patients may require renal replacement therapy. It is a late phenomenon that should not delay treatment if compartment syndrome is suspected.

Reduction of Reperfusion Injury
Surgeons and anaesthetists take all possible measures to reduce reperfusion injury by minimizing the duration of ischaemia through expeditious surgery and/or the use of shunts to maintain the blood supply to the distant organ while the operation is completed. In addition, attention to fluid balance, oxygenation, anaesthetic management and staged reperfusion may help to attenuate the effects of reperfusion.

PATHOLOGICAL FEATURES OF ARTERIAL DISEASE

A distinction is drawn between macrovascular disorders, which affect large vessels, and microvascular ones, which involve the distal parts of the arterial circulation – the smallest arteries and arterioles.

Atherosclerotic Occlusive Disease

This is the commonest cause of arterial disease in developed countries. It is also known as 'arteriosclerosis' or 'atheroma' and to lay people as 'hardening of the arteries'. Atherosclerosis is found in virtually 100% of adults from developed countries and is responsible for 50% of all deaths.

The prevalence of atheroma increases with age but it is not regarded as an intrinsic part of the ageing process.

Definition
The World Health Organization defines atherosclerotic occlusive disease as a variable combination of changes in the intima which include focal accumulations of lipid, complex carbohydrates, blood and blood products, fibrous deposits and calcium deposits associated with secondary changes in the media.

Development
It is still far from clear how atheroma develops. The initial lesion of atherosclerosis involves the intima and begins in childhood with the development of focal intimal thickening with an increase in smooth muscle cells and extracellular matrix known as fatty streaks. Migration of smooth muscle cells into the intima results in apoptosis and macrophage infiltration and calcification. Further accumulation of connective tissue, lipid-laden smooth muscle cells result in the formation of the fibrous plaque. More advanced lesions present with necrosis in the lipid-rich core and calcification.

Aetiology
Smoking
Tobacco smoking is the single largest risk factor for arterial disease, and the risk is directly related to the number of 'pack-years' smoked. Tobacco smoke contains many hundreds of different chemicals, and it is unclear which are directly toxic to vascular endothelium. In addition, smoking increases blood viscosity and activates leucocytes. Cessation of smoking is associated with a rapid reversal of the adverse rheological changes and a reduction in the risk of future vascular clinical events.

Diabetes
Both insulin-dependent and non-insulin-dependent diabetes greatly increase the risk of atheroma. Lesions develop earlier in life and progress more rapidly. The distribution of atheroma may also differ from that found in non-diabetic patients – it progresses from distal small vessels proximally. Both secondary increases in blood lipid levels and changes in endothelial cell metabolism may be involved.

Hyperlipidaemia
The normal plasma level of cholesterol varies between populations: in the UK, 5–6 mmol/L is usual. Many of those with arterial disease have much higher levels. The measured total cholesterol level has three main components:
- High-density lipoprotein (HDL)
- Low-density lipoprotein (LDL)
- Very low-density lipoprotein (VLDL)
  in addition to chylomicrons. *Triglyceride* measurement forms part of the complete lipid profile.

Treatment is aimed at reducing levels of harmful LDL and increasing the proportion of beneficial HDL.

Raised plasma levels result from:

- A high-fat diet
- A genetically determined reduction in the removal of lipid and lipoproteins from the circulation (primary hyperlipidaemia); hyperlipidaemia is one of the commonest inherited autosomal dominant conditions (approximately 1 in 500 of the UK population)
- Secondary hyperlipidaemia caused by a variety of other conditions – diabetes, hypothyroidism, excessive alcohol intake and drugs (thiazide diuretics and corticosteroids)

The Heart Protection Study[1] has clearly demonstrated that lipid-lowering therapy with statins (hydroxymethyl-glutaryl co-enzyme A reductase inhibitors) is indicated for all patients with peripheral arterial disease (PAD). There was a 24% reduction in myocardial infarction, stroke and revascularization in patients randomized to statin therapy. Furthermore, this effect is independent of original cholesterol levels. For patients with PAD, 5 years of statin therapy is estimated to prevent 70 major vascular events per 1000 patients treated. In summary, all patients with PAD should be treated with a statin irrespective of their age and cholesterol levels. The Transatlantic Intersociety Consensus Document (TASC II)[2] from 2009 recommends that all patients should aim to have levels of LDL <2.59 mmol/L and patients with disease in multiple vascular beds should aim at levels <1.81 mmol/L. Current guidelines recommend 80 mg of atorvastatin or equivalent dosages.

Inflammation

Humoral and cellular pathways are involved in the presence of inflammation observed in atherosclerotic lesions. Oxidized LDL enhances the secretary role of macrophages which release a variety of inflammatory molecules, leading to enhanced expression of various cell surface adhesion molecules, smooth muscle cells and macrophages. They also contribute to the production of reactive oxygen species, stimulate matrix metalloproteinases and induce tissue factor expression.

Infection

Chronic infection may contribute to the pathogenesis of atherosclerosis. *Chlamydophila pneumoniae*, cytomegalovirus (CMV), *Helicobacter pylori*, enterovirus, hepatitis virus, herpes simplex virus and HIV have all been implicated.

Anatomical Distribution

Atherosclerotic disease is recognized as being a systemic disorder, with all vascular beds affected. However, although atheroma can be found throughout the circulation, it does not necessarily lead to disease states. Significant atheroma also has a predilection for certain sites – the carotid bifurcation, the coronary arteries, the infrarenal aorta and the superficial femoral artery. In any one patient, not all may be affected equally or indeed at all.

Complications

An atheromatous plaque may cause:

- Narrowing or occlusion, which can result in ischaemia and infarction
- Thrombosis
- Athero-embolism due to plaque rupture, affecting the distal circulation
- Weakening of the arterial wall with aneurysmal dilatation
- Periarterial inflammation

Aneurysmal Disease

The term aneurysm denotes an abnormal localized dilatation of a blood vessel >150% normal diameter. Almost any artery may become aneurysmal, although the commonest large vessel is the infrarenal aorta (>3 cm), followed by the iliac (>1.5 cm) and popliteal arteries (0.8 cm). It is a chronic degenerative disease with life-threatening implications.

Classification

- Anatomical – Aneurysms may be localized (saccular) or diffuse (fusiform).
- Pathological – They may be *true*, i.e. lined by all three layers of the normal arterial wall, or *false/pseudo*, i.e. formed in the adventitia or completely outside the wall.
- Aetiological – See below.

Aetiology

Atherosclerosis

There is continuing controversy over whether aneurysmal disease is just another manifestation of atherosclerosis. However, many believe it to be a separate condition – medial degenerative disease. Nevertheless, there is no doubt that aneurysmal disease shares the same risk factors as atheromatous occlusive disease (although hypertension appears a more pertinent risk factor) and that aneurysmal and occlusive arterial disease often coexist. It is likely that they are caused by localized arterial wall injury superimposed on the degenerative age-related changes, haemodynamics, systemic risk factors and probably a genetically determined predisposition. There is a strong familial element in aneurysmal but not in occlusive disease. Furthermore, some patients who have never smoked exhibit widespread aneurysmal dilatation (arterial ectasia or arteriomegaly) without any evidence of peripheral, cerebral or coronary occlusive disease. Risk factors associated with aneurysmal disease also include age, male sex, hypertension, smoking, chronic obstructive pulmonary disease (COPD) and connective tissue disorders. Even with successful management of life-threatening aneurysms, the long-term survival is significantly lower, with only 67% of patients with an abdominal aneurysm repair surviving to 5 years, compared with 81% of the age-matched population, and 65% of patients with a thoracic aneurysm repair surviving to 5 years compared with 89% of the age-matched population.

Inflammation

In some patients, atherosclerosis, whether associated with aneurysmal dilatation or not, can lead to an intense peri-adventitial inflammatory and fibrotic response. The reasons are unclear, but clinical problems can consequently occur. Inflammation is a histological feature in all aneurysms. However, approximately 10% of abdominal aortic aneurysms (AAAs) have an excessive inflammatory element: the anterior wall is extremely thick, and structures such as the ureters are often surrounded, causing obstruction and hydronephrosis or caval occlusion (peri-aortitis). There is no evidence that such aneurysms are any more or less likely to rupture, but operative repair can be technically very difficult. Patients frequently complain of abdominal or back pain, and their erythrocyte sedimentation rate (ESR) is usually raised. On computed tomography, the thickened aortic wall is seen to pervade surrounding tissues. Steroid treatment has been advocated to reduce inflammation and oedema in order to relieve pain, ureteric obstruction and to make aneurysm repair more straightforward. There is no evidence that steroid treatment reduces, and it may even increase, the risk of rupture. Endovascular treatment of an inflammatory aneurysm has become the first-line treatment in anatomically suitable aneurysms due to the reduced peri-operative complication profile.

Dissection

Weakness of the aortic wall may result in an intimo-medial tear and allow blood to track under pressure through and/or outwith the various layers of the wall. This may lead to dilation of the vessel and aneurysm formation, which usually affects the thoraco-abdominal aorta. Causes of the defect include:

- Atherosclerosis, usually with hypertension
- Marfan's syndrome or Ehlers-Danlos type IV (see later) in which there is a structural defect in the biochemical nature of the media

Infection

The arterial wall is normally highly resistant to bacterial and other infections. However, certain organisms (see 'Arteritis' later), notably *Salmonella, Staphylococcus* and *Treponema pallidum*, have a particular ability to infect, and thus to weaken, the aortic wall, leading to the formation of a mycotic aneurysm and its rupture. Prior to World War II and the development of penicillin, syphilitic aneurysms were far commoner, and typically involving the proximal aorta and arch. Currently, in developed countries, mycotic aneurysms account for less than 1% of all aneurysms.

Aneurysm Complications

Aneurysms are treated to prevent or manage complications, the most notable of which is rupture. Other complications include thrombosis and distal embolization. Less frequently, aneurysms cause external compression or stretching of surrounding structures – the bronchus or recurrent laryngeal nerve (thoraco-abdominal) or the duodenum (infrarenal aorta).

Arteritis (Vasculitis)

Vasculitides are defined by the presence of leucocytes in the vessel wall with reactive damage to mural structures. Arteritis can cause macrovascular complications such as ischaemia and aneurysm. Other patients may present with Raynaud's phenomenon.

Aetiology

Vessels of any size may be affected. Inflammation may damage the vessel wall directly through effects on the endothelium and/or vasa vasorum or indirectly through immunological mechanisms.

A range of arteritides are attributed to immunologically mediated injury. They may or may not occur in association with arthritis, myositis and myocarditis as part of a defined disease such as systemic lupus erythematosus (SLE). In the majority, the inducing antigen is unknown. These hypersensitivity arteritides may be further classified on the basis of the histological changes in the arterial wall.

Pathological Features

Inflammation may be acute or chronic and associated with necrosis, fibrosis or granuloma formation in the vessel wall. The clinical features depend largely upon the size, type and anatomical distribution of vessel(s) affected, together with the chronicity and severity of the inflammatory process. Acute forms may have a sudden and dramatic onset, progressing to death, with all the lesions at the same stage of development. Chronic forms may have an insidious onset, a waxing and waning course, with lesions in various stages of progression and remission. Early diagnosis is important because many patients respond quickly to medical treatment but, if left untreated, have a poor prognosis (Table 27.1). Although there is no universally accepted classification of the arteritides, they may be grouped on the basis of aetiology, type of vessel affected and symptoms. There is an increasing tendency simply to use the term vasculitis.

The dominant feature may be:

- **Necrotizing:** Inflammation is associated with segmental necrosis of the vessel wall, which often contains a considerable amount of fibrin (fibrinoid necrosis).
- **Acute inflammatory:** There is a short history and usually an identifiable antigen, often a drug. Small veins, arteries and capillaries are affected by an acute inflammatory response. Lesions may progress rapidly (even to death), be self-limiting in response to withdrawal of antigen or may become chronic.
- **Chronic inflammatory:** Although these are characterized by a chronic inflammatory reaction, presumably in response to repeated exposure to an antigen, often the source is unknown.
- **Granulomatous:** Inflammation is associated with the development of granulomas, with or without the presence of giant cells.
- **Fibrosis:** Excessive fibrosis is found in the vessel wall.

TABLE 27.1 Investigation of Vasculitis.

Investigation	Results and comments
Acute-phase proteins • C-reactive protein (CRP) • Complement factors (C)	CRP, C3 and C4 usually elevated; useful for diagnosis and monitoring treatment
ESR	Usually elevated; less responsive than CRP
Autoantibodies • Antinuclear antibody • Anti-double-stranded DNA • Anticentromere • Extractable nuclear antigen • Anticardiolipin • Antineutrophil • Anti-citrullinated protein antibodies (ACPAs)	May be of primary pathogenic significance or may simply be secondary markers of tissue injury; most helpful in the diagnosis of defined connective tissue disorders such as SLE, scleroderma and CREST syndrome
Serum electrophoresis • Cryoglobulins	Serum immunoglobulins (Ig) are usually non-specifically elevated; monoclonal Ig (paraproteins) may be present; some paraproteins (cryoglobulins) precipitate on cooling and damage skin vessels
Urinalysis	High incidence of renal involvement in arteritis mandates examination of the urine for protein, blood, casts and red cells. Plasma creatinine as well as 24-hour urinary protein and creatinine clearance should be performed
Biopsy • Renal • Temporal artery	If positive may confirm arteritis and aid more precise diagnosis; negative biopsy does not exclude arteritis because lesions are focal and can be missed
Imaging • CT • MRI	May identify vasculitic lesions in deep organs
Echocardiography	Assesses myocardial and valvular function in patients with myocarditis, endocarditis, aortitis and coronary artery aneurysms (Kawasaki disease)
Angiography	Delineates the pattern of large-vessel disease; allows planning of arterial reconstruction (Takayasu's disease)

Surgical Arteritides

Vasculitides are classified predominantly by the size of the vessels affected. Recently, the presence of antineutrophil cytoplasmic antibodies (ANCAs) can further subclassify the disease.

Large-Vessel Vasculitis

Giant Cell or Temporal Arteritis

This is a chronic vasculitis affecting large and medium-size arteries. It mostly involves the cranial branches of the arteries originating from the aortic arch. The temporal and retinal arteries are frequently involved in this condition. Arm vessels may also be affected.

Clinical Features

Symptoms. In retinal artery disease, blindness is the leading symptom, which may cause presentation to a vascular surgeon with the mistaken diagnosis of a transient ischaemic episode from a lesion in the carotid artery. Scalp tenderness, claudication of jaw, tongue or with deglutition can also be presenting symptoms.

Physical Findings. Usual findings are:
- evidence of hypertension
- a tender, thickened temporal artery
- loss of vision

Investigation.
1. Bloods: A markedly elevated ESR (>50 mm/h) will be found.
2. Biopsy: The diagnosis is confirmed by removal of a segment of temporal artery, which shows a necrotizing arteritis with a predominance of mononuclear cells or a granulomatous process with multinucleated giant cells.
3. Alternative methods that aid in diagnosis and management include ultrasonography of the temporal artery, which shows a characteristic halo; or resolution of symptoms on commencement of high-dose steroids. Any patient with suspected temporal arteritis is commonly commenced on high dose corticosteroids prior to biopsy, and so extensive delay to biopsy may lead to normal histology.

Takayasu's Arteritis

This condition primarily affects the aortic arch (and its branches) in young women. It can affect the entire aorta or be localized.

Clinical Features

Symptoms. Most patients suffer a vague prodromal illness followed, after a variable period of time, by symptoms and signs of vascular occlusion – most commonly arm claudication, syncopal attacks and visual disturbance.

Physical Findings. These will depend on the arterial bed involved. Stenosis, occlusion, thrombosis, secondary atherosclerosis and aneurysmal dilatation of affected vessels are all seen.

Investigation and Management. Apart from an acute-phase response, there are no specific markers of the disease.

Primary treatment is with steroids and immunosuppressants, but vascular reconstruction is sometimes required.

Medium-Sized-Vessel Vasculitis

Polyarteritis Nodosa

This is a systemic necrotizing vasculitis that affects medium and small-vessel disease and which may lead to ulceration and gangrene of the digits or mesenteric ischaemia.

Kawasaki Disease

This occurs mainly in children, and is often associated with a mucocutaneous lymph node syndrome. It is most commonly noted in the coronary arteries.

Isolated Central Nervous System Vasculitis

This affects medium and small arteries over a diffuse area of the central nervous system with corresponding symptoms.

Small-Vessel Vasculitis

Churg–Strauss Arteritis

This involves mainly small arteries of the lung and skin but can also be generalized. It is often associated with vascular and extravascular granulomatosis. Patients classically present with asthma and an eosinophilia. The condition responds to steroid therapy.

A number of other small-vessel vasculitides have been described such as Wegener's granulomatosis, microscopic polyarteritis, hypersensitivity vasculitis, essential cryoglobulinaemic vasculitis and also vasculitides secondary to viral infections and connective tissue disorders.

Systemic Sclerosis (Scleroderma)

This condition commonly presents with Raynaud's syndrome (see later) many years before other features of the disease become apparent. It may progress to tissue loss with ulceration and gangrene of toes and fingers that may require amputation. The Calcinosis, Raynaud's, Oesophageal motility disturbances, Sclerodactyly, Telangiectasia (CREST) syndrome is a variant.

Systemic Lupus Erythematosus (SLE)

This condition may also present because of Raynaud's phenomenon. The reader is referred to appropriate medical textbooks for detailed description of this and other connective tissue diseases discussed in this section.

Miscellaneous Conditions

There are a number of other conditions that are associated with arterial disease.

Behçet's Disease

This condition is characterized by orogenital ulceration and vasculitis. It is associated with venous thrombosis and thrombophlebitis, as well as arterial aneurysm and occlusion.

Buerger's Disease (Thromboangiitis Obliterans)

This may be a form of atherosclerosis or, perhaps more likely, a type of inflammatory arteritis. Small, rather than large and medium-sized, arteries are affected. Veins may also become involved and develop thrombophlebitis. Femoral and popliteal pulses are often normal, but pedal pulses are absent. Young male smokers are almost exclusively involved, and there appears to be a genetic element in that the incidence is particularly high in certain ethnic groups. Symptoms of peripheral vascular insufficiency nearly always begin before the age of 30. Complete cessation of smoking allows collaterals to form and is associated with a good prognosis, but failure to refrain almost inevitably leads to major amputation.

Connective Tissue Disorders

There are four main connective tissue disorders requiring vascular surgery expertise.

Marfan's Syndrome

This is a familial autosomal dominant disorder in which the basic underlying defect is a mutation in the fibrillin gene (FBN 1) on chromosome 15; penetrance can be variable. The physical characteristics are:
- Long fingers
- High arched palate
- Lens dislocation
- Focal medial necrosis of the aorta, which may lead to aortic valve root dilatation and incompetence, dissection of the ascending aorta and thoraco-abdominal aneurysm formation

Ehlers–Danlos Syndrome

This is a familial disorder of collagen with multiple subtypes. Patients are 'double-jointed', have wide scars and carry a high mortality from aneurysm rupture. Types I and IV are of most concern, with type IV presenting with arterial, bowel or uterine rupture.

Loeys–Dietz Syndrome

These conditions are highly complex and require referral to tertiary centres. Intervention thresholds are in general at smaller diameters and most will undergo multiple interventions during their lifetime. Endovascular repair is felt to serve the patients poorly in the long term and investigations must be tailored to their age, co-morbidities and extent of disease.

Fibromuscular Dysplasia

This is characterized by arterial stenoses and dilatations and results in a typical 'string of beads' appearance on angiography. It most often affects the renal and carotid arteries in young women and is amenable to endovascular treatment.

Patient Assessment

History

Accurate recording of the nature, severity, onset and duration of symptoms is vitally important. Relevant past medical history and existing co-morbidities, with particular emphasis on cardiac disease (angina, myocardial infarction), hypertension (severity, duration, treatment and quality of control), cerebrovascular disease (transient ischaemic attacks (TIA), amaurosis fugax and stroke), renal disease (renal failure, requirement for dialysis) respiratory disease (COPD, emphysema, asthma) and diabetes is also mandated. History taking should aim at identifying the five key risk factors for peripheral vascular disease: smoking, hyperlipidaemia, diabetes, hypertension and family history. Nutritional status, baseline physical activity levels and overall fitness are also important and key determinants of treatment outcomes.

Systematic Enquiry

Ask the patient about the following:
- A history of allergy – particularly to iodine, which may be considered as a contrast medium for arteriography
- Drug therapy, past and present:
  - angiotensin-converting enzyme (ACE) inhibitors and non-steroidal anti-inflammatory drugs (NSAIDs), which may precipitate renal failure in patients with renal artery stenosis and borderline renal function
  - anticoagulant therapy, in case invasive investigations and/or surgery are being contemplated
- Symptoms of arterial disease elsewhere (arterial disease is nearly always multisystem) – e.g. a patient with leg ischaemia frequently has significant coronary artery and cerebrovascular disease which predispose to myocardial infarction and stroke.

Information may not be volunteered because the presenting features may supersede or mask disease elsewhere (claudication in the leg may limit exercise tolerance so that angina is not manifest, and, conversely, relief of leg pain may unmask cardiac pain).

Physical Findings

General

The examination begins the moment the patient enters the consulting room. An impression of general health, vigour and mobility are important in the management of arterial disease, especially if major surgery to prolong life or to improve its quality is to be considered.

Tobacco on the breath and/or staining of the fingers suggest recent heavy cigarette smoking.

Other relevant general findings are the presence of finger clubbing, anaemia, jaundice, lymphadenopathy, central cyanosis and degree of breathlessness, particularly the ability to lie flat on the examination couch (those with arterial disease often have a history of cardiorespiratory disease). Gouty tophi are infrequently found, but hyperuricaemia accelerates atheroma and is amenable to

treatment. Xanthomata or xanthelasma may suggest treatable hyperlipidaemia.

Weight loss and cachexia are not usually caused by arterial disease except when the mesenteric vessels are involved. They do, however, play a key role in patients' overall physiological reserve. If they are a striking feature, the cause should usually be sought elsewhere and nutritional status should be optimized prior to major surgical intervention.

Assess mental state and coherence. A previous stroke may be evident from paralysis of a limb, hemiplegia or speech disturbance and can indicate carotid artery disease. It must be remembered that the atherosclerosis is a systemic disorder and so small-vessel cerebrovascular disease is common and that cognition may be moderately impaired.

Walk with the patient and observe how he or she copes with a flight of stairs in order to determine the march tolerance and general level of fitness.

Cardiovascular Examination

Pulse rate and rhythm, in particular the presence or absence of atrial fibrillation, are established. Blood pressure should be recorded in both arms because subclavian artery (mainly left) disease is relatively common. Although minor differences of 10–15 mmHg are not diagnostically significant, they may affect the accuracy and interpretation of future blood pressure monitoring. Subclavian artery disease may also preclude the use of an axillofemoral graft. Supra-aortic pulses (carotid, subclavian, axillary) should be gently palpated and the presence of bruits sought. A prominent carotid pulse usually signifies a tortuous vessel rather than an aneurysm. The presence of a carotid bruit is not pathognomonic of stenosis and is unreliable, but its presence does increase the likelihood of a significant stenosis.

The heart and precordium are examined to elicit the presence of murmurs and evidence of left ventricular hypertrophy (displacement of the apex beat).

The abdomen must be fully uncovered from xiphisternum to the groin. Look for abnormal pulsations (Fig. 27.2). Note any scars. Palpation is gentle because both normal and aneurysmal aortas are often tender. The most important measurement in an aneurysm is width (maximal transverse diameter), not length, and allowance must be made for the thickness of the abdominal wall musculature and fat. It can

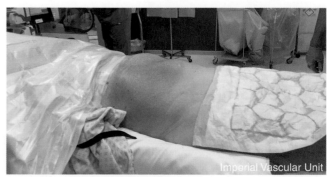

• **Fig. 27.2** A large abdominal aortic aneurysm is obvious on inspection of the abdomen in this thin patient.

be difficult to distinguish between the transmitted pulsation of an upper abdominal mass (including faeces in the transverse colon) which overlies the aorta and the expansile pulsation of an aneurysm. Positioning the patient so that the mass is no longer resting on the aorta may make the distinction obvious. Assessment of the possible presence of an aortic aneurysm, even by experts, is notoriously unreliable – sensitivity has been shown to be as low as 31%, and physical findings should be confirmed by ultrasound. The normal aorta bifurcates at the level of the umbilicus (L3–4), and abnormal pulsations below this area are usually iliac in origin. Aortocaval fistula is associated with a machinery murmur on auscultation, and stenoses of the aorto-iliac, mesenteric and renal arteries may produce a systolic bruit, but once again the sensitivity of auscultation is poor. The presence of scars indicative of previous surgery should be noted as this can be highly relevant when planning intervention.

Lower-limb pulses should be noted together with any accompanying bruits. The femoral pulse is usually easy to feel at the mid-inguinal point (below the inguinal ligament midway between the anterior superior iliac spine and the pubic symphysis). The popliteal pulse is felt on deep palpation in the popliteal fossa with the knee flexed to relax the popliteal fascia. It is usually difficult to feel; if it is very obvious, then the examiner should consider the possibility of a popliteal aneurysm. The posterior tibial pulse is felt between the medial malleolus and the Achilles tendon. The dorsalis pedis artery is a continuation of the anterior tibial and is felt on the dorsum of the foot just proximal to the groove between the first and second metatarsals, lateral to the tendon of extensor hallucis longus. In 10% of healthy people, it is congenitally absent, the dorsum of the foot being supplied by a perforating branch off the peroneal which may be felt 1 cm medial to the lateral malleolus at the ankle. Features of chronic ischaemia in the legs are loss of hair, pigmentation, ulceration, pallor or gangrene. Elevation of the severely ischaemic foot causes pallor and guttering of the veins. Dependency produces a reddish-blue appearance from the presence of desaturated blood within the skin – the sunset foot. Buerger's test for chronic limb-threatening ischaemia (CLTI, previously critical limb ischaemia or CLI) is assessment of the angle at which the leg becomes pale whilst the patient is lying flat. In the healthy patient, the leg should be pink at 90 degrees. In the presence of arterial disease, a sunset foot on dependence due to reactive hyperaemia is seen. Tissue loss is usually obvious, although lesions of the heel and between the toes are easily missed if examination is cursory.

Neurogenic Claudication

In a small proportion of patients with intermittent claudication, pedal pulses are palpable. Spinal or neurogenic claudication, where pain is caused by nerve root compression, must be considered especially if the patient complains of lower back pain. In this condition, pain often affects the thigh and the calf equally, is present on standing not just walking and is usually relieved only by sitting or lying down, not just by ceasing to walk. Straight leg raising may be impaired, and there may be subjective and objective neurosensory loss. There may be muscle wasting or reduced reflexes, and the femoral nerve stretch test may be positive. Arterial and neurogenic claudication sometimes co-exist and it is therefore important to establish which one is the predominant cause. An MRI scan of the lumbar spine when in doubt is recommended to exclude the presence of active nerve impingement prior to embarking on arterial revascularization.

Venous Claudication

Obstruction to venous outflow produces a bursting pain in the calf on walking. Unlike arterial and neurogenic claudication, the pain is usually only relieved by elevation, the leg is chronically swollen and there is usually a clear history of previous deep-vein thrombosis. Arterial pulses are almost always present even though it may be difficult to feel due to oedema.

Investigations

A careful history and examination will provide the majority of information required, especially symptom burden. The surgeon will also usually have at this point a fairly clear idea of the treatment options available.

Investigations should start with non-invasive testing where possible, aiming to obtain the most information, in the safest and most suitable way for the patient and for the least cost. There must also be a clear idea how the results of any particular test will affect the management. A significant proportion of patients do not require surgical intervention, either because their symptoms are mild, not vascular or because their general condition renders surgery too hazardous or unlikely to make a difference to their overall status and quality of life. In such patients, complex investigations are rarely indicated unless it is thought desirable to establish a baseline against which progression can be measured.

Although arteriography gives excellent anatomical information about the arterial circulation of the lower limb, it is expensive, invasive and not without hazard. In addition, although intra-arterial pressures can be measured at angiography, the investigation provides little haemodynamic information. Therefore, non-invasive sonographic studies that can be performed routinely and safely are preferred as a first-line imaging modality. These provide functional information through measurement of blood pressure, limb volume and flow velocity.

Risk-Factor Assessment

A major role of the vascular surgeon is to identify risk factors for arterial disease that influence primary and secondary prevention and optimize outcomes if intervention is to be considered (Box 27.2). Up to a fifth of patients with arterial occlusive disease are diabetic, although in up to half of these, the diagnosis may not have been made before the onset of vascular symptoms. A third to a half of vascular patients may have hyperlipidaemia requiring control with diet and/or medication. Other risk factors include hypertension, smoking, lack of exercise and obesity.

Reduction in blood cholesterol concentrations in patients with hyperlipidaemia and coronary artery disease can reduce death from myocardial infarction by up to a third. There is increasing evidence that careful glycaemic control in diabetics reduces the vascular complications of the disease, and treatment of even mild hypertension markedly reduces the risk of stroke. Cessation of smoking is associated with a reduction in vascular events and with increased long-term patency of arterial reconstruction. The approach to vascular disease should be adopting a healthier lifestyle change, including individual risk-factor control and also exercise. Vascular centres should offer risk-factor, lifestyle management and supervised exercise clinics as part of vascular patient care. Best medical therapy is crucial in improving outcomes of vascular patients, who have far poorer life expectancy than age-matched controls. International guidance now recommends an antiplatelet agent, high-dose statin and optimal blood pressure control for all arteriopaths.

Ultrasound

The principles of ultrasound investigation are discussed in Chapter 15.

Ankle:Brachial Pressure Index

This can be measured by detection of pulsation at the arm and foot vessels with a Doppler probe as the pressure is gradually reduced via cuff inflation, in a resting patient lying down.

Normal pedal pressure is usually 10–20 mmHg higher than brachial pressure, and the normal ABPI is around 1.1. An ABPI of less than 0.9 normally indicates a haemodynamically significant lesion (which may be asymptomatic); 0.5–0.8 is

associated with claudication; <0.5 with critical ischaemia and rest pain; and less than 0.3 often indicates tissue loss – ulceration or gangrene. There is considerable variation between patients, with proximal lesions and multilevel disease having a greater effect on the ABPI than isolated distal disease. For an individual, the trend in ABPI over time is more important than the absolute value. ABPI can also be used as surveillance post-intervention. After successful surgery or angioplasty, the ABPI should rise by at least 0.15; a subsequent similar fall suggests that re-occlusion has taken place.

Non-Compressible Vessels

Calcified crural vessels, most commonly but not exclusively found in diabetics, may not be compressible, and the ABPI is then falsely elevated. In these cases, toe pressures (using appropriate cuffs) can be obtained. Digital arteries tend to be affected less by calcification and therefore are more reliable.

Post-Exercise ABPI

After exercise, increased cardiac output and reduced peripheral resistance raise flow velocity to the point where pressure across the stenosis begins to fall. A reduction in ABPI after exercise may therefore unmask mild to moderate disease. Reactive hyperaemia may be used as an alternative to exercise when the general state precludes treadmill exercise. A cuff is placed on the thigh, inflated above systolic pressure for 5 minutes and then released. The temporary ischaemia distal to the cuff causes reactive vasodilatation which leads to a phase of hyperaemic flow when the cuff is removed. The fall in ABPI on reactive hyperaemia correlates well with that found after exercise, but treadmill testing has the added advantage of offering an assessment of the patient's overall fitness and of cardiorespiratory function.

Segmental Pressures

By placing cuffs around the upper thigh, lower thigh and calf, the level of lesions causing significant falls in pressure can be determined.

B-Mode Ultrasound

This procedure is principally used in vascular surgical practice to screen for, assess the size of and follow the time course of aneurysms, particularly in the abdominal aorta (Fig. 27.3).

Duplex Ultrasound

This has revolutionized vascular surgery and yields simultaneous anatomical and physiological information on flow in a variety of arteries safely, non-invasively and repeatedly. Duplex is used in many areas affected by occlusive and aneurysmal arterial disease (Fig. 27.4). Disadvantages include potential variation in scan interpretation which requires significant experience and is operator-dependent.

Assessment of Stenosis

When blood flows through an arterial stenosis, velocity increases. The high-speed jet can be localized on B-mode

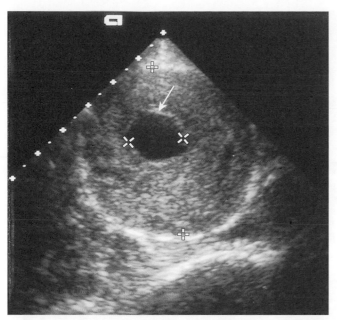

• **Fig. 27.3** A B-mode ultrasound scan, which demonstrates a transverse cross-sectional image of a large abdominal aortic aneurysm. The appearance has been linked to that of a fried egg. The bright circular band around the egg is the aneurysm wall; the white of the egg is the laminated thrombus within the aneurysm sac; and the yolk is the channel through the centre of the aneurysm where blood still flows (arrow).

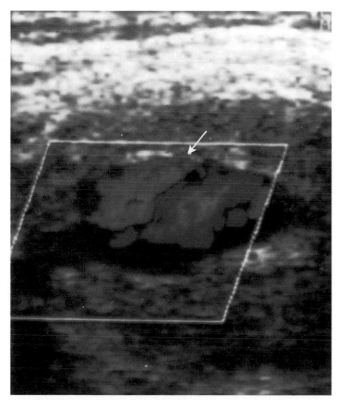

• **Fig. 27.4** A Colour Flow Duplex Scan of a Longitudinal Cross-Sectional Image of an Aneurysm The B-mode facility demonstrates the aneurysmal wall (arrow), while the colour Doppler indicates flow within the lumen; *red*, flow towards the ultrasound probe; *blue*, flow away from the probe. The appearance of red and blue flow within the aneurysm is indicative of turbulence.

ultrasound with the aid of colour flow mapping, and the precise velocity of the jet can be measured. The increase in velocity is proportional to the degree of stenosis and so, by comparing the velocities proximal (V_1) and distal (V_2) to the stenosis (V_1/V_2 ratio), an estimate of the degree of stenosis can be made. For example, in the internal carotid artery, a V_1/V_2 ratio greater than 4 together with a peak systolic velocity greater than 230 cm/s suggests a stenosis of greater than 70%. Similar assessments can be made at any other site where the artery lies superficially and can thus be insonated by the ultrasound beam. In many patients, reliable information can even be obtained from the aorto-iliac segments. Duplex can also be used to look for stenoses within arterial (vein) bypasses – graft surveillance. It is important, then, to determine which reporting method has been used, especially when comparing different scans, though cross-over tables have been produced.

Plaque Morphology

Duplex ultrasound also provides useful information about plaque composition. In the carotid artery, this may relate to a plaque's propensity to cause a stroke. Thus, the more lipid-rich and the less fibrous a carotid plaque, the more likely it is to be a source of atheromatous emboli which lodge distally to cause a stroke, TIA or amaurosis fugax (transient unilateral loss of vision secondary to occlusion of the retinal artery or its branches).

Plethysmography

This is the measurement of volume change: during systole, the limb expands with arterial inflow and during diastole, it contracts with venous outflow. Several types of instruments are available, but the simplest to use is the air plethysmograph (APG), also known as the pulse volume recorder.

Pneumatic cuffs are placed around the thigh, calf and ankle, and the cuff at the site to be assessed is inflated with air to a pressure of 60 mmHg so that the cuff is brought into light contact with the underlying leg. Any change in limb volume at that point produces changes in volume within the cuff such that the volume trace obtained closely resembles that of the arterial pressure wave. Air plethysmography is now more commonly used in the research assessment of the venous circulation.

CT Angiography

In vascular practice, CT angiography is most commonly used to examine the aorta in those with aneurysmal disease, occlusive disease or dissection (Fig. 27.5), the arch vessels and the lower limbs for stenosis or haemorrhage. Computer software systems can also generate three-dimensional volume-rendering reconstructions of the vasculature for planning purposes. It requires administration of intravenous contrast medium, which may precipitate pre-existing renal disease. Care should also be taken in patients with an iodine allergy.

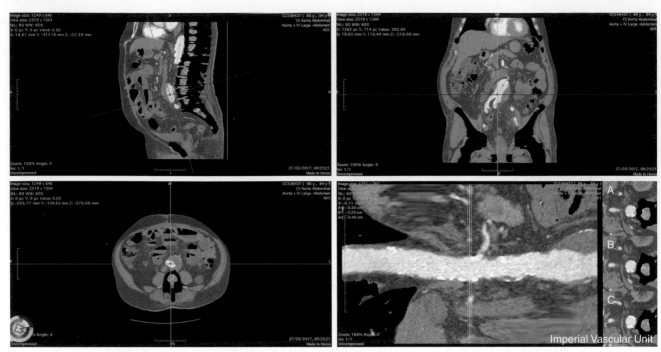

• **Fig. 27.5** Computed Tomography (CT) Scan Showing a Transverse Cross-Sectional Image of a Large Abdominal Aortic Aneurysm The examination has been performed with contrast so that the blood in the aneurysm appears white. The aneurysm is lined with a thin rim of thrombus. This particular aneurysm is an inflammatory one, as indicated by the marked thickening of the aortic wall. On the left-hand side, the ureter has become involved in the periaortic inflammatory processes, and there is a hydronephrosis.

Magnetic Resonance Imaging

By the use of different sequencing techniques, arteries and veins can be imaged with or without the injection of contrast medium. The use of MRI in cardiac imaging is relatively advanced, and by gating pictures to the electrocardiogram, real-time cine-loop images of the moving chambers and valves can be obtained. MR angiography (MRA) using gadolinium contrast has significantly improved the quality of the images. Recently MRA has been increasingly used for aortic surveillance especially in dissection patients and other thoracic pathologies.

Angiography

Despite the advances in non-invasive assessment described above, angiography remains the gold standard for many vascular pathologies providing simultaneous therapeutic endovascular solutions. Digital subtraction angiography (DSA) with intra-arterial administration of contrast medium, provides a 'roadmap' of the vasculature to be produced, by removing constant components of the image such as bones. However, it does require cessation of movement to ensure image quality (Fig. 27.6). It is invasive and access to the vessels is usually via a percutaneous approach. There are potential local access site complications including discomfort, infection, haematoma or pseudoaneurysm formation. Ultrasound-guided puncture is advised especially in highly calcified vessels or patients with unfavourable body habitus. Careful patient preparation is necessary (Box 27.3). Contrast allergy, impaired renal function and administration of certain drugs (e.g. metformin) need to be highlighted in advance and alternative imaging modalities considered. CT angiography and MRA are rapidly becoming credible noninvasive alternatives to DSA for diagnostic purposes.

TECHNIQUES

General Considerations

Vascular Prostheses
Synthetic Materials

Many of the techniques and prosthetic materials available in modern-day vascular surgical practice were not available as recently as 40 years ago. In particular, the development of durable, non-thrombogenic, sterile, prosthetic materials for the construction of arterial bypasses in the 1960s and 1970s was a major advance.

Prosthetic materials are used routinely in aorto-iliac surgery where the long-term patency of large-calibre, prosthetic reconstruction at a high-flow, high-pressure site is extremely good. The inner surface quickly becomes coated with protein, and at each end there may be some limited endothelial ingrowth. Externally reinforced grafts are coated with rings or a spiral of polypropylene. Many surgeons now use them routinely in order to overcome kinking or external compression, a particular hazard where a graft crosses a joint.

Biological tubular grafts obtained from cadavers (allografts or homografts) or animals (xenografts) and chemically treated

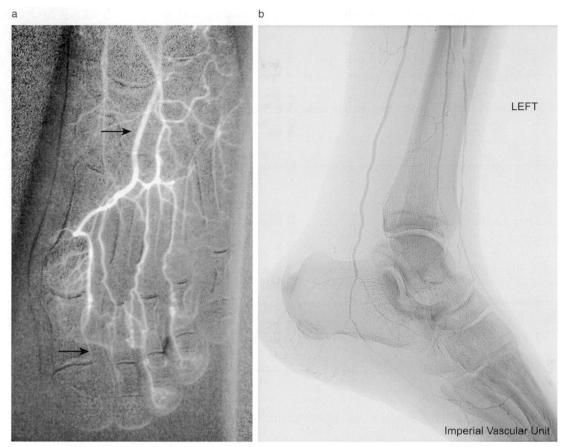

• **Fig. 27.6** Intra-arterial digital subtraction arteriogram showing filling of the plantar arch of the floor from the dorsalis pedis artery (arrow, upper). There is occlusion of the digital arteries to the great toe (arrow, lower) as a result of embolism from a proximal atheromatous plaque.

• BOX 27.3 Preparations for Angiography

- Informed consent
- Check for allergies to contrast/asthma
  - pre-intervention steroid administration
  - low iodine contrast
- Check for renal impairment
  - pre hydration with i.v. fluids
  - monitor fluid balance and U&E closely
  - stop nephrotoxic drugs
  - limit contrast load and consider alternative imaging
- Check for diabetes
  - stop metformin the day before

---

prostheses have been used since the late 1940s, but problems relating to availability, and concerns about cross-infection and late structural degeneration have limited their use. Nonetheless, bovine pericardium patches are commonly used.

Vein

Autologous vein (usually the great saphenous (GSV)) undoubtedly provides the best long-term results in medium- to small-calibre arterial reconstruction. The longer the graft, the more distal the distal anastomosis, and the poorer the run-off vessels, the greater the advantage. However, in a proportion of patients, the ipsilateral GSV is either unusable because of disease or has been removed for varicose vein or coronary bypass surgery. In such circumstances, vein can be harvested from other sites – the contralateral GSV, the small saphenous vein (SSV) or the arm. Pieces of vein can be spliced together to obtain the desired length for the bypass. Another advantage of autologous material is resistance to infection. A potential disadvantage is the relatively small size of arm and leg veins, which makes them generally unsuitable for aortic and iliac reconstruction. However, in exceptional circumstances, such as a grossly contaminated field, deep veins can also be harvested, spliced and panelled to form large-calibre conduits. In high-risk cases, the radial artery can also be harvested and used as a bypass conduit.

Use of Blood and Blood Products

Vascular operations are associated with greater blood loss than other surgical procedures, additionally contributed to by full anticoagulation. For these reasons, there is a particular requirement for effective and sometimes extremely rapid blood replacement. Interruption of the circulation to relieve occlusion or carry out bypass usually involves a temporary period of ischaemia for vital areas of the body. The combination of blood volume loss, ischaemia and reperfusion predisposes to coagulopathy, which may require correction with blood products such as fresh frozen plasma (FFP), cryoprecipitate and platelets.

Blood transfusion has its own shortcomings and complications. There is increasing enthusiasm for autotransfusion, which can be achieved in several different ways:

- **Predonation:** If the need for surgery can be predicted several weeks in advance, the patient can attend the blood bank and predonate their blood for their own later use. Although this overcomes problems with infection and incompatibility, the blood transfused still has the properties of that from the bank. This is seldom used due to storage and timing issues.
- **Isovolaemic haemodilution:** Blood is taken from the patient immediately before the operation and replaced with crystalloid; it may then be transfused back during the procedure. The advantage is that the retransfusion is of fresh whole blood. This is seldom used in practice.
- **Autotransfusion (cell saving):** Blood shed during operation can be collected by suction, washed and re-infused. This has become routine for major vascular interventions.

Pre- and Postoperative Management (see also Ch. 8)

Preoperative Management

The history obtained from the patient with arterial disease is the most important information to guide the surgeon and the team. Preoperative assessment (Box 27.4) should address three essential questions:

- Is vascular disease the cause of the patient's symptoms?
- What are the physiological effects or potential risks of the arterial segment affected?
- What is the operative risk?

Patients with vascular pathologies are usually older, with cardiorespiratory and renal comorbidities, are more likely to be diabetic and often have reduced physiological reserve. Multisystem disease (e.g. ischaemic heart disease, hypertension, COPD, renal impairment, diabetes) is the rule rather than the exception. Establishing the severity of symptoms and prognosis are essential as these are weighed against the risks of surgery or intervention. Preoperative assessment in conjunction with a focused anaesthetic review and risk-factor optimization are mandated prior to proceeding with major intervention. Pre-habilitation and early involvement of a vascular or care-of the-elderly physician and medical specialty teams is often required to ensure optimal perioperative outcomes. Elective in-hospital mortality rates for infrarenal aortic aneurysm repair, carotid endarterectomy and lower limb bypass are 1–3% for UK hospitals. Major amputation carries a 7–12% risk of in-hospital mortality.

Postoperative Management

Postoperative management (Box 27.5) varies according to the operative procedure. Careful monitoring of blood pressure is important after a carotid endarterectomy. Judicious management of the fluid balance is important after abdominal aortic aneurysm repair, with careful monitoring of the hourly urine output. Distal limb perfusion needs to be assessed frequently for signs of graft blockage or distal embolization (Fig. 27.7). Haematological parameters, electrolytes and indices of renal function need to be carefully monitored in all postoperative patients until normal diet has been resumed. All patients should be restarted on best medical therapy for atherosclerosis as soon as is appropriate: anti-platelet therapy, usually aspirin, high-dose statin, and antihypertensive medication. Some cases may require a period of formal anticoagulation, with variable rate unfractionated heparin, low-molecular-weight heparin (LMWH), warfarin or one of the direct oral anticoagulants (DOAC).

• BOX 27.5 Postoperative Management of the Vascular Patient

- Regular observations, particularly measurement of parameters assessing intravascular filling
- Observation of pulses distal to any reconstruction
- Neurological observations after CEA
- Wound or radiological puncture site observation
- Recommencement of anti-platelet treatment, prophylactic heparin or formal anticoagulation
- Objective measurement of ABPI if relevant

ABPI, Ankle:brachial pressure index; CEA, carotid endarterectomy.

• BOX 27.4 Preoperative Management of the Vascular Patient

- Check indication and side of operation (if relevant)
- Consent, with explanation of risks and benefits
- Measure ABPI where relevant
- Routine bloods and cross-match
- Consider beta-blockers
- Continue aspirin until day of surgery
- Thromboembolic prophylaxis with LMWH
- Antibiotic prophylaxis according to local protocol
- Intravenous hydration whilst nil by mouth

ABPI, Ankle:brachial pressure index; LMWH, low-molecular-weight heparin.

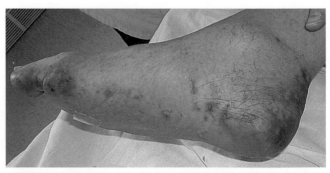

• **Fig. 27.7** Trash Foot Note patchy discolouration caused by a shower of small emboli.

Percutaneous Transluminal Angioplasty and Thrombolysis

Percutaneous Transluminal Angioplasty (PTA)

Vessel access is gained percutaneously via the modified Seldinger technique: needle puncture, guide wire through needle, sheath over guide wire. A wire is passed endoluminally through the site of stenosis or occlusion, i.e. lesion crossing. A PTA balloon catheter is advanced over the guide wire and the balloon is inflated to re-instate optimal flow within the diseased segment ensuring run-off is maintained. If there is significant balloon wasting or recoil in cases of high-grade stenoses or highly calcified plaques, a balloon expandable stent is deployed across the lesion acting as a metal scaffold to ensure patency (Fig. 27.8). For long arterial occlusions in patients unfit for bypass surgery, subintimal angioplasty recanalization can be attempted; this creates a false lumen within the subintimal layer through plaque disruption but does carry a risk of distal embolization.

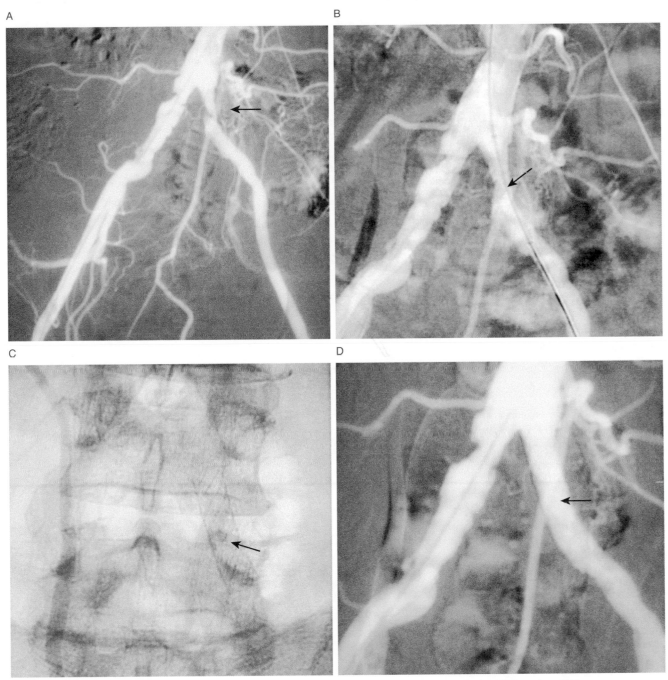

• **Fig. 27.8** Angiograms Showing Stages of Percutaneous Transluminal Angioplasty (A) There is a 90% stenosis of the left common iliac artery (arrow). (B) A guide wire (arrow) has been passed across the stenosis from a left common femoral arterial puncture, and the lesion has been stretched open by a 10 mm angioplasty balloon. (C) A metal stent has been positioned across the lesion (arrow) to prevent restenosis. (D) A final angiogram shows a widely patent left common iliac artery without residual stenosis.

Since PTA was first described, there have been major advances in technique and device availability for this less-invasive approach to revascularization. This has led to a reduction in open revascularization procedures overall, although the results for long-term durability are inferior to open bypass surgery.

Indications and Results

The TASC II document has categorized aorto-iliac and femoral lesions into four groups with specific evidence-based recommendations. For TASC A and B lesions, PTA should be attempted first, whereas TASC D lesions are best treated with open surgery. Controversy exists for TASC C lesions which can be treated by either approach after careful consideration and tailored for individual patient needs and according to each centre's experience. Figs 27.9 and 27.10 show the TASC II classification of aorto-iliac and femoral popliteal disease respectively.

Type A lesions

- Unilateral or bilateral stenoses of CIA
- Unilateral or bilateral single short (≤3 cm) stenosis of EIA

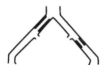

Type B lesions

- Short (≤3 cm) stenosis of infrarenal aorta
- Unilateral CIA occlusion
- Single or multiple stenosis totaling 3–10 cm involving the EIA not extending into the CFA
- Unilateral EIA occlusion not involving the origins of internal iliac or CFA

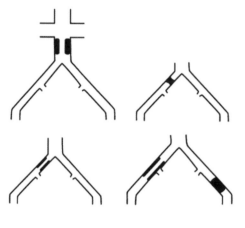

Type C lesions

- Bilateral CIA occlusions
- Bilateral EIA stenoses 3–10 cm long not extending into the CFA
- Unilateral EIA stenosis extending into the CFA
- Unilateral EIA occlusion that involves the origins of internal iliac and/or CFA
- Heavily calcified unilateral EIA occlusion with or without involvement of origins of internal iliac and/or CFA

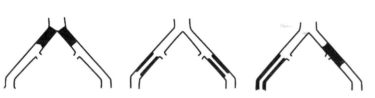

Type D lesions

- Infra-renal aortoiliac occlusion
- Diffuse disease involving the aorta and both iliac arteries requiring treatment
- Diffuse multiple stenoses involving the unilateral CIA, EIA, and CFA
- Unilateral occlusions of both CIA and EIA
- Bilateral occlusions of EIA
- Iliac stenoses in patients with AAA requiring treatment and not amenable to endograft placement or other lesions requiring open aortic or iliac surgery

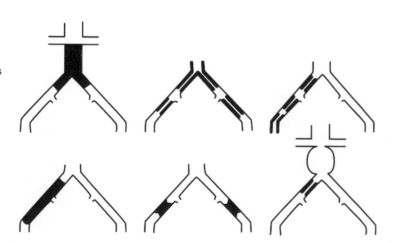

• **Fig. 27.9** TASC II classification of aort-iliac disease. (From Norgren L, et al. Inter-society consensus for the management of peripheral arterial disease (TASC II). J. Vasc. Surg. 2007; 45 (Suppl S), S5–67.)

Type A lesions

- Single stenosis ≤10 cm in length
- Single occlusion ≤5 cm in length

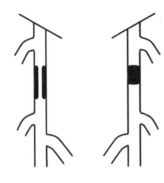

Type B lesions

- Multiple lesions (stenoses or occlusions), each ≤5 cm
- Single stenosis or occlusion ≤15 cm not involving the infrageniculate popliteal artery
- Single or multiple lesions in the absence of continuous tibial vessels to improve inflow for a distal bypass
- Heavily calcified occlusion ≤5 cm in length
- Single popliteal stenosis

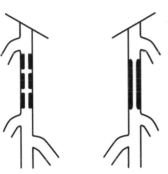
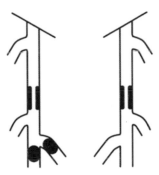

Type C lesions

- Multiple stenoses or occlusions totaling > 15 cm with or without heavy calcification
- Recurrent stenoses or occlusions that need treatment after two endovascular interventions

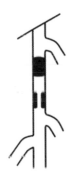

Type D lesions

- Chronic total occlusions of CFA or SFA (>20 cm, involving the popliteal artery)
- Chronic total occlusion of popliteal artery and proximal trifurcation vessels

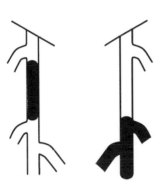

• **Fig. 27.10** TASC II classification of femoral popliteal disease. (From Norgren L, et al. Inter-society consensus for the management of peripheral arterial disease (TASC II). J. Vasc. Surg. 2007; 45 (Suppl S), S5–67.)

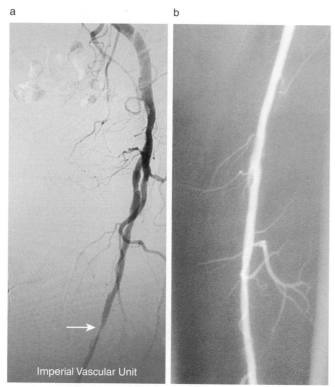

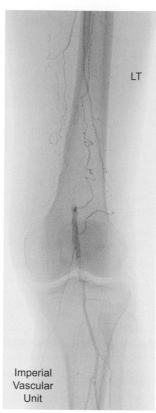

• **Fig. 27.11** Focal atheromatous plaque with attached thrombus in the right superficial femoral artery (arrow, (A)). This plaque had been the source of emboli to the toes and was treated successfully by angioplasty (B) and 6 months of anticoagulation with warfarin.

• **Fig. 27.12** SFA occlusion with reconstitution at the popliteal artery.

Aorto-Iliac Disease

The results of PTA are undoubtedly best in large, high-flow vessels, and it is often the treatment of choice in stenoses and occlusions of the aorto-iliac system.

Infra-Inguinal Disease

Recent developments in PTA, with the introduction of drug-eluding balloons and stents, have greatly expanded the treatment portfolio. However, limited level 1 evidence exists to guide the clinician. The BASIL trial (2005)[3] remains the only completed randomized study to date. Except in the uncommon case of a short stenosis of the superficial femoral artery (Fig. 27.11), the results of infra-inguinal PTA (usually performed for claudication) are disappointing. Some interventional radiologists strongly disagree with this view and claim good long-term success even after recanalization of long occlusions of arteries both above and below the knee. Fig. 27.12 shows a more complex occluded SFA with reconstitution at the popliteal artery. However, the BASIL trial indicates that the most durable results are seen in patients undergoing bypass procedures. Additional data from a meta-analysis of 20 000 patients by Wang et al. (2018)[4] supports this view.

Infra-popliteal intervention is technically demanding and high risk; as such it is reserved for severe disease with critical ischaemia and tissue loss (Critical Limb Ischaemia or Chronic Limb Threatening Ischaemia, discussed below).

The BASIL 2 and BASIL 3 studies, currently recruiting, are evaluating the outcomes of surgery versus PTA (BASIL 2) and PTA with different technologies (BASIL 3) for below the knee interventions.

Other Sites

Although the bulk of PTA is performed for lower limb ischaemia, the technique has been used in the carotid, renal and mesenteric arteries. The long-term outcomes of PTA and stenting in these areas remain to be defined. PTA is also successfully used to dilate stenoses within bypass grafts (graft surveillance), provided intervention is carried out at least 6 weeks following primary surgery.

Complications

Although percutaneous techniques are associated with less morbidity and mortality compared to open surgery, they are not without complications, and there is a significant early technical failure rate which depends on the clinical indications and the anatomical site. The main complications are related to the arterial puncture required to access the arterial tree: haematoma, false aneurysm formation, occlusion and thrombosis. Although many of these complications can be treated non-operatively, a proportion of patients require direct operative repair. Less commonly, angioplasty of a stenosed artery may lead to acute occlusion, worsening ischaemia and the need for emergency surgical revascularization or sometimes amputation.

Thrombolysis

Thrombolytic agents, such a streptokinase, urokinase and tissue plasminogen activator (TPA), differ from heparin and warfarin in that, rather than preventing clot formation, they actually lyse pre-formed thrombus. The technique involves infusing thrombolytic agents into the vessel to dissolve the clot to visualize the culprit lesion which can then be treated either surgically or by PTA. The exact indications for thrombolysis are difficult to define.

Complications

Thrombolysis is not without morbidity and mortality. Most complications are due to local or distant site haemorrhage, with an intra-cerebral bleed risk of approximately 1%. Thrombolysis is contraindicated after recent surgery and in the presence of active bleeding, significant peptic ulcer disease or a recent haemorrhagic stroke. It should be used with caution in the elderly population. Dissolution of clot can also lead to distal embolization, distal trashing and soft tissue damage. All patients undergoing thrombolysis should also be closely monitored for compartment syndrome.

Open Surgical Techniques

Endarterectomy

Endarterectomy was first described by Dos Santos in 1947. Before the advent of reliable prosthetic bypass materials, endarterectomy (open removal – coring out – of atheroma from inside a diseased artery) was the standard operative approach for occlusive arterial disease, especially in large-calibre vessels. However, the technique poses a number of challenges:

- It is technically demanding and maximally invasive.
- Unlike bypass surgery (see later), endarterectomy requires a very wide dissection of all, or almost all, of the length of the artery to be cleared.
- Arterial disease is generalized, and there are few instances where a diseased artery can be cleared to normal artery above and below the lesion; thus there is always a point of transition between the endarterectomised surface and the diseased intima of the adjacent vessel which, especially downstream, can form a ridge or a flap which is a focus for thrombosis, vessel occlusion and distal embolization.
- The technique involves the removal of intima and media, sometimes leaving only the adventitia, which can be very friable with a high risk of rupture and bleeding complications.

Closure of the vessel wall following endarterectomy often necessitates using a piece of vein or prosthetic material as a 'patch' in order to prevent narrowing of the lumen.

Endarterectomy is now much less frequently done except in certain specific sites, notably the carotid bifurcation and common femoral artery (Fig. 27.13).

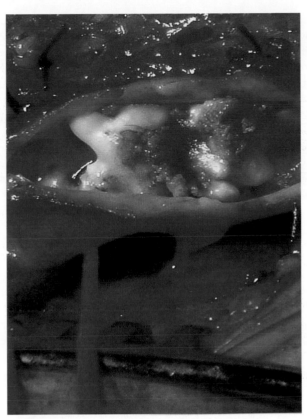

• **Fig. 27.13** Common Femoral Artery Exposed and Opened to Reveal 'Coral-Like' Plaque Which is Best Treated by Endarterectomy

---

CLINICAL BOX 27.1

Bypass Procedure

- Dissect out and control arteries above and below the occlusion
- Make a tunnel through the tissues to allow passage of the bypass
- Give systemic heparin
- Clamp arteries
- Construct proximal and distal anastomoses
- Flush out native vessels and the graft to expel any air or clot
- Complete anastomoses
- Remove clamps
- Re-establish flow
- Assess adequacy of graft flow and distal perfusion

Bypass Reconstruction

This is now the commonest procedure for occlusive arterial disease.

Technique

The technical aspects of the procedure are summarized in Clinical Box 27.1.

The indication for most bypass procedures currently performed in the UK is critical lower limb ischaemia, when failure to intervene and revascularize the leg often leads to amputation (25% by 1 year).

Bypass grafts are usually described in terms of their inflow, outflow and conduit (e.g. femoral to popliteal bypass with reversed vein). Bypasses can generally be grouped into those that are anatomical – the conduit follows more or less the same course as the native vessel (e.g. femoropopliteal) – and those that are extra-anatomical, where a different path is used (e.g. axillofemoral).

Embolectomy

There has been a steady decline in the proportion of patients developing acute ischaemia secondary to an embolus, as opposed to thrombosis from chronic atherosclerotic plaque. There are several reasons for this observation:

- A declining population of patients with valve damage and atrial fibrillation after rheumatic fever
- Increased use of warfarin and other anticoagulants in the management of atrial fibrillation
- Increased use of thrombolysis for myocardial infarction, which limits infarct size and the development of left ventricular mural thrombus

However, the prevalence of atrial fibrillation is actually increasing due to the increasing prevalence of old age, even if this is now well-managed.

Nevertheless, embolectomy is still frequently performed – especially in the arm, where an embolus has always been the commonest cause of acute ischaemia. Once the diagnosis of embolus has been reliably made on clinical assessment, perhaps supplemented by the use of angiography and normal pulses in the contralateral limb, the operation can be performed under local, regional or general anaesthesia. An embolectomy is also commonly performed intra-operatively or postoperatively following bypass procedures to treat graft, proximal/distal thrombosis.

Technique

The operation is summarized in Clinical Box 27.2.

Postoperatively, anticoagulation is continued. Investigations for a definite source of the embolus are required. An

---

CLINICAL BOX 27.2

Embolectomy Procedure

- Dissect out the relevant artery, usually the brachial in the arm or the common femoral in the leg, and control flow proximally and distally with tapes or plastic slings
- Give systemic heparin
- Open the artery via a transverse arteriotomy
- Pass balloon catheters (Fogarty) into the artery with the balloon deflated and then remove with the balloon inflated to extract the clot to establish inflow first and then outflow
- Establish the adequacy of clot extraction clinically, with intra-operative Doppler or by means of on-table angiography
- Close the arteriotomy with interrupted prolene if transverse (or with a patch of vein if there is concern about the artery being narrowed at that point)
- Re-establish flow and consider further procedure if not adequate

---

echocardiogram, 24-hour tape and imaging of major vessels should be performed and coagulation disorders excluded. In the absence of a proven source, a judgement must be made as to the appropriateness and duration of anticoagulation in collaboration with a haematology specialist.

Although most emboli lodge in the arm or leg, any arterial bed may be involved: e.g. the carotid artery, leading to stroke, or the superior mesenteric artery with bowel ischaemia. Only a small minority of emboli are the result of infective endocarditis or of tumour. However, it is routine to send a portion of the extracted clot for bacteriological culture and histopathological examination.

Sympathectomy

Limb Ischaemia

The sympathetic nervous system causes arteriolar constriction and, in the past, it was believed that by interrupting the sympathetic nerve supply to an ischaemic area, vasodilatation might improve the flow of blood. However, blood vessels in ischaemic tissues are already maximally dilated and, if sympathectomy does provide any benefit in severe distal ischaemia, it is likely that other mechanisms, such as alteration of pain perception, are responsible. With the increased use of arterial bypass for lower limb ischaemia, chemical sympathectomy is held in reserve for those with no revascularization options.

Hyperhidrosis

The sympathetic nervous system also innervates sweat glands. Upper limb (cervical or thoracic) sympathectomy is most often used for severe axillary and palmar hyperhidrosis if medical treatment fails. The operation used to be performed through the root of the neck but is now performed thoracoscopically. Lumbar sympathectomy is also of value in patients with severe plantar hyperhidrosis. The effect on sweat gland function is usually permanent. Repeated injections of botulinum toxin is an alternative for axillary hyperhidrosis. Cervical sympathectomy is less successful at this site compared to the palms.

The procedure is not without risks. Injuries to the pleura and great vessels are rare but can lead to major complications. Other complications include 'compensatory' increased sweating at other sites (trunk, thighs, face). Cervical sympathectomy carries a small risk of Horner's syndrome (drooping ipsilateral eyelids, constricted pupil and reduced facial sweating) and lumbar sympathectomy of sexual dysfunction.

Raynaud's Phenomenon

Cervical sympathectomy has been recommended for Raynaud's phenomenon (RP), but the long-term results in the hand are poor. Lumbar sympathectomy, however, may provide long-lasting relief in RP affecting the toes; the exact mechanism for this remains unclear.

Amputation

Indications

Ideally, no patient with critical ischaemia should undergo major limb amputation for peripheral vascular disease without assessment by a vascular surgeon. Arterial reconstruction, where possible, is by far the better option because of:

- Mortality – 10–20% for amputation
- Stump infection and ischaemia – both are common and, in up to 10%, lead to further amputation at a higher level; deep venous thrombosis and pulmonary embolus are also well-recognized complications
- Failed rehabilitation – 2 years later, less than two-thirds of below-knee and less than one-third of above-knee, unilateral amputees are independently mobile
- Financial cost – although a distal bypass operation for limb salvage may entail hospital expenditure in the region of £5000, a major limb amputation frequently costs 10 times as much once rehabilitation, artificial limbs and long-term care are considered

It is a medical, humanitarian and economic disaster to perform vascular reconstructive surgery which fails early. However, 50–75% of patients with critical limb ischaemia are dead within 5 years (mostly from cardiac and cerebrovascular events). Not all bypass procedures, therefore, are required to work for a prolonged period. Reconstruction should be attempted if there is at least a 75% chance of the bypass remaining functional for 2 years or to heal active ulceration. Sometimes, however, amputation is the only option in those with unreconstructable arterial disease and advancing tissue loss or with those with intractable pain or tissue loss and multiple co-morbidities who are deemed high-risk for major bypass surgery.

Level

Because rehabilitation is directly related to the amputation level, every effort should be made to preserve the knee if it is mobile, has adequate viable soft tissue coverage and there is a prospect of a prosthesis. Although numerous investigations have been proposed, there is not a single test which reliably predicts at which level an amputation will heal. Some patients will rehabilitate very well with an above knee amputation, and some will rehabilitate poorly with a below knee amputation. Level remains, therefore, largely a matter of clinical judgement. It is imperative that specialist rehabilitation and physiotherapy services are involved early in the care pathway as soon as the decision to amputate has been made. Fig. 27.14 shows a below knee amputation stump which is healing well.

Perioperative Pain

Preoperative. Many patients who require an amputation for critical limb ischaemia are in considerable pain. Adequate perioperative analgesia is vital for both humane reasons and because it hastens recovery and rehabilitation. The anaesthetist is usually closely involved in this aspect of care (see Ch. 8).

Postoperative. Phantom pain, a continuation or worsening of the pain experienced in the limb before amputation, often accompanied by a distressing sensation that the limb is still present, is common. Various treatments have been advocated such as electrical stimulation, pregabalin and gabapentin, low-dose amitriptyline and ketamine. There

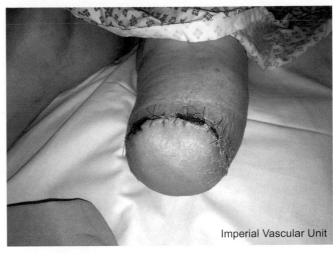

Imperial Vascular Unit

• **Fig. 27.14** Healing below knee amputation stump.

is some evidence that, if the patient is transferred to the operating room in a pain-free state, then the incidence of phantom pain is reduced. Epidural pain relief may achieve this end. Early work on postoperative nerve catheters has indicated that they are a useful adjunct.

Rehabilitation

Although an amputation might be considered a technically straightforward procedure, there are important surgical principles which have to be followed if the chances of stump healing are to be maximized. In addition to the surgical team, the successful postoperative rehabilitation of an amputee depends upon the close collaboration of other disciplines – physiotherapists, occupational therapists and prosthetists.

Management of Aneurysmal Disease

Abdominal Aortic Aneurysm (AAA)
Epidemiology and Aetiology

The prevalence of this condition has declined from 5% in 1991 to approximately 1.7% in 2014. It was, however, responsible for the death of 2113 men and 942 women in 2014 (0.7% of all deaths). The principal cause of death is rupture; distal embolization from aneurysm sac thrombus and less commonly, thrombotic occlusion can also lead to poor overall outcomes. The aetiology of aneurysmal disease is discussed earlier. Most patients are asymptomatic, although some may present with abdominal or back pain due to inflammation and compression of surrounding structures. Rarely, aneurysms may be present with life-threatening gastrointestinal bleeding secondary to an aorto-duodenal fistula.

Pathological Features

In keeping with the law of Laplace, an aortic aneurysm inevitably slowly expands, a process accelerated by hypertension and continued smoking. The rate of expansion is highly variable. Thus the lifetime rupture risk posed by a 5 cm AAA is considerably greater for someone aged 50 years than it is for someone over 75. Anterior ruptures are usually fatal, whereas rupture into the retroperitoneum can be managed with immediate surgery. The risk of rupture is related to the size of the aneurysm: the infrarenal aorta normally measures 1.5–2.0 cm in diameter and is considered to be aneurysmal when the diameter is larger than 3 cm. The reported annual risk of rupture varies widely but recent analysis suggests modern medical therapy and smoking cessation leads to rates of:

- 5.5–6 cm: 3.5% (i.e. 35% 10-year risk)
- 6.1–7 cm: 4.1%.
- >7 cm: 6.3%

Balancing the risks of surgery against those of rupture can be difficult in smaller aneurysms. The UK Small Aneurysm Trial[5] demonstrated that for stable AAAs of 4–5.5 cm diameter, surveillance was safer than surgery, as the rupture risk was approximately 1% per annum. This does not apply to saccular or mycotic aneurysms, rapidly expanding or symptomatic aneurysms and perhaps equivalent-sized AAAs in small females. Such patients should all be offered intervention. Currently, elective repair is normally offered to suitable patients if their AAA diameter is equal or above 5.5 cm, the rate of growth is more than 1 cm per year or if their aneurysm has become symptomatic.

Only one-third of patients with rupture reach hospital, and of those that are operated upon in highly-experienced centres, mortality still reaches 35%. Thus, the overall mortality for rupture is >80%, and possibly many other deaths occur from rupture of an undiagnosed, asymptomatic aneurysm.

Screening

The mortality for elective AAA repair in asymptomatic patients in vascular centres is less than 5%; early mortality is lower for endovascular versus open repair. It is therefore justifiable to detect and offer treatment to those whose aneurysm has reached threshold in an elective setting. Ultrasound-based screening of a target population has been introduced. Studies have shown that mass screening in men over the age of 65, and elective repair of asymptomatic aneurysms, can significantly reduce aneurysm-related mortality. The UK National Abdominal Aortic Screening Programme (NAAASP) was launched in 2008, screening all men over the age of 65 with a single ultrasound and has thus far screened 1.3 million men, with 4000 men referred for treatment of an aneurysm >5.5 cm (0.3%). Screening may be extended to first-degree relatives of known patients with AAA.

Clinical Features

In slim patients, the aneurysm itself as well as its transmitted pulsation may be visible on inspection. On palpation, there will be a pulsatile, expansile swelling in the midline of the abdomen, usually extending towards the left-hand side. However, it is important to appreciate that clinical examination alone, even when performed by an experienced vascular surgeon, may be unreliable for confirming the presence or absence of aneurysmal disease and for estimating the size of the aorta and aneurysm extent, especially in obese patients. Any suspicion of AAA should therefore prompt an ultrasound examination. Although AAA tenderness indicates actual or impending rupture, or the presence of an inflammatory component, this too is unreliable unless in experienced hands. There is an association between AAA and aneurysms elsewhere, so the examiner should specifically exclude the presence of femoral and popliteal aneurysms. The surface marking of the aortic bifurcation is at the level of the umbilicus, so any pulsation felt below this level is likely to denote the presence of iliac aneurysmal disease.

Management

Although, as described earlier, most AAAs gradually increase in size, the unpredictable nature of this disease mandates appropriate surveillance protocols, that are usually offered on an annual basis. Closer surveillance may be indicated for those approaching threshold.

Indications for Elective Repair. The decision to operate involves weighing the known risk of leaving the AAA in place against that of operation. The first depends upon:

- size
- presence of symptoms
- age and physiological state

Guidelines on size criteria for treatment of AAAs are given in Table 27.2. The risk of operation depends primarily upon the patient's cardiorespiratory status. Anaesthetists, cardiologists, vascular or care-of-the-elderly physicians can assist the surgeon in the decision-making process and subsequent rehabilitation for the patient. There is no benefit in repairing a small aneurysm at low risk of rupture in an elderly person with severe cardiorespiratory disease whose overall prognosis and life-expectancy is poor. Indeed, evidence suggests that those unfit for open surgery have poor prognosis even if the aneurysm is repaired (5-year survival of 28–46%), compared to those who are fit (66% and age-matched survival of 82% at 5 years).

27Technique. Procedure for infrarenal AAA repair is summarized in Clinical Box 27.3 and Emergency Box 27.1. Postoperative high-dependency critical care is routine

TABLE 27.2	Guidelines on Size Criteria for Treatment of Abdominal Aortic Aneurysms.
Criteria	**Treatment**
Symptomatic aneurysms regardless of size	Urgent surgery
Asymptomatic aneurysms of diameter <5.5 cm	Surveillance if increasing by <1 cm/year Elective surgery if increasing by >1 cm/year
Asymptomatic aneurysms of diameter >5.5 cm	Elective surgery

Procedure for Repair of Abdominal Aortic Aneurysm

- Open the abdomen through a long vertical midline or transverse incision
- Confirm the presence of an operable aneurysm and the absence of other disease which might affect prognosis, particularly colorectal cancer
- Dissect the neck of the aneurysm free by mobilizing the fourth part of the duodenum to the right with care to avoid injury to the left renal vein
- Dissect the iliac arteries free
- Administer a bolus dose of i.v. heparin, usually 3000–5000 units, and, after a delay of 1–2 minutes, clamp the iliac vessels first and then the aorta
- Open the aneurysm longitudinally, and deal with any back-bleeding from lumbar arteries or the inferior mesenteric artery by suture ligation
- Evacuate thrombus – most aneurysms are full of organized blood clots with only a small central lumen to allow blood flow
- Suture an appropriately sized graft end-to-end with non-absorbable sutures to the infrarenal neck of the aneurysm and then to the iliac bifurcation of individual iliacs
- Before the lower anastomosis is completed, thoroughly flush the arteries and the graft to expel any clot
- Restore flow to the legs, one side at a time to minimize the stress on the heart of the fall in blood pressure upon reperfusion; then evaluate haemostasis and lower limb perfusion
- Close the sac of the aneurysm and the posterior peritoneum over the graft to exclude it from the peritoneal cavity (inlay technique) and to separate the graft from the duodenum to minimize the risk of an aorto-duodenal fistula
- Close the abdomen in the standard manner

Management of Suspected Leaking Abdominal Aortic Aneurysm

- Take a history and examine to assess comorbidity and quality of life
- Establish i.v. access and consider colloid replacement to maintain systolic BP at 100 mmHg, although permissive hypotension is preferred; monitor O_2 and saturation. Accept a lower systolic pressure if the patient is cerebrating
- Arrange urgent blood tests and cross-match 8 units plus products
- Carry out ECG and rectal examination to exclude myocardial infarction or GI bleed (which may also lead to abdominal pain and collapse)
- Inform senior surgeon, anaesthetist, theatres and ICU
- Remain with patient and transfer directly to theatre
- Occasionally, a CT scan is appropriate to determine open or endovascular treatment

practice. Figs 27.15 and 27.16 show an operative picture of an open aneurysm repair.

Endovascular Treatment of Aneurysms. An alternative approach to aneurysm exclusion involves the deployment of an endovascular stent (metal scaffold with fabric lining) through a transfemoral approach (Fig. 27.17 and Clinical Box 27.4). Fixation of the stent relies on radial forces in the neck of the aneurysm just below the renal arteries and in the iliac vessels. Some endovascular devices contain metal hooks or barbs to aid in the fixation process. Metal struts can be placed supra-renally or infra-renally. Successful aneurysm exclusion mandates adequate proximal and distal stent landing zones that are disease-free. Aneurysms with a suitable neck-length of 15 mm, <60-degree neck angulation and favourable iliac arteries are suitable for endovascular repair.

Careful preoperative planning using CT reconstruction techniques allows accurate measurements to provide satisfactory sealing and treatment outcomes (Figs 27.18 and 27.19). Multiple endovascular devices have been developed to address more complex anatomies. The technical success rate in experienced centres is greater than 98%. The long-term durability of endovascular aneurysm repair (EVAR)

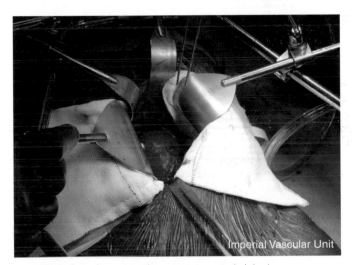

• **Fig. 27.15** Open intraoperative aneurysm repair. Intact aneurysm sac

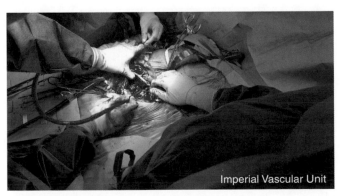

• **Fig. 27.16** Operative view of open aneurysm repair. Open aneurysm sac

is still uncertain and appears to be inferior to open surgical repair. This is due to patient selection, practices outside the manufacturers' instructions for use (IFU), incremental

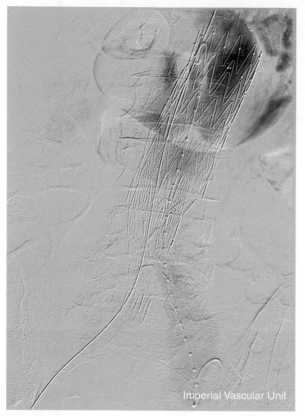

• **Fig. 27.17** Fluoroscopic Image of an Endovascular Stent Being Deployed Within an Abdominal Aortic Aneurysm. (Courtesy Imperial Vascular Unit)

gains in technology and surgical experience. Intermediate and long-term follow-up data have shown that the incidence of secondary interventions in patients with EVAR is approximately 10% per year. Long-term data exists only for first-generation devices, many of which are now considered obsolete. Endoleak, graft kinking, stenosis or thrombosis and device migration are causes for secondary interventions, emphasizing the need for lifelong surveillance. The minimally invasive nature of EVAR, advances in technology and device availability led many centres to adopt an EVAR-first approach to aneurysm repair. It was initially felt that surveillance after 5 years was unnecessary, but, due to a combination of unexpected patient longevity and improvement in surveillance technology, it has become evident that a significant number of endografts fail after 8 years post-implantation. This does not appear to have changed with new endografts, and may represent a fundamental consequence of lack in actual fixation with endovascular treatments. The latest National Institute for Health and Clinical Excellence (NICE) recommendations (2018) (still in consultation at the time of writing) recommend that endovascular repair is not cost-effective in preventing aneurysm rupture and therefore should not be offered to patients unless a hostile abdomen (multiple previous abdominal operations making open repair hazardous) is present; thus patients unfit for open repair should be treated conservatively.

Popliteal Aneurysm

Thirty percent of patients with an AAA also have a popliteal artery aneurysm (PAA), and 50% of patients with PAA have an AAA.

CLINICAL BOX 27.4

Standard EVAR

- Careful preoperative stent planning with CT reconstruction (Figs 27.18 and 27.19).
- Open the groins through a vertical or oblique incision centred on the femoral artery. Alternatively, percutaneous Seldinger technique with advanced closure devices.
- Isolate and control the CFA bilaterally.
- Careful front-wall puncture of the CFA with insertion of a soft J wire into the iliac vessels for side from which the main body (pre-planned) will be placed. All the following under fluoroscopy control:
- Temporary sheath placement (6Fr) over the wire.
- Wire replaced with hydrophilic soft tipped wire.
- Pigtail catheter fed over the wire.
- Procedure repeated for contralateral limb.
- Ipsilateral pigtail advanced with the wire to descending aorta.
- Ipsilateral wire exchanged for a stiff wire (e.g. Lunderquist or Meyer wire).
- Administer a bolus dose of i.v. heparin, usually 3000–5000 units.
- Exchange of sheath for EVAR device sheath over the wire.

- Placement of main body based on bony landmarks and orientation checked with anticipated angulation.
- C-Arm fluoroscopy adjusted to appropriate angulation to be perpendicular to renal arteries.
- Power pump angiography run via the contralateral pigtail catheter placed in distal descending aorta.
- Position of lowest renal arteries checked and marked.
- Careful deployment of EVAR main body.
- Check angiography to ensure appropriate placement compared to renal arteries.
- Cannulation of contralateral EVAR limb gate using hydrophilic wire and catheter combination.
- Check angiography for distal placement (iliac bifurcation) and marking of angiogram for each limb.
- Deployment of ipsilateral and contralateral limbs with extension as necessary.
- Ballooning of all seal and connection points.
- Final angiography to ensure no evident endoleaks and satisfactory appearances.
- Closure of arteriotomies with non-absorbable (Prolene) sutures and closure of groins.

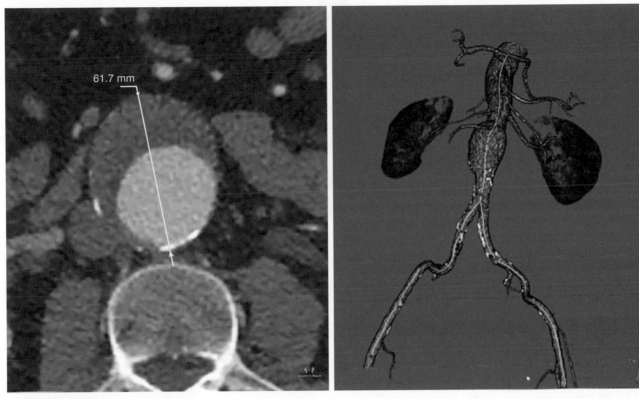

D Aneursym : 61.7 mm

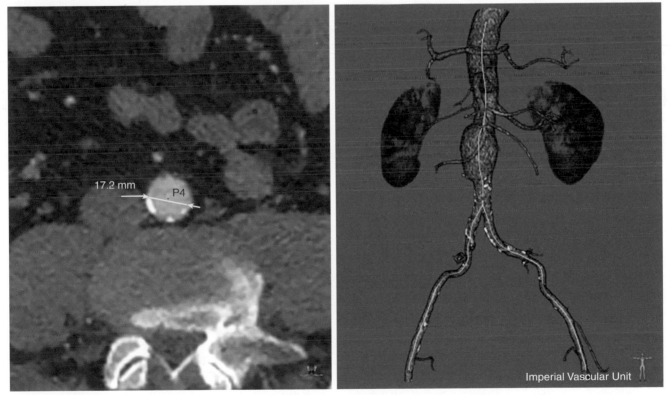

D P4 : 17.2 mm

• **Fig. 27.18** Example of image manipulation using CT images to plan EVAR stent graft.

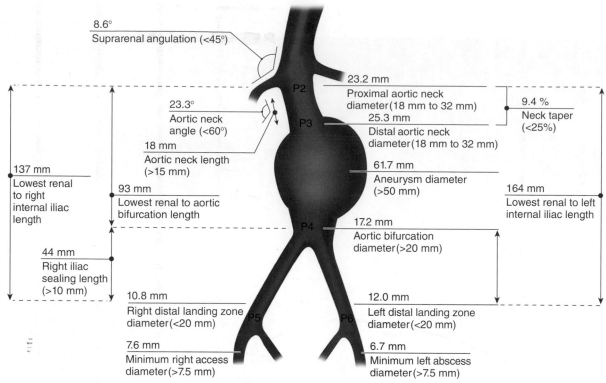

8.6°
Suprarenal angulation (<45°)

23.2 mm
Proximal aortic neck
diameter(18 mm to 32 mm)
25.3 mm

9.4 %
Neck taper
(<25%)

23.3°
Aortic neck
angle (<60°)

Distal aortic neck
diameter(18 mm to 32 mm)

18 mm
Aortic neck length
(>15 mm)

61.7 mm
Aneurysm diameter
(>50 mm)

137 mm
Lowest renal
to right
internal iliac
length

93 mm
Lowest renal to aortic
bifurcation length

164 mm
Lowest renal to left
internal iliac length

17.2 mm
Aortic bifurcation
diameter(>20 mm)

44 mm
Right iliac
sealing length
(>10 mm)

10.8 mm
Right distal landing zone
diameter(<20 mm)

12.0 mm
Left distal landing zone
diameter(<20 mm)

7.6 mm
Minimum right access
diameter(>7.5 mm)

6.7 mm
Minimum left abscess
diameter(>7.5 mm)

• **Fig. 27.19** Sample sizing sheet for EVAR stent graft.

Pathological Features

PAAs are predominantly atherosclerotic. Complications include thrombosis with or without distal embolization. Because the aneurysm itself is nearly always asymptomatic, presentation is usually as an emergency with the symptoms of acute limb ischaemia, unless an incidental diagnosis has been made on vascular examination.

Management

Emergency. Acute thrombosis of a PAA is associated with a high rate of limb loss because usually the distal calf vessels all thrombose simultaneously. Small thrombi from within the PAA may embolize to the crural and pedal vessels, which makes surgery technically challenging due to the loss of distal run-off. Thrombosis in a PAA is an accepted indication for thrombolysis either percutaneously or through surgical exploration. Despite this, 50% of those who present with an acute thrombosis of a PAA lose the affected limb.

Elective. Elective PAA repair should be offered to patients whose aneurysm diameter exceeds 2.5 cm or when a significant amount of thrombus has been detected on ultrasound. Symptomatic PAA with evidence of distal embolization should also be repaired in an expedited fashion. About 20% of patients have bilateral disease, so the other limb should be carefully examined and, if a PAA is found, repair should be offered once threshold is reached.

Technique. A reversed vein bypass is constructed from the superficial femoral artery above to the popliteal artery below the aneurysm. The PAA is tied off and thus excluded from the circulation. Endovascular stents can also be used if the anatomy is suitable for elderly patients who are deemed unfit for open surgery.

Thoraco-Abdominal Aortic Aneurysm (TAAA)

Epidemiology

Aneurysmal disease affects the infrarenal aorta in 90% of cases. However, with increased awareness and improved imaging techniques, particularly CT, it has become apparent that a greater proportion of aortic aneurysms than was previously thought (perhaps 15–20%) involve the suprarenal aorta and/or the thoracic aorta (Fig. 27.20). The risk of rupture appears to be similar to that of infrarenal aneurysms, although the treatment threshold is usually set at 6 cm due to the complexity of repair. The rate of rupture appears to significantly increase above 7 cm. Unlike in infrarenal aneurysms, there is little level 1 evidence to guide timing for intervention.

Management

Open TAAA repair is attempted in only a few centres in the UK, and the technique is highly specialized, requiring deep hypothermic arrest or left heart bypass. Blood loss is significant and the recovery is prolonged. Many patients are considered unfit to withstand the physiological perioperative insult. Thoracic endovascular aneurysm repair (TEVAR) is an attractive alternative treatment for isolated thoracic aortic aneurysms that do not involve the supra-aortic or visceral vessels. Hybrid repair, which involves open revascularization of the great or visceral vessels and stenting of the remaining

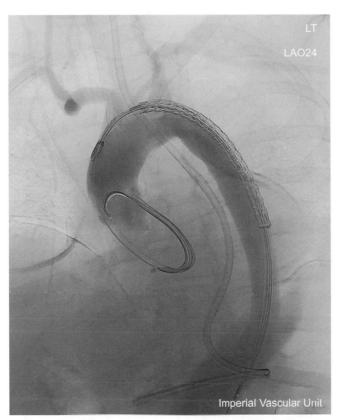

• **Fig. 27.20** Angiogram Showing Aneurysmal Dilatation of the Thoracic Aorta The guide wire is lying within the lumen (arrow). Angiography may underestimate the size of an aneurysm because it only demonstrates the lumen and not the large amount of thrombus that also usually lies within the aneurysm sac.

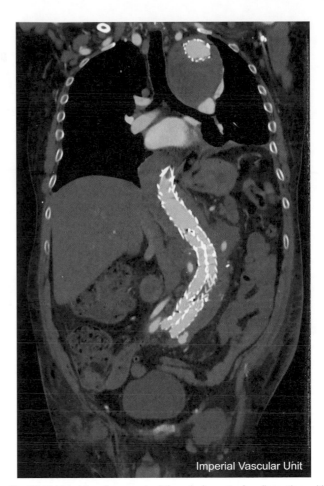

• **Fig. 27.21** Hybrid replacement of the whole aorta for dissection with visceral revascularization grafts, CT coronal plane.

aorta, is a viable alternative. The introduction of custom-made endovascular devices with fenestrations and branches tailored to individual patient anatomy have expanded the treatment options for TAAAs. These devices, however, are costly and take weeks to manufacture, precluding treatment of ruptured cases. The perioperative risks of paraplegia and stroke remain a concern. Treatment should be tailored to individual patient cardiorespiratory fitness and anatomical features. Figs 27.21–27.23 show CT reconstructions of a patient with a type 2 (whole aorta) thoracoabdominal aortic aneurysm with staged whole aorta replacement. Fig. 27.4 shows abdominal aortic stent placement after visceral revascularization.

False Aneurysm

Aetiology

Most false aneurysms are iatrogenic, the consequence of arterial puncture of the common femoral or radial artery, although increasing rates of knife crime present another source. Following trauma to the arterial wall, blood enters the perivascular space to form a haematoma which liquefies to create a fluid cavity into which arterial blood still circulates and which is walled off from surrounding tissues by a fibrous capsule.

Management

If a false aneurysm is small it may close spontaneously, provided that the patient is not anticoagulated; 50% of cases will experience spontaneous thrombosis. It is also possible to induce thrombosis by compression under ultrasound guidance, though this can be painful for the patient. Most false aneurysms can be treated successfully with thrombin injection into the sac, provided there is a narrow neck to the main artery, preventing embolization of thrombin into the circulation. However, if the aneurysm is very large, with a wide neck and continuing to expand, then surgical repair is necessary. This is usually a straightforward procedure – closure of the hole in the artery and obliteration of the sac.

Anastomotic False Aneurysm

A false aneurysm can also develop at the site of an anastomosis between the prosthetic material and the native artery. In these circumstances, the surgeon should always consider the possibility of infection. Such anastomotic aneurysms may require operative repair to prevent rapid expansion and rupture.

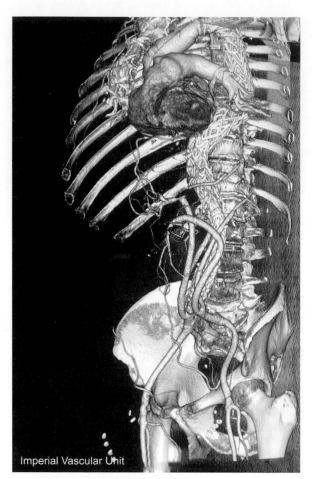

• **Fig. 27.22** Hybrid replacement of the whole aorta for dissection with visceral revascularization grafts, CT sagittal plane.

• **Fig. 27.23** Hybrid replacement of the whole aorta for dissection with visceral revascularization grafts, CT 3D reconstruction.

CHRONIC LOWER-LIMB ISCHAEMIA

Intermittent Claudication

Intermittent claudication (IC) of the lower limb is the mildest manifestation of chronic arterial insufficiency and affects approximately 5% of men over 60 years. In the majority of cases, it is the consequence of atherosclerotic narrowing or occlusion of the superficial femoral artery in the thigh.

Clinical Features

Symptoms

Arterial insufficiency causes ischaemic muscle pain on walking which is relieved by rest. It is often reproducible after walking the same distance. Symptoms are usually worse when walking on uphill. At rest, the blood requirement is met by the collateral circulation through the profunda femoris system which joins the popliteal artery below the blockage often just above the knee level. However, exercise produces a demand which cannot be met, and the calf muscles become ischaemic. With disease affecting the SFA only, thigh muscles are still perfused via the profundal femoris and the pain is usually felt only in the calf. If stenosis is more proximal (aorto-iliac), then pain affects the muscle groups in the calf and thigh and even the buttock if the blood flow to the iliac system is compromised.

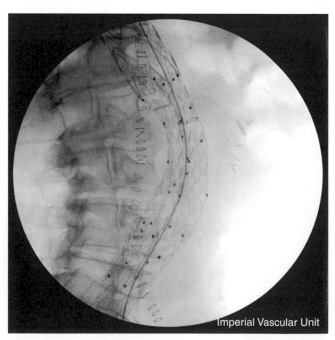

• **Fig. 27.24** d: Intra-opreative angiography of abdominal aortic stent placement after visceral revascularization using hybrid grafts.

Impotence is another presenting symptom (Leriche syndrome) seen with internal iliac involvement.

Physical Findings

On examination, the limb may be obviously ischaemic. Pulses are usually diminished or absent below the femoral.

Diagnosis

Other causes of lower limb pain should be excluded. Pain that radiates from the back, hip and knee joint usually indicates osteoarthritis. Venous outflow obstruction (venous claudication) may also be difficult to distinguish from true arterial claudication, especially if these conditions coexist. Pre- and post-exercise ABPIs is a reliable method for ruling out arterial insufficiency.

Management

Arterial claudication is common; patients should be reassured that, in 80% of cases, symptoms remain stable or improve with continuing exercise, risk factor modification, smoking cessation and best medical therapy. Anxious patients should be reassured that amputation is unlikely, with rates of less than 1–2% per year. Asymptomatic disease should not be intervened for and should be managed conservatively. However, certain patients are at risk of disease progression, including those who:

- present with severe claudication of less than 50 m
- have ABPI <0.5
- have multilevel or distal disease
- have diabetes
- continue to smoke

These patients need careful assessment, aggressive risk factor management and enrolment in a supervised exercise class. Arterial reconstruction via open or endovascular means should be offered when critical limb ischaemia develops or when the symptoms significantly impact on the patient's quality of life.

Medical Therapy

For many years the standard treatment for the majority of patients was advice to 'stop smoking and keep walking'. All patients should be:

- Encouraged to stop smoking
- Monitored and treated for hypertension
- Started on anti-platelet therapy
- Started on high-dose lipid-lowering therapy, irrespective of blood test status
- Monitored and treated for additional risk factors such as diabetes
- Told to exercise beyond the point of pain in order to develop collateral circulation.
- Referred to a supervised exercise programme (NICE guidance)

The majority accept this advice, are motivated and attempt to alter their lifestyle. However, a proportion of patients will not comply or will not accept their level of disability. In such cases, intervention may be considered, though these are the very patients whose interventions have a high risk of failure. Once intervention has commenced, the natural history of the condition changes, and treatment failure may lead to worsened outcomes rather than a return to baseline status. There are now robust guidelines to support supervised exercise regimes worldwide.

Percutaneous Transluminal Angioplasty

Intervention for claudication is controversial. There have been direct comparisons between PTA and best medical therapy (BMT). Where patients have been randomly allocated to one treatment or the other, PTA has not been shown to confer any additional long-term benefit. Even in the first 6 months, while BMT is taking effect, PTA of suitable lesions does not provide better short-term symptomatic improvement.

In the longer term, there are clear advantages to BMT because not only does it lessen symptoms bilaterally but it also increases longevity by reducing the risk of death from ischaemic heart disease, stroke and lung malignancies – by far the most frequent causes in this group. Furthermore, PTA costs £500–1000 per procedure and, although arguably less invasive than open operation, is associated with a 1–2% major morbidity rate, compared to a virtually non-existent complication rate with exercise. To some extent, comparisons between BMT and PTA are clinically inappropriate and the two procedures should be viewed as complementary and not competitive. The fundamental question is not in which patients should PTA be considered instead of BMT, but rather in which patients will PTA augment the results of BMT.

There is no doubt that the results of PTA are better in the aorto-iliac than in the femoropopliteal segment. If clinical examination suggests that aorto-iliac (inflow) disease is significantly contributing to symptoms, then angiography with a view to PTA should be considered. By contrast, if the femoral pulses are normal and the clinical diagnosis is one of femoropopliteal or infrapopliteal occlusion, routine investigation in greater detail is not indicated and is usually reserved for those with a threat to the limb or livelihood.

Operation

Contention also surrounds this option. As mentioned previously, the natural history is benign in terms of limb loss, and potential mortality or morbidity from intervention must be set against this. The paradox is that the patients who have the most to lose (due to relative youth) are the ones considered for the highest risk procedures.

Aorto-Iliac (Supra-Inguinal) Disease. There is a lower threshold for reconstruction in this segment because:

- The ability to compensate for aorto-iliac occlusion by formation of collaterals is not as good as it is for infrainguinal disease.
- The long-term results of aorto-iliac reconstruction are considerably better than in infra-inguinal bypass; more than 80% of aortobifemoral grafts for claudication are patent at 10 years.

- Bilateral claudication can be corrected by a single intervention.
- Iliac angioplasty and stenting offers durable and less invasive procedures with good outcomes.

Infra-Inguinal Disease. By contrast, there is much less enthusiasm for infra-inguinal bypass because:

- Compensation by collateral development is often good.
- At 5 years, less than 70% of femoropopliteal grafts are still patent.
- Bypass grafting leads to involution of collateral pathways; if the graft blocks, the patient nearly always returns to a worse level of ischaemia than that present before the operation. Additionally, the operation itself often eliminates small but important collateral vessels.
- Rest pain or acute limb ischaemia may develop after a failed graft and re-operation is therefore required; the long-term results of such procedures are much less impressive than those of primary reconstruction.

In 2005, the BASIL trial[3] questioned the approach of 'having a go first' with PTA and then proceeding to surgery as those patients with failed PTA have worse outcomes following surgery with an amputation-free survival of 60% versus 40% at 7 years. Careful patient selection is imperative.

There can be few experienced vascular surgeons who have not seen a patient die or lose a limb as a result of vascular reconstruction performed for claudication. In the UK, most adopt an extremely conservative approach, and less than 10% of infra-inguinal grafts are performed for claudication. A good aphorism is 'Vascular Surgery is a series of completely sensible and unavoidable operations, apart from the first'.

CRITICAL LIMB ISCHAEMIA OR CHRONIC LIMB-THREATENING ISCHAEMIA

Critical limb ischaemia (CLI), or chronic limb-threatening ischaemia (CLTI) is defined as rest pain requiring strong continuous (opiate) analgesia for a period of 2 weeks or more, and/or tissue loss, in association with an ankle pressure of less than 50 mmHg or toe pressure less than 30 mmHg. The inference is that, without intervention, a patient with CLTI will come to major amputation within weeks or months – epidemiological studies have shown that within 1 year, 30% of patients with CLTI undergo a major amputation and a further 25% are dead and 50% are dead in 5 years. In the over 80 years age group, a quarter are dead within 6 months.

Clinical Features

Symptoms

Rest pain is indicative of severe ischaemia, usually felt in the forefoot or digits, and the pain is typically worst at night and disturbs sleep. The reasons for this are:

- Metabolic rate in the foot is increased under the warm bedclothes.

- Cardiac output and blood pressure fall during sleep.
- A beneficial effect of gravity on pedal blood pressure is lost.

For these reasons, relief at night is often sought by hanging the leg over the side of the bed or walking about on a cold floor. Calf cramps at night are more likely to be due to dehydration or electrolyte imbalance.

Physical Findings

Constant pain in the foot with single-level arterial disease is uncommon and should instigate a search for other causes, as the arterial network is extremely adept at providing collateral pathways.

Ischaemic tissue is extremely sensitive to injury: even minor wounds fail to heal and ulceration follows. Ulceration is usually on the tips of the toes (Fig. 27.25). Minor damage quickly leads to infection, and bacterial toxins destroy yet more tissue. Frank gangrene then ensues and can spread extremely rapidly, especially in diabetics.

Relatively limited arterial occlusion may sometimes be sufficient to cause CLTI if cardiac function is suboptimal due to pump failure. For example, after myocardial infarction or another cardiac event, cardiac output and systolic blood pressure may fall to a point where even a small increase in peripheral vascular resistance cannot be overcome. Management is difficult because of the hazards of major intervention, and the outlook is poor. This is frequently observed in critical care patients requiring aggressive inotropic support to maintain an adequate blood pressure through vasoconstriction.

Management

Medical

In contrast to claudication, the presence of rest pain suggests that tissue loss is imminent. CLTI does not usually improve without revascularization, but medical measures have important complimentary roles:

- Assessment and treatment of heart failure, intercurrent infection and anaemia
- Control of diabetes
- Antibiotic therapy of local infection
- Pain relief
- Use of anticoagulants and occasionally prostacyclin-based drugs when tissue loss is minimal

All of these measures can ensure that an optimum condition is achieved before surgical intervention is performed.

Balloon Angioplasty

The majority view is that, in patients with early rest pain and/or minimal tissue loss (subcritical ischaemia), PTA may tip the balance just enough to salvage the limb when surgical reconstruction is not feasible. The belief that all patients with CLTI should, in the first instance, be managed with PTA and bypass reconstruction should be reserved for those who do not respond, has not been supported by randomized or cohort studies. Indeed, the results of the BASIL trial have highlighted significantly inferior outcomes for patients treated with surgery after unsuccessful PTA.

A

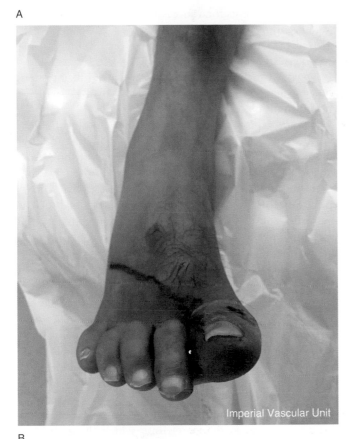

Imperial Vascular Unit

B

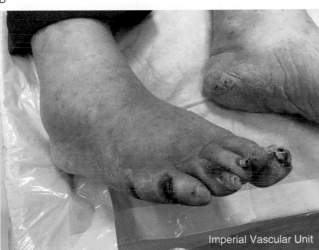

Imperial Vascular Unit

• **Fig. 27.25** Two examples of critical limb ischaemia with ulceration of the toes and sunset foot appearance which blanches on elevation.

Sympathectomy

This has a niche role to play in CLTI, as those with early rest pain may achieve some relief, and it may offer some benefit in those with unreconstructable disease. However, it will not heal extensive wounds.

Amputation

This is a last resort. Primary amputation can be the best option in the elderly frail patient with extensive tissue loss, but mortality is inevitably high (63% at 1 year in the over 80s).

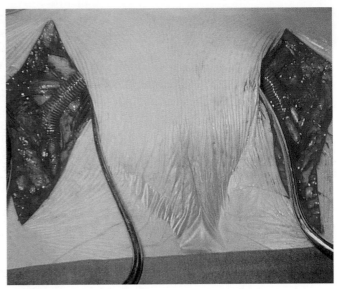

• **Fig. 27.26** An Operative Photograph Showing a Dacron Graft Carrying Blood from the Left to the Right Common Femoral Artery Below a Right Iliac Occlusion

Palliation

There are circumstances in which the patient and the family interests are best served by the provision of good quality end-of-life care.

Surgery

Bypass surgery and, to a lesser extent, local endarterectomy are the mainstays of treatment. Due to the frequently present multilevel disease and multiple co-morbidities, mortality rates for medical and vascular limb salvage surgery can reach 10%.

Aorto-Iliac Disease. In CLTI, this is usually associated with infra-inguinal disease. As already implied, the results of PTA and stenting are optimal at this site, as are the long-term results of open arterial reconstruction. In younger, fitter patients who are considered unsuitable for PTA, the gold standard treatment is via an aortobifemoral bypass graft. In those not fit for aortic surgery, an extra-anatomical bypass may be offered. For example, if there is an iliac occlusion on one side and a relatively disease-free vessel on the other, a femoro-femoral crossover graft (Fig. 27.26) is possible. An alternative is an axillobifemoral graft, where the inflow for the graft is taken from the axillary artery below the clavicle (Fig. 27.27). This avoids a laparotomy and the associated risks.

Femorodistal Bypass. This refers to arterial reconstruction below the inguinal ligament in which common femoral or superficial femoral arteries are the site of proximal anastomosis and the popliteal or tibial vessels are the site of distal anastomosis. A pop-pedal bypass is a variant form more distal disease (Fig. 27.28).

Technical aspects of limb salvage surgery. In general, the shorter the graft, the easier it is to construct and the better the patency.

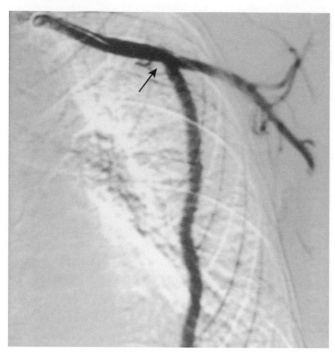

• **Fig. 27.27** Angiogram showing a graft using the left axillary artery as an inflow (arrow) in order to revascularize both legs below an aorto-iliac occlusion. The patient was not considered fit enough to undergo aortic surgery.

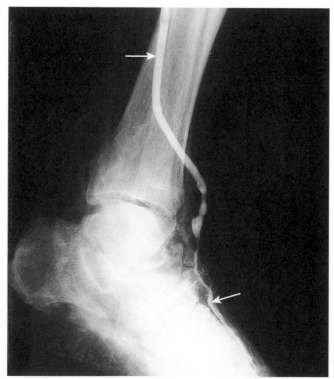

• **Fig. 27.28** An on-table angiogram to show flow of contrast from an in-situ femorodistal vein graft (upper arrow) into the dorsalis pedis artery (lower arrow) on the dorsum of the foot. The operation was carried out for critical limb ischaemia in a diabetic patient.

The requirements for a successful distal bypass are:
- good inflow
- a reliable conduit
- good outflow

Inflow is usually provided by the ipsilateral iliac system, and any iliac disease must be corrected by PTA with or without stent placement.

Conduit. There is no doubt that the autologous vein provides the best long-term results, especially if the distal anastomosis is below the knee. The patency of long prosthetic bypasses (PTFE or Dacron) can be improved by using a vein interposition cuff at the distal anastomosis. Different variations of this technique have been described such as the Miller cuff and the St Mary's boot. Vein grafts may be placed in a reverse manner or in situ (non-reversed). In the former, the vein is reversed to remove any obstruction to flow that may occur from intact valves. In the latter, the vein is not reversed and the valves are cut using a valvulotome. Although no significant difference in patency between the two techniques has ever been demonstrated, from a technical point of view there are advantages to the in situ technique when a long bypass to calf and foot vessels is to be constructed, from both a graft size viewpoint and location. However, in situ bypasses may be more prone to compression and infection following wound dehiscence as they are not anatomically tunnelled and are more superficial.

Outflow refers to the vessels into which the graft is to deliver blood. If the bypass is delivering blood to a dead-end, then thrombosis is inevitable.

Long-Term Patency. Femorodistal bypasses have a finite life expectancy and this should be explained to the patient. Advice should be given regarding symptoms and signs of graft occlusion. The chances of resurrecting a failed graft, particularly a vein graft, are often directly related to timing of diagnosis and subsequent treatment. The vein graft receives its blood supply from its venous vasorum, which have been disconnected from its native supply, so thrombosis and occlusion for >24 hours will result in a scarred endothelium which will likely re-occlude even if the thrombus is cleared.

All patients undergoing bypass surgery should be on anti-platelet therapy postoperatively. Anticoagulants are also used, especially with ultra-distal bypasses. Warfarin has been shown to improve long-term patency, but anticoagulation in an elderly population is not without hazard.

Graft Surveillance. It has been known for some time that certain grafts develop stenoses over time and that these predispose to occlusion. There is some evidence that, if this can be identified and corrective measures applied before thrombosis occurs, the long-term patency may be significantly improved. However, the Vein Graft Surveillance Trial[6] indicates that duplex ultrasound surveillance has no benefit over clinical review.

Failure can be classified as early, due to technical failures, mid-term, due to neo-intimal hyperplasia, and late, due to progression of native disease. Stenosis most frequently takes place either at the distal anastomosis or within the body of a vein graft. The cause of neo-intimal hyperplasia represents scarring where the intima has been damaged and which then impinges on the lumen to create a stenosis. If a tight stenosis is detected, a confirmatory angiogram is done and the lesion is corrected by either PTA or open surgical revision. Most stenoses develop within the first 18 months. Late failure is more often the result of disease progression in the native arteries proximal or distal to the bypass.

Management of Thrombosis in a Graft

The options are:

- *Surveillance* – if the leg is viable, consider no intervention and wait for collaterals to develop
- *Thrombolysis* – if successful, the underlying lesion which caused the graft to occlude can then be identified and corrected by either surgery or PTA
- *Thrombectomy* – mechanical removal of thrombus, followed by intra-operative angiography to identify the underlying lesion and surgical correction
- *Construction* of a new graft – some believe that in virtually all circumstances, the graft must be replaced by a new bypass in order to optimize long-term patency.

The Diabetic Foot

Clinical Features

Diabetics have a tendency to develop, often quite suddenly, severe ischaemia and infection in the feet which progresses to rapid tissue necrosis and limb loss. The reasons for this are as follows:

- Vascular disease – which, in diabetes, develops earlier in life and tends to be more extensive and distal – makes intervention, by means of either angioplasty or surgery, more difficult and technically demanding.
- Sensory neuropathy reduces or abolishes protective reactions to minor injury and to symptoms of infection and/or ischaemia.
- Retinopathy also leads to suboptimal visual inspection of the foot
- Autonomic neuropathy causes a lack of sweating and the development of dry, fissured skin which permits entry of bacteria.
- Motor neuropathy results in wasting and weakness of the small muscles, loss of the longitudinal and transverse arches of the foot, and development of abnormal pressure areas such as over the metatarsal heads (Fig. 27.29).

Management

Tissue loss is neuropathic or ischaemic, or more commonly, a combination of both (neuro-ischaemic). The principles of management are effective glycaemic control, wide debridement of necrotic tissue, drainage of pus and, if ischaemia is present, revascularization. Foot care is essential with involvement of a podiatrist and a foot and ankle surgical specialist. Early removal of calluses, skin moisturizing and protection

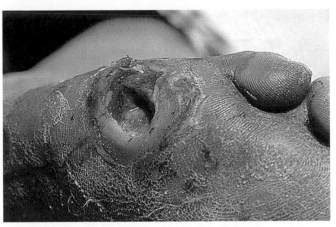

• **Fig. 27.29** Typical 'Punched-Out' Ulcer Over the Head of the 5th Metatarsal in a Patient with Diabetic Peripheral Vascular Disease and Neuropathy.

of the foot from injury are encouraged. Surgical correction of foot and ankle deformities should also be considered. The optimum management pathway is multi-disciplinary and holistic. It is key to remember that, like vascular disease, diabetes is a systemic disorder.

ARTERIAL DISORDERS OF THE UPPER LIMB

The arm is affected by ischaemia eight times less commonly than the leg because:

- atherosclerosis affects the leg more frequently
- the arterial supply of the leg in relation to muscle bulk is much poorer than that of the arm
- the ability of the arm to derive collateral supply appears superior

Unlike the leg, the commonest cause of ischaemia is embolism. Ischaemia can progress rapidly, and loss of any part of the upper limb has a devastating functional result. However, with widespread anticoagulation for heart arrhythmias, frequency of significant embolic events is reduced.

Thoracic Outlet Syndrome

Aetiology

Thoracic outlet syndrome (TOS) occurs when the lower trunk of the brachial plexus and/or the subclavian vessels are compressed as they pass over the first rib, a cervical rib or a cervical fibrous band which runs from the transverse process of the seventh vertebra towards the first rib. The majority of patients are female and aged between 20 and 40 years.

Clinical Features

Symptoms

The symptoms are predominantly neurological, typically pain, weakness, and/or paraesthesia over the ulnar aspect of the hand and forearm, often extremely vague and difficult to assess. Compression of the subclavian vein at the thoracic outlet may cause axillary vein thrombosis – Paget–Schrotter disease. Only 5% present primarily with arterial ischaemic symptoms, most commonly claudication or Raynaud's phenomenon (below). Turbulent flow caused by a subclavian stenosis may progress to post-stenotic dilatation of the subclavian artery, which in turn may develop into an aneurysm; thrombus within this may cause a distal embolism.

Physical Findings

A cervical rib can be palpable. On external rotation and hyperabduction of the shoulder, the radial pulse may be lost and the hand may go pale and numb (these signs are not specific because a significant proportion of healthy individuals will also lose the radial pulse on extreme shoulder positioning). Wasting of the small muscles of the hand is always pathological but can occur in a wide variety of conditions. Obvious digital ischaemia may be present after embolization (Fig. 27.30) but also occurs in Raynaud's phenomenon where it is, however, always bilateral.

Investigation

Plain Radiography

A plain radiograph of the neck may show a cervical rib (identifiable as the transverse process is downward pointing in the cervical vertebrae, but upward in the thoracic) (Fig. 27.31) or a prominent transverse process which suggests, but does not establish the presence of, a fibrous band.

MRA and MRV

This is now the investigation of choice in that compression of the nerve roots and the artery can be demonstrated, especially with a dynamic study in various positions.

Angiography

A fixed stenosis in the neutral position, especially when it is associated with post-stenotic dilatation or aneurysm, is always pathological and remains the clearest indication for arterial surgery. Stenosis present only on abduction is present in 10% of healthy individuals. Angiography of the subclavian from femoral access runs the slight (but present) risk of vertebral artery territory stroke.

Duplex Ultrasound

If present, a subclavian aneurysm together with any intraluminal thrombus can be identified, as can venous obstruction. Dynamic duplex with assessment of vessels with the arm in various positions can help diagnosis. As with angiography, 10% of the healthy population may show changes in blood flow in abduction and these should be interpreted with caution.

Venography

This investigation confirms venous obstruction and/or impingement; however, it is now rarely used.

Nerve Conduction Studies

These are useful in localizing the problem to the thoracic outlet and should be considered before operation, especially as it provides a baseline in case of recurrence or operative difficulties.

Management

Non-Operative

In the absence of objective neurological damage or arterial ischaemia, treatment is symptomatic by physiotherapy in an attempt to improve posture and strengthen the muscles of the neck and shoulder girdle.

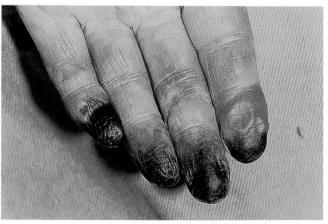

• **Fig. 27.30** Clinical photography showing extensive digital gangrene in a patient who had been treated medically for presumed Raynaud's phenomenon despite the fact that the symptoms had only ever affected one hand. More recently, gangrene had developed over only a few weeks. In fact, this patient had a cervical rib associated with a subclavian aneurysm containing thrombus which had been embolizing down into the digital arteries. The rib was excised, the subclavian aneurysm replaced with a PTFE graft, and the tips of the affected fingers amputated.

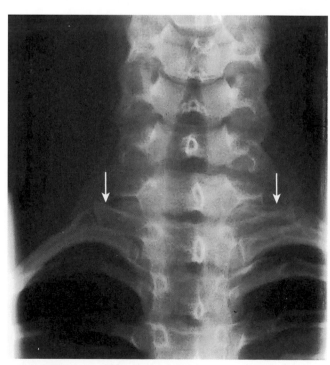

• **Fig. 27.31** Plain radiograph of the cervical spine showing the presence bilaterally of cervical ribs (arrows).

Surgery

Failure of conservative measures suggests the need for operative decompression. If a cervical rib or fibrous band is present, it can be excised via a supraclavicular approach. If not, many advocate excision of the first rib through a transaxillary approach; a few suggest this even if a cervical rib is present. A subclavian aneurysm is excised and replaced by a bypass graft.

When the symptoms are clear-cut and the diagnosis certain, the results of surgery are good. In other circumstances, when the surgeon and the neurologist are uncertain and operation is carried out as a diagnostic test or as a last resort, results and patient satisfaction can be poor.

ACUTE ISCHAEMIA OF A LIMB

Aetiology

The great majority of cases of acute limb ischaemia are caused either by embolism or by thrombosis at a site of previous atherosclerotic narrowing. Differentiation is of clinical importance because the management is quite different (Table 27.3). However, even the experienced vascular specialist may be unable to distinguish between the two with confidence, and it is not uncommon for a patient with established peripheral vascular disease to present with an embolus.

Embolism

Embolic material comes from:
- mural cardiac thrombus after a myocardial infarct
- left atrial appendix in atrial fibrillation
- vegetations from a heart valve in endocarditis or rheumatic disease
- thrombus from the aorta or other major vessel that is aneurysmal or atherosclerotic
- thrombus formed within a surgical graft

Embolic material tends to lodge at distal sites, which affects end-organ perfusion.

Thrombosis

Surgical thrombectomy alone rarely succeeds, because of early re-thrombosis; some form of arterial bypass or thrombolysis is usually necessary.

Clinical Features

Symptoms

Symptoms are often described as the six Ps:
- pulseless
- pain
- pallor
- 'perishing' cold
- paralysis
- paraesthesia

Physical Findings

These reflect the symptoms. The presentation of an acutely ischaemic limb may not fulfil all the 'six Ps' criteria at the time of presentation. The limb is usually pale and pulseless, with painful digits. Reduced sensation is not always easy to assess, especially in patients with peripheral neuropathy such as diabetics. Deterioration of sensory neurologic function is an indication of progressive ischaemia. Loss of pressure sensation, pain and temperature are late features of prolonged ischaemia. Loss of movement is a late feature. In embolic occlusion, events occur rapidly with early loss of motor and sensory function. In these circumstances, the diagnosis of ischaemia, as well as the need to act quickly, is usually obvious. In those with thrombosis, the presentation is often acute on chronic.

Management

Faced with the acutely ischaemic limb, the following questions must be addressed:
- Is the limb salvageable?
- Is the limb threatened?

The Non-Viable Limb

Features that indicate the limb is no longer salvageable include:
- fixed staining of tissues
- lack of blanching on pressure
- anaesthesia with rigid muscles – rigor mortis

Acute-on-chronic limb ischaemia may be the manifestation of another terminal illness such as cardiac failure or malignancy. To subject such a patient to amputation if his or her condition is pre-terminal is not good practice.

TABLE 27.3	Clinical Features of Acute Embolism and Thrombosis.	
Embolus	**Thrombosis**	
Ischaemia is of sudden onset and very severe because of lack of preformed collaterals	Onset often insidious and less severe because of the pre-existence of collaterals	
A potential source of embolus can usually be identified	No obvious source of embolus	
Hospital records may indicate the presence of previous normal pulses	Previous records indicate long-standing peripheral pulse deficit	
No history of arterial disease	History of arterial disease, e.g. myocardial infarction, stroke, peripheral vascular disease	
Normal pulses in contralateral limb	Absent or reduced pulses in contralateral limb	

In all circumstances, management focuses on whether it is appropriate to offer amputation or palliation. The wishes of the patient must be respected. If informed consent cannot be obtained, then the next of kin or other relatives should be involved in the decision making.

The Threatened Limb

Features of an ischaemic limb that is likely, in the absence of revascularization, to become non-viable include:

- loss of sensation
- loss of active movement
- pain on passive movement and when the calf muscles are squeezed

When these features are present, there is a 6-hour therapeutic window to re-instate flow and avoid irreversible nerve and muscle injury.

If embolism is obvious, embolectomy is performed, but if the diagnosis lacks certainty, an angiogram avoids a blind procedure; alternatively, on-table angiography can be performed. When a limb is threatened but a patient's general condition precludes long and complicated arterial surgery, amputation may be the only option.

Management is summarized in Emergency Box 27.2.

The Non-Threatened Limb

If sensation and movement are present and calf tenderness is absent, then the limb is not immediately threatened and it is safe to delay intervention. A period of medical optimization with intravenous fluid and heparin therapy may lead to spontaneous improvement as collateral circulation compensates for the compromised arterial segment. Angiography and reconstruction can then be performed at a later date. An alternative involves intra-arterial thrombolysis, but this requires 12–24 hours to complete, and often continues for up to 72 hours. Pharmacomechanical thrombolysis is another option but still requires some hours prior to flow re-instatement. It is imperative that the limb is assessed frequently as changes may occur rapidly and valuable time may be lost if revascularization is urgently needed.

EMERGENCY BOX 27.2

Management of a Limb Threatened by Acute Ischaemia

- Make cardiorespiratory assessment of the patient
- Provide O_2 therapy and BP optimization as necessary
- Provide analgesia
- Arrange blood tests (including clotting and cross-match), ECG and chest X-ray
- Keep nil by mouth and give i.v. fluids
- Start i.v. heparin – 5000 IU stat and 1000 IU/hour
- Arrange imaging – duplex ultrasound, arteriogram or on-table arteriogram depending on local availability
- Obtain consent
- Perform arterial reconstruction and consider fasciotomies

VASOSPASTIC DISORDERS (RAYNAUD'S PHENOMENON)

Understanding of this area has been hampered by the use of inconsistent terms. Here, standard European definitions are used:

- Raynaud's phenomenon (RP) is the general term which describes the clinical features of episodic digital vasospasm in the absence of an identifiable associated disorder
- Secondary Raynaud's syndrome (RS) is when the phenomenon occurs secondary to one of the conditions listed in Box 27.6.

Epidemiology and Aetiology

Raynaud's phenomenon is 10 times more common in women than in men and may, in its mild form, affect up to 25% of the young female population. An episode in the fingers typically occurs in response to cold and emotion, but other predisposing factors such as the oral contraceptive pill, certain migraine drugs and tobacco have been identified. The toes and other extremities may be involved, and there is increasing evidence that RP may be a manifestation of a total body microvascular disorder.

• BOX 27.6 Conditions Associated with Raynaud's Syndrome

Connective tissue disorders

- Systemic sclerosis (90%)
- Systemic lupus erythematosus (30%)
- Mixed connective tissue disease (80%)
- Dermatomyositis/polymyositis (20%)
- Sjögren's syndrome (30%)

Macrovascular disease

- Thoracic outlet obstruction
- Atherosclerosis
- Buerger's disease
- Radiation arteritis

Occupational trauma

- Vibration white finger (VWF)
- Chemical exposure, e.g. nitrates, polyvinyl chloride
- Repeated exposure to extreme cold

Drugs

- Cytotoxic drugs
- Ergotamine
- Beta-blockers
- Ciclosporin

Miscellaneous

- Malignancy
- Reflex sympathetic dystrophy
- Arteriovenous fistula

Clinical Features

There are three phases:

- pallor – because of digital artery spasm
- cyanosis – from the accumulation of deoxygenated blood
- redness (rubor) – reactive hyperaemia as blood flow returns.

Pain is unusual unless there are other complications, e.g. digital ulceration and gangrene.

Diagnosis

In the majority, the diagnosis of RP can be made on symptoms and physical findings; additional investigations are not required unless secondary RS is suspected. The proportion of patients who have an underlying disorder is uncertain; experts who run specialist clinics tend to collect the more intractable and severe examples, and, with adequate long-term follow-up, as many as 80% of all referred patients will eventually develop features of an underlying cause. Conversely, a general practitioner who sees a small number of mildly affected patients may only occasionally identify one with a defined connective tissue disease (CTD) (see Box 27.6). Only a minority have clear evidence of CTD on presentation. However, those with current tissue loss or scars from its previous occurrence must be assumed to have secondary RS, and a careful enquiry into the presence of isolated features of CTD should be made. Abnormal dilated nail-fold capillary loops, visible with an ophthalmoscope, are suggestive of, but not specific for, RS. Presentation for the first time in childhood or over the age of 30 increases the likelihood of RS. Eighty percent of those who present at over 60 years of age have an underlying disorder, although it is most often atherosclerosis. An asymmetrical distribution should also alert the vascular surgeon to the possibility of microembolization from a proximal lesion (TOS), and a full vascular examination should be done in all.

Management

Medical

Most often, reassurance about the usually benign nature of the condition, advice to stop smoking and to avoid exposure to cold are sufficient; chemical handwarmers and electrically heated gloves are available. There is controversy over whether the oral contraceptive pill should be discontinued, but hormone replacement therapy appears to be safe. Numerous drugs have been used, the best of which appears to be the calcium channel blocker nifedipine, although side-effects are relatively common. Vasodilators may also be useful. In those with severe attacks, admission to hospital for a 5-day infusion of prostacyclin may provide great symptomatic relief in the winter months and, for unknown reasons, the beneficial effects may last up to 6 weeks.

Surgical

Secondary Raynaud's syndrome caused by macrovascular arterial disease is nearly always unilateral and may progress rapidly to tissue loss in the hand if the underlying lesion is not identified and treated expeditiously. In RS in the hand, sympathectomy is associated with poor long-term results, but the procedure appears to be more useful in the feet. In the variant CREST syndrome, digits affected by severe ulceration or calcium deposits may require amputation, although every attempt should be made to preserve as much tissue as possible.

CEREBROVASCULAR DISEASE

Carotid Artery Disease

Pathological Features

In Europe, 1.4 million strokes occur per year and stroke leads to 1.1 million deaths annually. Overall, 10–15% of all strokes are secondary to previously asymptomatic internal carotid artery stenosis (>50%).

Clinical Features

Symptoms

Micro-embolization to the eye leads to ipsilateral transient loss of vision (amaurosis fugax), often described by the patient as a black curtain coming across the eyes, which usually lasts from a few seconds to a few minutes. A larger embolus may cause permanent blindness due to retinal infarction. Embolization to the middle cerebral artery leads to hemispheric symptoms, usually a contralateral hemiparesis and, if the dominant hemisphere is affected, loss of speech. A cerebral event which does not cause brain infarction and therefore does not leave residual symptoms and signs is termed a transient ischaemic attack (TIA).

A completed stroke progresses to brain damage with a residuum of neurological features.

Physical Findings

The neurological findings and their duration are consistent with the size of the area of brain affected.

Diagnosis and Investigation

CT or MRI scanning should be performed urgently. Carotid artery stenosis may be visualized by angiography (see Fig. 27.1), but this technique is associated with a 1–2% stroke rate and is therefore not used as a first-line investigation. Colour flow duplex scanning gives accurate and functional information on the presence and degree of stenosis, and an increasing number of centres primarily utilize this imaging modality prior to offering operative treatment. A preoperative CT brain scan is usually performed to identify the presence of pre-existing cerebral damage, rule out haemorrhage and exclude other pathology.

Management

Early Management

Immediate assessment in a specialist acute stroke unit should be arranged whenever possible. Urgent imaging is undertaken and thrombolysis with alteplase given if appropriate for ischaemic strokes within 4.5 hours of symptom onset. Mechanical thrombectomy is a more current alternative and offered within 6 hours of symptom onset. High-dose aspirin and statin is prescribed for ischaemic stroke and TIAs, whilst anticoagulation (heparin/warfarin) is used for acute venous stroke (cerebral venous sinus thrombosis). Nutritional support should be given. Antihypertensive treatment is used in hypertensive emergencies (encephalopathy, nephropathy, cardiac failure or infarct, aortic dissection or eclampsia) or with thrombolytic therapy (controlled to 185/110 or lower), as outcomes show a U-shaped curve with low and high blood pressure leading to worse outcomes.

Carotid Endarterectomy (CEA)

Indications. Two large randomized controlled trials and patient level data meta-analysis[7-9] have indicated that, in cases of amaurosis fugax, TIA or stroke within the last 6 months with good recovery plus an internal carotid artery (ICA) stenosis of 50% or greater, the risk of future stroke is significantly reduced by CEA. This should be carried out in conjunction with best medical therapy. The number needed to treat for >50% ICA stenosis to prevent one stroke is 13 and for >70% ICA stenosis is 6. Interestingly, the benefits of surgical intervention increases with age. Surgery should be performed within 2 weeks of developing symptoms whenever possible. The risks of surgery in patients with acute stroke (first 48 hours) and in those with completed stroke with poor recovery outweigh the benefits. Recent evidence from randomized trials indicate that most patients with asymptomatic lesions will not benefit from surgical intervention due to excellent outcomes from best medical therapy. However, certain patients with high-grade asymptomatic lesions do still benefit from endarterectomy – for example the young or those with progression despite treatment.

Technique. The major complication of CEA is a stroke. The benefits of the operation depend crucially upon a low perioperative stroke rate, which should be less than:
- 5% after previous symptoms
- 1% in those who are asymptomatic

Carotid Artery Stenting

Multiple trials have been undertaken comparing carotid artery stenting with CEA in both asymptomatic and symptomatic patients. The data indicate that the immediate complication rate from endovascular treatment in symptomatic patients is higher than that associated with CEA. Recent European guidelines[10] have highlighted that CAS has a higher risk of stroke (hazard ratio (HR) of 1.81) and death or stroke (HR 1.72) but a lower risk of MI (HR 0.44) and cranial nerve injury (HR 0.08). Finally, older patients fare worse with CAS, an important consideration with our ageing population. However, these results must be interpreted with caution as outcomes in stenting are closely associated with experience. More recent results from centres using a cerebral protection device (umbrella-like system in the distal internal carotid artery to prevent debris embolizing to the brain) and stents in addition to angioplasty are improved.

CAS has a role in hostile neck anatomy after previous neck surgery or irradiation, and high or tandem carotid lesions. It is likely that both carotid stenting and CEA will have a place in future treatment of carotid disease, especially with the advent of trans-carotid stenting with flow reversal techniques. Currently recruiting trials (ACST-2 and ECST-2) will hopefully provide further information.

Carotid Body Tumour

Pathological Features

These lesions are rare, commonly bilateral with a strong family history and arise in the carotid body or, less commonly, in one of the adjacent nerves such as the vagus. They are paragangliomas, but it is not clear what proportion have a malignant component. Lymph node deposits may be found in up to 25%, but distant metastases are extremely rare and local recurrence is uncommon.

Clinical Features

The usual presentation is a painless lump in the neck. It is frequently mistaken for a lymph node or a parotid lesion and may have been explored previously. The lump is not tender, is fleshy and, most importantly, can only be moved transversely in relation to the carotid sheath.

Diagnosis

A typical lump in the neck is investigated by either angiography, duplex scanning, CT or MRI. Angiography reveals a tumour blush and typical splaying of the internal and external carotid arteries into a wine glass shape (Fig. 27.32).

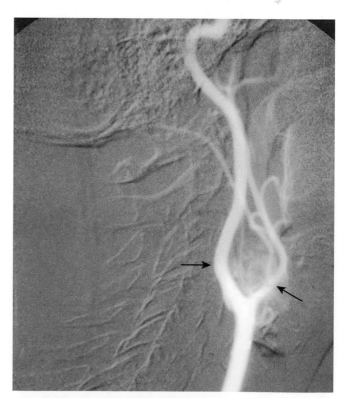

• **Fig. 27.32** Angiogram showing a 'blush' of contrast and splaying of the internal (left arrow) and external (right arrow) carotid arteries because of the presence of a carotid body tumor.

Other imaging gives more detailed information on the feasibility of resection. Few carotid body tumours are part of the multiple endocrine neoplasia (MEN) syndromes. Those are more likely to secrete active substances. If there is adequate suspicion, then levels of circulating catecholamines and thorough investigations should be sought prior to any intervention.

Management

Carotid body tumours should be excised because they grow locally: the larger the tumour, the more difficult the operation becomes. However, intervention runs the risk of arterial and nerve damage. Preoperative embolization of tumours to reduce vascularity during operation has not been met with success and hence is rarely performed. Radiotherapy is reserved for symptomatic treatment of an inoperable lesion.

VISCERAL ISCHAEMIA

Acute Mesenteric Ischaemia

This condition is discussed in detail in Chapter 13.

Chronic Mesenteric Ischaemia

The ability of the gastrointestinal circulation to develop collaterals ensures that the great majority of patients with arterial inflow obstruction are asymptomatic. It is generally believed that at least two of the three arteries which supply the gut (coeliac axis, superior and inferior mesenteric arteries) must be critically stenosed or occluded for symptoms to develop.

Clinical Features

A typical complaint is of severe abdominal pain after eating – mesenteric angina. Fear of eating develops, so that mesenteric ischaemia is always associated with significant weight loss. This presentation mimics many other abdominal disorders, and frequently the patient has had numerous inconclusive investigations before the diagnosis is finally made.

Apart from weight loss, which is universal, there are rarely any physical findings. Occasionally an epigastric bruit is present.

Diagnosis and Management

Although, in these slim patients, an experienced ultrasonographer or vascular scientist can often identify mesenteric disease on duplex scanning, the diagnosis can only be made with certainty on angiography.

Surgical revascularization is the mainstay of treatment, although balloon angioplasty and stent placement has an increasing role. The commonest operative approach involves taking a graft from the aorta or iliac vessels to the superior mesenteric artery and the coeliac axis. This is a major surgical undertaking and is associated with significant risk including death, but the long-term results are good. Conservative management may, in some cases, lead to a slow and painful death from progressive cachexia.

RENAL ARTERY DISEASE

Renal Artery Stenosis

Pathophysiological and Pathological Features

In most patients, renal artery stenosis (RAS) is asymptomatic and merely an incidental finding at postmortem or on angiography performed for another indication (Fig. 27.33). RAS leads to decreased renal perfusion and the release of renin from the juxtaglomerular apparatus. Renin converts angiotensinogen to angiotensin I, which is in turn converted to angiotensin II in the lung. Angiotensin II causes vasoconstriction and the release of aldosterone from the adrenal cortex. The renal excretion of sodium is reduced and blood pressure rises, which may, in the short term, return renal perfusion to normal. However, a progressive stenosis leads to worsening ischaemia, hypertension, loss of nephrons, atrophy and irreversible renal failure. The two main causes of RAS are atheroma (60%) and fibromuscular dysplasia (up to 40%). These two disease processes are quite different (Table 27.4). Less common causes include renal artery aneurysm thrombosis and embolism arteritis and trauma.

Clinical Features

Renovascular hypertension affects a large number of people. For example, in the UK, approximately 10% of the adult population is hypertensive, and in these, a renal cause is thought to be responsible for about 10% of cases. Suggestive features include onset before the third and after the

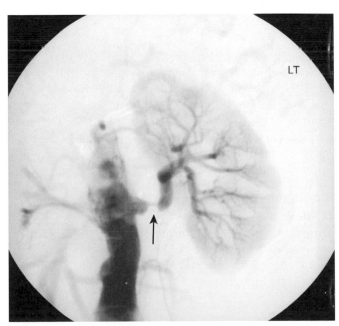

• **Fig. 27.33** Angiogram showing almost complete occlusion of the left renal artery from atherosclerosis (arrow). This was successfully treated by percutaneous placement of a stent.

<table>
<tr><td>**TABLE 27.4**</td><td colspan="2">**Comparison of Renal Artery Atherosclerosis and Fibromuscular Dysplasia.**</td></tr>
<tr><td>**Atherosclerosis**</td><td colspan="2">**Fibromuscular dysplasia**</td></tr>
<tr><td>60%</td><td colspan="2">40%</td></tr>
<tr><td>Males aged 60 years and over</td><td colspan="2">Females usually aged 40–60 years; may affect children</td></tr>
<tr><td>Stenosis at or within 1–2 cm of ostium</td><td colspan="2">Affects distal two-thirds of renal artery ± segmental branches</td></tr>
<tr><td>30% have aortic occlusive or aneurysmal disease</td><td colspan="2">Often multifocal</td></tr>
<tr><td>Part of generalized atherosclerotic disease</td><td colspan="2">'String of beads' on angiogram</td></tr>
<tr><td>10–20% may occlude in 3 years</td><td colspan="2">Occlusion uncommon</td></tr>
<tr><td>30% have bilateral disease</td><td colspan="2">Unknown aetiology</td></tr>
</table>

• BOX 27.7 Investigations of Patients with Renal Artery Stenosis

Technetium (Tc)-labelled DTPA or MAG3 scanning
- Poor take-up of radioisotope on affected side
- Reveals RAS if greater than 60%, especially after administration of an ACE inhibitor which exacerbates renal hypoperfusion

Colour flow duplex ultrasound
- Directly measures flow velocities in the renal arteries
- Very operator-dependent
- Probably not reliable at present

Renin levels
- Can be measured in general circulation or in renal vein
- High levels suggest renovascular hypertension but low sensitivity and specificity

MRI
- Provides images of the renal arteries without exposure to ionizing radiation
- At present there are still problems with expense, availability and software

DTPA, Diethylenetriaminepentaacetic acid; MAG3, mercaptoacetyltriglycine.

fifth decade and the presence of peripheral vascular disease. Hypertension is typically of abrupt onset, severe or malignant in nature and difficult to control with standard medical therapy.

Renal failure caused by RAS is much less common but it should always be considered in the differential diagnosis of renal failure, particularly when there is evidence of peripheral vascular disease. Deterioration of renal function after administration of an angiotensin-converting enzyme (ACE) inhibitor can form the trigger for clinical detection because these drugs prevent the adaptive responses described above. Discontinuation of the ACE inhibitor usually returns renal function to pre-treatment levels.

Diagnosis

It is important to make a precise diagnosis, but this can be difficult. Clinically, suspected RAS is usually confirmed by angiography. Although many other less invasive and expensive investigations have been advocated, none is sufficiently sensitive or specific as a screening test (Box 27.7). Occasionally, the clinical significance of the diagnosis of RAS can only be confirmed by reduction in blood pressure and/or improvement in renal function after its correction.

Management

Medical

Drugs can control all but the most severe forms of hypertension and may limit hypertensive nephropathy in the unaffected contralateral kidney. However, medical treatment cannot arrest progression of stenosis.

Surgical

Recent randomized trials have shown no benefit in renal revascularization in terms of blood pressure or renal function for atherosclerotic disease. The revascularization options are either endovascular with angioplasty +/- stenting or open bypass using vein.

Fibromuscular dysplasia appears to show improved treatment outcomes, and is usually dealt with by angioplasty.

If there is a small non-functioning kidney, nephrectomy may be the only option. Acute thrombosis of a chronically stenosed renal artery may not lead to renal infarction, because of the development of collateral capsular supply, and surgical bypass or PTA with stenting can sometimes be successful.

Renal Artery Aneurysm

This is an uncommon disorder that may lead to renovascular hypertension and renal failure. Rupture also occurs, and repair should be considered if the lesion exceeds 2 cm in diameter.

VASCULAR TRAUMA

Mechanisms

The commonest non-iatrogenic cause of injury to blood vessels in the UK is road traffic accidents (usually blunt injuries). Penetrating injuries – e.g. knife and gunshot wounds – are much less frequent. Iatrogenic injury to the brachial and common femoral arteries from angiography and angioplasty are by far the commonest. If the injury is caused by a sharp instrument such as a knife, the arterial or venous wound tends to be limited to the area of immediate injury and the remaining vessel is undamaged. In some, particularly high-velocity, missile wounds (see Ch. 36) or in blunt trauma, the extent of the injury is often more extensive, in terms of both the vascular injury and associated injuries in other systems.

Clinical Features

The two principal consequences of arterial injury are:

- Haemorrhage – external and obvious or internal and thus clinically unapparent until hypovolaemia develops. Blood loss tends to be greater if there is only partial rather than complete transection, because in partial transection, the laceration is held open by the continuity of part of the wall, whereas in complete transection, vasospasm and intimal retraction with thrombosis occur, which limits loss.
- Ischaemia – this is often severe because the injury is acute and the vasculature has previously been normal; therefore, there is little opportunity for collaterals to develop.

History and Symptoms

An obvious history of injury is common, but sometimes, in the context of multiple trauma, this may not be apparent. Otherwise the symptoms are those of acute vascular disruption.

Physical Findings

In young people, provided that the systolic blood pressure is above 100 mmHg, peripheral pulses should be readily palpable. Absent or diminished pulsation should immediately alert the clinician to the likelihood of vascular injury. In closed injury, an expanding haematoma may be palpable.

Doppler Examination

An audible Doppler signal may be present from a collateral circulation even if the artery is transected proximally.

Investigation

CT angiography should be considered in any instance where there is doubt about the diagnosis or where the site of injury is uncertain; additionally, it allows a road map and targeted treatment, and may be followed by endovascular repair or embolization (Fig. 27.34).

Management

As in any acutely ill patient, management begins with resuscitation (see Ch. 13). Immediate control of haemorrhage by direct pressure and then operation rapidly to restore normal flow are essential. The latter is achieved either by direct repair of the artery and accompanying large veins, if possible, or by means of a bypass graft. Because of the risk of infection, prosthetic materials should be avoided wherever possible.

All patients who sustain vascular trauma should receive appropriate antibiotics and, when indicated, tetanus

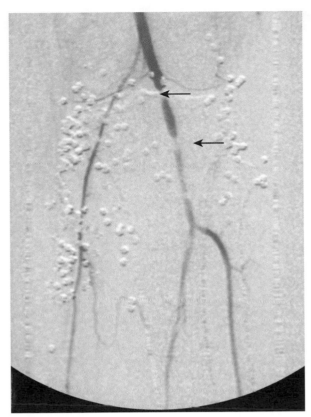

• **Fig. 27.34** This young man had a close-range shotgun wound of the knee. Although peripheral pulses were still present, the angiogram indicates severe multilevel injury to the popliteal artery (arrows). The vessel was reconstructed successfully with a vein graft, but unfortunately, because of extensive nerve injury, above-knee amputation was eventually required. Numerous shotgun pellets are also seen in the soft tissues.

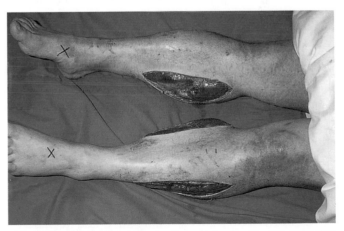

• **Fig. 27.35** Bilateral Fasciotomies Done Following Revascularization of Bilateral Severe Leg Ischaemia Note how the muscles are bulging through the skin incisions.

prophylaxis. The use of thromboembolic prophylaxis has to be decided on an individual basis and must be balanced against the risks of thrombosis versus those of haemorrhage. The risk of reperfusion injury is greatest in vascular trauma, and fasciotomy is frequently indicated for prevention (Fig. 27.35).

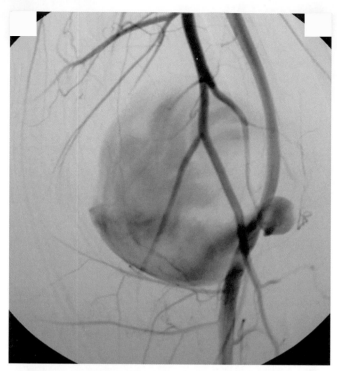

• **Fig. 27.36** Angiogram Showing a Large False Aneurysm of the Superficial Femoral Artery The course of the native artery is seen to deviate as a result of the mass effect of the false aneurysm.

ARTERIOVENOUS MALFORMATION

These types of malformation are congenital but not hereditary abnormalities, almost invariably present at birth, although they may not present for medical attention until much later in life. A number of rare syndromes are recognized including the Klippel–Trénaunay syndrome (KTS), characterized by a port-wine stain, varicose veins, bony and soft tissue hypertrophy involving the limb, which has an identified genetic abnormality in most patients (*PIK3CA*). Parkes–Weber syndrome is indistinguishable from Klippel–Trénaunay syndrome visually, but it is distinguished by the presence of multiple, microscopic, fast-flow arteriovenous shunts. Haemangiomas, by contrast, present a few days or weeks after birth and are much more likely to regress spontaneously. The more proximal an arteriovenous malformation (AVM) is in the circulation, the greater the transmitted flow. A proportion of malformations appear to be entirely venous. The terminology is often mixed when describing vascular malformations, with the term AVM being wrongly used to describe even pure venous malformations.

Clinical Features

Symptoms

Patients present at almost any age; onset of symptoms may be related to the appearance of the menarche, to pregnancy or to an episode of minor trauma. There is swelling, discoloration and/or bleeding which is usually not life-threatening; pain, high-output cardiac failure, limb hypertrophy and ulceration are less common.

Physical Findings

Lesions with an arterial component are usually pulsatile, a machinery-type murmur is heard on auscultation and, using a hand-held Doppler device, flow is easily detected in all phases of the cardiac cycle. Venous lesions engorge and empty with dependency and elevation, respectively.

Diagnosis

Appearance in later life requires distinction from malignant lesions such as sarcoma and metastatic deposits. Apart from biopsy to exclude malignancy in cases of doubt, the diagnosis is usually clinical.

Investigation

In venous lesions, phleboliths may be seen on plain radiographs. A chest X-ray allows assessment of cardiac size. Ultrasound, with or without venography, can be used to assess venous lesions. CT and particularly MRI (now the investigation of choice) give valuable information about deep extent when excision is contemplated. Angiography is invasive, should not be done for diagnostic purposes and is reserved for those lesions in which therapeutic embolization is under consideration.

Traumatic Arteriovenous Fistula

If, as a result of trauma, there is damage to an adjacent artery and vein, a fistula between them may develop.

Clinical Features

Symptoms include pain, swelling and sometimes other features of distal ischaemia. If the shunt is large, then, over some weeks and months, cardiac failure may develop.

There is often a thrill on palpation and, on auscultation, a machinery bruit throughout the cardiac cycle. Distal venous engorgement may develop.

Management

Surgical repair is indicated, but various endovascular techniques such as embolization and coverage of the fistulous opening in the artery with a covered stent may also be utilized.

False Aneurysm

As discussed above, arterial injury may lead to false or pseudo-aneurysm (Fig. 27.36). Treatment is by ultrasound-guided compression, thrombin, surgical repair, or, in certain circumstances, embolization with a coil or placement of a stent. Large false aneurysms causing compression of local structures may require an open surgical approach. Recently, combinations of stenting, coiling and thrombin injections have been used in experienced centres to deal with more complex pseudoaneurysms.

Management

AVMs may not require treatment except for counselling and reassurance for both the patient and, in children, the parents. When necessary, the principles are control of symptoms and prevention of complications with minimal intervention. Radiologists, cardiologists and vascular, orthopaedic, plastic and maxillofacial surgeons may all be involved in therapy.

Operation may occasionally be required to exclude malignancy. Complete excision provides good long-term control but is rarely feasible. The technique of dissection and ligation of feeding arteries is always associated with recurrence, compromises arterial access for interventional radiologists and should not be performed. Dissection and 'debulking' of the venous component can provide significant improvement in symptomatology and function, but often requires multiple stages and needs an experienced surgeon due to high risk of bleeding. Amputation is sometimes required as a last resort. Therapeutic embolization, in which the lesion is filled from within with thrombogenic coils, gel or onyx is another alternative but requires high skill and careful planning. It can be a useful bridge to surgery, reducing the intraoperative blood loss and the extent of surgery: however, it should be used with caution as it can lead to chronic pain symptoms secondary to inflammation. The risk of ischaemia in surrounding or distal vital tissues – inadvertent embolization of neural tissues, fingers and toes – is also a particular concern. Venous lesions can be treated by direct injection of sclerosant and/or partial excision of prominent veins once the normality of the deep venous system (sometimes absent or hypoplastic) has been assured.

VENOUS AND LYMPHATIC DISORDERS

Venous Disorders

The venous system is a high capacitance, low pressure, low flow, highly complex fluid dynamics system. The majority of the blood in the human body resides in the venous system at any time. The venous system is affected by conditions that cause clotting within it. This may in turn have consequences for the return of blood from the tissues and input from the arterial side. In addition, anatomical abnormalities (e.g. venous valves or scarring) may interfere with the fluid dynamics of the venous circulation and impair tissue nutrition, especially oxygenation, in the periphery.

Anatomical and Physiological Considerations (Fig. 27.37)

Superficial veins in the limbs and head and neck drain the skin. They contain valves which permit central flow but oppose reflux. The deep venous system comprises all channels within the investing (deep) fascia. In the limbs, these contain valves similar to those in the superficial veins. Communication between the superficial and the deep veins is provided by veins which perforate the investing

fascia – reflux in these is also prevented by valves. However, direction of flow is more complicated than has originally been appreciated. In the trunk, the deep veins are without valves (with venous return prompted by respiratory pressure changes), thereby creating a central pool in which changes in pressure are uniformly distributed. Changes in central venous volume and pressure are one of the major methods by which cardiac output is maintained.

The detailed physiology of the veins of the lower limbs, whose function is much influenced by the upright posture of humans, is considered below.

Pathological Features

Thrombosis

The fluidity of blood within veins is dependent on:
- Free flow, although stagnation is probably only an accessory factor to other causes of thrombosis
- Normal composition
- An intact endothelial surface. All vessels, but veins in particular, contain plasminogen activators which initiate the lysis of fibrin and so cause the dissolution of small accumulations of fibrin

These three factors were first invoked as the underlying causes of venous thrombosis by the German pathologist Virchow (Box 27.8, Table 27.5).

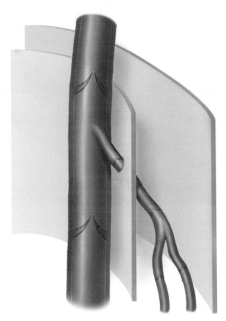

• **Fig. 27.37 The Superficial and Deep Venous Systems** The superficial vein passes through deep fascia to the deep venous system. A valve exists between the superficial and deep vein, permitting one-way passage of venous blood from superficial to deep systems.

• BOX 27.8 Virchow's Triad

Venous thrombosis occurs when there is:
- Stasis
- Increased viscosity of blood
- Endothelial trauma

TABLE 27.5	Factors in the Development of Venous Thrombosis (Virchow's Triad).	
Factor	Causes	Effects
Stasis	Obstruction Varicosity	Encourages aggregation of platelets and margination of leucocytes
Increased viscosity of blood	Increased platelets (thrombocytosis) Cell surface factors (malignancy) Surgery and trauma	Affects factors? Reduced fibrinolysis
Endothelial trauma	Direct injury	Provides point for adherence of platelets

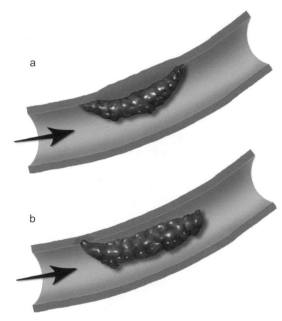

• **Fig. 27.38** Pathogenesis of Venous Clotting (A) Thrombophlebitis – blood clotting in vein secondary to inflammation of endothelium of the vein; (B) phlebothrombosis – blood clotting in vein due to stasis or factors other than inflammation.

Clotting of blood within a vein takes two clinico-pathological forms (Fig. 27.38):

• *Thrombophlebitis*, in which there is a strong element of endothelial trauma, either from a physical cause, or inflammation, or both

• *Venous thrombosis*, which may have a local (usually trauma) or general precipitating cause, but acute inflammation is not initially present

Although these are two distinct pathological entities, there may be an element of overlap in an individual case. The first is more common in superficial vessels and the second in the deep system, but essentially both result in a blood clot in a vein.

The pathological distinction between the two types is of clinical importance. In thrombophlebitis, the clot is deposited on damaged endothelium and is therefore attached to the vein wall throughout its (damaged) length. Spread takes place proximally (downflow) but usually only to the point of the next venous confluence where flow, if sufficient, will prevent further propagation. In venous thrombosis, the clot is loosely attached to the vein wall at the point of origin and extension proximally is as a free-floating mass (propagated thrombus) which may be of considerable extent and can easily become detached to pass proximally into the heart and lungs (pulmonary embolus) and can cause sudden death by obstruction of cardiac output. In both types of thrombosis (and in contrast to thrombosis in an artery), resolution takes place largely by fibrinolysis and the action of lysosomal enzymes secreted by leucocytes. The lumen is usually re-established (re-canalized) so that blood flow is restored. Crucially, the presence of a clot (superficial or deep) produces a pro-thrombotic state, with significant rates of further thromboses (both local and at distant sites).

However, there may be a varying amount of damage to the wall of the vein (and its delicate valves), so that it undergoes some fibrous replacement with loss of elasticity. In consequence:

• Valves are destroyed or rendered incompetent
• The vein can become dilated, predisposing to stagnation.
• The vein can become scarred with the formation of webs and fibrotic stenoses

The effect of this on venous function in the lower limb is considered later.

Recanalization is a variable entity, and is difficult to predict.

Varicose Veins

A vein is said to be varicosed when it becomes dilated and tortuous. Veins anywhere in the body can be affected but for practical purposes this common condition affects the lower limbs, as primary upper limb varicosities are uncommon and often related to complicated disease pathways.

Anatomy

Venous drainage of the lower limb is by both the deep and superficial systems.

• Superficial veins lie in the subcutaneous tissue, i.e. external to the deep fascia.
• Deep veins are within the enveloping deep fascia and drain all structures within the fascial compartments, the most important of which are the muscles.

The two systems are connected by communicating veins, each of which contains a valve that permits flow only from the superficial to the deep system. There are upwards of 100 perforators in each leg, of which only a small number are of clinical importance. The two major ones are:

• The entry of the long saphenous vein into the common femoral vein at the saphenous opening in the groin – the sapheno-femoral junction

- The junction of the short saphenous vein with the popliteal vein in the popliteal fossa – the short sapheno-popliteal junction

Other communications are found along the line of the subsartorial canal (mid-thigh, medially – the so-called Hunterian perforator) and on the medial aspect of the leg – Cockett's perforators. Perforators also exist on the lateral aspect of the leg and thigh, but they are clinically less significant. A poorly recognized superficial-to-deep communication is via the perineal veins which drain from the superficial system in the thigh, via the vulva and peri-vaginal plexus, to both the internal iliac and ovarian veins.

The major deep veins follow the same paths as the arteries, and below the knee are known as their venae comitantes. Above the knee, the veins join up to form a single companion trunk, the superficial femoral vein. This is then joined by the profunda vein just distal to the inguinal ligament to form the common femoral vein, into which the long saphenous vein drains before it (the CFV) becomes the external iliac vein at the level of the inguinal ligament. The valves in the deep system prevent reflux.

Venous Physiology in the Lower Limb

The energy required to propel blood from the heart to the periphery is generated by left ventricular contraction. In the erect position, the return of blood to the right side of the heart from the lower limbs is assisted by:

- Inspiration, which lowers intrathoracic pressure
- The muscle pumps of the thigh, calf and feet – of the two, this mechanism is by far the more important

Contraction of the muscles in the relatively rigid compartments deep to the investing fascia causes intra compartmental pressure to rise. Furthermore, the veins and venous sinuses in the muscles are directly compressed by the muscular contraction. Blood is expelled and directed proximally by the one-way valves. The valves in the perforating veins prevent its escape into the superficial system. This sequence can be illustrated by measurement of venous pressure in a superficial vein on the dorsum of the foot. With the patient horizontal and at rest, pressure is around 15 mmHg. On standing, but without muscle activity, blood continues to flow towards the heart but the pressure is increased to around 100 mmHg – an amount equivalent to the hydrostatic effect of a column of blood from the right atrium to the dorsum of the foot. Contraction of the muscles in the calf and foot (e.g. by rising on tiptoe, or shifting weight from one leg to the other) pumps blood towards the heart – the one-way valves prevent reflux into both the superficial system and distally. Relaxation of the muscles results in a transient fall in pressure to 40 mmHg, which then allows blood to flow in from the superficial veins via the perforators. This principle explains gravitational oedema – relative hypertension in the venous system due to lack of usage of the calf muscle pump due to immobility and extended periods sitting or standing still.

As seen in the cardiac pump, failure of the leg muscle pump, the valves or the presence of obstruction, impairs the normal fall of superficial venous pressure on exercise and causes an accelerated return to resting pressure upon standing.

The common factor in the production of venous disease in the lower limbs is loss of valvular competence in the:

- Superficial system – leading to cosmetic tortuosities (varicose veins) without disturbance of pump function
- Communicating veins – resulting in deep-to-superficial incompetence (DTSI) with reflux of blood and high pressures in the superficial system on exercise. Pressures transferred to the superficial system by contracting calf muscles in the presence of DTSI can be significantly greater than the pressure generated in the standing individual with incompetent superficial veins alone. However, the direction of flow in the perforating veins is a source of international controversy.
- Deep valves – which raises the pressure in the deep system

It is not known which comes first – the dilatation of veins leading to the valves not meeting and becoming incompetent, or the incompetent valves leading to reflux and dilation of the veins.

Epidemiology

Varicose veins are extremely common, possibly the most common disease in humans. The prevalence of incompetent veins is around 30–40% of the population, with a female: male ratio of 3:1, but varices are less common in the young (<20 years). Symptomatic varicose veins are less common. The symptoms involved are aching, pain, heaviness and itching

The major complications of chronic venous hypertension are swelling, chronic inflammation and damage to the skin. This may eventually go on to ulceration and even malignancy – the eponymous 'Marjolin's ulcer', which is an aggressive, ulcerating, squamous cell carcinoma arising in an area of chronic ulceration. The cost of a venous ulcer is enormous both in terms of quality of life and economic cost (approximate cost of healing one 50p-coin-sized venous ulcer is £8000). A large proportion of venous patients are of working age and the venous diseases cause significant quality of life impairment and work disruption.

It is a progressive disease, with approximately 6% of patients advancing through the clinical stages of the disease per year.

Classification and Aetiology

It is customary to classify varicosities into:

- Primary – there is venous reflux only, where the varicosities appear without an obvious underlying cause
- Secondary – where the varicosities occur because of some other cause: obstruction, or thrombo-inflammatory destruction of valves in both the communicating and deep veins

Primary Varicose Veins

The exact mechanism by which valve failure occurs is still disputed. It was originally assumed that a valve or valves in a communication between the deep and superficial systems became incompetent from above downwards, followed by progressive proximal to distal destruction of the valves in the superficial system exposed to increased hydrostatic pressure. For example, in the long saphenous system, first sapheno-femoral valve incompetence, followed by dilation of the vein itself and thus valve failure throughout its length. Studies with Doppler ultrasound, however, have suggested that branches of the long saphenous vein (LSV) may become incompetent without or before incompetence at the sapheno-femoral junction. In addition, use of the saphenous vein for cardiac and arterial surgery suggests that its muscular wall makes it resistant to dilation when pressure is raised. Evidence from genetic studies in lymphoedema has suggested that valve structure creation can be turned off and on in mice.

There is little doubt that there is a familial component but, this apart, there is no convincing hypothesis of cause. A contributing factor is thought to be multiple pregnancies – possibly through hormonal effects on the muscle of the vein wall – as progesterone and oestrogen cause relaxation of smooth muscle.

Secondary Varicose Veins

These are less common than the primary type but are still frequent in some groups, such as women who have had multiple or complicated pregnancies. Causes are:

- Deep or, less commonly, superficial venous thrombosis with recanalization and consequent deep and/or deep-to-superficial valve destruction
- Obstruction with venous hypertension – e.g. injury to a proximal vein, or obstruction by a tumour, obesity (weight of the abdominal pannus on the iliac venous tree).
- Congenital or acquired arteriovenous fistulae, with increased pressure and flow being transmitted from the arterial side of the circulation

Secondary varicose veins are associated with the syndrome of chronic venous insufficiency, which is considered later.

Secondary Effects

Peri-Venous Tissue Changes

Chronic venous hypertension causes characteristic changes in the skin and subcutaneous tissues of the lower limb. A rise in pressure at the venular end of the capillary loop to a value greater than the plasma oncotic pressure – normally 25 mmHg (about 34 cmH$_2$O) – causes:

- Accumulation of interstitial oedema fluid which, at least initially, may be compensated for by increased removal by greater lymph flow
- Impaired delivery of oxygen to cells, which predisposes the skin to break down from minor trauma – thus causing ulceration
- Egress of plasma and red cells into the surrounding tissue

Skin Changes

The changes in the skin and subcutaneous tissues seen in chronic venous hypertension are described collectively in the term lipodermatosclerosis (LDS). It is characterized by:

- Inflammation – caused by extrusion of plasma proteins, which are recognized as foreign by the macrophages and against which an immune (inflammatory) response is mounted. This is sometimes misdiagnosed as infection (bacterial cellulitis) and inappropriately treated with antibiotics. It should, however, be recognized that trauma to the skin can become secondarily infected. Thus the 'sterile inflammation' is complicated by bacterial inflammation (cellulitis). This has practical implications in that the sterile inflammation will not respond to antibiotics. Usually, however, non-infective inflammation responds to anti-inflammatory agents.
- Pigmentation – secondary to the extrusion of red cells and their subsequent destruction by macrophages. Hemosiderin, the end-product of the breakdown of haemoglobin, is brown and causes the brown pigmentation characteristic of LDS.
- Thickening of the subcutaneous tissues – oedema and patchy fibrosis.
- Atrophy of the skin – often with depletion of normal pigment cells and white dermal patches – 'atrophie blanche'.

Microscopic assessment of lipodermatosclerosis shows additional changes which stem from the venous hypertension and poor cellular nutrition:

- Dilation and tortuosity but a decrease in the number of capillaries
- Trapping of white cells within capillary loops
- Peri-capillary deposition of a cuff of fibrin
- Increased numbers of extravasated leucocytes

All of these may play a role in the progression of the disorder. The dilated capillaries may be more permeable, so exacerbating the oedema. The fibrin cuff has been thought to reduce diffusion and so interfere with nutrition. However, this is currently regarded as unlikely and more probably a secondary phenomenon. Tissue oxygenation is certainly reduced. White cell activation associated with the release of cytokines, proteolytic enzymes and free radicals could result in further damage. Finally, tissue repair is inhibited by the physical presence of extravasated fibrinogen and by alpha-2-macroglobulin which binds growth factors, so making them unavailable (trap hypothesis).

This progressive fibrosis and inflammation leads to the 'inverted champagne bottle' appearance which further impairs the venous system by disrupting and damaging the venous pump system leading to poor outflow.

A further, though uncommon, event is for squamous carcinoma to develop in a long-standing ulcer – Marjolin's ulcer, named after the French surgeon, Jean Nicolas Marjolin, who first described the condition in 1828.

Calf Perforating Veins – 'Perforators'

Normally, during walking or running, the superficial veins in the lower limbs drain the skin into the deep veins via perforating veins (a.k.a. 'perforators') in both the calf and thigh – here we are not considering the sapheno-femoral and popliteal junctions as 'perforators'. The load on these perforators is increased in proportion to the incompetence in the superficial system – usually from either the sapheno-femoral or sapheno-popliteal junctions. With increased load they dilate. The superficial incompetence may be of an order that causes the perforating vein/s to dilate beyond the point where their valves are competent. At this stage, the significant pressures generated by the calf muscles during ambulation are transferred retrogradely through these now incompetent calf perforators to the skin where the changes of chronic venous hypertension can develop. After the superficial incompetence has been addressed surgically, the load is removed and the perforators usually decrease in diameter to the point where they once again become incompetent. However, this may not occur and the patient can be left with chronic isolated calf-perforator incompetence and the consequences of the chronic venous hypertension. It is common for clinicians to miss this and, worse, if recognized, to feel that nothing can be done for these patients except for them to wear support stockings for life with the consequence that they may well develop chronic recurrent leg ulceration. This is unfortunate as this source of incompetence may be successfully addressed surgically, by either endovenous or open methods, thus providing the tormented patient with relief and even cure. Duplex Doppler scanning will confirm the diagnosis – see later.

The pathological and other features of ulceration are considered in more detail later.

Clinical Features

History and Symptoms

The symptoms of varicose veins may vary considerably. Because both varicose veins and leg symptoms are common, it is important to realise that they may neither be causal nor even related. This is key in managing expectations of patients.

A Family History. This is obtained in more than a third of patients and is often coupled with onset at a relatively young age. In secondary varices, there may be a history of deep-vein thrombosis (see later) although absence of this does not exclude such an event having taken place.

Patients with varicose veins may ascribe symptoms to them which, in fact, have other causes. Common symptoms which can be associated with varicose veins (some of which may have alternative causes) are listed in Table 27.6.

Discomfort. Aching is traditionally regarded by patients as a symptom they should have and may dominate their complaints – even though in fact they are more concerned about the unsightliness. Relief of discomfort on elevation or through the use of an elastic stocking is common although non-specific. Patients who have incompetent or obstructed deep veins may complain of discomfort of a bursting type on exercise. This will become more pronounced if a tourniquet is placed around the patient's thigh at a pressure higher than that in the superficial venous system (but, of course, lower than arterial pressure) – *Perthe's* test.

TABLE 27.6	Symptoms of Varicose Veins and Alternative Explanations.	
Symptom	**Alternative causes**
Ugly appearance	Obesity
	Vascular disorders
Aching	Simple fatigue
	Musculoskeletal disorders in limb or trunk (sciatica, arthritis of hip or knee)
Pain on exercise	Arterial claudication
	Spinal claudication
Ankle swelling	Oedema of other cause – cardiac, renal, lymphoedema
Restless legs	Neurological disorder
Pigmentation and depigmentation	Skin disorders
Eczema	Skin disorders
Attacks of superficial phlebitis	Systemic causes – neoplasia – thromboangiitis obliterans
Ulceration	See Table 27.14
Bleeding into the subcutaneous tissues	Blood disorders with reduced clotting ability or increased bleeding tendency

Pain. Pain may follow the development of a skin complication such as ulceration and will increase when complicated by cellulitis. Blood clot within a vein excites a non-bacterial inflammatory response – superficial venous thrombosis (superficial thrombophlebitis) – and is accompanied by acute pain along the line of the affected vein. Infection of a vein – e.g. where a cannula is present to administer intravenous fluids – may even cause thrombosis by initially damaging the wall of the vein.

Bleeding Varices. Varices may bleed:
- Into the subcutaneous tissues. This is usually minor and causes only discomfort and bruising.
- Externally, from the rupture of a varix. This is usually precipitated by minor trauma. If the patient remains upright, there can be considerable blood loss because the haemorrhage is at high pressure. Deaths from such bleeding, which is in effect from the right side of the heart, still occur annually. However, they are rare – presumably because the patient has the insight to apply pressure and/or assumes the horizontal position (voluntarily or otherwise), thus reducing the pressure and allowing a thrombus to plug the leak.

'Venous eczema'. Early inflammation gives rise to itching. This may lead the patient to scratch and further damage the skin – and this may become infected, causing bacterial cellulitis. Venous eczema may be seen in patches in relation to prominent varicosities and especially in the legs

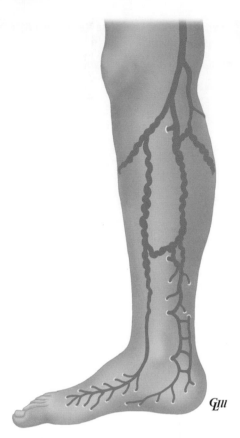

• **Fig. 27.39** Variceal Pattern in Long Saphenous System

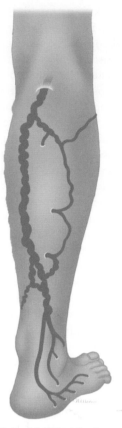

• **Fig. 27.40** Variceal Pattern in Short Saphenous System in Leg

(i.e. below the knee where the venous pressure in the superficial system is higher than in the thigh).

Ulceration. This is often painless, although episodes of inflammation caused by infection may change this. Additionally, the raw wound can be extremely painful during dressing change.

Upon completion of taking a history from a patient it is important to have developed some idea of the severity of the symptoms and whether they are related to their varicose veins or are the consequence of another disorder.

Signs in the Lower Limbs

Variceal Pattern. The initial examination is in the upright position with the groin and foot fully exposed. The pattern of varices (Figs 27.39 and 27.40) is usually easily recognized as being in the territory of either the long saphenous (most common (Fig. 27.41)) or the short saphenous vein (next most common), or both (unusual in primary varices). However, the patterns seen cannot, on their own, be used to make an anatomical diagnosis – because of the intercommunication between the two systems. Unusual variations in the distribution of varices suggest a possible pelvic obstruction; if associated with apparent enlargement of the limb and port wine stains of the skin, there is the possibility of an arteriovenous malformation or of the rare *Klippel–Trénaunay syndrome* – a complex developmental anomaly with multiple venous malformations, fistulae and overgrowth of the limb and which is associated with hypoplasia

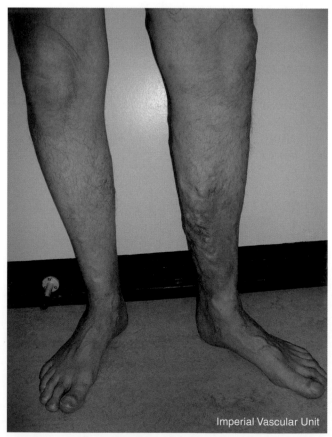

Imperial Vascular Unit

• **Fig. 27.41** Leg Showing Varicosities Within the Distribution of the Long Saphenous Vein and Skin Changes Above the Medial Malleolus.

of the deep veins, or even *Parkes–Weber syndrome* which has arterio-venous fistulae. The clinical manifestations of ovarian vein insufficiency are usually brought on by pregnancy, where the combination of raised progesterone levels (which causes smooth muscle cell relaxation) and the bulky uterus produce dilation in the vein and thus valvular insufficiency. Vulvar and lower-limb varicosities can be impressive. The condition usually recedes after delivery but may persist and treated varicosities may recur. Patients with significant ovarian vein incompetence may also have pelvic congestion syndrome – cyclical lower abdominal discomfort. These symptoms may be debilitating to the extent that treatment of the underlying condition (ovarian vein incompetence) is considered – by endovenous embolization.

With the patient supine and on raising the leg, varices either disappear completely or reduce significantly in size. An exception is when there is obstruction to venous outflow from the limb, causing secondary varices. The variceal pattern then includes the groin and adjacent abdominal wall.

Blow-Outs. These are localized dilations and may be visible and palpable along either saphenous vein. They are sometimes associated with a palpable defect in the deep fascia and the presence of an incompetent perforating vein. A pronounced dilation is sometimes seen at the site of major incompetence between the deep and superficial systems: e.g. a saphena varix in the groin, which must be distinguished from a femoral hernia (see Ch. 30); and a mass of tortuous vessels in the popliteal fossa. Blow-outs may also be seen in relation to incompetent medial calf perforators and should alert the clinician to their presence. Treating them (see later) may cure the patient of unpleasant manifestations of chronic venous hypertension including inflammatory sclerosis and lipodermatosclerosis (LDS).

Oedema. This is associated with primary varices, pits readily and is typically seen at the site of the grip of an ankle sock. Gross oedema, except when associated with ulceration, is more likely to have a secondary or multiple causes: cardiac disease, renal disease, or lymphoedema. Other causes of leg enlargement are lipoedema and primary cyclic oedema syndrome. In lipoedema, there is a primary (usually familial) thickening of the subcutaneous tissues of the lower limbs, but sparing the feet – most frequently seen in women. Untreated lymphoedema leads to fat deposition in the lymph-fluid filled spaces causing lipoedema. The condition can be associated with a seemingly inexplicable, local tenderness. In primary cyclic oedema syndrome, there is an idiopathic cyclic swelling of the legs, again, almost exclusively seen in females. As its name implies, the cause is unknown.

Skin and Subcutaneous Tissues. In mild varices, the skin is usually normal. However, where there has been long-standing superficial venous hypertension, whether caused by superficial reflux alone or associated with damage to the deep system, the characteristic changes of lipodermatosclerosis develop (see above and Fig. 27.42).

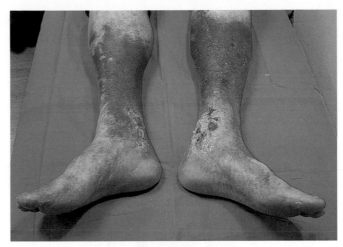

• **Fig. 27.42** Extensive bilateral lipodermatosclerosis and dark brown pigmentation (from the deposition of haemosiderin) with an area of ulceration as a result of long-standing deep venous incompetence.

General Examination

This may reveal underlying causes to explain symptoms and signs in patients who present with varices, particularly heart failure and musculoskeletal or pelvic disease in the elderly. Examination of the peripheral arterial system (skin temperature, nutritional changes and peripheral pulses) is essential to distinguish venous from arterial disorders, or to assess the relative contribution of each to a complication such as ulceration.

Clinical Tests of Valve Function

Clinical tests can be useful but have been superseded by the gold standard investigation, duplex ultrasound. Percussion of the column of blood in a vein with the patient standing – the 'tap test' – causes upward transmission of a palpable wave, especially when the vein is distended. In a varicose vein that has incompetent valves along its length, the wave is also transmitted downward. This procedure is most useful in the long saphenous system.

The Trendelenburg test (Fig. 27.43) is done by elevating the leg to 45 degrees to empty the superficial veins by gravity and this may be assisted by stroking them from distal to proximal. A tourniquet is then lightly applied to the leg (the degree can only be learnt by practice but, in essence, it should be tight enough to prevent reflux of blood in the superficial system but sufficiently light not to impair arterial flow to the limb) just distal to the sapheno-femoral junction and the patient asked to stand. If there is isolated sapheno-femoral valve incompetence, the varicosities remain empty for at least 15–30 seconds and then gradually refill as blood continues to flow in from the arterial side of the circulation. The test is repeated with release of the tourniquet immediately on standing when, in the presence of significant venous insufficiency, reflux from the deep system will cause rapid filling of the varicose veins. Finally, if the veins fill at once even with the tourniquet in place, the sequence is repeated, moving the tourniquet down the limb until the

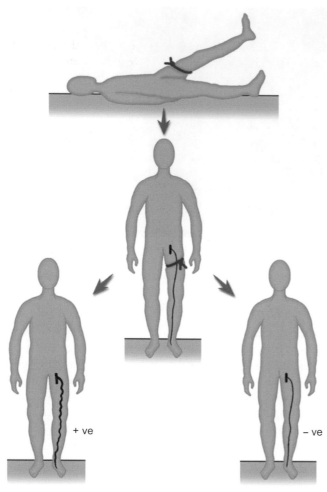

• **Fig. 27.43** The Trendelenburg Test.

lowest point of DTSI is found. If there is still rapid filling when the compression is below the level of the termination of the popliteal vein (just below the knee), then it is likely that there are incompetent perforating veins in the calf. However, localization of these is not usually successful by this simple clinical procedure.

The Trendelenburg test may be done with finger pressure alone rather than a tourniquet (the true Trendelenburg test uses finger pressure), but experience is required; a precisely applied tourniquet is preferable.

Investigations

The investigations described below are for localization of incompetent deep-to-superficial communications and for identification of valvular insufficiency in deep veins.

Continuous Wave Ultrasound

The Doppler directional probe (see Ch. 7) generates continuous waves which are reflected after striking their target. The reflected waves are then perceived by a sensor and transformed into a visual signal or sound. If the target is moving (as with the red cells in blood) on reflection, the frequency of the waves is altered – thus flow can be assessed. This

principle is used to detect points of incompetence such as at the sapheno-femoral junction. With the probe just distal to this point, flow upwards in the saphenous vein is accelerated by compressing the calf or a prominent varix. Release of compression in the presence of competent valves causes a sharp cut-off of the signal. However, if there is incompetence, reflux occurs and generates a new signal. The test can be repeated at other sites of suspected DTSI such as the popliteal fossa (short sapheno-popliteal junction) and on the medial aspect of the leg where there are perforating veins. However, the accuracy of this investigation, except at the sapheno-femoral junction, is poor and other investigations, such as duplex ultrasound Doppler scanning, provide more accurate information.

Duplex Ultrasound Scanning

Duplex ultrasound scanning is commonly used in the assessment of venous conditions and many surgeons use it routinely. It provides a combination of ultrasound imaging of the vessel and Doppler detection of the direction of flow. The underlying principles of assessment of flow are similar to those for the hand-held continuous-flow instrument. The advantages are:

- Valves at these junctions and in the deep veins can be seen.
- The anatomy, particularly at the sapheno-femoral and sapheno-popliteal junctions, can be clearly shown.
- Reflux is demonstrated by the reversal of the direction of flow, using the same principle as continuous-flow Doppler. Colour-coding the direction of flow improves the precision with which reflux can be detected. More than 0.5s of reflux is considered pathologic.

Modern, easily-portable machines enable surgeons to manage their patients in clinics and theatre more confidently. This has led to a significant drop in the incidences of recurrence due to tactical treatment failure.

Venous Pressure and Volume Studies

The physiology of the venous muscular pump has been discussed in a previous section. Dynamic changes in volume of the leg are measured by various techniques, known collectively as plethysmography. They are not used in routine investigation but are extensively used in research to help delineate disease and can be helpful when clarifying complex recurrence after surgery or after deep venous stenting.

Radiological Imaging

Since the advent of reliable duplex scanning, invasive, contrast-based radiological investigations are rarely indicated. They are still occasionally used in complicated cases where duplex investigation has been inconclusive.

CT Venography

This excellent X-ray and contrast-using study allows assessment of abdominal components of the venous tree which are often blocked from ultrasound by bowel gas. It utilizes a special delayed protocol to allow careful venous assessment.

MR Venography

This is an alternative cross-sectional imaging solution, perfect for young patients due to its lack of ionizing radiation. Images can be obtained with and without contrast, but are better with contrast.

Ascending Venography

This is used to show the anatomy of the deep veins. Contrast medium is injected into a dorsal vein on the foot and, encouraged by the application of a tourniquet at the ankle, fills the deep system. It can be outlined in even more detail by application of a further venous tourniquet above the knee (Fig. 27.44). The technique can help to:

- Identify sites of incompetent communicating veins (perforators) in the calf or thigh, although it does not necessarily reveal all of them
- Demonstrate pathology in the deep veins caused by thrombosis – persistent occlusion or valvular incompetence. Its use is reserved for difficult problems associated with deep venous insufficiency

Descending Venography

This is used to quantify and investigate reflux. Contrast is injected proximally in the IVC, to show the pattern and extent of reflux in the lower limbs.

Multiplanar views are vital in venography, due to the complexities of the low pressure venous system. Pressure gradients performed during venography may also provide key information.

Intravascular Ultrasound

The development of small 360-degree ultrasound probes that can fit on a 4Fr and 6Fr (1–2 mm) catheter have provided an option for non-contrast and 360-degree assessment of the iliac veins. This is crucial for the placement of venous stents.

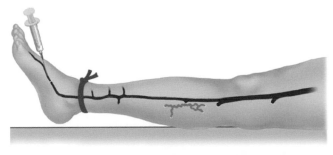

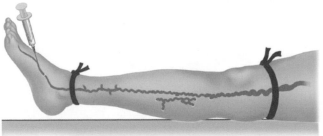

• **Fig. 27.44 Ascending Venography** The deep venous system is outlined in more detail by applying a tourniquet above the knee.

Management of Primary Varices

By definition, these are varices in the superficial system with no evidence of disease in the deep venous system.

Once it is reasonably certain that the symptoms and signs in the leg are associated with the varices, there are four management options: compression hosiery, foam sclerotherapy, endovenous ablation or surgery. The 2013 NICE guidelines have extensively investigated the effectiveness and economics of these interventions. This has led to a hierarchy of:

1. endovenous ablation,
2. foam sclerotherapy,
3. surgery and
4. compression hosiery.

It must be recognized, however, that the principle aim of venous intervention is symptom relief, and that technical success does not necessarily equate to symptom relief and vice versa.

Compression Hosiery

The indications are:

- those who refuse other forms of treatment
- most pregnant women.
- high-risk patients (high thrombotic risk) with limited disease or high-risk patients with extensive disease
- skin changes
- deep venous incompetence

The type of support and the choice are given in Table 27.7. It is important that any garments used should produce linear graduated compression, with the highest compression just above the malleoli and pressure decreasing towards the knee. Badly fitted support stockings or those which do not achieve graduated compression may produce more annoyance than relief and can, on occasion, cause damage to the

TABLE 27.7	Choice of Support Garment.		
Indication	Class	Pressure applied (at ankle, mmHg)[a]	Garment
Young patients; mild symptoms	I	14–17	Compression tights
Severe varices; early skin changes	II	18–24	Graduated compression: elastic stockings
Advanced skin changes; ulcer	III	25–35	Heavy-duty elastic stockings or initially elastic bandaging

[a]The compression pressure quoted is obtained by measuring the elastic tension at different sites on the stocking and deriving pressure from Laplace's equation: pressure = tension × radius. Methods for measuring the pressure under the stocking when it is in use are also available.

skin. Poor choice of stockings increases the frequency of non-compliance (which is in the region of 30%). Patients should be instructed to apply compression hose before they rise in the morning and to remove them only before retiring. They should be replaced every 3 months. Costs are approximately £30–£150 per pair. Bespoke manufacturing is available, as are adjustable Velcro and zippered neoprene wraps, which are more easily taken on and off, though at higher cost.

Foam Sclerotherapy

The principle of foam sclerotherapy is to produce sterile chemical inflammation in a vein with a sclerosant – obliteration of the lumen follows. Commonly used sclerosant solutions are sodium tetradecyl sulphate 1–3% (Fibro-Vein) and polidocanol (ScleroVein) – the latter is not licenced in the UK. Both of these are detergent based sclerosants. Previously, sclerotherapy was found suitable only for isolated varices without a large truncal reflux; if this exists, recurrence rates are high. However, in recent years, ultrasound-guided injection of foamed sclerosants (mixed with air via a three-way tap or microfilter – the Tessari method) has been demonstrated to increase the success rate. Recurrence rates are significantly higher than with other techniques; however, the intervention costs are very low and can be completed in virtually all patients. Furthermore, though vanishingly rare (four reported cases worldwide), with foam sclerotherapy there is a documented risk of stroke. Initially believed to be secondary to bubble propagation, recent work has shown that intra-cardiac bubbles after any venepuncture are common, but without sequelae. Trans-oesophageal echocardiography demonstrates that 25% of the population at large has an asymptomatic patent foramen ovale. Therefore, if a physical bubble embolus was the cause, rates of symptoms would be much higher. It is likely that the cause of migraines and transient visual effects seen is possibly endothelin-1 (produced by the vein on treatment). This is limited by abiding by maximum volume guidance.

Further uses for sclerotherapy are:
- Obliteration of isolated incompetent perforating veins
- Vulvar varices which persist after pregnancy – but these patients should first be investigated for underlying ongoing pelvic and/or ovarian vein incompetence as, if present, recurrence is likely
- Treatment of telangiectasia (thread veins/spider veins/star-burst veins, etc.) by micro-injection sclerotherapy (MIST) – this is sought by patients for cosmetic reasons

A common and frequently bothersome complication of injection sclerotherapy is skin-staining, in up to 30%. It usually fades over up to 2 years. The risk of this occurring is thought to be diminished by careful attention to adequate compression of the injected varices, but there is no objective evidence. Various compression regimes are used throughout the world, from none to compression for up to 6 weeks. Early evidence suggests that good treatment technique is the best management. Some patients may suffer with 'coagulum' – trapped liquefied haematoma which can be painful.

Relief is with targeted aspiration. Potential complications are listed in Table 27.8. All are uncommon, but their possibility means that sclerotherapy should not be undertaken lightly and only after adequate training (Fig. 27.45) shows an injection of foam and (Fig. 27.46) shows the resultant ultrasound image.

Surgery

The indications and contraindications for surgery are given in Table 27.9. The aim is to interrupt by ligation the major points of incompetence between the superficial and deep venous systems and, if appropriate, to remove the varices for both functional and cosmetic reasons. The two most common operations are sapheno-femoral and sapheno-popliteal ligation (Fig. 27.47) both of which can be done using day-care facilities, ideally under local anaesthetic blockade and tumescent anaesthesia. The procedure should be combined with removal of the saphenous trunk down to the knee by stripping, i.e. passing a flexible guide

TABLE 27.8	Complications of Sclerotherapy.	
Cause	**Reason**	**Outcome**
Subcutaneous injection	Inexperience; failure to check reflux of blood into syringe	Pain, skin necrosis, ulceration
Intra-arterial injection	Failure to observe arterial pressure in syringe	Possible loss of limb from arterial thrombosis
Sclerosant entering deep veins	Inadequate compression	Deep-vein thrombosis
Escape of sclerosant into general circulation	Inadequate compression	Anaphylaxis, haemolysis

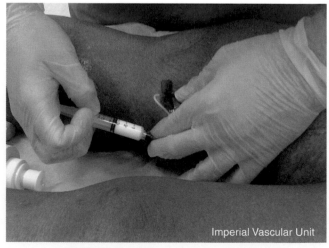

Imperial Vascular Unit

• **Fig. 27.45** Injection of Foam Sclerotherapy.

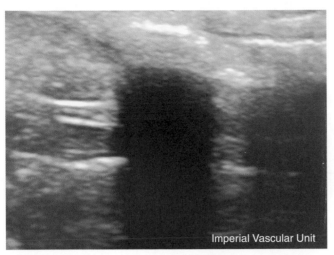

• **Fig. 27.46** Resultant Ultrasound Imaging After Foam Sclerotherapy.

TABLE 27.9	Indications for Surgery in Primary Varicose Veins.	
History or physical finding	**Indication**	**Contraindication**
Pain	Definite if established as not due to another cause	Doubt as to cause
Phlebitis	Varicose veins the only cause	Other conditions not excluded
Bleeding	Episode of considerable bleeding to exterior	Minor bleeding: systemic blood disorder not excluded
Skin and subcutaneous changes, including eczema	To alleviate itch and prevent cellulitis and ulceration	Deep venous disease must be excluded
Ulceration	Adjunct to healing	Surgery not able to correct venous hypertension

down the lumen of the vein, securing it to the divided vein and forcibly removing the vein subcutaneously. This not only improves the cosmetic result but also reduces recurrence, because the incompetent low resistance reservoir is removed. 'Neovascularization' is the most common cause of recurrence in these patients. This is the presence of a network of small veins enmeshed in scar tissue that leads to recurrent reflux either in a recurrent (or bifid) GSV or previously competent anterior thigh vein. Previously, this was thought to be due to inadequate technique or inadequate tributary ligation. However, this recurrence pattern is seen in all surgical trials throughout the world and is resistant to all attempts at prevention (including implantation of prosthetic patches to block tissue regrowth) but is not

seen in endovenous ablation. It therefore must be a normal consequence of this form of treatment. The presence of neovascularization does not necessarily equate to clinical or symptomatic recurrence.

If, in addition to sapheno-femoral or sapheno-popliteal incompetence, other incompetent sites have been identified, these too are ligated. Variceal channels are avulsed through small 'stab incisions' to give a pleasing cosmetic result – these incisions can be as small as 1 to 2 mm in length but sometimes need to be enlarged to accommodate larger varicosities. These incisions are sufficiently small to allow closure with Steri-Strips alone – no sutures are necessary, but may lead to improved cosmesis.

The incidence of recurrence after surgery for primary varices is up to 30% at 5 years in randomized controlled trials. It must be remembered that varicose veins are a progressive condition, and that not all recurrence is symptomatic or needs treatment. The commonest causes of recurrence are:

- Progression of disease (not truly recurrence)
- Poor operative technique, including failure to adequately ligate the sapheno-femoral junction, and strip the long saphenous vein to the extent that the Hunterian (mid-thigh) perforator is not removed (treatment failure)
- Failure to recognize concomitant short saphenous incompetence (tactical failure)
- Failure to recognize incompetent perforators (tactical failure)

Recurrent primary varices require careful investigation, including, most importantly, duplex ultrasound assessment.

Endovenous Ablation

Since the advent of endovenous ablation in 2001, there has been a sea change in venous treatment with the development of treatment catheters that utilize thermal energy to achieve obliteration of the great or small saphenous vein by denaturing the vein wall. The energy utilized is either radiofrequency or LASER energy or steam administered from a catheter placed within the lumen of the vein. The catheter is inserted percutaneously under ultrasound guidance and the procedure is carried out under local anaesthesia in 95% of cases and does not need a formal operating theatre.

Postoperative pain and bruising are reduced compared to surgery with equivalent long-term durability with data out to 5 years available. These techniques are now first-line treatment in the NICE guidelines (2013).

The catheter tip is placed 1–2 cm from the deep junction, leading to a different pattern of recurrent disease. The anterior thigh vein appears to be a common cause of recurrence at 5 years, with up to 32% refluxing at 5 years, though not all are symptomatic.

Multiple different laser wavelengths are now available, starting from 810 nm and now standard care in many places is 1540 nm. Longer wavelengths have reduced pain profiles, with equivalent long-term durability. Radiofrequency ablation has been shown to be less painful than laser treatment. Non-thermal ablation techniques including mechanochemical ablation (MOCA) and glue occlusion have emerged in

A

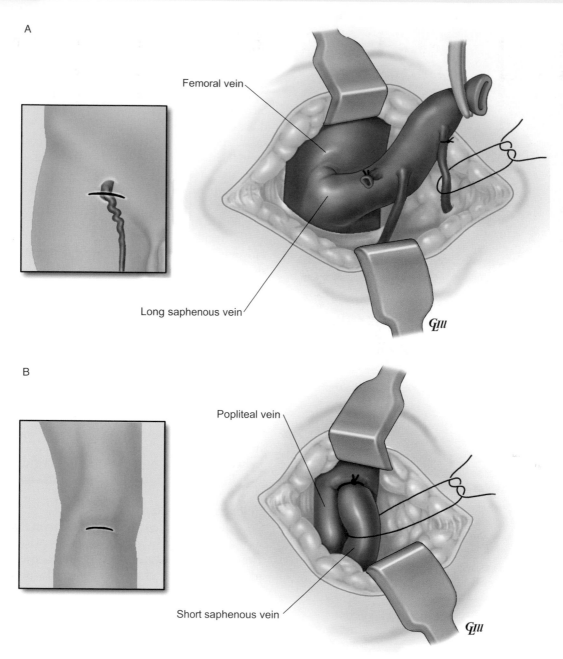

Femoral vein

Long saphenous vein

B

Popliteal vein

Short saphenous vein

• **Fig. 27.47** Operations for (A) sapheno-femoral and (B) sapheno-popliteal ligation.

the last 5 years and have been shown to have equivalent technical success with reduced procedural pain.

Ideally, the vein surgeon should have all the above methods available in her/his surgical armamentarium. A combination of patient preference, anatomical pathology and fitness for anaesthesia will then allow the most appropriate choice to be made. Fig. 27.48 shows an occluded GSV after ablation.

It is imperative that patients are given realistic expectations of varicose vein treatment during the informed consent procedure. Problems after varicose vein surgery (Box 27.9) are a common cause of medical negligence claims (due to the high number of procedures completed per year

– 40 000 in the NHS per annum) but are largely avoidable with careful attention to detail during the history, investigation, consent, operative and postoperative periods. Since the advent of the vascular surgery specialty and endovenous ablation, this appears to be reducing.

Venous Thrombosis

Thrombosis may develop in superficial or deep veins anywhere in the body through any one or a combination of the three events which constitute Virchow's triad (see Table 27.5). This can occur in a wide range of circumstances.

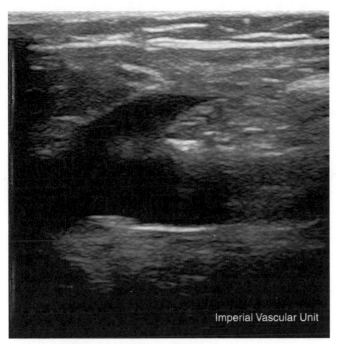

• **Fig. 27.48** Occluded GSV After Endovenous Ablation.

Imperial Vascular Unit

TABLE 27.10	Major Antecedents of Deep-Vein Thrombosis.	
Factor	**Circumstances**	
Immobilization (venous stasis)	Bed rest during serious illness or injury Long-distance air travel Unconsciousness	
Changes in clotting	Contraceptive pill – oestrogen containing Injury and operation Pregnancy/childbirth Malignant disease Hyperviscosity (e.g. polycythaemia) Antithrombin III, protein S and protein C deficiency Other thrombophilias	
Effects on vein wall	Trauma – accidental or from cannulation Extrinsic compression – inflammation, tumour, bony abnormality	

Superficial Venous Thrombosis (Thrombophlebitis)

Aetiology

There are three main causes:

- stasis – e.g. varicose veins
- local trauma and inflammation – may be of any type but in surgical practice is frequently the result of i.v. therapy
- generalized hypercoagulability – e.g. malignancy and thromboangiitis obliterans

Stasis is frequently a contributing factor to the other two. Recent studies have shown a significant association between superficial (SVT) and deep venous thrombosis (DVT) – 10% of patients with SVT develop DVT within 45 days despite anticoagulation, and this is not necessarily at geographically close sites.

Clinical Features

An inflammatory response (thrombophlebitis) to the thrombus is produced in the vein wall and surrounding tissues – this is frequently associated with pain. There may be

fever and, if the process is a pyogenic one, rigors, as bacteria are shed into the general circulation.

An obvious cause, such as an intravenous cannula and infusion, may be present. There is usually a red line along the skin over the vein – this is tender and firm to the touch.

Management

If there is a precipitating factor, this should be removed.

It is recommended that SVT be treated with 6 weeks of therapeutic anticoagulation. Studies have shown good results with low-molecular-weight sub-cutaneous injections. Recently, direct oral anticoagulants have become a viable alternative.

Spreading thrombophlebitis with systemic features may require blood culture and antibiotic therapy – and occasionally there is suppuration for which drainage is necessary. In recurrent attacks of migratory phlebitis, a search should be instituted for either arterial disease or an underlying malignancy – classically, carcinoma of the pancreas, though the pick-up rate is low.

Deep-Vein Thrombosis (DVT)

Although thrombosis in the deep veins of the lower limb draws most attention (because of its frequency and potentially serious consequences) the process is not limited to this part of the circulation and can occur anywhere in the deep venous system. The causes are summarized in Table 27.10 and follow the pattern of Virchow's (see Table 27.5).

Axillary–Subclavian Vein Thrombosis

Aetiology

Only 2% of deep-vein thromboses occur in these vessels. The subclavian vein, along with the artery and nerves to the upper limb, pass through the so-called thoracic outlet which is bounded anteriorly by the subclavius muscle (attached to the inferior border of the clavicle) and first rib postero-inferiorly. This space can be narrowed by poor posture (e.g. carrying a heavy rucksack for prolonged periods), exercise (butterfly swimming and weight-lifting are good examples), trauma (fractured clavicle), etc. Narrowing of this already narrow space may lead to obstruction of venous return and precipitation of venous thrombosis. Further anatomical causes in the area are cervical ribs and hypertrophy of the scalenus anterior muscle. The condition is more frequent in men and is often associated with physical exercise which involves the shoulder girdle – the so-called Paget–Schrötter syndrome (effort thrombosis of upper extremity), which was described independently by Paget in 1875 and Schrötter in 1884. Forcible abduction of the shoulder may cause intimal damage which is a starting point for thrombosis. Thrombophilia is another underlying cause – from use of the contraceptive pill and congenital deficiencies (in antithrombin 3, protein C and protein S deficiencies and other blood clotting disorders which cause hypercoagulability). Finally, the common use of axillary/subclavian vein catheters for i.v. therapy commonly cause thrombosis from irritant solutions, local trauma or bacterial infection. It is said that DVT in the upper limb carries a 10% incidence of pulmonary embolus.

Clinical Features

History. There may or may not be an obvious precipitating cause. The onset is fairly rapid (2–3 days) with the development of swelling of the upper limb, dragging pain and heaviness. Not infrequently, the limb will take on a dusky-blue colour due to venous congestion.

Physical Features. The limb is obviously swollen from the axilla to the fingers. The oedema initially pits readily but may become firm. Dilated (collateral) veins coursing over the shoulder girdle are seen, unless obscured by obesity or oedema.

Investigation

The diagnosis is usually obvious. However, subsequent investigation for an underlying cause may be required once the acute condition has subsided. It is important to obtain a baseline chest X-ray for anatomical reasons. D-Dimer assessment may help in those patients without clear cut signs. Additionally, the gold standard for diagnostic investigation is duplex ultrasonography.

Management

The limb should be elevated to minimize the development of induration from prolonged oedema and to make the patient more comfortable. As the swelling subsides, elastic support is substituted for elevation. Anticoagulant therapy, initially with heparin and thereafter with oral agents, is continued until the limb has returned to normal. There is a risk of post-thrombotic syndrome. Patients should be anticoagulated for 6 months, and there is a reasonable chance of recurrence thereafter without anticoagulation.

Thrombolytic therapy with tissue plasminogen activator (t-PA) is increasingly used but should be used with extreme caution because of the potentially devastating complication of haemorrhage, especially cerebral (<1%). If thrombolysis is considered and offered, it should be offered as a package with decompression of the thoracic outlet with first rib resection on the appropriate side. After successful thrombolysis, venoplasty to ensure patency and rib resection on the next available list is key. Stenting without removal of the mechanical cause is contraindicated.

First rib resection has significant morbidity attached, but does allow patients to stop anticoagulation in the future as the precipitating cause has been treated.

Lower-Limb DVT

This is the condition that has attracted most attention because of its frequency and well-established relation to surgical procedures, particularly in the elderly. However, because of the factors outlined in Table 27.10, it is not confined to the surgical patient: those with serious illnesses who require or are traditionally associated with immobilization, those with congestive heart failure and those with malignant disease are also at high risk. There is mounting evidence that the incidence of DVT amongst people travelling on long-haul flights may be higher than realized.

Anatomical Considerations

The deep venous system of the lower limb has already been described – it comprises all the venous channels within the investing deep fascia. In clinical practice, lower-limb thrombosis in the deep system commonly includes thrombus in the pelvic veins, in particular, the external iliac and common iliac veins, either in isolation or in continuity with thrombus which originates in the leg. For both diagnosis and management, it is helpful to qualify a lower-limb DVT by referring to the particular segment or segments of vessel involved, e.g. a popliteal vein thrombus or an iliofemoral vein thrombus – the latter carries a higher risk of life-threatening pulmonary embolus.

Aetiology and Epidemiology

All the factors given in Table 27.10 apply to DVT in the legs. Of particular importance in the postoperative patient are:
- Immobility during the operation and postoperatively
- Techniques of anaesthesia that promote muscular flaccidity and low rates of blood flow – prolonged general anaesthesia with paralysis and assisted ventilation
- Posture of the patient on the table – continuous pressure on the calves of the supine patient, the position used for hip replacement or lithotomy position
- Application of partial or full limb casts
- Venous obstruction in the pelvis during a surgical procedure
- Increased tendency to clotting following surgical or other injury
- Other thrombogenic changes in endothelial cell and leucocyte function after injury – this area is still under study

The incidence of DVT has been thoroughly studied in the postoperative patient with whom this account is chiefly concerned. Table 27.11 shows an average incidence of DVT of 30% in patients undergoing general surgical procedures. However, the detection techniques used in previous studies are not as accurate as current compression duplex ultrasound, with high false positive rates. Additionally, the ubiquitous use of thromboprophylaxis for surgical patients has significantly reduced that risk. The incidence varies widely with age. Advancing age is associated with a rise, although this may partly reflect the type of surgery that is required, e.g. an incidence of more than 60% in hip replacement. The high figures do not necessarily reflect the need for therapy, in that small thrombi can undergo spontaneous lysis. The majority of thromboses in everyday life are asymptomatic and never known about.

Risk Factors for DVT in Surgical Patients. The risk of DVT associated with various surgical procedures has been indicated in Table 27.11. Additional factors for individual patients are shown in Figure 27.49. In practice it is important to remember that the following increase risk:

- age – particularly over 40
- obesity
- operation for malignant disease
- a previous episode of DVT or pulmonary embolism

TABLE 27.11	Percentage Risk of Postoperative Deep-Vein Thrombosis Without Prophylaxis.	
Circumstance	Average risk (%)	Reported range (%)
General surgery		
– Abdominal	30	3–50
– Malignancy		40–70
Urology		10–50
– Open prostatectomy	40	
– Transurethral resection	10	
Vascular operations		
– Femoro-popliteal bypass	10	
– Aorto-iliac	5	
Traumatic operations in orthopaedics		
– Trauma	35	
– Hip fracture		40–60
– Tibial fracture		40–50
Elective orthopaedic procedures		
– Hip replacement	50	40–60
– Knee replacement	80	50–90
Immobilized patients with major medical illness (no surgery)	20	10–30

- consumption of the contraceptive pill within 30 days of a surgical procedure and for 2 weeks after. However, the increase in risk is relatively small

Pathological Considerations

Origin. Seventy-five percent of thromboses originate in the calf, particularly the soleal sinusoids, and in the valves of the calf veins; the remaining 25% are isolated to the proximal femoral or iliofemoral veins. Approximately 30% of thrombi in the calf spread in continuity to the popliteal and superficial femoral vein segments.

Natural History. As already indicated, many small calf vein thrombi undergo spontaneous lysis. When propagation occurs and occlusion of a main trunk such as the tibial or popliteal vein takes place, the thrombus is initially free-floating but, after a relatively short time, becomes adherent to the vessel wall and the process of organization begins with either lysis or the replacement of fibrin by fibrous tissue, or a combination of the two. The subsequent events are described in the section on the postphlebitic limb.

The possibility of a portion of clot becoming separated and a pulmonary embolus occurring is at its greatest while the clot remains free-floating and continues to acquire thrombus.

Clinical Features

Symptoms. Particularly in the postoperative patient, there are rarely any complaints while the thrombus is confined to the small veins. Extension into the main vessels may cause the patient to become symptomatic with calf pain and swelling.

Signs. Physical signs, particularly in the early stages, are also minimal and the accuracy of clinical diagnosis is no greater than 50% when compared with objective methods.

- **Calf tenderness:** If possible, the knee should be flexed, the calf muscles relaxed and systematic bimanual palpation of each calf should take place up to the popliteal fossa. It is important to identify areas of tenderness, particularly in the soleal and gastrocnemius muscle masses. The consistency is compared in both limbs because the affected calf may feel more solid or less floppy than the normal one.
- **Oedema:** Ankle oedema in a limb that has not been the site of surgery and was not swollen before the operation should arouse suspicion. Spread onto the dorsum of the foot almost always means that, if venous thrombosis is responsible, the popliteal segment is involved.
- **Distension of superficial veins:** Unilateral distention may be present because blood has been diverted from the (blocked) deep system to the superficial but can also occur in association with hyperaemia or local infection.
- **Superficial thrombophlebitis:** This can occur independently of DVT in the postoperative patient but may be associated with a DVT. A tender cord-like thickening is usually easily palpable over the course of the normal or varicosed superficial vein. The overlying skin is erythematous and the site itself often very tender.
- **Limb discoloration:** A diagnosis should have been made long before the limb has become so oedematous and engorged with venous blood as to produce what has long been known as *phlegmasia caerulea dolens* – inflamed blue

RISK ASSESSMENT FOR VENOUS THROMBOEMBOLISM (VTE)

All patients should be risk assessed on admission to hospital. Patients should be reassessed within 24 hours of admission and whenever the clinical situation changes.

STEP ONE

Assess all patients admitted to hospital for level of mobility (tick one box). All surgical patients, and all medical patients with significantly reduced mobility, should be considered for further risk assessment.

STEP TWO

Review the patient-related factors shown on the assessment sheet against **thrombosis** risk, ticking each box that applies (more than one box can be ticked).

Any tick for thrombosis risk should prompt thromboprophylaxis according to NICE guidance.

The risk factors identified are not exhaustive. Clinicians may consider additional risks in individual patients and offer thromboprophylaxis as appropriate.

STEP THREE

Review the patient-related factors shown against **bleeding risk** and tick each box that applies (more than one box can be ticked).

Any tick should prompt clinical staff to consider if bleeding risk is sufficient to preclude pharmacological intervention.

Guidance on thromboprophylaxis is available at:

National Institute for Health and Clinical Excellence (2010) Venous thromboembolism: reducing the risk of venous thromboembolism (deep vein thrombosis and pulmonary embolism) in patients admitted to hospital. NICE clinical guideline 92. London: National Institute for Health and Clinical Excellence.

http://www.nice.org.uk/guidance/CG92

This document has been authorised by the Department of Health
Gateway reference no: 10278

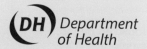

• **Fig. 27.49** Department of Health Risk Assessment for Venous Thromboembolism. (© Crown copyright 2010, 301292 1p March 10.)

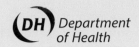

RISK ASSESSMENT FOR VENOUS THROMBOEMBOLISM (VTE)

Mobility – all patients (tick one box)	Tick		Tick		Tick
Surgical patient		Medical patient expected to have ongoing reduced mobility relative to normal state		Medical patient NOT expected to have significantly reduced mobility relative to normal state	
Assess for thrombosis and bleeding risk below				**Risk assessment now complete**	

Thrombosis risk

Patient related	Tick	Admission related	Tick
Active cancer or cancer treatment		Significantly reduced mobility for 3 days or more	
Age > 60		Hip or knee replacement	
Dehydration		Hip fracture	
Known thrombophilias		Total anaesthetic + surgical time > 90 minutes	
Obesity (BMI >30 kg/m^2)		Surgery involving pelvis or lower limb with a total anaesthetic + surgical time > 60 minutes	
One or more significant medical comorbidities (eg heart disease;metabolic,endocrine or respiratory pathologies;acute infectious diseases; inflammatory conditions)		Acute surgical admission with inflammatory or intra-abdominal condition	
Personal history or first-degree relative with a history of VTE		Critical care admission	
Use of hormone replacement therapy		Surgery with significant reduction in mobility	
Use of oestrogen-containing contraceptive therapy			
Varicose veins with phlebitis			
Pregnancy or < 6 weeks post partum (see NICE guidance for specific risk factors)			

Bleeding risk

Patient related	Tick	Admission related	Tick
Active bleeding		Neurosurgery, spinal surgery or eye surgery	
Acquired bleeding disorders (such as acute liver failure)		Other procedure with high bleeding risk	
Concurrent use of anticoagulants known to increase the risk of bleeding (such as warfarin with INR >2)		Lumbar puncture/epidural/spinal anaesthesia expected within the next 12 hours	
Acute stroke		Lumbar puncture/epidural/spinal anaesthesia within the previous 4 hours	
Thrombocytopaenia (platelets< 75x10^9/l)			
Uncontrolled systolic hypertension (230/120 mmHg or higher)			
Untreated inherited bleeding disorders (such as haemophilia and von Willebrand's disease)			

• **Fig. 27.49, cont'd**

painful (leg). This is where the obstruction to venous outflow is so severe as to impair arterial inflow. This, combined with arterial spasm induced by thrombophlebitis in the co-axial deep veins, may produce *phlegmasia alba dolens* – inflamed white painful (leg) (see 'white leg' later).

- **Pain on dorsiflexion of the ankle (Homans' sign):** This much-quoted sign of pain in the calf on passive dorsiflexion of the ankle is, as its originator always maintained, unreliable in the diagnosis of DVT. However, as most DVT patients are ambulant, and actively contracting the calf muscle repeatedly, the risk of embolization is largely theoretical. If the clot is mobile enough that a reduced pressure wave propagates it, then it would have propagated in any case.

Diagnosis

All postoperative patients should be regarded as at risk of DVT and pulmonary embolus. This implies that, whatever procedure has been undertaken, the legs should be examined at least daily and that minor, unexplained, fluctuations in temperature should arouse suspicion. It is also important to ensure that the method of prophylaxis in use is being adhered to. Screening in high-risk groups is appropriate.

Many of the mechanical problems which can mimic DVT, such as a ruptured popliteal cyst or a tear of the fibres of the gastrocnemius, are rarely relevant in the postoperative patient. However, the diagnosis can be confounded by local trauma within the limb itself, such as surgery to varicose veins or hip replacement. Objective methods are then required to exclude thrombosis. Oedema from fluid overload, or cardiac or renal failure, causes bilateral swelling. Haemorrhage into the limb may occur in a patient on anticoagulants, after an arterial puncture or direct arterial surgery, or even spontaneously after muscle strain.

Investigation

The techniques used for the investigation of the peripheral veins have been described above.

Duplex Scanning. The vessel and the flow rate through it are both visible and, in skilled hands, the accuracy of diagnosis is greater than 90%.

^{125}I Fibrinogen Uptake Tests. Fibrinogen labelled with iodine-125 is taken up by an actively growing thrombus and can be detected as a hot-spot by a scintillation counter. It is, however, not applicable in surgery that involves the limb below the inguinal ligament and is unhelpful in detecting thrombus above the mid-thigh and in the iliac segment. ^{125}I scanning is about 70–75% accurate but may take up to 5 days to establish a diagnosis if accretion to the thrombus is slow. It is now regarded as a research tool only, except in special circumstances.

CT Venography. Like CT of the pulmonary arteries, CT venography can provide excellent anatomical and disease extent data for lower and upper limb DVTs. It is non-invasive but with a significant contrast load (approx. 75–100 mL). This has excellent sensitivity, especially in the thorax,

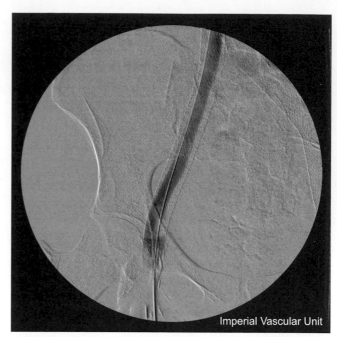

Imperial Vascular Unit

• **Fig. 27.50** Venogram of Pelvis and Iliac Vein Showing Venous Stent and Inline Flow.

but the radiation dose and contrast are significant downsides. Additionally, the sensitivity may pick up subclinical pulmonary emboli.

Venography. Many of the above techniques were developed because of the invasive nature of venography. Until the development, fairly recently, of non-irritant radio-opaque materials, the contrast agent used could itself cause thrombosis and, if extravasation occurred, tissue necrosis. With the development of low-osmolality contrast material these risks have effectively disappeared. There are, however, other disadvantages:

- The discomfort associated with needle insertion and the bursting sensation on injection of the contrast medium
- The time and expense involved in any radiological technique

Because up to 50% of patients with DVT have involvement of both limbs, venography should be performed bilaterally. Thrombi show up as contrast-lucent filling defects (Fig. 27.50). The segment(s) involved can be defined and the upper limit outlined. It is difficult to recognize the age of a thrombus on venography but very fresh clot can be seen to float in the lumen. Although invasive, the method is more than 90% accurate and is the last court of appeal should the diagnosis remain in doubt after other investigations. It is also useful in the context of thrombolysis of interventional management.

Management

It is a prerequisite in most clinical situations that an accurate diagnosis be reached before treatment is begun, particularly where that treatment may have undesirable side-effects. However, when there is a clinical likelihood of a DVT, treatment should not be withheld while awaiting confirmatory imaging. Low-molecular-weight heparin can usually be administered quite safely in most patients and then stopped if the duplex scan proves negative. Warfarin or a direct oral anticoagulant is not commenced until the diagnosis is proven.

Once the diagnosis is established treatment aims to:
- Prevent extension
- Reduce the chance of pulmonary embolization and death
- Limit the short- and long-term morbidity in the limb
- Take measures to avoid late recurrence of thrombosis

Anticoagulant Therapy. International guidelines on anticoagulation therapy in the context of venous thrombo-embolism currently aim to reduce the risk of death or fatal pulmonary embolus.

- Thrombus confined to the calf:

Spontaneous lysis is common. Guidance suggests that anticoagulation is not necessary from a mortality viewpoint. However, many clinicians would anticoagulate in order to try and reduce the risk of post-thrombotic syndrome. An appropriately measured and fitted below-knee support stocking and avoidance of sitting with the legs dependent are important supplementary measures. These do not prevent post-thrombotic syndrome but may help with symptom control.

About 20% of thrombi which begin in the calf extend proximally. If a decision is made to withhold anticoagulants, it is important to continue monitoring the limb with serial duplex ultrasounds. Therefore, the treatment options are 3 months of anticoagulation or serial imaging to identify progression.

- Thrombus in tibial, popliteal, superficial femoral and iliofemoral veins:

Immediate anticoagulation is essential, provided there is not an absolute contraindication. Although heparin has been used for the treatment of DVT for more than 40 years, controversy still exists on the optimum dose and the duration of treatment.

Traditionally, heparin (unfractionated) is administered by continuous i.v. infusion at a rate governed by a protocol designed to achieve an activated partial thromboplastin time ratio of 2. Unfortunately, due to individual patient variability, it is often out of target range (up to 50% of the time), both high and low.

Current advances in once-daily LMWH and DOACs allow once daily dosing with ambulant patients often on an outpatient basis. Warfarin is still the mainstay of long-term treatment due to familiarity and reversal agent availability. However, warfarin is patient dependent and causes hypercoagulability initially prior to achieving therapeutic levels. This means bridging therapy with LMWH is essential. This is usually for 10 days of the warfarin loading, as the international normalized ratio (INR) drops below 2 (the standard target range is 2–3) after initially achieving it (Box 27.10).

Patients with active cancer are treated with LMWH as this has a reliable treatment profile, important as tumours are prone to spontaneous bleeds, and also has a tumour lysis function.

• BOX 27.10 Calculation of the International Normalized Ratio (INR) for Anticoagulant Therapy with Warfarin

Measurement – the time for fibrin clot to appear in citrated plasma after the addition of thromboplastin reagent and calcium – prothrombin time (PT)
Standardization – all thromboplastin reagents are given an international sensitivity index (ISI) as recommended by the World Health Organization
Calculations

$$Prothrombin ratio = \frac{patient\ PT}{control\ PT}$$

$$INR = prothrombin ratio \times ISI$$

Extensive iliofemoral DVTs, however, may still require longer in-patient treatment for elevation, symptom relief and investigation, depending on patient symptomatology.

To reduce discomfort and potential morbidity, the leg should be elevated during the early days of treatment and intermittent compression pumps (inflatable leggings that repeatedly squeeze the legs) applied whenever not walking. After initial management, high-grade compression hosiery is of significant symptomatic benefit, but does not prevent post thrombotic syndrome.

Management of a suspected lower-limb DVT is summarized in Clinical Box 27.5.

Complications of Anticoagulant Therapy
Bleeding
Bleeding may occur:
- subcutaneously or into joint spaces
- intra-cerebral
- urinary tract or gut
- from wounds or puncture sites

Early warning signs include the development of extensive areas of spontaneous bruising or ecchymoses in pressure areas which can only be detected by regular observation. Daily urine testing can reveal microscopic haematuria; however, this can also be caused by recent catheterization. In the

CLINICAL BOX 27.5

Management of a Suspected Lower-Limb DVT

- Adopt a high index of clinical suspicion
- Administer LMWH or dabigatran at a therapeutic dose immediately
- Arrange duplex scan to confirm
- Elevate limb and fit compression stocking when mobilizing
- Load with warfarin (while continuing LMWH) or continue dabigatran therapy
- Exclude thrombophilia or pelvic mass

LMWH, Low-molecular-weight heparin.

postoperative patient, bleeding from surgical wounds and raw areas may occur. Careful control of therapy is important but it must be said that the risk of bleeding does not correlate well with the tests used to monitor anticoagulation, often due to the time delay between the time of taking the test and the result being available.

Heparin-Induced Thrombocytopenia (HIT)

This is a well-recognized but uncommon complication which ironically causes thrombosis. When heparin is continued for more than 4 or 5 days, regular platelet counts should be done. A mild transient decrease in platelet count is not associated with complications: however, a precipitous drop is. Bleeding is rare despite the low platelet count. Unlike other causes of thrombocytopaenia, HIT leads to arterial and venous thrombosis via an unknown pathway. It occurs in 50% of those not treated with a non-heparin anticoagulant such as fondaparinux (a heparinoid).

Continuing Management

The risk of recurrent thrombosis is greatest in the first 3 months after an acute episode. When extensive DVT has occurred, some would advocate a minimum of 6 months of oral anticoagulant therapy is prescribed, though this does not have extensive evidence to back it.

One DVT increases the patient's risk of further DVTs significantly. Two DVTs would lead to a recommendation of lifelong anticoagulation as the risk of further DVTs is so significant.

Anticoagulant therapy does not alter the effect of established thrombus in causing damage to the deep veins. To try to reduce the long-term local impact, patients should be discharged with instructions to wear graduated high-compression stockings – 25 to 36 mmHg. These should be worn continuously during oral anticoagulant therapy and duplex assessment of venous function carried out at the end of this period is extremely useful to assess the need for longer-term compression hosiery.

Alternative Methods.

- Thrombolysis:

  Seldom used in modern management of a DVT, its use is more appropriate in spontaneous extensive iliofemoral thrombosis where the limb itself is threatened (see 'White leg/*phlegmasia alba dolens*'), and where pulmonary embolus is a danger. In DVT after operation, thrombolytic therapy has little place because of the risk of haemorrhage.

- Surgery:

  Removal of the thrombus by surgery (usually by the use of a balloon catheter passed through a small incision or percutaneously) is now seldom used. The remaining indication is threat to life or limb and failure to respond to non-operative management. It invariably leads to re-occlusions due to repeat thrombosis.

- Catheter-directed thrombolysis:

  Recently, catheter-directed thrombolysis has become the gold standard for clot dissolution and extraction. This follows the same principle as arterial catheter-directed thrombolysis and leads to good results at the risk of bleeding. Mechanical device adjuncts are available in various guises which aim to speed up the removal of clot and therefore reduce the exposure time to thrombolytics. No definitive evidence exists of their superiority or cost-effectiveness; however, they are increasing in usage.

Prophylaxis Against DVT and Pulmonary Embolus (PE). Increased emphasis has been placed on the prevention of DVT and PE in hospitalized patients. PE is one of the major causes of avoidable hospital death. DVT is a cause of significant morbidity – see earlier. NICE has issued guidance on this important subject (see Further reading below). All patients admitted to hospital should be assessed at the time of admission for both the risk of venous thromboembolism (VTE) and the risk of bleeding. If appropriate, VTE prophylaxis is offered using one or more of the methods available (Table 27.12), but pharmacological prophylaxis should not be given if the risk of bleeding exceeds the risk of VTE. The assessment of risk for both VTE and bleeding is shown in Fig. 27.49. The assessment should be repeated at 24 hours after admission and whenever there is a significant change in the patient's condition.

The methods of prophylaxis available (see Table 27.12) are of two types:

- **Mechanical:** preservation of calf muscle flow and emptying of veins in the leg
- **Pharmacological:** alterations in the dynamics of the clotting mechanism designed to discourage venous thrombosis but not lead to bleeding.
  - Mechanical:

  These techniques are less effective overall than pharmacological ones but are advocated for surgical patients. Intermittent inflation of sleeves around the legs causes increased venous flow during (and after) operation. Low-compression graduated stockings should also be used, unless there is an arterial compromise.

  - Pharmacological:

  These techniques interfere in different ways with normal blood coagulation. Their relative merits must be balanced against the possibility of causing excessive or uncontrollable bleeding, their time course of action and their ease of administration.

Unfractionated heparin given subcutaneously at either 8- or 12-hour intervals is most effective when the dose is calculated for each individual and based on a known response in preoperative APPT, or heparin levels. Calcium heparin is said by some to be more effective than sodium heparin when each is administered at a dose of 5000 units. The use of unfractionated heparin reduces the incidence of DVT by up to 60% in general surgery and up to 50% in most orthopaedic procedures. Prophylactic low-dose heparin also lowers the frequency of both fatal and non-fatal pulmonary emboli. Unfractionated heparin has been largely replaced by LMWHs (see below), although it is still used in patients with renal failure.

Method	Efficacy	Disadvantages
Mechanical		
Physiotherapy by leg exercises	No proven effect	None
Early mobilization	No proven effect although useful for other reasons	None
Graduated compression stockings	Probably minor influence	Must be good quality and individually fitted
Intermittent calf compression	Known reduction	Cumbersome
Pharmacological		
Oral anticoagulants	Known reduction, especially orthopaedics	Takes time to be effective Needs careful control Increased bleeding risk
Unfractionated heparin	Successful in general surgery Ineffective in orthopaedics Used in renal failure	8- to 12-hourly injections
Low-molecular-weight heparin	Known reduction	Risk of thrombocytopenia
Dabigatran ctexilate	Proven in orthopaedics	Expense
Rivaroxaban	Proven in orthopaedics	Expense
Fondaparinux	Proven in orthopaedics	Injections Expense

TABLE 27.12 Prophylaxis of Deep-Vein Thrombosis (Especially Postoperative).

Low-molecular-weight heparins cause a more specific antithrombotic effect through their ability to inhibit factor Xa. Furthermore, in experimental models, they produce less bleeding for an equivalent antithrombotic effect. A similar or greater reduction in the incidence of venous thrombosis has been demonstrated in general surgical patients using a single daily dose begun the day before operation. A reduced dose is used in renal patients.

Warfarin given in appropriate dosage clearly reduce the risk of thrombosis but they also carry a higher potential for bleeding complications unless their administration is very carefully controlled. The agent must be started several days before operation to prolong the prothrombin time so that the INR is approximately 2. A modification of this is to start the warfarin on the evening of surgery and to aim to bring the INR to a similar level by the fifth postoperative day.

Direct oral anticoagulants – Dabigatran etexilate is a direct thrombin inhibitor that can be taken orally and is used as VTE prophylaxis in orthopaedic surgery. Rivaroxaban, edoxaban and apixaban are oral factor Xa inhibitors with excellent and reproducible treatment profiles. DOACs are now first-line treatment for DVT prophylaxis postoperatively and long-term treatment of DVT in many cases.

Fondaparinux is a factor Va inhibitor given subcutaneously as an alternative to LMWH in orthopaedic surgery. Unlike LMWH, there is no risk of heparin-induced thrombocytopenia.

Aspirin: recent studies have suggested that aspirin has an equivalent thromboprophylaxis efficacy to the DOACs in orthopaedic joint replacement patients.

• VTE prophylaxis algorithms:

As the complexity of decision-making in VTE prophylaxis has become greater, NICE have designed algorithms for different clinical situations. Those for elective and non-elective orthopaedic surgery and for non-orthopaedic surgery are available at https://pathways.nice.org.uk/pathways/venous-thromboembolism. Similar algorithms for other situations can be found in the guidance (see 'Further Reading').

Duration of Prophylaxis

Pharmacological prophylaxis is normally continued for the duration of the inpatient stay. Continuing self-administration at home of a single daily subcutaneous dose of LMWH or use of the oral rivaroxaban for 5 weeks postoperatively is recommended in high-risk patients, such as after hip replacement surgery.

Pulmonary Embolism in DVT

The life-threatening complication of DVT is pulmonary embolism (PE). This is where the thrombus becomes detached, is carried proximally and lodges in the pulmonary artery or its branches, thus obstructing right heart output.

Aetiology

The great majority of pulmonary emboli occur after surgical procedures complicated by the development of DVT. However, DVT and consequent PE can occur in immobilization for any cause. Other causative factors are shown in Table 27.12. PEs may also occur without a peripheral DVT in certain cases.

Epidemiology

In England and Wales (population *c.* 60 million) there are approximately 25 000 deaths a year from PE. In the 1960s, prior to the use of heparin prophylaxis, 6 in every 1 000 patients undergoing total hip replacement died as a result of PE. Currently, with the use of prophylactic measures as documented above, the fatal PE rate in hip surgery patients is 0.1%. In pelvic operations for malignancy, this rises to 1% despite prophylaxis. The mortality of untreated symptomatic PE, however, remains at 30%. Following massive PE, of those who die, 50–70% do so in the first hour.

Physiological and Pathological Considerations

Embolism occurs when either the whole or the proximal propagated part of a free-floating clot detaches from the wall of a vein. The event may be spontaneous or stripping of the attachment may occur as a result of an acute rise in venous pressure such as occurs during a Valsalva manoeuvre on defaecation. The clot is swept proximally into the pulmonary artery and, if sufficiently large to be arrested in the main stem or across the bifurcation of the vessel, reduces cardiac output so much that death results instantly or within a very short time. Lodgement in branches produces a volume of lung tissue that is initially ventilated but underperfused – the so-called 'ventilation-perfusion mismatch' that can be detected on certain special investigations. There is arteriolar spasm in the involved segment, thus reducing inflow and causing infarction. If the block to the pulmonary circulation is large, pressure in the right heart rises. Subsequently, the segment becomes consolidated as a consequence of haemorrhagic infarction. If the patient survives, the clot can lyse (50% within 2 weeks) and the circulation will be restored. Alternatively, or even when there has been initial but incomplete lysis, organization and fibrosis take place with a pulmonary scar detectable up to a year later on perfusion studies. Repeated emboli may, by this mechanism, cause the development of pulmonary artery hypertension and right heart failure.

Clinical Features

Symptoms. Symptoms may be sudden in onset and without warning. However, in retrospect, a swollen ankle or leg may have been present, and it is a source of chagrin to notice this for the first time while trying to save the life of a patient with acute circulatory collapse. Small emboli may not cause any symptoms. Those that involve up to half of the pulmonary circulation give rise to symptoms confined to the lung. Greater involvement causes additional cardiac and systemic effects. Pre-existing pulmonary disease increases the effects of a given amount of obstruction.

- **Chest pain.** Infarction of the lung causes well-localized pleuritic pain over the affected segment, worse on inspiration or coughing. A large embolus may be associated with crushing substernal rather than pleuritic pain and rapidly followed by cardiac arrest.
- **Dyspnoea** may be present but is not a striking feature except in very large emboli.
- **Haemoptysis** may follow within minutes or hours in those who survive but is usually confined to blood streaking of the sputum.
- **Transient or prolonged loss of consciousness** implies a large embolus with circulatory effects.

Signs.

1. Circulatory
   With a large embolus there is:
   - Arterial hypotension, usually with a pale, vasoconstricted skin, although sometimes with cyanosis
   - Raised jugular venous pressure
   - Tachycardia and, in large emboli, gallop rhythm
   - Dysrhythmias

2. Respiratory
   Examination of the chest may show:
   - pleural friction rub with associated crackles (*syn.* crepitations) and
   - later, signs of consolidation will appear

3. General
   There may be evidence of DVT in the lower limbs, but detachment of the whole or the greater part of the clot from a relatively proximal vein may mean that the limb is normal.

Investigation

Plasma D-Dimer. This is the first investigation, a negative test effectively ruling out a pulmonary embolus (sensitivity 99%). However, false positives are common after surgery and further confirmatory investigation is necessary.

Chest X-Ray. In small emboli there may be no abnormality on chest X-ray. If infarction has occurred, a wedge of consolidation with its apex centrally located may be present or there may be evidence of areas of reduced vascularity – loss of vascular markings.

Pulmonary Radioisotope Ventilation/Perfusion (V/Q) Scans. Technetium-99m-labelled albumin given intravenously may demonstrate areas of underperfusion of the lung. A normal ventilation/perfusion (V/Q) scan excludes a significant PE. Other causes of underperfusion (such as previous PE) may confuse the clinical picture but in an abnormal scan, there is an approximately 75% chance that a recent embolus is present. Specificity is greatly enhanced if ventilation is simultaneously assessed by the inhalation of xenon-133: there is a mismatch between perfusion (decreased) and ventilation (initially maintained).

- Multislice CT scan
  This is the investigation of choice because it is generally readily available and is non-invasive. Multislice scanners reliably detect even small emboli (sensitivity 83%, specificity 96%), though these may not be clinically significant.
- Electrocardiography
  In a small to moderate-sized PE, the ECG is frequently normal. A large embolus, which produces dilation of the right heart, causes tall and peaked P waves in lead II, right axis deviation, right bundle branch block and T-wave inversion in precordial leads. Large emboli can produce changes which are difficult to distinguish from inferior myocardial infarction.
- Blood gas analysis
  Reduction in pO_2 occurs if cardiac output is profoundly depressed and/or a large volume of lung is underperfused. Dyspnoea increases the elimination of carbon dioxide and the pCO_2 is therefore also reduced. This situation is uncommon except in collapse/consolidation of the lung (see Ch. 18) and, given the clinical circumstances, provides confirmatory evidence of PE.
- Investigation of possible DVT
  Provided the patient is in a stable circulatory state the usual investigations are undertaken.

Diagnosis

It is important to be aware that the finding of a normal ECG, chest X-ray and negative duplex scan (excluding DVT) does not exclude a diagnosis of PE. If there is any clinical suspicion, the patient should be anticoagulated pending diagnostic confirmation with CT angiography or V/Q scan.

Other events may present a clinical picture very similar to that of a large embolus:

- Myocardial infarction – usually with the features of left rather than right ventricular failure
- Massive fluid overload – generalized features are present in addition to right heart failure
- Severe sepsis
- Haemorrhage – the jugular venous pressure is low
- Tension pneumothorax
- Cardiac tamponade
- Aortic dissection

Management

Resuscitation. When cardiac arrest is thought to have occurred, the standard techniques need to be instituted in an attempt to establish adequate cardiac output and also to reach a diagnosis which is used to guide further treatment. In unstable patients, long-acting anticoagulants should not be used in anticipation of further intervention. A loading dose of 10 000 units of heparin should be given intravenously.

Continuing Treatment.

- Resuscitation successful

An adequate cardiac output to sustain systemic perfusion is achieved. A continuous heparin infusion is begun at 25 units/kg per hour. Assuming progress is maintained, a similar regimen to that described for the management of venous thrombosis is followed and the patient is subsequently changed to oral anticoagulation for a minimum of 6 months.

- Resuscitation unsuccessful

Hypotension and an inadequate cardiac output persist. The options are:

- Establish cardiopulmonary bypass and remove the clot at open operation
- Right heart catheterization and regional administration of a thrombolytic agent such as alteplase
- Pulmonary artery catheterization and suction removal of the clot – a method which can be combined with thrombolysis
- Systemic thrombolysis

In the past, dramatic, occasionally successful, transthoracic embolectomies without cardiopulmonary bypass were described. However, without the availability of bypass, patients who survive to reach operation would also get to the preferable alternatives of thrombolysis or direct suction. Alteplase thrombolysis has been shown to be beneficial in a randomized controlled trial[11] with a significant survival advantage. This therapy should be adopted more widely.

Management of a suspected PE is summarized in Emergency Box 27.3.

EMERGENCY BOX 27.3

Management of a Suspected Pulmonary Embolism

- Assess arterial blood gases (on air)
- Measure plasma D-dimer
- Arrange portable chest X-ray and ECG (to help exclude other pathologies)
- Start oxygen
- Administer therapeutic i.v. heparin or subcut. LMWH
- Arrange multislice (or spiral) CT or V/Q scan to confirm diagnosis
- Consider streptokinase thrombolysis
- Arrange venous duplex or MRI (venous phase) scan as indicated to assess lower-limb and pelvic veins
- Prescribe long-term anticoagulation
- Consider use of IVC filter

LMWH, Low-molecular-weight heparin.

Recurrent Pulmonary Emboli

If treatment of the DVT is rigorous, survival after PE may not be followed by recurrence. However, further episodes of circulatory collapse, dyspnoea and chest pain are not infrequent. Extension of underperfusion or infarction in the lung can be confirmed by further isotope scanning or pulmonary angiography.

Management involves:

- Making sure that anticoagulation with heparin has been achieved and is at a therapeutic level
- Consideration of interruption of the venous pathway above the most proximal level of thrombosis

The methods available for interruption are:

- Surgical plication either by sutures or clips – now rarely used
- Percutaneous insertion of a filter into the vena cava below the renal veins. These filters can usually be removed (percutaneously) a few weeks later when the patient has been stabilized. However, this rarely occurs. Use of filters has greatly reduced in recent years due to an appreciation of the complications of placing a thrombogenic implant into a thrombogenic patient's venous system.

Indications for IVC filter insertion are:

- Recurrent PE despite adequate anticoagulation
- PE with contraindication to anticoagulation

White Leg

Extensive venous thrombosis in the lower extremity can produce a clinical syndrome known as 'white leg' – historically known as *phlegmasia alba dolens* – inflamed white painful (leg); so-named because it was originally thought that the condition had an inflammatory element.

Aetiology

Rapid thrombosis along the whole length of the deep venous system and into the iliac segment so obstructs drainage that arterial input is reduced. Furthermore, thrombophlebitis in the coaxial deep veins induces arterial spasm. The condition used to be common in the puerperium but is now more often seen in those with generalized hypercoagulability, e.g. in malignancy, sometimes occult.

Clinical Features

Symptoms. Pain and swelling in the whole limb are the dominant features. Systemic disturbance is often quite considerable.

Signs. The affected limb is:
- Grossly swollen up to the inguinal ligament, and oedema may spread onto the abdominal wall
- Cool and white because of reduced arterial input
- Often without arterial pulsation at the ankle from swelling, which makes it difficult to feel, but also because arterial pressure in the limb is reduced
- Characterized by dusky cyanosis at the tips of the toes

The last suggests that necrosis is about to supervene, but, in fact, this is limited to the skin (see later).

Management

The initial treatment is that of any DVT, with anticoagulants and limb elevation. Thrombolysis is advocated with better results with early administration. However, it is doubtful if the results are improved over those of standard therapy, in that what appears to be a limb that requires major amputation (so-called venous gangrene) turns out, on continued non-intervention, to have only very limited loss of tissue in the skin and subcutaneous layers of the toes. However, fulminant venous gangrene is often a terminal event.

Once the acute episode is over, investigation of venous function follows the lines already outlined.

Post-Thrombotic Syndrome (PTS)

These and other terms are used to describe a limb in which there is damage to the deep veins, their valves and the valves in the communicating veins with the production of:
- Raised static pressure in the deep veins.
- Transmission of this hypertension to the superficial system.
- In addition, the soft tissue supportive structure is compromised and scarred.

Aetiology and Pathological Features

The most common cause is a previous DVT. However, there is also the group of primary deep venous insufficiency that may have a similar clinical picture.

Pathological features are of venous hypertension (described earlier) in the superficial tissues. Damage to the deep valves is usually secondary to a DVT with recanalization; however, rarely, there may be congenital absence of valves in the deep system.

Clinical Features

History

There may be a history of DVT, although its absence does not mean that an asymptomatic DVT did not occur in the past. One-third of patients with a DVT go on to suffer from PTS. Over some years, the patient will have noticed the development of increased aching on exertion, ankle and calf oedema, venous eczema and ulceration. A bursting feeling on walking is relatively common. Otherwise the symptoms are the same as for other causes of venous hypertension (see earlier).

Signs

The findings are of venous insufficiency as already described. Oedema is often quite marked and, although predominantly venous and compressible, may, with time, develop a lymphoedematous component, and then onto lipoedema, which is firm and non-pitting.

Investigation

From the foregoing definition it is clear that it is essential to establish the status of the whole venous tree. The methods of achieving this have already been outlined. Both deep and superficial incompetence may coexist. Great care should be taken in excluding any obstructive component in the deep veins before treating superficial venous incompetence.

Management

The potential for limb morbidity in patients with advanced changes of venous hypertension is often poorly recognized by clinicians.

Prophylaxis

Adequate prophylaxis and treatment of DVT and the subsequent use of effective well-tailored high-compression garments can be expected to dramatically reduce the development of the chronic changes of deep venous insufficiency. However, this is poorly tolerated by patients, and in fact has not been shown to reduce the rates of PTS in a randomized trial.

Treatment

Superficial Incompetence Only. If clinical and other tests show that this is the cause, improvement up to complete cure can be produced by standard treatment with treatment of incompetence, and obliteration of varices. Long-term use of support hose is a valuable supplement.

Deep-Vein Incompetence with Superficial Incompetence. In those patients without deep venous obstruction, treatment of superficial incompetence is the first stage of treatment. A long-term below-knee stocking is important (above knee offers no clinical benefit but is sometimes better tolerated): the compression should be graduated, with a value of 36 mmHg at the ankle; ankle, calf and leg-length measurements should only be taken after oedema has been reduced to ensure an accurate fit. This requires regular repeat measurements. Techniques of venous stenting and venous bypass for obstruction and for incompetent valve reconstruction have been developed, but require careful patient selection and diligent follow-up. With these in place, outcomes can be equivalent to arterial bypass, though the evidence is limited to small case series.

Leg Ulceration

Epidemiology

Eighty to eighty-five percent of leg ulcers are of venous origin, although, particularly in the elderly, an arterial element may be co-causative. Ten percent are entirely the consequence of arterial disease. It is probable that approximately 1% of the population have, or have had, a leg ulcer and that at any one time 30–40% of ulcers are active. Approximately 70% of those with active ulcers are over 70 years of age and there is a prevalence of 2% in the over-80s. Females exceed males by a factor of three, perhaps reflecting the risks of pregnancy and childbirth.

It has been estimated that management of leg ulceration caused by venous disease costs the NHS in the UK approximately £1 billion a year.

Aetiology

Oedema from venous hypertension and raised pressure at the venular end of the capillary loop, skin and subcutaneous hypoxia, and an episode of minor trauma are the usual antecedents of ulceration. The higher the burden of incompetent veins the more likely ulcers are. Once an ulcer is established, healing of the poorly nourished skin is difficult, and granulation tissue and a fibrous base develops. Chronic recurrent inflammation causes scarring (fibrosis), which in turn impairs arterial input and venous output – this is a further impediment to healing. Secondary infections by skin flora such as *Staphylococci* are common and may cause painful spreading cellulitis.

Other causes of leg ulceration may have to be taken into consideration; these are given in Table 27.13. Venous hypertension is, however, by far the commonest cause.

Clinical Features

Venous ulcers occur most commonly just above the medial malleolus. They are usually oval in shape, flat and without a raised edge, look relatively healthy and have a granulating base usually covered with a thin layer of fibrin. Weeping eczematous change may be seen in the surrounding skin which often arises from the use of inappropriate local applications. The tissues are indurated and there may be scarring in the adjacent paper-thin skin where healing has occurred in the past. Concomitant infection, with either surrounding erythema or extensive cellulitis, may be present, but is not ubiquitous.

A venous ulcer (Fig. 27.51) is recognized easily when it is situated in the typical position close to the medial malleolus, surrounded by pigmentation and oedema. However, venous ulcers also occur on the lateral side of the leg and on the foot, principally the dorsal surface. The circumferential size of the lesion does not indicate its cause, and venous ulcers may be multiple.

Diagnosis

An exact diagnosis must precede management. Apart from the obvious distinctions that have to be made from the conditions shown in Table 27.13, a venous ulcer must be differentiated from an ischaemic one because the treatment is so different. The features that permit this are shown in Table 27.14. Awareness of the association of ulceration with diabetes mellitus is well understood, but the association with rheumatoid arthritis, systemic sclerosis (scleroderma), sickle cell anaemia and other generalized diseases is less well recognized. The more elderly the patient, the more likely there are to be multiple aetiological factors.

It is rare in hospital practice to see an ulcer which has not been 'treated' for some considerable period of time elsewhere, often without adequate determination of the cause – particularly the nature of the venous component which may be easily treated. The recently completed EVRA trial[12] had to exclude 25% as the ulcers were >6 months old by time of referral.

TABLE 27.13	Causes of Ulceration of the Leg.
Underlying cause	**Mechanism**
Venous disease	Superficial venous hypertension – hypoxia, oedema, trauma
Arterial disease	Reduced inflow – hypoxia
Trauma	Skin loss, infection, persistent pressure in prolonged bed rest
Rheumatoid arthritis (often with an added arterial or venous component)	Autoimmune inflammation in subcutaneous tissues (vasculitis)
Pyoderma gangrenosum	
Systemic sclerosis	Inflammation of skin and subcutaneous tissues – cause unknown
Malignant disease	Squamous-cell carcinoma (usually de novo but occasionally associated with long-standing varicose veins and ulceration) Malignant melanoma Basal cell carcinoma
Diabetes mellitus	Neuropathy; possibly an arterial component with skin infarction Lesions more frequent at pressure points – ball of foot and heel
Blood disorders	Microvascular thrombosis in sickle cell disease and spherocytosis

Management

Most venous ulcers which are correctly diagnosed and treated respond readily to conventional treatment, but even relatively small lesions can take up to 3 months to heal. More chronic lesions – the result of inappropriate or inadequate

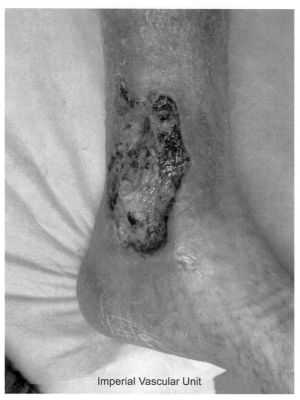

• **Fig. 27.51** Untreated Venous Ulcer Overlying the Medial Malleolus Note the covering of slough and lack of granulation tissue.

initial assessment and treatment – require a more precise and rigorous regimen:

Step 1 is to establish that arterial supply is adequate using clinical examination and ABPI. If ABPI is <0.8, modified compression in a specialist environment is needed.

Step 2 is to establish if there is correctable superficial venous hypertension. If this is so, surgical intervention as early as possible is indicated in addition to compression therapy. It should not be delayed for ulcer healing.

Step 3 If there is mixed superficial and deep incompetence, providing there is no deep venous obstruction, again surgical intervention and compression therapy is indicated.

Most venous ulcers heal if the patient is confined to bed with the foot elevated to at least the level of the heart so that venous hypertension is abolished, the micro-environment improved and healing promoted. However, bed rest is costly, debilitating for patients and has a high risk of VTE and therefore usually an inappropriate method. Therefore the usage of compression therapy is the gold standard.

It can be achieved by:

- *Bandaging* – usually multilayer and dependent on the skill of the nurse or doctor who applies it. Four-layer bandaging (Charing Cross method) has been used successfully for many years – it aims to produce a pressure of up to 40 mmHg at the ankle and 16 mmHg in the upper calf. This method requires a certain degree of skill that may not be readily acquired, though it does represent the gold standard for compression therapy. Short-stretch bandaging is an alternative and effective method that is increasingly used these days. Here, a bandage is used that is designed so that it cannot be overstretched

TABLE 27.14 Distinctive Characteristics of Venous and Arterial Ulcers.

	Venous	Arterial
History	Previous deep-vein thrombosis; varicose veins	Intermittent claudication; ischaemic heart disease; hypertension; diabetes
Pain	Occurs only in severe oedema, secondary bacterial infection, thrombosis, varicose veins	Nearly always present; worse at night; relieved by dependency
Site	Usually near medial malleolus but do occur on lateral side of leg	Common on toes, heel, foot and lateral aspect
Size/development	Variable but increases slowly if untreated	Variable but increases rapidly
Oedema	Common and worse at end of day	Uncommon unless the leg is dependent and patient immobile
Skin appearance	Pigmentation and atrophy; white patches; induration of subcutaneous tissues	Shiny, thin, atrophic nails
Skin temperature	Usually warm	Cool
Skin colour	Normal or slight cyanosis accentuated by dependency and improved by elevation	Pallor made worse by elevation and slow to recover; cyanotic on dependency
Appearance of ulcer	Shallow flat margin; looks healthy; no deep invasion	Often involves deep fascia; tendon may be exposed
Foot pulses	Present, although can be difficult to feel because of oedema	Reduced or absent

and thus cannot produce too high a compression force. Venous ulceration is a condition of the elderly, often with coexisting arterial disease, and it is therefore vital to check the ABPI. Compression therapy is contraindicated if the ABPI is less than 0.8.

- *Fitted elastic hosiery* with known compression – more expensive but does not require great expertise to apply; inappropriate if ulcers are very wet. The stockings can be off the shelf, bespoke or fitted with zips to aid donning. Differing compression strengths are available. The stockings must be changed every 100 washes due to elastic fatigue. They are often poorly utilized by patients.
- *Compressive neoprene wraps* with known compression – more expensive but allows easy donning and easy washing. These now have more widespread availability.

Step 4, which runs concurrently with steps 2 and 3, is local management of the lesion. The ulcer should be kept clean with regular saline cleanses, more frequently if there is substantial exudate (exacerbated by not elevating the limb and/or poor compliance regarding the wearing of support hose). The inappropriate use of topical agents, including impregnated bandages, should be avoided. Dressings are kept simple, and pharmacologically active substances applied only for specific and logical reasons – which means hardly ever. If the underlying causes are treated, then bland dressings are all that is required. Saline-gauze dressings are effective at cleansing ulcers but do need to be changed regularly, i.e. before they dry out, otherwise removal is painful and any delicate, rejuvenating epithelial layer will be removed. Non-adherent dressings offer a much better alternative. Antibiotics are not appropriate; all leg ulcers are colonized with bacteria and most will yield a positive culture which frequently shows multiple organisms, a so-called 'Garden of Eden' bacteriological culture. Systemic therapy is indicated only if there is spreading cellulitis or significant pain; topical applications are ineffective in controlling contamination unless the causes of the ulcer are dealt with. Often clinicians fear ulcers are infected due to green exudate on dressings, which merely indicate Pseudomonas colonization of the dressings due to infrequent dressing changes – the ulcer improves with a single dressing change rather than the single dose of antibiotics given. New chemical debridement techniques such as Prontosan allow for decolonization and rapid improvement of wounds without the need for surgery, antibiotics or painful soaks (potassium permanganate).

Surgical Measures in Ulceration

Occasionally, severely contaminated long-standing ulcers with infected granulation tissue at the base may benefit from surgical debridement. However, compression therapy should not be delayed for this. Once measures have been undertaken to reverse the pathophysiological processes, if the surface area of the ulcer is relatively large, consideration may be given to skin-grafting to decrease the patient's hospital stay or number of clinic visits. Either split-skin or pinch grafts are used, but these sadly often fail.

LYMPHATIC DISORDERS

Anatomical and Physiological Considerations

The lymphatic system comprises a network of capillaries and vessels lined by endothelial cells. The capillaries allow the absorption of protein-rich interstitial fluid across their walls and the vessels possess valves to prevent lymph reflux. Lymphatic vessels run alongside the venous system but drain directly to lymph nodes where the lymph fluid is filtered through lymphoid tissue. This permits phagocytosis of cellular and bacterial debris. In addition, lymph nodes provide a setting for immunological response to foreign antigens. The efferent lymphatic vessels eventually drain into the central venous system. The fluid dynamics seen in the lymphatic system are remarkable – fluid drainage against gravity despite extreme low pressure.

Pathological Conditions

These include lymphadenopathy (node enlargement), lymphangitis and lymphoedema.

Lymphadenopathy

Lymphadenopathy may occur as the result of local infection or tissue injury, or as a feature of malignancy – either metastatic tumour (e.g. breast cancer, malignant melanoma) or lymphoma. Node enlargement may be detected on examination or imaging such as ultrasound, CT or MR scanning. Open biopsy or fine-needle aspiration cytology of an enlarged node should provide a pathological diagnosis when required and allows appropriate treatment, e.g. radiotherapy or cytotoxic chemotherapy for lymphoma. Excision of local and regional nodes with a primary cancer (e.g. breast, colon, stomach) is described as a radical operation, gives prognostic information by staging the tumour and may also improve local control and survival for some cancers. For excision, the nodes must either be dyed, tagged with radioisotopes or large enough to clearly feel – otherwise they represent a small fatty structure in other fatty structures.

Acute Lymphangitis

Acute lymphangitis, or inflammation of the lymphatic vessels, occurs typically with streptococcal infections, when tender red lines may be seen and palpated in the dermis. There is associated regional lymphadenopathy – e.g. groin or axilla. Penicillin therapy combined with rest and elevation is usually effective.

Lymphoedema

Oedema is an excess of fluid between tissue cells. Lymphoedema is the swelling which results from the accumulation of interstitial fluid as a consequence of failure of the lymphatic system to drain it.

Classification and Aetiology

The condition is classed as either primary (disorder of the lymphatic system itself) or secondary (some other condition outside the lymphatic system which interferes with drainage).

Primary Lymphoedema

The subject is not well understood. The following factors are probably of importance:

- Very few patients are born with a hypoplastic lymphatic system, usually in the lower limb *(congenital hereditary lymphoedema)*.
- Obliteration of lymphatic channels by fibrosis of unknown cause may develop at or after puberty.
- Obstruction of a group of lymph nodes (e.g. in the pelvis) may also occur for the same reason.
- Hyperplastic tortuous lymph channels can sometimes be shown at lymphangiography (see later), suggesting another type of congenital disease (often associated with capillary naevi); the defect may be in the valves of the lymphatics.

Primary lymphoedema is six times more common in women than men. Cases of primary lymphoedema may be referred to as 'Lymphoedema Congenita', 'Lymphoedema Praecox', and 'Lymphoedema Tarda'. These terms are more descriptive than diagnostic, reflecting the stages in life when they manifest themselves clinically.

Secondary Lymphoedema

In Western countries the causes are:

- Surgical removal of a group of lymph nodes – either in the axilla (mastectomy for breast cancer) or the groin (usually for malignant melanoma, less commonly for other malignancies)
- Radiotherapy for malignancy – usually both factors (surgical removal and radiotherapy) are involved – it is not common for surgical excision alone to cause lymphoedema
- Malignant invasion of lymphatics and nodes
- Chronic venous disease, which may, particularly if recurrent infections occur, cause secondary lymphoedema in addition to the hydrostatic oedema that is present because of raised venous pressure. The lymphoedema of chronic venous disease is caused by constrictive fibrosis of the lymph channels induced by chronic inflammation.
- Cellulitis itself is an infection of the soft tissue, which results in damage to the lymphatic system – this is why there is often a recurrent cycle of cellulitis in some patients.

In developing and tropical countries intra-lymphatic infection is the commonest cause:

- *Filariasis* caused by the worm *Wuchereria bancrofti* induces fibrosis in the lymphatics. The incubation period after the initial mosquito bite may be up to 18 months, and the condition should therefore be borne in mind in those who have returned from tropical to temperate climates.
- Silica particles enter through the skin of those walking barefoot on silica-rich soils; lymphatic drainage is interfered with, and secondary infection of cuts further damages the partially obstructed lymphatics and nodes.

Functional Classification

An alternative approach combines developmental lymphatic abnormalities with an acquired element (probably repeated infection). The lymphoedema that follows is either:

- obliterative – from progressive intimal thickening
- obstructive – from developmental abnormalities in proximal nodes and possible fibrotic replacement
- valvular – from the presence of incompetence

Pathophysiological and Pathological Features

The interstitial space contains not only water and electrolytes but also proteins (mostly albumin), other large molecules, cellular debris and sometimes bacteria. Most of the water and electrolytes are reabsorbed at the venular end of the capillary loop. The rest enter the lymphatics and pass to the nodes and thence to the thoracic duct. In consequence, if lymph flow is obstructed, there is an increase in their concentration in the interstitial space. This stagnant fluid may:

- Be invaded by granulations and become organized into fibrous tissue
- Provide an ideal culture medium for pathogenic bacteria and so cause recurrent episodes of cellulitis which further aggravates interstitial fibrosis and destruction of lymph channels

Clinical Features

Although either primary or secondary lymphoedema may occur in any part of the body drained by lymphatics, the common clinical presentation is in the limbs – chiefly the lower – and the description that follows relates mainly to this. However, many of the principles apply elsewhere.

Primary Lymphoedema

Symptoms

There is often a family history, particularly on the female side, though this may be confused with one of venous disease. The most typical presentation is a teenage girl with the insidious and apparently spontaneous onset of unilateral swelling of the dorsum of the foot and the ankle. At first, the swelling is most obvious in warmer weather and tends to disappear with a night's rest, but once it has been present for some time, it fails to resolve completely. Pain is usually absent, but discomfort is associated with heaviness as the swelling increases. Oedema gradually becomes more marked and frequently ascends into the calf and from the dorsum of the foot forward to the toes. Onset in older patients is often similar and may occur at a more proximal level in the limb, for example the thigh, without foot and calf swelling. The skin remains healthy for many years and, in contrast to venous disease, complaints of pigmentation and ulceration are rare unless they develop because of recurrent cellulitis.

Signs

In half the patients, at initial presentation, the oedema is unilateral but, if bilateral, one limb frequently shows more advanced changes. The early oedema principally accumulates on the dorsum of the foot and initially pits on pressure. The pitting oedema and involvement of the dorsum of the foot distinguishes lymphoedema from lipoedema (or lipodystrophy), which is a non-pitting condition of the subcutaneous fat of the lower limbs where the foot is spared. Even at a late stage, there is frequently an element of removable fluid even though fibrosis may also have taken place. With more extensive oedema, this is uniformly distributed from the calf down into the toes. The skin is nearly always intact but may show visible and palpable thickening.

Dilation of dermal lymphatics and subsequent fibrosis gives rise to fine dermal papillae (especially over the toes) known as papillomatosis.

Secondary Lymphoedema

Symptoms

There may be a history suggestive of the underlying cause, and the onset of oedema may be closely related to this. Rapidity of onset may more closely mimic an acute venous thrombosis, with which secondary lymphoedema may occasionally coexist. Episodes of infection are more common in secondary disease.

Signs

The clinical appearances are similar to those of primary lymphoedema. When chronic venous disease is the cause, the features of venous hypertension will usually be apparent.

Investigation

The diagnosis is not usually in doubt, but distinction of primary from secondary lymphoedema – and, in both, detection of a cause – may require further investigation.

Distinction Between Lymphoedema and Venous Disease

Ultrasonography excludes disease of the deep and superficial veins.

Distinction Between Obliterative and Obstructive Disease

A bolus injection of technetium-labelled rhenium/sulphur colloid (lymphoscintigraphy) into the web space of the foot produces slow clearance from the tissues and minimal uptake of isotope in the draining lymph nodes in obliterative

disease. A CT scan may also indicate a lack or absence of nodes draining the area involved.

Management

Non-Operative

Management consists of:
- Reduction of oedema – elevation, distal-proximal massage (MLD – manual lymphatic drainage), mechanical pneumatic compression devices (Lymphopress)
- Neuromuscular stimulation devices
- Continuous support with compression garments such as elastic stockings
- Prophylaxis against infection – control of fungal infection, good skin hygiene and prevention of inadvertent skin trauma – scratching and wearing of shoes

Ongoing encouragement and support is often required, as patients consider that non-operative management implies that 'nothing can be done for me'. The authors have found referring patients to the Lymphoedema Support Network website useful in their long-term management (www.lymphoedema.org). There is also a section on the condition lipoedema which, as discussed, is distinct from lymphoedema.

Surgical

There is no current treatment that will reliably restore function to the lymphatic system.

Anastomotic and bridging procedures include:
- Improvement of lymphatic drainage in obstructive lymphoedema – microvascular anastomosis between lymphatics and veins
- Provision of lymphatic bridges by anastomosis of an isolated loop of ileum without its mucosa to a lymph node just distal to an obstruction.
- Implantation of silicon tubing to provide drainage channels
  Debulking operations are:
- Removal of the skin and thickened subcutaneous tissue with free split-skin grafting of the raw area
- Removal of much of the involved tissue with a dermal flap buried beneath the deep fascia which it is hoped will provide new lymphatic pathways for drainage
- Liposuction

Symptomatic relief and cosmetic improvement may come from any of the above procedures. Selection is difficult and the operations are technically challenging and usually complicated by significant blood loss. Liposuction is the least invasive. The removal of large amounts of tissue is debilitating and has high morbidity.

Differential diagnosis of an acutely swollen limb is summarized in Emergency Box 27.4.

Bacterial Cellulitis as a Complication of Lymphoedema

The condition is both a complication of lymphoedema and a cause of secondary forms. It is common and frequently misdiagnosed.

Aetiology

Organisms, usually beta-haemolytic streptococci though occasionally a synergistic combination, gain entry either through an apparently inconsequential injury or an insect bite. More commonly, there is a history of chronic fungal infection in the web spaces of digits.

Pathological Features

The condition is usually a self-limiting subcutaneous cellulitis but necrosis of skin and fascia can occur.

Clinical Features

Symptoms

The onset is usually with an acute influenza-like illness, with shivering and occasional rigors. Later, progressive swelling and erythema develop and spread with varying degrees of rapidity. If a limb is involved, it is acutely painful.

Signs

The area involved is red, hot and tender. Swelling is increased. The regional lymph nodes, if they are present, are also tender.

Management

Early recognition and prompt antibiotic treatment in association with methods designed to reduce the oedema rapidly and enhance lymphatic drainage may reduce the immediate complication of skin necrosis and reduce the likelihood of further obliteration of lymphatics. A simple but effective initial antibiotic option is high-dose flucloxacillin 2 g 6-hourly. The initial site of entry should be dealt with concomitantly, e.g. fungal infection in the web space.

Once the acute phase has subsided, the patient may be mobilized and oedema reduced by a high-compression support hose. Six weeks of oral erythromycin is recommended for prophylaxis.

FUTURE DIRECTIONS

Many of the techniques described in this chapter have been developed only over the last 20–30 years. This rapid pace of technological advance continues, particularly that of minimally invasive and endovascular techniques – for example, the repair of abdominal aortic aneurysms by a stent–graft placed percutaneously through the femoral artery without the need for an abdominal incision. More complex aneurysms can now be treated with hybrid repairs combining open surgery and stenting or with fenestrated custom-made stents. Laparoscopic intra-abdominal arterial surgery, although rarely practised, has also a role in certain cases and in experienced centres. With further improvements in technique and technology, stenting of a carotid artery stenosis may also evolve further.

Equally impressive have been the advances in non-invasive imaging. High-quality, real-time, colour flow duplex ultrasound techniques have already revolutionized the imaging of arteries and veins. New ultrasound contrast media may allow certain vessels such as the renal and mesenteric arteries, previously inaccessible to ultrasound diagnosis, to be imaged with increasing ease and accuracy.

However, with the advances seen in vascular surgery has come the realization that they may not come with the same longevity of the procedures they replace, and that performing high-risk surgery with costly devices may not be in the patient's best interests. Therefore, the holistic approach of the vascular surgeon and establishing the appropriate intervention is paramount. With these factors in mind, open arterial surgery and reconstruction will be required for many years to come. Indeed, skills to remove implanted stent grafts are vital for today's surgeon – Fig. 27.52) shows a removed stent graft.

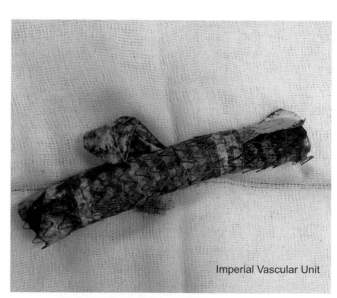

Imperial Vascular Unit

• **Fig. 27.52** Removed stent graft post implantation.

Despite years of research and the production of lab grown human and animal grafts, the major advances anticipated in graft development have yet to materialize. Autologous vein remains the ideal conduit. Research into gene therapy and growth factors continues apace, and is expected to play an important role in prevention and/or treatment of vascular disease in the future.

The landscape of vascular surgery has changed, with an ageing but fitter population leading to a relative increase in peripheral vascular disease in later life, balanced against a reduction in tobacco consumption. With the advent of excellent best medical therapy, this has led to a reduction in the conventional vascular patients; however, diabetes is expanding in prevalence, leading to patients presenting later with more complex disease patterns.

References

1. Heart Protection Study Collaborative Group. MRC/BHF Heart Protection Study of cholesterol lowering with simvastatin in 20,536 high-risk individuals: a randomised placebo-controlled trial. *Lancet*. 2002;360:7–22.
2. Norgren L, Hiatt WR, Dormandy JA, et al. Inter-Society Consensus for the Management of Peripheral Arterial Disease (TASC II). *Eur J Vasc Endovasc Surg*. 2007;33(suppl 1):S1–75.
3. Adam DJ, Beard JD, Cleveland T, et al. Bypass versus angioplasty in severe ischaemia of the leg (BASIL): multicentre, randomised controlled trial. *Lancet*. 2005;366:1925–1934.
4. Wang J, Shu C, Wu Z, et al. Percutaneous Vascular Interventions Versus Bypass Surgeries in Patients With Critical Limb Ischemia: A Comprehensive Meta-analysis. *Ann Surg*. 2018;267:846–857.
5. The UK Small Aneurysm Trial Participants. Mortality results for randomised controlled trial of early elective surgery or ultrasonographic surveillance for small abdominal aortic aneurysms. *Lancet*. 1998;352:1649–1655.
6. Davies AH, Hawdon AJ, Sydes MR, Thompson SG, VGST P. Is duplex surveillance of value after leg vein bypass grafting? Principal results of the Vein Graft Surveillance Randomised Trial (VGST). *Circulation*. 2005;112:1985–1991.
7. North American Symptomatic Carotid Endarterectomy Trial Collaborators, Barnett HJM, Taylor DW, et al. Beneficial effect of carotid endarterectomy in symptomatic patients with high-grade carotid stenosis. *N Engl J Med*. 1991;325:445–453.
8. European Carotid Surgery Trialists' Collaborative Group. Randomised trial of endarterectomy for recently symptomatic carotid stenosis: final results of the MRC European Carotid Surgery Trial (ECST). *Lancet*. 1998;351:1379–1387.
9. Guay J, Ochroch EA. Carotid endarterectomy plus medical therapy or medical therapy alone for carotid artery stenosis in symptomatic or asymptomatic patients: a meta-analysis. *J Cardiothorac Vasc Anesth*. 2012;26:835–844.
10. Naylor AR, Rantner B, Ancetti S, et al. *European society for vascular surgery (ESVS) 2023 clinical practice guidelines on the management of atherosclerotic carotid and vertebral artery disease*. European Journal of Vascular and Endovascular Surgery; 2022.
11. Goldhaber SZ, Haire WD, Feldstein ML, et al. Alteplase versus heparin in acute pulmonary embolism: randomised trial assessing right-ventricular function and pulmonary perfusion. *Lancet*. 1993;341:507–511.
12. Gohel MS, Heatley F, Liu X, et al. A Randomized Trial of Early Endovenous Ablation in Venous Ulceration. *N Engl J Med*. 2018;378:2105–2114.

Further Reading

Bergan JJ. *The Vein Book*. 2nd ed. Amsterdam: OUP Academic Press; 2014.

Browse NI, Burnand KG, Irvine AT, et al. *Diseases of the Veins*. London: Arnold; 1999.

Dieter RS, Dieter RA. *Venous and Lymphatic Diseases*. New York: McGraw-Hill Medical; 2010.

England T, Nasim A. *ABC of Arterial and Venous Disease*. 3rd ed. Chichester: Wiley-Blackwell; 2014.

Hands L, Ray-Chaudhuri S, Sharp M, Murphy M. *Vascular Surgery (Oxford Specialist Handbook in Surgery)*. Oxford: OUP; 2007.

Hallet JW, Mills JL, Earnshaw J, Reekers JA. *Comprehensive Vascular and Endovascular Surgery*. 2nd ed. Philadelphia: Mosby Elsevier; 2009.

Loftus I, Hinchliffe R. *Vascular and Endovascular Surgery: A Companion to Specialist Surgical Practice*. 6th ed. Philadelphia: Elsevier Saunders; 2018.

National Institute for Health and Clinical Excellence. *Venous Thromboembolism: Reducing the Risk*; 2010. Available online. Accessed 24 January 2011 from http://guidance.nice.org.uk/CG 92/QuickRefGuide/pdf/English.

NICE clinical guidance. *Stroke: Diagnosis and Initial Management of Acute Stroke and Transient Ischaemic Attack (TIA)*; 2008. Available online: https://www.nice.org.uk/guidance/ng89/ resources/department-of-health-vte-risk-assessment-tool-pdf-4787149213.

Sidawy AN, Perler BA. *Rutherford's Vascular Surgery and Endovascular Therapy*. 9th ed. Philadelphia: Elsevier; 2018.

Thompson MM, Fitridge R, Boyle J. *Oxford Textbook of Vascular Surgery*. 1st ed. Oxford: OUP Oxford; 2016.

28

Common Urological Conditions

CHAPTER OUTLINE

Introduction

Urology deals with diseases and disorders of the male genitourinary and female urinary tracts. Urologists have been responsible for the introduction of many new techniques. These include the development and widespread use of endoscopes, lithotripsy, prosthetic stents, laparoscopic surgery including robotic surgery and high-intensity focused ultrasound (HIFU).

KIDNEYS AND URETERS

Anatomy

Kidneys and Ureter Embryology

The definitive kidney, also called the metanephros, appears in the fifth week of gestation. It develops from two sources: (1) the metanephric mesoderm, which provides the excretory

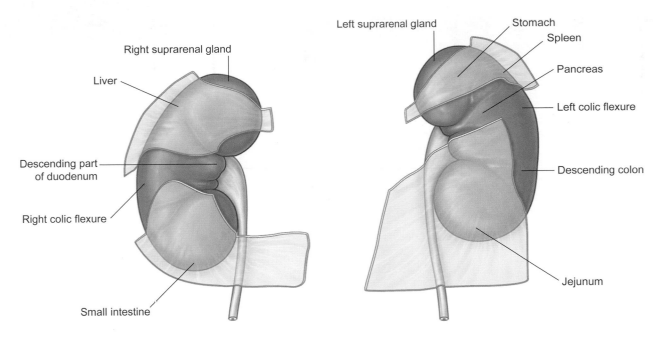

• **Fig. 28.1** Structures Related to the Anterior Surface of the Kidneys (Drake R, Vogl AW, Mitchell AWM,. Gray's Anatomy for Students, 4th ed. Philadelphia: Elsevier; 2019.)

unit and (2) the ureteric bud, which gives rise to the collecting system. The ureteric bud is an outgrowth of the mesonephric duct close to its entrance to the cloaca. It gives rise to the ureter, the renal pelvis, the major and minor calyces and 1 to 3 million collecting tubules.

Nephrons are formed until birth, when approximately 1 million are in each kidney.

Urine production develops around the 10th week of gestation, soon after the differentiation of the glomerular capillaries.

Clinical Anatomy

The kidneys measure 11 cm long, 6 cm wide and 4 cm thick and lie retroperitoneally on the posterior abdominal wall. The right kidney lies slightly lower than the left kidney. Posteriorly, lies the diaphragm, the quadratus lumborum, transversus abdominis and the 12th rib. Anteriorly, the right kidney is related to the liver, the second part of the duodenum and the ascending colon. Anterior to the left kidney, there is the stomach, the pancreas and its vessels, the spleen and the descending colon (Fig. 28.1).

The kidneys lie in a fatty cushion called the perinephric fat which is contained in the renal fascia. The renal pelvis anatomy can vary considerably and may lie completely outside of the kidney or be buried in the renal hilum. The pelvis divides into two or three major calyces, each of which divides into a number of minor calyces.

The ureters are 25 cm long and comprises the pelvis of the ureter, the abdominal, pelvic and intravesical portions. The abdominal part of the ureter lies on the medial edge of psoas major (L2–L5 level). They then cross into the pelvis at the bifurcation of the common iliac artery in front of the sacroiliac joint. The right ureter is crossed by the gonadal right colic and ileocolic vessels. The left ureter is crossed by the gonadal and left colic vessels. The pelvic part of the ureter runs on the lateral wall of the pelvis in front of the internal iliac artery to just in front of the ischial spine. It then turns forward and medially to enter the bladder. The intravesical ureter passes obliquely through the wall of the bladder and both the oblique angle and the vesical muscle act as a sphincter.

Blood Supply

The renal artery derives directly from the aorta whilst the renal vein drains directly in the inferior vena cava. The left renal vein passes anterior to the aorta, immediately below the origin of the superior mesenteric artery. The right renal artery passes behind the inferior vena cava.

The ureter receives segmental blood supply from the aorta, the renal, gonadal, internal iliac and inferior vesical arteries.

Lymphatic Drainage

Lymphatics drain into the para-aortic lymph nodes.

Kidneys and Ureters

Symptoms Arising from the Kidney and Ureter
Systemic

Fever

Acute infections in the urinary tract often present with fever. Acute pyelonephritis is often associated with a high fever (40°C). In infants and children, there may not be any associated urinary symptoms. Chronic pyelonephritis is not associated with fever. Swinging pyrexia can be a feature of renal carcinoma.

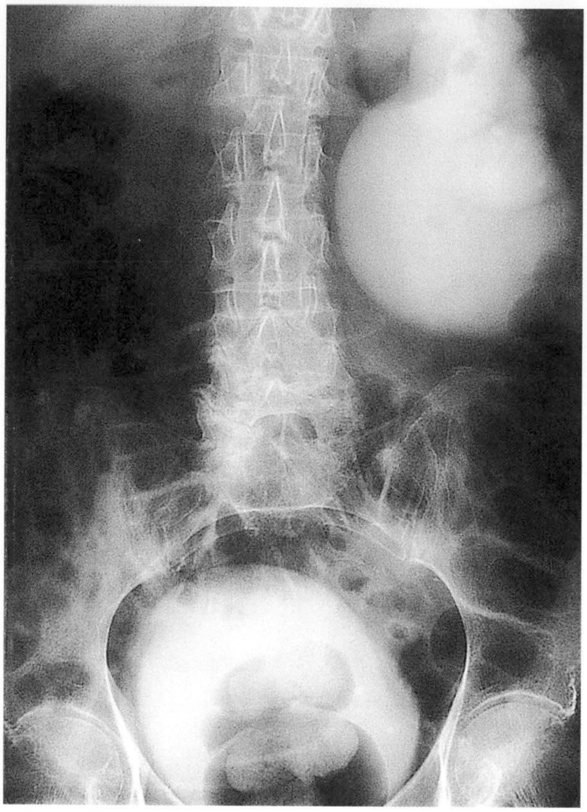

• **Fig. 28.2** An intravenous urogram showing a congenital obstruction of the left pelviureteric junction.

General Malaise and Weight Loss

These are often seen – as in diseases of other systems – with cancer or chronic infection. They may also be features of chronic kidney disease.

Pain

Pain may be perceived at the surface directly over the area of involvement: local renal pain is felt in the flank and costovertebral angle. It is typically a dull, constant ache and related to distension of the renal capsule. However, many renal diseases progress slowly and may not be associated with such pain until some secondary event occurs to cause acute capsular distension. Examples are cancer, tuberculosis, polycystic disease, staghorn calculi and hydronephrosis secondary to congenital pelviureteric junction obstruction or chronic bladder outflow obstruction (Fig. 28.2).

Pain may also be experienced further away from the site of origin. Such pain is often called 'referred'; it being felt at a location distant from the origin of the stimulus. Thus the severe pain of ureteric colic, which occurs in waves, and is often associated with vomiting, may be felt in the testicle (T11 to T12). A stone in the lower ureter may cause pain referred to the scrotal wall (L1) and the bladder.

Oliguria and Anuria

A reduced or absent urine output may be caused by underperfusion of the kidney as a result of hypovolaemic shock from blood, water and electrolyte loss or in sepsis. Bilateral ureteric obstruction and injury to a solitary kidney are other causes.

• BOX 28.1 Causes of Haematuria

Systemic

- Anticoagulants
- Sickle cell disease
- Bacterial endocarditis (emboli)
- Henoch–Schönlein purpura
- Cyclophosphamide

Nephrological

- Mesangial IgA disease
- Glomerulonephritis
- Renal infarcts
- Urinary infection
- Tuberculosis
- Polycystic disease

Urological

- Carcinoma of kidney
- Urothelial tumours
- Stones
- Schistosomiasis
- Benign prostatic

CLINICAL BOX 28.1

Haematuria Diagnosis and Investigation

- Haematuria may be painful or painless.
- Painful haematuria is usually associated with an infection but may result from stones, carcinoma in situ of the bladder, self-induced foreign bodies or urethral trauma.
- Painless haematuria is a sinister sign and most likely due to renal or bladder cancer. Other conditions are shown in Box 28.1.
- A cystoscopy investigation and ultrasound scan are mandatory.

Anaemia and its Symptoms

These are invariable in chronic kidney disease, but also occur as a result of renal tumours, chronic infection and recurrent or persistent haematuria.

Local

Haematuria

Haematuria always requires full investigation as this can be a sign of cancer (Clinical Box 28.1). The additional presence of proteinuria and abnormal red-cell morphology on microscopy are more suggestive of a renal cause. Common causes of haematuria are shown in Box 28.1.

Clinical Examination of the Upper Urinary Tract

Tongue

Because water and electrolyte disturbance are common in urological disease, the tongue should be examined for dryness and at the same time the breath smelt for the characteristic ammoniacal, fishy smell of uraemia.

Inspection

Patients with uraemia may have a yellow tinge and may have scratch marks from uraemic pruritus.

In children, inspection of the child as whole may give an impression of whether the child is happy and has normal growth and development, or may be suffering with a serious condition. Inspection of the abdomen may reveal the suggestion of a renal mass, which may be seen in the upper abdomen, or inferred from fullness or oedema in this area. The latter might imply a perinephric infection.

Palpation

The patient should lie supine on a firm surface. Bimanual examination of the kidney is performed by placing a hand in the costovertebral angle to lift the kidney while feeling the kidney with the other hand anteriorly. On deep inspiration, the kidney moves downwards and can be trapped and palpated between the two hands. The right kidney lies lower than the left, as it is positioned beneath the liver, and it is sometimes possible to feel the lower pole even if it is normal. The left cannot usually be felt unless it is enlarged or displaced.

Enlargement of the kidney suggests the possibility of polycystic disease, a renal cyst, tumour or hydronephrosis.

Percussion

Renal masses are frequently soft and difficult to feel. They can often be more easily outlined by percussion.

Auscultation

A bruit may be heard over the upper abdomen. Possible causes are renal artery stenosis, aneurysm of the renal artery and an arteriovenous fistula.

Investigation

A combination of haematological, biochemical, bacteriological, radiological, isotopic and endoscopic examination is often needed to achieve an accurate, rapid, cost-effective determination of the probable diagnosis and requirements for treatment.

Examination of the Urine

Technique

A timed urine collection may be required for assessment of renal function (see 'Creatinine clearance', later), proteinuria or the excretion of substances associated with stone formation.

In order to investigate a urinary tract infection, it is best to examine a freshly voided specimen taken midway through the act of micturition. Specimens collected from women who have not undergone any special preparation and who void into disposable plastic cups show a 95% concordance with a catheter specimen. In addition, genital cleaning makes little difference to the bacterial count. The most important factor is rapid transport of specimens to the laboratory.

Urine is usually collected into a clean polystyrene cup and then transferred without spillage to a sterile universal container.

In younger children, a plastic bag is attached around the urethral meatus. In girls, catheterization with a fine catheter is appropriate, although, in either sex, suprapubic needle aspiration is easy to perform, particularly if hydration is adequate and the bladder full. The suprapubic area is cleansed; local anaesthetic is injected to raise an intradermal wheal 1–2 cm above the pubic symphysis. A 10-mL syringe with a 22-gauge needle is inserted perpendicularly through the abdominal wall into the bladder, maintaining gentle suction with the syringe so that the urine is aspirated as soon as the bladder is entered.

Three consecutive early morning urines are required for the investigation of tuberculosis.

Colour and Appearance

Overtly bloody urine is usually unmistakable. However, red urine can result from:
- betacyanin excretion after beetroot ingestion
- phenolphthalein and other laxatives can colour the urine red
- myoglobinuria, the result of muscle trauma
- haemoglobinuria after haemolysis

Chemical Tests

Chemically impregnated reagent strips permit the simultaneous rapid performance of a number of tests, including the presence of blood, protein, ketones, glucose, nitrites and leucocyte esterase. These tests can be useful for screening and show good correlation with more-extensive laboratory examination. Positive tests for nitrites and leucocytes have a high predictive value for urinary infection and treatment should be started immediately, before culture results are available.

Microscopy

Examination of the centrifuged urinary sediment allows identification of red blood cells (which always requires further investigation), white blood cells, bacteria and casts. Cytological examination for malignant cells is also possible.

The presence of more than five white blood cells per high-powered field is abnormal (pyuria) and, if associated with bacteria, indicates a urinary infection. Sterile pyuria – white blood cells but without bacteria – occurs in:
- tuberculosis of the urinary tract
- urinary stones
- recent instrumentation/presence of an indwelling catheter
- recovery from urinary infection

Culture

Culture enables the organism present to be identified and early predictions made of which antibiotics may be effective in treatment.

Serum Creatinine Concentration and Creatinine Clearance

Creatinine in serum is the end-product of the metabolism of creatine in skeletal muscle, which takes place at a fairly steady rate. The molecule is filtered through the glomerulus and its clearance is approximately equal to the glomerular filtration rate (GFR). The serum creatinine concentration remains within the normal range until approximately 50% of renal function has been lost.

Kidney function used to be estimated by measuring creatinine clearance, which required a 24-hour urine collection in addition to serum creatinine estimation. This has been replaced by a calculated estimate of glomerular filtration (eGFR) (see Box 28.2).

Serum Urea Concentration

The amount of urea in the blood is also related to the GFR. However, it is more influenced by factors external to the kidney, for example:

- Dietary protein intake
- Endogenous sources of nitrogen in the gut such as a gastrointestinal haemorrhage
- Rate of urine production, which is the outcome of a number of factors including the state of hydration

Approximately two-thirds of renal function must be lost before a significant rise in the serum urea concentration takes place. The measurement is less specific as an index of renal function than is creatinine clearance.

Serum Calcium Concentration

The level of serum calcium should be routinely measured in patients with renal stones to identify hyperparathyroidism and alterations in vitamin D metabolism in those with chronic kidney disease. Calcium concentration may also be elevated in patients with renal-cell carcinoma, either as part of a paraneoplastic syndrome caused by the secretion of parathyroid hormone-like substance, or from bone destruction by secondary deposits.

Serum Alkaline Phosphatase

The concentration may be elevated as part of a paraneoplastic syndrome in renal-cell carcinoma or from bone deposits in patients with genitourinary or other cancer.

Imaging

Abdominal Plain X-Ray

A plain abdominal radiograph is frequently called a KUB (kidneys, ureters, bladder). It is always the first film to be examined before reporting on subsequent contrast studies and can avert pitfalls (Fig. 28.3). It is often used in the follow up of renal stones and can yield a great deal of information (Fig. 28.4).

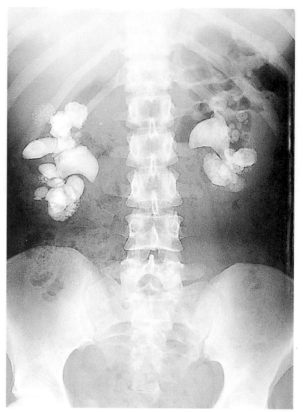

• **Fig. 28.3** Plain Film of the Abdomen (KUB) Bilateral renal calculi, which could be mistaken for an intravenous urogram, are shown.

X-Ray Contrast Studies

Water-soluble preparations that contain iodine can be administered by several routes, including directly into blood vessels. All procedures which use intravascular contrast media carry a small but definite ($\approx$5%) risk of an adverse reaction. Most are minor and include nausea, vomiting, itching, rash or flushing. Cardiopulmonary adverse reactions are rare (1:40 000), but may be life-threatening or fatal. The contraindications to the use of intravascular contrast to image the urinary tract are shown in Box 28.3.

Patients with relative allergic contraindications can be given corticosteroids. However, there is little evidence to indicate conclusively the prophylactic use of corticosteroids is efficacious.

Intravenous Urogram (IVU)

IVU was the most frequently used contrast investigation, but has largely been replaced by a combination of ultrasound and CT scanning. Many of the items shown in Fig. 28.5 may also be elicited or confirmed by urography and additional information also obtained (Fig. 28.6).

Those with chronic kidney disease are unable to excrete the usual dose of contrast media at a concentration sufficient to provide an image, and a larger than usual dose is required. It is usual to restrict fluids before an IVU so as to concentrate the urine, but this should not be done in diabetics.

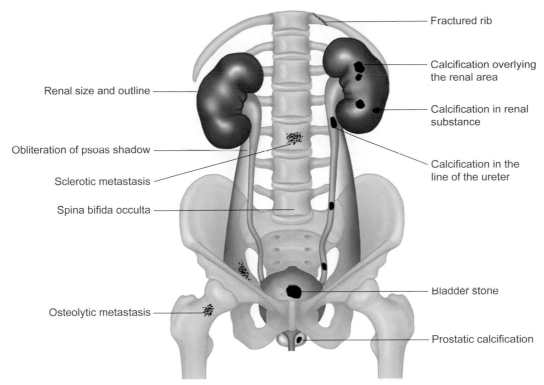

• **Fig. 28.4** A Guide to the Interpretation of a Plain Abdominal X-Ray

Renal size and outline

Obliteration of psoas shadow

Sclerotic metastasis

Spina bifida occulta

Osteolytic metastasis

Fractured rib

Calcification overlying the renal area

Calcification in renal substance

Calcification in the line of the ureter

Bladder stone

Prostatic calcification

Retrograde Ureterography

A cystoscopy and the placement of a ureteric catheter are required. Radio-opaque contrast medium is then introduced directly into the renal pelvis or ureter, via the ureteric catheter.

Antegrade Pyelography

Contrast medium is introduced either through a nephrostomy tube (nephrostogram) or by direct injection into the renal pelvis via a percutaneous needle puncture.

Arteriography

Arteriography (Fig. 28.7) is most frequently done to evaluate:
- Possible causes of renovascular hypertension
- Anatomical suitability of potential live related kidney donors
- Vascular anatomy before surgery

It has for the most part been superseded by magnetic resonance angiography.

Arteriographic techniques can also be used for therapy. Arteriovenous fistulae and bleeding vascular renal tumours can be embolized, and renal artery stenoses dilated.

Micturating Cystourethrography

This is performed to determine the presence of vesicoureteric reflux. Contrast medium is introduced into the bladder via a urethral catheter that is then removed. Dynamic X-ray studies are made during voiding, and contrast may be seen to reflux up the ureter(s) (Fig. 28.8). The urethra is also delineated and an assessment of residual urine can be made.

Ultrasonography

Ultrasound is used in the upper urinary tract to:
- Determine the size of the kidneys and look for the presence of pelvicalyceal dilatation, which may be due to obstruction in patients with chronic kidney disease, acute stone disease, acute/chronic malignant obstruction
- Distinguish between solid and cystic renal masses
- Identify non-opaque renal stones

Ultrasonography cannot provide detailed visualization of the calyces and pelvis, nor does it outline a non-dilated ureter or provide functional information about the upper urinary tract.

Computed Tomography

The principal uses of CT are:
- Diagnosis and staging of tumours (Fig. 28.9)
- Delineation and diagnosis of retroperitoneal masses

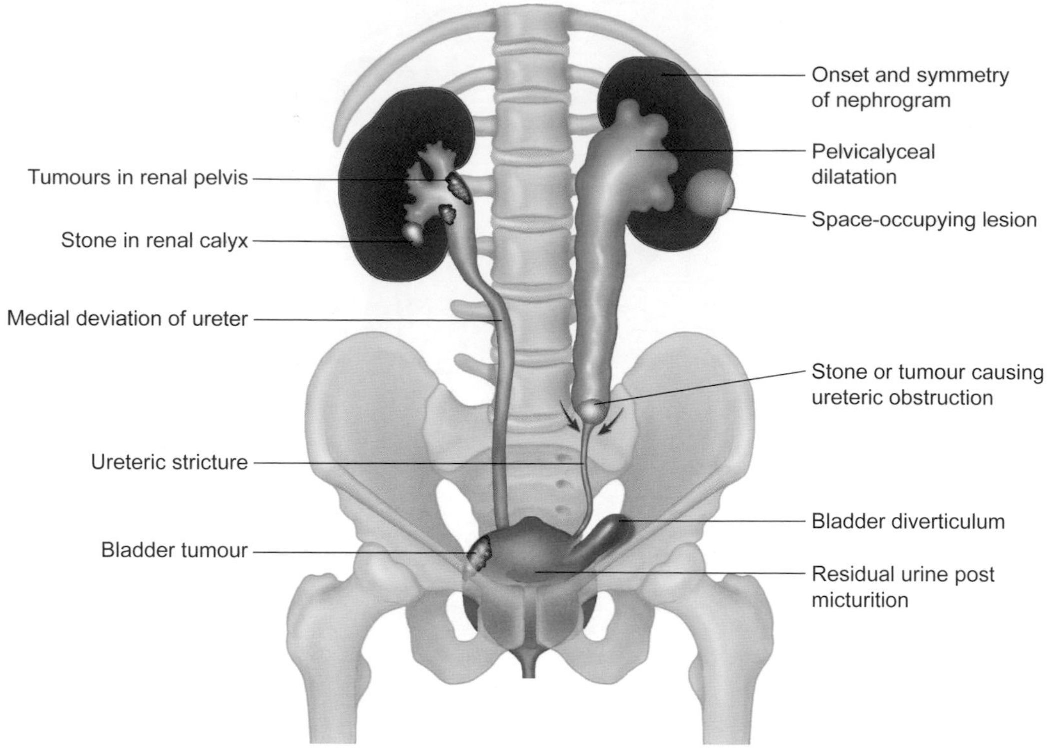

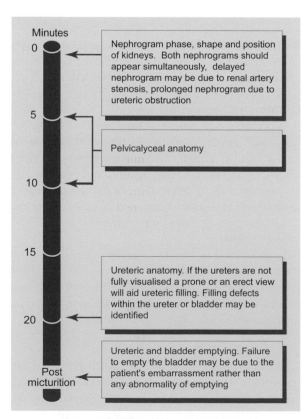

Onset and symmetry
of nephrogram

Pelvicalyceal
dilatation

Space-occupying lesion

Tumours in renal pelvis

Stone in renal calyx

Medial deviation of ureter

Stone or tumour causing
ureteric obstruction

Ureteric stricture

Bladder diverticulum

Bladder tumour

Residual urine post
micturition

• **Fig. 28.5** A Guide to an Interpretation of an Intravenous Urogram (IVU)

Minutes

0

Nephrogram phase, shape and position
of kidneys. Both nephrograms should
appear simultaneously, delayed
nephrogram may be due to renal artery
stenosis, prolonged nephrogram due to
ureteric obstruction

5

Pelvicalyceal anatomy

10

15

Ureteric anatomy. If the ureters are not
fully visualised a prone or an erect view
will aid ureteric filling. Filling defects
within the ureter or bladder may be
identified

20

Post
micturition

Ureteric and bladder emptying. Failure
to empty the bladder may be due to the
patient's embarrassment rather than
any abnormality of emptying

• **Fig. 28.6** Additional Information of an IVU

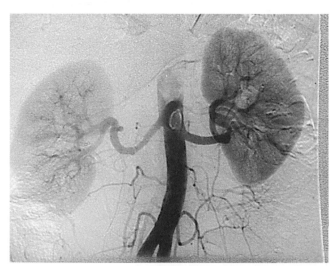

• **Fig. 28.7** A Normal Renal Angiogram Showing Single Arteries to
Both Kidneys

- Identification and classification of renal trauma
- Identification of urinary tract stones
- Delineation of renal pelvis and ureter (CT urogram)

Magnetic Resonance Imaging

The main advantages of MRI and contraindications to its
use are given in Box 28.4. New contrast medium such as
gadolinium are beginning to improve the imaging ability of MRI, particularly in the interpretation of prostate
architecture.

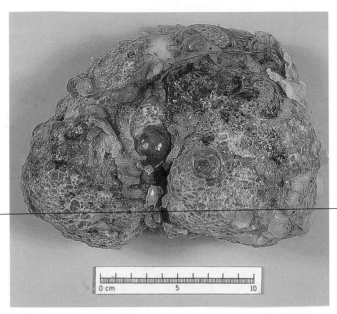

• **Fig. 28.12** A Polycystic Kidney

- Vomiting and diarrhoea
- Jaundice
- Weight loss
- High fever
- Unexplained screaming attacks

General Examination Commonly reveals hypertension. There may be features of chronic kidney disease. The kidneys are large and irregular (Fig. 28.12). Occasionally, there is hepatomegaly from cystic involvement of that organ.

Diagnosis. A definitive diagnosis can be made by ultrasound, which shows the pelvis of each kidney elongated and attenuated by the smooth surface of adjacent cysts. Ultrasonography confirms the presence of multiple cysts in the kidneys and other organs. This investigation should be used to screen children who are the offspring of parents known to have the condition.

Management

In the majority, the disease is progressive and ultimately necessitates renal replacement by dialysis and/or transplantation (see Ch. 12). Failure to control hypertension accelerates the loss of kidney function.

Urinary Tract Infection

Urinary tract infection is the most common bacterial infection in humans of all ages. It is more common in females than males. The incidence and sequelae of urinary infections, their diagnosis and treatment all vary with age. By the time adolescence is reached, 1% of boys and 5% of girls will have had a urinary tract infection.

Infection in Children

Aetiology and Pathological Features

Organisms that ascend from the urethral meatus are usually Gram-negative faecal flora. *Escherichia coli* and *Proteus* spp. are the commonest. Vesicoureteric reflux, or other anatomical abnormalities, may be associated with an increased risk of infection in children. If infection ascends to the growing kidneys (up to the age of 5 years) and is repeated, renal damage occurs with progressive scarring (the outcome of healing of a cortical abscess) and the development of chronic kidney

disease and hypertension. Infection is one of the few preventable forms of chronic kidney disease.

Clinical Features

The younger the child, the less specific the symptoms (see Box 28.5). Older children and adults may complain of:
- loin pain
- increased urgency and frequency
- burning on micturition
- haematuria
- enuresis

Specific signs are absent, but there may be some tenderness in one or both renal angles.

Investigation

Bacterial Culture

Urine should be obtained for dipstick testing (see earlier) and for culture and antibiotic sensitivities before antibiotic therapy is begun.

Imaging

Any child with an infection must be thoroughly investigated to find out if there is an anatomical abnormality.

Ultrasound identifies congenital abnormalities, dilatation of the renal pelvis and ureter, urinary stones and renal scarring.
Micturating cystourethrography is done, after the urine has been made sterile, to identify and quantitate vesicoureteral reflux, scarring and the adequacy of bladder emptying (see Fig. 28.8).
DMSA renography is the best way of identifying renal scarring.

Management

Infants and Children with a Normal Ultrasound and Micturating Cystogram

A single course of an appropriate broad-spectrum antibiotic (amoxicillin, trimethoprim and cephalosporins are among the most effective) should be given for 5–7 days. Thereafter, follow up for a year with monthly urine specimens for bacterial analysis. Because of the risk of renal scarring in infants, prophylactic low-dose antibiotics are given until the age of 2 years. In older children, prophylaxis is limited to 6 months. Clinical recurrence requires further antibiotic therapy and full investigation.

Children with Vesicoureteric Reflux and/or Renal Scarring

The treatment of the acute episode is as above. Thereafter, prophylaxis up to the age of 5 years is essential. Ultrasound examination of the kidneys is done at yearly intervals. A direct cystogram is done up to the age of 2 years if the reflux has not resolved. An indirect cystogram using MAG3 renography is performed annually up to the age of 5 years. The reflux resolves spontaneously in 80% and, in consequence, there has been a move away from its surgical correction. Indications for surgery are not clearly defined but include:

- recurrent infection in the presence of antibiotic prophylaxis
- persistent loin pain or fever
- poor compliance with prophylaxis
- progressive scarring

Acute Pyelonephritis

Aetiology

Commonly caused by aerobic Gram-negative bacteria which ascend from the urethra and genital tract; haematogenous infection is infrequent. Once infection is established in the bladder, its ascent to the kidney is the consequence of:

- microbial virulence
- presence of vesicoureteric reflux
- quality of ureteric peristalsis

Clinical Features

Symptoms are:

- high fever, sweating and often vomiting
- dull ache in the loin
- increased frequency
- dysuria
- haematuria
  The only specific sign is loin tenderness.

Investigation

Urine

This is turbid and contains protein and blood. Organisms, red cells, white blood cells and debris may be seen on direct microscopy. Culture is essential.

Blood

Apart from routine investigations, a blood culture may identify the pathogen responsible.

Imaging

Plain X-Ray. Plain x-ray of the abdomen may show renal enlargement or obliteration of the renal outline by perirenal oedema or the presence of a radio-opaque stone.

Ultrasonography. May identify a radiolucent stone but, more importantly, may show dilatation of the renal pelvis, which suggests an obstruction that needs urgent intervention (Fig. 28.13).

CT. May help rule out other causes of pain and show renal stones and/or confirm obstruction

Management

There is no need to wait for the results of bacterial culture and sensitivity tests. Antibiotic therapy should begin at once. The majority of infections are caused by organisms that are sensitive to trimethoprim, amoxicillin, cephalosporins,

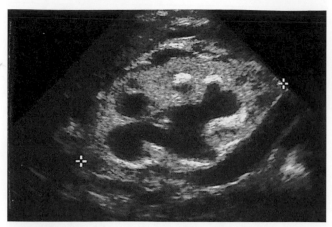

• **Fig. 28.13** Ultrasound Examination Showing Dilatation of the Renal Pelvis, a Result of Ureteric Obstruction

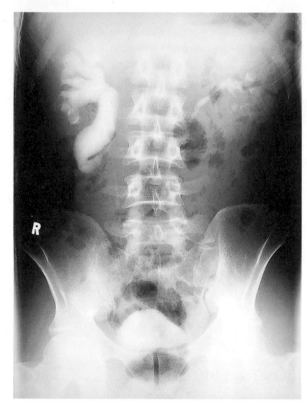

• **Fig. 28.14** An IVU Showing Reflux Nephropathy The right kidney is shrunken and scarred with calyceal clubbing.

quinolones or aminoglycosides. The urine is re-cultured a week after treatment is complete to ensure that the infection has been eradicated.

Once the acute episode has settled, any correctable precipitating cause is dealt with.

Reflux Nephropathy

Patients may present with recurrent loin pain especially on micturition. Reflux is largely a radiological diagnosis based on the finding of shrunken kidneys with an irregular outline because of cortical scarring – the end result of cortical abscesses. The calyces are clubbed (Fig. 28.14).

Clinical Features

The symptoms are those of:
- urinary tract infection
- chronic kidney disease
- hypertension

There are no specific signs. Most patients are hypertensive, while some are normotensive due to the development of a salt (Na^+)-losing nephropathy.

Management

Existing infection must be eradicated and recurrence prevented by long-term continuous antimicrobial prophylaxis. If hypertension is associated with unilateral disease, a nephrectomy may be indicated. Reflux may resolve spontaneously and so follow-up is indicated. Subureteric orifice injection therapy or ureteric re-implantation may be needed if resolution does not occur.

Renal Abscess

Aetiology and Pathological Features

There are two causes:
- Haematogenous spread – usually of *Staphylococcus aureus* – from a distant site. The condition is common in drug abusers and diabetics. Abscesses are usually multiple and in the cortex.
- Acute pyelonephritis, often with obstruction, causes medullary abscesses which are more common.

Clinical Features

Symptoms

There may be a history of recurrent urinary tract infection or parenteral administration of therapeutic (insulin) or other non-therapeutic substances. The patient is often acutely ill with high fever and loin pain.

Signs
- flank tenderness
- palpable mass
- erythema of the skin of the loin
- obvious pyuria

Investigation

This is as for acute pyelonephritis. Ultrasonography can identify a renal abscess, but it is difficult to distinguish this from a cystic-necrotic renal carcinoma and therefore a CT may be required.

Management

Management is with systemic antibiotic therapy. Percutaneous drainage of any collections seen on ultrasound is carried out.

Perinephric Abscess

Aetiology and Pathological Features

The majority of perinephric abscesses result from rupture of a renal abscess into the perinephric tissue. They therefore lie between the renal capsule and perirenal fascia. A large

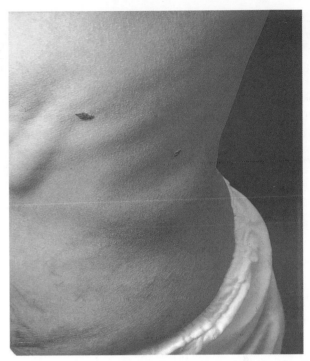

• **Fig. 28.15** A Perinephric Abscess Pointing Posteriorly Over the Iliac Crest

collection may point posterolaterally over the iliac crest (Fig. 28.15). The organisms are the same as those found in renal abscesses. There may be an underlying infected hydronephrosis (pyonephrosis).

Clinical Features

The onset tends to be similar to renal abscess. The patient has a fever and complains of loin pain.

Signs are of:
- tenderness over the affected kidney
- large mass
- pleural effusion on chest examination

Investigation

Blood

There will be a marked leucocytosis.

Imaging

Plain X-ray of the abdomen shows a soft-tissue mass in the flank with obliteration of the renal and psoas shadows. A stone in the renal pelvis may be seen. Because of spasm of the lumbar muscles, there is often a scoliosis with the concavity towards the affected kidney. Gas – produced by coliform or other organisms – may be seen in the renal collecting system or around the kidney.

Ultrasonography may demonstrate a hydronephrosis as well as delineating the extent of the abscess.

CT is the best investigation to confirm the diagnosis and show the details of the mass and presence of associated stones (Fig. 28.16).

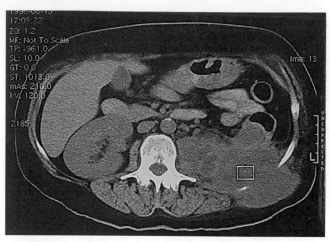

• **Fig. 28.16** A CT Scan of a Patient with a Perinephric Abscess and Pyonephrosis

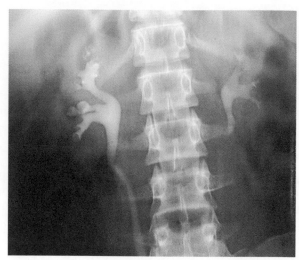

• **Fig. 28.17** A Tuberculous Abscess Cavity in the Upper Pole of the Right Kidney in a Patient who Presented with an Epididymal Swelling

Management

Percutaneous drainage under ultrasound guidance may be adequate, but an open operation is sometimes required. Nephrectomy is often needed because of underlying kidney disease.

Complications

Renal damage can develop as a sequelae of renal abscess formation. Ureteric stenosis, because of periureteric fibrosis, is a common sequel. If the kidney has not been removed, the patency of the ureter should be assessed after 1 month.

Renal Tuberculosis

Epidemiology

The condition is on the increase in the UK. There are three known reasons:

- Migration from or traveling to developing countries where the disease is endemic
- Tuberculosis in patients with AIDS
- Tuberculosis in drug users

More importantly, however, renal tuberculosis is reappearing in those that do not meet these criteria.

Aetiology and Pathological Features

The organism reaches the genitourinary tract by haematogenous spread from a focus in the lung, which is often asymptomatic. The kidney is usually the primary site, and other genitourinary organs become involved by shedding of bacteria into the urine. The progress of the disease is slow; in a patient who is otherwise well, it may take many years to destroy the kidney. Involvement of the renal pelvis and ureter may lead to stricture and hydronephrosis. Infection of the bladder wall causes progressive fibrosis and ultimately a shrunken bladder.

Clinical Features

The slow evolution of the disease means that, in a patient with an involved kidney, years may elapse before symptoms occur, although occasionally there may be a dull ache in the flank and haematuria. Spread to the bladder may cause increased frequency and pain on moderate bladder distension and at micturition. Rarely, the first presentation is when the patient discovers a painless epididymal swelling.

There are no specific signs.

Investigation

Urine

The finding of persistent pyuria without pyogenic organisms on ordinary culture is an indication to collect a first morning specimen on at least three separate occasions for culture for mycobacterium. Although a negative result does not exclude the disease, a positive one – which is obtained in a high percentage of samples – is confirmatory. If there is strong presumptive evidence for the presence of tuberculosis, but a negative result, cultures should be repeated, because not only is it necessary to be certain that genitourinary tuberculosis is present, but also the antimicrobial sensitivity must be determined before treatment is begun.

Imaging

Chest X-ray may show evidence of tuberculosis.

An IVU or, more commonly today, a CT Urogram may demonstrate calcification in the kidney, an abscess cavity or dilated calyces (Fig. 28.17). Absence of function is a consequence of complete destruction – auto-nephrectomy.

Management

Management is by combination of antimicrobial therapy. Treatment usually consists of 2 months of isoniazid, rifampicin, pyrazinamide and ethanbutol, and then 4 months of isoniazide and rifampicin. During this treatment, repeated examination by ultrasound is required to make sure that a ureteric stricture does not develop as the tuberculous lesions heal (Fig. 28.18).

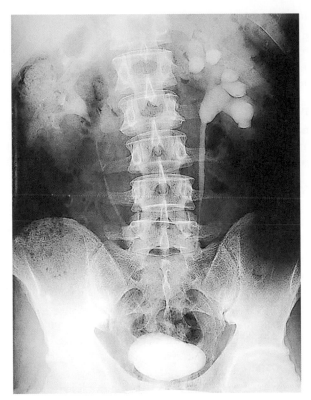

• **Fig. 28.18** An IVU Which Demonstrates a Left Ureteric Stricture After Treatment for Renal Tuberculosis

Renal Trauma

Injury to the kidney is not uncommon with 30% of severe abdominal trauma involving the kidney(s). However, it rarely results in an urgent life-threatening problem.

Aetiology and Pathological Features

Blunt trauma follows road traffic accidents and sporting injuries and may be accompanied by fracture of the 11th and 12th ribs and injuries to the liver and spleen.

Penetrating injuries by knives, bullets and a diagnostic biopsy may, in the first two instances, be associated with other abdominal and thoracic damage. A universal classification of renal trauma according to the American Association for the Surgery of Trauma is given in Box 28.6

Clinical Features

No symptoms may be attributable to the kidney, especially in multiple trauma. An otherwise well patient may complain of loin pain and haematuria.

Signs of renal trauma are:
- haematuria
- bruising over the ribs posteriorly
- evidence of penetrating injury
- tenderness and guarding in the loin
- hypotension

• **BOX 28.6** **Classification of Renal Injuries**

- Grade I Renal contusion
- Grade II Laceration <1cm
- Grade III Laceration >1cm or/and haematoma contained within perirenal fascia
- Grade IV Involvement of collecting system or/and segmental renal or vascular injury
- Grade V Renal hilum injury or/and shattered kidney

- expanding mass
- localized bruit from an arteriovenous fistula

Investigation

Imaging

1. *Plain X-ray* may show fractures of the 10th, 11th or 12th ribs.
2. *CT* scan with contrast is now the investigation of choice. It will accurately assess:
   - absence of function on the affected side but a normal contralateral kidney
   - absence of function and no contralateral kidney
   - the extent of injury
   - lacerations
   - extravasation
   - surrounding haemorrhage
   - vessel injury
   - non-renal injuries

CT angiography has largely replaced invasive investigations, but therapeutic angiography may be required in the following circumstances:
- non-function on CT
- persistent severe haematuria which might require embolization
- presence or development of a bruit
- late development of hypertension in a patient who has recovered from an injury

Management

Some factors influencing management are given in Clinical Box 28.2.

Any patient with a renal injury should be at rest in bed and have the usual observations. All urine passed is examined to assess and follow the degree of haematuria.

Penetrating Injury

Depending on the type of injury (e.g. gunshot or knife) and the findings on CT scanning, surgical exploration may be required for non-renal damage. Other injuries take priority and the kidney is explored only if there is evidence on preoperative evaluation or at operation of major damage. Nephrectomy may be inevitable. Most renal injuries, however, can be managed conservatively or by interventional radiological embolization.

CLINICAL BOX 28.2

Factors Influencing Management of Renal Trauma

- Only 2% of patients with blunt renal injuries, but up to 55% with penetrating injuries, will require exploration
- Nearly all patients with renal gunshot wounds have associated intra-abdominal injuries, compared with 12% with stab wounds posterior to the anterior axillary line
- Urine dipstick testing should be obtained early
- Radiographic imaging should not delay urgent surgery
- CT scanning provides optimal definition of the injury and is the investigation of choice. It also detects other abdominal injuries
- Ureteric and renal pelvic injuries are usually the result of a penetrating injury

Closed Injury

Treatment is initially non-operative with careful continued assessment. Prophylactic antibiotics are administered. Unless one of the more severe injuries listed in Box 28.6 is present, most injuries resolve, although a period of stay in hospital may be required. The incidence of later surgical intervention to manage complications is also increased but, in contrast to early exploration, nephrectomy is less commonly needed, especially in the era of interventional radiology.

Persistent Haematuria or Arteriovenous Fistula

Selective arterial embolization of the site is the management of choice.

Renal Tumours

Tumours of the kidney account for approximately 2% of all malignancies. Benign solid tumours are less frequent and include oncocytoma and angiomyolipoma.

There are four types of malignant tumour, apart from the very rare fibro- and liposarcomas:

- nephroblastoma (Wilms' tumour)
- adenocarcinoma
- transitional cell carcinoma of the renal pelvis
- squamous carcinoma of the renal pelvis

1. Nephroblastoma (Wilms' Tumour)

This is the commonest genitourinary neoplasm in infants and second only to brain tumours as a cause of death in this age group. Sex distribution is equal, there is a peak incidence at 2 years and the tumour is bilateral in 5%.

Pathological Features

It is an undifferentiated embryonic tumour which contains primitive glomeruli and tubules as well as irregular areas of collagen, cartilage, bone and adipose tissue. Spread is by direct infiltration of the kidney and surrounding structures, by lymphatics and by the bloodstream to the liver, lungs, long bones and brain.

Clinical Features

There is often failure to thrive, and a thin, ill infant or child presents with a visible abdominal mass. The majority present with a mass, half have hypertension and one-third have haematuria.

Investigation

Imaging

Ultrasonography demonstrates a solid renal mass. CT or MR scanning is required for staging.

Management

In all patients, a radical nephrectomy (a procedure in which, through an open, abdominal approach, the kidney, perirenal soft tissue and adjacent lymph nodes are removed as a block and the renal vessels divided as close to their origin as possible) is done. The renal vessels are ligated early in the operation to reduce the risk of escape of malignant cells during manipulation.

Treatment with neo- and adjuvant chemotherapy and/or radiotherapy depends on the stage of the disease.

Prognosis

For localized tumours, there is a 5-year survival of over 90%, but this falls in the presence of anaplastic histology, lymph node metastases and/or metastases to solid organs.

2. Renal Adenocarcinoma

Epidemiology and Pathological Features

The peak incidence is in the fifth generation, and the condition is commoner in men. It is further sub-classified into clear-cell carcinoma (80%), papillary (10–15%), chromophobe (5%), and other rare subtypes (≤1%) (collecting duct and medullary cell). In clear-cell adenocarcinoma, the tumour arises from the renal tubules, is usually well-encapsulated and contains areas of haemorrhage and necrosis. On histological examination, it consists of columnar or cuboidal cells with clear cytoplasm and dark nuclei. Papillary carcinoma also arises from the renal tubules, whilst chromophobe arises from the cortical portion of the collecting duct. Spread is by local infiltration and chiefly by the blood to distant organs. There may be direct growth into the renal vein and vena cava. Paraneoplastic syndromes may occur (Table 28.1).

Staging

TNM staging is used, based on the preoperative investigations, operative findings and the histological examination of the excised tissues. T stages are shown in Table 28.2 and N and M stages in Table 28.3.

Clinical Features

Twenty percent of tumours are detected on ultrasound examination during the course of investigations for non-specific symptoms or for features that suggest a paraneoplastic syndrome.

TABLE 28.1 Paraneoplastic Syndromes in Renal Cell Carcinoma.

Event	Cause
Raised ESR	Changes in plasma proteins
Anaemia	Depressed erythropoiesis and haemolysis
Polycythaemia	Erythropoietin secretion
Hypercalcaemia	Tumour secretion of parathormone-like substance
Raised alkaline Phosphatase Concentration	Secretion from the tumour
Pyrexia	Circulating pyrogens
Hypertension	Secretion of renin
Amyloid deposition	Unknown
Peripheral neuropathy and myopathy	Unknown

TABLE 28.2 T Component of TNM Staging of Carcinoma of the Kidney.

Stage	Findings
T1a	Tumour <4 cm
T1b	4–7 cm limited to kidney
T2	Tumour >7 cm limited to kidney
T3	Tumour extends into major veins or invades adrenal or perinephric tissue but not beyond Gerota's fascia
T4	Tumour invades beyond Gerota's fascia

TABLE 28.3 N and M Components of TNM Staging of Carcinoma of the Kidney.

Stage	Findings
NX	Regional lymph nodes cannot be assessed
N0	No regional lymph node metastases
N1	Metastases in a single lymph node <2.0 cm in diameter
N2	Metastases in single lymph node 2–5 cm in greatest diameter or multiple lymph nodes, none >5 cm in greatest diameter
N3	Metastases in lymph node >5 cm in greatest diameter
M0	No distant metastases
M1	Distant metastases

Symptoms

Specific symptoms are not common, but there are some which are semi-specific:
- aching loin pain
- episodes of acute pain – caused by haemorrhage into the tumour and sometimes of sufficient severity for the patient to present as an emergency
- haematuria (60%)
- symptoms of paraneoplastic syndromes (see Table 28.1)
- pathological fracture

Signs

A loin mass may be the only finding unless there is clinical evidence of distant metastases. By the time that the classical triad of loin pain, loin mass and haematuria is present, the tumour is usually advanced.

Investigation

Urine

Haematuria should be sought. Significant proteinuria may indicate involvement of the renal vein.

Blood

Analysis should be done for any of the paraneoplastic syndromes. Hypercalcaemia or a raised alkaline phosphatase does not necessarily imply metastatic disease.

Imaging

Chest X-ray may show typical 'cannonball' metastases.

IVU demonstrates a space-occupying lesion, best seen in the nephrogram phase, and also calyceal distortion.

Ultrasonography can distinguish between a cyst and a solid tumour and is an effective way of identifying involvement of the renal vein and the vena cava.

CT scan is the most precise way of staging the tumour (see Tables 28.2 and 28.3; Fig. 28.19).

Renal angiography is less commonly used but is essential in bilateral tumours or a tumour in a solitary kidney. This allows an operative plan to be made.

Management

Surgery

Radical nephrectomy is the primary treatment in the absence of metastatic disease, or in the presence of low volume metastatic disease. Laparoscopy (with or without robotic assistance) is generally used both for removal of the whole kidney and more limited resections of small peripheral tumours (partial nephrectomy). Large tumours and those with tumour tissue invading the renal vein or inferior vena cava are generally not suitable for a laparoscopic approach, necessitating open surgery.

Smaller renal tumours can be managed with partial nephrectomy, or less commonly with other minimally invasive techniques including cryoablation and radiofrequency ablation.

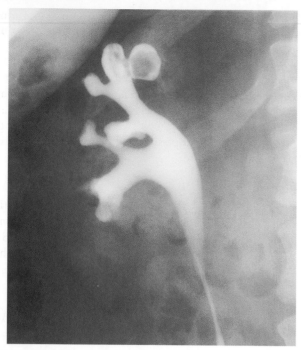

• **Fig. 28.19** An IVU Showing Multiple Transitional-Cell Carcinomas of the Right Renal Pelvis

Non-Operative Treatment

In symptomatic patients who are unsuitable for surgical treatment, embolization of the renal artery is effective in controlling pain and haematuria.

Radiotherapy to the primary tumour is ineffective but may help in reducing the pain of a bony metastasis. Endocrine therapy and chemotherapy are both ineffective. Treatments for patients with metastatic disease include sunitinib and sorafenib (tyrosine kinase inhibitors), bevacizumab (a mono-clonal antibody against vascular endothelial growth factor) and everolimus (mTOR inhibitor). Nivolumab (mono-clonal antibody blocking the interaction between Programmed Cell Death Protein (PD)-1 and its ligand PD-L1) has recently been used in metastatic disease and is showing improved effectiveness compared with previous treatment regimens.

Prognosis

Seventy percent of those with T1 clear-cell tumours survive for 5 years, and prolonged survival has been reported after removal of secondary deposits. However, there may be long intervals between the presentation of the primary and of metastases. Very rarely, secondary deposits may regress after removal of the primary. The use of newer biological therapies has significantly lengthened the survival of patients with metastatic disease.

3. Carcinoma of the Renal Pelvis

Carcinoma of the renal pelvis accounts for 10% of all renal tumours, and may be bilateral in up to 25% of cases.

Aetiology and Pathological Features

Ninety percent are derived from the transitional epithelium (urothelium) and are likely to be associated with similar tumours elsewhere in the urinary tract. However, urothelial tumours of the bladder are 60 times more common than those of the renal pelvis.

Ten percent of tumours in the renal pelvis are squamous carcinomas – a consequence of metaplastic change – and are almost invariably associated with stones. The aetiological factors for transitional cell cancer are similar to those for the same lesion in the bladder.

Clinical Features

These are loin pain and haematuria.

Investigation
Cytology

Malignant urothelial cells may be present in the urine.

Imaging

An IVU may show a filling defect in the calyces or renal pelvis (see Fig. 28.19), which must be distinguished from a non-opaque renal calculus by ultrasound. CT scanning with urographic phase is the best to provide details of the upper tracts and presence of filling defect. It also provides further information about the primary tumour and to exclude metastatic disease.

Management

Management is by removal of the kidney and ureter together with a cuff of bladder mucosa around the ureteric orifice. The reason for such radical surgery is the possibility of the occurrence of a further tumour. In the bladder, it is simple to diagnose a recurrence/occurrence of tumour by cystoscopy, but the ureteric stump cannot be so easily examined.

Renal-preserving approaches include endoscopic ablation with laser (via ureteroscopy) for smaller tumours, and endoscopic resection through a percutaneous nephrostomy tube has been attempted for larger tumours. Instillation of chemotherapeutic agents directly into the renal pelvis has been attempted.

Prognosis

In localized transitional-cell tumours of the renal pelvis the outlook is good, but squamous-cell carcinoma of the renal pelvis has a poor prognosis.

Stone Disease
Epidemiology

The incidence and site of occurrence of urinary stones vary in different parts of the world and in different parts of the

UK. Renal stones are more common in affluent communities whereas bladder stones remain common in developing countries. In the UK, the incidence of upper urinary tract stones varies from 15 per 100 000 in the north of England (Burnley) to 47 per 100 000 in the south-east (Canterbury). There are similar differences in the type of stone between countries: uric acid stones make up only 5% of the total in the UK, but this rises to 40% in Israel.

Aetiology

In the majority of instances aetiology is unknown.

Metabolic Disorders

Conditions that alter the composition of the urine, chiefly (but not exclusively) to increase its calcium content, are shown in Box 28.7.

Other Causes

The commonest of these is infection with the urea-splitting organism *Proteus*. The result is the production of ammonia, an alkaline urine and triple phosphate stones (staghorn calculi) (see Fig. 28.3), which are a mixture of calcium, magnesium and ammonium phosphate. Other factors are dehydration and immobilization.

Characteristics of Stones

These are given in Table 28.4.

Clinical Features

Symptoms

These depend on the size and position of the stone and the presence or absence of infection. The patient may be asymptomatic or give a history of occasional haematuria or dysuria. In cystine stones, there may be a family history, and, in all stones, there may have been previous episodes. A stone lodged at the neck of a calyx or at the pelviureteric junction causes renal colic, in which there are waves of increasing pain in the loin often superimposed on a background of continuous nagging pain at the same site. Radiation downwards into the groin or scrotum/labia or vagina *(Loin to Groin)* is indicative of a stone in the ureter.

Physical Findings

Tenderness may be found in the loin and, if found, may well indicate infection, superimposed on obstruction, when pyrexia is also likely. In the presence of a non-obstructing, or only partially obstructing, stone clinical examination is often normal.

Differential Diagnosis

Pain in stone disease is notorious for causing diagnostic confusion with other acute abdominal conditions, some of which require urgent surgical management (Box 28.8). The presence of haematuria on dipstick may help direct the diagnosis. Urgent imaging, preferably non-contrast CT, will

---

• BOX 28.7 Metabolic Causes of Urinary Tract Stones

Hypercalcaemia and hypercalciuria

- Hyperparathyroidism
- Idiopathic hypercalciuria
- Hypervitaminosis D
- Disseminated malignant disease
- Myeloma
- Prolonged immobilization
- Sarcoidosis
- Milk alkali syndrome
- Cushing's disease
- Hyperthyroidism

Increase in other substances

- Cystinuria (tubular transport defect for cystine, lysine, ornithine and arginine)
- Xanthinuria
- Primary hyperoxaluria
- Secondary hyperoxaluria (ileostomy)
- Hyperuricuria (gout; chemotherapy for leukaemia)
- Indinavir therapy

TABLE 28.4 Characteristics of Stones.

Stone	Incidence	Colour	Appearance	Radio-opacity
Calcium oxalate (mulberry stone)	80%	Pale yellow-brown	Sharp projections	Opaque
Triple phosphate[a] (magnesium ammonium phosphate – struvite stone often causing a staghorn calculus)	10%	Chalky white	Soft	Opaque
Uric acid	5%	Light brown	Facetted	Lucent
Cystine[b]	2%	Yellow-brown	Smooth	Moderately opaque
Xanthine	Rare	Yellow-brown		Lucent

[a]Often associated with infection with urea-splitting organisms, e.g. *Proteus*.
[b]Often a family history and/or episodes of repeated stone formation.

- Appendicitis
- Cholecystitis
- Diverticulitis
- Pyelonephritis
- Leaking aortic aneurysm

help establish the diagnosis and avoid delay in management and rule out other alternative conditions.

Investigation

Any patient who has formed a renal stone may have a 50% chance of producing another. It is important to identify metabolic or structural abnormalities because appropriate management may reduce the risk of recurrence.

Urine

- Culture and sensitivity, measurement of pH and screening for cystine.
- Two 24-hour collections with the patient on a normal diet for measurement of calcium, uric acid, oxalate and citrate concentrations.

Blood

Concentrations of the following are measured:

- urea
- creatinine
- electrolytes
- total protein
- calcium
- alkaline phosphatase
- urate
- phosphate

In a patient with a stone causing complete obstruction and with superimposed infection *(pyonephrosis)*, the bladder urine may be sterile. Urine will therefore be obtained, for culture, by the insertion of a percutaneous nephrostomy, which will also relieve the obstruction.

Imaging

A patient who presents with acute symptoms and signs and a suspected stone must have an urgent imaging. Non-contrast CT KUB is the investigation of choice.

The diagnosis can be firmly established, the size of the stone determined, together with the degree of obstruction, the likelihood of the stone passing spontaneously and the need for hospital admission.

Non-Operative Management

Asymptomatic Stone

Small (<5 mm), asymptomatic, non-obstructing renal pelvis stones can often be managed conservatively. The frequency of follow-up and threshold for intervention will depend on development of attributable symptoms (e.g. pain, UTIs) and patient age and co-morbidities.

Acute Episode

The pain of ureteric colic is severe and is treated with diclofenac and, if necessary, narcotic analgesics and antispasmodics such as Buscopan. Stones less than 0.5 cm in diameter will usually, but not always, pass spontaneously. Development of uncontrolled pain, vomiting and/or pyrexia will necessitate a change from conservative to active management. Whilst the majority of patients have no detectable underlying metabolic abnormality, some stone types are more commonly associated with a pre-disposing metabolic abnormality. The common stone compositions include calcium oxalate (>80%), triple phosphate (5–20%), uric acid (5–10%), mixed calcium phosphate + oxalate (10%), whilst pure calcium phosphate, cysteine and xanthine are rare (≤1%).

Oxalate Stones

The commonest abnormality detected is idiopathic hypercalciuria. Low oxalate diet and a high fluid intake to dilute urine calcium concentration is often recommended. Low calcium diet is usually unsuccessful as that increases oxalate absorption and hence a normal intake of calcium is recommended.

Attempts to reduce urine calcium excretion with bendrofluazide have only been shown to reduce calcium stone formation after prolonged periods of therapy.

Cystine Stones

Cystinuria is an inherited defect of amino acid transport involving cystine, ornithine, lysine and arginine. Cystine is relatively insoluble, particularly in acid urine, and this can lead to stone formation. Because its excretion is relatively constant, the stones can be both dissolved and prevented by maintaining a high fluid intake throughout the 24 hours and alkalinizing the urine. The latter can be achieved with either sodium bicarbonate or potassium citrate, or a combination of both. If this fails, treatment with penicillamine, which produces a more soluble cystine–penicillamine complex, is sometimes successful. However, it may be associated with the development of skin rashes and the nephrotic syndrome.

Uric Acid Stones

Uric acid is less soluble in acidic urine and, as a result, patients with chronic diarrhoea or an ileostomy are more likely to produce uric acid stones. They can be dissolved or prevented by increasing the fluid intake and alkalinization of the urine. In addition, allopurinol (100 mg three times a day) should be given to those with an elevated serum level.

Triple Phosphate Stones

These are composed of magnesium, ammonium and phosphate. They are formed as a result of urease-producing infections than can break urea to form ammonia. The prevention of recurrent phosphate stones associated with infection is dependent on three factors:

- complete removal of the initial stone(s)
- correction of any anatomical abnormalities of urine drainage
- maintenance of sterile urine

The latter can be achieved with long-term low-dose antibiotic therapy. If this proves difficult, treatment with a urease inhibitor (acetohydroxamic acid) should be considered.

Surgical Management

Indications for Intervention

Urgent ureteric stent insertion or percutaneous nephrostomy drainage is required when:

- fever does not resolve after 24 hours of appropriate antibiotic therapy in a patient with an obstructed kidney
- severe pain persists in spite of the medical management outlined previously
- obstruction of a solitary kidney is present

The nephrostomy track can be used at a later stage for endoscopic stone destruction or removal. An indwelling stent can be inserted antegradely to establish drainage down the ureter before treatment by lithotripsy (see later).

Intervention in Persistent Stone

Major advances have been made in the management of stones over the past 25 years by techniques other than open surgery. The indication for open stone surgery is extremely rare in contemporary urology.

Fragmentation of the stone in situ can be achieved with:

- extracorporeal transcutaneous techniques (extracorporeal shock wave lithotripsy, ESWL)
- direct application of shock waves or laser to the stone by a probe inserted through a semi-rigid or flexible ureteroscope retrogradely (endoscopically) or percutaneously via a dilated nephrostomy tract (percutaneous nephrolithotomy, PCNL)

Removal (without fragmentation) can be achieved either endoscopically or percutaneously, in selected cases.

DISORDERS OF THE URETER

Congenital Anatomical Abnormalities

Ureteric Duplication

Incomplete duplication is much more common than complete ureteric duplication and occurs in approximately 1% of individuals. Complete duplication is present in about 1 in every 500–600 individuals. The extent of incomplete ureteral duplication may vary from a bifid renal pelvis (which could be considered as a normal variant) to two separate ureters joining with each other at some point during their course. A complete duplication results in two separate ureters with two separate ureteric openings in the bladder. The orifice of the upper-segment ureter always enters the bladder more medial and caudal to the lower-segment orifice *(Weigert-Meyer rule)*. The ureter from the lower part of the kidney is more likely to be associated with vesicoureteric reflux, as the orifice of this ureter is more lateral and cephalic. As the orifice of the ureter from the upper pole is more caudal, it can be located in an ectopic position which may open at the level of the bladder neck, urethra, vestibule or vagina and may result in either obstruction or incontinence.

Clinical Features

Duplication of the ureters is commonly asymptomatic. Vesicoureteral reflux into the lower moiety can result in infection, haematuria or flank pain.

Management

Asymptomatic duplications do not require any treatment. If one of the moieties of the kidney is non-functioning and causing symptoms, a hemi-nephroureterectomy is the procedure of choice. In cases of complete duplication, with preservation of renal function, vesicoureteral reflux is managed with either re-implantation or injection of inert material into the submucosa to prevent reflux. An ectopic ureter can either be re-implanted or a hemi-nephroureterectomy can be performed, depending on the function of that portion of the kidney.

Congenital Obstruction at the Pelviureteric Junction

The pelviureteric junction (PUJ) is the most common site of obstruction in the upper urinary tract.

Aetiology

In the congenital type, intrinsic abnormalities of the PUJ are the most common cause of obstruction. They result from an aperistaltic segment at the level of the PUJ, resulting in a functional obstruction to the passage of urine. In some cases, valve-like processes and polyps have been found.

Extrinsic abnormalities are seen in about one-third of patients with PUJ obstruction. Aberrant (lower pole) renal vessels may cause obstruction, especially when they cross in front of the PUJ or when the ureter appears to be trapped between two such vessels. PUJ obstruction occurs in approximately 1:1 500 births. It is more common in males and is bilateral in 5% of cases. Obstruction is acquired as a result of stricture formation following surgery for stones, trauma or tuberculosis.

Clinical Features

Symptoms

The typical clinical presentation has changed since the advent of widespread antenatal sonographic screening. A significant number of babies with antenatal hydronephrosis are subsequently found to have a PUJ obstruction.

Symptoms in infants and children are:

- abdominal mass
- urinary tract infection
- haematuria
- failure to thrive

Symptoms in adults are:

- intermittent loin pain, sometimes associated with alcohol and caffeine consumption
- urinary infection
- haematuria following mild trauma
- symptoms of stones

Signs

In infants and children, the sole sign is abdominal mass.
In adults, signs are:

- loin tenderness
- rarely, abdominal mass

It can be an incidental finding during the course of investigation for another condition

Investigation

To diagnose PUJ obstruction, both anatomical and functional studies of the kidney are required.

Ultrasound

Anatomical information of the kidney can be obtained by ultrasound examination. Ultrasound examination reveals dilatation of the pelvicalyceal system and also demonstrates the state of the renal cortex.

Nuclear Isotope Scan

MAG3 scan will assess the relative function of the kidney, confirm obstruction and monitor progress of the patient on surveillance as well as after definitive treatment.

Management

Options for management include:

- surveillance
- surgical reconstruction, pyeloplasty (robotic, laparoscopic, open)
- endoscopic incision (endopyelotomy)
- retrograde balloon dilatation
- percutaneous balloon dilatation

Most PUJ obstructions are now discovered antenatally and hence are asymptomatic. Management is decided on the basis of anatomical and functional information provided by different scans. After birth, the kidneys are observed by repeated scanning with ultrasound and/or isotope renography.

Indications for surgery

These are:

- deterioration of renal function
- worsening of renal dilatation
- thinning of renal cortex
- the presence of symptoms, pain, haematuria or infection

For primary PUJ obstruction, if operative intervention is required, surgical reconstruction is the method of choice. The most common surgical technique is the *Anderson–Hynes pyeloplasty* which disconnects the pelvis from the ureter,

reduces the size of the pelvis but requires re-anastomosis of the ureter to the pelvis. A *Culp pyeloplasty* is useful for those with a small extrarenal pelvis. Re-anastomosis of the ureter is not required (Fig. 28.20). Laparoscopic and robotic surgery are routinely used.

Disorders That May be Either Congenital or Acquired

Megaureter

Aetiology

The underlying cause of the congenital variety is the same as that of PUJ obstruction, but the muscular imbalance in megaureter is at the ureterovesical junction. The ureter proximal to this becomes dilated and hypertrophied. The condition may be bilateral, and a secondary hydronephrosis may develop with the formation of stones.

Secondary megaureter may be caused by schistosomiasis or bladder outflow obstruction.

Pathophysiology

Classification on the basis of reflux and the presence of obstruction to flow is shown in Box 28.9 and is used to guide management. Very rarely, reflux and obstruction may coexist. A combination of ultrasound scanning, micturating cystograms and renography permits appropriate categorization.

Clinical Features

Symptoms of megaureter are:

- incidental finding during investigation for another condition
- loin pain
- urinary infection

Management

Non-obstructed, non-refluxing megaureters do not require treatment.

Congenitally obstructed megaureters should be re-implanted after the narrowing at the distal end has been removed. Those with reflux are treated along the lines of management of vesicoureteric reflux. A secondarily obstructed megaureter requires treatment of its cause.

Vesicoureteric Reflux

Aetiology and Pathological Features

Primary reflux is the result of a defective valvular mechanism at the ureterovesical junction; when compared with a normal ureter, the intramural course is short and more horizontally directed. The condition is bilateral in 50%, and 90% of affected patients are female. There is a familial incidence. As the ureterovesical junction matures, reflux may cease spontaneously.

Secondary reflux may occur because of bladder outlet or urethral obstruction or in neurogenic bladders.

Inflammatory conditions of the bladder wall (schistosomiasis, tuberculosis) can hold the ureteric orifice open.

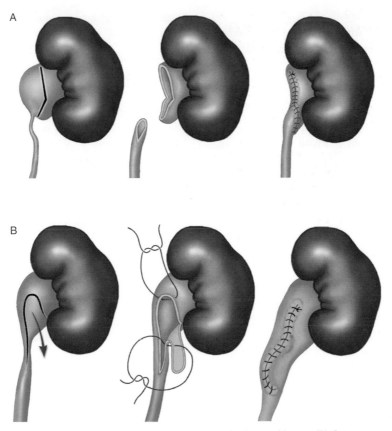

• **Fig. 28.20** Pyeloplasty operations: (A) Anderson–Hynes; (B) Culp

Congenital
- Non-refluxing or refluxing
- Non-obstructed or obstructed

Secondary
- Non-refluxing or refluxing
- Non-obstructed or obstructed

Clinical Features

In primary reflux, the onset is in the first decade. Symptoms may include fever, lethargy, anorexia, nausea and vomiting. There is often mild haematuria, but the main symptoms are those of recurrent urinary infections. Older children may complain of pain in the loin or on micturition. In secondary disease, the onset is later, and again symptoms of infection predominate.

There are no specific signs.

Investigation

Ultrasound is often normal but may show ureteric dilatation or renal scarring.

Micturating cystogram. Cystoureteric reflux is best demonstrated at the time of micturition (see Fig. 28.8).

Isotope scanning. A DMSA scan can be used to identify current renal damage.

Management

The majority of patients can be satisfactorily managed by antibiotic therapy. Long-term therapy to suppress infection is necessary up to the age of 5 years. The incidence of renal scarring after this age is very low. Surgical re-implantation of the ureter is indicated when medical management fails to suppress the development of new urinary infections or there is non-compliance with antibiotic treatment. The injection of inert, non-absorbable substances around the ureteric orifice to prevent reflux offers a non-surgical option to treat this condition.

Ureterocele

Ureterocele is a cystic dilatation of the terminal portion of the ureter and may occur in either a normally placed ureter or rarely in an ectopic one. They occur in approximately 1:1000 births. This usually involves the upper-segment ureter of a duplex system. They may become very large and occupy most of the available space in the bladder.

Clinical Features

Some patients are asymptomatic. When symptoms do occur, they are usually secondary to complications, such as:
- obstruction of the bladder outlet
- infection
- loin pain

Signs are minimal. An ectopic ureterocele in a female may present as a vaginal tumour at birth or in childhood. Occasionally, they may present at the urethral meatus.

Diagnosis

The diagnosis is made on an ultrasound which shows a rounded swelling in the bladder associated with a dilatation of the ureter – hydroureter.

Management

Asymptomatic ureteroceles do not need treatment. If the ureter is dilated or there is a stone, the ureterocele can be transected endoscopically. The cut is made on the inferior surface because this makes reflux less likely. Ectopic uretero-celes require a hemi-nephroureterectomy.

Acquired Conditions

Ureteric Injuries

Aetiology

Open injuries occur from gunshot or stabbing. A closed avulsion of the ureter from the renal pelvis may follow rapid deceleration. However, surgical injuries during abdominal or pelvic operations are the commonest cause. The ureter is at particular risk if it is displaced from its usual anatomi-cal position by the condition under treatment. Operations most frequently associated with ureteric injuries are listed in Box 28.10.

Pathological Features

One or both ureters may be ligated. The kidney stops secret-ing once the intraureteric pressure has risen to the filtra-tion pressure. In consequence, dilatation of the renal pelvis is mild and, if the condition goes untreated, atrophy of the kidney takes place. Less commonly, the lumen is incom-pletely obstructed by inclusion in a stitch, in which case the kidney continues to secrete and hydronephrosis develops, often with accompanying infection. Alternatively, the ure-ter is divided or suffers a crushing injury. The latter may be ischaemic. Urine then leaks to the exterior or into the retroperitoneal tissues and, less commonly, the peritoneal cavity.

Clinical Features

The injury may be recognized at the time of surgery. If not, bilateral ligation will be recognized very soon. Leak usu-ally presents around the fifth postoperative day but may be delayed for 10–14 days if it results from ureteric ischaemia. The features are:

- Bilateral ligation – immediate postoperative anuria
- Unilateral ligation – either absence of clinical features or, if there is proximal infection, fever and persistent loin pain
- Division – urine appears from the drain, the wound or the vagina
- Retroperitoneal leakage of sterile urine leads to abdominal distension secondary to ileus and intraperi-toneal leakage to signs of free fluid in the peritoneal cavity
- Retro- or intraperitoneal leakage of infected urine is associated with the features of peritonitis and generalized sepsis

Investigation

In the early stages of complete obstruction, CT urogram shows a nephrographic effect – contrast medium outlines the whole kidney, but little change in radiodensity is seen in the renal pelvis or ureter. In incomplete obstruction or transection, there is some delay in excretion, and ure-teric dilatation on the side of the injury down to the site of damage is usually seen with contrast extravasation. If, however, this is not identified, retrograde ureterography may help.

Management

Prevention

A CT scan should be done before any operation in which the ureters are at risk, particularly if there is the possibility of ureteric displacement.

Treatment

If recognized late, a nephrostomy is indicated to drain the kidney and divert the urine away from the injury. The inser-tion of a ureteric stent may be possible. A surgical repair can be planned at a later stage.

If the injury is recognized at the time of surgery, ligatures should be removed, the crushed area resected, the cut ends should be spatulated and a primary tension-free anasto-mosis performed over a ureteric stent (Fig. 28.21B). Other techniques include:

- Re-implantation of the damaged ureter into the bladder (Fig. 28.21D)
- Use of the bladder flap (Boari) to replace the damaged segment (Fig. 28.21C)
- Anastomosis of one ureter to the other (Fig. 28.21A)
- Replacement of the ureter by small intestine

• BOX 28.10 Operations Most Frequently Associated with Ureteric Injuries

Gynaecological
- Hysterectomy
- Ovarian cystectomy
- Repair of vesicovaginal fistula
- Anterior colporrhaphy

General surgery
- Sigmoid colectomy
- Abdominoperineal resection of the rectum
- Repair of aortic aneurysm

Urology
- Excision of bladder diverticula
- Ureterolithotomy
- Ureteroscopy

Retroperitoneal Fibrosis

Aetiology

There are two forms: idiopathic and secondary. In the first, as its name implies, the cause is not known. Secondary retroperitoneal fibrosis may follow:
- Treatment with methysergide
- Extravasation of urine
- Retroperitoneal sepsis
- Aortic or iliac aneurysms
- Radiotherapy
- Most commonly, retroperitoneal spread of malignant disease – cervix, ovary, testis, prostate and lymphomas

Pathological Features

In the primary idiopathic form, one or both ureters become encased in and obstructed by a retroperitoneal plaque of fibrous tissue between the pelviureteric junction and the pelvic brim, although involvement may be more extensive.

Clinical Features

Symptoms are non-specific but include backache, low-grade fever and malaise, as well as those of hypertension, renal failure or anuria. The physical findings are also non-specific and related to the renal failure or hypertension.

Investigation

ESR is invariably raised.
Ultrasound may show upper urinary tract dilatation.
CT scanning shows upper urinary tract dilatation, with medial deviation of one or both ureters, and is useful to define the extent of the retroperitoneal mass.
Bilateral retrograde ureterography often results in complete anuria from ureteric oedema and should be avoided.

Management

Treatment is either with long-term stenting or surgical ureterolysis. A definitive diagnosis of possible underlying causes can only be made by histological examination of tissue from the retroperitoneum. This can be achieved by percutaneous biopsy or by open biopsy, ureterolysis can be done at the same time. To prevent recurrence of obstruction, both ureters are either wrapped in omentum or brought laterally and intraperitoneally to distance them from the fibrotic mass. Idiopathic retroperitoneal fibrosis does respond to treatment with steroids, but long-term therapy is required.

Ureteric Stone

Aetiology and Site of Lodgement

These stones originate in the kidney and migrate downwards. Arrest is likely at the three sites of relative narrowing: the pelviureteric junction, the pelvic brim where the ureter crosses the iliac vessels and the transmural (bladder) ureter.

Clinical Features

Ureteric stones almost always cause ureteric colic, and they account for one of the most frequent urological presentations in the Accident and Emergency Department.

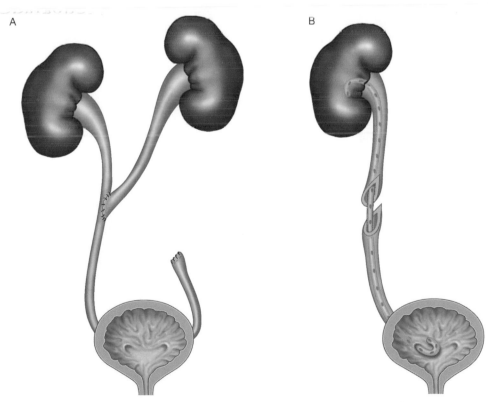

• **Fig. 28.21** Techniques Which May Be Used for Repair of an Injured Ureter

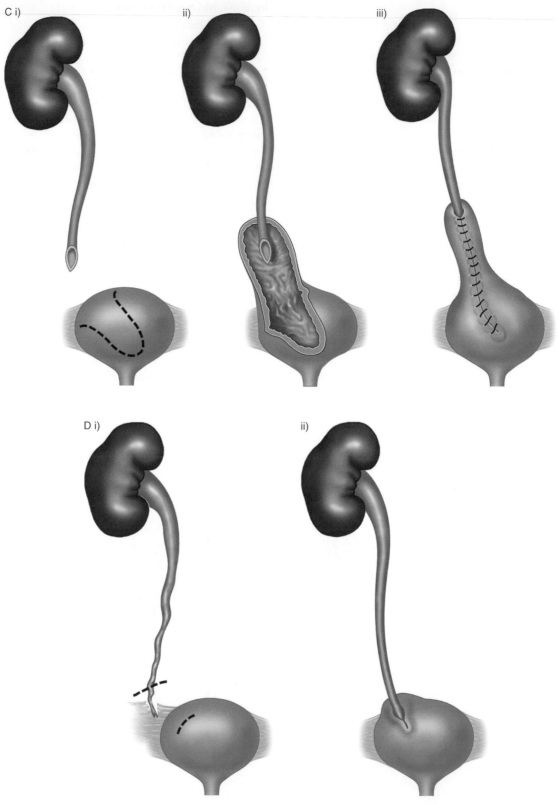

C i) ii) iii)

D i) ii)

• **Fig. 28.21** Cont'd

Symptoms

The patient is in severe pain, which is intermittent and radiates from the loin to the groin and sometimes into the testicle, scrotum or labia. Vomiting frequently occurs and the patient is unable to find any comfortable position or to lie still. The urine may be bloodstained.

Signs

Fever suggests the presence of a pyonephrosis. The abdomen is tender with slight guarding. An impacted stone may be complicated by paralytic ileus, which produces a silent distended abdomen.

Investigation

Urine

Examination of the urine is carried out for red blood cells and bacterial culture.

Imaging

A plain abdominal X-ray may show a calcified opacity lying in the course of the ureter. A non-contrast CT KUB scan should always be done urgently to confirm the diagnosis and to assess the degree of obstruction and the likelihood of the stone passing spontaneously; 90% of stones less than 0.5 cm in diameter will do so (Fig. 28.22).

Management

The primary management is relief of pain, although the majority require only non-steroidal anti-inflammatory agents. Some may require stronger opiate analgesia.

Indications for Intervention

These are:
- evidence of infection
- recurrent or persistent pain
- failure of the stone to progress downwards
- deterioration of renal function
- obstruction in a solitary kidney

Methods of Intervention

In an emergency, intervention is by either percutaneous nephrostomy or the passage of a ureteric stent, retrogradely, to bypass the obstruction (Fig. 28.23).

Definitive treatment is by:
- Extraction – snaring small stones in the lower 5 cm of ureter in a basket passed retrogradely up the ureter
- Extracorporeal fragmentation by shock wave lithotripsy (ESWL)
- In situ fragmentation with lithotripsy or laser via a ureteroscope

Urinary Diversion

Decompression or drainage of the urinary tract is frequently employed in urological practice. It is now usually done under radiological control or endoscopically, rather than at open operation.

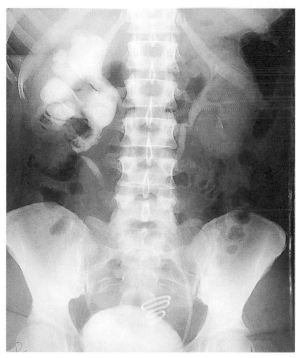

• **Fig. 28.22** An IVU Showing Clubbed Calyces Secondary to Ureteric Obstruction

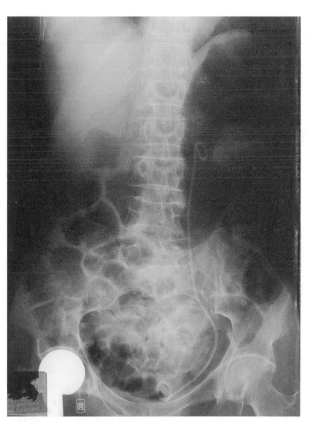

• **Fig. 28.23** Double Pigtail Catheter Providing Drainage of the Renal Pelvis and Stenting of the Left Ureter

Nephrostomy

In nephrostomy, a drainage tube is passed through the kidney into its pelvis. It is employed to decompress and drain a kidney that is obstructed. Decompression may also be needed after operations such as reconstruction of the pelvi-ureteric junction or percutaneous nephrolithotomy (PCNL) An external drainage bag can be avoided if it is possible to intubate an obstruction or suture line by placing a ureteric stent across it so that one end lies in the renal pelvis and the other in the bladder (see Fig. 28.23). The technique is frequently used before lithotripsy, to prevent fragments of stone causing ureteric obstruction.

Other Forms of Urinary Diversion

Surgical diversion of urine to the exterior is required if the bladder is removed or is so congenitally deformed *(exstrophy)* or diseased meaning that adequate function is impossible. Diversion is most frequently achieved by using an isolated segment of ileum into which the ureters are implanted. The segment acts as a conduit *(ileal conduit/urostomy)* to bring the urine to the abdominal wall (Fig. 28.24). Intestine can also be used to make a new bladder with an anastomosis to the urethra/bladder neck *(neo-bladder)* or to a continent external opening on the abdominal wall, which the patient catheterizes intermittently *(Mitrofanoff)*. Rarely, the ureters may be implanted into the intact sigmoid colon. However,

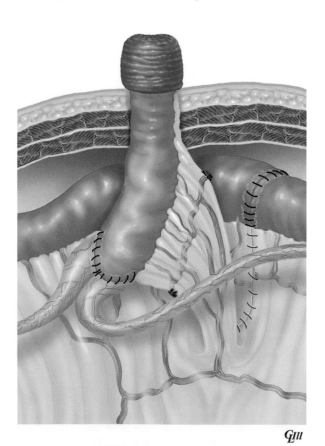

• **Fig. 28.24** An Ileal Conduit

that technique often leads to ascending urinary infection and chronic pyelonephritis. This procedure has now been superseded by the creation of a pouch in the sigmoid colon *(Mainz II)*. This has lower incidence of complications.

THE LOWER URINARY TRACT

Symptoms in the Lower Genitourinary Tract
Bladder Pain

This may be sharp or dull and is located in the midline of the lower abdomen. Rapid overdistension of a previously normal bladder causes severe pain, but if the distension is gradual over weeks or months, pain is absent.

Prostatic Pain

This is a dull ache that may be felt in the lower abdomen, the rectum, perineum and anterior thighs.

Urethral Pain

This is usually felt at the tip of the penis and ranges from a mere tickling discomfort to severe and sharp pain exacerbated by passing urine.

Scrotal Pain

Pain may be referred to the scrotum as in renal colic. Similarly, pain arising from the scrotal contents may be referred to the groin or abdomen. Most scrotal pain is the result of stretching of the tunica albuginea; if this happens acutely, pain is severe, but slow distension, as in a tumour, causes a dragging sensation or a dull ache, or no symptoms at all.

Disorders of Micturition

Increased frequency may occur during the day and the night *(nocturia)* and may be a response to an excess fluid intake or failure of the kidneys to concentrate the urine, as occurs in diabetes insipidus, hypercalcaemia, chronic kidney disease and diseases which produce a high solute load such as diabetes mellitus.

Urological causes of increased frequency are:
* urinary infection
* incomplete bladder emptying
* detrusor overactivity
* small capacity bladder
* bladder cancer.
* previous treatment with radiotherapy

Dysuria. The term describes a burning sensation during the passage of urine. It may occur throughout micturition or just at its end (terminal dysuria). Infection with inflammation of the urethra is the commonest cause.

Urgency. This is a repeated desire to pass urine but with little to show for it other than pain related to the urethra or the penile tip. Infection is likely.

Intermittency. The urine stream is interrupted during micturition. The symptom is associated with bladder stones, ureteroceles and benign prostatic obstruction.

- True – a fistula between the urinary tract and the exterior
- Giggle – in young girls, provoked by bouts of unrestrained mirth
- Stress – leakage during a transient increase in abdominal pressure such as caused by coughing or laughing
- Urge – a desire to pass urine of such severity that the patient is unable to reach the toilet: it may be associated with urinary infection, bladder stones, detrusor instability or bladder cancer
- Dribbling or overflow – there is a continual loss of urine from a chronically distended bladder

Hesitancy. This is the need to wait before the urine stream begins. Prostatic obstruction to urine flow and stricture are causes.

Incomplete Emptying. This is, as the phrase implies, a feeling that the bladder has not emptied at the end of micturition. Prostatic disease and detrusor dysfunction are possible causes.

Terminal Dribbling. This is a progressive reduction in the rate of urine flow at the end of the urine stream and is associated with prostatic obstruction.

Post-Micturition Dribbling. This is leakage after the patient believes that micturition is complete and is associated with detrusor overactivity, prostatic obstruction, urethral diverticula or the failure to empty the urethra manually after micturition.

Incontinence. Can be of five types (Box 28.11).

Abnormal Urine Stream. The stream may be:
- Slow – prostatic obstruction or detrusor insufficiency
- Split – often associated with a urethral stricture

Examination

A significantly distended bladder is visible and palpable in most patients when examined in the supine position. Dullness to percussion in the midline of the abdomen above the pubic symphysis nearly always means bladder distension in a male.

The external genitalia are often not examined, because of embarrassment. The foreskin, glans penis and urethral meatus must be examined for meatal stenosis, phimosis, anatomical abnormalities such as hypospadias, penile tumours and warts. The scrotal contents are examined with the patient both supine and standing to aid identification of a varicocele.

Rectal Examination

In the UK, it is traditional to examine the male in the left lateral position. The purpose is to identify abnormalities within the anal canal and rectum and to determine the size, contour and consistency of the prostate. A similar position is used in the female but is usually preceded by a vaginal examination with the patient supine and the knees flexed. In the latter, oestrogenization of the perineum, urethral prolapse, urethral

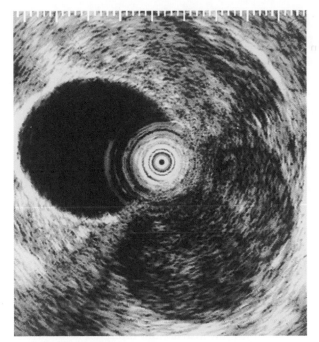

• **Fig. 28.25** Transrectal Ultrasound Scan Showing Benign Enlargement of the Prostate

diverticula and gynaecological abnormalities of the vagina, cervix, uterus and its adnexa can be detected.

Investigation
General

Bacteriological and biochemical investigation for the upper urinary tract are also relevant to the lower tract.

Imaging
Urethrography

Water-soluble contrast medium is introduced into the urethra via a catheter to outline urethral strictures, urethral diverticula and urethral injuries.

Ultrasonography

Transabdominal, transvaginal and transrectal routes are available (Fig. 28.25). The techniques provide precise information on:
- residual urine
- bladder tumours
- prostatic size
- nature of prostatic enlargement – benign or possibly malignant

Transrectal ultrasound (TRUS) guidance also improves the accuracy with which a prostatic biopsy is obtained during the investigation for prostatic malignancy.

CT and MRI are the most accurate way of assessing the presence of lesions, depth of invasion (staging) of bladder cancer and staging of prostate cancer.

Bladder Function
Urinary Flow Rate

The patient voids into a device which records the rate of accumulation of the expelled urine (flow meter). The total

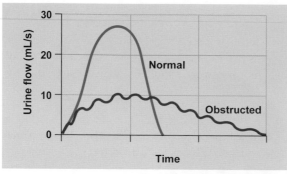

• **Fig. 28.26** Measurement of Urinary Flow Rate Using a Flow Meter

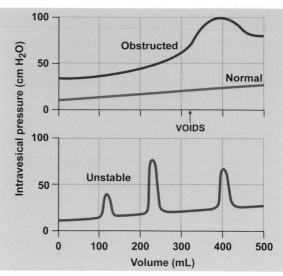

• **Fig. 28.27** Urodynamic Pressure Studies Showing Obstructed and Unstable Reponses

voided, which should ideally be greater than 150 mL, and the peak and mean flows, as well as voiding time are recorded (Fig. 28.26). The peak flow is inversely related to the likelihood of being obstructed, for example a peak flow less than 12 mL/s indicate a 90% probability of having bladder outflow obstruction, though it is important to note that urinary flow study cannot differentiate between obstruction and poor bladder contractility due to detrusor failure.

Urodynamics

This investigation is more invasive. Urethral catheterization with a filling catheter and a pressure transducer is required. A further pressure transducer is placed in the rectum to measure intra-abdominal pressure. Subtraction of pressures recorded by the two catheters is done automatically and gives a true detrusor pressure, which is measured both during bladder filling and on micturition (Fig. 28.27). After micturition, residual volume is measured by emptying the bladder through the filling catheter.

Endoscopy

A flexible cystoscope passed under local anaesthetic, or a small rigid cystoscope using sedation or general anaesthesia, is used. The whole of the urethra and bladder can be examined and ureteric catheters inserted.

DISORDERS AND DISEASE OF THE BLADDER

Congenital Abnormalities

Exstrophy of the Bladder (Ectopia Vesicae)
Epidemiology and Aetiology

The incidence is approximately 1:50 000 live births, with male and females being equally affected. The cause is unknown. The bladder does not infold, so that its mucosa is exposed as a flat plate on the surface of the abdomen.

Pathological Findings

There is failure of development of the anterior wall of the urogenital sinus and of the lower abdominal wall. The abnormality is associated with:
- wide separation of the symphysis pubis
- epispadias – failure of dorsal closure of the urethra
- inguinal hernia
- imperforate anus

A secondary problem is the development of adenocarcinoma of the bladder, if the exposed bladder mucosa remains exposed and is not removed or reconstructed.

Management

The bladder and penis are reconstructed in stages after a pelvic osteotomy to allow approximation of the symphysis pubis. The insertion of an artificial sphincter is usually necessary to maintain continence. Urinary diversion and excision of the deformed bladder may be required. Continence can be achieved in 80% of cases.

Urachal Extrophy

The incidence is much less than bladder extrophy. Failure of the urachus to close results in a urachal fistula with leakage of urine from the umbilicus at birth.

Persistence of the mid-part of the urachus produces an urachal cyst palpable in the midline below the umbilicus, which may undergo malignant change.

Infections of the Lower Urinary Tract

Acute Cystitis

It is most commonly caused by Gram-negative bacteria. Other pathogens and other conditions that cause an allergic or chemical cystitis, as well as radiation induced cystitis, can give similar symptoms. Bacterial infection is more common in women than men due to the shorter urethra. The presence of 10^3 CFU/mL in mid-stream voided urine from a woman with typical symptoms of cystitis is diagnostic. In men 10^4 CFU/mL is required for diagnosis.

Clinical Features

Frequency, dysuria, lower abdominal pain, urgency, haematuria and pyrexia all occur to a varying degree.

Mild suprapubic tenderness may be present, and the urethral meatus may be inflamed. Apart from these, specific signs are absent unless there is evidence of underlying disease.

Investigation

Urine

It is essential to send a urine specimen for culture and sensitivity before antibiotic therapy is begun. In females, a high vaginal swab should be sent for analysis to exclude *Candida, Trichomonas* and other vaginal pathogens, because such infections may precipitate an attack of cystitis.

Imaging

Patients who present with visible haematuria must have both upper tract imaging and a cystoscopy, which are also indicated when the MSU shows no bacterial growth. Carcinoma in situ of the bladder may present with cystitis-like symptoms.

Management

An episode requires a high fluid intake and antibiotic administration (e.g. amoxicillin), which may need to be modified once the results of urine culture and bacterial sensitivities are available. A further MSU is required if symptoms do not resolved. Further investigations may be required if the infection does not resolve or recurs frequently

Chronic Cystitis

The cause is usually inadequate treatment and investigation of an acute attack. Postmenopausal women are prone to recurrent episodes of cystitis and may benefit from topical or systemic oestrogen replacement therapy. Ten percent of patients who receive pelvic irradiation suffer from haemorrhagic cystitis without bacterial infection. Most cases subside spontaneously during the 12–18 months after completion of therapy, although it may lead to bladder fibrosis and a small contracted bladder.

Interstitial Cystitis

This occurs most frequently in women who have storage voiding symptoms and negative urine cultures. Many develop severe bladder pain, frequency, urgency and incontinence.

Tuberculosis of the Bladder

In those who present with intractable symptoms that resemble cystitis and have a sterile pyuria, repeated examinations of early morning urine should be carried out to identify the tubercle bacillus.

Management

Antimicrobial therapy as described earlier. The treatment of contracted bladder is considered later.

Schistosomiasis (Bilharzia)

Epidemiology and Aetiology

The blood fluke *Schistosoma haematobium* is endemic in the Middle East and the Nile valley and other rivers and lakes of eastern and southern Africa. Human infestation is acquired by contact with infected water. Adult worms produce ova in the pelvic and vesical veins. The ova migrate through the bladder wall into the urine, which is passed into the irrigation ditches, where miracidia penetrate the water snail. These develop into cercaria which again can pass through human skin to repeat the cycle (Fig. 28.28).

Pathological Features

The eggs in the bladder wall cause an inflammatory reaction, which goes on to fibrosis, calcification and secondary infection. Stone formation and squamous carcinoma are secondary consequences. The ureters may be involved directly or may become secondarily dilated because of the small, thick-walled and fibrotic bladder.

Clinical Features

Symptoms

In acute presentations, pyrexia, itching, dysuria, frequency and haematuria are seen (Katayama fever). In those who are in a chronic state, frequency, haematuria and episodes of infection resistant to treatment are usual.

Investigation

Urine Examination and Bladder Biopsy

Eggs can be identified in either the urine or on bladder biopsy.

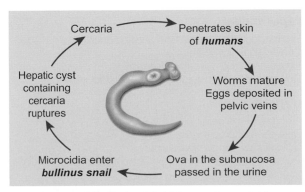

• **Fig. 28.28** Life Cycle of *Schistosoma haematobium*

Imaging

Ultrasound may show dilated ureters, stone formation or a small contracted bladder.

Cystoscopy. There is a small bladder, and there may be small sandy patches around the ureteric orifices because of calcified granulomas. Areas of squamous malignancy may be obvious.

Management

Medical treatment is with the drug praziquantel. Surgery may be required to reconstruct the ureters and a small contracted bladder.

Bladder Trauma

Because of its anatomy, the bladder may rupture into either the peritoneal cavity or the extraperitoneal space. The differences in cause between the two forms of rupture are summarized in Box 28.12.

Intraperitoneal Rupture

Clinical Features

Symptoms

Usually, there is a history of injury. Patients with a very full bladder have often consumed large quantities of alcohol, and a clear history may be difficult to obtain. There is usually also severe lower abdominal pain – modified by the patient's clinical state – and anuria.

Signs

These are as follows:
- If the urine is sterile, increasing abdominal distension, discomfort and peritonism
- If the urine is infected, features of peritonitis
- Attempted micturition results in the passage of a few millilitres of bloodstained urine
- Urethral catheterization is easy, but urine is not forthcoming, although there may be a little blood

Management

The abdomen is explored, the bladder injury repaired and the bladder drained with a catheter. An abdominal drain is left in for a few days.

BOX 28.12 Causes of Bladder Rupture

Intraperitoneal
- Blunt abdominal trauma with a full bladder
- Penetrating injury (rare)
- Gross overdistension at endoscopy
- During endoscopic surgery on the bladder vault

Extraperitoneal
- Fracture of the pelvis
- Resection of prostate
- Difficult lower abdominal surgery
- During repair of a direct hernia with bladder in the medial aspect of the sac

---

Extraperitoneal Rupture

Trauma is the main cause – a fracture of the pelvis, or during transurethral resection of the prostate or bladder tumours.

Clinical Features

There is a history of injury, either accidental or surgical. Symptoms are:
- Lower abdominal pain, although this may be masked by the effects of pelvic fracture
- Inability to micturate or, at most, a few drops of blood-stained urine

Urine and blood extravasated into the perivesical space cause the following:
- Tender suprapubic thickening
- Palpable mass (occasionally)

Management

Extravasation of urine after transurethral resection of the prostate or of a bladder tumour usually responds to a period of urethral catheterization. For severe injuries, which are a consequence of pelvic fracture, suprapubic drainage of the bladder and drainage of the retropubic space may be required.

Bladder Tumours

The bladder, like the rest of the urinary tract, is lined with transitional-cell epithelium. Because it acts as a store for urine, and any carcinogens that may be present, it is the commonest site for the development of malignant urinary tract tumours. Benign tumours of the urothelium are exceedingly rare, as are benign tumours of the bladder muscle (detrusor). Malignant rhabdomyosarcomas of the detrusor muscle occur in childhood. However, the great majority of bladder tumours arise from the urothelium. Ninety-five percent of these are transitional-cell carcinomas (TCC). Carcinoma in situ (CIS) refers to flat areas of epithelium composed of cells with anaplastic features and disorderly pattern of growth without extension into the bladder lumen compared to papillary TCC that can extend into the lumen of the bladder. Squamous-cell tumours occur more commonly with schistosomiasis, and in patients who have long-term catheters, and adenocarcinomas are associated with untreated bladder exstrophy or a urachal remnant.

Epidemiology

Urothelial cancer has a male predominance, although the incidence in females is increasing, which is likely to be related to the increased incidence of cigarette smoking in this group. The highest incidence of bladder cancer is in the sixth and seventh decades.

Aetiology

Chronic irritation and carcinogenic chemicals are associated with the development of the disease.

Chronic irritation may be caused by:

- schistosomiasis
- exstrophy with persistent infection and physical trauma
- stones
- recurrent or chronic infections
  Carcinogens include:
- tobacco smoke – nearly 40% of bladder cancers can be directly attributed to smoking
- products of the chemical industry – aniline dyes, printing, rubber processing, pesticides

Because of the known association with the above industries, there are now regular surveillance programmes, which use cytological examination of the urine. If a worker in an industry that is known to have a high-risk develops bladder cancer, both the victim and dependents may be entitled to compensation.

Clinical Features

Symptoms

The great majority of patients present with painless haematuria. A small proportion have urinary infections. A few tumours are found coincidentally in patients who undergo a cystoscopy for other reasons or a lesion identified incidentally on imaging. Advanced cases have lower abdominal pain, severe dysuria, strangury and incontinence of bloodstained urine. Similar irritative findings are found in patients with carcinoma in situ. As noted above, these symptoms must be distinguished from bacterial cystitis.

Signs

Unless the disease is advanced, abnormalities are usually absent. A careful bimanual examination may reveal a mass in the bladder wall, but if the diagnosis is established by other means (usually endoscopically), then bimanual examination is better done under anaesthesia to help stage the lesion.

Investigation

Urothelial tumours are often multifocal. Any patient who presents with symptoms suggestive of a urothelial tumour requires full investigation of the urinary tract, which includes:

- Urine microscopy and culture for evidence of haematuria and infection
- Cytological examination of the urine – most likely to be positive in those with carcinoma in situ or high-grade TCC tumours
- Assessment of renal function
- Imaging: IVU used to be used to search for other tumours in the renal pelvis, ureter or bladder (Fig. 28.29), although small tumours were difficult to detect. CT urogram scanning is more accurate and gives additional information about the primary tumour stage and shows other synchronous lesions or metastatic disease and is now used instead of IVU
- Endoscopic examination of the urethra and bladder: endoscopy identifies the number, position and macroscopic type of urethral or bladder tumours and obtains tissue for histological examination of both the tumours and apparently normal mucosa

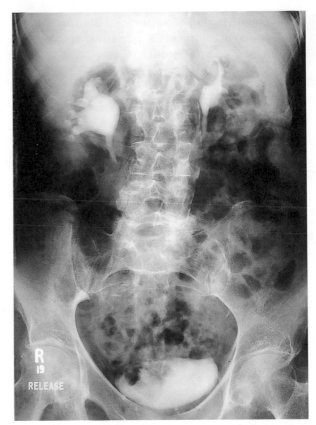

• **Fig. 28.29** Intravenous Urogram Showing a Large Filling Defect in the Right Side of the Bladder as a Result of a Tumour

- Bimanual examination (rectum and abdomen in the male; vagina and abdomen in the female) to assess spread of tumour beyond the bladder wall
- CT chest abdomen and pelvis as well as FDG PET CT scan may be used to exclude distant metastases
  In tumours which show histological evidence of invasion into bladder muscle, a CT or MRI scan is essential to determine the stage of the disease (see later) and the need for more radical treatment.

Histological Grading

Histological grades that were traditionally used are the 1973 WHO classification as below:

- Carcinoma in situ – this is a high-grade lesion
- Well-differentiated – Grade 1 (G1)
- Moderately-differentiated – Grade 2 (G2)
- Undifferentiated – Grade 3 (G3)

Most tumours contain a mixture of cell types. Grade is assigned based on the worst pattern of differentiation.

The 2004 WHO classification grouped tumours into either low- or high-grade urothelial carcinomas.

Tumour Staging

The TNM classification is used.

Tumour category is best assessed by histological examination of the resected specimen (pT category). The depth of penetration into or through the bladder wall is used as the criterion for the T component. A tumour is nominally

TABLE 28.5	Local Staging of Superficial Bladder Cancer from Histological Examination of the Resected Specimen.
Stage	Histological findings
pT(CIS)	Carcinoma in situ
pTa	Papillary carcinoma with basement membrane intact
PT1	Tumour has penetrated the basement membrane

TABLE 28.6	Local Staging of Bladder Cancer that is No Longer Superficial.
Stage	Findings
T2	Superficial muscle is involved
T2a	Through superficial muscle
T2b	Into deep muscle
T3a	Through deep bladder muscle into fat (microscopic)
T3b	Extending beyond muscle into fat (macroscopic) but bladder still mobile
T4a	Adjacent structures involved
T4b	Fixed to pelvic wall

TABLE 28.7	Nodal Staging in Bladder Cancer.
Stage	Findings
N0	No nodes involved
N1	Single regional node <2 cm
N2	Multiple regional nodes <5 cm
N3	At least one node >5 cm

TABLE 28.8	Management of Superficial Bladder Cancer.
Stage	Treatment
pT(CIS)	Endoscopic removal of local areas and intravesical BCG
pTa	Transurethral resection (TUR)
PT1	TUR
	For recurrence – repeated resection and intravesical BCG. or mitomycin
pT1 with poorly differentiated tumour (G3)	BCG and TUR
PT2	Radical surgery or radiotherapy

regarded as superficial (pTa) if it has not penetrated the basement membrane and pT1 when invades basement membrane (Table 28.5). Tumours that have invaded the bladder wall to a greater degree are pT2–pT4, and their classification is based on a combination of histological and bimanual examination (Table 28.6).

Node category. Lymphatic nodal spread from bladder cancer is to nodes on the surface of the bladder, the internal iliac and para-aortic nodes and then more distally. The classification is shown in Table 28.7.

Management

Treatment depends on the grade and stage of the tumour, as well as on the patient's fitness and preferences. At the initial endoscopic examination, the tumour is resected as far as possible, with deeper areas of resection being sent separately for histological examination to assess spread into the bladder muscle. Random biopsies of apparently normal bladder mucosa should also be obtained, as these may show changes of dysplasia or carcinoma in situ and provide useful prognostic information on the likelihood of recurrence. The treatment of superficial cancer (pTiS–pT1b) is summarized in Table 28.8. pT2 to pT4 tumours, unless they have advanced nodal involvement or distant metastases (N3 or M1), are managed by radical resection, radical radiotherapy or systemic chemotherapy, or a combination of these modalities. Radical cystectomy (cysto-prostatectomy in the male) is followed by urinary diversion. The simplest form of urinary diversion is the ileal conduit (see earlier). However, orthotopic neobladder reconstructions have been developed, such as the Studer pouch, to allow voiding through the urethra with no need for a stoma or external appliance. With T2 disease, there is a 5% improved survival rate with the addition of neo-adjuvant chemotherapy.

Surveillance

Once a diagnosis of urothelial carcinoma has been made, regular lifelong follow-up may be required, depending on the grade and stage of the tumour; 50% of patients will develop further tumours (unless they presented with a low-grade single pTa, G1 tumour).

Prognosis

Five-year survivals are summarized in Table 28.9; 95% of those with pT1a tumours survive 5 years.

Bladder Diverticula

A diverticulum is a protrusion of mucosa through the bladder muscle (Fig. 28.30).

TABLE 28.9	Survival in Bladder Cancer.	
Stage	Grade	5-year survival (%)
pTiS		75
pT1A	1	95
pT1B	1	72
PT1	3	39
pT2		45
pT3		39
pT4		5

TABLE 28.10	Classification of Bladder Fistulae.	
Type	Origin	Condition
Bladder to exterior	Congenital	Extrophy of bladder Urachal fistula
Bladder to vagina	Acquired	Injury (prolonged obstructed labour)
		Hysterectomy
		Cancer
		Radiotherapy
Bladder to colon	Acquired	Diverticular disease
		Cancer
		Radiotherapy
Bladder to small intestine	Acquired	Crohn's disease
		Radiothorapy
Bladder to rectum	Acquired	Post-prostalectomy
		Carcinoma of rectum
		Radiotherapy for prostatic cancer
		Laser therapy to the prostate
Bladder to uterus	Acquired	Malignancy of either organ
		Caesarean section
		Radiotherapy

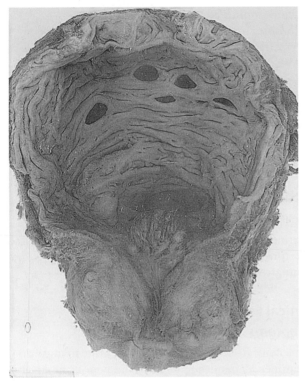

• **Fig. 28.30** Bladder Showing the Opening of Multiple Diverticula

Aetiology and Pathological Features

The majority are acquired and associated with bladder outflow obstruction.

Diverticula are often multiple, not surrounded by muscle fibres and therefore unable to empty when the detrusor contracts. Stagnation of urine in a diverticulum or the urinary tract leads to infection, stone formation and squamous metaplasia with the possibility of tumour. A tumour in a diverticulum has a worse prognosis than one in the intact bladder because invasion into surrounding tissues occurs earlier.

Clinical Features

Uncomplicated single or multiple diverticula are usually asymptomatic and found coincidentally during the course of investigation of a patient with bladder outflow obstruction. Complications lead to haematuria, dysuria and frequency.

There are no signs which are specific to the condition but infection may cause local tenderness.

Investigation and Management

Diverticula are frequently seen on ultrasound (with a full bladder), CT urography and at cystoscopy.

Bladder outflow obstruction should be relieved. If diverticula do not cause problems thereafter, treatment is not required. Persistent infection is an indication for removal.

Bladder Fistulae

A fistula is an epithelium-lined track between one hollow viscus and another or between a viscus and the exterior. Bladder fistulae are classified in Table 28.10.

Vesicovaginal Fistula
Aetiology and Pathological Features

The commonest cause of vesicovaginal fistula, in developing countries, is prolonged obstructed labour and ischaemic necrosis, by the descending fetal head, of the anterior vaginal wall and bladder. In developed countries, they more often occur as a result of complications of gynaecological surgery, pelvic malignancy and irradiation damage to the vagina and bladder following treatment for cervical cancer.

Clinical Features

There is a constant leak of urine through the vagina.

There may be features of the underlying cause apparent. Examination of the vagina shows urine trickling down from the vault, and the fistula may be thickened and palpable.

Investigation

CT and MRI Scanning

These imaging techniques are used to assess pelvic and urinary tract disease following previous treatment for pelvic malignancy.

Dye Test

If there is doubt about the source of leakage, a swab is placed into the vagina and methylene blue inserted into the bladder via a urethral catheter. Blue staining of the swab in the vagina confirms the presence of vesicovaginal fistula. A swab soaked in clear urine suggests a uretero-vaginal fistula. Patients with a vesicovaginal fistula often have multiple fistulae. The dye test should be repeated without the swab and the vagina examined directly using a Sims' speculum.

Management

Very few fistulae close spontaneously, however prolonged the bladder drainage.

Fistulae Caused by Irradiation or Malignancy

Urinary diversion is most appropriate because the tissues are unsuitable for repair and, in the case of malignancy, life expectancy may be short. In women with a long-life expectancy, a continent urine diversion or Mainz II pouch may be appropriate, depending on the degree of radiation tissue damage.

Obstetric and Post-Traumatic Fistulae

Repair should not be attempted within 3 months, to allow control of infection and revascularization of the ischaemic tissues. For postoperative fistulae, an immediate repair is done if the problem is noted at the time of surgery or within 10 days

Fistulae from Bladder to Gut (Enterovesical Fistulae)

These are usually between the large bowel and the bladder.

Clinical Features

The patient complains of:
- recurrent urinary infections
- bubbles in the urine (pneumaturia)
- faecal material in the urine (uncommon)
  Signs are non-specific but include those of cystitis.

Investigation and Management

The diagnosis is not usually in much doubt, but a barium enema or CT with bowel contrast often identifies the site and extent of underlying disease. This is usually diverticular disease or, more rarely, carcinoma of the large bowel.

Management is by resection of the abnormal bowel and closure of the bladder.

Neuropathic Bladder

This term is used to describe bladder dysfunction of neural origin. The neurophysiology of bladder function is incompletely understood, and clinical classifications are therefore the most useful in therapy and widely used. Three types are recognized:
- acute atonic bladder
- chronic atonic bladder
- hyperreflexic bladder

Aetiology

The causes may be divided into congenital and acquired. The latter can be further divided into trauma, cord compression, primary central nervous system disease and spinal cord disease secondary to that elsewhere.

Pathological Features

Whatever the type of neuropathy, the secondary effects are:
- urinary stasis with dilatation of the upper urinary tract
- recurrent ascending infection
- progressive loss of renal function
- secondary stone formation

Clinical Features

Symptoms

These range from painless retention of urine to uncontrolled incontinence, frequency, urgency and poor urine stream. In long-standing neuropathy, there may be systemic symptoms of chronic kidney disease.

Signs

There is commonly evidence of other neurological involvement from the underlying cause. A full neurological examination is essential. Depending on the clinical nature of the neuropathy, the bladder may be distended with a trickle of overflow or empty with urine constantly emerging from the urethral meatus.

Investigation

Urine

Because of the likelihood of infection, bacterial culture is carried out repeatedly.

Renal Function

Standard techniques are used.

Ultrasonography

Upper urinary tract dilatation and bladder emptying can be assessed.

Urinary Flow Studies

These are an essential part of the diagnosis and management of the neuropathic bladder. The patient with a full bladder voids into a machine which measures both the volume voided and the maximum flow (Q_{max} in mL/s). The pattern of voiding can also be observed. Voided volumes of <150 mL may lead to erroneous results. The maximum flow rate varies depending on sex and age. For example, a normal maximum flow rate in men <40 years is ≥21 mL/s, whereas in women <50 years, a flow ≥25 mL/s is expected.

Pressure Flow Studies

Bladder and intra-abdominal pressure (usually via a rectal probe) are measured simultaneously. The abdominal pressure is automatically subtracted from the bladder pressure to give detrusor pressure. The bladder is filled at a standard rate and the detrusor pressure measured. Rises in pressure during filling are recorded, as is the detrusor pressure at maximal urine flow. After completion of voiding, the residual urine can be measured. Bladder emptying can be recorded using a video system. A video pressure flow study can be done by adding fluoroscopy and contrast imaging of the bladder during filling and voiding.

Management of Clinical Types of Neuropathy

The general aims of treatment are to restore continence and preserve renal function.

Acute Atony

This condition typically occurs after spinal cord injury in the stage of spinal shock (see Ch. 29) and may last up to 3 months. The internal involuntary sphincter remains closed and the detrusor inactive so that the bladder is distended and empties by overflow. This situation should, however, be avoided because it results in delay of return of function to the bladder-spinal reflex centres (sacral 2, 3 and 4). Intermittent urethral catheterization, performed by either the patient or a carer four to five times a day, prevents distension. The eventual result is an automatic bladder which empties involuntarily every 2 or 3 hours or a bladder from which the urine can be expelled by manual compression.

Chronic Atony

The cause is either a peripheral neuropathy or long-standing outflow obstruction. The former is usually irreversible, and either intermittent self-catheterization or urinary diversion should be considered. It may be possible to correct the latter without producing incontinence (see 'Prostatic hyperplasia'). Urodynamic studies are essential in assessing residual detrusor function and the likelihood of the bladder being able to empty once the obstruction is relieved.

Hyperreflexia

Uninhibited high-pressure detrusor contractions are found on urodynamic studies but are not diagnostic of systemic neuropathy. Other features which may be found are:

- detrusor sphincter incoordination
- high voiding pressure
- significant residual volume
- poor and intermittent flow rate

The bladder assumes a fir tree appearance on CT urography, IVU or cystography (Fig. 28.31).

Management includes:

- Bladder conditioning – the patient is asked to delay voiding for longer and longer periods
- Anticholinergics – these are usually used in combination with bladder conditioning and are effective in mild to moderate cases
- Intravesical botulinum toxin injection – considered if anticholinergics failed. Will likely require repeating at intervals when the effect wears off
- Clam ileocystoplasty – an opened segment of small bowel is sutured into the opened bladder. This decreases the bladder pressure and increases the bladder volume. The reduction in bladder pressure results in poor bladder emptying, and intermittent self-catheterization is usually necessary
- Urine diversion if indicated

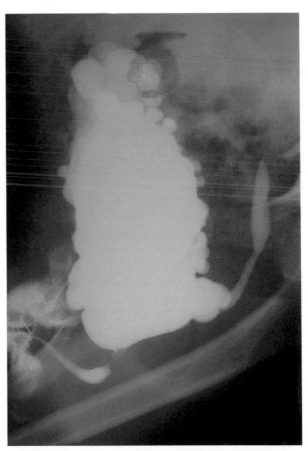

• **Fig. 28.31** Fir Tree Appearance of a Neuropathic Bladder

Incontinence

Incontinence is the involuntary passage of urine from the urethra and occurs as a result of either sphincter weakness or bladder overactivity.

The most common cause of stress incontinence in women is descent of the bladder neck so that any sudden increase in abdominal pressure acts only on the bladder and not the sphincter mechanism. In men, it results from a prostatectomy or, more rarely, damage to the sphincter during endoscopic transurethral resection.

Clinical Features

Symptoms

Stress incontinence results in involuntary loss of urine whenever intra-abdominal pressure is raised – by coughing, sneezing or exercise. Symptoms of detrusor instability include frequency, urgency, urge incontinence, nocturia and bed-wetting. Not all of these symptoms may be present.

Signs

Patients with detrusor overactivity may have evidence of a neuropathy. Stress incontinence may be demonstrable when the patient coughs or strains.

Investigation

Urine Examination

Bacterial culture is essential. Cytology should be obtained because the clinical features of detrusor instability can be mimicked by carcinoma in situ of the bladder. The two conditions can coexist.

Urodynamic Studies

Patients with symptoms of detrusor overactivity may have normal urodynamic findings.

Management

Stress Incontinence

Conservative treatment includes:
- weight loss
- pelvic floor exercises
- pelvic floor stimulation
- local or systemic oestrogen therapy
- ephedrine 15–30 mg t.d.s. (at least 3 months' treatment is usually required)

In men, pelvic floor exercises and ephedrine are worth a trial. Failure to respond requires surgical therapy with the insertion of an artificial sphincter or injection of inert substances into the sphincter area.

In women who have failed to respond to a conservative regimen, surgical treatment aims to elevate the bladder neck by a retropubic approach (colposuspension) or a transvaginal approach inserting an inert sling to support the urethra (transvaginal or transobturator)

Detrusor Overactivity

Whether or not detrusor overactivity has been identified by urodynamic studies, the majority of patients respond to bladder training. After a full explanation of the condition, the patient is asked not to pass urine for increasingly lengthy periods. An accurate fluid chart of input and output and of the timing of micturition is also kept. In the few patients who fail to respond, anticholinergic agents are of value (e.g. oxybutynin hydrochloride or tolterodine), but they must not be used in patients with a history of glaucoma. Another agent that that can be used is a β adrenergic agonist (Mirabegron).

THE PROSTATE

The gland is subject to hormonal influences throughout life. In utero, it is stimulated by maternal oestrogen, and an alteration in the androgen–oestrogen balance may be responsible for the enlargement of the prostate which occurs in later life. During the active sexual period, androgenic stimulation predominates. Testosterone produced by the testes, adrenals and the peripheral conversion of other steroids is converted in the prostate by the enzyme 5α-reductase to dihydrotestosterone, the most active androgen within the prostate.

Clinical Assessment

Rectal examination allows direct assessment of the size, shape, consistency and other features of the gland by digital palpation through the anterior wall of the rectum.

The normal gland has the following characteristics:
- It is soft to firm.
- It has a well-defined median sulcus.
- It is not tender.
  Abnormalities are as follows:
- Increased size causes the prostate to bulge backwards into the rectum so that the finger inserted through the anus passes a posterior overhang. The median sulcus becomes less obvious.
- Changes in consistency are either diffuse or localized. A very hard and irregular gland is characteristic of prostatic cancer but can occur in other conditions.
- Tenderness is present in inflammation.

It is notoriously difficult to accurately judge absolute prostatic size via rectal examination.

Diseases of the Prostate

The prostate is subject to three major disorders:
- infections
- benign prostatic hyperplasia (BPH)
- carcinoma of the prostate

Infections

There are three clinical entities of prostatitis:
- acute bacterial prostatitis
- chronic bacterial prostatitis
- chronic pelvic pain syndrome that further sub-classify into inflammatory and non-inflammatory

Acute Bacterial Prostatitis

Aetiology

This condition is more common in patients with diabetes mellitus. *Escherichia coli*, *S. aureus* and *Neisseria gonorrhoeae* are the common organisms. *Chlamydia* may also be found in the young and is often sexually transmitted. The route by which these organisms reach the prostate is unknown, but some instances may be by retrograde spread from the urethra.

Clinical Features

There is general malaise with fever, rigors, dysuria and frequency. Pain is felt in the perineum, the rectum and the suprapubic and sacral areas. Rectal examination reveals an acutely tender but soft prostate.

Investigation and Management

Bacterial culture of urine should be performed and, if possible, fluid obtained from the urethra after gentle prostatic massage, if the patient allows.

Management is with bed rest and appropriate antibiotic therapy. If *Chlamydia* is identified, a full sexual history will be needed and any contacts treated.

Chronic Bacterial Prostatitis

Aetiology

This condition may arise as a result of a blood-borne infection or failure adequately to treat an episode of acute prostatitis. The prostate becomes the site of chronic inflammation with fibrous tissue formation.

Clinical Features

There are symptoms of generalized ill health, frequency, dysuria, haematuria, haematospermia and perineal discomfort.

Rectal examination reveals a tender, hard and sometimes slightly irregular prostate. The prostate may also feel normal.

Investigation and Management

Culture of expressed prostatic secretion or post-massage urine usually does not result in a growth of bacteria, but white blood cells are present.

The condition is difficult to eradicate. Long-term antibiotic therapy with a quinolone antibiotic, trimethoprim or tetracycline may be of value, whilst alpha-adrenergic blocking agents can be used to relax the smooth muscle of the prostate.

Chronic Pelvic Pain Syndrome

These patients do not have prostatic infection but suffer from chronic pelvic pain and require symptomatic relief.

Benign Prostatic Hyperplasia

This condition is present in almost all men over the age of 40. Benign prostatic hypertrophy (BPH) occurs in 75% of men in the eighth decade, and 20% of men over the age of 40 will require treatment during their lifetime for bladder outflow obstruction.

Aetiology and Pathological Features

The cause of BPH is unknown, but the condition is generally regarded as a consequence of fluctuating levels of both androgen and oestrogen (and consequently the ratio between them) at different times of life. The effect is to produce hyperplasia of the glandular cells of the central zone with associated myoepithelial and fibrous tissue development. The cells involved vary in their proportionate contribution in any one patient. Perhaps because of this, the condition is variably referred to as benign prostatic hyperplasia and benign prostatic hypertrophy, but both are subsumed under the shorthand BPH. The hyperplastic central zone cells displace the peripheral zone so that a pseudocapsule is formed. Hyperplasia also variably compresses the urethral lumen, but this has little relationship to the overall size – glands of less than 40 g can cause as much trouble as those in excess of 100 g. The main relevance of the size of the prostate is that it may affect the type of treatment given.

Clinical Features

The patient may present in one of four ways:
- prostatic obstruction (bladder outflow obstructive symptoms)
- acute retention of urine
- chronic retention of urine
- acute on chronic retention of urine

Prostatic Obstruction

This may present with lower urinary tract symptoms (LUTS), which include:
- hesitancy
- poor stream
- intermittency
- terminal dribbling
- increased frequency during the day or at night
- nocturia
- urinary tract infection

The last two symptoms are due to incomplete bladder emptying. In addition, patients with bladder outflow obstruction frequently have detrusor overactivity and may therefore complain of urgency, urge incontinence and postmicturition dribbling. Not all patients with LUTS have benign prostatic hypertrophy. Not all patients with benign prostatic hypertrophy have outflow obstruction. The interrelationship of these phenomena – LUTS, benign prostatic hypertrophy and bladder outflow obstruction – is best illustrated by a Venn diagram (Fig. 28.32).

Acute Retention of Urine

Forty percent of patients who present in this way do not have a preceding history of prostatic outflow obstruction.

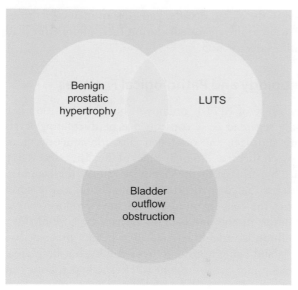

• **Fig. 28.32** The Inter-Relationship Between Benign Prostatic Hypertrophy (BPH), Lower Urinary Tract Symptoms (LUTS) and Bladder Outflow Obstruction (BOO)

The episode may be precipitated by anticholinergic drugs, diuretics (including alcohol), prolonged voluntary suppression of micturition, constipation, urinary tract infection and surgery for conditions outwith the urinary tract.

Symptoms are a sudden inability to pass urine and, after a very short period, acute severe suprapubic pain because of distension of what has usually been a previously normal bladder.

Signs. The patient is in severe pain and frequently unable to stay still. The bladder is palpable and tender in the midline above the pubis and below the umbilicus. Rectal examination may reveal an enlarged prostate, but the gland is pushed down by the overfull bladder so that the size may be exaggerated.

Chronic Retention

Symptoms. Chronic retention is painless. The patient may be ill from the metabolic effects of back pressure on the kidneys. There is characteristically the passage, at frequent intervals, of small quantities of urine and of rising on a number of occasions at night. Bed wetting may be a feature.

Signs. The patient's clothes and underwear may be wet and smell of urine. Apart from the systemic features of chronic kidney disease, there is a visible suprapubic swelling, dull to percussion. A search is made for any neurological abnormality because a painless bladder enlargement from such a cause may be confused with BPH and chronic retention.

Rectal examination shows the same general features as those of acute retention.

Investigation

Lower Urinary Tract Symptoms (LUTS)

Urine is taken for culture. Renal function tests in the form of U&Es are sent. Only in the presence of urinary blood or abnormal renal function should upper-tract ultrasound be performed. In the absence of these, patients perform a micturition flow test. Ninety percent of people with a flow rate of less than 12 mL/s have a degree of bladder outflow obstruction characterized by a peak maximum detrusor pressure in excess of 50 mmHg. Bladder ultrasound residual post-micturition is performed and transrectal ultrasound of the prostate to assess the size of the gland and look for the possibility of a middle lobe.

Management of Prostatic Obstruction

Not all men require treatment in the absence of marked outflow obstruction demonstrated by very poor flow and high post-micturition residuals or upper-tract dilatation. In the absence of bothersome lower urinary tract symptoms, a period of watchful waiting to see whether patients have become more symptomatic or quiescently obstructed can be justified. Medical treatment includes alpha-adrenergic blocking agents and these are subdivided into selective and non-selective alpha blockers. These drugs have an effect on all prostates of all sizes. 5α-reductase inhibitors are effective in the treatment of benign prostatic hypertrophy, and are more effective in men with larger prostates (>30 g). They block the conversion of testosterone to dihydrotetoterone and cause a reduction in volume of the prostate over a 12-month period on the drug of between 20 and 30%. 5α-Reductase inhibitors can improve lower urinary tract symptoms and also reduce the risk of presenting with acute urinary retention by as much as 50%. The combination of 5α-reductase inhibitors and alpha-adrenergic blockers offers better outcomes than either alone

Minimally Invasive Surgical Treatments

Surgical Treatment

The treatment of choice for prostates with an estimated weight of less than 100 g is transurethral surgical treatment of the prostate. Traditionally, this is performed using an endoscope and radio-frequency diathermy loop. Prostatic chips are resected – this is called transurethral resection of the prostate (TURP), although other transurethral surgical methods are available. These include transurethral incision of the prostate where the bladder neck is incised, usually at the 5 or 7 o'clock position from the ureteric orifice to the verumontanum. This is a good alternative where the prostate is not enlarged and the bladder neck is the cause of obstruction.

Transurethral laser therapy of the prostate is the commonest alternative surgical method using either green light laser, to desiccate and destroy the prostatic tissue, or the holmium laser to enucleate the adenoma. Transurethral vaporization of the prostate is radio-frequency diathermy using a corrugated diathermy ball to desiccate tissue rather than dissect tissue.

For large glands in excess of 100 g, holmium laser enucleation (HoLEP) or an open Millin's retropubic prostatectomy may be the best treatment. The latter is usually performed through a lower midline or Pfannenstiel incision. The prostatic capsule is incised and the obstructing adenoma is enucleated.

The advantages of transurethral prostatectomy are:
- Absence of wound infection
- Significant reduction in pain
- Less frequent urinary infection
- Postoperative incontinence reduced
- Lower incidence of general complications such as chest infection, deep-vein thrombosis and pulmonary embolus
- Hospital stay and early mortality are reduced
  Complications are:
- Bleeding – primary, reactionary or secondary haemorrhage
- Absorption of irrigation fluid into the systemic circulation which can cause hyponatraemia with epileptiform fits and cardiovascular collapse (the TUR syndrome). This is uncommon with bipolar saline resection
- Failure to void
- Urinary infection
- Epididymo-orchitis
- Incontinence
- Erectile dysfunction

Retrograde ejaculation is an inevitable sequela of transurethral prostatectomy about which patients must be warned.

Prognosis. The majority (90%) of patient with outflow obstruction are satisfied with the outcome of TURP. With mixed symptoms, only 70% of patients are completely satisfied with the result of a prostatectomy. The main reasons for this are that, where both bladder outflow obstruction and detrusor overactivity conditions co-exist, the detrusor overactivity did not resolve after prostatectomy.

Acute Retention of Urine

The patient is in severe pain, and catheterization is required (Emergency Box 28.1). It is commonly managed with urethral catheterization, though a suprapubic route can be used. The advantages of a suprapubic catheter include:
- Lack of damage to the urethra
- Urethral stricture from an indwelling catheter does not occur
- False passages are avoided
- Ease of introduction in a patient with a large prostate
- Trial of voiding is simple
- The operative field is left clear for a subsequent TUR

Suprapubic catheters should be inserted under ultrasound guidance to avoid the risk of bowel or vascular injury at the time of insertion.

Because 40% of patients with acute retention have no previous history of outflow obstruction, it is reasonable to allow them to attempt to void after clamping the suprapubic catheter. Those who are able to void usually had residual

---

EMERGENCY BOX 28.1

Acute Retention of Urine

- This is a urological emergency. The aim of treatment is to relieve pain. If a urethral catheter is to be used, it should be the smallest, softest self-retaining catheter, e.g. 12-Fr Foley.
- If retention is due to blood clot, then a large (22-Fr) three-way catheter, to allow irrigation, should be used. The volume of urine drained (<700 mL) is a good predictor of the likelihood of spontaneous voiding when the catheter is removed.
- A short course of an alpha-adrenergic blocker, e.g. alfuzosin, may aid initiation of voiding.
- Insertion of a catheter by the suprapubic route has significant advantages (see main text).
- If it is not possible to insert a catheter, do not persevere. Call for more senior help.
- Only those trained in their use should utilize a catheter introducer.
- A rectal examination with the bladder distended will give misleading information as to the prostate size.
- Acute urinary retention will significantly increase the level of serum prostate-specific antigen, misleadingly suggesting a diagnosis of carcinoma of the prostate.

---

urine of less than 700 mL when initially catheterized and may avoid a prostatectomy in the short term. Patients who revert back into retention require a prostatectomy.

Chronic Retention

The treatment is by prostatectomy. The only indication for preoperative catheter drainage is in patients with impaired renal function secondary to back pressure on the kidneys (high pressure retention). Catheterization eventually leads to the development of a urinary infection, which increases the morbidity and mortality of a subsequent operation and is difficult to eradicate in a large floppy bladder. Bladder catheterization may result in diuresis leading to dehydration, hypotension and further impairment of renal function, so close monitoring of the patient's weight, blood pressure, pulse, fluid input and urine output is required. Once renal function has improved and stabilized, definitive surgery can be undertaken.

Carcinoma of the Prostate

Epidemiology

This tumour is the most common malignancy to affect men. The disease increases with age and is rarely discovered under the age of 50, with the incidence peaking in men in their 70s. Examination of serial sections of the prostate of men who have died from other causes has demonstrated that 29% of those aged between 50 and 60, 49% of men in the age group 70–79 and 67% of those aged 80–89 had unsuspected prostate cancer. Not all are clinically apparent and, even when identified, they may not express the same malignant potential. At one extreme are those tumours which are found only at death, whilst at the other there are rapidly progressive tumours with invasive and metastatic potential. In between there are tumours with intermediate degrees of aggression and long periods of local growth only. However, the availability of screening techniques and advances in diagnostics, have led to a significant over-diagnosis and subsequent treatment of the many men discovered. The same dilemma exists about treatment: diagnosis does not necessarily imply progression or a need to treat.

Aetiology

Prostate cancer appears to have multi-factorial causal factors. There is a genetic relationship to males within a family who have had the disease, as well as a relationship to the female line in a family who have had breast cancer. There are genetic studies showing predisposition to the disease with certain genetic phenotypes including *BRCA1&2*. There is also increasing evidence in relation to diet in that it is a disease of the developed countries. In populations who have a predominately vegetarian diet, the incidence is low; when these individuals adopt a Western diet, the incidence increases to that in developed countries.

Pathological Features

Tumours are usually adenocarcinomas, arising in the periphery of the gland in 70% of cases. The tumour spreads along neuronal pathways, via the lymphatic and via the blood (principally to bone). Tumours may locally invade into the peri-prostatic tissue, and spread by lymphatics to the obturator nodes, presacral nodes, as well as to the iliac and para-aortic nodes.

Clinical Features

The commonest presentation of prostatic cancer is now due to 'screening' with prostate-specific antigen (PSA) rather than presenting with symptoms. However, clinical features may include the following.

Symptoms

These include:
- Bladder outflow obstruction (see above), though such symptoms are usually from a benign prostatic enlargement appearing coincidentally in a man with prostate cancer.
- Metastatic disease – bone pain, leg swelling from lymphatic obstruction
- Renal failure from bilateral ureteric obstruction

Signs

These include:
- A nodule in a palpably benign gland
- Hard irregular prostate on rectal examination, sometimes with perirectal and periprostatic thickening
- Ankle and leg oedema
- Other signs of metastases

The disease may only be discovered at an incidental rectal examination or on histological examination of prostatic tissue removed during a transurethral prostatectomy for clinically benign disease.

Investigation

Histological diagnosis is required in the vast majority of cases and this is performed using either transrectal ultrasound guided biopsy or, now more commonly, transperineal biopsy. Tumours may be discovered in the tissue from a TURP for bladder outflow obstruction as noted above.

Other investigations include:
- Routine evaluation of renal function
- Serum alkaline phosphatase concentration – elevated in patients with bone metastases

Serum Prostate-Specific Antigen Concentration

PSA is a protein secreted by prostatic cells and may be elevated in benign prostatic hypertrophy, inflammatory change of the prostate and in malignant prostatic disease. Twenty percent of men with prostate cancer have a normal PSA. Further understanding and usage of PSA has shown clinical value in the serum free to serum total PSA ratio, with a percentage below 10% indicating a higher risk of cancer. There is a small group of patients who have non-PSA expressing tumours and these are often poorly differentiated. PSA velocity and density can also be useful to increase the accuracy of prostate cancer detection.

PCA3 is a relatively new genetic marker which is measured from secreted prostatic cells in urine. The specimen is produced after the first void following vigorous prostatic massage. Shed prostatic cells are spun down and a risk index is given. An index above 35 is indicative of a high risk of cancer and a PCA3 below 35 indicates low risk. This test is still not in common use as the risk of cancer can still be as high as 20% in low-risk patients. It may have a role in finding more aggressive cancers.

Gleason Grade

Histopathological grade is classified using the Gleason system. The histopathologist scores two separate areas of cancer with a grade from 1 to 5, with 1 being benign and 5 being highly malignant. However, most pathologists have dispensed with the 1 annotation. Most prostate cancers are between 3 and 4, with few poorly differentiated Gleason 5 cancers. A joint Gleason score is described by giving the predominant grade first and the less predominant second. Thus, Gleason 4+3 will have a more predominant 4 pattern as opposed to a 3+4 where the moderate 3 grade is more predominant. The Gleason score, the sum of the two grades, has a high concordance with the risk of metastasis, margin positive status and disease recurrence. In order to try to relate the histological diagnosis to clinical risk, and therefore outcome, there is increasing use of a new Grade Group system (grade groups 1–5).

There is also the further histological pre-cancerous classi-fication of prostatic intraduct neoplasia (PIN). The original understanding was that the presence of PIN increased the likelihood of finding cancer in subsequent biopsies. More recent evidence, however, showed the risk to be similar to cancer pick up rate without PIN. The presence of *Atypical Small Acinar Proliferation* (ASAP) increases the risk of find-ing subsequent cancer by >40%.

Ultrasonography

Abdominal ultrasound may identify unilateral or bilateral hydronephrosis because of ureteric involvement. Transrectal ultrasound has been used both as an aid to diagnosis and for staging prostate cancer, but unfortunately it is not particu-larly accurate in either and so is rarely used.

MRI Scanning

MRI screening has advanced over the past years to include multiple parameters that allows for better accuracy in detecting significant prostate cancer. It also allows for accurate local staging that will guide the future treatment. This better detection rates has helped avoid unnecessary biopsies.

Bone Scanning

Radioisotope bone scan can detect areas of increased bone activity irrespective of their cause (Fig. 28.33). Confir-matory X-rays may need to be taken of areas of increased isotope uptake. Bone metastases from carcinoma of the prostate are sclerotic (osteoblastic). Bone scintigraphy is required in all patients who present with a PSA of greater than 10 (may vary depending upon local guidelines) or who present with poorly differentiated disease (Gleason 4+3=7 or above). There is no indication for bone scan in well- to moderately-differentiated disease with a PSA of less than 10. The chances of a positive scan are extremely low.

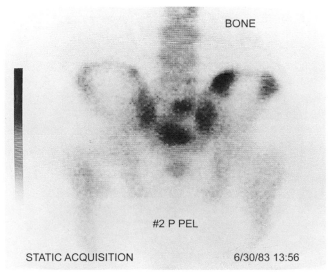

BONE

#2 P PEL

STATIC ACQUISITION   6/30/83 13:56

• **Fig. 28.33** A Bone Scan Showing Multiple Hot Spots Caused by Metastatic Carcinoma of the Prostate

Choline PET/ PSMA PET

Promising modalities in the detection of metastatic disease. The accuracy of PSMA PET CT scan is higher than choline-based scans.

Staging

Staging is by the TNM classification, given in Table 28.11.

Management

The management of prostate cancer can largely be divided by stage into those with organ-confined disease and those who present with metastatic disease.

Management of Organ-Confined Prostate Cancer

The widespread use of PSA testing over several decades, the patient outcome data after radical prostatectomy and histological specimen analysis has led to an improved understanding about the variable natural history of pros-tate cancer. Whilst it remains one of the commonest cancers in men, the number of men who die from the dis-ease is relatively small in relation to its overall incidence. Recent studies have questioned the validity of PSA screen-ing and its value in reducing prostate cancer mortality and have emphasized the considerable potential cost to the patient. It has become clearer from a number of stud-ies that active surveillance has a clear rationale, based on the fact that patients with moderate to well-differentiated disease of small volume, i.e. involving a small percent-age of cores involved or of any one core, together with a

TABLE 28.11	Staging of Prostate Cancer.
Stage	**Findings**
T1a	An incidental finding of tumour with low biological potential for aggressive behaviour in a prostate removed for clinically benign disease
T1b	An incidental finding of a tumour with potentially biological aggressive behaviour found in a prostate removed for clinically benign disease (high-grade or diffuse)
T1c	Tumour identified because of an elevated serum prostate-specific antigen
T2a	Tumour invoking half a lobe or less
T2b	More than half a lobe but not both
T2c	Both lobes
T3	Tumour extends through capsule and may involve seminal vesicle
T4	Tumour fixed, invasive of adjacent structures other than seminal vesicle

low-presenting PSA, are very unlikely to develop progressive disease, particularly in men over the age of 65. Based on recent studies, active surveillance is a very good option for these men. The role of active surveillance becomes less clear in younger men. Longer follow-up needs to be established to relate the actual risk of progression over time in such individuals. There is a trend to treat with curative intent in men under the age of 55 – that is by radical prostatectomy or radiotherapy. There is still a rationale, however, for closely monitoring those patients who have small volume tumours of low grade, histological Gleason score, low PSA and low PSA ratio scores. In these patients, such active surveillance may result in a deferral of treatment, with a deferral of accompanying side effects, rather than not requiring treatment.

The term 'watchful waiting' is used when elderly or infirm men present with the disease and are considered unlikely to benefit from primary treatment either in the form of surgery, radiotherapy or other modalities. Such patients should be monitored and treatment can be instituted if the disease progresses, usually in the form of androgen manipulation.

Primary Management Strategies for Prostate Cancer

- No treatment, with assessment of progress
- Endocrine therapy
- Radiotherapy
  - conformal external beam
  - external beam proton therapy
  - seed implant brachytherapy
- Surgery
  - robotic-assisted
  - laparoscopic
  - open – perineal or retropubic
- HIFU (high-intensity focused ultrasound)
- Cryoablation

No Treatment

Men with asymptomatic low-stage, low-grade disease may be offered Active Surveillance. This is an active process with follow-up with regular observation of PSA, repeat MRI scans and possible repeat prostate biopsies. It is performed in men who are still young and fit enough to benefit from treatment, but who may be able to avoid the side effects of such treatment. The aim is to be able to intervene in those men whose disease is changing, so that they can still undergo treatment with curative intent, with one of the treatments outlined below. This is different to Watchful Waiting, which is performed in those with significant comorbidities. This is an infrequent monitoring of men with the aim of controlling symptoms when they arise.

In this group, early treatment by hormone therapy provides a slight survival advantage and reduction in morbidity from disease progression in men who have asymptomatic advanced localized or metastatic prostate cancer.

Endocrine Therapy

Most of the cells of the prostate are dependent on the male hormone testosterone for their multiplication. Ninety percent of circulating testosterone is produced by the testes under the influence of luteinizing hormone (LH), which is in turn controlled by the hypothalamic secretion of luteinizing hormone-releasing hormone (LHRH; Fig. 28.34). The remaining 10% of testosterone is produced by the adrenals and by peripheral conversion of other steroids. Eighty percent of patients with symptomatic prostate cancer respond subjectively and 60% respond objectively to androgen suppression or ablation. The mean duration of response is 1–2 years. Once the tumour is no longer hormone-responsive, the mean survival was 6 months, until the advent of new treatments such as abiraterone and enzalutamide, and the use of chemotherapy.

Androgen suppression. This is only used in men with locally advanced or metastatic disease, or as a neo-adjuvant treatment with external beam radiotherapy. LHRH

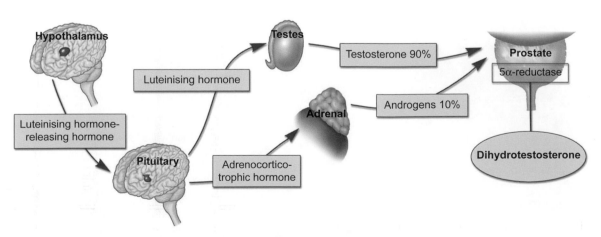

• **Fig. 28.34** Hormonal Control of the Prostate

analogues initially stimulate the pituitary, but, after approximately 7 days, the pituitary receptors become blocked and downregulation occurs. Serum testosterone falls to castrate levels. These substances are long-acting and are administered subcutaneously every 1 or 3 months. Because of the initial stimulation of the pituitary, an anti-androgen should be given for a few days before, and 2–3 weeks after, the analogue is given to prevent a flare response.

Androgen ablation is by bilateral subcapsular orchidectomy and removes the testosterone-producing part of the testicle. There is no difference in response between orchidectomy and LHRH analogue therapy, and the choice of treatment should lie with the patient.

Radiotherapy

Radiotherapy is effective in controlling the pain of bony metastases. It is also very effective in the treatment of the primary if it is thought that the tumour is confined to the prostate. There have been no worthwhile randomized controlled trials to compare radiotherapy with radical surgery, although comparative data suggests that the efficacy is similar. Low dose-rate prostate brachytherapy, in which radioactive seeds are placed throughout the prostate with the aid of a template and ultrasound guidance, is used for patients with low to intermediate risk disease.

Surgical Treatment

Radical Prostatectomy

It is used for disease that is believed to be localized to the prostate and is widely undertaken in the USA and Europe. The use of so-called 'keyhole surgery' (laparoscopic and robotic-assisted laparoscopic) is increasingly overtaking open procedures around the world. Some concerns about radical prostatectomy include:

- The purpose of the operation is to remove the whole of the prostate with its confined cancer; this is not always accurately assessed before surgery.
- Morbidity includes incontinence, erectile dysfunction and anastomotic strictures.

HIFU and Cryoablation

These are no longer used for whole gland treatment of prostate cancer as the long-term results are inferior to standard treatment options.

Chemotherapy

When patients with metastatic disease fail to respond to endocrine therapy, chemotherapy may be considered. Recent trial data supports the use of chemotherapy early on in fit patients with metastatic disease rather than waiting for endocrine therapy to fail.

Prognosis

In men with prostate cancer confined within the capsule who undergo radical prostatectomy, approximately 81% have 10 years progression-free survival, whereas only 25% of those who have metastatic disease at presentation are expected to survive 5 years with current therapy.

THE MALE URETHRA

Congenital Abnormalities

These are:
- urethral valves
- hypospadias
- epispadias

Urethral Valves

Pathological Features

Folds of urothelium develop in the posterior urethra in utero to form a valve-like obstruction to the passage of urine. Gross dilatation of the prostatic urethra (Fig. 28.35), distension of the bladder and ureters and hydronephrosis result. Severe renal impairment follows. With increasing use of antenatal ultrasound, many boys with urethral valves are diagnosed in utero by antenatal screening.

Clinical Features

The bladder may be palpable, and the infant constantly dribbles urine. The development of a urinary infection may draw attention to the problem before end-stage renal failure develops.

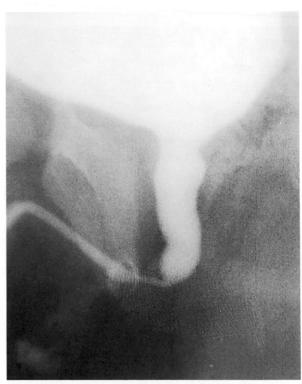

• **Fig. 28.35** Urethral Valves Causing Bladder Distension and Dilatation of the Prostatic Urethra

Management

When diagnosed in utero, a stent can be inserted to drain the baby's bladder into the amniotic cavity, so preserving renal function. Endoscopic division of the valves is required, sometimes with urinary diversion to improve renal function.

Hypospadias

Aetiology

The two genital folds on the ventral aspect of the phallus fail to fuse and form the anterior urethra of the male. The meatus is therefore displaced posteriorly for a variable distance. Hypospadias is classified according to where the opening lies (Fig. 28.36). Other genital abnormalities, such as failure of testicular descent, are often present, and there may be a family history.

Clinical Features

Apart from the abnormal opening of the urethra, the foreskin is hooded and the penis is bent (chordee) ventrally because of secondary fibrosis in the area of the absent urethra.

Management

Surgical repair, usually utilizing the foreskin, is carried out at around the age of 1 year

Epispadias

This is extremely rare. The urethra opens on the dorsum of the penis. This is often associated with exstrophy of the bladder. No clear embryological mechanism has been formulated. Complex repair is required.

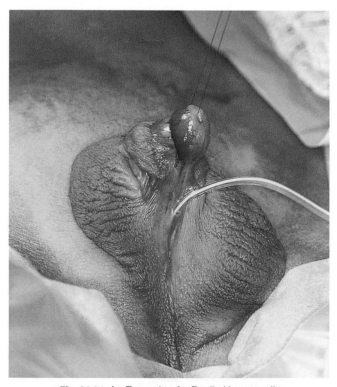

• **Fig. 28.36** An Example of a Penile Hypospadias

Urethral Injury

Aetiology

The male urethra is more frequently injured than that of the female. The most common cause is instrumentation of the urethra by a catheter or cystoscope. Up to 30% of pelvic fractures are associated with urethral damage, and 10% of urethral trauma, beyond the pelvic floor, is caused by a fall-astride injury.

Clinical Features

History

A urethral injury should always be suspected in a patient who has been injured and who presents with any of the following:
- blood at the urethral meatus
- haematuria
- anuria

Signs

Physical examination may reveal a palpable bladder. Lower abdominal tenderness is always present in a patient with a pelvic fracture and does not necessarily imply bladder or urethral damage. In fall-astride injuries, there may be bruising and swelling in the perineum. In rupture of the membranous urethra, the prostatic area is said to be boggy and the prostate high-riding. However, anyone who has attempted to perform a rectal examination in a man with a fractured pelvis realises how difficult this physical sign is to elicit.

Investigation

It is unwise to make repeated attempts to pass a urethral catheter. If the diagnosis is in doubt, urethrography using water-soluble contrast media is done.

Management

The urethral injury takes low priority in the overall management of patients subjected to severe multiple trauma.

Anterior Urethral Injuries

If the rupture is complete, the perineal haematoma is evacuated and a primary repair done. If incomplete, either a well-lubricated soft, small urethral catheter should be passed by an experienced urologist and left in situ for 10 days or a suprapubic catheter inserted.

Posterior Urethral Injuries

Either a suprapubic catheter should be inserted or a urethral catheter should be railroaded into the bladder (Fig. 28.37). This allows alignment of the divided ends, and, if a stricture develops, subsequent management may be easier. Posterior urethral injuries can also be simultaneously repaired during open reduction and internal fixation of pelvic fractures.

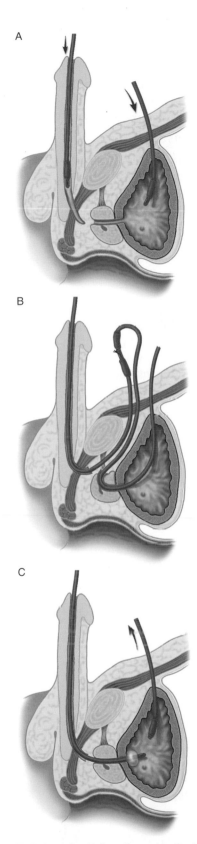

A

B

C

• **Fig. 28.37** A Technique for Railroading a Urethral Catheter in a Patient with a Ruptured Urethra

Congenital
- Meatal stenosis

Traumatic
- Urethral catheterization
- Cystoscopy
- Transurethral resection
- After rupture of urethra

Inflammatory
- Gonorrhoea
- Non-specific urethritis
- Long-term urethral catheter

Complications

These are as follows:
- urethral stricture
- incontinence
- erectile dysfunction (neurogenic and vascular)

Urethral Stricture

Aetiology

Strictures may be congenital, traumatic or inflammatory (Box 28.13).

Clinical Features

There may be a history related to the underlying cause. The patient complains of difficult and incomplete micturition with a poor stream. There is a thin, divergent urine stream with terminal dribbling. The bladder may be palpable.

Investigation and Management

Urine flow rate is reduced and prolonged with intermittent peaks signifying temporarily improved flow due to abdominal strain. Urethrography demonstrates the site, length and number of strictures.

The treatment of choice is direct endoscopic incision or a urethroplasty, depending upon the site, aetiology and length of the stricture.

PENIS

Phimosis

Definition and aetiology

This is inability to retract the foreskin.

Congenital

It is not usually possible to retract the foreskin without the application of undue force until the age of 2–3 years because the inner surface of the foreskin adheres to the glans. Active treatment may be required in recurrent balanitis or UTI in the form of circumcision.

Acquired

This is the result of:
- recurrent infections (balanitis) of which diabetes mellitus is a known contributor
- underlying tumour of the glans penis

Clinical Features

The preputial orifice is white and scarred and indurated, presenting symptoms including secondary intractability of the foreskin, irritation at or bleeding from the preputial orifice, dysuria and, occasionally, acute urinary retention.

Management

Treatment is by circumcision. The operation should not be carried out until infection is under control.

Paraphimosis

Aetiology and Pathological Features

The foreskin contains fibrous tissue, often because of previous attacks of inflammation, usually as a result of forceful retraction of the prepuce. It normally cannot be retracted, but, if this occurs either by manipulation or during sexual intercourse, the fibrous band encircles the penis in the subcoronal area to cause congestion of the glans.

Clinical Features

There may be a suggestive history. Pain in the glans is usually moderate to severe, and there may be difficulty on micturition.

It is not possible to reduce the retracted foreskin. The glans is oedematous. A tight band may be palpable in the subcoronal area.

Management

A penile block with lidocaine (lignocaine) followed by gentle pressure and traction, will usually result in reduction. Failure necessitates a dorsal incision of the constricting band. Patients should subsequently be circumcised if it is a recurrent problem.

Circumcision

Indications

Indications are:
- religious ritual circumcision – Muslims, Arabs and Jews
- phimosis
- paraphimosis
- recurrent balanitis
- preputial injuries

Complications

The operation should not be undertaken lightly. Complications include:
- primary or secondary haemorrhage
- secondary infection

- meatal ulceration and stenosis because of the absence of protection by the foreskin
- injury to the glans
- over-radical excision with scarring
- unsatisfactory cosmetic outcome
- glans hypersensitivity followed by hyposensitivity

Peyronie's Disease

Aetiology and Pathological Features

The cause of this condition is unknown but believed to be traumatic. There appears to be an increased incidence in patients with Dupytren's contracture.

The corpora cavernosae develop a fibrous thickening which results in bending or angulation of the penis when erect. Circumferential fibrosis may result in distal flaccidity during an erection.

Clinical Features

The penis is angulated during erection, which may make intercourse impossible or painful (Fig. 28.38). The degree of angulation can be assessed by inducing an artificial erection with an injection of intracavernosal prostaglandin E1.

Management

The penis can be straightened, but made shorter, by excising a wedge from the corpora opposite to the maximum angulation. Resuturing the excised edges straightens the penis. Other techniques include plication of the opposite side or vein grafting of the scarred fibrotic area.

Priapism

Classified into high flow (arterio-venous fistula) or low flow (ischaemic). Ischaemic priapism is defined as persistent and painful erection of the penis.

Aetiology and Pathological Features

The great majority (80%) have no underlying cause. Those known are summarized in Box 28.14, and some relate to episodes of blood sludging. If detumescence does not take

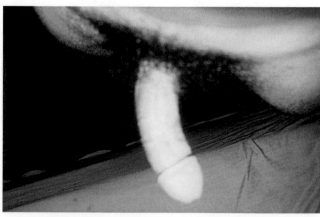

• **Fig. 28.38** Peyronie's Disease with Penile Bending

place within 8 hours, venous and arterial thrombosis ensues with fibrosis in the corpora and permanent erectile failure.

Management

Because of the risk of irreversible damage to the erectile apparatus, this is a urological emergency. Aspiration of the thick viscid blood from the corpora may be sufficient. The use of an alpha agonist such as phenylephrine, injected directly into the corpora at the correct dose and with appropriate monitoring, may be very effective. If that fails, a shunt is created between the corpora cavernosa and the glans penis, the corpora cavernosa and the corpora spongiosa or the corpora cavernosa and the saphenous vein.

Carcinoma of the Penis

Aetiology

The occurrence of the disease mainly in the uncircumcised and elderly suggests that poor standards of sub-preputial hygiene allow the accumulation of carcinogens, but there is no direct evidence for this. The tumour is a squamous carcinoma. It is now rare in developed countries.

Clinical Features

There is an offensive bloody discharge issuing from beneath a non-retractile foreskin. Inguinal lymphadenopathy is invariably present as a result of either infection or secondary spread. An early carcinoma is shown in Fig. 28.39.

Management

This depends on the extent of the disease. Treatment options include:

- wide excision with skin resurfacing
- partial amputation
- radical amputation with block dissection of inguinal lymph nodes
- radiotherapy
- chemotherapy

TESTIS, EPIDIDYMIS AND CORD

Undescended Testis

Epidemiology

Both testes are undescended in 30% of premature infants: at term, this has fallen to 3%; and at 1 year 1%. Spontaneous descent after 1 year is exceedingly rare.

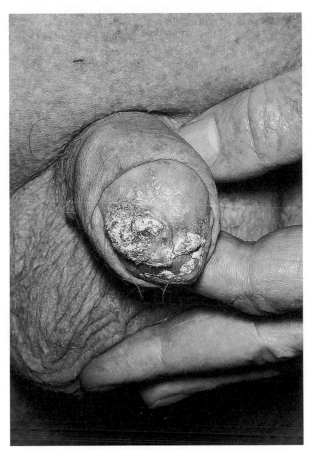

• **Fig. 28.39** An Early Carcinoma of the Penis Involving Only the Glans

Aetiology

The cause is failure of migration along the normal line of descent. In an ectopic testis, the testicle deviates away from the line and may lie in front of the penis in the superficial inguinal pouch, in the perineum or in the thigh. The cause is not known.

Clinical Features

An empty scrotal sac or hemiscrotum at 1 year indicates that the testicle is:

- proximal to the external inguinal ring (undescended)
- truly absent
- retractile – the cremaster muscle reflex pulls the organ up towards the inguinal canal
- ectopic

A retractile testis can usually be coaxed into the scrotal sac, or will enter spontaneously if the child is asked to crouch. An ectopic testicle may be palpable in the areas described above but cannot be brought into the scrotum. An incompletely descended testis may be palpable at the external ring or in the neck of the scrotum. A testicle in the inguinal canal is impalpable.

Complications

Complications are:

- infertility – inevitable in bilateral and common in unilateral undescent, and frequent in those who have had undescent treated

- torsion
- trauma
- inguinal hernia
- malignant disease – 8-fold increase in the risk of cancer

Investigation

If the testicle is not palpable, ultrasonography, CT, MRI and laparoscopy are useful investigations to determine whether the testicle is truly absent and, if not, where it is situated.

Management

The aim is to bring the testicle with its blood supply into the scrotum as early as possible, usually at the age of 1. Boys who present with a well-developed undescended testis before puberty should undergo an orchidopexy, an operation to bring the testicle and its blood supply into the scrotum and fixed in a dartos pouch. However, if the testis is poorly developed, an orchidectomy is advised. Beyond puberty, orchidectomy should be done. A testicular prosthesis can be placed in the scrotum, if desired.

Torsion

Aetiology and Pathological Features

Torsion is a recognized complication of testicular maldescent. The episode occurs any time between birth and early adolescence but is uncommon thereafter. A horizontally lying testicle with a long mesorchium and cord within the vaginal sac, so that the testis hangs like the clapper of a bell, is most prone to torsion. This anatomical arrangement is usually bilateral, so that both testes are at risk. The twist deprives the organ of its blood supply; if untwisting does not take place within 6 hours, ischaemia is irreversible, gangrene develops and the testis either suppurates or atrophies. As such, testicular torsion is one of the few urological emergencies requiring urgent access to the operating theatre.

Clinical Features

There may be a history of previous episodes of testicular pain. The pain may be initially felt in the iliac fossa or over the cord and is often associated with vomiting.

The testicle is extremely tender, swollen and drawn up in the scrotum. The unaffected testicle may have a horizontal lie.

Other conditions which must be considered are:
- torsion of an appendix of the testis
- acute epididymo-orchitis
- idiopathic scrotal oedema

Investigation

Urinalysis will reveal a sterile, acellular urine.
Ultrasonography will demonstrate the absence of blood supply to the affected testicle, but this should not delay the definitive management of scrotal exploration.

Management

Treatment of testicular torsion is, for the reasons given earlier, a surgical emergency.

Non-Operative

It may be possible to de-rotate the testis, although this is very painful and does not offer definitive treatment.

Surgical

The testis is de-rotated and fixed with non-absorbable sutures. The unaffected testis is dealt with at the same operation. A gangrenous testis should be removed.

Orchitis and Epididymo-Orchitis

Aetiology and Pathological Features

Primary orchitis is rare except in association with mumps. The testis is often secondarily infected from epididymitis, which originates by retrograde spread from the prostate and seminal vesicle; a blood-borne infection is the alternative source. A surgical procedure on the lower urinary tract, such as a TUR, may also be a precipitating factor. The organisms are usually *N. gonorrhoeae*, *E. coli* and *Chlamydia*, depending upon the age of the patient. Chronic infection or a discharging sinus may be the consequence of tuberculosis.

Clinical Features

There may be a preceding history of an operation or of dysuria, frequency and haematuria. Pain in the scrotum is acute, and the patient is conscious of swelling. Fever and rigors are not uncommon.

The epididymis is acutely tender and enlarged, although it may be difficult to distinguish it from the equally tender testis. Overlying redness and oedema may be present.

Investigation

Blood count. Leucocytosis is present.
Blood culture. A positive culture is useful to direct antibiotic treatment, although this should be started on an empirical basis before the result is available.
Urinalysis. This will reveal a pyuria, and the organism may be revealed by culture. Urine PCR can detect chlamydia.
Urethral swab. *Chlamydia* can also be diagnosed in this way.
Ultrasonography. Increased blood flow may be demonstrated.

Management

In a young sexually active man, the commonest infecting organism is *Chlamydia*. Bed rest, scrotal elevation and doxycycline is appropriate. Other antibiotics may be needed according to cultures. In such cases, the partner should also be investigated and treated.

Epididymitis caused by other organisms such as *E. coli*, should be treated accordingly. Ciprofloxacin offers good penetration of the epididymis.

SCROTAL SWELLINGS

A non-inflammatory swelling of the scrotal contents may be a:
- testicular tumour
- epididymal cyst (spermatocele)

- varicocele
- hydrocele
- hernia

Clinical Examination

The following points enable distinctions to be made:
- If it is possible to get above the swelling and palpate a normal cord, the swelling is not a hernia.
- If there is a cough impulse in the groin or, with the patient lying flat, the scrotal mass disappears or is reducible, the swelling is a hernia.
- The testicle lies anteriorly and the epididymis posteriorly; gentle palpation establishes where the swelling lies and therefore its origin.
- Hydroceles transilluminate.
- Varicoceles are more apparent with the patient standing and typically feel like a bag of worms in severe cases.

Hydrocele
Aetiology

These may be congenital or acquired. Congenital hydroceles follow failure of obliteration of the processus vaginalis. Peritoneal fluid can then enter the scrotum. The great majority of acquired hydroceles are of unknown origin, but 10% are associated with tumour or infection of the testicle.

Clinical Features

An infant presents with a large scrotal sac, and the hydrocele is easily demonstrated by transillumination.

In adult life, there is a firm painless transilluminable swelling which it is possible to get above.

Management

The majority of congenital hydroceles resolve spontaneously by the age of 3, but persistence beyond this time requires operative treatment by division and ligation of the processus. In acquired hydrocele, an ultrasound scan will identify any underlying cause. If the hydrocele is symptomatic, surgery may be required.

Epididymal Cysts and Spermatoceles

These may be single or multiple and are usually related to the head of the epididymis. They lie posterior or superior to the testicle and may transilluminate.

Management

Asymptomatic cysts do not require treatment. Surgical excision may be required in symptomatic cases.

Varicocele
Aetiology and Pathological Features

The venous valve at the junction of the left spermatic vein with the renal vein may be incompetent or becomes so. It is rare for the same to take place on the right where the vein enters the IVC. Very occasionally, a tumour in the kidney with extension along the renal vein may be present. Varicocele is a common finding in men presenting with subfertility but is equally common in men requesting vasectomy for contraception. A left-sided varicocoele is present in 20–25% of men. The veins of the pampiniform plexus become enlarged and tortuous.

Clinical Features

There is a dragging sensation in the scrotum, which is worse in hot weather and on prolonged standing. Subfertility may be apparent.

Physical examination reveals the 'bag of worms', which becomes more obvious if the patient stands. A cough impulse is present in the same position. The left testicle may be smaller than the right. Smaller varicocoeles may only become obvious on Doppler ultrasound examination

Management

Treatment is required for those with symptoms and possibly for those with subfertility. The procedures of choice are embolization of the testicular vein under radiological control or microvascular open ligation

Testicular Tumours

Benign, interstitial cell and Leydig cell tumours of the testis are exceedingly rare. Malignant tumours are uncommon (1–2% of all neoplasms in males) but do occur in young adults with an otherwise long life expectancy. In the age range 20–35 years, testes tumours are the most common solid malignancy. The psychological effects of a diagnosis of malignancy are, in consequence, considerable.

Aetiology and Epidemiology

Maldescended testes – particularly those retained within the abdomen – have a 40% greater chance of malignant change than does a normal testis. Otherwise the cause is unknown. The overall incidence is 2–3 per 100 000 of the population per year. They are rare before puberty. Germ cell tumour account for 90% of testicular tumours; of these, about 45% are seminoma with a peak incidence at 30–40 years, and a similar incidence (42%) are non-seminomatous germ cell tumours (NSGCT) with a peak incidence at 20–30 years (see below). Lymphomas, which are often bilateral, occur in the 60–70-year age range.

Pathological Features

Classification of germ cell tumours is as follows:
- seminoma
- NSGCT (Fig. 28.40)
- mixed – these consist of both seminomatous and non-seminomatous elements but should be treated as NSGCT.

The further subdivision of NSGCT is shown in Box 28.15.

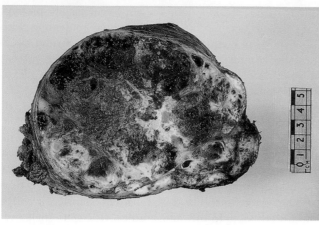

• **Fig. 28.40** A Malignant Teratoma Showing Cystic Degeneration and Haemorrhage

---

• BOX 28.15 Teratomatous tumours of the testis

- Differentiated (TD) – teratoma differentiated
- Intermediate (MTI) – malignant teratoma intermediate
- Undifferentiated (embryonal) carcinoma (MTU) – malignant teratoma undifferentiated
- Trophoblastic (chorionic) carcinoma (MTT) – malignant teratoma trophoblastic

---

TABLE 28.12	Royal Marsden Hospital Staging System.
Stage	**Details**
I	Tumour confined to testis
IM	Rising concentrations of serum markers with no other evidence of metastasis
II	Abdominal node metastasis
A	≤2 cm in diameter
B	2–5 cm in diameter
C	>5 cm in diameter
III	Supradiaphragmatic nodal metastasis
ABC	Node stage as defined in stage II
M	Mediastinal
N	Supraclavicular, cervical or axillary
O	No abdominal node metastasis
IV	Extralymphatic metastasis
Lung	
L1	≤3 metastases
L2	≥3 metastases, all ≤2 cm in diameter
L3	≥3 metastases, one or more of which are ≤2 cm in diameter
H+, Br+, Bo+	Liver, brain or bone metastases

Clinical Features

Symptoms

Ten percent of patients give a history of previous orchidopexy, and in 5%, the tumour is bilateral. There is often a recent history of trauma, although this is not a cause but merely draws the patient's attention to the presence of a lump. The most frequent complaint is of a painless swelling which causes a dragging sensation in the scrotum. In one-third, the swelling is painful. Patients with a choriocarcinoma may develop gynaecomastia. Others present with symptoms from secondary deposits such as backache, haemoptysis, shortness of breath or neurological complaints.

Signs

These include:
- a hard lump in the body of the testis
- diffuse testicular enlargement
- absence of tenderness on gently squeezing the testicle
- hydrocele

Investigation

Tumour Markers

They include alpha-fetoprotein (AFP) and beta-human chorionic gonadotrophin (β-hCG) and lactate dehydrogenase (LDH). Non-seminomatous components secrete both AFP and β-hCG. Lactic dehydrogenase correlates with tumour burden. Pure seminomas do not secrete AFP; 15% have β-hCG. Seminomas may secrete placental alkaline phosphatase (PLAP) though it is mainly used in pathological testing. Tumour markers should be measured preoperatively and postoperatively. Persistently raised post-orchidectomy tumour markers indicates the presence of residual disease.

Imaging

Ultrasound. If it is not possible to determine the nature of the mass in the testicle clinically, ultrasound is particularly helpful. The normal testis has a homogeneous appearance. Malignant tumours are inhomogeneous, may be cystic and may be associated with speckled calcification (microlithiasis).

CT scan. A CT scan of the chest and abdomen is done to identify pulmonary deposits and retroperitoneal and supraclavicular lymphadenopathy. Regular repeated examination is required postoperatively as part of a surveillance schedule.

Staging

Tumour stage and its pathological subtype have considerable influence on management (see below). The Royal Marsden Hospital Staging System is summarized in Table 28.12.

Management

Patients with testicular tumours should be dealt with in specialist centres. There is no doubt that the earlier the diagnosis, the better the results. Improvements in therapy mean that the majority of testicular tumours should be regarded as curable.

Surgery

Orchidectomy is done through an inguinal incision allowing at least 10 cm of spermatic cord to be excised. Operations through the scrotum also have a high incidence of tumour implantation. In order to reduce the risk of disseminating malignant cells by manipulation of the testis, the cord is mobilized and clamped before the testis is delivered from the scrotum. In men with a small or atrophic contralateral testis, or a history of subfertility, a biopsy from the contralateral testis should be taken. Up to 5% of men will have carcinoma in situ involving the other testis.

Adjuvant Management

The management options of seminoma and NSGCT are given in Table 28.13. If chemotherapy is to be used, the patient should be advised to store semen prior to the chemotherapy. Patients with testicular tumours are often subfertile, and chemotherapy may result in irreversible germ cell damage.

Prognosis

The prognosis depends on the extent of metastasis and level of tumour markers.

Seminoma

For those who have metastatic disease, the 5-year survival is approximately 90% if there are no visceral metastasis beyond the lung. The 5-year survival falls to 70% if there are visceral non-pulmonary metastasis.

Non-Seminomatous Germ Cell Tumours

The 5-year survival in the presence of lymph node and/ or pulmonary metastasis is approximately 90%. If the tumour markers are moderately elevated (AFP = 1000–10 000 ng/mL or HCG = 5000 – 50 000 mIU/L), the 5-year survival falls to 80%; it falls to 50% if markers were significantly elevated (AFP >10 000 ng/mL or HCG >50 000 mIU/L) or there are non-pulmonary metastasis.

ANDROLOGY

Infertility

Ten percent of couples have difficulty in conception. In approximately one-third, the problem lies with the male and in a further one-third, there are contributory factors from both. Unless the male is found to be azoospermic (a complete absence of sperm), investigations of both partners should proceed simultaneously. The purpose of investigation is to give the couple a prognosis on the likelihood of conception. Couples who have been trying for more than 5 years with regular unprotected intercourse are unlikely to conceive without assisted conception.

Clinical Features

History

Relevant questions include:
- age of both partners
- length of time trying to conceive
- previous children of both
- frequency of intercourse
- whether intercourse is taking place in the vagina

A previous medical history of orchitis, sexually transmitted infections, inguinal or scrotal surgery, testicular injury or fallopian tube injury or disease, such as pelvic inflammatory disease, should be sought. The occupation of both may be of significance, as may their general health and social habits (drug and alcohol intake).

Physical Examination

In the male, testicular and epididymal size should be assessed, the presence of a vas on both sides confirmed and gynaecomastia excluded.

In the female, further examination is usually performed by a gynaecologist and is not further considered here.

Investigation

Semen Analysis

This is the most useful investigation. The patient should abstain from intercourse for at least 2 days, and the specimen

---

TABLE 28.13 Supplementary Management of Seminoma and Teratoma After Orchidectomy.

Stage	Seminoma	Teratoma
I	Pelvic and para-aortic irradiation for relapse	Surveillance
		Platinum-based chemotherapy for relapse
IIa & b	Irradiation	Platinum-based chemotherapy
		Radical retroperitoneal lymphadonectomy for residual disease
IIC	Platinum-based combination chemotherapy	Platinum-based chemotherapy
		Radical retroperitoneal lymphadenectomy for residual disease

should be produced by masturbation into a sterile container and examined within 1 hour of production. The measurements provided by the laboratory and their normal values are shown in Table 28.14.

If white blood cells are found, a further semen specimen should be cultured for bacteria. The mixed agglutination reaction (MAR) test screens for antisperm antibodies and should be <50%.

Endocrine Analysis

Measurements of testosterone and prolactin are only required if a patient complains of lack of libido. In those with small testes, the FSH concentration in the blood should be measured. If it is elevated and the patient has azoospermia, no further action is required as no treatment is available.

Management

In patients with oligospermia, it may be possible to separate out the most actively motile sperm and use these for artificial insemination. Azoospermia and a normal FSH suggest a diagnosis of testicular obstruction, which may be amenable to surgical correction.

Treatment of varicocele may improve both the sperm count and motility but not necessarily conception. Infected semen is an indication for treatment with antibiotics as for prostatitis. In the presence of antisperm antibodies, there is some evidence that treatment with prednisolone improves pregnancy rates, but using high-dose steroids has significant risks and side-effects.

It is possible to directly aspirate sperm from the epididymis or extract viable sperm from a testicular biopsy. These sperm can be directly implanted into an ovum (Intra Cytoplasmic Sperm Injection – ICSI). These techniques are used in cases of severe oligospermia and azoospermia.

Impotence

A better term is erectile dysfunction. The definition is the inability to achieve and maintain an erection for completion of satisfactory intercourse. There is a predominantly organic

cause in approximately 80% of men, but the fact that they cannot have penetrative sex introduces an additional psychological element.

Aetiology

Organic

Organic factors are:
- generalized atherosclerosis
- diabetes mellitus
- multiple sclerosis
- post pelvic surgery (bladder, prostate, rectum/colon)
- post pelvic radiotherapy
- pelvic fracture with urethral injury
- endocrine dysfunction
- anti-hypertensive therapy
- corporeal venous dysfunction
- other drugs

Psychogenic

The psychodynamics are poorly understood and probably multifactorial.

Clinical Features

Organic

The findings are those of the underlying cause.

Psychogenic

In this form, the following are more likely to be present:
- age less than 50
- non-smoker – smokers may have vascular disease
- absence of neurological or endocrine disorder
- no anti-hypertensive therapy
- presence of nocturnal and early morning erections
- erections with different partners
- erection is often present up to the time of attempted penetration

Investigation

These are required only in the following situations:
- The patient presents with lack of libido, when measurements of serum testosterone and prolactin concentrations are required.
- Young patients with impotence as a result of pelvic trauma, to ensure that there is not a correctable arterial problem.

Management

Those with obvious psychogenic causes may benefit from psychosexual counselling. Correctable organic disease should be treated.

Therapies are as outlined below:
- Sildenafil, vardenafil and tadalafil are members of type 5 phosphodiesterase inhibitors which prevent the breakdown of cyclic GMP, a second messenger for smooth muscle relaxation. They improve erectile ability sufficiently to allow intercourse to take place in approximately 60% of men with organic disease.

TABLE 28.14	Semen Analysis.
Measurement	Normal value
Volume	2–6 mL
Sperm concentration	More than 50 million/mL
Sperm motility	More than 60%
Abnormal sperms	Not more than 30%
White blood cells	None
Mixed agglutination reaction (MAR)	Negative

- Intraurethral prostaglandin E1. A small pellet of prostaglandin is inserted into the anterior urethra in men with organic erectile dysfunction – 66% achieve an erection satisfactory for intercourse.
- Intracavernosal prostaglandin E1. The patient administers an injection of prostaglandin E1 directly into the corpora cavernosa – 80% of men with organic erectile dysfunction achieve an erection.
- Vacuum erection devices. These consist of a plastic cylinder placed around the penis. By creating a vacuum within the cylinder, the penis becomes erect. The erection is maintained by placing a rubber constriction device around the base of the penis prior to removal of the cylinder.

- Penile prostheses. These are of two types: a semi-malleable and an inflatable. They are inserted at operation into both corpora cavernosa. They should only be considered when other treatments have failed.

Complications

Complications are:
- Phosphodiesterase inhibitors – facial flushing, headache, gastro-oesophageal reflux, visual disturbances
- Intraurethral prostaglandins – penile pain and discomfort
- Intracavernosal prostaglandin – penile discomfort, penile fibrosis, prolonged erection
- Vacuum devices – penile oedema and bruising
- Penile prostheses – pain, infection, extrusion

Further Reading

Mundy AR, Fitzpatrick J, Neal DE, George NJ. *The Scientific Basis of Urology*. 3rd ed. London: Informa Healthcare; 2010.

Reynard J, Brewster S, Briers S. *Oxford Handbook of Urology*. 3rd ed. Oxford: OUP; 2013.

Tanagho EA, McAninch JW. *Smith's General Urology*. 17th ed. New York: McGraw-Hill Medical; 2008.

29

Common Neurosurgical Conditions

Neurosurgery involves the treatment of medical and surgical conditions affecting the brain, spinal cord and peripheral nerves. Historically, neurosurgery has been based upon fundamental principles of decompressing neural tissue with the aim of preserving function and preventing deterioration but, as our understanding of neuroscience progresses, neurosurgeons have explored novel domains including neuromodulation (e.g. deep brain stimulation) and restorative therapies (e.g. peripheral nerve repair).

Basic Clinical Principles

Being a tertiary specialty, modern neurosurgical assessment is often undertaken after a diagnosis has been reached, usually via some form of advanced imaging. However, treatment decisions are often based around the concept of clinico-radiological correlation and therefore, a sound understanding of clinical neurological assessment forms a crucial part of accurate decision making.

Clinical Assessment

As with any other field in medicine, a systematic approach to assessing a patient begins with assessment of the airway, breathing and circulation (ABC). In cases of trauma, additional consideration must be given to cervical spine immobilization and the systematic approach should follow Advanced Trauma Life Support (ATLS) primary survey protocol (Box 29.1). This systematic approach is all the more important as many neurosurgical patients present in coma, which may necessitate swift life-saving interventions.

Following acute stabilization, a history and examination can be conducted, although both may be limited in situations where a patient is in coma. In such cases, collateral histories should be sought from family members, bystanders and paramedic staff. Examination should focus on assessment of the level of consciousness (see next), followed by an assessment of the upper limbs, lower limbs and cranial nerves and, if appropriate, higher cognitive function.

Assessment of the Level of Consciousness

The Glasgow Coma Scale (GCS) (Box 29.2) is now universally used. It consists of three domains (eye opening, verbal response, motor response) which deteriorate as coma deepens. The score for each component is recorded and the total for the patient obtained. A fully conscious patient scores 15 points, whilst one who is completely unresponsive, or indeed dead, scores 3. Coma is considered to be 8 points or less, and usually correlates with a need for securing a definitive airway *via endotracheal intubation*. A detailed tutorial on how to assess the GCS, from the original group in Glasgow, can be found at www.glasgowcomascale.org. Changes can be easily noted on a chart, and the scale is simple enough to be reproduced accurately by a range of healthcare professionals and a score of 8 or less correlates with severe brain injury.

An extremely useful adjunct to the GCS is the size and reactivity of the pupils to light. 'Fixed and dilated' pupil(s) may be a sign of raised intracranial pressure and uncal herniation causing compression of the oculomotor (III) nerve, although other local injuries to the orbit/globe (and mydriatic agents) may cause similar signs or preclude assessment.

Investigations

Computed Tomography

CT has revolutionized diagnostic neurology since its introduction in the mid-1970s. It allows imaging of brain, skull bones, soft tissues and spinal column and has become the first-line of investigation for many conditions treated by neurosurgeons. Modern technology enables 3D reconstruction of the bony skeleton and non-invasive cerebral angiography (CTA).

Magnetic Resonance Imaging

In recent years, the use of MRI has moved on from a purely diagnostic tool to one that has augmented our understanding of normal and abnormal brain function. Unlike CT, soft tissues (the neural tissue of the brain and spinal cord) can be imaged and it has now become the gold standard for imaging of the brain and spinal cord. Like CT, MR can be used for non-invasive angiography (MRA) and venography (MRV). It can also be used for characterizing tissue properties such as through diffusion-weighted imaging (DWI) and MR spectroscopy. It can identify white matter tracts (diffusion-tensor imaging or DTI) and areas of eloquent brain (functional MRI or fMRI) that are useful adjuncts in the planning of brain tumour surgery. In addition to identifying, localizing and characterizing structural abnormalities of the brain and spinal cord, it has a growing role in prognostication in situations such as severe traumatic brain injury.

Digital Subtraction Angiography

Contrast medium is injected into the cerebral or spinal arteries to see and delineate the blood vessels and associated aneurysms and arteriovenous anomalies. The blood supply of a tumour can also be visualized. Although diagnostic invasive angiography is declining in use whilst that of CT and MR angiography increases, therapeutic angiography to treat cerebral aneurysms, arteriovenous malformations (AVMs) and embolize tumours prior to surgery to reduce intraoperative blood loss is being used more frequently. Invasive angiography is also being used in acute stroke to retrieve clots in large vessels (thrombectomy).

Lumbar Puncture (LP)

LPs provide a means of sampling CSF from the lumbar cistern and are used to diagnose subarachnoid haemorrhage (xanthochromia and a bilirubin peak on spectrophotometry) if CT scanning is non-diagnostic and meningitis (pus cells on microscopy and bacteria on Gram stain or culture). It may also be used therapeutically to drain CSF in communicating hydrocephalus. LP should only be performed after imaging to rule out a space-occupying lesion or decreased CSF volume around the brainstem.

Electrophysiology

Recording of electrophysiological (especially epileptic) activity from the brain can occur via electrodes in the scalp (electroencephalography or EEG), on the surface of the brain (electrocorticography or ECoG) or even within the brain (stereoelectroencephalography or SEEG). Nerve conduction studies and electromyography are important in the diagnosis of peripheral nerve and radicular lesions.

The Monro–Kellie Doctrine: The Central Tenet of Cranial Neurosurgery

Although initially investigated by Alexander Monro and George Kellie, it is Harvey Cushing who is credited with describing the doctrine as we know it today: with an intact skull, the sum of the volume of brain, blood and CSF is constant. The introduction of another mass (tumour, haematoma, CSF) causes a decrease in the original three components, until a certain point when compensatory mechanisms fail, resulting in elevated intracranial pressure, perturbed perfusion of the brain and therefore damage to neural tissue (Fig. 29.1). Although an oversimplification, much of neurosurgery and neurocritical care can be understood through an appreciation of this basic principle.

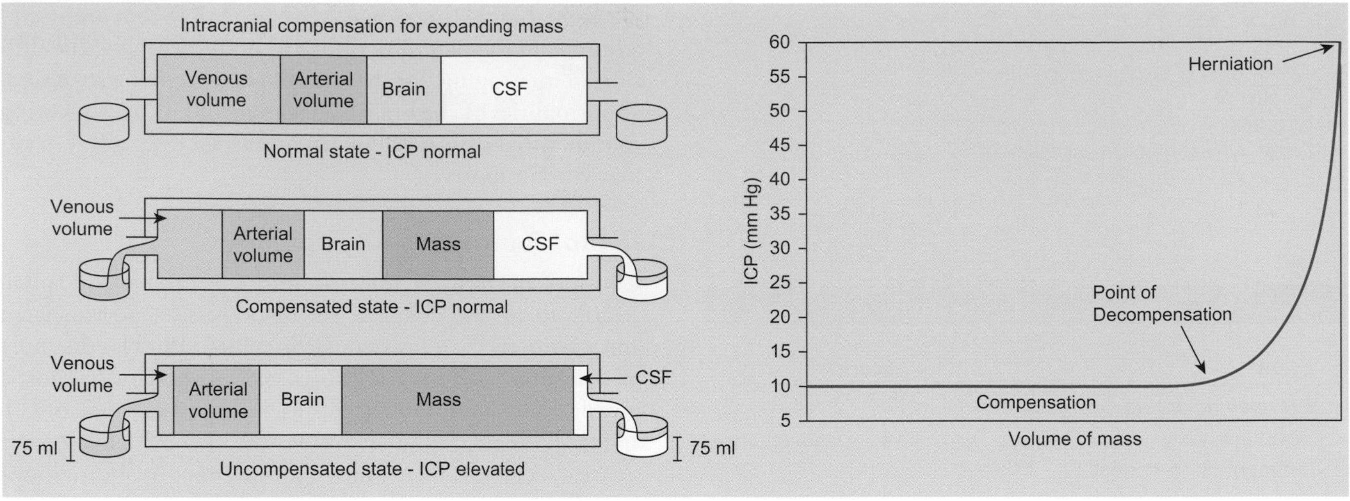

• **Fig. 29.1** The Monro–Kellie Doctrine

Cranial and Spinal Trauma

Traumatic Brain Injury

Traumatic brain injury (TBI) is a leading cause of death and disability and places a huge demand on individuals and society. Incidence of ED visits related to TBI in the United States is estimated at 800/100 000 per year and mortality of about 17/100 000 per year, with similar figures applying to Europe.

Pathophysiology

Traumatic brain injury (TBI) can be categorized into primary and secondary, a description of the timing of cellular damage. Primary brain injury occurs immediately on impact. Movement of the brain within the skull results in tearing of neurons and blood vessels. The severity of injury is dependent on the force of impact. Injury to neural tissue can be diffuse or focal. Focal injury can occur at the site of impact (coup injury) or diametrically opposite to the point of impact (contrecoup injury), both of which are caused by the impact of the brain on the skull. Common sites for contusions (bruising) in the brain include the base of the frontal temporal lobes. Diffuse injury is caused by rotational and shearing forces and has a predilection for the interface between the grey and white matter, the corpus callosum and brainstem.

Secondary brain injury results from ongoing cellular insult caused by hypoxia, cerebral ischaemia, inflammation, infarction and infection and is potentially avoidable. Injury to the brain results in oedema and swelling, which may cause a rise in ICP, resulting in a concomitant decrease in the perfusion pressure to the brain as the cerebral perfusion pressure (CPP) is determined by the difference between mean arterial pressure (MAP) and ICP. The body compensates by raising the arterial blood pressure to maintain perfusion. Usually, the phenomenon of autoregulation regulates blood flow to the brain across a range of arterial pressures but this mechanism is disrupted in TBI, resulting in further increases in

cerebral blood volume and therefore ICP, further reducing CPP and leading to a self-perpetuating situation resulting in secondary damage (Fig. 29.2).

Although preventative strategies (e.g. helmets and seatbelts, each of which were popularized in the UK by neurosurgeons Hugh Cairns and John Gillingham, respectively) have played a significant role in reducing primary brain injury, little can be done to reverse this damage. The mainstay of neurosurgical and neurocritical care management of TBI lies in treatments designed to reduce secondary brain injury.

Other causes of raised pressure include:
- Expanding intracranial haematoma.
- Epilepsy. The brain uses glucose and oxygen abundantly when a seizure is taking place, and ischaemia develops rapidly if they are not controlled.
- Hydrocephalus. This can occur due to mass lesions in the posterior fossa, intraventricular haemorrhage causing obstructive hydrocephalus or brain injury with communicating hydrocephalus.

Clinical Assessment and Management

Resuscitation. Initial resuscitation, according to ATLS principles, includes cervical spine immobilization, and assessment and treatment of the airway, breathing and circulation (see Box 29.1). Head injury patients commonly have multiple other injuries and a compromised airway can kill a patient much more quickly than an expanding intracranial haematoma. Following this systematic approach should also ensure adequate ventilation, preventing cerebral hypoxia, and circulatory support, preventing cerebral ischaemia by maintaining cerebral perfusion pressure.

Further assessment includes:
- A brief history, including the time of injury, mechanism and factors that may affect the extent of injury (e.g. speed of vehicle, seatbelt, helmet, etc, for road traffic accidents).
- Examining the head for lacerations and signs of skull and base of skull fractures (e.g. battle sign, Racoon eyes, CSF rhinorrhoea/otorrhoea).

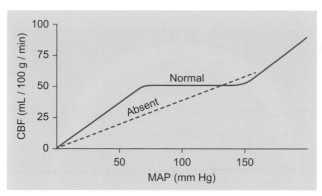

• **Fig. 29.2** Intracranial pressure is normally kept constant by autoregulation. This is disrupted in traumatic brain injury and autoregulation is lost. This results in an increase in intracranial pressure. CBF, Cerebral blood flow; MAP, mean arterial pressure.

• Assessment of the Glasgow Coma Score (GCS), pupillary response and lateralizing limb neurology.
• CT scanning is essential to identify injuries that may require neurosurgical intervention. The National Institute for Health and Care Excellence (NICE) provide clear and useful guidelines regarding which patients should be scanned and when. In major trauma, in addition to a CT scan of the head, CT of the cervical spine, chest, abdomen and pelvis may also be undertaken to assess for other injuries.

Based on this assessment, patients can be broadly divided into categories of severity, based on the Mayo classification (Table 29.1) or based on the GCS (13–15 is mild, 9–12 is moderate and 3–8 is severe).

Management

Once the acute resuscitation has been completed and imaging performed, key management steps include:
• Measurement and correction of coagulopathy, especially if a patient is known to be on anticoagulant medication. Local protocol should be followed and may include a combination of prothrombin complex concentrate (PCC), fresh frozen plasma (FFP) and vitamin K.
• Anti-epileptic medication either to treat or prevent seizures. The use of seizure prophylaxis and choice of antiepileptic agent for seizure treatment are highly variable, although common options include phenytoin and levetiracetam.

Acute Surgical Intervention

The decision-making process for acute surgical intervention is based upon a combination of the patient's presenting features and CT scan findings. Indications for acute intervention may include:
• Acute extradural (Fig. 29.3A), subdural (see Fig. 29.3B) or intracerebral haematomas: may require emergency craniotomy to remove the clot and prevent life-threatening herniation.
• External ventricular drain (EVD) insertion: as part of the treatment strategy to control intracranial pressure, a drain may be inserted into the ventricles to drain CSF.

TABLE 29.1	Mayo Classification of Traumatic Brain Injury.
Classification	**Criteria**
Moderate-severe (definite)	Death
	Loss of consciousness >30 minutes
	Antegrade amnesia >24 hours
	GCS score <13 in the initial 24 hours
	Intracerebral, subdural, epidural or subarachnoid haemorrhages; cerebral or haemorrhagic contusion, penetrating TBI (dura penetrated) or brainstem injury
Mild (probable)	Loss of consciousness – momentarily to <30 minutes
	Post-traumatic anterograde amnesia – momentarily to <2–4 hours
	Depressed basilar or linear skull fracture (dura intact)
Symptomatic (possible)	None of the 'moderate-severe' or 'mild' criteria apply
	One or more of the following present: blurred vision, confusion (mental status changes), dizziness, headache, nausea or focal neurological symptoms

Adapted from http://practicalneurology.com/2018/04/single-isolated-concussion-part-i-definitions-classification-and-prognosis/

• Decompressive craniectomy (either hemispheric (see Fig. 29.3C) or bifrontal (see Fig. 29.3D)): a significant portion of bone is removed to allow space for the brain to swell. This is often performed in the first few days of admission for refractory elevated ICP following a period of ICP monitoring. A large recent multicentre randomized trial, the RescueICP study[1] has shown that decompressive craniectomy effectively reduces death at 6 months from 49% to 27% compared to ongoing medical care but increases the proportion of patients in a vegetative state or with severe disability.
• Elevation of depressed skull fracture: to prevent intracranial haemorrhage, mass effect, CSF leak and infection. It is often necessary if the depression is greater than the thickness of the skull.
• Repair of base of skull fractures causing CSF leak.

Neurocritical Care Management

Irrespective of whether surgical intervention occurs, severe TBI patients should be cared for on a dedicated neurocritical care unit, using established protocols designed to reduce cerebral metabolic demands and optimize perfusion in order to prevent secondary brain injury. These often follow a tiered approach, based on the ICP monitoring (Fig. 29.4).

A

B

C

D

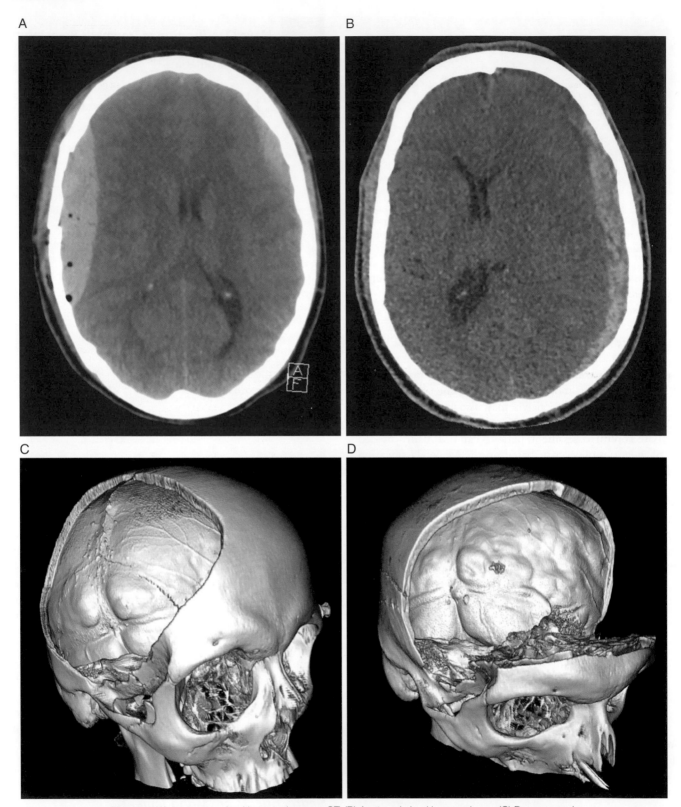

• **Fig. 29.3** (A) Acute extradural haemorrhage on CT. (B) Acute subdural haemorrhage. (C) Decompressive craniotomy (hemispheric). (D) Decompressive craniotomy (bifrontal).

Outcome After Head Injury

The best prognostic indicator for outcome is the patient's best GCS score after resuscitation. The consequences of even mild head injury can be very significant with patients suffering from poor memory, personality changes, physical disability, epilepsy and depression either alone or in combination, which can have a significant impact on work and social life. Families may be wrecked by the difficulties of caring for these people. Intensive rehabilitation with physiotherapy, speech therapy, occupational

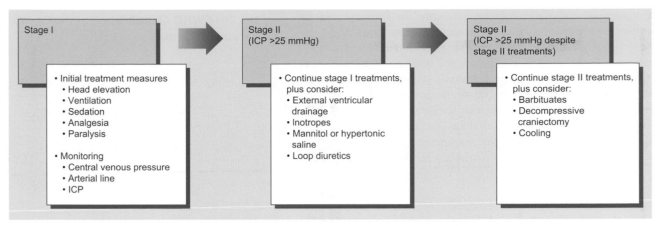

• **Fig. 29.4** Neurocritical Care Management of Traumatic Brain Injury.

therapy and psychological help started soon after injury may reduce the difficulties and improve functional outcomes.

Chronic Subdural Haematoma

Subdural collections can be acute or chronic. Although trauma is clearly a significant factor in the aetiology of acute subdurals, it may only play a minor role in the aetiology of chronic subdurals. Chronic subdurals are far more common than acute subdurals and commonly occur in the elderly.

Pathogenesis

Chronic subdural haematoma (CSDH) is common in conditions of cerebral atrophy, notably old age and alcoholism and in patients on anticoagulant/antiplatelet medication. Minor trauma leads to a small amount of insignificant bleeding in the subdural space. As this blood breaks down, it is thought that an inflammatory process results in the collection expanding rather than being reabsorbed. Chronic subdural haematoma in infants should always raise suspicion of non-accidental injury.

Diagnosis

Usually a hypodense or isodense crescentic collection on CT scan.

Treatment

If symptomatic, these can be treated by burr hole craniostomy or mini-craniotomy, with thorough irrigation with warmed saline. The use of a subdural or subgaleal drain has been shown to reduce recurrence. Although steroids reduce recurrence, the Dex-CSDH study[2] has shown that they result in worse functional outcomes and therefore should not be used.

Spinal Trauma

In the assessment and management of traumatic spinal injuries, one must consider both the bony injury and injury to the neural tissue of the spinal cord or cauda equina nerve roots.

Initial Clinical Assessment

As with traumatic brain injury patients, the ATLS approach must be used in the initial management of patients, including cervical spine immobilization and assessment and management of the airway, breathing and circulation. Securing a definitive airway and ventilation is particularly important in patients with a high cervical spine injury affecting diaphragmatic innervation as these patients can rapidly develop respiratory distress. They can also develop neurogenic shock due to loss of sympathetic outflow. Neurogenic shock is refractory to fluid replacement therapy so early inotropic support is crucial to preventing hypotension and secondary injury to both the brain and spinal cord. At this stage, a gross neurological examination should also be conducted, if the patient is awake, to ensure all four limbs are moving.

Current major trauma protocols often involve CT imaging of the whole spine to identify bony injuries. When a spinal injury is identified on imaging, as a safety mechanism, the patient should be immobilized using a hard cervical collar, flat bed rest and movement only via a log roll. A detailed neurological examination should be undertaken to assess whether there is neurological injury – this has been standardized via the American Spinal Injury Association (ASIA) International Standards for Classification of Spinal Cord Injury assessment scale. If there is any neurological injury, consideration should be given to obtaining an MRI scan of the spine to identify if there are disc fragments, bone fragments or epidural haematomata requiring urgent decompression.

Management

Initial management should be supportive, to ensure adequate oxygenation and perfusion of the injured cord to prevent secondary injury. Vasopressive support should be given expeditiously to ensure mean arterial pressure is maintained above 85 mmHg. Current evidence does not support a role for steroids in patients with traumatic spinal cord injury.

If there is neurological injury, studies such as the STAS-CIS study[3] have shown that early decompression (<24 h after injury) confers better neurological outcomes than delayed decompression. By analogy with traumatic brain injury, opening and expanding the dura may also improve outcomes for significantly disabled patients. Consideration must be given to whether the injury requires instrumented stabilization at the same time – the surgical decision making for this is nuanced and can be achieved, in general principles, via anterior, posterior or 360-degree fixation.

For spinal injuries without neurological deficits, management options include conservative management, non-operative immobilization to allow the fracture to heal (a hard cervical collar for cervical spine or thoracolumbar support orthoses for thoracic and lumbar spine fractures) or instrumented fixation.

Longer-term management, especially for spinal cord injury patients, is centred around rehabilitation and enablement, although there is much hope in both electrical stimulation and regenerative therapies for spinal cord injuries such as stem cell and olfactory ensheathing cell therapy to improve function.

Tumours of the Brain and Meninges

The incidence of brain tumours in the UK is about 18/100 000 per year, with an age-standardized mortality of 8.7/100 000 per year. Although brain tumours account for only 2% of all primary tumours in the UK, they are responsible for 7% of life years lost before the age of 70 and cause about 3000 deaths every year.

Pathology

Most classification systems begin by classifying tumours by their location (supratentorial in 80–85% vs infratentorial in 15–20%) and as either extra-axial (commonly benign and arising from the meninges, e.g. meningiomas) or intra-axial (more likely to be malignant, the most common forms being metastatic tumours and tumours of astrocytic origin).

Histologically, they are graded according to a World Health Organization (WHO) grading system into grades I to IV, progressing from benign to malignant. The 2016 update to the WHO Classification of Tumours of the Central Nervous System expands upon this purely histological classification by incorporating molecular subtypes. Some of the important tumour types are depicted in Table 29.2.

Clinical Features

Brain tumours can present as follows:
- Raised ICP: Classical history is of a few weeks progressively worsening headaches, worst in the mornings and associated with nausea and vomiting. Examination of the fundi may reveal papilloedema. Raised ICP may be caused by the tumour mass, vasogenic oedema or compression of the CSF pathways resulting in obstructive hydrocephalus.
- Seizures: Patients presenting with seizures of late onset should be investigated.

TABLE 29.2	The 2016 WHO Classification of the Central Nervous System.
Diffuse astrocytic oligodendroglial tumours	Melanocytic tumours
Other astrocytic tumours	Lymphomas
Ependymal tumours	Histiocytic tumours
Other gliomas	Germ cell tumours, e.g. germinoma
Choroid plexus tumours	Tumours of the sellar region
Neuronal and mixed neuronal-glial tumours	Metastatic tumours
Tumours of the pineal region	
Embryonal tumours, e.g. medulloblastomas	
Tumours of the cranial and paraspinal nerves, e.g. Schwannoma	
Meningiomas	

- Focal neurological deficit: influenced by the site of the tumour (Fig. 29.5).
- Rarely, tumours are picked up incidentally when patients are scanned for another reason such as trauma.

Investigation

Tumours are often identified on a non-contrast CT scan, but this is insufficient for diagnostic purposes. A gadolinium-enhanced MRI scan should be performed as a minimum, although other sequences, such as diffusion-weighted imaging and MR spectroscopy, may be helpful in delineating the pathology. Surgical planning may be aided by specific sequences such as 3D volumetric T1 post-contrast sequence for neuronavigation and DTI/fMRI to identify eloquent areas of brain that should be avoided during the approach or resection.

If metastases are suspected, staging of (or finding) the primary is required, usually via a CT of the chest, abdomen and pelvis and close coordination with oncologists. Certain tumours (e.g. ependymoma) also require evaluation of the rest of the neuraxis (i.e. MRI whole spine with contrast) to look for drop metastases.

Management

Immediate management should start with the ABC approach. In the acute period, steroids (usually dexamethasone, with gastric protection) may be required to reduce the surrounding oedema and antiepileptics if the patient presented with a seizure. Rarely, emergency surgery, such as a craniotomy to debulk the tumour or external ventricular drainage/shunting to treat hydrocephalus, may be required

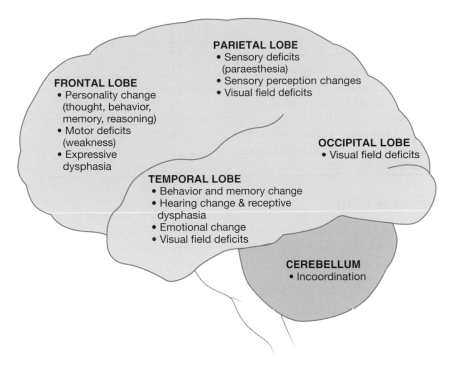

PARIETAL LOBE
- Sensory deficits (paraesthesia)
- Sensory perception changes
- Visual field deficits

FRONTAL LOBE
- Personality change (thought, behavior, memory, reasoning)
- Motor deficits (weakness)
- Expressive dysphasia

OCCIPITAL LOBE
- Visual field deficits

TEMPORAL LOBE
- Behavior and memory change
- Hearing change & receptive dysphasia
- Emotional change
- Visual field deficits

CEREBELLUM
- Incoordination

• **Fig. 29.5** Focal Neurological Deficit Depending on the Site of Tumour

but most cases are able to wait to be discussed at a multidisciplinary team meeting in order to offer the optimal management strategy. Patients and their relatives should be involved in the planning of an individualized strategy. Options may include combinations of the following:

Surgery

The aim of surgery is usually to obtain tissue to get a diagnosis and to reduce the mass effect caused by the tumour. Certain tumours are amenable to complete curative resection (e.g. meningioma) but, for high-grade tumours (e.g. glioblastoma), the aim is to resect as much tumour as possible without causing or worsening the neurological deficit. Many techniques have been developed to optimize this balance. Extent of resection has been shown to affect prognosis and this can be maximized using neuronavigation, fluorescence (commonly 5-ALA) and intraoperative ultrasound/MRI. Functional brain can be preserved by using advanced imaging such as DTI and fMRI, and awake surgery, in which the patient remains awake during the resection and function is assessed by cortical stimulation and mapping. Common risks of surgery include infection, bleeding, seizures, neurological deficit, stroke, CSF leak and a small risk to life.

Stereotactic Radiosurgery (SRS)

This involves the placement of a stereotactic frame and application of focused high-dose single fraction of radiation to a specific area of the brain. Whilst SRS is non-invasive and does not require a general anaesthetic, there are limitations including the lack of tissue for histological diagnosis and size limitations (usually 3 cm in maximum diameter). SRS is useful for small, difficult to resect meningiomas, acoustic neuromas and metastases.

Oncological Therapy

This may include chemotherapy, conventional (intensity-modulated) radiation therapy and emerging therapies such as proton beam therapy and immunotherapy. The gold standard adjuvant treatment regimen for glioblastoma is referred to as the Stupp protocol, which involves a combination of chemotherapy using temozolamide and radiation therapy. Even with optimal management, median survival for glioblastoma is around 14–16 months with only a quarter of patients surviving 2 years from diagnosis.

Best Supportive Care

In patients who are not candidates for surgical or oncological therapy, it is important to optimize symptoms through good supportive and palliative care.

Paediatric Tumours

Brain tumours are the most common solid tumours in children and the second most common form of cancer, with an incidence of approximately 2–5 cases per 100 000. The intracranial distribution is different compared with adults, 40% occurring above the tentorium and 60% below.

Posterior fossa tumours, such as medulloblastomas, pilocytic astrocytomas and ependymomas are most common. The principles of classification are identical to those used for adult tumours. Again, the approach to treatment of paediatric tumours is multidisciplinary with combinations of surgery, chemotherapy, radiotherapy and immunotherapy being employed. Presentation with symptoms and signs of obstructive hydrocephalus is likely.

Cerebral Haemorrhage and Stroke

Cerebral haemorrhage makes up a large part of neurosurgical practice, much of which is related to trauma. This chapter focuses on the management of spontaneous cerebral haemorrhage, which can be classified by its location. The two most common locations are:

- Intracerebral haemorrhage: Within the brain substance
- Subarachnoid haemorrhage: In the subarachnoid space (which may include the ventricular system)

Intracerebral Haemorrhage (ICH)

This accounts for 10–20% of all strokes and is associated with the highest mortality and morbidity. The haemorrhage is most often deep within the cerebral substance and is usually associated with hypertension.

Clinical Features

The most common site in adults is within the basal ganglia and thalamic region. Presentation is often with sudden-onset headache, neurological deficit and possibly coma. CT scans reveal a hyperdense haematoma within the brain parenchyma (Fig. 29.6A). In most patients, a CT angiogram and/or delayed MRI scan should be performed to exclude other causes such as aneurysms, AVMs, amyloid angiopathy and bleeding into tumours.

Surgical Intervention

Surgical intervention is not usually indicated for basal ganglia or thalamic ICH. A pooled analysis of results from the UK-based Surgical Trial in Intracerebral Haemorrhage (STICH) trials[4,5] suggests that early surgical intervention, via craniotomy and evacuation of the haematoma, may have a role for large (>30 mL), superficial (<1 cm from the cortical surface) clots where the patient has a GCS between 9 and 12. Newer preliminary studies suggest that minimally invasive evacuation of haematoma and washout with thrombolytic agents may also have a role.

Cerebellar haemorrhage may need surgical intervention due to compression of the fourth ventricle (causing obstructive hydrocephalus), necessitating insertion of an external ventricular drain. In cases where the clot is large, brainstem compression can also occur, necessitating a posterior fossa craniectomy and evacuation of haematoma.

Subarachnoid Haemorrhage (SAH)

Spontaneous SAH has an incidence of about 10–15 per 100 000 population per year. Common causes include aneurysm rupture (75–80%) and bleeding from an arteriovenous malformation (5%); a cause is not found in 10–15%. Risk factors include smoking and hypertension.

Clinical Features

The characteristic presentation is of a severe, sudden-onset (thunderclap) headache, associated with photophobia and neck stiffness. This may be preceded by a headache for 2–3 days (sentinel headache). A decreased level of consciousness or focal neurological deficit may also occur. At presentation, patients may be graded by clinical (WFNS) or radiological (Modified Fisher) scoring systems (Table 29.3).

Management

- Resuscitation: A, B, C, D
- Establish diagnosis: Options include:
  a. CT scan: Modern CT scans may be up to 98% sensitive if performed within 24 h of the ictus (see Fig. 29.6B)
  b. Lumbar puncture: Performed if the CT scan is negative but there remains clinical suspicion from the history. Needs to be performed at least 12 h after the ictus to allow time for the haemoglobin to be broken down into bilirubin. Can stay positive for 2–4 weeks following the initial bleed
  c. CT or MR angiography (non-invasive) or digital subtraction angiography (invasive) to identify cause of haemorrhage (see Fig. 29.6C)
- Treatment: Considered in two parts:
  a. Securing the aneurysm: Traditionally this was done by placing a small titanium clip across its neck by open craniotomy. Alternatively, the aneurysm may be filled with platinum coils or be by-passed using stents or flow diverters by endovascular techniques. The ISAT trial[6] suggested that the mortality and morbidity following endovascular coiling of an aneurysm following rupture is significantly less than that for surgical clipping, although the results of long-term follow-up for this cohort are rather more controversial. Coiling has now become the treatment of choice for most aneurysms in most centres, although some aneurysms are better treated by open clipping. Most cases should be discussed in a multidisciplinary format (consisting of neurovascular neurosurgeons and interventional neuroradiologists) before treatment.
  b. Managing the complications: There are numerous potential complications that must be looked for and addressed in these patients, including:
    i. Rebleeding: Before the aneurysm is secured, there is a risk of rebleeding, which is about 4% per day in the first 48 h and 1% per day for the next 2 weeks. Pending expeditious treatment, patients should be placed on bed rest, given laxatives to prevent excessive straining and have their blood pressure controlled to a maximum systolic blood pressure of 140 mmHg.
    ii. Vasospasm/delayed ischaemic neurological deficit: The risk of vasospasm and resultant ischaemia is highest between days 3 and 14 after the initial bleed. Vasospasm is prevented through the historic 'triple H' strategy of hypervolaemia, haemodilution and hypertension, involving treatment with 60 mg nimodipine every 4 h for 21 days and generous (3 L/day) fluid replacement. If a patient develops a new neurological deficit attributable to vasospasm, treatment involves augmentation of blood pressure using vasopressors on an intensive care unit; other less established therapies include intra-arterial delivery of calcium channel blockers and angioplasty/stenting of affected vessels.

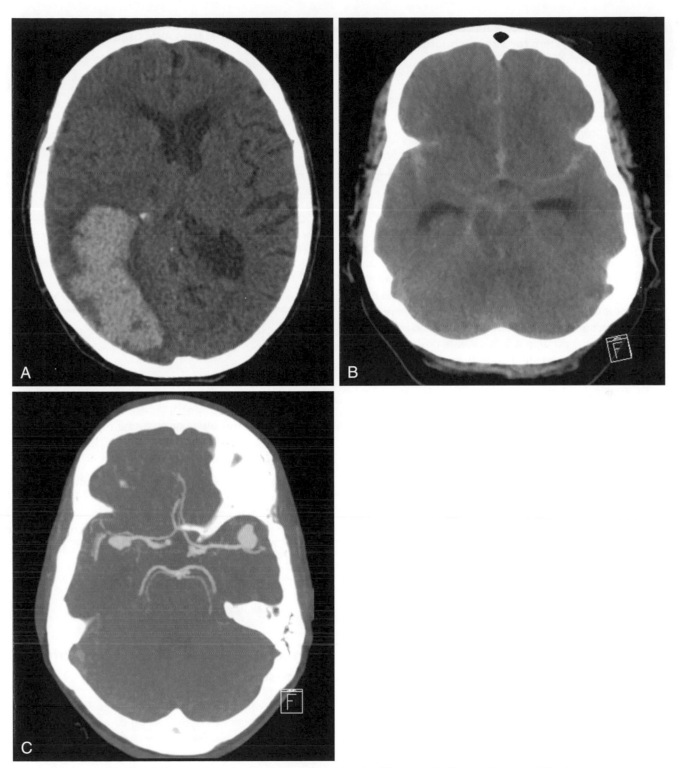

• **Fig. 29.6** CT scans of spontaneous haemorrhage showing (A) intracerebral haemorrhage and (B) subarachnoid haemorrhage. (C) CT angiogram, revealing bilateral middle cerebral artery aneurysms.

iii. Hydrocephalus: Can often be acute, necessitating emergency insertion of an external ventricular drain. Some patients may develop delayed hydrocephalus requiring permanent CSF diversion via a ventriculoperitoneal shunt.

iv. Electrolyte disturbances: Sodium abnormalities, especially hyponatraemia secondary to the syndrome of inappropriate antidiuretic hormone

(SIADH) are common. Daily electrolyte profiles are mandatory.

v. Seizures: If present, should be managed with antiepileptics. Many can be used but levetiracetam tends to be the agent of choice in the first instance.

vi. Cardiac complications: About half of patients with SAH may have electrocardiographic abnormalities, some of which may be identical to that of an acute

TABLE 29.3	World Federation of Neurological Surgeons Grading System for Subarachnoid Haemorrhage (WFNS) Scale.		
Glasgow Coma Score	Motor Deficit	Grade
15	Absent	1
13–14	Absent	2
13–14	Present	3
7–12	Present or absent	4
3–6	Present or absent	5

TABLE 29.4	Spetzler-Martin AVM Grading Scale.	
Spetzler-Martin AVM Grading Scale	Points
Size	
0–3 cm	1
3.1–6.0 cm	2
> 6 cm	3
Location	
Noneloquent	0
Eloquent[a]	1
Deep venous drainage	
Not Present	0
Present	1
AVM Total Score	1–5

[a]Eloquent locations: areas of sensorimotor, language, visual, thalamus, hypothalamus, internal capsule, brainstem, cerebellar peduncles and deep cerebellar nuclei
The lower the score, the better the outcome.

myocardial infarction such as T-wave inversion and ST segment elevation/depression. Patients may also develop a neurogenic stress cardiomyopathy and neurogenic pulmonary oedema requiring vasopressive and ventilatory support in the intensive care unit.

An AVM, if superficial and in a suitable position, can be surgically excised. However, if deep or in an area of vital function, it can be treated by embolization or stereotactic radiosurgery. Treatment decisions are individualized but often based around the Spetzler-Martin grading system (Table 29.4).

Ischaemic Stroke

The role for neuroendovascular specialists in the management of ischaemic stroke is growing due to the rapidly increasing evidence for mechanical thrombectomy in acute stroke.

Decompressive Craniectomy

Thus far, the established role for neurosurgery is in acute malignant middle cerebral artery (MCA) infarction, where, in the right setting, a decompressive hemicraniectomy may be performed. Three landmark studies (DECIMAL,[7] DESTINY[8] and HAMLET[9]) showed that decompressive craniectomy effectively reduces mortality but increases the proportion of patients with a severe disability. Current NICE guidance suggests that decompressive craniectomy should be considered when the following criteria are met:

- Age ≤60
- Clinical deficits suggestive of MCA infarction with National Institute of Health Stroke Score (NIHSS) >15
- Decrease in the level of consciousness to give a score of 1 or more on item 1a of the NIHSS
- Signs on CT of an infarct of at least 50% of the middle cerebral artery territory, with or without additional infarction in the territory of the anterior or posterior cerebral artery on the same side, or infarct volume greater than 145 cm^3 as shown on diffusion-weighted MRI
- Within 72 hours of symptom onset

Surgical intervention may also be warranted for ischaemic stroke in the cerebellum as the oedema can cause obstructive hydrocephalus (necessitating insertion of an external ventricular drain) or brainstem compression (necessitating a posterior fossa craniectomy).

Mechanical Thrombectomy

Several recent studies have established the role for mechanical thrombectomy in ischaemic stroke. This is currently limited to patients with established large vessel (middle cerebral artery or internal carotid artery) occlusion, within 6 hours of stroke onset, although more recent studies such as the DAWN and DEFUSE-3 studies[10,11] have shown that, with careful selection using advanced imaging, patients may benefit from mechanical thrombectomy up to 16–24 hours after symptom onset.

Congenital Anomalies and Paediatric Neurosurgery

With better intrauterine diagnosis, congenital anomalies of the central nervous system can be detected early in pregnancy. If remediable, the need for early post-delivery or even pre-delivery treatment can be anticipated and arranged.

Spinal Dysraphism

A group of conditions where the neural tube fails to close, a process that normally takes place during the first 25 days of fetal development. It affects 2/1000 live births (2–3/100 if found in a sibling). It is commonly associated with other abnormalities such as hydrocephalus.

Conditions vary from asymptomatic spina bifida occulta to open myelomeningoceles:
- Spina bifida occulta: A bony defect where the spinous process is absent, usually with no clinical significance. However, if a tuft of hair, sinus, dimple or mark on the skin overlying the defect is present, it may be associated with underlying defects.
- Meningocele: A CSF-filled cavity formed by outpouching of the posterior wall of the neural tube through the space formed by the bony defect.
- Myelomeningocele: The CSF space has parts of the spinal cord or roots within it. The skin covering the defect may break down, allowing cord and roots to become externalized, and CSF to leak. As a consequence, meningitis often occurs and can be life-threatening.

Presentation

- Skin defects over the lumbar spine
- Neurological deficit, including weakness in the legs, diminished pain response and bladder dysfunction
- Identification of associated pathology, including Chiari II malformation, lipomas, cord tethering and sinuses Investigations include ultrasound and MRI.

Management

Spina bifida occulta may not require any treatment. A meningocele associated with a CSF leak should be repaired immediately due to the risk of CNS infection. In the absence of a leak, excision can be delayed or may not be necessary at all. Surgical intervention in myelomeningocele aims at replacing the neural tissue into the spinal canal and closing the communication between the CSF space and the outside world. Surgical closure can be life-saving in preventing meningitis but may not improve neurological deficit, including paraplegia and loss of sphincter control. There have been recent advancements in prenatal surgery for myelomeningocele, with the landmark MOMS trial[12] suggesting that it reduced the requirement for CSF diversion and improved motor outcomes; this needs to be balanced against maternal and fetal risks.

Encephaloceles

In this condition, fusion of the neural tube fails at the cranial end. Meninges and brain herniate through the defects in the skull, most commonly in the occipital region and frontonasal areas. They are surgically corrected with great care as they often contain vascular structures.

Craniosynostosis

Premature fusion of one or more cranial sutures causes excessive compensatory growth perpendicular to the fused suture (Virchow's Law). Craniosynostosis is usually classified as syndromic (e.g. Apert, Pfeiffer or Crouzon Syndromes associated with autosomal dominant mutations in the

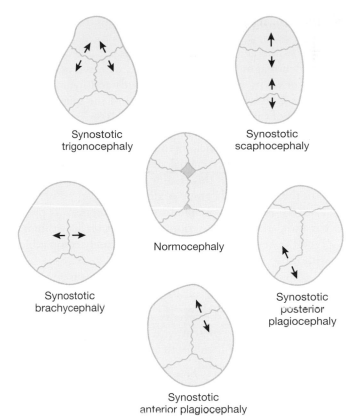

• **Fig. 29.7** Types of Craniosynostosis (From https://en.wikipedia.org/wiki/Craniosynostosis)

fibroblast growth factor receptor genes) or non-syndromic. A second classification is phenotypic (based on the number and nature of fused sutures). Some common examples are shown in Fig. 29.7.

Clinical Manifestation

- Craniofacial deformity
- Other features of specific syndromes
- Raised intracranial pressure causing cognitive and developmental deficits

Treatment

Surgery aims to reconstruct the cranial and facial skeleton, partly for cosmetic reasons but primarily to reduce raised intracranial pressure and improve neurodevelopmental/cognitive outcomes. Complex craniofacial deformities require an individualized multidisciplinary team approach, often centralized to a small proportion of neurosurgical centres. Brain growth is the main stimulus for the growth and shaping of the skull and therefore any corrective surgery should be performed early (between 4 and 12 months of age), while the brain is still growing.

Chiari Malformation

Downward displacement of the posterior fossa structures causes an anatomical malformation at the medullary spinal junction. The reason for this is unknown, but there are multiple types:

- Type I: The cerebellar tonsils lie below the level of the foramen magnum. This is associated with syringomyelia (cyst or cavity within the spinal cord) and hydromyelia (excess CSF within the central canal of the spinal cord) in 50% of cases and hydrocephalus in 10%.
- Type II: Structures including the medulla, cerebellar vermis and fourth ventricle herniate through the foramen magnum. The lower cranial nerves and upper cervical roots are displaced. This is almost exclusively associated with the spina bifida group of disorders.
- Type III: A cervico-occipital myelomeningocele is present and parts of the posterior fossa structures lie within it.
- Type IV: Severe anatomical deformity rarely compatible with life.

Clinical Presentation

This is influenced by the severity of herniation and varies with age. Infants may present with lower cranial nerve palsies and respiratory difficulties that may become life threatening. Ataxia, motor and sensory deficits may be more predominant features in childhood. Patients with mild forms of type I will present in adulthood and commonly suffer from headaches, exacerbated by rises in intracranial pressure from straining or coughing and may have upper limbs signs and symptoms (paraesthesia/weakness/altered temperature sensation) attributable to a syrinx.

Investigations

MRI of the brain and spine to look for an abnormality of the medullary spinal junction and disorders commonly associated with Chiari malformation such as syringomyelia, hydrocephalus and spina bifida.

Treatment

Surgical treatment is aimed at managing hydrocephalus, if present, with ventriculo-peritoneal shunts, or at decompressing the foramen magnum to allow more space for the contents of the posterior fossa. This may involve removing the posterior arch of the C1 and the posterior rim of the foramen magnum. Some surgeons advocate keeping the dura intact whilst releasing tight fibrous bands, whereas others advocate a more radical approach of opening the dura, coagulating the tonsils and performing an expansion duraplasty.

Spasticity

Spasticity can be caused by a number of different aetiologies with diplegic cerebral palsy probably the most common cause. If spasticity causes functional problems, such as with locomotion and contractures, treatment initially involves a combination of physiotherapy, orthoses, Botox injections and systemic drugs to reduce tone. Neurosurgical treatment

of spasticity is usually considered only in severe cases and may involve:

- Intrathecal baclofen pump insertion: A catheter in the lumbar CSF space, connected to an abdominally implanted programmable pump filled with baclofen (a muscle relaxant), which requires periodic refilling.
- Selective dorsal rhizotomy: Usually performed via a laminectomy at the level of the conus medullaris, this procedure involves deliberate division of 50–70% of the dorsal lumbosacral rootlets to reduce tone.

Hydrocephalus

Literally translated as water on the brain, this refers to an abnormal build-up of CSF.

Physiology

CSF is made by ultrafiltration through the choroid plexus, mostly in the lateral ventricles. It passes via the foramen of Munro to the third ventricle and through the aqueduct to the fourth ventricle. It then leaves the ventricular system and passes into the subarachnoid space through the foraminae of Luschka and Magendie and is reabsorbed into the bloodstream through the arachnoid granulations over the surface of the hemispheres. The CSF spaces contain a total of about 125 mL of CSF and about 625 mL of CSF is made daily, resulting in a fivefold turnover of CSF every day.

Types and Causes

Communicating

In this type, CSF can reach the subarachnoid space but is not absorbed. Often caused by infection, subarachnoid haemorrhage or trauma that can interfere with CSF reabsorption at the level of the arachnoid granulations. Idiopathic intracranial hypertension (IIH) and normal pressure hydrocephalus (NPH) are syndromes associated with communicating hydrocephalus.

Non-Communicating (Obstructive)

Blockage prevents CSF reaching the subarachnoid space. Causes include:

- Intraventricular haemorrhage
- Congenital anomalies (e.g. aqueductal stenosis or Dandy–Walker malformation)
- Mass effect from tumours, haematomas

Clinical Features

Presentation depends on the age of the patient and the cause.

In infants, features are:
- failure to thrive
- enlarging head
- tense fontanelle
- failure of up-gaze (setting sun sign)

In adults, features are:
- Typical features of raised intracranial pressure such as headaches, nausea and vomiting often worse in the mornings, decreased consciousness level, papilloedema
- Associated clinical signs of the cause – coma after head injury, subarachnoid haemorrhage or meningitis
- In IIH, features may include visual disturbance, which necessitates urgent treatment

In the elderly, NPH presents with Hakim's triad of symptoms:
- dementia
- ataxia
- urinary incontinence

Diagnosis and Management

A CT or MRI scan will show the enlarged ventricles and may reveal a cause. In communicating hydrocephalus, lumbar puncture can be attempted safely, allowing pressure measurement and diagnostic or therapeutic drainage of CSF.

Temporary drainage can be achieved by intermittent ventricular tap in infants or by external ventricular drainage.

Permanent drainage is achieved by inserting a shunt, which most commonly connects the lateral ventricle to the peritoneal cavity – a ventriculoperitoneal shunt. Shunts may also originate in the lumbar CSF space and may connect to the pleural cavity or right atrium. Modern shunt systems may have programmable valves – the settings can be changed via an external magnet to optimize drainage. Shunts are a common cause of readmissions in neurosurgery and may require revision due to infection, underdrainage (or blockage) or overdrainage. On presentation with suspected shunt dysfunction, assessment should include clinical examination, assessment of the GCS, fundoscopy to check for papilloedema, routine laboratory blood tests and investigation to look for other sources of infection, CSF sampling from the shunt reservoir, CT scan of the head and 'shunt series' X-rays to check for fracture or disconnection of the distal tubing.

In addition to shunting, non-communicating hydrocephalus may be treated by endoscopic third ventriculostomy (ETV) or endoscopic septum pellucidotomy to bypass an obstruction, which, in neonates, is sometimes combined with cauterization of the choroid plexus to improve outcomes. Importantly, ETV obviates the need for shunt tubing and all of its potential complications, although careful patient selection is essential as the ETV may sometimes fail. The ETV success score, based on age, aetiology and whether or not there was a previous CSF shunt, is often used to predict the chances of success.

Spinal Degenerative Disease

Degeneration of the vertebra and intervertebral discs results in pain, deformity and neurological deficit. The lumbar, cervical and thoracic regions are affected in descending order of frequency.

Lumbar Disc Prolapse

An acute disc prolapse occurs when the nucleus pulposus of the intervertebral disc herniates through the surrounding annulus fibrosis causing compression of the nerve roots (when the protrusion is posterolateral) or compression of the cauda equina (when the protrusion is central). This causes acute back pain radiating down the leg, which is made worse by coughing or straining. The distribution of pain and neurological deficit are dependent on the nerve root that is compressed (its dermatome/myotome). A posterolateral disc prolapse affects the nerve root of the level below (e.g. an L4/5 lateral disc prolapse will compress the transiting L5 nerve root).

Classical presentations of sciatica do not need urgent imaging in the first instance (unenhanced MRI of the lumbosacral spine) unless there are red flag signs suggestive of cauda equina syndrome (see later).

Management
Conservative
Numerous patients present with back pain and sciatica and the majority get better spontaneously over a period of weeks. Conservative management options should include analgesic medications (usually a course of NSAIDs), physiotherapy, regular exercise and weight loss. Other options may include neuropathic pain agents (e.g. gabapentin or pregabalin) and nerve root injection.

Surgery
If conservative management has failed, then surgery is indicated. This involves removing the prolapsed disc, commonly by fenestration (widening of the space between two laminae) and partial discectomy under the operating microscope. Minimally invasive techniques, including via the use of endoscopes, may lead to a reduction in postoperative recovery time and hospital stay, with some patients going home on the day of surgery.

Cauda Equina Syndrome

Occasionally, a large central disc prolapse, usually at L5/S1, compresses the cauda equina and causes a combination of symptoms that must never be ignored (Box 29.3). This condition is a surgical emergency and an urgent MRI scan must be obtained in the presence of these symptoms. Decompression must take place urgently to prevent permanent sphincter disturbance.

> ● BOX 29.3 Cauda Equina Syndrome
>
> - Back pain
> - Saddle anaesthesia
> - Bilateral sciatica
> - Urinary retention

Lumbar Canal Stenosis

With increasing age and degenerative change, there is a general narrowing of the spinal canal by bony overgrowth, facet joint and ligamentous hypertrophy. This gradually interferes with the blood supply to and function of the cauda equina nerve roots, leading to neurogenic claudication. This can be differentiated from arterial claudication by the presence of poor distal leg perfusion in the latter. Neurogenic claudication is only relieved by sitting, lying down or stooping forward, whereas arterial claudication can be relieved by just standing still.

Clinical Features

- Aching, numbness and occasionally weakness of the legs on walking, sometimes less than 100 m, relieved by rest.
- There are usually few clinical signs unless the patient is walked beyond the distance where symptoms develop.

Investigation and Management

MRI scanning will show a narrow spinal canal. Surgical treatment is by decompressive laminectomy.

Cervical Degenerative Disease

Acute disc prolapse or spondylosis due to chronic bony distortion can result in narrowing of the canal and consequent damage to the cervical spinal cord (myelopathy) or roots (radiculopathy), due to direct pressure and vascular compromise.

Clinical Features

Spinal cord compression causes an isolated myelopathy or a mixed myeloradiculopathy with radicular signs at the level of compression and myelopathic signs below. Nerve root compression causes an isolated radiculopathy without myelopathic signs.

Signs of radiculopathy:
- Pain and paraesthesia in affected dermatome
- Weakness and muscle wasting in affected myotome
- Hypotonia
- Reduced or absent reflexes
- Fasciculations

Signs of myelopathy:
- Weakness below the level of the lesion
- Often presents with gait disturbance
- Hypertonia: Spasticity (as opposed to the rigidity seen in Parkinson's Disease)
- Brisk reflexes, ankle clonus, positive Hoffman's reflex and extensor plantar response
- Can progress to sphincter dysfunction

Investigation and Management

If imaging is required, an unenhanced MRI scan is the first investigation of choice.

Whether the problem is myelopathy or radiculopathy, there are two surgical approaches to the cervical spine–anterior and posterior. Anteriorly, an anterior cervical discectomy can be performed to decompress either the spinal cord or nerve root. Posteriorly, a laminectomy or laminoplasty can be performed to decompress the spinal cord or a foraminotomy may be performed to decompress a nerve root. Certain patients may require instrumented fusion to maintain spinal stability following decompression.

The main aim of surgical decompression, especially in myelopathy, is to prevent further deterioration, although improvement can be seen in certain cases. Therefore, patients with myelopathy should be decompressed expeditiously to preserve as much function as possible.

Thoracic Degenerative Disease

Thoracic degenerative disease is uncommon, probably because the thoracic spine is less mobile. Thoracic disc prolapses do occur and usually cause a chronic myelopathy. The treatment is surgical decompression, sometimes through an anterior approach (thoracotomy). CT is desirable in addition to MRI as thoracic discs are often calcified.

Spinal Tumours

Spinal tumours other than metastases are far less common than those in the brain. They are often classified according to their anatomical site into extradural, intradural extramedullary and intradural intramedullary. They usually present with localized back pain and neurological deficits.

Investigation and Management

Investigation is usually by MRI and, with intradural lesions, pre- and post-contrast sequences should be obtained. CT scans may also be useful for extradural tumours as they can help with assessment of the integrity and stability of the bony skeleton and whether the tumour is lytic or sclerotic, the former being more likely to require fixation surgery in addition to decompression.

Management

Dependent on the location and the underlying diagnosis.
- Extradural metastatic spinal cord compression: This should be managed with patient immobilization and they should be started on high-dose dexamethasone with gastric protection. A multidisciplinary decision should be taken about whether the appropriate definitive management should involve surgical decompression or radiotherapy. Surgery is often reserved for single level metastases causing acute neurological deficits that may be reversed in patients with a good prognosis; instrumented fixation may also be required to maintain stability of the spinal column. If radiotherapy is being considered, an assessment must be made about whether the spine is stable or requires immobilization in an orthosis.

- Intradural (extramedullary and intramedullary) tumours: Surgical resection is associated with significant risk of neurological deficit. Asymptomatic lesions may therefore be followed up by surveillance imaging and resected if there is evidence of growth or neurological compromise. Surgical resection involves a laminectomy, durotomy and resection, usually with the aid of an ultrasonic aspirator. Intraoperative neurophysiological monitoring using somatosensory and motor evoked potentials (SSEP/MEP) is becoming the standard of care for intramedullary tumours to minimize risk of neurological deficits.

Peripheral Nerve Lesions

Although inflammation of various causes can cause peripheral neuropathy, the disorders of relevance to neurosurgery are structural, e.g. trauma and entrapment.

Trauma

Injury may be by traction (e.g. an avulsion of a root of the brachial plexus when the arm is distracted in relation to the body) or by division in a penetrating wound. These can be classified according to Seddon's classification into neurapraxia (a temporary interruption of conduction due to stretching which is often reversible), axonotmesis (loss of axon and myelin integrity but preservation of the connective tissue framework which may recover following Wallerian degeneration and axonal regrowth) and neurotmesis (loss of whole nerve fibre integrity, which is not reversible without surgical intervention).

Entrapment

Nerves that pass through bony or fibrous tunnels are affected (e.g. the median nerve in the carpal tunnel at the wrist and the ulnar nerve at the elbow).

Clinical Features

Loss of function (of lower motor neuron type) and anaesthesia follow trauma. Patients may also develop dysaesthesia, neuropathic pain and autonomic dysfunction in the affected limb region. Entrapment causes pain and tingling in the distribution of the nerve, with muscle wasting if there is motor denervation.

Investigation and Management

Further investigation is not required in obvious traumatic division, but a traction injury may require neurophysiological studies to confirm whether or not the injury is complete and therefore unlikely to recover. In entrapment, the symptoms and signs are often imprecise, and nerve conduction studies are required for confirmation.

Repair of traumatic division can be primary in a clean wound but is better delayed if there is contamination. Entrapment neuropathies are treated by surgical decompression.

Infections

Intracranial Abscess

Intracranial abscesses occur in 2–3 per million population. Although relatively uncommon due the advent of antibiotics, they are serious and life-threatening. They can occur in the form of intracerebral abscess or subdural/extradural empyema.

Pathophysiology

In spontaneous infection, 45% of patients' spread occurs directly from the sinuses, infected dental caries or chronic otitis media/mastoiditis. Trauma accounts for a further 10% as fracture of the skull base provides a route for infection; 25% result from haematogenous spread from a distant focus. The source is unknown in 15% of cases.

Neurosurgical interventions are perhaps the biggest risk factor for intracranial infections, although advances including laminar flow and perioperative antibiotic prophylaxis have reduced postoperative infections.

The organism varies according to the source:
- Direct invasion from the sinuses or middle ear: *Streptococcus milleri, Bacteroides fragilis, Streptococcus pneumoniae, Escherichia coli*
- Haematogenous: *Staphylococcus aureus, S. milleri, S. pneumoniae*
- In immunocompromised patients: *Candida, Aspergillus, Nocardia, Toxoplasma, Listeria*
- Trauma: *S. aureus*
- Postoperative: *S. aureus, Staphylococcus epidermidis*

Clinical Presentation

Patients with intracranial abscesses present in a similar way to any others with a space-occupying lesion including headache, vomiting, reduced GCS, focal neurological deficit and seizures.

Certain features raise suspicion of an abscess:
- Signs of systemic infection: temperature, raised inflammatory markers
- Signs of the source of infection: bacterial endocarditis, sinusitis, mastoiditis
- Immunocompromised patients

Investigations

CT or MRI with pre- and post-contrast sequences: These often show well-circumscribed ring-enhancing lesions once an abscess has formed, although, if performed earlier, they can be less well delineated. An MRI with diffusion-weighted imaging is often very helpful as the dense pus restricts diffusion, which can help differentiate abscesses from brain tumours (Fig. 29.8).

Management

- Urgent abscess drainage can be undertaken via image-guided burr hole aspiration. Recurrent abscesses may require surgical excision.

A

B

C

D

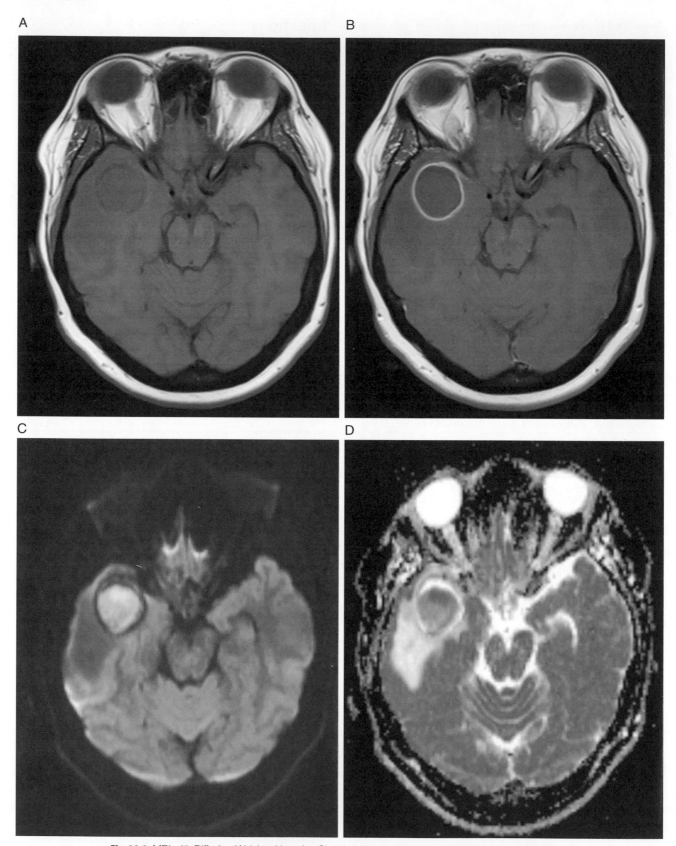

• **Fig. 29.8** MRI with Diffusion-Weighted Imaging Showing Intracranial Abscess. MRI sequences showing an intracranial abscess in the right temporal lobe. (A) T1-weighted imaging. (B) T1-weighted imaging with contrast enhancement showing the classical 'ring enhancing' lesion. (C) Diffusion weighted imaging (DQI) and (D) apparent diffusion coefficient (ADC) maps. The combination showing bright signal on DWI and dark signal on ADC indicate restricted diffusion secondary to the highly cellular pus at the centre of the abscess.

- Investigation of potential infective sources: Common investigations include CT scans to assess for sinusitis, echocardiography for endocarditis and orthopantomogram (OPG) for dental infection. Body CT with contrast can be done in the sick patient if no source is found.
- Antibiotic therapy: Initially, broad-spectrum antibiotics with central nervous system penetration (e.g. ceftriaxone or meropenem), which can later be rationalized based on the results of the microbial culture and sensitivities.

Meningitis

A diffuse infection of the meninges is actually far more common but shares the same causes as brain abscess. Features include fever, headache, neck rigidity, seizures, decreased consciousness level or confusion. Meningism can be elicited on examination by Kernig's and Brudzinski's signs.

Diagnosis is by lumbar puncture, which, in the case of bacterial meningitis, may reveal elevated white cells, a micro-organism on gram stain or culture, elevated protein and low glucose (compared to a paired serum glucose sample). Antibiotics form the mainstay of therapy; surgical intervention is rarely necessary.

Spinal Infection

Infections in the spine often begin with discitis, which can then spread to the adjacent vertebral bodies (osteomyelitis) and into the spinal canal (epidural abscess), causing spinal cord or cauda equina compression.

Pathophysiology

Intervertebral discs are particularly prone to haematogenous spread of infection (e.g. from bacterial endocarditis), due to the valveless Batson's paravertebral venous plexus, which allows retrograde flow when intrathoracic and intra-abdominal pressure is elevated. Risk factors include co-morbidities such as diabetes and immunocompromise. Recent surgical intervention is a risk factor for direct inoculation, especially in the presence of metalwork. The majority of infections are pyogenic, although, in some areas, a significant proportion may be spinal tuberculosis. Clinical presentation is most commonly with back/neck pain and systemic signs of infection, although patients may present or develop focal neurological deficits caused by spinal cord or nerve root compression. Careful neurological examination must be undertaken.

Investigations:
- Pre- and post-contrast MRI of the spine
- Blood cultures
- CT-guided biopsy/aspiration of paraspinal collections

Management

The majority of spinal infections may be treated non-surgically. In the absence of neurological deficit or significant spinal deformity, antibiotics should be started and can be rationalized following culture of organisms from peripheral blood or radiologically-guided biopsies of the discitis/ paraspinal collections. Indications for neurosurgical intervention include acute epidural abscess causing neurological deficits (which requires urgent decompression and evacuation of the epidural abscess) and progressive deformity (which may be managed initially by immobilization in a brace and later with instrumented fusion if needed once the infection has settled).

Functional Neurosurgery

As technology advances, the remit of indications for functional neurosurgery is rapidly expanding. In a specialty where regenerative or disease modifying therapies have been sparse, functional neurosurgery holds much promise.

Deep Brain Stimulation/Ablative Therapy

Deep brain stimulation (DBS) has firmly established itself as part of the treatment options for movement disorders (Parkinson's disease, tremor, dystonia) but its scope is expanding to include disorders such as epilepsy, neuropathic pain, cluster headache and psychiatric disorders (Tourette's and obsessive-compulsive disorder). DBS involves the insertion of electrodes deep into the brain via small burr holes, which are then connected to an implantable pulse generator (IPG/battery), often placed in the chest wall, similar to a cardiac pacemaker. Different disorders have different nuclei that are targeted, with the aim of improving signs, symptoms, function and quality of life.

DBS originated from both animal research and clinical evidence that ablative techniques (e.g. thalamotomy/pallidotomy) led to symptom improvement in movement disorders and such techniques may still be used in patients not eligible for DBS, for example if very elderly with essential tremor or older, more palliative cases of Parkinson's disease and in resource-poor settings where programming visits for DBS and IPG changes may not be feasible. Although radiofrequency thermocoagulation continues to be successfully practised by the senior authors (EP and TA), novel non-invasive lesioning techniques such as stereotactic radiosurgery and MRI-guided focused ultrasound are popularizing ablative procedures.

Epilepsy

Despite optimal medical therapy, a significant proportion of patients will continue to have seizures. Some of these may be candidates for neurosurgical intervention:
- Vagal Nerve Stimulation: Involves wrapping an electrode around the vagus nerve, connected to an IPG and battery on the anterior chest wall. The mechanism of action is not well understood but about 50% experience improvement in seizure frequency at 5 years.
- Resective Surgery: Resective surgery is most commonly indicated for medically-refractory focal seizures and mesial temporal lobe epilepsy. Pre-surgical evaluation requires a thorough multidisciplinary work-up including

advanced imaging (MRI, SPECT) and electrophysiology (video-EEG and stereo-EEG or electrocorticography) to try and identify a focus for the seizures. Surgical resection must be approached with care so as to not cause any neurological, cognitive or behavioural deficits. Outcomes are classified according to the Modified Engel classification which looks at seizure severity, duration and frequency.

• Deep brain stimulation.

Pain

Trigeminal Neuralgia

If initial medical therapy for trigeminal neuralgia fails, surgical treatments may be considered. These include percutaneous procedures such as radiofrequency ablation or glycerol injection into Meckel's cave under radiological guidance. If there is MRI evidence of a neurovascular conflict of the trigeminal nerve and the anterior inferior cerebellar artery or another vessel at the nerve root entry zone, microvascular decompression, involving placing non-stick Teflon between the nerve and vessel, may be considered. In appropriately selected patients, up to 70% can remain pain-free 10 years after the operation. The operation involves a craniotomy behind and below the ear and hemifacial spasm due to facial nerve vascular compression can be treated similarly.

Other Pain Syndromes

Medically refractory neuropathic pain syndromes may also be amenable to neurosurgical treatments, such as spinal cord stimulation, dorsal root ganglion stimulation, DBS, ablative procedures such as dorsal root entry zone lesioning for brachial plexus avulsion, upper cervical anterolateral cordotomy for nociceptive cancer pain or intrathecal delivery of narcotic/analgesic agents. Appropriate patient selection is key to achieving good outcomes.

References

1. Hutchinson PJ, Kolias AG, Timofeev IS, et al. Trial of decompressive craniectomy for traumatic intracranial hypertension. *N Eng J Med*. 2016;375:1119–1130.
2. Hutchinson PJ, Edlmann E, Bulters D, et al. Trial of dexamethasone for chronic subdural hematoma. *N Eng J Med*. 2020;383:2616–2627.
3. Fehlings MG, Vaccaro A, Wilson JR, et al. Early versus delayed decompression for traumatic cervical spinal cord injury: results of the Surgical Timing in Acute Spinal Cord Injury Study (STAS-CIS). *PLoS One*. 2012;7:e32037.
4. Mendelow AD, Gregson BA, Rowan EN, et al. Early surgery versus initial conservative treatment in patients with spontaneous supratentorial lobar intracerebral haematomas (STICH II): a randomised trial. *Lancet*. 2013;382:397–408.
5. Mendelow AD, Gregson BA, Fernandes HM, et al. Early surgery versus initial conservative treatment in patients with spontaneous supratentorial intracerebral haematomas in the International Surgical Trial in Intracerebral Haemorrhage (STICH): a randomised trial. *Lancet*. 2005;365:387–397.
6. Molyneux A. International Subarachnoid Aneurysm Trial (ISAT) of neurosurgical clipping versus endovascular coiling in 2143 patients with ruptured intracranial aneurysms: a randomised trial. *Lancet*. 2002;360:1267–1274.
7. Vahedi K, Vicaut E, Mateo J, et al. Sequential-design, multicenter, randomized, controlled trial of early decompressive craniectomy in malignant middle cerebral artery infarction (DECIMAL Trial). *Stroke*. 2007;38:2506–2517.
8. Jüttler E, Schwab S, Schmiedek P, et al. Decompressive surgery for the treatment of malignant infarction of the middle cerebral artery (DESTINY). *Stroke*. 2007;38:2518–2525.
9. Hofmeijer J, Kappelle LJ, Algra A, et al. Surgical decompression for space-occupying cerebral infarction (the Hemicraniectomy After Middle Cerebral Artery infarction with Life-threatening Edema Trial [HAMLET]): a multicentre, open, randomised trial. *Lancet Neurol*. 2009;8:326–333.
10. Albers GW, Marks MP, Kemp S, et al. Thrombectomy for stroke at 6 to 16 hours with selection by perfusion imaging. *N Eng J Med*. 2018;378:708–718.
11. Nogueira RG, Jadhav AP, Haussen DC, et al. Thrombectomy 6 to 24 hours after stroke with a mismatch between deficit and infarct. *N Eng J Med*. 2018;378:11–21.
12. Adzick NS, Thom EA, Spong CY, et al. A randomized trial of prenatal versus postnatal repair of myelomeningocele. *N Eng J Med*. 2011;364:993–1004.

Further Reading

Greenberg MS. *Handbook of Neurosurgery*. 8th ed. New York: Thieme; 2016.

Hasegawa H, Crocker M, Minhas PS. *Oxford Case Histories in Neurosurgery*. 1st ed. USA: Oxford University Press; 2013.

Johnson RD, Green AL. *Landmark Papers in Neurosurgery*. 2nd ed. Oxford: Oxford University Press; 2014.

Lyndsay KW, Bone I, Fuller G. *Neurology and Neurosurgery Illustrated*, 5th ed. Churchill Livingstone; 2010.

30

Hernia

CHAPTER OUTLINE

No disease of the human body, belonging to the province of the surgeon, requires in its treatment a better combination of accurate, anatomical knowledge with surgical skill than hernia in all its variations.

SIR ASTLEY PATON COOPER (1804)

General Considerations

A hernia is a protrusion of a viscus or other structure beyond the normal coverings of the cavity in which it is contained. It may occur between two adjacent cavities such as the abdomen and thorax or into a subcompartment of a cavity – so-called internal hernias. The most frequent hernias are external ones of the abdominal wall in the inguinal, femoral and umbilical regions, and the account that follows concentrates chiefly on these.

Epidemiology

The first record of a hernia is in the Egyptian Papyrus Ebers (1550 BC) when it was regarded as a social stigma. Abdominal hernias are common. They occur at all ages and in both sexes and account for approximately 10% of the general surgical workload. Their relative frequencies are given in Table 30.1.

Classification

Hernias are best classified as congenital or acquired.

Congenital

In congenital hernias, there is a pre-formed sac which occurs as a consequence of the ordered or disordered process of intrauterine development – the patent processus vaginalis is a good example.

Acquired

There are two types of acquired hernia:

Primary hernias occur at natural weak points, such as those where:

- Structures penetrate the abdominal wall, e.g. the femoral vessels passing into the femoral canal
- Muscles and aponeuroses fail to overlap normally, e.g. the lumbar region
- Fibrous tissue normally develops to close a defect, e.g. at the umbilicus

Secondary hernias develop at sites of surgical or other injury to the wall which normally constrains the contents of a body cavity (usually the abdomen), e.g. after laparotomy or penetrating injury.

Aetiology

The two main factors predisposing to hernia are increased intracavity pressure and a weakened abdominal wall. In the abdomen, the raised pressure occurs as a result of:

- Cough – chronic obstructive airways disease
- Straining to pass urine – benign prostatic hyperplasia or carcinoma
- Straining to pass faeces – constipation or large-bowel obstruction
- Abdominal distension – which may indicate the presence of an intra-abdominal disorder
- Change in abdominal contents – e.g. ascites, encysted fluid, benign or malignant tumour, pregnancy, fat.
  A weakened abdominal wall occurs in:
- Advancing age
- Malnutrition – either of macronutrients (protein, calorie) or micronutrients (e.g. vitamin C)
- Damage to, or paralysis of, motor nerves
- Abnormal connective tissue (e.g. collagen and elastin) metabolism.

TABLE 30.1	Relative Frequency of External Abdominal Hernias.
Type of hernia	Incidence (%)
Epigastric	1
Umbilical	3
Incisional	10
Inguinal	78
Femoral	7
Other (rare)	1

Often, multiple factors are involved. For example, the presence of a patent, congenitally formed sac may not cause a hernia until an acquired abdominal wall weakness or raised intra-abdominal pressure allows abdominal contents to enter the sac. Heavy lifting and socio-occupational factors may make pre-existing hernias more symptomatic, but contradictory evidence exists regarding their role as causative factors in their own right.

Anatomical Features

A hernia consists of:
• a sac,
• its coverings and
• its contents.

The sac comprises a mouth, neck, body and fundus (Fig. 30.1). The coverings of a hernia refer to the overlying layers, which are attenuated as the hernia emerges. Working from the outermost layer inwards, these are as follows:
• skin
• subcutaneous fat
• aponeurosis
• muscle
• endo-cavity fascia
• endothelial lining – peritoneum in the abdomen

The contents of hernias vary, but most intracavity viscera have been reported. In the abdomen, the commonest contents are the small bowel and the greater omentum. Other possibilities include:
• the large bowel and appendix
• Meckel's diverticulum
• the bladder
• the ovary with or without the fallopian tube
• ascitic fluid

Natural History and Complications

The natural history of hernia development is progressive enlargement, not spontaneous regression. A notable exception is congenital umbilical hernia in neonates, where the orifice may close over the years following birth. With the passage of time, all acquired hernias enlarge and the frequency and severity of symptoms may change.

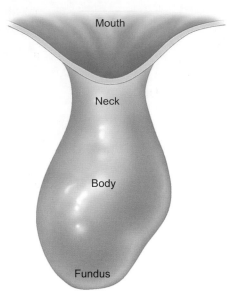

• **Fig. 30.1** Hernial Sac

Hernias may be reducible, irreducible, obstructed, strangulated or inflamed.

Reducible Hernia

In this type of hernia, the contents can be returned from whence they came, but the sac persists. The contents do not necessarily reappear spontaneously, but do so when assisted by gravity or raised intra-abdominal pressure.

Irreducible Hernia

The contents cannot be returned to the body cavity in this type of hernia. The causes of irreducibility are:
• Narrow neck with rigid margins often in association with a capacious sac (e.g. femoral, umbilical)
• Adhesion formation between the contents and the sac (usually long-standing hernias)

Irreducible hernias have a greater risk of obstruction and strangulation than reducible ones.

Obstructed Hernia

The obstructed hernia contains intestine in which the lumen has become occluded. Obstruction is usually at the neck of the sac but may be caused by adhesions within it. If the obstruction is at both ends of the loop, fluid accumulates within it and distension occurs (closed loop obstruction). Initially the blood supply to the obstructed loop of bowel is intact, but, with time, this becomes impeded and strangulation (see later) supervenes.

The term 'incarcerated' is sometimes used to describe a hernia that is irreducible but not strangulated. Thus, an irreducible, obstructed hernia can also be called an incarcerated one.

Strangulated Hernia

Ten percent of groin hernias present for the first time with strangulation. The blood supply to the contents of the hernia is cut off. The pathological sequence is: venous and lymphatic occlusion; tissue fluid accumulation (oedema) causing further swelling; and a consequent increase in venous pressure. Venous haemorrhage develops, and a vicious circle is set up, with swelling eventually impeding arterial inflow. The tissues undergo ischaemic necrosis. If the contents of the sac of an abdominal hernia are not bowel, e.g. omentum, the necrosis is sterile, but strangulation of bowel is by far the most common and leads to infected necrosis (gangrene). The mucosa sloughs and the bowel wall becomes permeable to bacteria, which translocate through it and into the sac and from there to the bloodstream. The infarcted, friable intestine perforates (usually at the neck of the sac) and the bacteria-laden luminal fluid spills into the peritoneal cavity to produce peritonitis. Septic shock ensues with circulatory failure and death.

Inflamed Hernia

The contents are inflamed by any process that causes this in the tissue or organ that is not normally herniated, e.g.:
- acute appendicitis
- Meckel's diverticulitis
- acute salpingitis

It may be impossible to distinguish an inflamed hernia from one that is strangulated.

Special Types of Hernia

Sliding Hernia (Hernia en Glissade)

This hernia is one in which an extraperitoneal structure forms part of the wall of the sac (Fig. 30.2). Five percent of all hernias are sliding, and indirect inguinal hernias account for the majority. On the right, the caecum and ascending colon are involved, whereas on the left, the sigmoid and descending colon are found in the sac. A portion of bladder may slide into a direct inguinal hernia. The incidence of sliding hernias increases with age and the duration of the hernia. Failure to recognize a sliding hernia at operation may result in damage to the structure involved.

Richter's Hernia (Fig. 30.3)

In this type of hernia, only a portion of the circumference of the intestine (usually the small bowel) is trapped. The danger of this hernia is that the knuckle of bowel may become ischaemic without the development of obvious clinical features of obstruction (see 'Femoral hernia').

Hernia-en-W – Maydl's Hernia

This complicated disposition of intestine in an inguinal hernia is easier to illustrate (Fig. 30.4) than to describe. If strangulation occurs, the loop affected is within the abdominal cavity.

Clinical Features

Symptoms

There may be a history of factors predisposing to increased intracavity pressure (e.g. cough, ascites – see 'Aetiology').

Local symptoms include:
- A lump which varies in size, may disappear when recumbent and reappear and enlarge on straining

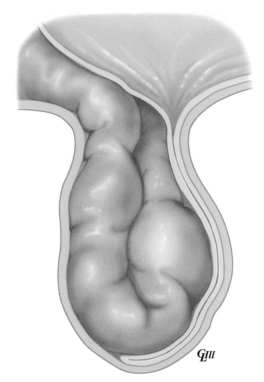

• **Fig. 30.2** Sliding Hernia

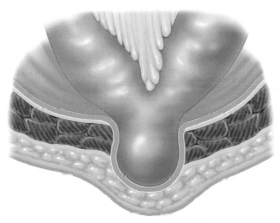

• **Fig. 30.3** Richter's Hernia

- Pain – local aching discomfort or dragging sensation, but sometimes sharp

Symptoms of complications may be:
- Intestinal obstruction – colic, vomiting, distension and absolute constipation. The obstruction may not always be complete and results in diarrhoea rather than constipation
- Strangulation – in addition to symptoms of intestinal obstruction, constant pain over the hernia, fever, tachycardia

Signs

The patient should first be examined in the supine position and then, in all external abdominal hernias, standing. The area of the swelling is palpated to determine the exact position

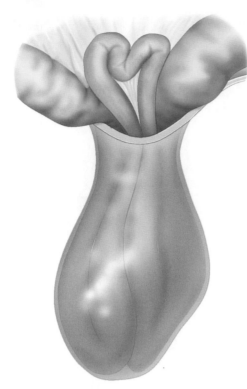

• **Fig. 30.4** Maydl's Hernia

TABLE 30.2	Other Causes of Lumps that Must Be Differentiated from Abdominal Wall Hernias.
Tissue	**Lump**
Skin	Sebaceous or epidermoid cyst
Fat	Lipoma
Fascia	Fibroma
Muscle	Herniation through sheath; tumour
Artery	Aneurysm
Vein	Varicosity
Lymphatic	Enlarged lymph node
Gonad	Ectopic testis/ovary

and then its physical characteristics. A Valsalva manoeuvre is useful for assessing hernias of the anterior abdominal wall and to look for evidence of diastasis of the recti muscles. The lump's distinguishing features are reducibility and an expansile cough impulse – the lump gets bigger and more tense. On standing, bulges become more obvious and can be made additionally prominent by coughing.

When the patient lies down, it is possible to test for reducibility – if the swelling can be returned to the abdominal cavity it is said to be reducible. Control of the hernia is the ability to prevent its reappearance by digital pressure over the point at which reduction occurred. The patient is asked to cough: if the hernia does not reappear, it has been controlled and the neck of the sac accurately located.

Other hernial sites should be examined, as bilateral and simultaneous hernias are common. Other causes of a lump that may be confused with abdominal wall hernias are shown in Table 30.2. A general physical examination is essential and includes a search for predisposing causes such as benign prostatic hyperplasia and colorectal cancer.

Signs Associated with Complications

Irreducibility. Locally there is a painless lump that does not reduce.

Obstruction. The hernia is tense, tender and irreducible. There may be distension of the abdomen and the other features of intestinal obstruction.

Strangulation. Signs are as for an obstructed hernia, but tenderness is more marked. The overlying skin may be warm, inflamed and indurated.

Investigation

Hernia is a clinical diagnosis.

Imaging

Ultrasound is being increasingly used to assess hernias that are difficult to define clinically, e.g. an early groin hernia.

CT and MRI have a role in the diagnosis of rare pelvic hernias (e.g. obturator hernia). They may also be helpful in the preoperative assessment of large incisional (or other) hernias where multiple defects may be present. In addition, CT or MRI scanning will exclude recurrent malignant disease in patients who have had previous cancer surgery and abdominal aortic aneurysm disease in those with connective tissue disorders.

Herniography. This technique, which involves the injection of contrast medium into the peritoneal cavity and subsequent X-ray, is now obsolete in most highly developed nations. It may rarely be used in infants to identify a clinically undetectable contralateral hernia in the groin.

Laparoscopy

Unexpected hernias are sometimes discovered at the time of laparoscopy, but it should not be considered a diagnostic modality.

Exploratory Operation

In some infants with a convincing history from the mother, a hernia is not found on clinical examination. Exploratory operation can then be justified.

Principles of Management

The natural history of a hernia is one of progressive enlargement. The cumulative risk of irreducibility, obstruction and strangulation increases with time. Strangulation is a relatively rare event for both inguinal and incisional hernias. For these reasons, surgical opinion now is that, with very few exceptions, surgeons should have a detailed discussion with each patient of the risks and benefits of both operative and non-operative management. Although operative intervention serves to relieve the patient's symptoms and to eliminate the occurrence of sequelae of a hernia, the risks have to be carefully weighed against the status quo. There is a particularly strong argument in favour of operation in those hernias that have a high incidence of strangulation if the patient is fit enough for surgery, i.e.:

- inguinal hernia with a narrow neck
- femoral hernia
- those that have become irreducible

Conversely, watchful waiting is appropriate in elderly, co-morbid patients with asymptomatic inguinal or incisional hernia that have minimal impact on quality of life.

Advances in anaesthesia have made elective inguinal hernia surgery safe and they may be successfully repaired under local anaesthesia. Only a small number of patients may have associated disorders that make an operation inappropriate or may decline it. Trusses are rarely used.

Presenting or predisposing conditions such as benign prostatic hyperplasia or obstructive airways disease may need treatment before the hernia is dealt with. In addition, in certain defined circumstances, preoperative preparation is necessary:

- Large hernias that warrant repair require particularly diligent preoperative preparation in order to minimize the risk of the operation and to ensure a favourable long-term outcome.
- Weight reduction should be encouraged.
- Smoking is strongly discouraged.
- Treatment of intercurrent disease (e.g. hypertension, diabetes) is essential.
- Optimization of cardiorespiratory fitness through exercise is encouraged.
- For giant hernias, when viscera are in a hernia sac for long periods of time, they lose the 'right of domicile' in the abdominal cavity; replacing them suddenly into the abdomen is associated with the dangers of abdominal compartment syndrome – renal failure, respiratory compromise, compression of the inferior vena cava and paralytic ileus. These complications may be averted by preparing the patient with abdominal wall expansion through botulinum toxin into the lateral abdominal wall muscles and/or therapeutic pneumoperitoneum, where the abdominal cavity is inflated by repeated intraperitoneal injections of air over the 2 weeks before operation, up to a total of 2.5 L.

Most elective operations are now usually done as either day or short-stay procedures, and patients are encouraged to resume normal activities as soon as possible. Groin hernias may be repaired by a laparoscopic approach, which has marginal benefits in reduction in pain and early return to work. Giant abdominal hernias are a major surgical undertaking.

Strangulation is a surgical emergency which still carries a high mortality rate, particularly if, for any reason, operation is delayed.

Surgical Techniques

Herniotomy is the removal of the sac and closure of its neck. It is the first step in nearly every hernia repair and, in some instances (e.g. infant inguinal hernia – see later), may be all that is required.

Herniorrhaphy involves some sort of reconstruction to:
- Restore the anatomy if this is disturbed
- Increase the strength of the abdominal wall
- Construct a barrier to recurrence

The first of these is usually possible by suture. The second and third may be achieved with local tissue, but the insertion of prosthetic material is also widely used.

Mesh for Hernia Repair

Meshes have been demonstrated to dramatically reduce the rate of hernia recurrence in all types of hernia repair. There are over 200 different types/brands of meshes on the market, indicating that there is no 'perfect' mesh, ideal for use in all circumstances. There are multiple different classification systems for categorizing the different meshes available, but no one system is universally accepted.

Meshes can be broadly divided into those that are made of synthetic materials and those that are derived from processed tissues (human or animal). Synthetic meshes are most commonly made of non-absorbable polymers (e.g. polypropylene, polyester, PTFE). Some synthetic meshes are made of polymers that are absorbable and the time taken for the polymer chains to degrade (can range from weeks to years) influences the characteristics of the implant. Combinations of polymers can be used to create partially absorbable meshes. Some meshes have antiadhesive coatings on one side and are intended for intraperitoneal use.

Meshes derived from processed tissue are commonly referred to as 'biologic' meshes. They can be derived from human cadavers (allografts) or animals (xenografts). Porcine and bovine sources are most common and can include dermis, pericardium and intestinal submucosa. They are normally very expensive and are restricted for use in special circumstances, such as contaminated fields.

Obstruction and Strangulation

The patient nearly always requires treatment of the associated obstruction of the gut.

Non-operative treatment can be considered in:
- Infants
- Obstructed hernia with a short history – presentation within 2 hours of onset in a hernia that was previously reducible and with no signs to suggest strangulation

The patient is put in the head-down position and an ice pack may be applied; then an attempt is made to reduce the hernia by taxis, which consists of gentle manipulation of the swelling in the direction of the hernial orifice. Considerable experience is required. There is no place for vigorous manipulation, which carries the obvious danger of damage to the bowel or reduction en masse – reduction of the sac and its contents but with persistent trapping of the latter so that strangulation progresses.

Urgent operation is needed in the great majority of obstructed or strangulated hernias. The hernial sac and its contents are exposed and the constriction or other cause of obstruction relieved. Further surgery may be required to remove ischaemic bowel or omentum. For the reasons given above, strangulated bowel implies bacterial translocation, and antibiotics are administered.

Outcome
Mortality

For elective repair, the overall mortality is less than 0.5% but increases with age to approximately 0.5–1% for those over 60 years. For emergency operations, it is 10 times greater. It is a sobering observation that the mortality for strangulated obstructing hernia has remained unchanged at around 20% for the last 50 years. Death is dependent on:

- Age – older patients have a higher incidence of intercurrent disease.
- Contents of the sac – gangrenous intestine (present in 10% of strangulated hernias) is associated with a 40% mortality rate.

Morbidity

The overall complication rate is high. Any of the complications that beset surgery can occur during or after operations for hernia. Specific to the procedure are:

- Persistent wound pain – often ascribed to a neuroma which forms after damage to or division of the ilio-inguinal or other nerve
- Cutaneous anaesthesia – division of a nerve
- Recurrent hernia.
- Seroma – an accumulation of serous fluid at the site of the hernia

The rate of recurrence is between less than 1% and 10% for primary hernias (depending on the type) and 5–30% for recurrent hernias. Recurrence is associated with:

- Age – the older the patient, the more likely is the hernia to recur
- Presence or absence of predisposing factors
- Site – high with incisional hernias; inguinal greater than femoral
- Size – the larger the hernia, the more likely it is to have distorted the surrounding anatomy
- Emergency or elective operation – the former being more likely to be associated with recurrence
- Operation on a recurrent hernia – more difficult and more likely to fail
- Experience of the surgeon
  See later for further consideration of recurrent hernias.

SPECIFIC HERNIAS

Inguinal Hernia

Inguinal hernias account for 80% of all external abdominal hernias. They occur at all ages, but are most common in

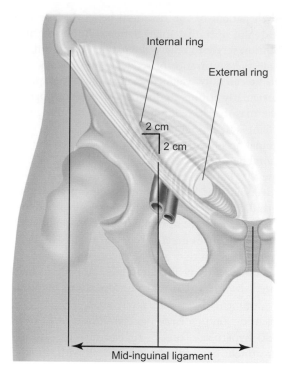

• **Fig. 30.5** The Inguinal Canal

infants and the elderly. Inguinal hernias are 20 times more common in men than in women, and more frequently occur on the right side.

Anatomy

The inguinal canal (Fig. 30.5) runs in an antero-inferior direction from the internal to external inguinal rings and, in the male, is the path taken by the testis to reach the scrotum. In that sex, therefore, it contains the spermatic vessels and the vas deferens; in the female it only contains the round ligament. The internal ring lies 2 cm or slightly more above and 2 cm lateral to the mid-inguinal point – that point on the inguinal ligament midway between the anterior superior iliac spine and the symphysis pubis. To find it, the femoral artery is identified as it passes deep to the mid-inguinal point and the fingers are moved upwards and laterally. The medial aspect of the ring is bounded by the inferior epigastric branch of the femoral artery. The external ring is just above the pubic crest and tubercle to which the inguinal ligament is attached. In infants, the internal and external rings are directly one behind the other but, during growth, they move apart.

The inguinal region and canal, particularly in the male, is a vulnerable area for the formation of hernia, but this is to some extent offset by contraction of the abdominal muscles, which compresses together the anterior and posterior walls of the canal and allows descent of the conjoint tendon to act as a partial shutter.

It is further thought that the cremaster muscle bunches the cord up into the canal, so acting as a plug.

TABLE 30.3	Differences Between an Indirect and a Direct Inguinal Hernia.	
	Indirect	**Direct**
Patient's age	Any age but usually young	Older
Cause	May be congenital	Acquired
Bilateral	20%	50%
Protrusion on coughing	Oblique	Straight
Appearance on standing	Does not reach full size immediately	Reaches full size immediately
Reduction on lying down	May not reduce immediately	Reduces immediately
Descent into scrotum	Common	Rare
Occlusion of internal ring	Controls	Does not control
Neck of sac	Narrow	Wide
Strangulation	Not uncommon	Unusual
Relation to inferior epigastric vessels	Lateral	Medial

Classification

Indirect Inguinal Hernia

This passes through the internal ring lateral to the inferior epigastric artery and along the canal to emerge at the external ring above the pubic crest and tubercle. Its coverings are the attenuated layers of the cord.

Direct Inguinal Hernia

This hernia bulges through the posterior wall of the canal medial to the inferior epigastric artery and is therefore not covered by the layers of the cord.

Pantaloon Hernia

This is a combination of both an indirect and a direct inguinal hernia.

Aetiology

Indirect Hernia

In an indirect hernia, there is a congenital sac or potential sac which is the remnant of the processus vaginalis. If the processus does not close, then an indirect hernia occurs in early life, but other factors may lead to it reopening at any age. Indirect hernias are 20 times more common in men than in women. Sixty percent occur on the right (possibly contributed to by damage to the motor nerves of the abdominal muscles at open appendicectomy), 40% on the left and 20% are bilateral.

Direct Hernia

This is an acquired lesion. For reasons unknown, though contributed to by accessory factors such as the wear and tear of advancing age, repeated straining and raised intra-abdominal pressure, the posterior wall of the inguinal canal becomes attenuated. Direct hernia is therefore a condition of later life and is rarely seen under the age of 40.

Clinical Findings

In both indirect and direct hernias, the cough impulse that can be seen or palpated must be distinguished from normal diffuse bulging in the inguinal region, particularly in individuals of spare build. The principal differences between the two types of hernia on clinical examination are summarized in Table 30.3.

In addition to the features outlined in Table 30.3, an indirect hernia that extends beyond the external ring appears above and medial to the pubic tubercle, in contrast to a femoral hernia (see below) which is below and lateral to that bony point. The pubic tubercle can be found either by feeling laterally along the pubic crest from the upper border of the symphysis pubic or by following the adductor longus tendon from the medial side of the thigh to its origin from the body of the pubis. The tubercle is directly above.

One of the most useful methods of distinction between the two kinds of inguinal hernia is that a reducible indirect hernia can be completely controlled with a fingertip placed firmly over the internal ring.

For the clinical features and management of an infantile inguinal hernia, see Chapter 9.

Other Causes of Groin Swelling

Although inguinal hernias are relatively easy to diagnose, there are a considerable number of other causes of swelling in this area that may require consideration when a lump is encountered. These include:

- femoral hernia
- hydrocele
- encysted hydrocele of the cord or of the peritoneovaginal canal
- undescended or ectopic testis
- lipoma of the cord
- epididymal cyst

Management

The general principles of hernia management have been given above. Most adult inguinal hernias are repaired by open operation under local or general anaesthesia as a day-case procedure, although the number of hernia repairs performed laparoscopically is increasing, because of the perceived benefits in bilateral or recurrent cases, and also in response to patient choice. Laparoscopy is the operative modality of choice for women due to improved recurrence rates and the ability to cover both inguinal and femoral canals with the same piece of mesh. Elderly patients and those with serious medical problems require in-patient care. Open and laparoscopic operations usually mean the insertion of a non-absorbable prosthetic mesh.

Open Mesh Repair

The mesh repair of inguinal hernia is the most common general surgical operation performed in the UK. The method involves the following steps:

- An oblique skin incision is made in the groin, 2 cm above the medial half of the inguinal ligament.
- Fat and Scarpa's fascia are divided to expose the external oblique aponeurosis, superficial ring and the inguinal ligament inferiorly.
- The aponeurosis and superficial ring are opened, avoiding damage to the ilio-inguinal nerve to allow access to the cremaster-covered cord and hernia sac. The cord is lifted off the posterior canal wall and pubic tubercle – 'dislocation'.
- The cremaster is opened to allow separation of the hernia sac from the cord structures. An indirect (lateral to inferior epigastric vessels) sac emerges through the deep inguinal ring, superior, lateral and anterior to the cord structures. A direct sac emerges through the posterior wall of the canal, medial to the inferior epigastric vessels.
- Indirect sacs are usually opened, the contents reduced, and the sac tied at its neck. Excess sac is then excised. Direct sacs are less often excised – rather they are reduced with closure of the defect with suture, or, if the neck is wide, reduced with a plication stitch. Very large sacs or long inguino-scrotal sacs may be divided in the groin and transfixed at the neck, with the distal part left in situ.
- The posterior wall of the inguinal canal is then repaired by placement of a prosthetic mesh. This is placed over the whole posterior wall, with the formation of a window to transmit the cord structures without constriction. The mesh is fixed along its inferior edge to the inner part of the inguinal ligament, and to the conjoint tendon and pubic tubercle by suture, glue or, in some cases, self-adherent meshes.
- Closure is by repair of the external oblique aponeurosis, followed by suture of the fat and skin.

Laparoscopic Repair

Mesh repair may be performed laparoscopically. This method is associated with less postoperative pain and more rapid return to normal activity. There are two main approaches to this method, TAPP (trans-abdominal pre-peritoneal) and TEP (totally extra-peritoneal):

- TAPP repair involves the insertion of a camera and instruments through all layers of the abdominal wall after insufflation of the peritoneal cavity. The hernia is then approached by incising the peritoneum from inside, creating a pocket between abdominal wall and peritoneum, reducing the hernial sac into the abdomen, and placing a mesh between the peritoneum and abdominal wall, covering the hernial orifice. The peritoneal incision is then closed to prevent contact between mesh and bowel.
- TEP repair does not involve breaching the peritoneum. Instead, a space is created between the peritoneum and the abdominal wall using a balloon which is introduced into this space. When inflated, the balloon peels the peritoneum off the abdominal wall. The balloon is then removed and the space maintained by gas insufflation. Camera and instruments may then be inserted, and the hernia sac reduced from within, and a mesh placed over the defect to prevent recurrence.

The wounds are smaller, less painful and allow earlier mobilization compared with open repair. There is less exposure and handling of nerves and there is therefore a lower incidence of pain, paraesthesia and anaesthesia complications. The planes in which dissection and mesh placement occur make the laparoscopic method preferable in recurrent hernia repair if an open approach has been used previously, avoiding the need to operate on already scarred and distorted tissues. Both groins may be approached with minimal increase in the trauma of access, and therefore there is clear benefit in cases of bilateral inguinal hernia.

These procedures, however, carry a higher risk of major visceral or large vessel injury (small bowel, bladder and external iliac vessels in particular), although such injuries remain rare. The operation costs of laparoscopic procedures are higher and general anaesthesia is required. Few surgeons would attempt laparoscopic repair in very large inguinal hernias. The recurrence rate in laparoscopic repairs is dependent upon the case volume of the surgeon and, in the general population, may be higher than with open mesh repair.

Specific Complications

- Urinary retention
- A scrotal haematoma may follow extensive dissection
- Damage to the ilio-inguinal nerve produces an area of anaesthesia over the pubic tubercle, scrotum or labia

Outcome

Recurrence rate for inguinal hernia is one of the most hotly debated subjects in general surgery. With selection of patients only after adequate evaluation of contributing factors and with good technique, recurrence rates for groin hernias should be low. The recurrence rates seen in national registries is more widely quoted as 2–10% for primary hernias and higher in the management of recurrence. However, such rates should be balanced against the population under study, the technique used and the quality of follow-up.

Recurrent Inguinal Hernia

Even with what seems to be optimal operative technique, hernias recur. Factors involved in recurrence include:

- Predisposing causes – those with uncorrectable precipitating factors (such as connective tissue disorders) or on high-dose steroid therapy which interferes with healing
- Type of hernia – indirect hernias have a 1–7% recurrence rate but direct hernias reach 4–10%
- Type of operation – repairs under tension do not heal with adequate protection against recurrence
- Postoperative wound infection

Management of Recurrence

Recurrent inguinal hernias should be considered for repair in order to avoid the same complications that occur in primary hernias, which are even more likely when recurrence has taken place. Because of scarring, the dissection can be difficult; in the male, orchidectomy is occasionally performed to allow closure of the deep ring. Recurrent hernias are best managed by using a different approach than the primary repair; for example if previous open primary repair, recurrence should be repaired laparoscopically and vice versa. If laparoscopy is contraindicated for some reason, open pre-peritoneal repair is an acceptable option.

Femoral Hernia

With femoral, the local pain the patient may not mention, while to the tiny lump in groin she does not call attention

ON STRANGULATED FEMORAL HERNIA – ZACHARY COPE, 1947

Femoral hernias are acquired downward protrusions of peritoneum into the potential space of the femoral canal (Fig. 30.6). They account for 7% of all hernias but, in that they are four times more common in women than in men, they constitute 33% of groin hernias in females (5% in men). They are most common in late middle age and the multiparous and, unlike inguinal hernias, are rare in children. Bilateral hernias occur in 20%.

Anatomy

The femoral canal is a 1–2 cm gap medial to the femoral sheath and femoral vein which contains a lymph node and fat. Its anterior (inguinal ligament), medial (lacunar part of the inguinal ligament) and posterior (pectineal part of the inguinal ligament) boundaries are rigid (see Fig. 30.6). This narrow femoral ring produces a considerable risk of incarceration of any hernia that passes through it.

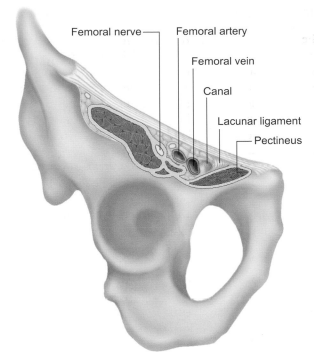

• **Fig. 30.6** Femoral Canal

Aetiology and Pathological Features

As mentioned above, the hernia is acquired. The wide pelvis of the female and the laxity of ligaments after repeated pregnancy are contributory factors, as is weight loss. As the sac develops, it passes forwards through the saphenous opening, whose well-defined lower edge directs it upwards to lie over the inguinal ligament in the subcutaneous plane.

The narrow canal makes a femoral hernia the one most likely to result in a Richter's hernia (30% of strangulated femoral hernias), although strangulation of an omental plug also takes place.

Clinical Features

History

The patient is typically a middle-aged or elderly female, often of thin build, who complains of an intermittent lump low in the groin. However, a major problem is that she may not have noticed the lump and the first clinical presentation is with strangulation (see later), which occurs in 20%.

Signs

In a small hernia, a cough impulse is only rarely detected. A larger hernia may be seen to bulge on straining just below the medial part of the inguinal ligament. An irreducible hernia is a lump whose consistency varies according to its contents, which may extend upwards across the inguinal ligament. In consequence, it can be difficult to distinguish from an inguinal hernia, but the upper medial border of

TABLE 30.4	Inguinal Swellings Which May Resemble a Femoral Hernia.
Condition	**Findings**
Inguinal hernia	Swelling is above and medial to the pubic tubercle
Saphena varix	Compressible Palpable thrill on coughing
Enlarged lymph node	Usually multiple Not fixed on deep aspect and therefore more mobile Seek cause – infection, tumour, lymphoma
Lipoma	Soft but not reducible
Femoral artery aneurysm	Expanding pulsation Bruit
Psoas abscess	Fluctuant Lateral to femoral artery Associated swelling in the iliac fossa
Ectopic testis	Empty scrotum

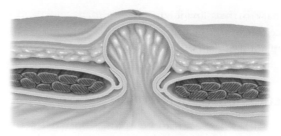

• **Fig. 30.7** Umbilical Hernia

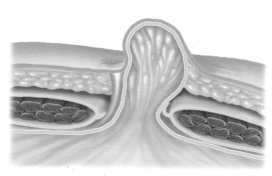

• **Fig. 30.8** Para-Umbilical Hernia

a femoral hernia is always below and lateral to the pubic tubercle. The other conditions that should be taken into consideration when a femoral hernia is diagnosed are shown in Table 30.4.

Strangulation

In contrast to a strangulated inguinal hernia, in a strangulated femoral hernia there are often no localizing symptoms and signs and the lump is often small, unimpressive and overlooked by the patient (and perhaps the clinician). The classic presentation is that of small-bowel obstruction. However, the clinical features of this may be modified by the presence of a Richter's hernia which only partly obstructs the lumen of the gut so that the symptoms and signs are more like those of gastroenteritis. This, combined with the difficulty in finding the hernia, makes for a late diagnosis, sometimes only after the gut has perforated and there is spreading peritonitis.

Management

All femoral hernias should be repaired without delay because of their high risk of strangulation. A truss has no place in management because it cannot control the hernia. The principles are given above. In elective operations, repair is usually by direct incision over the hernia, excision of the sac and sutured closure of the femoral canal or a laparoscopic approach. For operation on a patient with obstruction or strangulation, it may be necessary to open the abdomen to find the segment of gut that has been trapped should it reduce before it can be dealt with.

Umbilical Hernia

Congenital (Infantile) Umbilical Hernia

This condition is considered in Chapter 9.

Adult Umbilical Hernia

Only a small minority of adult umbilical hernias are the outcome of the persistence of a congenital defect.

Aetiology and Anatomical and Pathological Features

Two types of hernia occur with overlapping but different aetiological factors of clinical importance.

True Umbilical Hernia (Fig. 30.7)

In this condition, the protrusion is through the umbilical scar, everting the umbilicus, whose attenuated fibres are at the apex of the hernial sac. The cause is often secondary to an increase in the volume of contents of the abdominal cavity – e.g. due to obesity, ascites or large benign or malignant intra-abdominal tumours.

Para-Umbilical Hernia (Fig. 30.8)

The weakest area of the umbilical scar is at the superior aspect between the umbilical vein and the upper margin of the umbilical ring. It is at this point that a para-umbilical hernia develops. The emerging sac displaces the umbilical scar, which lies below and slightly to one side.

These hernias are more common than true umbilical hernias and typically are found in the obese middle-aged patient. Women are affected five times more frequently than men. Generalized inadequacy of the musculofascial layers of the abdominal wall and repeated pregnancy are important contributory factors.

The neck of the hernia is often narrow. In consequence, tissues that enter have great difficulty leaving; adhesions form and the hernia becomes irreducible. The sac progressively acquires more contents and may become very large. The contents are usually omentum, often with small bowel or transverse colon. Frequently, the sac becomes loculated when adhesions form between the omentum and the peritoneum. Not surprisingly, these hernias are at risk of strangulation.

Clinical Features

True Umbilical Hernia

Symptoms. These are often present where there is an underlying cause of ascites or there may merely be gross obesity. Very rarely, the patient will give a history which dates back to infancy or childhood.

Signs. Ascites may be obvious. The umbilicus is attenuated and sometimes paper-thin. Evidence of underlying malignancy should be sought both in the abdomen as a whole and at the umbilical opening, where a nodule or nodules may be palpable.

Para-Umbilical Hernia

Symptoms. There is local pain and a swelling at the navel. Non-specific gastrointestinal symptoms are common, and features of recurrent intestinal obstruction may have occurred.

Signs. The umbilicus assumes a crescent shape. Inspection and palpation reveal a swelling just above the umbilicus whose centre (in contrast to true umbilical hernia) is not attached to the apex of the protrusion. However, in grossly obese patients, the swelling may not be obvious to the naked eye and moreover, is barely palpable. In others the hernia may be enormous. Usually it is reducible (at least in part) and there is a cough impulse. If reduction is possible, the palpable defect can be of any size, from one fingertip to admitting the fist.

Conditions that may be confused with a para-umbilical hernia include:
- cyst of the vitello-intestinal duct (rare)
- cyst of the urachus (also rare)
- metastatic tumour deposit

Management

True Umbilical Hernia

Any underlying cause should be sought and dealt with. In the rare event that nothing is found and the hernia is causing symptoms, it is treated as a para-umbilical hernia.

Para-Umbilical Hernia

Symptomatic hernias require treatment. There is a high risk of strangulation, and repair should be advised, even in the absence of symptoms. The usual procedure is to mobilise the sac and its contents, return the latter to the abdomen, close the neck and repair the abdominal wall. In the absence of contamination the use of permanent synthetic mesh to reinforce the repair is advised. In contaminated settings, simple suture repair with delayed absorbable sutures is recommended. Overlapping fascial (Mayo) repairs are obsolete.

Strangulated Umbilical Hernia

The patient with severe abdominal pain and vomiting and a soft non-tender umbilical hernia is a diagnostic trap. The loculated nature of the hernia allows a strangulated portion of bowel (often of the Richter's type) to go unnoticed clinically. In other instances, the local features of strangulation may be obvious. The operative approach is as for an elective case, and the strangulating contents are dealt with according to their state.

Epigastric Hernia

Anatomy

The linea alba is the raphe formed by the junction of the rectus sheaths and the decussation of their fibres across the midline; it extends from the xiphoid process to the symphysis pubis. In its upper half, it is 1–3 cm wide and fibrous, but below the umbilicus it is a narrow cord.

Pathological Features

The linea may be attenuated because of a congenital weakness in its lattice structure. Small neurovascular bundles that penetrate are also points of diminished resistance. Herniations of extraperitoneal fat through the linea usually occur in its upper half. They are found in 1% of the population from adolescence onwards. Males are three times more commonly affected than females, and the protrusions are multiple in 20% of cases. The initial extraperitoneal fat protrusion may be followed by the formation of a peritoneal sac, and omentum may enter this (intestinal contents are rare). Extraperitoneal fat or omentum is frequently incarcerated and may strangulate.

Clinical Features

Symptoms

Three-quarters of epigastric hernias are asymptomatic and found incidentally on physical examination. When symptoms are present, they are of two types:
- Local pain – often exacerbated by physical exertion
- Ill-defined pain – epigastric in site, often worse after meals (abdominal distension may strangulate the contents), and the clinical picture may mimic that of peptic ulceration

Signs

The hernia may be visible if the patient is placed in an oblique light. The swelling is palpable in the midline and is usually tender and irreducible.

A patient who presents with vague upper-abdominal symptoms and in whom an epigastric hernia is found should be fully investigated for the possibility of peptic ulcer, gall-bladder or pancreatic disease before symptoms are attributed to the hernia.

Management

Patients with symptomatic hernias are offered repair. The herniated fat is excised. If a sac is present, the contents are reduced and the sac excised. The fascial defect is closed by suture. Any coincidental defects are similarly dealt with at the same time. Even small hernias may have a lower recurrence rate with the use of mesh reinforcement.

Incisional Hernia

An incisional hernia is one that occurs through the wound of a previous operation. It has the same features as a hernia that is caused by non-surgical injury to the abdominal wall.

Incisional hernias are seen in up to 20–30% of midline laparotomy incisions at 2 years postoperatively on CT scans and the risk of developing a symptomatic incisional hernia is life-long. Such hernias comprise 10% of the total number seen.

Aetiology

Partial dehiscence of all or part of the deeper fascial layers occurs, but the skin remains intact or eventually heals. An incisional hernia is a postoperative complication and, like all such complications, its cause can be considered in terms of three factors: preoperative, operative and postoperative.

Preoperative Factors

- Age – the tissues of the elderly do not heal as well as those of the young
- Malnutrition – protein-calorie malnutrition, vitamin deficiency (vitamin C is essential for collagen maturation) and trace metal deficiency (zinc is required for epithelialization)
- Sepsis – worsens malnutrition and delays anabolism
- Uraemia – inhibits fibroblast division
- Jaundice – impedes collagen maturation
- Obesity – predisposes to wound infection, seroma and haematoma
- Diabetes mellitus – predisposes to wound infection
- Steroids – have a generalized proteolytic effect
- Peritoneal contamination (peritonitis) – predisposes to wound infection

Operative Factors

- Type of incision – vertical incisions are more prone to hernia than are transverse ones.
- Technique and materials – tension in the closure impedes blood supply to the wound; badly tied knots can work loose; closure with rapidly absorbable suture material fails to support the abdominal wall for a sufficient time to permit sound union. The size of bites of tissue taken when closing the linea alba may be important and suture length to wound length ratios >7:1 are associated with the lowest incidence of hernia development.
- Type of operation – operations involving the bowel or urinary tract are more likely to develop wound infection.
- Drains – a drain passing through the wound often results in a hernia.

Postoperative Factors

- Wound infection – equal in importance with the wrong choice of suture material. There is enzymatic destruction of healing tissues; inflammatory swelling raises tissue tension and impedes blood supply; 5–20% of wound infections result in a hernia.
- Abdominal distension – postoperative ileus increases the tension on a wound; stitches may cut out.
- Coughing – generates wound tension.

Approximately 40% of incisional hernias occur with a documented episode of wound infection.

Pathological Features

Most incisional hernias develop within 1 year of an operation, but the risk of hernia development remains life-long. Once a hernia has formed, mechanical forces ensure that it inexorably enlarges.

Incisional hernias are extremely variable. They may be wide- or narrow-necked; often, as contents accumulate, adhesions develop in the sac, and just deep to the neck, so that the hernia becomes irreducible. Strangulation is a relatively rare event, particularly with wide-necked hernias. The sac can assume huge proportions, eventually housing much of the normal intraperitoneal contents.

Clinical Features

Symptoms

There may have been a stormy convalescence from a surgical procedure. The complaint is of a bulge in the scar. As the hernia enlarges, patients may complain of difficulty with mobility, micturition and defaecation, which are dependent upon functioning rectus abdominis muscles in the midline for generating core stability and raised intra-abdominal pressure. The hernia may give rise to local discomfort. The overlying skin may become thin and atrophic; eventually, ulceration and even rupture can occur. Strangulation is rare but a surgical emergency.

Signs

Examination reveals a readily apparent, usually reducible, hernia with a cough impulse at the site of an old scar. If the hernia is complex, many fibrous bands may be felt passing between the margins of the defect. When the patient is lying flat, these hernias are deceptively small, but any manoeuvre that raises intra-abdominal pressure produces the hernia in all its glory.

Management

Even small symptomatic hernias should be considered for repair early. In asymptomatic hernias, non-operative management has been performed, but there remains the risk of developing symptoms and a small but not negligible risk of intestinal obstruction, strangulation and skin ulceration. All management options and their associated risks and benefits should be discussed, even in older patients. Protracted observation simply allows the hernia to increase in size, and subsequent repair is rendered more difficult and hazardous. The surgical technique depends upon the size of the defect, but essentially comprises excision of the sac, closure of the defect and reinforcement of the abdominal wall with a prosthetic mesh.

Laparoscopic repair of incisional hernias is performed by gaining access to the peritoneal cavity to allow insufflation, followed by insertion of camera and instrument ports away from the hernia. This is not always easily achieved because of intra-abdominal adhesions. The hernia is reduced carefully by division of adhesions between contents and sac; this is the time at which injury to the bowel most easily occurs. The defect (or defects) are isolated with sufficient clearance on all sides, to allow satisfactory mesh placement. Many surgeons advocate closure of the defect with sutures placed either laparoscopically or transfascially via a suture grasper. Commonly, a mesh is placed with one side coated with an anti-adhesive layer facing the bowel, to minimize adhesion of bowel to mesh. The mesh is placed and secured with tacks and/or sutures intraperitoneally, with generous overlap of the edges of the defect.

Repair of very large incisional hernias involving much of the anterior abdominal wall are rarely undertaken laparoscopically because of the difficulty in securing adequate overlap of the mesh over the defect.

Outcome

The results of surgery are not as good as for primary hernias. Small incisional hernias have a recurrence rate of 2–5%, whereas in large ones, it is 10–20%. Common postoperative problems include seroma formation, which may require surgical intervention, chronic pain and a mesh sensation in the abdominal wall that limits activity or reduces quality of life.

Parastomal Hernia

Parastomal hernia are an important subtype of incisional hernia. They are very common and usually develop within the first 2 years of index surgery, although the risk may be lifelong. It has been estimated that up to 80% of patients with an end colostomy may be affected, with lower incidences for ileostomies, urostomies and loop stomas. Symptoms may include pain, bowel obstruction, skin irritation and difficulty with stoma bag adhesion. Signs are usually a bulge immediately adjacent to the stoma, although this can be difficult to palpate in the obese. The majority of parastomal hernias are managed non-operatively by expert stoma care nurses, but up to one-third of patients may require surgical intervention. Unlike other hernia types, there is no

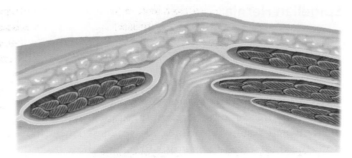

• **Fig. 30.9** Interparietal Hernia

obviously superior technique for repair. Surgeons have been reticent to operate due to high rates of recurrence and complications, regardless of the approach or technique used. Re-siting of the stoma has been similarly unsuccessful with high rates of parastomal hernia at the new stoma site and incisional hernia development at the old stoma site. Prevention may be the best strategy and many surgeons have recommended the use of prophylactic mesh when constructing the stoma, although the adoption of prophylactic mesh has not been widespread.

Rare but Clinically Important Hernias

The following hernias comprise only 1% of the total, but they are considered because their recognition is of clinical importance.

Interparietal Hernia (Fig. 30.9)

The hernial sac lies between the layers of the abdominal wall. The cause may be congenital, when there is an associated abnormality of testicular descent, or acquired in an area of weakness in the lateral aspect of the deep inguinal ring and inguinal canal (when the sac usually communicates with a concomitant indirect inguinal hernia). The classification of such hernias is based on the anatomical location of the sac:
• properitoneal (20%)
• interstitial (60%)
• superficial (20%)

Clinical Features

The properitoneal type of hernia is impalpable. The interstitial and superficial types often present with a small swelling above and lateral to the inguinal canal and deep ring. Such insignificant local features are ignored by patients, and 90% of these hernias present with intestinal obstruction that culminates in strangulation. The key to early diagnosis is to consider this type of hernia in any patient with the features of intestinal obstruction (simple or strangulating) with a palpable mass lateral to the deep ring and an abnormally placed testis.

Management

Operation (usually an emergency laparotomy for strangulating obstruction of unknown cause) reveals the hernial sac, which is excised and the fascial defect repaired.

Spigelian Hernia

This is an interparietal hernia in the line of the linea semilunaris (the lateral margin of the rectus sheath, running from the tip of the ninth costal cartilage to the pubic crest). The hernia is usually at the level of the arcuate line, below which all aponeurotic layers are reflected anterior to the rectus muscle. The cause is related to the aponeurotic arrangement, which results in an area of weakness where fibres from the transversus aponeurosis fuse with those from the internal oblique. The hernial sac emerges and enlarges like a mushroom deep to the external oblique.

Clinical Features

Symptoms

Symptoms are:
- Local pain that is worse on straining
- Lump
- Non-specific lower-quadrant discomfort which needs to be investigated in its own right
- Features of obstruction or strangulation

Signs

Signs are:
- Tenderness at the site of the hernial orifice
- Lump which may be difficult or even impossible to feel

Investigation and Management

Recently, CT scans have proved useful in the demonstration of these hernias in patients with convincing histories but who lack clinical signs. Repair is as for other hernias – excising the sac, closing the defect and reinforcing the repair with mesh.

Obturator Hernia

In this condition, herniation occurs along the obturator canal, which carries the obturator nerve and vessels out of the pelvis (Fig. 30.10). It is most commonly seen in frail old ladies. The hernia starts as a pre-peritoneal plug and gradually enlarges, taking a sac of peritoneum with it. A loop of bowel may enter the sac and reduce spontaneously. Eventually, a knuckle fails to reduce. Further loops can then be incorporated. A Richter's strangulation is common.

Clinical Features

Symptoms

Lying deep to the pectineus, these hernias are largely asymptomatic until complicated by intestinal obstruction or strangulation. There is often a past history of intermittent symptoms of obstruction. In about 50%, there may be the complaint of pain along the upper medial side of the thigh which radiates down to the knee, caused by pressure on the obturator nerve. Though present, this symptom is often not elicited.

Signs

There are rarely any signs, except those of obstruction or strangulation. The diagnosis is made either on CT of the

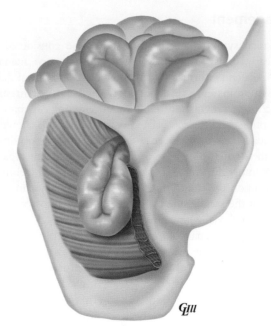

• **Fig. 30.10** Obturator Hernia

abdomen and pelvis in those who present with small bowel obstruction or at the time of laparotomy for small-bowel obstruction of unknown cause. With pressure on the obturator nerve, the patient holds the leg flexed to reduce the pain. In 20% of patients, the hernial sac protrudes medially around the pectineus and presents as a palpable swelling in the femoral triangle. Rectal and especially vaginal examination can reveal a swelling in the region of the obturator foramen.

Management

If discovered at laparotomy, the intestine is reduced, the sac withdrawn and the defect closed. If the diagnosis is made clinically, an elective procedure by the retropubic, pre-peritoneal approach can be done.

Lumbar Hernia

Such hernias may be:
- congenital
- acquired primary
- acquired secondary – the result of surgical incision

Acquired hernias through an incision for lumbar approach to the kidney are not uncommon; however, with the decline in open renal surgery, they are becoming less common.

Acquired Primary Lumbar Hernia

Hernias that occur through anatomical weak points in the lumbar region – the superior and inferior lumbar triangles (Fig. 30.11) – are uncommon.

Clinical Features

Most present with a bulge or lump in the flank, associated with an aching discomfort. There is usually a cough impulse

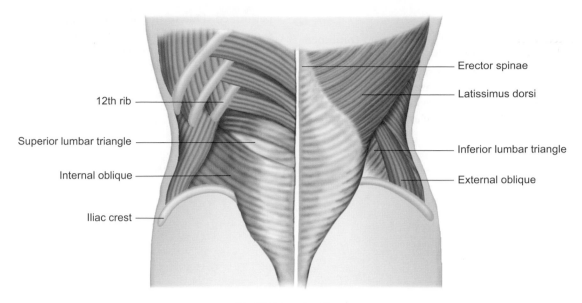

• **Fig. 30.11** Lumbar Hernia

and the mass is reducible. The contents are most often small and large bowel – very rarely the kidney. Some 20% become incarcerated and 10% strangulate.

An irreducible lumbar hernia must be distinguished from:
- lipoma
- soft-tissue tumour
- haematoma
- tuberculous cold abscess
- renal tumour

Management

Primary hernias are managed by direct closure of the defect. Large incisional hernias require a mesh prosthesis.

Sciatic Hernia

A sciatic hernia is the protrusion of a pelvic peritoneal sac through the greater or lesser sciatic foramen (Fig. 30.12).

Clinical Features

Patients present with discomfort and a swelling in the buttock, and there may be symptoms of sciatic nerve compression. If the hernia is large, there is a reducible mass in the gluteal area, made larger on standing. Herniation of the ureters can cause urinary symptoms. There is an appreciable risk of strangulation.

Management

Treatment is by excision of the sac and closure of the defect by a transabdominal or transgluteal approach.

Perineal Hernia

These may be:
- congenital
- primary acquired
- incisional

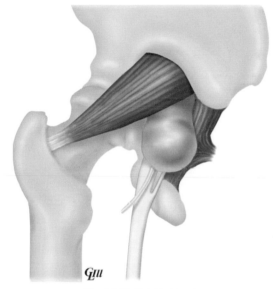

• **Fig. 30.12** Sciatic Hernia

Primary acquired perineal hernias occur in middle-aged, multiparous women. Their broad pelvis and the muscle-weakening effect of childbirth result in herniation through the pelvic floor. Incisional perineal hernia follows abdominoperineal excisions of the rectum, usually for rectal cancer. The recent trend for wider excisions incorporating the levator muscles and increased use of neoadjuvant chemoradiotherapy with its attendant adverse effect on wound healing has led to an increase in the incidence of this once rare hernia.

Clinical Features

There is usually a perineal swelling and discomfort when sitting. A soft mass is found in the perineum, which is usually reducible. The wide neck has elastic margins. These hernias rarely have dangerous complications.

Management

Repair can be via abdominal, pelvic or combined approach. In the case of small hernias, laparoscopic abdominal approaches with mesh repair are feasible. For larger hernias now seen more commonly, the hernia may be better approached from below, the sac dissected free and reduced into the abdominal cavity. Mesh repair can still be performed. Due to the history of radiotherapy treatment, some advocate the use of tissue flaps for perineal hernia repair, which may be undertaken in combination with the use of mesh. There are numerous different flaps described, but the optimal flap is uncertain and will often depend upon surgeon preference and previous surgical history of the patient.

31

Principles of Plastic Surgery

Derived from the Greek 'plastikos' meaning to mould or to give shape, the specialty of plastic surgery is perhaps more accurately described as one of reconstructive surgery. The layperson's perception of plastic surgery is one of cosmetic surgery, which represents a facet of the specialty, though aesthetic goals along with restoration of form and function underpin the basic principles of the specialty. Unlike other surgical specialties, there is no specific territory of the body which is the monopoly of plastic surgery. Although a degree of subspecialization has developed recently, the plastic surgeon might be regarded as the last of the general surgeons in treating a great variety of problems in many sites (although in general, body cavities are excluded). Some of the techniques used in the current era of plastic surgery have been in use for many years; for example, the forehead flap was described first almost 3000 years ago in India but it remains the go-to flap for nasal reconstruction. The greatest advances in reconstructive techniques have been driven by warfare and the need to reconstruct increasingly complex battlefield injuries both in the short-to-medium term after the injury but also in the longer term.

The aetiology of defects requiring reconstruction may be congenital or acquired through trauma, degeneration, neoplasia or iatrogenic conditions. As a result, the plastic surgeon works alongside other surgical specialities (Table 31.1) in order to minimize the risk of wound-related problems by: (1) obliterating anatomical dead space, (2) importing well-vascularized tissue to optimize wound (or bone) healing, (3) performing functional reconstructions and (4) restoring anatomical form.

Plastic Surgery Techniques

Plastic surgery is an innovative speciality that continues to develop new solutions for complex problems. Whilst flaps and skin grafts have been used for hundreds of years, advances in vascular anatomy knowledge and surgical technique have led to the development of modern microsurgery and perforator flaps. Advances in immunology have enabled successful face and limb transplants (vascularized composite allotransplantation (VCA)). In parallel, rapid advances in technology and biomaterials have led to the development of novel reconstructive techniques, for example, acellular dermal matrices for breast and abdominal wall reconstruction. However, the greatest advances, arguably, have arisen from advances in anaesthetic practice and monitoring, which have facilitated surgeons in performing increasingly complex surgical procedures requiring bespoke reconstructive solutions.

The choice of techniques available to the plastic surgeon are many and traditional teaching espoused using a 'reconstructive ladder' by performing the simplest procedure in the first instance before proceeding to more complicated techniques. However, reconstructive decision making has changed as the more complex techniques (e.g. microsurgery) can now be performed routinely and reliably. Indeed, successful reconstructive surgery has facilitated our surgical colleagues in other specialities to undertake increasingly complex cases. In the broadest terms, the decision of which reconstructive technique to use are determined by: (1) what is appropriate for the patient who is being treated and (2) what are the requirements of the wound being reconstructed? Rather than choosing a 'simple' technique, the modern approach is to offer the technique that will produce the 'best' result in terms of reliable wound healing and restoration of form and function.

TABLE 31.1	Plastic Surgery Involvement With Other Specialties
Specialty	**Procedure**
Neurosurgery	Cranioplasty, transcranial tumour resection, external-internal carotid artery bypass
Otorhinolaryngology	Head and neck reconstruction
Cardio-thoracic surgery	Chest wall reconstruction for cancer, sternal reconstruction, pectus excavatum repair
Breast surgery	Breast reconstruction after breast conservation or mastectomy
Upper gastrointestinal (GI) surgery	Free jejunal flaps for oesophageal reconstruction
Hepatobiliary surgery	Hepatic artery anastomoses for living related/paediatric liver transplants
Gynaecology	Gynaecological reconstruction
Lower GI surgery	Perineal reconstruction after pelvic exenteration/sacrectomy
Orthopaedic surgery	Hand surgery, lower limb trauma, osteomyelitis surgery, bone sarcoma reconstruction
Urology	Hypospadias/epispadia repair and reconstruction for bladder exstrophy

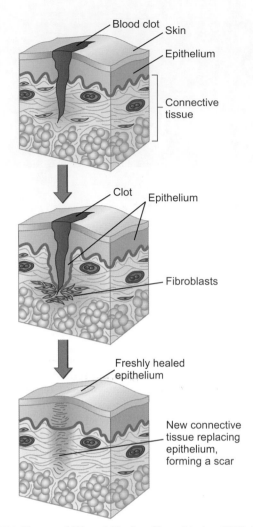

• **Fig. 31.1** Stages of Wound Healing (From Mosby, 2022. Mosby's Medical Dictionary, 11th ed. St. Louis: Elsevier.)

Wound Healing

Wound healing is the most fundamental process that underlies, and permits, all surgical interventions. All healing proceeds through discrete physiological stages that are subject to local and systemic control and that are co-ordinated carefully at a molecular level to facilitate normal wound healing. Dysregulation of these processes can lead to adverse healing characterized by fibrosis. The phases of normal wound healing are: (1) haemostasis and haematoma formation, (2) inflammation, (3) proliferation and (4) re-modelling (Fig. 31.1).

Haemostasis: Vascular injury causes vasoconstriction and platelet aggregation to form a thrombus by activation of the extrinsic clotting cascade.

Inflammation: Influx of neutrophils (24 h) followed by macrophages (2–3 days) caused by release of platelet derived growth factor (PDGF) and transforming growth factor β (TGF-β) from activated platelets.

Proliferation (3 days–3 weeks): Characterized by the recruitment and activation of fibroblasts by TGF-β to produce type III collagen to cause wound contraction and associated with angiogenesis and re-epithelialization.

Remodelling (up to 1 year): Replacement of type III collagen with type I and re-organization of type I collagen along tension lines to increase tensile strength.

Failure of normal wound healing can occur as a result of both local and systemic factors and, where possible, the causative factor should be treated.

Healing by Primary Intention (Surgical Wound Healing)

Tension-free wound closure using appropriate sutures and meticulous approximation of the skin edges, in eversion, results in the best possible scar. In addition to sutures, a variety of technologies exist for achieving skin closure, such as skin glues, staples (absorbable or metallic) or negative pressure wound therapy (NPWT) systems that splint the wound in the early postoperative period (e.g. PICO).

Healing by Secondary Intention

Maintaining an optimal wound healing environment by wound toilet, appropriate dressing choice, vigilance for infection and optimization of the systemic factors that affect wound healing will allow most wounds to heal by secondary intention. This process is characterized by the generation of

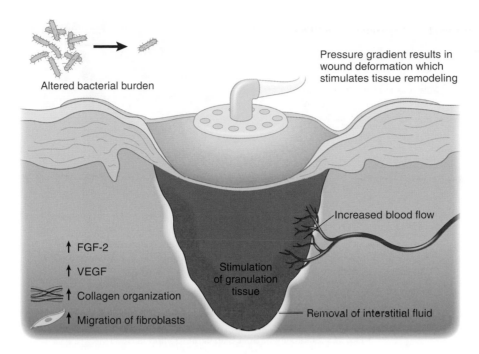

- **Fig. 31.2** Mechanism of Action of NPWT *FGF*, Fibroblast growth factor; *NPWT*, negative-pressure wound therapy; *VEGF*, vascular endothelial growth factor. (From Hasan MY, Teo R, Nather A. Negative-pressure wound therapy for management of diabetic foot wounds: a review of the mechanism of action, clinical applications, and recent developments. Diabet Foot Ankle. 2015;6:27618.)

granulation tissue from the base of the wound and re-epithelialization, which occurs as a result of migration of keratinocytes from the wound edge. Healing by secondary intention takes longer than primary intention and generates a significant healthcare burden with regards to dressing management; however, in appropriate cases it remains the technique of choice to achieve healing. Adjuncts, such as NPWT, can be used to expedite this process. The resultant scars from healing by secondary intention have poorer aesthetic outcomes and there is a greater risk of hypertrophic scarring.

Scar Management

Dysregulation of normal wound healing processes results in adverse scar formation, which may be either hypertrophic or keloid in nature. Hypertrophic scars develop soon after surgery but remain confined to the limits of the original wound. They are common, have no racial preponderance, can be improved by surgery but often improve with time. Conversely, keloid scars are characterized by growth extending beyond the margins of the original wound, they can occur at any time after surgery/injury and can occur after even quite minor trauma. They are symptomatic (itch), can be worsened by surgery and are commoner in people with dark skin. There is also often a family history of keloid scarring in individuals who develop it.

The mainstay of scar management is non-surgical and where surgery is considered, the timing of intervention in relation to the maturity of the scar is key. Unless there is an overwhelming need to protect vital structures (eyes, mouth), surgery should only be considered once the scar has matured fully.

Non-surgical modalities for scar management aim to modulate the oxygenation and vascularity of scars and, in doing so, reduce the inflammatory/proliferative component of the scar. This may be mechanical (massage, compression therapy, silicone therapy), pharmacological (steroid injection, anti-histamine, neuropathic agents) or ablative (radiotherapy or LASER therapy) in nature. Surgical intervention includes scar revision techniques to interrupt the scar (usually for hypertrophic scars or those crossing joint lines/adjacent to vital structures) or scar excision (intra- or extra-lesional) for keloid scars. The latter may be performed with adjunctive intra-lesional steroid injection, compression therapy or radiotherapy

Negative Pressure Wound Therapy

NPWT is well established as a method of aiding wound closure or temporizing wounds as a bridge to definitive reconstruction. NPWT works by exerting mechanical forces on the wound, altering the biochemical milieu of the wound environment and reducing bacterial contamination (Fig. 31.2). A non-adherent foam is placed in the wound and negative pressure applied either continuously or intermittently. NPWT dressings should not be applied directly to heart, brain, exposed vasculature or grossly infected tissues.

Skin Grafts

A graft is defined as tissue moved from one part of the body (donor site) to a recipient area without its blood supply. It is, therefore, reliant upon establishing a new blood supply from the recipient bed to survive, and examples of wound

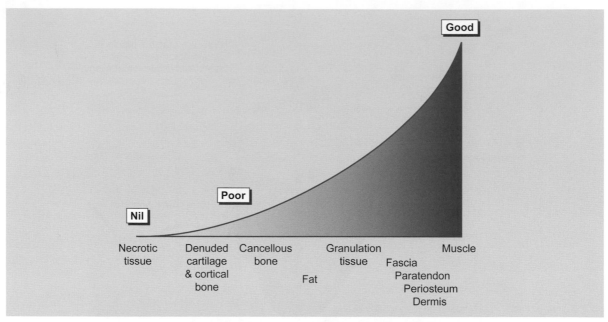

• **Fig. 31.3** Suitability of Split Skin Graft to Various Beds

beds that will *not* provide such a blood supply include bone (without periosteum), cartilage (without perichondrium), tendon (without paratenon) or necrotic/avascular tissue (Fig. 31.3).

Skin grafts include the epidermis and a part of the dermis (split-thickness) or they can include the entire dermis (full-thickness). Following application to a wound bed, skin grafts stick to the bed by fibrinous adhesion and obtain oxygen and metabolites by the process of serum imbibition (direct absorption into the graft). Establishment of a blood supply occurs by direct physiological anastomoses between blood vessels in the graft and those in the bed (inosculation) and in-growth of blood vessels down new vascular channels (neo-vascularization) or existing channels (re-vascularization). By 5 days after application it is usually evident whether a skin graft is starting to establish its own blood supply, although the complete process can take up to several weeks to complete. Graft loss can occur for several reasons: namely, haematoma beneath the graft (minimized by meshing or cutting fenestrations in the graft), infection, inadequate immobilization of the graft to its bed permitting shear, positioning the graft on an unsuitable bed incapable of nourishing the graft or technical error (placing the graft upside down!). The spectrum of ability of different tissues to receive a graft is shown in Fig. 31.4. Most wounds older than 48 hours will be covered by granulation tissue, whose vascularity will be related to that of the underlying tissue.

Split-Thickness Skin Grafts

Split-thickness skin grafts are taken with either hand-held graft knives or by powered dermatomes, both of which cut the superficial layers of the skin 150–300 μm thick (see Fig. 31.4). As a large number of epithelial remnants are left behind at the donor site, these will, in the same manner as a bad graze, heal within 2 weeks, provided they are kept free from infection.

'Take' also depends on stability of the graft. Shearing forces which disrupt in-growing capillary loops must be avoided by immobilizing the skin graft. This can be achieved with tie-over dressings, external splintage or use of an NPWT placed on top of the skin graft.

Common donor sites include the lateral thigh and buttock but, when required, skin can be harvested from any area. Donor sites heal by secondary intention and can be dressed with a variety of alginate or adherent dressings that remain in situ for 2 weeks, although time to healing may be increased significantly in elderly patients. Large areas of skin graft, required in major burns for example, can be harvested by re-using donor sites but these tend to heal with alteration of pigmentation and, occasionally, with hypertrophy.

Split-thickness skin grafts lack dermal constructs and for this reason they undergo significant secondary contracture after they have stuck to a recipient bed, and the thinner they are, the greater the secondary contracture. Consequently, they are less suitable for use on the face or adjacent to vital structures.

The coverage of split-thickness skin grafts can be increased by meshing them at increasing ratios to stretch them out. This has the added advantage of allowing drainage of underlying fluids and/or haematoma through the wound.

Full-Thickness Skin Grafts

Full-thickness skin grafts are composed of the epidermis and the full-thickness of the dermis. As these grafts contain dermis, they are less prone to secondary contracture. The donor site is closed primarily and examples of donor sites for full-thickness grafts include: supra-clavicular fossa, neck, abdomen, groin, medial arm and behind or in front

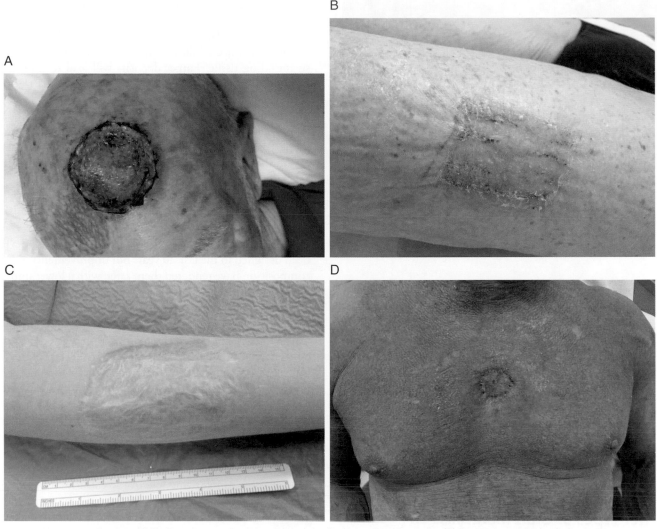

• **Fig. 31.4** (A) Early post-operative appearance of split skin graft to the scalp. (B) Appearance of a healed split skin graft donor site. (C) Mature split skin graft. (D) Early postoperative appearance of a full thickness skin graft (FTSG).

of the ear. Consequently, full-thickness grafts are only suitable for smaller areas of coverage and are reserved for areas such as the head and neck or hand, where it is important to minimize the risk of secondary contracture. The colour and texture of the standard post-auricular graft is not ideal for all facial areas, and one should consider other donor sites such as redundant upper-eyelid skin, pre-auricular and supraclavicular skin to achieve optimum facial skin matching.

Cultured Skin and Skin Substitutes

Although not in common usage, there has been considerable clinical experience in the culture of keratinocytes isolated by trypsin from a small split skin graft. These are allowed to proliferate into large sheets of cells on a substrate of fibroblasts. However, such ultrathin layers of cells when applied as a graft are not sufficiently robust to withstand wear and tear and are subject to high infection rates with subsequent graft loss. These cultured epithelial autografts are seldom used alone for coverage. The fundamental problem is that replacement of epidermis alone is insufficient for full-thickness defects and that the complex dermal structure cannot regenerate or be cultured in the same way. A variety of dermal substitutes exist in the market that gained initial popularity in the surgical management of burn injuries and chronic wounds but now are used more frequently for implant-based breast reconstruction and ventral hernia repairs. These substitutes may contain synthetic elements, for example, nylon or silicone, or may be acellular xenografts. Examples include:

- Biobrane (Dow Hickman/Bertek Pharmaceuticals, Sugar Land, Texas, USA) – a Silastic sheet with nylon mesh seeded with porcine collagen and used principally for superficial partial-thickness skin loss.
- Transcyte (Advanced Tissue Sciences, Inc., La Jolla, California, USA) – silicone sheet on collagen-coated nylon mesh seeded with neonatal fibroblasts.
- Integra (Integra Life Sciences, Plainsboro, New Jersey, USA) – a bilaminar sheet of bovine collagen and shark chondroitin 6-sulphate neodermis with an overlying

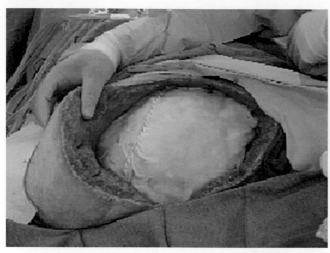

• **Fig. 31.5** Abdominal Wall Reconstruction with Surgimend

Silastic sheet which is removed and replaced with thin split autograft following revascularization of the neodermis at 3 weeks.
• Acellular dermal matrices: can be derived from human cadaveric skin (AlloDerm, LifeCell, Woodlands, Texas, USA), porcine skin (Strattice, Allergan, USA) or bovine (Surgimend, Integra Life Sciences, USA). The most common clinical indications for use are in stabilizing wounds and creating a vascularized bed for skin grafting, to achieve lower pole coverage in implant-based breast reconstruction or abdominal wall reconstruction, particularly in the context of failed/infected hernia repairs with prosthetic mesh (Fig. 31.5).

Other Types of Graft Materials

Other tissues available as free grafts for deep tissue defects, contour defects and functional restoration include bone, cartilage, nerve, tendon and fat. Bone is usually harvested from the ilium or rib and cartilage from the ear concha or the rib. For bridging gaps in nerves, a cutaneous nerve such as the sural nerve may be sacrificed, and for tendon reconstruction vestigial tendons such as palmaris longus and plantaris are used (fascia lata is a reasonable substitute in their absence).

Fat Grafting

Fat harvested from any area of abundance can be reinjected to treat small to moderate contour defects. This technique was popularized by Sidney Coleman and consists of: (1) fat harvest using liposuction techniques, (2) fat preparation by centrifugation or washing and (3) fat grafting. Fat harvest is performed by pre-infiltration of the donor site with a very dilute adrenaline solution and local anaesthetic. A variety of harvest systems exist that are either manual or motorized. The collected fat is processed by either centrifugation or washing to remove fat debris, blood and oil to leave a residual pellet containing adipocytes and mesenchymal stem cells. The fat is then injected in multiple planes at the recipient sites and care must be taken to deposit very small amounts over a large area to build up the volume. This is to allow the injected fat to acquire a blood supply from the surrounding tissue. Larger deposits will lead to poor graft take, nodules of fat necrosis and oil cysts. Patients must be counselled that fat grafting usually requires multiple stages as fat retention with each round of grafting is typically less than 50%. Fat grafting is used routinely for adjusting aesthetic outcomes in breast reconstruction but is also used commonly for adding volume to the facial skeleton (either aesthetic or reconstructive).

Prostheses

Not only has an enormous range of implantable devices been designed in the last 20 years but improvements in their composition have rendered them safer, with a lower implant failure rate.

Silicone, the most commonly used implant material, is a polymer of silica and oxygen that can take on different physical characteristics from a thin oil to a hard block depending on its degree of polymerization. It is relatively inert but after implantation, such as in a breast prosthesis or small joint replacement, is characteristically enveloped in a capsule of fibrous tissue of variable thickness lined with smooth mesothelium. An abnormally thick capsule may distort a breast prosthesis and, as yet, this phenomenon is unable to be predicted or prevented.

Other materials used as a bone substitute, either to restore contour such as following loss of the calvarium or for skeletal replacement, include acrylic bone cement and (more commonly) metal such as stainless steel, chrome cobalt and titanium. The recent discovery that bone will produce a very tight bond on a molecular level with titanium even when the latter extends through skin or mucosa has generated 'osseo-integrated' implants as studs on which artificial teeth and, more recently, external facial prostheses, such as a nose or ear, can be securely attached.

Flaps

Where a skin graft is not appropriate or a more durable construct is necessary, or indeed when aesthetics dictate, a defect should be resurfaced with a flap. A flap is defined as a composite block of tissue that is moved from a local, regional or distant donor site with its blood supply (vascular pedicle) to a recipient bed. Flaps may be classified by their geography (local, regional or free flaps), composition (fasciocutaneous, myocutaneous, muscle only, bone or any combination thereof) or geometry (rotational, transposition, advancement).

The Blood Supply to the Skin

The earliest flaps were simply skin and subcutaneous fat designed without appreciation of the underlying blood supply (random pattern flaps), so that their length and mobility were restricted. The evolution of perforator flap surgery came from a better understanding of how the skin received its blood supply from three main sources: direct cutaneous arteries, muscular perforators and via tributaries of the vascular plexus within the underlying deep fascia and fascial septa (Nakajima classification, Fig. 31.6A). This has allowed for the design of more reliable and anatomically predictable flaps.

Blood Supply to Flaps

The fundamental principle that underlies all flap surgery is an understanding of the blood supply to anatomical territories and muscles. This 'angiosome' concept was first defined by Ian Taylor and classifies the vascular territory of named blood vessels as anatomic, dynamic and potential. This is perhaps best exemplified when considering the blood supply to the anterior abdominal wall in raising a deep inferior epigastric artery perforator (DIEP) flap (Fig. 31.7). In the broadest terms, the anatomic zone represents that territory that is directly perfused by the source vessel/perforator (zone 1), the dynamic zone represents that adjacent territory that is perfused by the opening of 'choke vessels' between adjacent angiosomes (zone 2/3) and the potential territory represents that territory that can only be perfused by the source vessel through the utilization of vascular delay techniques (zone 4).

The pattern of vascular supply to muscle flaps is different to that of fasciocutaneous flaps.

The Mathes and Nahai classification (see Fig. 31.6B) describes the vascular supply to muscle flaps according to the number of vascular pedicles supplying that particular muscle and the dominance of these pedicles. A dominant pedicle is one which can provide blood supply to the entire muscle in isolation:

- Type 1: have a singular pedicle, e.g. tensor fascia lata, gastrocnemius, recus femoris
- Type 2: have a single dominant pedicle and multiple secondary pedicles, e.g. gracilis, temporalis, trapezius
- Type 3: have a dual dominant blood supply, e.g. rectus abdominis, gluteus maximus, serratus anterior
- Type 4: have multiple segmental pedicles, e.g. Sartorius or tibialis anterior
- Type 5: have a single dominant pedicle and segmental supply allowing for the muscle to be raised on either, e.g. latissimus dorsi, pectoralis major

The Cormack and Lamberty classification (see Fig. 31.6C) describes the pattern of supply to fasciocutaneous flaps:

- Type A: pedicled flaps based on multiple, longitudinal perforating vessels, e.g. lower limb pedicled flaps
- Type B: flaps perfused by a single fasciocutaneous perforator, e.g. scapular/parascapular flaps and the anterolateral thigh flap (ALT)
- Type C: flaps perfused by multiple perforators arising from a deep named blood vessel running in an intermuscular septum, e.g. the radial forearm flap

- Type D: as per type C but including bone, e.g. the distal radius raised with the radial forearm flap

Free Tissue Transfer

Reconstructive microsurgery using free tissue transfer is now the standard of care for reconstructing a variety of complex defects. The field of microsurgery continues to evolve, find novel applications and refine existing processes. As a result, free tissue transfer is now a predictable and reliable method of reconstruction with low failure rates. This has been driven as much by technological advances as it has by anaesthetic and perioperative advances.

The stages of any free tissue transfer procedure include (see Fig. 31.7):
1. Elevation of the flap, islanding it on the vascular pedicle.
2. Preparation of the recipient bed and dissection of suitable, healthy recipient vessels.
3. Detachment of the flap followed by anastomosis of flap vessels to recipient vessels.
4. Inset of flap and closure of donor site.

Success rates from free tissue transfer vary slightly depending on the precise defect being reconstructed; for example lower limb trauma and previous irradiation of the recipient site may increase failure rates slightly. However, these risks can be mitigated by meticulous planning, intraoperative decision making and surgical teamwork. The same principles are applied to replantation surgery and, indeed, vascularized composite tissue allotransplantation (VCA).

Perforator Flaps

A perforator flap is one in which the cutaneous perforator supplying a skin territory is dissected back to its source vessel. The vascular anatomy of these flaps is highly variable and dissection of the perforator often follows an intramuscular route. However, the advantage of perforator flaps is the reduction in donor site morbidity attributable to muscle harvest with the flap. The best example of this is the evolution of breast reconstruction from using free transverse rectus abdominis musculocutaneous (fTRAM) to DIEP flaps, which leave behind the rectus abdominis muscle and so reduce the risk of developing a hernia or abdominal bulge. Other examples of perforator flaps include the ALT, anteromedial thigh flap (AMT), superior or inferior gluteal artery perforator (SGAP/IGAP), thoracodorsal artery perforator (TDAP) or medial sural artery perforator (MSAP) flaps.

Supermicrosurgery

The term supermicrosurgery refers to vascular anastomoses performed on vessels less than 1 mm in diameter. The term was first applied to physiological lymphatic surgery techniques such as lymphaticovenous anastomoses (LVA) (Fig. 31.8) but has also been applied to perforator-to-perforator anastomoses, for example, in patients undergoing free flaps for salvage of the diabetic foot. Super microsurgery requires

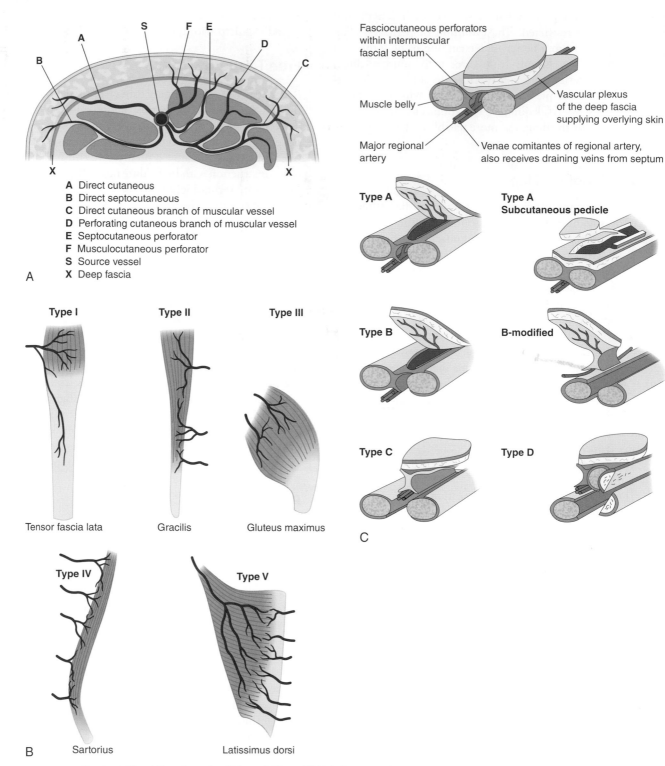

A
A Direct cutaneous
B Direct septocutaneous
C Direct cutaneous branch of muscular vessel
D Perforating cutaneous branch of muscular vessel
E Septocutaneous perforator
F Musculocutaneous perforator
S Source vessel
X Deep fascia

B
Type I — Tensor fascia lata
Type II — Gracilis
Type III — Gluteus maximus
Type IV — Sartorius
Type V — Latissimus dorsi

C
Fasciocutaneous perforators within intermuscular fascial septum
Muscle belly
Major regional artery
Vascular plexus of the deep fascia supplying overlying skin
Venae comitantes of regional artery, also receives draining veins from septum

Type A
Type A Subcutaneous pedicle
Type B
B-modified
Type C
Type D

• **Fig. 31.6** Blood Supply to the Skin and Flaps (A) Nakajima classification. (B) Mathes and Nahai classification. (C) Cormack and Lamberty classification. (A, From Hallock, G.G., 2003. Direct and indirect perforator flaps: the history and the controversy. Plast Reconstr Surg. 111, 855–865; B, from Mathes, S.J., Nahai, F., 1981. Classification of the vascular anatomy of muscles: experimental and clinical correlation. Plast Reconstr Surg. 67, 177–187; C, from Kalaskar, D.M., Butler, P.E., Ghali, S., (Eds.), 2016. Textbook of Plastic and Reconstructive Surgery. UCL Press, London.)

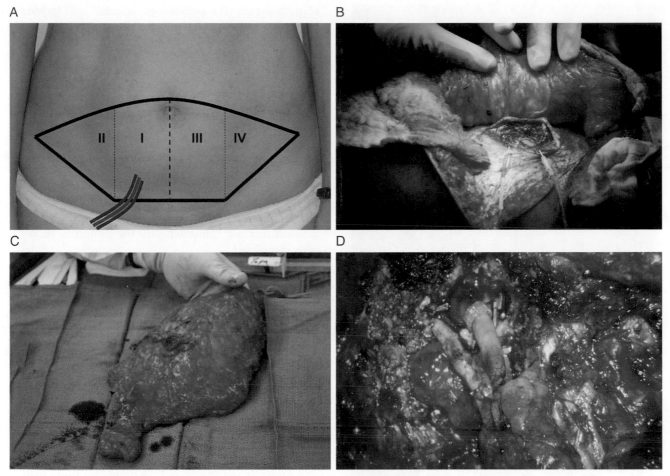

• **Fig. 31.7** Stages of a Free Flap: Performing a Deep Inferior Epigastric Artery Perforator (DIEP) Flap for Breast Reconstruction (A) Perfusion zones of a right medial row DIEP flap. (B) DIEP flap raised on two perforators. (C) DIEP flap *ex vivo* during the ischaemic interval. (D) Microvascular anastomoses of the DIEP flap vessels to the internal mammary artery and vein recipient vessels. (A, From Lipa JE. Breast reconstruction with free flaps from the abdominal donor site—TRAM, DIEAP, and SIEA flaps. Clin Plast Surg. 2007;34(1):105–121, Fig. 1.)

the use of higher magnification microscopes and superfine microsurgical instruments but also meticulous surgical planning and technique.

Vascularized Composite Tissue Allotransplantation (VCA)

VCA represents a highly novel surgical technology, which is still very much in its infancy. To date, approximately 90 VCAs have been performed world-wide and tissues that have been transplanted include: bilateral hand (Fig. 31.9), face, skull, penis and scrotum, abdominal wall and uterus. Whilst the technical success of these procedures is clear, the longer-term sequelae of immunosuppression, in patients who do not have life-threatening conditions, have demanded caution and careful patient selection in performing these procedures. The immunosuppression regimes that have been used traditionally for VCA are similar to those used for solid organ transplantation; however, given the highly variable antigenicity of composite tissues, more novel, biological regimens

(chimerism) are being increasingly used to attempt to induce tolerance.

Tissue Expansion

A tissue expander (which consists of an empty silicone balloon connected by a tube to a filler valve) is implanted subcutaneously adjacent to a defect at an initial operation. Over a period of weeks or months, the expander is inflated by serially injecting saline percutaneously into the filler valve, thereby distending the overlying skin. When enough skin has been generated, the expander is removed and the surplus skin used for reconstruction (Fig. 31.10). Tissue expansion causes characteristic changes in the structure of the overlying skin such as thinning of the dermis, greater angiogenesis, realignment of collagen fibrils and secretion of hormonal and growth factor mediators. In contrast, it results in a thickening and hyperkeratinization of the epidermis.

Tissue expansion is ideally suited to late burn scar reconstruction, where there may be a paucity of normal skin, and in the treatment of congenital melanocytic naevi in

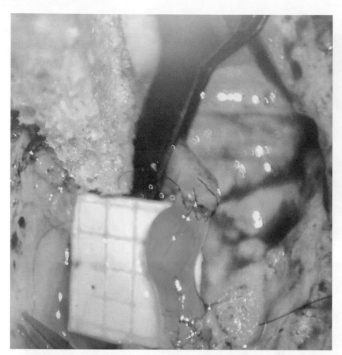

• **Fig. 31.8** Lymphaticovenous anastomosis (LVA) for lymphoedema treatment showing patent blue uptake in the lymphatic channel to help identify lymphatic channels for LVA.

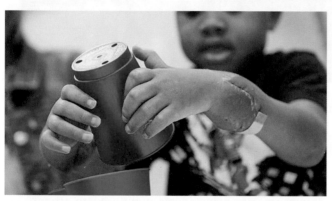

• **Fig. 31.9** Vascularized Composite Tissue Allotransplantation (VCA)

children. The great advantage is that the skin adjacent to the defect is most likely to match that of the area to be reconstructed, providing a good aesthetic match. This is particularly important in certain areas where the skin has very specific properties, such as the hair-bearing scalp. Recent advances in tissue expansion pertain to the development of osmotic tissue expanders and air expanders, which contain cylinders capable of self-expansion thereby obviating the need for percutaneous saline injection.

The method appears to be seductive in its simplicity, but in practice there is a 30–40% complication rate including infection, erosion of skin and extrusion.

Common Reconstructive Referrals

The scope of plastic surgery is broad and plastic surgeons may be asked to consult across a variety of clinical contexts including the extremes of age and a diverse range of pathologies. The commonest referrals will include the management of skin infections, complex/chronic wounds, trauma (hand, burn, lower limb, facial and bite injuries), reconstruction following cancer excision and congenital abnormalities.

Acute Referrals

Trauma

Trauma has become a multidisciplinary specialty, and the plastic surgeon is an integral member of the trauma team. The assessment of all trauma patients must follow established management precepts, such as Advanced Trauma and Life Support (ATLS). Life-threatening injuries always take priority and the need for plastic surgical intervention is sometimes not identified until the secondary survey has been completed.

Assessment of traumatized tissues must include examination of the injury to assess for contamination, sepsis, the presence of underlying fractures, damage to associated vital structures and a thorough neuro-vascular examination. Findings must be documented clearly and serial examination may be required to detect evolving changes.

Wound Management

The viability and perfusion of injured tissues must be established in order to assess the feasibility of replantation or revascularization. The extent of devitalized tissue may not be evident in the acute setting, particularly in the context of lower limb and/or degloving injuries. Therefore, examination under anaesthesia may be required on more than one occasion to establish the full extent of the soft tissue injury and to define the reconstructive need. The index debridement should aim to remove all debris and devitalized tissue back to healthy bleeding tissue. If there is any doubt about tissue viability, the patient should be returned to theatre for further examination and debridement.

Hand Trauma

Examination and diagnosis of hand injuries requires an in-depth knowledge of hand anatomy. Due to the compactness of structures in the upper limb, even small penetrating injuries can result in significant damage to nerves, tendons and blood vessels. Similarly, infections of the upper limb must not be underestimated and can result in significant loss of hand function. Stiffness as a result of injury and/or surgery to the hand can cast a long shadow over functional recovery and close collaboration with hand therapy teams is necessary for even the smallest of injuries.

Burn Injuries

Burns should be managed along established burn injury protocols such as the Emergency Management of Severe Burns (EMSB). Early identification of an airway burn or inhalational injury is vital in permitting pre-emptive intubation and ventilation rather than attempting this when the airway is lost and the patient is in respiratory failure. The key to identification is in the history of the burn injury (type of

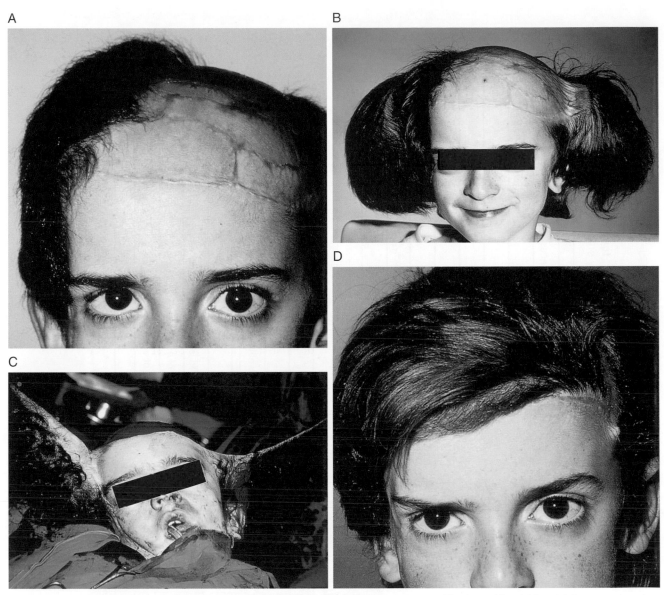

• **Fig. 31.10** Reconstruction of Hair-Bearing Scalp (A) Following a compound fracture of the right parietal bone with loss of the overlying scalp, a large scalp flap was used to repair this wound. The skin graft used to cover this flap's donor site has left an obvious area of alopecia. (B) Following insertion and inflation of two tissue expanders. (C) At operation the expanders have been removed and scalp flaps have been raised in the expanded skin prior to excising the skin graft. (D) 6 weeks after completion of the reconstruction.

burn, burn in an enclosed space) and examination of the upper and lower airways (singed facial hair, blistering of the oropharyngeal mucosa, altered voice or stridor). Once airway (A) and breathing (B) have been secured, assessment moves onto the circulatory system (C) by clinical examination (including examination of peripheral perfusion in limb injuries) and adjuncts to examination such as vital observations, urinary catheterization and invasive monitoring as required. Estimation of fluid requirements in the early period after a burn injury are guided by formulae such as the Parkland formula (fluid in 1st 24 hours = weight (kg) × 2–4 mL Hartmann's × total body surface area (TBSA %) burn injury). This represents the requirement from the time of the burn injury, and the first half of this volume should be delivered in the first 8 hours after injury and the second half over the proceeding 16 hours. Fluid status should be re-assessed frequently and these estimates may need to be adjusted according to clinical and physiological parameters. The patients GCS (D) should be documented and exposure (E) performed to assess the extent and depth of the burn injury. The TBSA of burn injury is assessed using a Lund and Browder chart or Wallace's rule of 9s (Fig. 31.11) taking into account the age of the patient. The depth of the burn injury is assessed by clinical examination and features such as blistering and loss of capillary refill and sensation indicate a deeper burn. Burns are classified as partial (superficial or deep dermal) or full thickness in nature. Care must be taken with circumferential burns on the neck, thorax or limbs as they can impair circulation and ventilation and may require escharotomy to release the burnt tissue.

Lund and Browder chart for calculating the percentage of total body surface area burnt

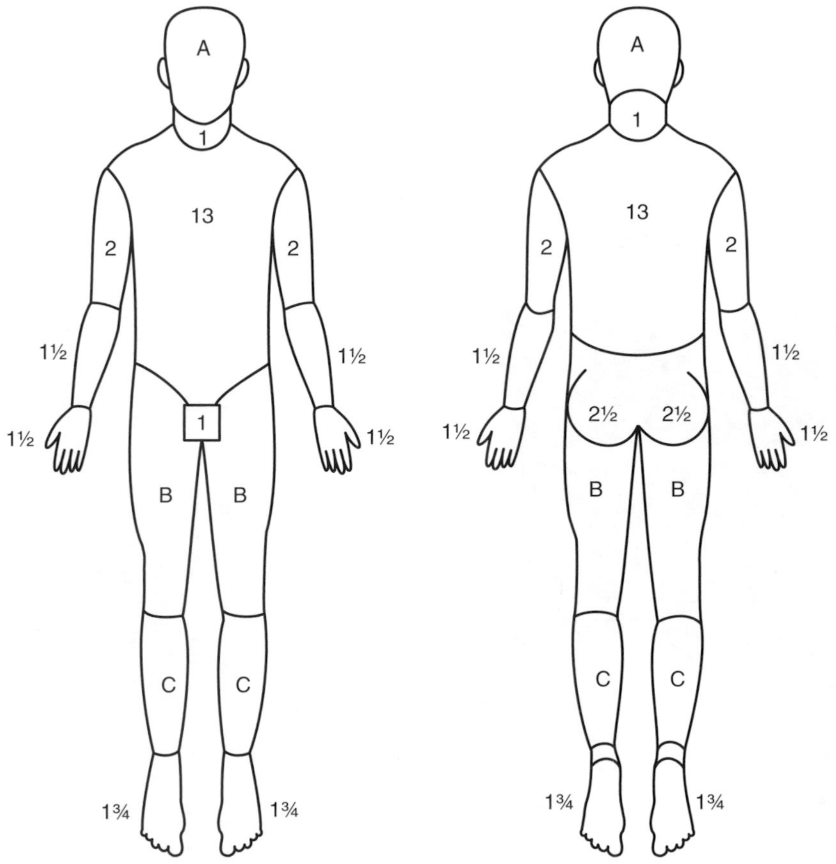

Region	Partial thickness (%) [NB1]	Full thickness (%)
head		
neck		
anterior trunk		
posterior trunk		
right arm		
left arm		
buttocks		
genitalia		
right leg		
left leg		
Total burn		

NB1: Do not include erythema

Area	Age 0	1	5	10	15	Adult
A = half of head	9½	8½	6½	5½	4½	3½
B = half of one thigh	2¾	3¼	4	4½	4½	4¾
C = half of one lower leg	2½	2½	2¾	3	3¼	3½

Therapeutic Guidelines Limited is an independent not-for-profit organization dedicated to deriving guidelines for therapy from the latest world literature, interpreted and distilled by Australia's most eminent and respected experts.

Published in eTG complete, March 2008. ©Therapeutic Guidelines Ltd. www.tg.org.au

A

• **Fig. 31.11** (A and B) Lund and Browder chart and assessment of burn depth.

	Description	Capillary refill?	Sensation?
Epidermal	Bright red/pink Heals within 7 days.	Present (fast)	Yes
Superficial dermal	Pale pink. Often blistered. Heals within 14 days	Present	Yes – very painful
Mid-dermal	Dark pink	Sluggish	May be present or absent
Deep	Blotchy red (from haemoglobin that has leaked out of damaged capillaries)	Absent	Absent
Full thickness	White, waxy or leathery appearance	Absent	Absent

B

Fig. 31.11, cont'd

Prophylactic antibiotics are not indicated for burn injuries but the patient's tetanus vaccination status must be established and a booster given if in doubt. Early nutritional supplementation is essential as patients with burn injuries have a highly catabolic metabolism and, where possible, this should be given enterally. Physiotherapy should be instituted early to minimize the effect of joint contractures both from injury but also from immobilization.

Clear guidelines exist for referral of patients with burn injuries to the appropriate burns service. For example, patients with complex burn injuries (extremes of age, anatomically sensitive area, concomitant airway/inhalational injury or suspicion of non-accidental injury (NAI) or adults with greater than 15% TBSA or children with greater than 10% TBSA) warrant referral to a burns centre.

Acute surgery for burn injuries may be prophylactic, in the case of escharotomy, or required to remove all non-viable burnt tissues. Where debridement is performed, it should be done in a stable patient with appropriate anaesthetic/intensive care facilities in place, under general anaesthesia with blood products and monopolar diathermy available. Debridement should proceed with maximal dermal preservation and minimal blood loss.

Secondary burn surgery for release of contractures or resurfacing should be performed, ideally, at a time when scars are matured. Exceptions to this are when the burn scar threatens vital structures (eyes or mouth), in which case surgery may need to be performed before scar maturation has occurred.

Lower Limb Trauma

Lower limb trauma should be managed along established ATLS protocols and by the standards set by the British Orthopaedic Association Standards for Trauma 4 (BOAST 4). The energy transfer sustained during injury will ultimately determine the long-term outcome of the injured limb and assessment should document the degree of soft tissue loss, the underlying skeletal injury and the distal neurovascular status. Lower limb reconstruction aims to support and facilitate bone healing after skeletal fixation and therefore optimal management requires close collaboration and communication between orthopaedic and plastic surgery teams. Ideally, the initial debridement should be performed jointly. This should involve meticulous debridement of soft tissues, followed by removal of all devitalized bone fragments and delivery of the bone ends out of the wound for debridement and toilet of the bone ends and medullary canals. Skeletal fixation and definitive soft tissue coverage should be performed in a timely manner and at the same operative sitting. Insertion of metalware prior to definitive soft tissue coverage increases significantly the incidence of metalwork infection and osteomyelitis. Only in low-energy injuries can local reconstructive options be used with any degree of reliability and usually a free flap anastomosed to the lower limb vessels outside of the zone of trauma is required to provide definitive coverage.

Elective Referrals

Congenital Abnormalities

Birth defects result from failure of a variety of development processes, including formation, fusion, separation and regression of parts. This can affect any part of the body but most commonly involves the hands, craniofacial skeleton and genitourinary systems. Patients are best managed in the context of a multidisciplinary team as these children, particularly if their deformity has arisen as part of a syndrome,

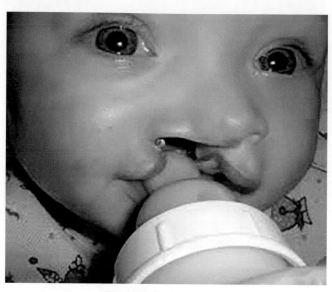

• **Fig. 31.12** Orofacial Clefting

have complex medical needs affecting multiple systems. The timing of surgical interventions must be considered carefully in the context of the child's global developmental needs. Common conditions seen in clinic include:

- Hands: syndactyly, polydactyly, trigger thumb, clinodactyly, brachydactyly, hypoplastic thumbs, radial/ulnar dysplasias
- Genitourinary: hypospadias, bladder exstrophy, epispadias and ambiguous genitalia secondary to hormonal abnormalities
- Craniofacial: craniosynostoses (premature fusion of cranial sutures), orofacial clefting including cleft lip and/or palate (Fig. 31.12), encephaloceles, plagiocephaly without synostosis, cryptotia, microtia, aplasia cutis

Cancer Reconstruction

The plastic surgeon is an integral part of the multidisciplinary team for the treatment of skin, breast, head and neck, sarcoma, gynaecological and lower gastrointestinal cancers. Improvements in local and systemic treatment modalities have heralded significant advances in survival for most cancers. This has driven the development of more radical surgical approaches to achieve cure, particularly in the context of recurrent or oligometastatic disease. The role of the plastic surgeon is to facilitate clear resection margins by being able to reconstruct complex defects reliably to enable timely wound healing and commencement of adjuvant therapies along with restoring reasonable quality of life for patients.

Breast reconstruction: for those women in whom mastectomy is indicated, the standard of care is mastectomy with immediate reconstruction (implant-based or autologous). The first-line flap for autologous reconstruction is the DIEP flap and where this is not feasible, other autologous options include the transverse upper gracilis

(TUG) flap, SGAP/IGAP flaps or the latissimus dorsi (LD) flap. Reconstructive outcomes are superior with immediate, rather than delayed, breast reconstruction. Autologous breast reconstruction is a staged procedure with the first stage aiming to recreate the breast mound/volume by flap transfer. Subsequent stages are performed 4–6 months later and may include lipofilling to address contour deformities, contralateral breast reduction/mastopexy to improve symmetry and nipple reconstruction. Implant-based reconstructions used to require the use of tissue expansion to expand the breast pocket to the desired volume prior to exchange of the expander for a fixed-volume implant. However, the introduction of acellular dermal matrices has allowed surgeons to achieve immediate cover of the lower pole of the implant, therefore obviating the need for tissue expansion. However, implants for breast reconstruction have been reported to be associated with higher complication rates attributable to adjuvant therapies such as radiotherapy and chemotherapy.

Skin cancer: The management of skin cancers remains the mainstay of general plastic surgical practice. Plastic surgery techniques allow the removal of skin cancers with suitable margins and reconstruction of the defect to achieve the best possible functional and aesthetic outcomes. The most common tumour types encountered are basal cell cancers (BCCs), squamous cell cancers (SCCs) and melanomas. The management of skin cancers involves the treatment of pre-malignant lesions, treatment of the primary tumour, assessment and monitoring of regional nodal basins and vigilance for the development of metastatic disease.

Head and neck cancers: Defects of the aerodigestive tract and/or facial skeleton from tumour excision are perhaps the most complex defects to reconstruct and occur in a challenging patient population. Restoring of function is of the utmost importance and the goal of aerodigestive tract reconstruction is to allow swallowing and speech. Common flaps used for oropharyngeal reconstruction include the ALT, MSAP or radial forearm free flaps, or indeed, local options such as the facial artery myomucosal (FAMM) flap. Reconstruction of the hypopharynx may involve the use of either a tubed ALT flap or a free jejunal flap and this may be performed in combination with a pedicled pectoral flap, particularly in a previously irradiated neck, to provide more robust soft tissue cover. Reconstruction of the facial skeleton after excision of a maxillary sinus tumour or a tumour involving the mandible (Fig. 31.13) may require free flaps that include bone. Common donor sites for such flaps include the fibula, the scapular/parascapular flaps and the deep circumflex iliac artery (DCIA) flap.

Perineal reconstruction: This may be required for the management of either gynaecological or colorectal tumours. Perineal reconstruction can be performed, mostly, using regional flaps such as the gracilis, pudendal artery perforator flaps, gluteal perforator flaps or even the rectus

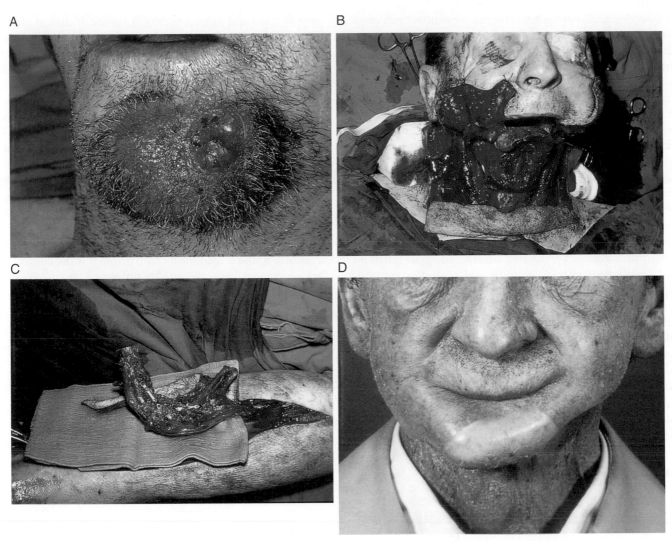

• **Fig. 31.13** An Example of Complex Intra-Oral Reconstructive Surgery (A) An advanced carcinoma of the floor of the mouth, invading the chin. (B) Defect following bilateral neck dissection and resection of chin skin, mandible from angle to angle, floor of mouth and anterior tongue. (C) Free flap raised for reconstruction. A fibular flap will reconstruct the mandible with some overlying skin, vascularized through its deep fascial attachment, which will replace the floor of mouth. Two osteotomies have been made in the bone, which has been plated in a design to conform with the resected mandible. (D) Four months following surgery there is good bony union. External skin cover was achieved with an axial skin flap from the upper chest (deltopectoral flap).

abdominis myocutaneous flap. The latter particularly is one of the workhorse flaps used for perineal reconstruction following pelvic exenteration and/or sacrectomy. Most of these patients will have had previous radiotherapy. The goal of perineal reconstruction is to reconstruct the pelvic floor and fill the dead space in the pelvis with healthy vascularized tissue to facilitate wound healing in the zone of radiotherapy and prevent perineal herniation. In female patients, vaginal reconstruction can also be considered.

Sarcoma: The reconstruction of these defects can be extremely challenging due to the extent of resection and functional demands of reconstruction, particularly in sarcomas arising from bones. Plastic surgeons may be required to reconstruct large bone defects using vascularized bone flaps or stable axial joints such as the sacro-iliac

joint. Functional muscle reconstruction may also be required for limb salvage in patients undergoing radical compartmentectomies. One of the primary concerns of reconstruction in soft tissue sarcoma is to achieve primary, durable wound healing that can tolerate adjuvant radiotherapy and mitigate the risks of radiotherapy-related wound healing complications.

Pressure Ulcers

These wounds are caused by pressure necrosis of tissues in an immobilized and often debilitated patient. In those patients who are temporarily incapacitated and subsequently become ambulant, the prognosis is good and the defects can be managed conservatively. The majority of ulcers, however, occur in paraplegic patients in tissues over bony prominences subject to chronic pressure when a combination of poor-quality and insensate tissues, poor general nutrition and, occasionally, poor motivation exacerbate the situation.

Prevention is the best solution to pressure ulcer management and this can be achieved through the identification of risk factors for developing pressure ulcers, for example, through scoring systems such as the Waterlow score. The mainstays of management are to ensure robust pressure relief through the use of the correct bedding and mattresses, frequent turning or re-positioning to re-distribute pressure and meticulous skin care. Secondarily, management is directed at reversing those metabolic or physiological factors that may contribute to the development of pressure ulcers and optimizing patients for surgery. Examples of this include rigorous glycaemic control, adequate nutrition and supplementation of vitamins and co-factors for healing. The management of sepsis is achieved primarily by the debridement of necrotic or devitalized tissues and this can be achieved either at the bedside or in theatre depending on the extent of the wound. Again, due to often complex medical needs and co-morbidities, pressure ulcers are best managed by a dedicated MDT. Surgery should only be performed in cases where all the reversible courses of ulceration have been addressed, the patient has been optimized medically and is motivated to prevent a recurrence of the pressure ulcer.

Aesthetic Surgery

In cosmetic surgery, patients will seek to enhance their appearance or maintain a youthful appearance through non-surgical and surgical means. A thorough clinical assessment of the patient is essential in order to identify any psychiatric disorders that may be driving the quest for surgery, such as body dysmorphic disorder (BDD). Aesthetic goals and expectations should be discussed frankly and the surgeon should be candid about what is feasible and achievable. Complications must be explained and patients given appropriate information in order to make a decision. The British Association of Aesthetic Plastic Surgeons (BAAPS) has outlined standards for practice that recommend processes for consultation, 'cooling off', performing aesthetic procedures and following up these patients. In carefully selected and counselled patients, excellent results can be achieved in what is a very diverse and challenging branch of the specialty. The techniques that are often used in aesthetic practice are often identical to those used for reconstruction but the context in which they are being delivered is different.

Further Reading

Barret-Nerin J, Hemdon DN. *Principles and Practice of Burn Surgery.* New York: Informa Healthcare; 2004.

McGregor AD, McGregor IA. *Fundamental Techniques of Plastic Surgery: and Their Surgical Applications.* 10th ed. London: Churchill Livingstone; 2000.

Settle JAD. *Principles and Practice of Burns Management.* Edinburgh: Churchill Livingstone; 1996.

Thorne CH, Bartlett SP, Beasley RW, Aston SJ, Gurtner GC. *Grabb and Smith's Plastic Surgery.* 6th ed. Boston: Lippincott Williams & Wilkins; 2006.

Warwick D, Dunn R, Melikyan E, Vadher J. *Oxford Specialist Handbooks in Surgery – Hand Surgery.* Oxford: OUP; 2009.

32

Skin Disorders

Introduction

Skin is our largest organ and most humans carry around over 3 kg of it. It is waterproof, insulates us and guards us against extremes of temperature, damaging sunlight and dangerous chemicals. The surgeon's role is often in the diagnosis of skin conditions and importantly determining whether benign or malignant. This is done through a combination of skilful history-taking, examination and biopsy. The skin should be examined using the naked eye: the characteristics of the individual lesion(s) and their distribution are key to making the diagnosis. The whole skin surface must be examined even if the patient presents with an apparently solitary lesion, and careful consideration should be made of the need to examine the mucous membranes and the skin appendages, including nails and hair. It is also important to examine the regional lymph nodes draining the area of involvement, particularly in suspected neoplastic conditions.

Skin conditions may be benign or malignant. Other conditions encountered include inflammatory rashes, perhaps triggered by drugs or a physical stress such as surgery, so a broader understanding of dermatological conditions is essential.

Embryology and Anatomy

There are three layers to the skin (Fig. 32.1):
- epidermis
- dermis
- subcutis

Epidermis

The epidermis originates from the embryonic ectoderm, in contrast to the other two deeper layers which are of mesodermal origin. Some epidermal structures – the pilosebaceous unit and nail matrix (see later) – migrate inwards during development and are anatomically located in the dermis. Similarly, some cells of mesodermal origin, such as melanocytes which are of neural crest origin, migrate outwards to the epidermis and are located within the basal cell layer.

The interface between the epidermis and dermis is convoluted – the dermal projection of the epidermis is a rete peg and the upwardly projecting portion of the dermis is the papillary dermis (Fig. 32.2). Between the epidermis and dermis there is a basement membrane zone which is traversed by anchoring fibrils, which are important in adherence of the two structures.

Epidermal Cells

The *keratinocyte* is the predominant cell of the epidermis. The epidermis is made up of stratified keratinizing squamous epithelium, the layers of which can be identified histologically and represent stages of the maturation of cell division of the keratinocytes. The cells mature progressively as they migrate from the basal layer towards the surface. Initially, in the basal-layer keratinocytes, keratin filaments appear in the cytoplasm. As the cells mature further, the cytoplasm becomes progressively replaced by keratin – a structural protein which is surrounded by a phospholipid envelope that was the original cell membrane. As the cells within each division migrate towards the surface, they flatten and, by the time they reach the surface, they form a laminated structure – the stratum corneum (see Fig. 32.1). This serves as a physiological barrier to chemical and microbiological invasion from without, as well as to fluid and salt loss from within. The epidermal transit time from the basal layer to stratum corneum is about 28 days. Disruption of this smooth transition occurs in inflammatory conditions of the epidermis such as psoriasis, and also as a result of actinic (sun-induced) damage to the basal cell – a process known as dyskeratosis which makes the affected epidermis unstable.

Melanocytes are cells of neural crest origin which produce the ultraviolet (UV) radiation-absorbing pigment melanin.

They are located along the basement membrane between the basal keratinocytes and have a dendritic shape with multiple root-like projections. Different racial groups have the same number of melanocytes, but there is a difference in the amount and type of melanin produced: Celtic races, for example, produce predominantly phaeomelanin, a yellow-red pigment which gives poorer UV protection than brown-black eumelanin. Increased melanin production can be stimulated by UV light and the cytokines released by

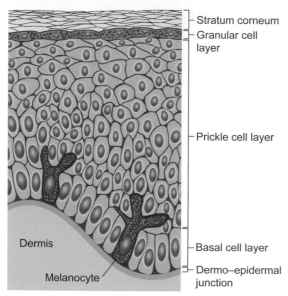

• **Fig. 32.1** Structure of Normal Epidermis

inflammatory processes. Melanocytes distribute their melanin granules to the surrounding basal cells through their dendrites. Once these granules are taken up by the basal cells, they are dispersed through the cytoplasm to absorb UV radiation, which protects the nuclei, as well as deeper cells, from UV damage. Thus, melanin has a key role in preventing malignant change to basal cells and photodamage to the underlying collagen: individuals who produce phaeomelanin, which is less photoprotective, will burn rather than tan and are more vulnerable to developing UV-induced skin tumours and wrinkling.

Immunocompetent cells are of a number of classes: Langerhans cells are derived from bone marrow and are closely related to the macrophage. They are located just above the basal layer of keratinocytes in the so-called suprabasal layer. They express HLA receptors on their surface and are central to the presentation of antigens to other immunocompetent cells. They also, in their own right, release cytokines such as interleukin-2. Their prime importance is in immunosurveillance of the skin and mediation of the cutaneous immune response.

Lymphocytes are present in small numbers in the normal epidermis – mainly T lymphocytes of both CD4 and CD8 subsets. The T lymphocytes are derived from the thymus, which also, like the epidermis, is of ectodermal origin, and it is believed that they migrate through the epidermis as part of their surveillance of immune function. The interaction between Langerhans cells and lymphocytes makes the epidermis an important component of the body's immune system. This can be disturbed in some inflammatory conditions of the epidermis which are T-cell mediated: e.g.

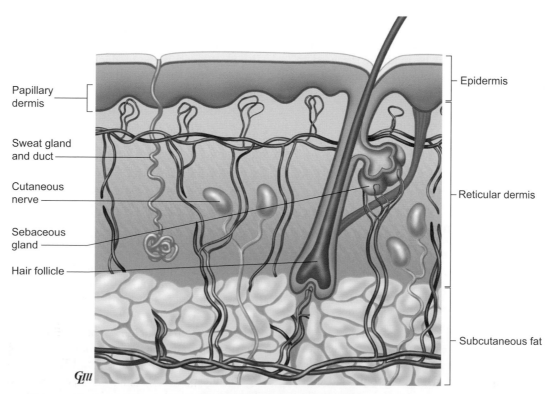

• **Fig. 32.2** Structure of Normal Skin

psoriasis in which T lymphocytes release lymphokines into the epidermis, resulting in keratinocyte proliferation. In the cell-mediated (type IV) reaction, such as that seen to adhesives used in wound dressings, the colophony allergen is presented by an antigen-presenting cell, such as a Langerhans cell, to a T lymphocyte, setting off the cascade of events which result in allergic contact eczema.

The epidermal immune system may be suppressed in various ways. UV light can suppress type IV reactions in the skin. Some skin diseases, such as atopic eczema, are associated with local immunodeficiency and patients are prone to cutaneous infections with *Staphylococcus aureus*. The cutaneous immune system may also be suppressed during systemic diseases such as diabetes mellitus, HIV and leukaemia.

Merkel cells, like melanocytes, are of mesodermal origin derived from the neural crest. They function as mechanoreceptors to help sense touch, and so are found particularly on the digital pads of the fingers.

Dermis

The major component of the dermis is connective tissue, composed mainly of collagen fibres within an amorphous ground substance. The papillary dermis is the uppermost layer of the dermis, intertwined with the rete ridges of the epidermis. Below this, the reticular dermis is less cellular and contains more densely packed collagen and elastic fibres (see Fig. 32.2). The dermis contains blood vessels which derive from a deep vascular plexus, sweat glands, nerves, lymphatics and muscle fibres associated with a pilosebaceous unit (see later).

Dermal collagen is produced by fibroblasts which lie between the collagen bundles. It forms a mesh-like network which provides a supportive framework for skin structures, and gives the skin strength and elasticity. Changes in collagen occur with ageing and from UV light, both of which make collagen less flexible and less able to provide support for other structures. Wrinkles result, and purpura may also follow from the increased fragility of blood vessels.

Dermal blood vessels arise from a deep arterial plexus which then subdivides and, finally, a capillary loop which supplies the dermal papillae. Blood then drains through a papillary venous network and back into the subcutaneous vessels.

Lymphatic channels can be recognized within the dermis. Their obstruction or failure causes cutaneous lymphoedema.

Dermal nerve fibres are:
- Afferent for cutaneous sensation
- Efferent vasomotor and also to the sweat glands, both of which help regulate body temperature; there is also a supply to the erector pili muscle

Sweat glands are of two types:
- Eccrine glands are present throughout all skin and secrete an aqueous fluid.
- Apocrine glands occur in the intertriginous areas of the axillae and groin and also the scalp – their secretion is greasy.

Pilosebaceous units are a combination of a hair shaft, hair follicle and a sebaceous gland. Attached to the hair shaft are muscle fibres of the pili erector muscle. The keratin of the hair shaft is derived from a germinal layer of the hair bulb which lies deep in the dermis. The hair follicle is richly supplied by nerves and blood vessels. The sebaceous gland produces an oily secretion, sebum, which is discharged into the hair follicle via the pilosebaceous duct.

Nail matrix produces the specialized keratin of the nail plate which grows out beneath the proximal nail fold (Fig. 32.3). The plate is closely adherent to the underlying nail bed. Melanocytes can be present in the nail matrix, causing linear pigmented striae within the nails, as well as providing a starting place for melanoma. On either side of the nail plate are the lateral nail folds. The nail plate can grow into the soft nail fold, giving rise to an ingrowing nail; if the nail folds become infected, this is termed paronychia (Fig. 32.4).

Subcutis

The subcutis, which predominantly contains loose adipose tissue and elastin, serves to attach the skin to underlying muscle and bone as well as supplying it with blood vessels and nerves.

Principles of Investigation: The Biopsy

Histological examination is required to confirm diagnosis, especially where there is uncertainty on clinical grounds. Small lesions may be completely excised (an excisional

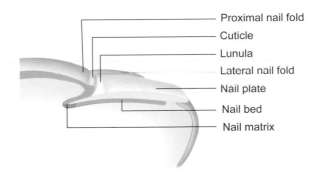

• **Fig. 32.3** Sagittal View of the Nail Anatomy

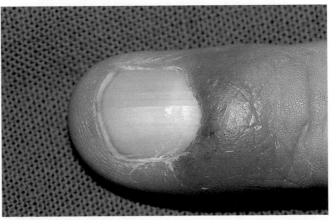

• **Fig. 32.4** Paronychia Showing Loss of Cuticle and Swelling of Nail Fold biopsy), larger ones may be removed initially in part (an incisional or punch biopsy) before definitive therapy is decided on. When taking a biopsy from a rash, a relatively fresh representative lesion should be biopsied, and the biopsy should be taken across the edge of a lesion. It is important to provide adequate material for histological interpretation, which usually means a full-thickness biopsy including epidermis, dermis and a small amount of subcutis. Mapping biopsies may be required for some conditions such as angiosarcoma. Skin surgery is usually performed under local anaesthetic.

Full-Thickness Skin Biopsies

Any incision into collagen (i.e. through the dermis) leaves a scar on healing, and this must be explained to the patient beforehand. Hypertrophic and keloid scarring is always a possibility, especially for surgery on the upper trunk and shoulders, and the risk is higher in patients with Fitzpatrick type V and VI skin tones. Full-thickness skin biopsies may be incisional or excisional, and a variety of techniques can be used including:

- **Punch biopsy** (Fig. 32.5). A small sharp tool, not dissimilar to an apple-corer, is used to obtain a cylindrical sample of full-thickness skin. This technique is often used to obtain an incisional biopsy for diagnostic purposes. Very small punch biopsies can heal well by secondary intention; otherwise, primary closure is achieved with interrupted sutures.

- **Ellipse biopsy** (Fig. 32.6). Using a scalpel, an ellipse-shaped full-thickness biopsy is obtained of the skin. This technique is often used to perform excisional biopsies, e.g. of a melanoma, or when good-sized samples of the subcutis as well as the more superficial skin is required. The wound is closed with sutures which are left in situ for 5–20 days, depending upon the site of the surgery, size of wound and other wound-healing factors.

For larger wound defects a variety of techniques are used to close wounds, including skin grafts and rotation flaps.

Principles of Therapy

Neoplastic lesions must be excised according to oncological principles to ensure optimal treatment, and the sample submitted for histological examination to confirm the diagnosis and to check that the margins taken were adequate.

A variety of therapeutic surgical techniques may be used: punch and ellipse biopsies as described earlier, and also these methods below which, in experienced hands, have the advantage of removing superficial skin lesions without damaging collagen.

Curettage. A ring or spoon-shaped curette is used to remove the epidermal lesion, by drawing the curette under the lesion, e.g. seborrhoeic keratoses.

Shave Biopsy. A scalpel or razor blade is used to remove a superficial skin lesion in a single piece of unfragmented

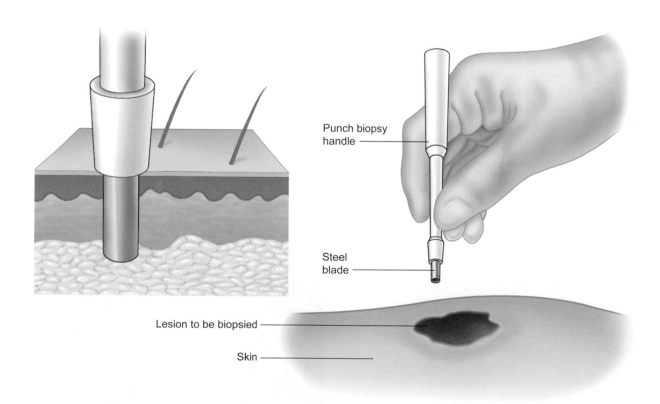

Punch biopsy handle

Steel blade

Lesion to be biopsied

Skin

• **Fig. 32.5** Punch Biopsy Technique. The sharp instrument is driven into the skin to obtain a cylindrical section of skin. Inset: the sample obtained is of full-thickness skin down to subcutis.

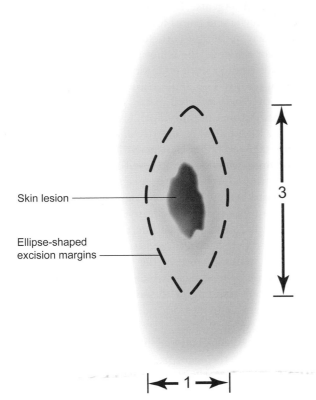

Skin lesion

Ellipse-shaped excision margins

3

1

• **Fig. 32.6** Ellipse biopsy of skin showing the planned excision margins for a pigmented lesion, with the 3:1 ratio typically used to ensure a thin linear scar after suturing.

tissue, e.g. a benign intradermal melanocytic naevus which catches on clothing.

Snip Excision. Sterile scissors are used to remove pedunculated skin lesions, e.g. skin tags. Haemostasis is then achieved to the resultant erosion using cautery or by applying direct pressure.

Cryosurgery. This can also be used to treat superficial lesions such as viral warts (see later) satisfactorily. Patients should be warned of the likelihood of pain and blistering after this treatment, and, especially in patients with pigmented skin types, of the risk of pigmentary changes. Injudicious use of this method may result in deeper tissue injuries, such as digital nerve or extensor tendon damage when used on the dorsal aspects of the fingers.

Lasers. Lasers can be used to treat benign vascular and pigmented lesions. The emission wavelength of the laser can be matched to the absorption spectrum of the pigment present, e.g. haemoglobin or melanin. Carbon dioxide lasers are more destructive, but are precise and give immediate haemostasis and vaporize a lesion; they have a role in ablative therapy especially in *in-transit* melanoma.

DISORDERS OF THE SKIN

The skin is the body's largest organ – by weight, up to 15% of body mass. It is, along with the mucosal surface of the gastrointestinal tract, with which it is continuous, the interface between the external and internal environment and has a number of important functions in protection and in the maintenance of homeostasis. It is extensively exposed to agents which are actually or potentially noxious, including chemicals, carcinogens and pathogenic organisms. Also, it is at constant risk of physical trauma and subject to a large number of endogenous diseases such as eczema, lichen planus and psoriasis and may be involved in systemic problems such as vasculitis and granulomatous diseases (e.g. sarcoidosis). The prevalence of skin disorders in the UK is summarized in Box 32.1.

INFECTIONS

The skin is constantly exposed to infectious agents. Protection is afforded by the physical barrier of the stratum corneum and the very effective immunological barrier of the epidermis.

Host defences may be breached as a result of:
- Physical injury, e.g. trauma or surgery to the skin
- Endogenous skin diseases, e.g. eczema or venous ulceration
- Immunosuppression, e.g. HIV, drugs or leukaemia
- Pathogenic organisms that are able to penetrate the normal skin defence mechanisms, e.g. fungal and candidal infection

Viral Infections

Human Papillomaviruses

These are a group of RNA viruses, and more than a hundred subtypes have been identified so far. The skin manifestation is a wart, these can be common type, plantar or genital.

Epidemiology and Aetiology

Warts are common, and most people suffer infection at some stage. They are mostly prevalent in children, where they are probably acquired from direct contact or from communal recreational facilities such as swimming pools. Genital (including perianal) warts are usually found in adults, and are most commonly, though not exclusively, acquired as a result of sexual contact so that they may coexist with other sexually transmitted infections.

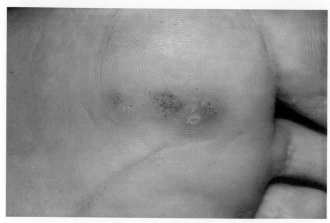

• **Fig. 32.7** Viral warts (verrucae) on the sole, demonstrating thrombosed capillaries which clinically appear as 'black dots'.

History

Cutaneous warts may present suddenly with rapid growth or more gradually creep up on their hosts over many weeks, even years. Itching may be a feature. Larger lesions can become painful, especially if they are on pressure points such as the heel or ball of the foot. Lesions can be of cosmetic concern when on exposed sites such as the hands or face.

Clinicopathological Features

The virus infects the basal keratinocytes of the epidermis, resulting in increased proliferation of these cells. In stratified squamous epithelium, this gives rise to hyperkeratosis and a hard wart is seen. The characteristics of a wart are loss of the normal dermatoglyphics of the skin and thrombosed capillaries that are seen as small black dots which bleed if the overlying hard skin is pared away (Fig. 32.7). On mucosal surfaces the wart is softer – a fleshy papilloma.

Management

Prevention

Vaccines have been produced against HPV subtypes 16 and 18, which together are associated with 70% of cervical cancers, and are also associated with many cases of anal cancer. HPV immunization of girls aged 12–18 years is routine in the UK and the vaccination of boys aged 12–13 was introduced in 2019–2020. The currently used vaccine, the Human Papillomavirus Quadrivalent (Types 6, 11, 16, and 18) Vaccine, Recombinant (tradename Gardasil), protects against HPV subtypes 6, 11, 16 and 18. HPV types 6 and 11 cause 90% of genital warts. These developments open up the future possibility of a vaccine against the HPV types (e.g. 1 and 2) more typically involved in cutaneous warts on the hands and feet.

Natural History

Spontaneous resolution is the rule once natural immunity has developed, but this takes longer in adults than in children, so that infection can last for many years. The multiplicity of treatment options for management of viral warts reflects the relatively poor efficacies of these individual treatments.

Keratolytic Agents. The use of local keratolytic agents such as salicylic acid paints for hand and foot warts remains the mainstay of therapy, particularly in children. Even when cure is not achieved, the removal of excessive keratin helps to limit discomfort until resolution occurs.

Cryotherapy. The application of liquid nitrogen can destroy the virus-infected tissue, which then sloughs off. Early resolution in individual lesions may follow, but there is a high rate of recurrence and treatment is painful.

Curettage and Other Destructive Measures. Physical ablation of larger warts can be achieved by curettage, diathermy or laser therapy, but they also have significant recurrence rates.

Immunotherapy. Immunotherapy aims to stimulate the body's immune system to effectively eliminate the virally infected cells, e.g. diphencyprone, a potent contact allergen which, in expert hands, is used to induce localized eczema associated with clearance of the warts; and imiquimod, a topical immune modulator which binds to cell-surface toll-like receptors resulting in the secretion of numerous pro-inflammatory cytokines, including interferon-α, resulting in clearance of the warts.

Cytotoxic Agents. Podophyllin (a compound preparation which contains the agent podophyllotoxin) is particularly helpful in treating genital warts. Its application must be closely monitored, however, because it causes soreness and is teratogenic and therefore must not be used during pregnancy. Bleomycin has also been successfully used by injecting intralesionally.

Special Problems with Genital Warts (syn. *Condylomata acuminatum*). It is important, when assessing a patient with genital warts, to ensure that they have not also acquired any other sexually transmitted disease. In addition to podophyllin and imiquimod, these warts may be treated with physical destruction or excision under general anaesthesia. Excision has the benefit of providing histology as dysplasia and even squamous cell carcinoma (SCC) may be present, especially in immunocompromised patients.

Molluscum contagiosum
Aetiology and Pathological Features

This is caused by a pox virus. The individual lesions are smooth and dome-shaped; they have a characteristic central depression or umbilication and, if squeezed, a central white core can be expressed called the molluscum body. Florid molluscum contagiosum may occur in immuno-suppressed patients, particularly those with HIV infection. When patients acquire immunity to the virus, the lesions disappear.

Management

Early resolution of individual lesions can be induced by minor trauma such as cryotherapy or superficial diathermy; imiquimod has also been used to good effect.

Herpes Viruses

There are two types of infection:

• Herpes simplex is due to a number of subtypes of herpes simplex viruses (HSV).

• BOX 32.2 Herpes Simplex and Zoster

Herpes simplex

- Subtype 1 – onset in childhood and usually orofacial
- Subtype 2 – onset in adults and usually genital
- Attacks may be precipitated by UV light, or an illness, e.g. upper respiratory infection

Herpes zoster

- Caused by activation of dormant varicella-zoster (chickenpox) virus
- Distribution is characteristically dermatomal and unilateral – more widespread infection suggests immunosuppression, e.g. HIV infection
- Can present with unilateral abdominal pain before skin lesions appear
- Rarely recurs but may be complicated in the long term by severe post-herpetic neuralgia
- Antiviral drugs reduce the acute pain and duration of herpes zoster and should always be given

- Herpes zoster is due to varicella-zoster virus (VZV). The distinction is summarized in Box 32.2.

Herpes Simplex

This condition can affect any area of the skin; however, it is most commonly seen close to the mucous membranes of the lips in HSV type 1 and the genitalia in HSV type 2. The patient notices a prodromal tingling of the skin followed by the eruption of clusters of small vesicles. The active lesions are infectious, and surgeons need to take care to avoid direct contact, as this can result in a herpetic whitlow on a finger.

Herpes Zoster

This is caused by VZV; the primary widespread infection is chickenpox. The virus then lies dormant in the dorsal root ganglia of the CNS and is reactivated along peripheral nerves to produce vesicles and pustules in a dermatomal distribution, known as shingles or herpes zoster. Its relevance for surgeons is that herpes zoster can be triggered by stresses such as surgery. Additionally, the prodromal phase, before the development of vesicles, gives rise to pain in the skin of the affected dermatome which may cause diagnostic difficulties by mimicking other nerve lesions such as sciatica, or an acute abdomen. Treatment with aciclovir or valaciclovir shortens the duration of the attack.

Bacterial Infections

Staphylococcal Infections

Aetiology, Pathological Features and Management

Staphylococcus aureus (SA) can cause primary skin infections such as impetigo, furunculosis and acute paronychia. Diabetic patients are particularly susceptible. Since the 1950s, the majority of strains of *S. aureus* have been resistant to many commonly used antibiotics such as penicillin; from the mid-1990s, there has been an increasing incidence of methicillin-resistant SA (MRSA) such that it is now endemic in British hospitals. Despite intensive infection control interventions, 8% of SA infections are resistant to methicillin. Community acquired MRSA (CA-MRSA) infections are also increasingly seen. CA-MRSA can cause skin and soft tissue infections in healthy young people; most strains are sensitive to non-beta lactam antibiotics e.g. vancomycin. Panton–Valentine leukocidin (PVL) is a toxic substance produced by nearly all CA-MRSA strains which is associated with an increased virulence.

Impetigo

This condition mainly affects the face and is much more common in children than in adults: presentation is as flaccid blisters underneath the stratum corneum which rupture early on, so giving rise to a raw eroded base. Impetigo is contagious, and infected children should be kept away from school. Swabs are taken to determine the antibiotic sensitivities of the organism. Both staphylococcal and streptococcal bacteria may cause the condition. If the lesions are localized, topical antibiotics such as fucidic acid or mupirocin are effective, dependent on sensitivities. If lesions are more widespread, they are treated with systemic flucloxacillin.

Furunculosis

This term describes a group of conditions characterized by staphylococcal infection of the hair follicles. Staphylococcal folliculitis is a pyoderma localized to the hair follicle and can be either superficial or deep. A furuncle (boil) is a deep-seated inflammatory nodule which develops around a hair follicle from a preceding, more superficial folliculitis. A carbuncle is a more-extensive and even deeper infiltrating inflammation which occurs in thick and inelastic skin – commonly on the back of the neck.

The acute lesions of furunculosis are characterized by pain and tenderness of the infected area and soft tissue. Localization of pus gives rise to abscesses. The natural history of the lesions is for the pus to discharge and this to be followed by resolution. Treatment of the early soft-tissue phase is with systemic antibiotics. If a deep abscess forms, then surgical drainage is indicated. Carbuncles and ecthyma represent infective gangrene of the deep tissues. The subcutaneous tissues become painful and indurated and drain to the surface through sinuses. Surgical debridement may be necessary, in addition to a course of antibiotics.

Paronychia

This is the term given to inflammation of the nail fold. Infection is usually acquired through loss of the cuticle of the proximal nail fold, sometimes the consequence of a self-inflicted injury at manicure. Paronychia may be acute when caused by *S. aureus* infection, or chronic when the result of *Candida* infection whose acquisition is difficult to determine (see Fig. 32.4). Treatment is by surgical debridement – which may have to include the nail – under local anaesthetic.

Streptococcal Infections

Streptococcus pyogenes (beta-haemolytic streptococcus Lancefield group A) causes dermal infections of two types:
- Erysipelas – infection in the deep dermis but not the subcutaneous tissues
- Cellulitis – full-thickness infection of the skin with involvement of the subcutaneous tissues

The presentation of both may be that of the systemic features of severe sepsis, with rigor and fever, but without initial overt evidence of skin involvement. The earliest cutaneous sign is erythema. The leg and face are most commonly affected, although any site may be involved. The infection spreads through the tissue by the release of toxins, giving rise to a brawny erythema spreading across the skin with a sharp well-demarcated edge (Fig. 32.8). If left untreated, the infection will eventually resolve, but there is a significant mortality from overwhelming toxaemia and septicaemia.

The treatment of choice for streptococcal cellulitis is bed rest with intravenous antibiotics. The majority of streptococci are sensitive to penicillin, and this is the agent of choice. The fever usually settles within 24–48 hours, and the erythema and swelling subside slowly. Streptococcal cellulitis can complicate chronic skin conditions such as venous leg ulceration and lymphedema. When this occurs, treatment with antibiotics may have to be prolonged to prevent early relapse.

Necrotizing Fasciitis

Necrotizing fasciitis is an acute, uncommon but potentially fatal, soft tissue infection. It occurs in healthy individuals but the majority (70%) have an underlying immunosuppression e.g. diabetes. It may be caused by a single bacterium or a synergistic combination of different bacteria.
- Type I infections are, by definition, polymicrobial
- Type II infections: *Streptococcus pyogenes* is the commonest organism isolated (15%)
- Type III infections comprise gas gangrene and these are usually caused by *Clostridium perfringens*

The commonest causative organisms are group A streptococcus, *S. aureus* (including MRSA), *Vibrio vulnificus*, *Clostridium perfringens* and *Bacteroides fragilis*. An ill-defined erythema develops which rapidly becomes necrotic. The patient complains of severe pain and with high fever and the other features of systemic inflammatory response out of proportion to the local skin findings. A high index of suspicion is required as diagnosis can be difficult resulting in delayed treatment. The infection spreads quickly in the fascial plane and involves both skin and subcutaneous tissues. Urgent CT or ultrasound scanning may confirm the diagnosis and help to define the extent of the disease, but these should not delay definitive surgical treatment. Urgent surgical debridement of the affected tissues is required together with intravenous antibiotics (e.g. linezolid with meropenem or piperacillin/tazobactam). Antibiotic treatment may be

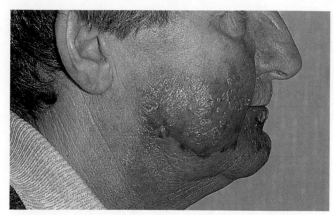

• **Fig. 32.8** Erysipelas Showing Indurated Red Plaque Spreading Across Face

modified once bacteriological culture results are available. Repeat operation is often required and may require extensive debridement, including creation of colostomy in pelvic infections, Fournier gangrene. Transfer to a plastic surgical unit for reconstructive surgery is often required once the infection has been treated.

Venous Ulceration

Ulceration in the gaiter area of the leg is common in patients with post-thrombotic venous hypertension and is also seen with advanced varicose veins. These ulcers may become secondarily infected and cause surrounding cellulitis. The condition and its treatment are described in detail in Chapter 27.

Fungal Infections

Superficial Mycoses

These infections are due to fungi that can only invade fully keratinized tissues. The clinical appearance depends on the severity of the inflammatory reaction to the fungi. When mild, the lesions are red and scaly; when severe, boggy areas of inflammation may arise; when present on the scalp or beard, this is known as a kerion (Fig. 32.9). It is important to recognize this to prevent inappropriate surgical intervention as these lesions can best be treated medically with appropriate systemic antifungals. Mycological examination of the tissue conducted by direct microscopy is used to confirm the diagnosis.

TUMOURS

The skin is exposed to chronic irritation and carcinogens. Tumours of the skin, as with any other tissue, can be benign or malignant. The latter may be primary or secondary.

A number of premalignant conditions can be identified and are discussed below. Tumours that derive from the epidermis (ectodermal) have different clinical features from those of the dermis (mesodermal).

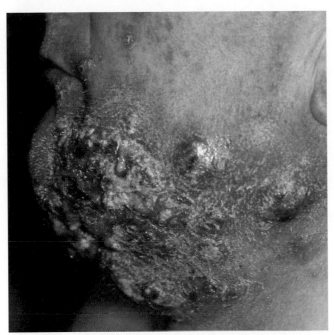

• **Fig. 32.9** Kerion in the Beard Area Due to *Trichophyton verrucosum* Treatment is with systemic antifungal therapy: this lesion resolved without scarring after treatment with oral terbinafine.

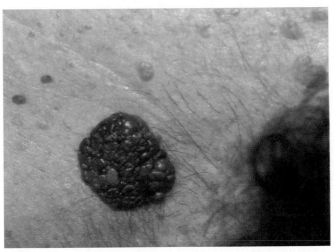

• **Fig. 32.10** Large, Deeply Pigmented Seborrhoeic Keratosis with Greasy, Cerebriform Surface Close by, several smaller skin-coloured seborrhoeic keratoses may also be seen.

Benign Tumours of the Epidermis

Seborrhoeic Keratosis/Wart (syn. Basal Cell Papilloma)

These lesions are common in the elderly.

Clinical Features

History

These are rough lesions which may catch on clothing; this or other trauma may cause minor bleeding. The appearance is unattractive, and cosmetic distaste is a common reason for presentation.

Physical Findings

Raised, well-circumscribed lesions which may occur anywhere on the body, although the trunk is the most common site. They are initially flat with varying amounts of pigmentation. The surface is waxy with superficial clefts and fissuring (Fig. 32.10).

Management

The differential diagnosis between deeply pigmented papillomas from malignant melanoma can be difficult; if there is doubt, elliptical excision biopsy is indicated with a 1-mm margin.

However, if the diagnosis is certain, shaving back the lesion or curettage and cautery give a satisfactory cosmetic result with the additional benefit of providing a specimen for histological confirmation of the diagnosis.

Skin Tags

These lesions are usually found in sites where skin surfaces rub together and the skin is therefore chronically irritated. There is loose connective tissue core covered by epidermis which may be pigmented.

Skin tags are irritated by clothing and bleed, as well as causing local symptoms in areas such as the skin surrounding the anus. Patients often present to request removal. The diagnosis is obvious to the naked eye.

Management can be conservative with reassurance or surgical excision and cautery.

Solar (Actinic) Keratoses

These scaling red macular (flat) lesions are typically clustered on sun-exposed areas of the skin, often on a background of collagen damage known as solar elastosis. The basal epidermal cells are dysplastic: clinically, this results in the skin surface changing from smooth to scaly with excessive keratin. Induration or pain can occur if the lesion becomes invasive. Actinic keratosis is viewed as a premalignant lesion because there are atypical keratinocytes present in the epidermis. In the presence of actinic keratosis, the risk of developing SCC is approximately 10% at 10 years. Treatment ranges from surveillance, 5-fluorouracil creams, photodynamic therapy to curettage.

Management

Isolated superficial lesions are dealt with by cryotherapy. If there is any induration, curettage and cautery are used and the fragments sent for histological examination. Where there is a high suspicion of SCC, lesions should be excised to avoid ambiguous histology. Close follow-up is indicated when the histological diagnosis is uncertain.

Extensive areas of sun damage with multiple solar keratoses are better managed topically with application of cytotoxic creams such as 5-fluorouracil or immunomodulators such as imiquimod to stabilize the epithelium; this has to be done under close supervision.

Keratoacanthoma

This lesion arises from squamous epithelium. It is most common on exposed areas of the body and is thought to result from minor trauma. As its name suggests, it has a central keratin plug with a surrounding collar of acanthotic thickened epidermis (Fig. 32.11).

Clinical Features

The lesion is characterized by rapid onset and growth. It then enters a static phase, which may last 3–4 months before spontaneous resolution. The appearance of the lesion by itself can be very difficult to distinguish from an SCC (see later), although the latter usually grows progressively but less rapidly. The same difficulty also occurs on histological examination, but carcinoma always invades the deeper dermis. Treatment is by excision with a margin of surrounding skin; if there is any remaining doubt about the diagnosis, careful follow-up is indicated.

Other Benign Skin Tumours

Benign Pigmented Skin Lesions

Freckles (syn. Ephelides)

Freckles are areas of the epidermis where melanocytes produce more melanin, usually in response to ultraviolet light. The number of melanocytes is normal, and they are quite stable.

Lentigo (Plural Lentigines)

Lentigines are areas of the epidermis where the number of melanocytes is increased and melanin production is excessive. They are found in areas of chronic sun exposure and hence are most common on the face, hands and shoulders. If seen in young patients, they are the sites of solar damage, and the patient should be advised against unnecessary exposure to the sun.

Melanocytic Pigmented Naevus: 'Moles'

The term naevus (plural naevi) is not necessarily confined to melanocytic skin lesions; it may equally refer to blood vessels (vascular naevi). The more correct generic term is a hamartoma. Essentially, there is an abnormal collection of a normal skin constituent: in this case, melanocytes. Congenital melanocytic naevi are rare, often darkly pigmented and may be hairy or papillary. Melanocytic naevi may occur anywhere on the skin – including the nail bed, where they give rise to a linear pigmented stria. According to the clinical and histological features, melanocytic naevi can be subdivided into five types:

- Junctional – at the dermo–epidermal interface (clinically brown and flat)
- Intradermal – entirely within the dermis (clinically skin-coloured and raised)

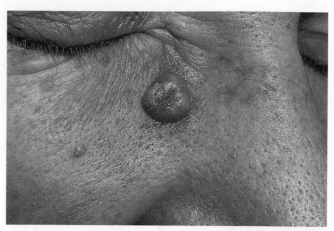

- **Fig. 32.11** Keratoacanthoma on Cheek Showing Central Keratin Plug with Surrounding Acanthotic Collar

- Compound – features of both junctional and intradermal (clinically brown and raised)
- Blue – deep dermal with considerable pigmentation which gives rise to their colour (blue-black and flat)
- Spitz naevus – reddish brown in colour, usually on the face or limbs of children and young adults; they are benign (but see later)

Most moles which are not present at birth will develop in the second or third decade. A Spitz naevus may undergo rapid growth and for this reason is often removed to exclude malignancy. Histological examination shows large cells which are pleomorphic and can be very difficult to distinguish from those of malignant melanoma. Skilled histological assessment is necessary.

Dermatofibroma

This is a tumour (often multiple) of dermal connective tissue which contains histiocytes and is of unknown cause. They are more common in women than in men. A small intradermal nodule is present. Pigmentation is usual, and the overlying epidermis is tethered to the lesion, giving a puckered appearance if the lesion is squeezed.

As the lesion matures, it changes from red-brown to pale, although often with a retained surrounding halo of pigmentation. A slow increase in size may occur, and excision may be necessary, especially with the darker lesions, to exclude other malignant pathologies. It is more important to differentiate benign dermatofibromas from more advanced and aggressive neoplasms that may appear similar to dermatofibromas in some cases.

Dermatofibrosarcoma protuberans (DFSP) is a rare locally aggressive neoplasm that can be mistaken for a benign dermatofibroma. DFSP requires a wide excision margin as it has a tendency to recur but has only a small risk of metastatic spread.

Benign Abnormalities of the Blood Vessels

Haemangiomas are distinguished by the size of the blood vessel that is involved.

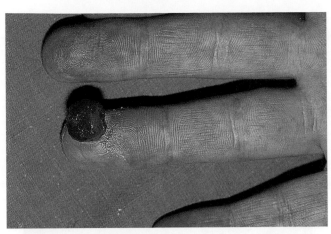

• **Fig. 32.12** Pyogenic Granuloma on Finger Showing Friable Vascular Tumour

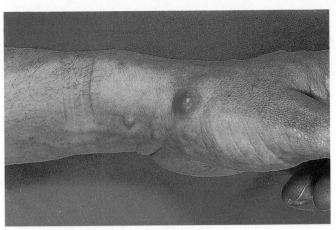

• **Fig. 32.13** Neurofibroma on Wrist, Showing Soft Fleshy Swelling

Pathological Features

Capillary haemangiomas are common and may give rise to salmon pink discoloration on the surface of the skin. The back of the neck is a common site. Other variants include the port wine stain on the face, which may be associated with ipsilateral intracranial haemangiomata, giving rise to epilepsy (Sturge–Weber syndrome). Strawberry naevi may appear in infancy and grow with age before resolving spontaneously by the early teens. Campbell de Morgan spots appear as small cherry papules on the trunk, are very common and of no significance, although they can become increasingly numerous with age and give rise to cosmetic embarrassment. Pyogenic granulomas are exuberant granulation tissue, an exaggerated healing response to minor trauma, and are usually found on the finger or the lip (Fig. 32.12). In spite of their name, the lesions are not infective in cause. They are friable and bleed readily. Glomus tumours appear as small vascular blebs on the skin. They have a generous nerve supply and are tender, especially if they occur within a confined space such as the nail bed.

Neurofibromas

These are benign tumours of the fibroblasts of the nerve sheath. The usual presentation is as a solitary lesion in the area of a peripheral nerve. On clinical examination, they are soft and fleshy (Fig. 32.13).

Schwannomas are benign tumours arising from the Schwann cells around the peripheral nerves, are much firmer nodules than neurofibromas and are closely tethered to an identifiable nerve. Pressure on the tumour may cause pain in the area of distribution of the nerve. Cutaneous neurofibromas can be managed conservatively or with careful excision if symptomatic.

Some patients have multiple neurofibromas, which form part of the syndrome of neurofibromatosis with associated cafe-au-lait spots and axillary freckling. There are sometimes Schwannomas of the larger cranial nerves and phaeochromocytomas. There are three clinically and genetically distinct forms of neurofibromatosis, neurofibromatosis types 1 and 2 (NF1 and NF2) and Schwannomatosis. NF1 is due to a mutation on chromosome 17q (neurofibromin protein) and NF2 is a mutated 22q (merlin protein). They are both autosomal dominant but with variable phenotypes. There is also a high spontaneous mutation rate. In Schwannomatosis, there are multiple non-cutaneous Schwannomas with absence of bilateral vestibular Schwannomas.

Benign Appendage Tumours

Skin appendages, such as sweat glands and hair follicles, are a source of benign tumours. Non-specific tumours such as syringomata or trichofolliculomas are not usually diagnosed clinically but only retrospectively following excision of a nondescript skin nodule. A cylindroma is of hair follicle origin and gives rise to a fleshy nodule. They usually occur on the scalp and may become very large, giving rise to what in the past was labelled a turban tumour.

Cysts

A cyst is an epithelium lined cavity usually filled with thick products of epithelial secretion or of cell breakdown which have undergone degeneration. The most common type originates from the hair follicle.

Epidermoid and Pilar Cysts

These are sometimes incorrectly termed sebaceous cysts. Epidermoid cysts have walls derived from the follicular infundibular epithelium, so they are found anywhere on the body where hair follicles occur. Many are solitary but multiple lesions occur. They range in size from a few millimetres to several centimetres. The cyst is located in the deep dermis but is connected to the superficial epithelium through the pilosebaceous duct. A blocked duct may be visible on the surface as a central black punctum. Clinically, they are soft and are mobile over deeper structures. Pilar cysts have walls derived from the outer root sheath of the hair follicle, and are almost invariably found on the scalp.

Epidermoid and pilar cysts are not usually painful unless they are injured with disruption of the contents into the surrounding dermis, where they cause an intense inflammatory reaction. When this occurs, the area swells and becomes tender.

Uninflamed cysts are excised; care must be taken that all abnormal epithelial elements are removed, or recurrence is likely. If the cyst has become inflamed, then the contents are best drained and the inflammation allowed to subside, at which point the whole cyst can be excised.

Dermoid Cysts

Congenital

These are rare and arise from abnormalities of development where epithelial remnants occur. They are found in lines of embryological fusion; the midline of the neck, the scalp and the face are common sites. The contents of the cysts include ectodermal structures of hair and sebaceous glands in addition to keratin.

Implantation Dermoid

In this condition, a usually insignificant injury drives a fragment of dermis into the subdermal layer from where its secretions cannot escape. The fingertip is the commonest site (e.g. rose gardeners), although they may occur at any site of injury.

Lipomas

This is strictly a growth of fat deep to the skin proper. The overlying skin is normal, and the lump can be moved in relation to it. Fluctuation can be elicited, although the lesion is not cystic. The histological appearance is of a mass of adipose tissue with thin fibroid septa. The size varies, and penetration into muscles can occur. Treatment is by excision, particularly if the lipoma increases in size or becomes tender as this raises clinical suspicion of a liposarcoma. Liposarcomas can be differentiated from lipomas on histology and a core needle biopsy is recommended if there is clinical concern.

Premalignant Conditions of the Epidermis

Bowen's Disease

This is characterized by a well-circumscribed scaly plaque (Fig. 32.14) most commonly on the lower legs, although it can occur anywhere on the body including the anus. The clinical appearance is similar to a solitary patch of psoriasis. Histological examination shows full-thickness epidermal dysplasia sometimes amounting to carcinoma *in situ*. The condition is potentially malignant, although progression is slow.

Management

A variety of methods can be used to treat the condition, including curettage and cautery, the use of topical cytotoxic

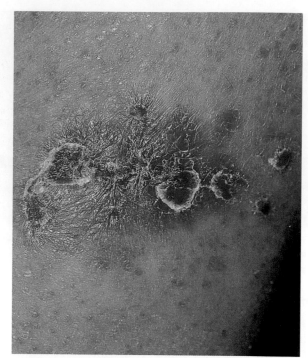

• **Fig. 32.14** Bowen's Disease on Leg Showing Psoriasiform Plaque

drugs, excision, cryotherapy and, sometimes, superficial radiotherapy. The choice depends on the size of the lesion, its site and the age of the patient.

Leucoplakia

In this condition, a fixed white plaque is seen on mucous membranes. The differential diagnosis is from lichen planus – a common inflammatory condition of the skin and mucous membranes – which has a more lace-like appearance, and *Candida* where the white plaques can be brushed off from the surface mucosa. Oral candidiasis usually occurs in immunocompromised patients, in diabetics or in those on systemic corticosteroid therapy. If there is any doubt, the plaque should be biopsied to exclude dysplasia and, if positive, the area ablated by cryotherapy or laser.

Paget's Disease of the Nipple

This is discussed in Chapter 26.

Lentigo Maligna

This is a rare plaque-like condition which tends to develop in late middle age, most commonly on the cheek, and increases slowly in size with time. Initially, the plaque is uniformly pigmented, but as the lesion develops, irregular pigmentation occurs which is the early superficial spreading phase of a malignant melanoma (Fig. 32.15). If left untreated, the melanoma advances and enters a deep invasive phase with the same risk of metastases as melanoma elsewhere.

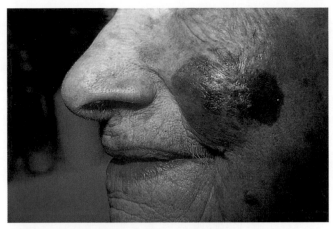

• **Fig. 32.15** Lentigo Maligna on Cheek Showing Plaque with Variation in Pigmentation

Management

Smaller lesions should be excised. There is a problem here with lesions that occupy a large surface area, and excision is not usually possible without grafting. A graft is unsightly, and the condition may be managed expectantly by close and regular follow-up. Action is taken if there is a change in appearance.

Non-Melanoma Skin Cancer

Classification

There are two commoner clinical types of carcinoma, both of which arise from keratinocytes:
- basal cell carcinoma (BCC)
- squamous cell carcinoma (SCC)

A variety of factors predispose the epidermis towards these malignancies:
- exposure to the sun
- immunosuppression
- hereditary disorders, e.g. xeroderma pigmentosum, a condition of failure of DNA repair

Non-melanoma skin cancer (BCC and SCC) are one of the commonest types of malignancy. BCC is the most common (80%), with approximately 20% being SCC. The incidence of BCC and SCC increases with age. There is a female preponderance in those under 40 years of age but later in life, the sex distribution is roughly equal.

The vast majority are related to UV light exposure. For SCCs, the major pattern is chronic long-term exposure. For BCCs, the pattern of sporadic exposure with episodes of burning is more important. Patients on immunosuppression after organ transplant have a significantly increased incidence of SCC; risk factors include length of immunosuppression, ethnic origin and associated sunlight exposure. Human papilloma virus DNA is found in the majority of transplant recipient SCCs. In addition to this increased risk, transplant recipients have higher risk tumours which are more likely to develop locoregional recurrences following treatment.

Basal Cell Carcinoma

This generally arises in sites exposed to the sun. Ninety percent of lesions are on the face.

Classification

There are four clinical types:
- nodulocystic – the most common (60%)
- pigmented
- superficial spreading
- morphoeic or sclerotic

Pathological Features

Basal cell carcinomas cause local invasion and destruction of surrounding tissues. They penetrate into subcutaneous tissue and can erode into vital structures such as the orbit and brain. Histologically, the tumour cells have strongly basophilic nuclei and little cytoplasm. Cells at the periphery of the tumour give rise to a palisade pattern reminiscent of normal basal cells. Metastases are extremely rare.

Clinical Features

A **nodulocystic** lesion has fluid-filled spaces and initially presents as a small translucent or pearly nodule which eventually breaks down, usually as the result of minor trauma, to produce an ulcer – a rodent ulcer characterized by a rolled pearly edge with surface telangiectasia (Fig. 32.16).

A **pigmented form** has characteristic pearly nodules around the edge (Fig. 32.17).

Superficial spreading carcinoma is a scaly plaque, usually on the trunk, with epidermal atrophy; pearly translucent nodules can usually be seen around the periphery of the lesion (Fig. 32.18).

Morphoeic or **sclerotic lesions** heal by fibrosis and scarring and may be multifocal; they do not look at all like cystic basal cell carcinomas, do not have pearly nodules but appear as a rather depressed plaque of sclerotic skin (Fig. 32.19). Superficial and morphoeic have the highest tendency to recur after excision due to subclinical lateral spread.

Management

It is important that the tumour is treated adequately on the first occasion to render recurrence unlikely. Treatment depends on the site and size of the lesions at the time of diagnosis. In accordance with the British association of dermatology guidelines, standard excision with 4-mm margins is adequate in 98% of cases of BCC. Curettage is only suitable for lesions less than 1 cm and may result in poor cosmesis. Larger lesions or those in difficult anatomical locations may require plastic surgery involvement or be treated with radiotherapy. Whilst these tumours are radiosensitive, radiotherapy often results in higher rates of local recurrence and worse cosmetic outcomes than surgical excision. Mohs micrographic surgery may also be considered. Superficial lesions can be treated with topical immunomodulators such as imiquimod, topical chemotherapeutic agents such as 5-fluorouracil, photodynamic therapy or cryotherapy.

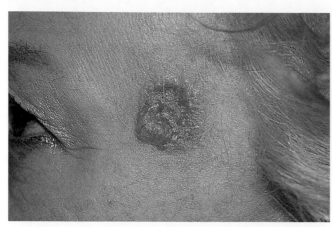

• **Fig. 32.16** Cystic Basal Cell Carcinoma on Temple Showing Central Breakdown and Ulceration

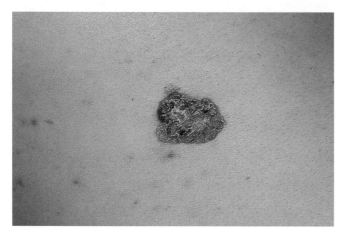

• **Fig. 32.17** Pigmented Basal Cell Carcinoma Showing Pigmentation of Lesion

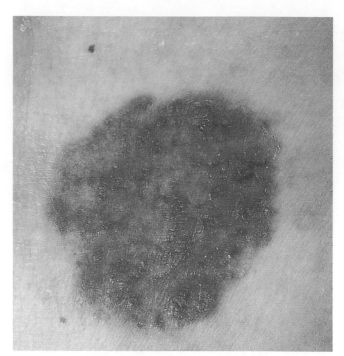

• **Fig. 32.18** Superficial Basal Cell Carcinoma on Back Showing Spreading Flat, Red Plaque

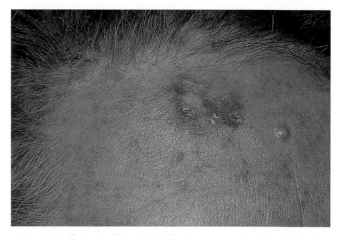

• **Fig. 32.19** Sclerotic Basal Cell Carcinoma on Forehead Showing Depressed White Plaque

Squamous Cell Carcinoma

Aetiology and Pathological Features

Older age groups than those with basal cell carcinoma are usually affected and lesions are also most commonly found on skin repeatedly exposed to ultraviolet light. Industrial carcinogens are also important in their development (ionizing radiation, arsenic and chronic exposure to coal tar and mineral oils). They can also arise as a consequence of chronic inflammation, e.g. within chronic leg ulcers. Smokers are prone to squamous cell carcinomas of the lip. The origin of the tumour is within the epidermis, and the cells show some degree of maturation towards keratin formation. Occurrence may be *de novo* or in pre-existing skin lesions such as active solar keratoses, leukoplakia or Bowen's disease. SCC invades the dermis and deeper tissues such as bone and cartilage. Metastasis to distant sites via both the lymphatics and the bloodstream takes place, although the second is usually a late and uncommon complication of the disease. Lesions of the lip (Fig. 32.20) and ear are prone to spread early.

Clinical Features

The usual presentation is with either an enlarging painless ulcer with a rolled indurated margin or a papillomatous

appearance with areas of ulceration, bleeding or serous exudation from secondary infection on the surface. An unexplained area of ulceration or thickening of the lip must be biopsied at once to establish a diagnosis.

Management

SCC of the skin can spread to the lymph nodes or result in distant metastases. Risk of metastasis is determined by tumour site, depth, size and histologic features, as well as patient characteristics and comorbidities.

Most lesions are small, and, for those less than 2 cm, local excision with 4-mm margins is adequate. With lesions >2 cm in recurrent lesions or in high-risk patients, such as those on immunosuppression, 6-mm margins are required. Especially in the face, this may require reconstruction by

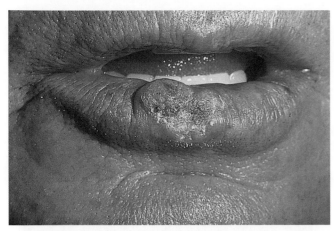

• **Fig. 32.20** Squamous Cell Carcinoma on Lower Lip Showing Infiltrated Keratinized Lesion with Ulceration

grafting or flap procedures. Where extensive surgery seems likely, radiotherapy can be considered, although long-term sequelae include radiodermatitis, and an unattractive white, avascular scar may make this choice inappropriate for exposed areas such as the face. Tumours on the lip and ear must be treated vigorously as high-risk lesions from the outset.

Malignant Melanoma (syn. Melanoma)

This is a highly malignant tumour derived from melanocytes (Box 32.3).

Epidemiology and Aetiology

Malignant melanoma can arise *de novo* or from a pre-existing melanocytic naevus, especially in fair-skinned people of Northern European origin. The highest incidence in the world is in northern and western Australia, perhaps because of the historic relatively high level of UV light exposure to people of Northern European origin. Melanoma is the 19th commonest cancer worldwide and its incidence is increasing more rapidly than for any other cancer, with a 128% increase in incidence since 1990. Over the last decade, the mortality rates for melanoma in Britain for men have increased by 14% but have remained relatively stable in women. The cause for this is unknown but may reflect a tendency for women to present at an earlier stage. These figures reflect the rising melanoma incidence seen but are much less pronounced than would be predicted from the incidence figures.

Pathological Features

All skin areas are vulnerable, although the most commonly affected sites are the lower extremities in women and the trunk in men. Tumours may also arise in the choroid of the eye and in the mucosal membranes. The classification of spread is dealt with below under 'Management'. However, the pathways are:
- Direct extension into the underlying dermis and thence to the subcutaneous tissues
- Satellite nodules – around the lesion caused by tumour deposits in the draining lymphatics
- To regional lymph node basin
- Haematogenous spread to distant organs

Clinical Classification

There are five clinical types of malignant melanoma:
- Superficial spreading melanoma (70%) (Fig. 32.21)
- Lentigo maligna
- Nodular melanoma (Fig. 32.22)
- Acral lentiginous melanoma (Fig. 32.23)
- Amelanotic melanoma (Fig. 32.24) – a lesion where the malignant melanocytes are not producing melanin; this is uncommon

Clinical Features That Suggest a Melanoma

Most patients present with a new skin lesion or a change in the character of a pre-existing naevus. The features are summarized in Box 32.4.

Other Presentations

Malignant melanoma can also present with metastases – localized lymph node enlargement or distant spread such as cerebral deposits.

Prophylaxis

Public awareness campaigns are an important part of the management of the disease. Patients should be persuaded to check their skin regularly for moles that change and should then come early to their doctor if there is concern. Avoidance of unnecessary exposure to the sun by the use of hats, clothing and effective barrier creams is an important message to communicate to the public and should, in the long term, reduce the incidence of both malignant melanoma and other epidermal cancers.

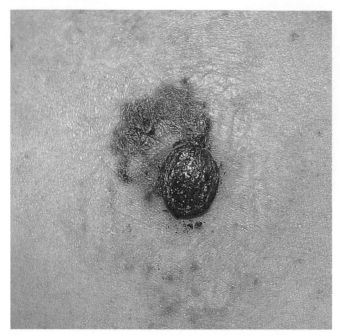

• **Fig. 32.21** Superficial Spreading Malignant Melanoma It shows asymmetry, irregular border and variation in colour with a raised nodule developing.

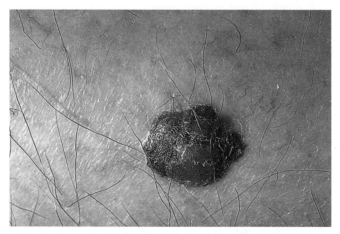

• **Fig. 32.22** Nodular Malignant Melanoma Showing Raised, Deeply Pigmented Tumour

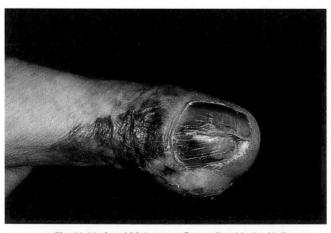

• **Fig. 32.23** Acral Melanoma Spreading Under Nail

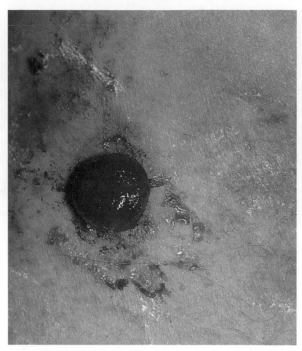

• **Fig. 32.24** Amelanotic Malignant Melanoma on Neck Showing Raised, Non-Pigmented Tumour

---

• **BOX 32.4** **Changes in Pigmented Lesions Indicative of Malignant Melanoma**

American Cancer Society Checklist

A Asymmetry of lesion
B Irregular border
C Irregular colour
D Diameter >6 mm

Glasgow Seven-Point Checklist

Major Features	Minor Features
1. Change in size	4. Diameter of lesion >7 mm
2. Change in shape	5. Inflammation around lesion
3. Change in colour	6. Bleeding of lesion
	7. Itch/altered sensation

One major feature indicates removal of lesion.

A feature of both checklists is the presence of a changing lesion which identifies it as being different from other pigmented lesions on the patient.

Patients with a greatly increased risk of melanoma are those with a giant (20 cm or more) congenital pigmented naevus and those with a strong family history of melanoma. Patients who have had a previous primary melanoma or who have >100 typical moles or >2 atypical moles have a moderately increased chance of developing melanoma. Individuals with fair skin and poor tanning ability or freckling should also be advised to take great care with sun avoidance and protection.

Management and Prognosis

Suspicious Lesions

Any questionable lesion on either history or physical examination must always be completely excised with a 1-mm margin down to subcutis and sent for histological examination. A more difficult decision is when a patient presents with multiple naevi which are showing variation in the evenness of pigmentation within lesions and between lesions. Patients with this so-called 'atypical naevus syndrome' have a higher than normal risk of developing melanoma. They should be managed by careful photography of the lesions to act as a reference for future change. Any suspicious lesions should be excised and examined microscopically.

Establishing the Diagnosis

Initial management is by local full thickness skin excision. It is essential to have a clear peripheral and deep margin. The specimen is then assessed histologically to confirm the diagnosis and to assess depth of invasion.

Histological classification is in two ways:

- Breslow thickness (which has become the widely adopted best criterion for assessment) – measurement of penetration of malignant cells in millimetres from the granular cell layer of the epidermis through to the deepest invading melanocyte (Fig. 32.25). Tumours less than 0.76 mm at the time of primary excision carry an excellent prognosis, but those that have penetrated further have a poorer prognosis proportionate to depth. Although the inverse relationship between thickness and survival is generally linear, there are occasional melanomas that do not follow the rule. Tumour thickness is the most important prognostic factor but others such as age, sex, size of lesion, mitotic index and tumour-infiltrating lymphocytes need to be considered.
- Clark's classification – grades the tumour on the depth within the dermis of malignant invasion (Table 32.1).

TNM classification is also based on tumour thickness but includes other variables such as ulceration and mitotic rate (see American Joint Committee on Cancer (AJCC) 8th Edition, https://cancerstaging.org/references-tools/deskreferences/pages/default.aspx).

It must be emphasized that malignant melanoma is a curable disease if treated at an early stage.

Treatment

The treatment paradigm of melanoma is rapidly advancing and becoming increasingly complex. Surgery is still the main stay of therapy in early disease but, for the first time, there are now new effective adjuvant therapies with proven survival benefits. All patients with histology-proven melanoma should be discussed in a dedicated multidisciplinary team meeting.

Wide Excision

The main aim of a wide excision of melanoma after a diagnostic excision is to prevent the cancer recurring at the site of origin, and to maximize long-term survival. The functional

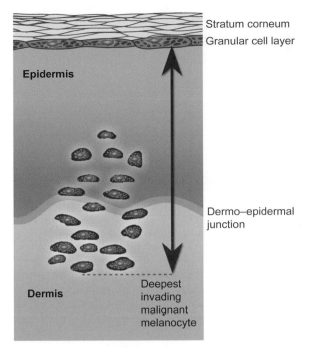

• **Fig. 32.25 Breslow Classification** The pathologist measures the thickness of the tumour in millimetres as the distance from the granular cell layer of the epidermis to the deepest invading melanoma cell.

TABLE 32.1	Clark's Classification of Levels of Malignant Melanoma.
Level	**Definition**
I	Lesion confined to epidermis (melanoma in situ)
II	Invasion into upper (papillary) dermis
III	Occupation and expansion of papillary dermis by melanoma cells
IV	Invasion into deeper (reticular) dermis
V	Invasion into subcutaneous fat

5-year survival figures fall steadily with deeper layers

and cosmetic impact of surgery on an individual patient, are major secondary considerations when planning a further excision. The recommended margins are dependent on Breslow thickness (Table 32.2). Depending on the margins required and site of the tumour, skin grafting or flaps may be required

Sentinel Lymph Node Biopsy

Patients with melanomas greater than 0.8 mm should have investigation for lymph node involvement with clinical examination and a sentinel lymph node biopsy (SLNB) at the time of their wide local excision.

Treatment of Nodal Disease

If involved lymph nodes are found clinically or radiologically, patients should be offered a lymph node dissection. For SLNB-positive nodes, patients should be offered close

TABLE 32.2	Re-excision Margins Related to Breslow Thickness.
T1 Lesions 0–1 mm thick	1 cm
T2 Lesions 1–2 mm thick	1–2 cm (Depending upon site and pathological features)
T3 Lesions 2–4 mm thick	2–3 cm (Depending upon site and pathological features)
T4 Lesions >4 mm thick	3 cm

From Marsden, J., et al. UK guidelines for management of melanoma. Br. J. Dermatol. 2010; 163: 238–256.

surveillance with ultrasound, with completion lymph node dissection reserved for rare instances where further surveillance is not possible, or when the patient presents with palpable nodal disease. Regional lymph node metastasis is one of the most significant prognostic factors for tumour recurrence and survival in malignant melanoma. The accurate detection of lymph node metastases is necessary to correctly stage patients, determine surgical treatment strategies and identify patients who may benefit from adjuvant therapies.

Immunotherapy

Two new immunotherapy treatment options are now available for patients with resected melanoma, with NICE recently licensing adjuvant immunotherapy within the Cancer Drugs Fund. These new treatments are nivolumab and pembrolizumab. These are anti-PD-1 monoclonal antibodies that work as immune checkpoint inhibitors allowing the T-cells to recognize and attack the cancer cells. They have shown improved recurrence-free survival in the CheckMate 238 (https://doi.org/10.1016/S1470-2045(20)30494-0) and KEYNOTE-054 (https://doi.org/10.1016/S1470-2045(21)00065-6) trials. This means patients have beneficial adjuvant treatment options after SLNB but they must have their nodal disease completely resected by either sentinel lymphadenectomy or lymph node dissection to be eligible.

In patients with advanced disease, other systemic agents are also available. Ipilumimab is another immune checkpoint inhibitor that targets CTLA-4, and can be used on its own or in combination with nivolumab, increasing efficacy but also toxicities. BRAF inhibitors are targeted agents used in those with BRAF mutations. Treatment is limited by the development of resistance, though the combination of BRAF and MEK inhibitors delays the development of this.

Adjuvant therapy in melanoma

There have been several significant advances in the treatment of adjuvant melanoma. Two recent trials for resected stage III melanoma have resulted in both NICE and FDA approvals. The first of these is Checkmate 238 which compared immunotherapy agents nivolumab, an anti-PD1 antibody, with ipilimumab, an anti-CTLA-4 antibody. This showed nivolumab to have significant improvement in recurrence free survival (RFS) with the further benefit of reduced toxicity.

The second, the Combi-AD trial for patients with BRAF mutant melanoma, V600K or V600E, compared combination therapy with dabrafenib, a BRAF inhibitor and trametinib, a MEK inhibitor versus placebo. The combination treatment showed improved RFS, distant metastases-free survival and overall survival.

This has led to these agents being the current standard of care and the optimal adjuvant treatment strategy should be personalized for that particular patient, after discussion and consideration of the BRAF mutational status, and the wishes of the patient in conjunction with their medical oncologists.

Treatment of advanced melanoma

Patients with advanced disease may also be treated with either anti-PD1 immunotherapy or BRAF and MEK inhibitors. In addition, ipilimumab can be used on its own or in combination with nivolumab increasing treatment efficacy but also toxicities.

Oncolytic viral therapy is another treatment option in patients with injectable disease. This novel class of drug uses native or genetically modified viruses to directly cause tumour cell lysis and stimulate an antitumour immune response. Talimogene laherparepvec (TVEC) is a genetically modified type I herpes simplex virus. It is presently the only oncolytic virus approved by the FDA and NICE with an indication for advanced melanoma based upon improved durable response rate in a randomized, phase III trial.

The potential future directions for treatment of melanoma, which are being investigated in trials, include adjuvant treatment for high risk stage II melanoma, neoadjuvant treatment of advanced melanoma, and adoptive cell transfer therapies, which include CAR-T (chimeric antigen receptor T cell) and TIL (tumour infiltrating lymphocyte) therapy.

Treatment of In-Transit Disease

Other surgical options are available for the treatment of *in-transit* disease. Lesions can be removed under local anaesthetic with either a scalpel or CO_2 laser. Patients with a high burden of disease within a limb can also be offered an isolated limb perfusion in specialist centres. This procedure is performed under general anaesthetic as a single treatment. It enables the delivery of cytotoxic treatment (high-dose melphalan and TNF-α) directly to the limb that could not be tolerated as systemic therapy. Where available, other injectable therapies such as talimogene laherparepvec (T-VEC), a recombinant herpes simplex, may be considered for the irresectable disease, as it has been proven to be helpful in attaining locoregional control with direct and indirect antitumour effect. Finally, electochemotherapy, whereby chemotherapy given locally or systemically (e.g. bleomycin) in conjunction with electroporation of in transit lesions, has a proven benefit as regards palliation and local control.

Malignant Tumours of the Dermis

These are rare. The dermis is of mesodermal origin, and therefore malignant tumours are classified as sarcomas. They initially present as small nodules which increase in size and may become tender.

Kaposi Sarcoma

This is a type of haemangiosarcoma which used to be a relatively rare disease and was found most commonly as a small purple nodule usually on a lymphoedematous leg either of an elderly person of central European Jewish extraction or in sub-Saharan Africa. More recently, however, it has become recognized as an opportunistic tumour in immunosuppressed patients, especially those with HIV infections, in association with herpes simplex virus type 8 infection. In this context, there are a variety of clinical presentations. The most usual is that of a small purple nodule (Fig. 32.26), but a dusky purple plaque or with mucosal involvement is not uncommon. The treatment is usually surgical excision for small discrete lesions and radiotherapy for larger ones.

Other Malignancies of the Skin

Lymphoma

Most cutaneous lymphomas are T-cell in origin and, as they present with diffuse scaly plaques which may look like a cutaneous fungal infection (hence they are also known as mycosis fungoides), they rarely present to surgeons. B-cell lymphomas, however, may present with a solitary nodule or cluster of nodules, and the diagnosis is made on biopsy.

Merkel Cell Cancer

This is a rare but aggressive cancer that arises from the neuroendocrine cells of the skin. Histologically, it appears in the dermis and subcutis. The lesions consist of sheets and nodules of small hyperchromatic epithelial cells with high rates of mitosis and apoptosis. Lymphovascular invasion is commonly seen. Pre-existing infection with Merkel cell polyomavirus is seen in up to 80% of cases. It most commonly presents in sun-damaged areas of the skin. Treatment is with surgical excision with margins >1 cm. Adjuvant radiotherapy should be considered to reduce the rates of local recurrence. In patients presenting with lymph node metastases, 5-year survival is less than 50%.

Secondary Carcinoma

The skin may be the site of distant spread of internal carcinoma. Sometimes solitary nodules arise in the skin that are the result of blood-borne metastases or direct involvement through the lymphatics. Biopsy of the lesion

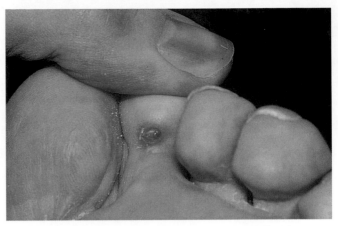

• **Fig. 32.26** Kaposi Sarcoma Showing Purple Nodule

usually provides a clue to the site of the primary disorder. Solitary nodules may occur in cancers that are known to spread with single metastases such as thyroid and renal carcinoma.

Cutaneous Signs of Internal Malignancy

The skin is well recognized as a marker for non-metastatic signs of internal malignancy:

- Pruritus may be a presenting feature of myeloproliferative malignancies, particularly in young people – polycythaemia vera, lymphoma
- Deep jaundice from obstruction of the bile duct – carcinoma of the head of the pancreas
- Increased pigmentation – ACTH secretion in carcinoma of the bronchus
- Finger clubbing – colonic/bronchial carcinoma
- Unusual annular erythemas such as erythema gyratum repens – carcinoma of the bronchus
- Tylosis (diffuse keratinous thickening) with palmar plantar hyperkeratosis – carcinoma of the oesophagus
- Acanthosis nigricans (a velvety papillomatous appearance in the intertriginous areas of the axillae and groin and around the neck) – upper gastrointestinal tumours
- Acquired ichthyosis – any internal malignancy

Further Reading

Bolognia JL, Jorizzo JL, Rapini RP. *Dermatology.* 2nd ed. St Louis: Mosby Elsevier; 2007.

Burns T, Breathnach S, Cox N, Griffiths CEM, eds. *Rook's Textbook of Dermatology.* 8th ed. Oxford: Wiley-Blackwell; 2010.

Buxton PK, Morris-Jones R. *ABC of Dermatology (ABC series).* 5th ed. London: BMJ Books; 2009.

Calonje JE, Brenn T, Lazar AJ, McKee PH. *Pathology of the Skin: with Clinical Correlations.* 4th ed. Philadelphia: Mosby Elsevier; 2011.

Du Vivier A. *Atlas of Clinical Dermatology.* 3rd ed. Edinburgh: Churchill Livingstone; 2002.

Wolff K, Johnson RA. *Fitzpatrick's Color Atlas and Synopsis of Clinical Dermatology.* 6th ed. New York: McGraw-Hill Medical; 2009.

33

Sarcoma

Introduction

Soft tissue lumps may be benign or malignant and with malignant soft tissue tumours classified into over 100 subtypes. Classification is essential as each subtype of soft tissue tumour has different biological behaviour, treatment requirements and outcomes. Malignant tumours of mesodermal origin (soft tissue) are known as sarcomas (Fig. 33.1). The mesoderm includes adipose, muscle, connective, neural, vascular and lymphatic tissues. Sarcomas are a group of rare tumours that account for less than 1% of all malignant tumours. They affect all regions of the body, but commonly the trunk and extremities. Benign soft tissue lesions vastly outnumber malignant lesions, at a ratio of 150:1. This makes appropriate work up and treatment essential. Sarcomas affect men and women in roughly equal proportions. They affect all age groups, but some tumours types are more common at specific age ranges (Table 33.1). The most common means of metastasis for sarcomas is via the haematogenous route (via the bloodstream) and therefore the lungs are the most common site of metastasis. In this section we aim to discuss the classification of soft tissue neoplasms, the principles of diagnosis including clinical presentation, initial investigations, pathology, staging and lastly the treatment options. Figs. 33.2 to 33.7 show examples of soft tissue tumours.

Classification

Soft tissue tumours (STT) are classified according to tissue differentiation and cell morphology (Fig. 33.8). This is based on histological classification determined by light microscopy augmented with the use of immunohistochemistry and cytogenetics. Table 33.2 shows part of the WHO classification of soft tissue tumours. They are divided by cell line of differentiation and whether the tumour is thought to be benign, locally aggressive, rarely metastatic or malignant.

Clinical History

The most common mode of STT presentation is as a painless mass. In nearly all cases sarcomas are thought to arise de novo and not from preexisting benign lesions. Like most problems in clinical medicine, the investigation of a soft tissue lump should start with a full history, including when the lump first appeared. Has the lump changed since it first appeared? Rapid growth may suggest a malignant process; however slow growth does not exclude it. Are there multiple lumps present? Are there associated local symptoms such as pain, radiating nerve pain or paraesthesia? (For example, pain with activity is often associated with haemangiomas or benign nerve sheath tumours). Are there systemic symptoms such as night sweats or weight loss? A history of trauma can result in myositis ossificans or may be incidental bringing the mass to the attention of the patient. A history of previous cancer and treatment may be relevant as some cancers may metastasize to the soft tissues or recur locally and treatment with radiotherapy is a risk factor for some sarcomas, e.g. angiosarcoma. A past medical history should be taken, both to ascertain the risk of development of specific STT subtypes and to help stratify operative risk by identifying co-morbidities and performance status.

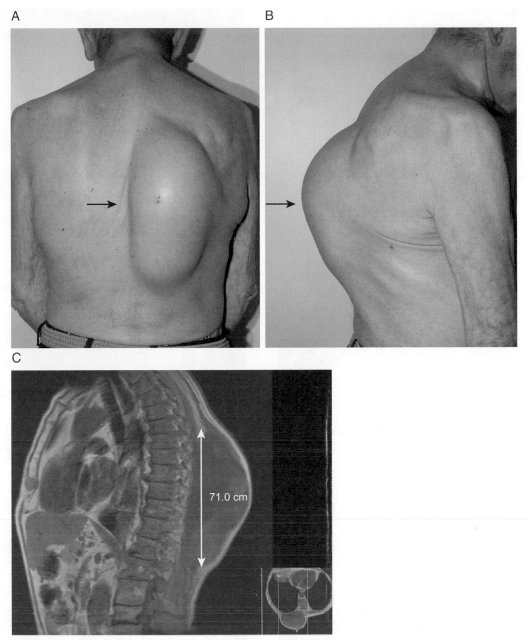

• **Fig. 33.1** Large Spindle Cell Sarcoma of the Deep Thoracic Tissue. (A B) Posterior and lateral views, (C) MRI lateral view.

Lifestyle factors such as smoking, diet and exercise have not been linked to soft tissue sarcoma (STS). For retroperitoneal and visceral sarcomas, a full gastrointestinal history should be taken including pain, early satiety, altered bowel habit and per rectum (PR) bleeding.

It must also be remembered that not all lumps are STT. Many will be infective (abscesses), lymphatic (lymphoma, lymph node metastases from other cancers), anatomical or bony lesions and normal variant anatomy.

Pathogenesis

The pathogenesis of STT is complex. Cancer is a genetic disease. Alterations in certain genes due to transcription, deletion or duplication errors can result in increased activity in cell growth genes (oncogenes) or dysfunction of cell growth regulating genes (tumour suppressor genes). These genetic errors can be inherited as familial cancer syndromes or sporadic, arising de novo with no prior family history.

Most sarcomas are sporadic. Two studies of childhood sarcomas found the rate of sarcomas associated with Li-Fraumeni syndrome to be 3%; however, this number was higher in children under 3 years of age.[1–2] Familial gastrointestinal stromal tumour (GIST) is associated with less than 1% of all GISTs. In a study of sporadic sarcomas, 50% of tumours reviewed had at least 1 of over 70 known gene mutations.[3] A single translocation error is thought to be responsible for dysregulated cell growth in 15–20% of mesenchymal tumours, i.e.

TABLE 33.1	Sarcoma Subtypes Peak Incidence
Sarcoma Subtype	Peak Incidence (years)
Rhabdomyosarcoma	Most common STS <14
Osteosarcoma	Most common BS children/ adolescents
Ewing's sarcoma	10–19s
Synovial sarcoma	30–40s
Malignant phyllodes tumour	50–60s
Liposarcoma	60–70s
Leiomyosarcoma	>70s
Angiosarcoma	>70s
Fibroblastic sarcoma	>70s

BS, Bone sarcoma; *STS,* soft tissue sarcoma.

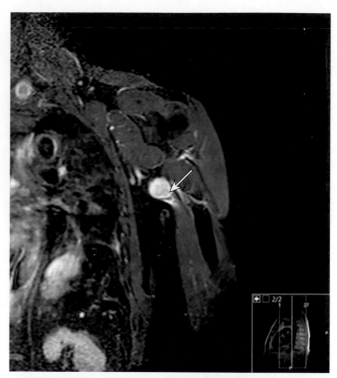

• **Fig. 33.3** Schwannoma of the Brachial Plexus

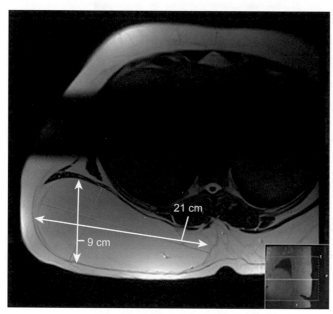

• **Fig. 33.2** Massive Superficial Lipoma Back

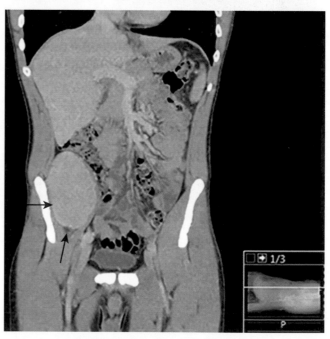

• **Fig. 33.4** Solitary Fibrous Tumour Iliacus

the COL1A1-PDGFB fusion gene in dermatofibrosarcoma protuberans. Other sarcomas are associated with more non-specific complex karyotypes where multiple abnormalities are common, i.e. pleomorphic sarcoma and myxofibrosarcoma.

Sporadic Cancers Carcinogenesis

- *Stem cell cancer theory:* This model[4] suggests that sarcomas, if not all cancers, have a hierarchy of cells within them. Most cancers are made up of a heterogenous group of cells. Cancer stem cells (CSC), like regular stem cells, have the ability to self-replicate as well as give rise to differentiated cells (progeny). It is not clear whether these cells originate from mesenchymal stem cells and lose the ability to regulate or come from differentiated mesenchymal cells and gain stem cell–like properties. Some evidence supports the theory that these stem cells may be responsible for relapse and metastasis. In Ewing's sarcoma, a subgroup of cancer cells were found to express CD133, the main stem cell marker found on the cell surface. These cells were found to be capable of differentiation into adipogenic, chondrogenic and osteogenic lineages. In rhabdomyosarcoma, CD133 expression has been associated with differentiation, chemo-resistance and worse overall survival in mouse models.

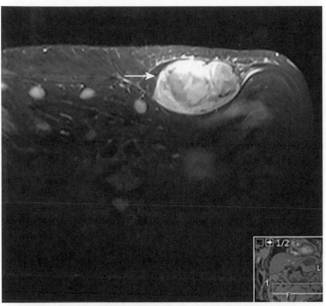

• **Fig. 33.5** Desmoid Fibromatosis of Abdominal Wall

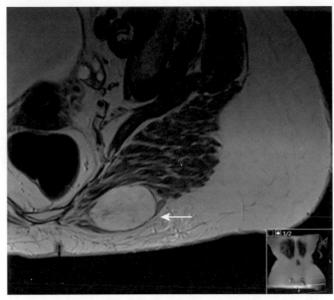

• **Fig. 33.7** Myxoma Gluteus Maximus

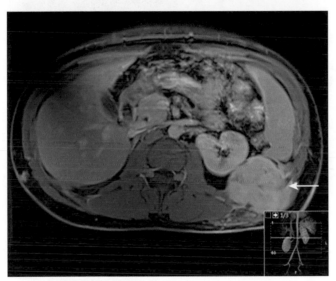

• **Fig. 33.6** Malignant Peripheral Nerve Sheath

- *Two-hit theory:* Knudson[5] suggested that dominantly inherited cancers entail a germline mutation. The patient therefore had one mutated allele at birth and one normal allele of a gene from each parent. For tumour genesis to occur, a second somatic mutation needed to occur. This explains why the penetrance of some inherited cancers is not 100%. In non-hereditary cancers the same two defects need to occur but both are acquired. This theory was first described with retinoblastoma and the RB1 gene, a sarcoma which often affects young children.

Risk Factors for Sarcoma

- *Radiation therapy:* Treatment of other cancers such as lymphoma or breast cancer are associated with the development of angiosarcoma and radiation-induced sarcomas with an average time to onset of 10 years.

- *Viruses:*
  - Human herpes virus 8 (HHV8) has been linked to Kaposi sarcoma but usually only manifests in patients who are also immunosuppressed such as HIV or transplant patients.
  - Rous sarcoma virus (RSV) was the first oncogenic virus to be discovered over 100 years ago. It was originally noted that sarcoma extract from domestic chickens could be transmitted to other fowl through a filter too fine to allow cells or bacterium to pass. The RSV is a retrovirus which contains the Scr gene, an oncogene which triggers uncontrolled growth in the host cell. This was the first oncogene discovered and paved the way for further discoveries such as the rat sarcoma virus and the Ras gene.
- *Lymphoedema*: Chronic lymphoedema from all causes is associated with angiosarcomas and lymphangiosarcomas. Congenital lymphoedema present at birth and associated with an autosomal dominant familial condition is called Milroy disease. These patients are at a greater risk of this subset of sarcomas.
- *Pregnancy*: Desmoid-type fibromatosis, a benign condition, frequently presents in women during or after pregnancy.
- *Chemicals*: Vinyl chloride (a chemical for making plastics), arsenic, phenoxyacetic acid and dioxin have been linked to angiosarcoma of the liver.

Familial Cancer Syndromes (Inherited)

- *Gardner syndrome:* This syndrome is associated with a defect in the adenomatous polyposis coli (APC) gene, a tumour suppressor gene which helps regulate beta-catenin. Beta-catenin stimulates genes which result in cell division. Gardner syndrome is a type of familial

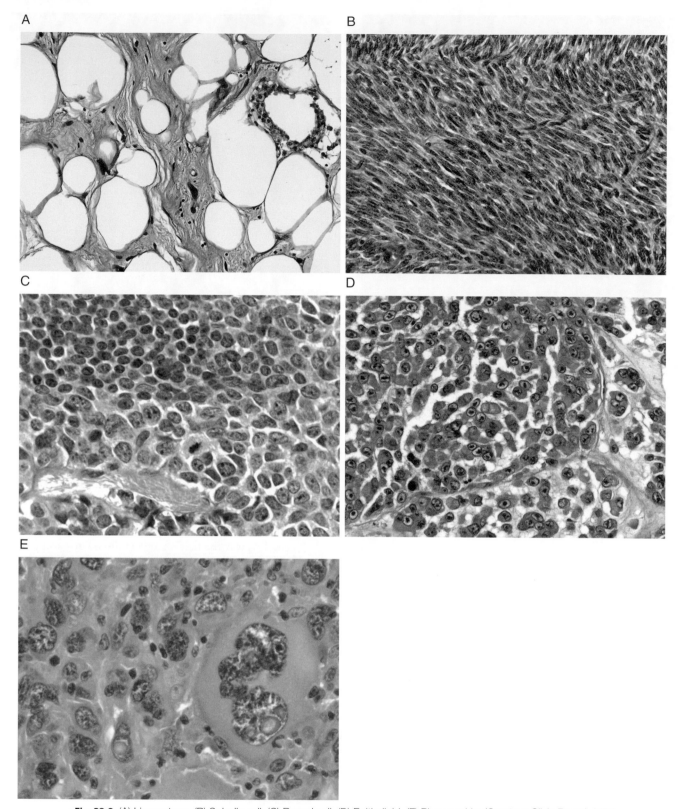

• **Fig. 33.8** (A) Lipomatous. (B) Spindle cell. (C) Round cell. (D) Epithelioid. (E) Pleomorphic. (Courtesy Silvia Bagué, MD.)

adenomatous polyposis (FAP), a disease of the colon causing hundreds of polyps and a high risk of colon cancer, with extracolonic manifestations including desmoid tumours (Fig. 33.9), sebaceous cysts, fibromas and osteomas. Desmoid tumours can be intra- or extraperitoneal.

• *Neurofibromatosis:* This causes many benign tumours that form on nerves anywhere in the body called neurofibromas. It is caused by a defect in the NF1 gene. Five percent of patients will develop a sarcoma, either a malignant peripheral nerve sheath tumour (MPNST), GIST or a rhabdomyosarcoma.

TABLE 33.2   WHO Classification of Soft Tissue Tumours[a]

Tissue of Origin	Benign	Intermediate (Locally Aggressive)	Intermediate (Rarely Metastasis)	Malignant
Adipocytic	Lipoma	Atypical lipomatous tumour	-	Dedifferentiated liposarcoma
	Lipomatosis			Myxoid liposarcoma
	Angiolipoma			Pleomorphic liposarcoma
	Extrarenal angiomyolipoma			Liposarcoma, not otherwise specified (NOS)
	Hibernoma			
Fibroblastic/ myofibroblastic	Nodular fasciitis	Palmar/plantar fibromatosis	Dermatofibrosarcoma protuberans (DFSP)	Adult fibrosarcoma
	Proliferative fasciitis	Desmoids-type fibromatosis	Fibrosarcomatous DFSP	Myxofibrosarcoma
	Proliferative myositis	Lipofibromatosis	Pigmented DFSP	Low-grade fibromyxoid sarcoma
	Myositis ossificans	Giant cell fibroblastoma	Solitary fibrous tumour	Sclerosing epithelioid fibrosarcoma
	Elastofibroma		Solitary fibrous tumour, malignant	
	Ischaemic fasciitis		Inflammatory myofibroblastic tumour	
	Fibroma of tendon sheath		Low-grade myofibroblastic sarcoma	
	Fibrous hamartoma of infancy		Myxoinflammatory fibroblastic sarcoma	
	Fibromatosis colli		Atypical myxoinflammatory fibroblastic tumour	
	Juvenile hyaline fibromatosis		Infantile fibrosarcoma	
Fibrohistiocytic	Tenosynovial giant cell tumour	-	Plexiform fibrohistiocytic tumour	-
	Deep benign fibrous histiocytoma		Giant cell tumour of soft tissue	
			Tenosynovial giant cell tumour, localized and diffuse	
Smooth-muscle	Leiomyoma	-	-	Leiomyosarcoma (excluding skin)
Perivascular	Glomus tumours	-	Malignant glomus tumour	-
	Myopericytoma			
	Angioleiomyoma			
Skeletal-muscle	Rhabdomyoma	-	-	Embryonal rhabdomyosarcoma
				Alveolar rhabdomyosarcoma
				Pleomorphic rhabdomyosarcoma
				Spindle cell rhabdomyosarcoma

TABLE 33.2	WHO Classification of Soft Tissue Tumours—cont'd			
Tissue of Origin	**Benign**	**Intermediate (Locally Aggressive)**	**Intermediate (Rarely Metastasis)**	**Malignant**
Vascular	Haemangioma	Kaposiform Haemangioendothelioma	Retiform haemangioendothelioma	Epithelioid haemangioendothelioma
	Arteriovenous malformation		Papillary intralymphatic angioendothelioma	Angiosarcoma
	Epithelioid haemangioma		Composite haemangioendothelioma	
	Angiomatosis		Pseudomyogenic haemangioendothelioma	
	Lymphangioma		Kapsoi sarcoma	
Gastrointestinal stromal (GIST)	Benign GIST	-	GIST, uncertain malignant potential	GIST, malignant
Nerve sheath	Schwannoma	-	-	Malignant peripheral nerve sheath tumour
	Melanotic schwannoma			Epithelioid malignant nerve sheath tumour
	Neurofibroma			Malignant triton tumour
	Perineurioma			Malignant granular cell tumour
	Granular cell tumour			Ectomesenchymoma
Tumours of uncertain differentiation	Acral fibromyxoma	Haemosiderotic fibrolipomatous	Atypical fibroxanthoma	Synovial sarcoma
	Intramuscular myxoma		Angiomatoid fibrous histiocytoma	Epithelioid sarcoma
	Juxta-articular myxoma		Ossifying fibromyxoid tumour/malignant	Alveolar soft-part sarcoma
	Deep angiomyxoma		Mixed tumour NOS/malignant	Clear cell sarcoma of soft tissue
	Pleomorphic hyalinizing angiectatic		Myoepithelioma	Extraskeletal myxoid chondrosarcoma
	Ectopic hamartomatous thymoma		Myoepithelial carcinoma	
			Phosphaturic mesenchymal tumour, benign	Desmoplastic small round cell tumour
			Phosphaturic mesenchymal tumour, malignant	Extrarenal rhabdoid tumour
				PEComa NOS, malignant
Undifferentiated sarcomas				Undifferentiated spindle cell sarcoma
				Undifferentiated pleomorphic sarcoma
				Undifferentiated round cell sarcoma

Continued

Tissue of Origin	Benign	Intermediate (Locally Aggressive)	Intermediate (Rarely Metastasis)	Malignant
				Undifferentiated epithelioid sarcoma
				Undifferentiated sarcoma NOS

ªOnly partial list of STT provided
PEComa, Perivascular epithelioid cell neoplasm/NOS, Not otherwise specified.
From Fletcher CDM, Bridge JA, Hogendoorn PCW, Mertens F. WHO Classification of Tumours of Soft Tissue and Bone (WHO Classification of Tumours), 4th ed. vol. 5: Lyon, France: IARC Publications; 2013.

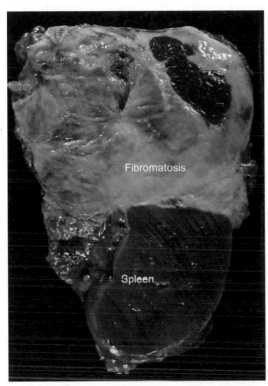

• **Fig. 33.9** Intra-Abdominal Fibromatosis Surrounding Spleen (May be associated with Gardner's syndrome.) (Courtesy Silvia Bagué, MD.)

- *Li-Fraumeni syndrome:* Related to a defect in the TP53 gene and is associated with a high risk of breast cancer, leukaemias, brain tumours and sarcomas in 10% of sufferers.
- *Retinoblastoma:* Caused by a defect in the RB1 gene and causes ocular tumours in children and adults. These patients have a higher risk of soft tissue and bone sarcomas.
- *Gorlin syndrome:* Caused by a defect in the PTCH1 gene, patients have a high risk of developing basal cell skin cancers as well as an increased risk of fibrosarcoma and rhabdomyosarcoma.
- *Familial gastrointestinal stromal tumours (GIST):* Associated with KIT, PDGFRA and 4q12 gene mutations resulting in multifocal GISTs developing from hyperplasia of the interstitial cells of Cajal. These cells serve as pacemakers which create slow wave action potentials that lead to contraction in smooth muscle.

Examination

Initial clinical examination should start with a general assessment of the patient for evidence of weight loss or cachexia along with performance status and fitness.

Extremity/Truncal Sarcoma (Fig. 33.10)

The lesion should be palpated specifically to determine if it is superficial or deep. Ways to describe a lump are listed in Box 33.1. Guidelines for urgent referral for ultrasound assessment in the UK are any patient presenting with a lump with any of the following criteria:

- lesion >5 cm
- rapid growth
- deep to fascia
- fixed or immobile
- painful
- recurrence after excision

It must be remembered, however, that most soft tissue lesions, whether benign or malignant, generally present as painless masses. Sarcomas may cause pain when compressing or involving local nerves. *Tinel's tap test* is often positive over nerve sheath tumours such as Schwannomas, causing an electric shock-type pain in the distribution of the affected nerve, which can be exacerbated by biopsy. Around 30% of sarcomas present as small superficial lesions. Some specific characteristics may help narrow down the differential diagnosis. Vascular malformations may be compressible or have associated thrills or bruits. Ganglion cysts may transilluminate with a pen torch. Regional lymph node beds should be checked, but malignant spread in this way is uncommon in most soft tissue sarcoma subtypes. Large pelvic or proximal limb masses may cause peripheral oedema by compressing lymphovascular structures.

Retroperitoneal/Visceral Sarcomas (Figs. 33.11, 33.12)

A careful abdominal examination, including PR examination if appropriate, should be performed. Retroperitoneal sarcomas (RPS) are often large and easily palpable by the time they are clinically detected (Fig. 33.13). Positive findings include palpable mass, abdominal distension and tenderness.

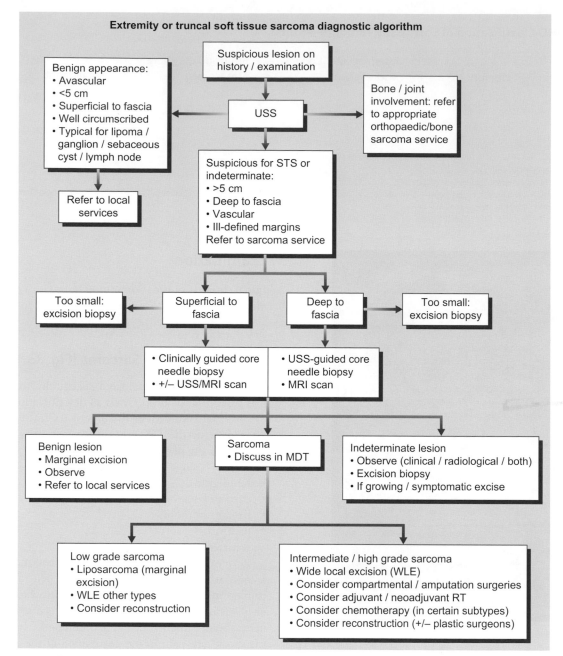

Extremity or truncal soft tissue sarcoma diagnostic algorithm

Suspicious lesion on history / examination

Benign appearance:
• Avascular
• <5 cm
• Superficial to fascia
• Well circumscribed
• Typical for lipoma / ganglion / sebaceous cyst / lymph node

USS

Bone / joint involvement: refer to appropriate orthopaedic/bone sarcoma service

Refer to local services

Suspicious for STS or indeterminate:
• >5 cm
• Deep to fascia
• Vascular
• Ill-defined margins
Refer to sarcoma service

Too small: excision biopsy

Superficial to fascia

Deep to fascia

Too small: excision biopsy

• Clinically guided core needle biopsy
• +/– USS/MRI scan

• USS-guided core needle biopsy
• MRI scan

Benign lesion
• Marginal excision
• Observe
• Refer to local services

Sarcoma
• Discuss in MDT

Indeterminate lesion
• Observe (clinical / radiological / both)
• Excision biopsy
• If growing / symptomatic excise

Low grade sarcoma
• Liposarcoma (marginal excision)
• WLE other types
• Consider reconstruction

Intermediate / high grade sarcoma
• Wide local excision (WLE)
• Consider compartmental / amputation surgeries
• Consider adjuvant / neoadjuvant RT
• Consider chemotherapy (in certain subtypes)
• Consider reconstruction (+/– plastic surgeons)

• **Fig. 33.10** Extremity or Truncal Soft Tissue Sarcoma Diagnostic Algorithm *MDT,* Multidisciplinary team; *RT,* radiotherapy; *STS,* soft tissue sarcoma; *USS,* ultrasound scan.

• **BOX 33.1** | **Descriptive Characteristics for a Lump**

• Tenderness
• Site
• Size
• Surface
• Shape
• Edge
• Consistency
• Fluid thrill
• Pulsatility
• Mobility and movement with inspiration
• Whether you can get above the mass

The consistency of the mass, firm or soft, can be noted and the degree of fixation to surrounding tissues can be assessed. Very immobile masses may suggest a more difficult operation. Raised intra-abdominal pressure may lead to hydroceles, varicoceles or hernias or compression of the stomach or duodenum leading to early satiety. If the diagnosis is in question, all regional lymph nodes should be assessed as lymphoma can also present with large retroperitoneal and visceral masses. Endocrine tumours and germ cell tumours may also present with large retroperitoneal masses, and before a biopsy is considered, work-up should be performed to rule them out. Particular care should be taken to rule out a functioning endocrine tumour prior to any biopsy, to avoid precipitating.

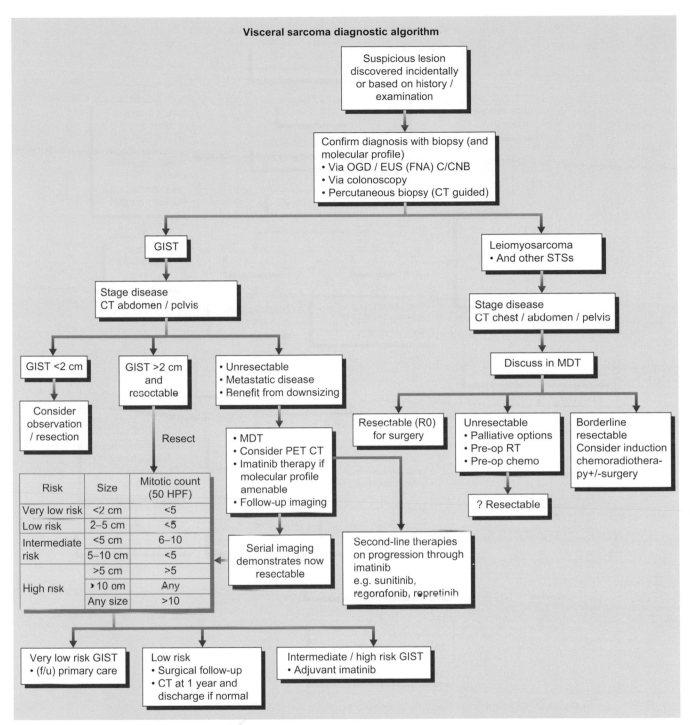

Visceral sarcoma diagnostic algorithm

Suspicious lesion discovered incidentally or based on history / examination

Confirm diagnosis with biopsy (and molecular profile)
• Via OGD / EUS (FNA) C/CNB
• Via colonoscopy
• Percutaneous biopsy (CT guided)

GIST

Leiomyosarcoma
• And other STSs

Stage disease CT abdomen / pelvis

Stage disease CT chest / abdomen / pelvis

GIST <2 cm

GIST >2 cm and resectable

• Unresectable
• Metastatic disease
• Benefit from downsizing

Discuss in MDT

Consider observation / resection

Resect

• MDT
• Consider PET CT
• Imatinib therapy if molecular profile amenable
• Follow-up imaging

Resectable (R0) for surgery

Unresectable
• Palliative options
• Pre-op RT
• Pre-op chemo

Borderline resectable
Consider induction chemoradiotherapy+/-surgery

? Resectable

Risk	Size	Mitotic count (50 HPF)
Very low risk	<2 cm	<5
Low risk	2–5 cm	<5
Intermediate risk	<5 cm	6–10
	5–10 cm	<5
High risk	>5 cm	>5
	>10 cm	Any
	Any size	>10

Serial imaging demonstrates now resectable

Second-line therapies on progression through imatinib e.g. sunitinib, regorafenib, repretinib

Very low risk GIST
• (f/u) primary care

Low risk
• Surgical follow-up
• CT at 1 year and discharge if normal

Intermediate / high risk GIST
• Adjuvant imatinib

• **Fig. 33.11** Visceral Sarcoma Diagnostic Algorithm *EUS,* Endoscopic ultrasound; *FNA,* fine-needle aspiration; *GIST,* gastrointestinal stromal tumour; *HPF,* high-power field; *MDT,* multidisciplinary team; *OGD,* upper endoscopy; *RT,* radiotherapy; *CNB,* core needle biopsy.

Performance Status/Co-Morbidities

Performance status is a way of determining if someone is in reasonable health and may help guide whether a patient is likely to be able to benefit or even tolerate treatments such as surgery or chemotherapy. This is determined by a person's ability to perform normal activities of daily living (ADLs). The WHO performance score is measured from 0 to 5, with zero being fully active, one unable to do strenuous activity, two able to self-care but unable to work, three confined to bed, four completely disabled and five dead. People with low performance status are more likely to experience adverse effects of treatment and poorer overall survival. Co-morbidity describes the effect of all other diseases on a patient other than the primary disease being treated. Several scoring systems are used to predict future mortality. The Charlson co-morbidity index predicts 10-year mortality for patients with a range of conditions including diabetes, heart disease, cancer and liver disease. Combining both performance and co-morbidity status helps to select appropriate treatment for patients. Assessment by specialists in Elderly Medicine may also be helpful.

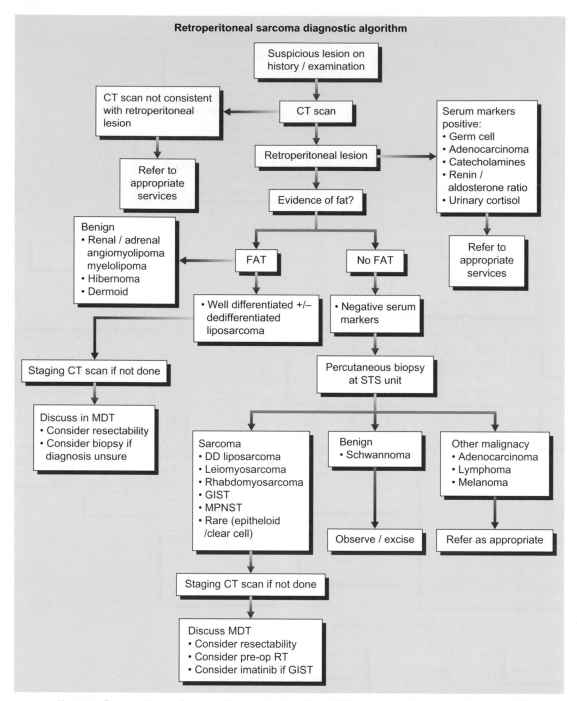

Retroperitoneal sarcoma diagnostic algorithm

Suspicious lesion on history / examination

CT scan

CT scan not consistent with retroperitoneal lesion

Refer to appropriate services

Retroperitoneal lesion

Serum markers positive:
• Germ cell
• Adenocarcinoma
• Catecholamines
• Renin / aldosterone ratio
• Urinary cortisol

Refer to appropriate services

Evidence of fat?

FAT

No FAT

Benign
• Renal / adrenal angiomyolipoma myelolipoma
• Hibernoma
• Dermoid

• Well differentiated +/− dedifferentiated liposarcoma

• Negative serum markers

Percutaneous biopsy at STS unit

Staging CT scan if not done

Discuss in MDT
• Consider resectability
• Consider biopsy if diagnosis unsure

Sarcoma
• DD liposarcoma
• Leiomyosarcoma
• Rhabdomyosarcoma
• GIST
• MPNST
• Rare (epitheloid /clear cell)

Benign
• Schwannoma

Other malignacy
• Adenocarcinoma
• Lymphoma
• Melanoma

Observe / excise

Refer as appropriate

Staging CT scan if not done

Discuss MDT
• Consider resectability
• Consider pre-op RT
• Consider imatinib if GIST

• **Fig. 33.12** Retroperitoneal Sarcoma Diagnostic Algorithm *GIST,* Gastrointestinal stromal tumour; *MDT,* multidisciplinary team; *MPNST,* malignant peripheral nerve sheath tumour; *RT,* radiotherapy; *STS,* soft tissue sarcoma.

Age

As previously mentioned in Table 33.1 sarcomas affect all age groups, but specific types vary with age.

Distribution

Sarcomas can affect any region of the body; however, the abdomen and thigh are the most common sites, with lower extremity lesions being twice as common as upper extremity lesions. Table 33.3 shows the distribution of sarcomas compared to anatomical sites.

Sarcomas vary by location, the most common lesions in descending order are:
• Lower extremity: liposarcoma / undifferentiated pleomorphic sarcoma (UPS)/fibrosarcoma/myxofibrosarcoma/ leiomyosarcoma
• Upper extremity: UPS/liposarcoma/myxofibrosarcoma/ fibrosarcoma/leiomyosarcoma
• Retroperitoneal: liposarcoma / leiomyosarcoma / UPS / GIST / MPNST
• Visceral: GIST/leiomyosarcoma/liposarcoma/UPS
• Trunk: UPS/liposarcoma/myxofibrosarcoma/MPNST

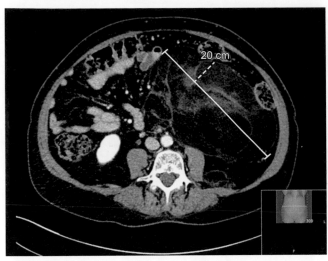

• **Fig. 33.13** Dedifferentiated Liposarcoma of the Retroperitoneum

TABLE 33.3	Distribution of Sarcomas by Anatomical Sites	
Site	**Percentage**	
Head and neck	10%	
Upper limb and girdle	15–20%	
Retroperitoneal/ intraperitoneal	15–20%	
Chest/abdominal wall	10%	
Lower limb and girdle	40%	

• **BOX 33.2** **Sarcomas Which May Potentially Spread Via Lymphatics**

- Synovial sarcoma
- Clear cell sarcoma
- Rhabdomyosarcoma
- Epithelioid sarcoma
- Angiosarcoma
- Undifferentiated pleomorphic sarcoma

Mode of Metastatic Spread

Soft tissue sarcomas which are large, greater than 5 cm, deep to the fascia, high grade (discussed later) and locally recurrent at presentation have a higher risk of metastasis. Most sarcomas preferentially spread via the blood stream (haematogenous route) and therefore commonly spread to the lungs. Rare sites of metastatic disease include skin, soft tissues, bone, liver and brain. Some exceptions include leiomyosarcomas of the retroperitoneum which can metastasize to the liver and round cell/myxoid liposarcomas which can metastasize to the retroperitoneum, abdomen, bone and paraspinal soft tissues. Sarcomas can spread rarely via the lymphatics as well as via the blood stream and these are listed in Box 33.2. Numbers range from less than 5 to 15%. Visceral sarcomas such as

GISTs are often contiguous with the abdominal cavity; therefore metastasis can occur throughout the peritoneal cavity, termed peritoneal sarcomatosis, and the liver.

Radiology

Imaging in soft tissue masses often requires a multimodal approach.

Plain Radiographs

Plain X-rays are easily available and cheap. They may confirm the presence of a mass and identify lesions of bony origin or abnormal calcification of soft tissues such as myositis ossificans or calcified phleboliths (haemangiomas). They are more useful in extremity lesions. Chest X-ray may be used in staging and surveillance.

Ultrasound Scan

An ultrasound scan (USS) is relatively inexpensive and accessible. It is useful as a first-line investigation particularly for superficial lesions. It can confirm the size of the lesion, whether it is superficial or deep to the fascia, whether it is a solid mass or cystic and if it has vascularity (Fig. 33.14). This is useful in determining the differential for the mass and determining whether further investigation is required. USS can assist in obtaining a biopsy particularly if lesions are near important structures, e.g. blood vessels. The main disadvantages are that USS requires a skilled operator and there can be intra-observer variability.

Magnetic Resonance Imaging

MRI is the modality of choice for diagnosis and local staging of soft tissue masses in the extremities, head, neck and trunk (Fig. 33.15). Recently, whole body MRI has been useful for the staging and surveillance of paediatric patients due to the reduction in radiation exposure it provides compared to staging CT scans. MRI is useful in assessing the full extent and relationship of masses to nerves and blood vessels and can delineate between muscle, fat and bone. It is less useful than CT at identifying soft tissue calcification. MRI often cannot provide specific diagnosis but can narrow down the differential and favour a benign or malignant entity. It can, however, be diagnostic in the case of lipomas, ganglion, cysts, peripheral nerve sheath tumours and haemangiomas. Soft tissue sarcomas tend to appear encapsulated and respect anatomical planes. They often have a heterogenous appearance.

Computer Tomography

CT has a primary role in the evaluation of visceral and retroperitoneal suspected STS (Fig. 33.16). It can also be used for patients who have a contraindication to an MRI scan. CT is as effective as MRI at determining tumour involvement of muscle, bone and neurovascular structures. It can

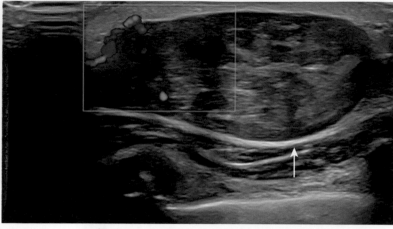

• **Fig. 33.14** Heterogenous Solid Lesion with Associated Vascularity (Solitary Fibrous Tumour) on USS

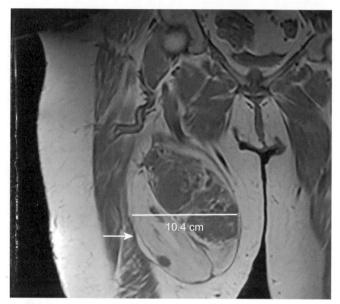

10.4 cm

• **Fig. 33.15** MRI Showing Large Atypical Lipomatous Tumour of Sartorius

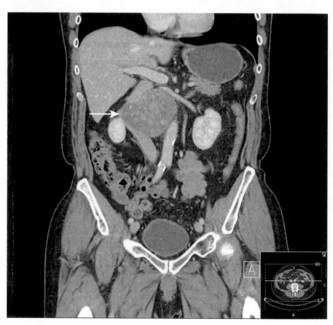

• **Fig. 33.16** CT Showing Leiomyosarcoma of the Inferior Vena Cava

be used to stage high-risk patients and the response to treatment. CT chest can be used to stage patients with high-risk lesions (intermediate or high grade, deep and >5 cm). The National Comprehensive Cancer Network (NCCN) guidelines suggest chest X-ray (CXR) or CT for extremity or trunk STS. CXR is inexpensive and limits the radiation dose to patients in screening for lung metastases.

CT may be overly sensitive and identify lesions which are benign or require unnecessary biopsy or lung resection at worst. The requirement for CT chest can be decided based on high-risk lesions, i.e. greater than 5 cm, deep to fascia and high grade. The rate of pulmonary metastasis in low-grade lesions is reported as between 6 and 9%. CT chest is recommended for visceral/retroperitoneal as there may be local extension, diaphragmatic involvement, and to complete staging as lung is a common site of metastaic disease on RPS. Abdominal and pelvic CT are recommended in round cell/myxoid liposarcomas as well as epithelioid sarcomas/angiosarcoma and leiomyosarcomas.

Response to systemic therapy can be monitored using the response evaluation criteria for solid tumours (RECIST). This uses a decrease of at least 30% in the sum of measured longest diameters of target lesions to define a partial response to treatment or an increase of 20% as disease progression. The modified Choi et al. criteria[6] was invented to monitor a response to imatinib therapy for GISTs. They used a decrease in attenuation of target lesions after contrast enhancement of 15% or more as well as a change in size to define partial response.

Positron Emission Tomography

Positron emission tomography (PET)-CT using fluorode-oxyglucose (FDG) may delineate between benign soft tissue tumours and sarcomas, particularly high-grade sarcomas; however, it is less reliable with low- or intermediate-grade sarcomas and is therefore not recommended in the initial work up of STS. PET-CT is a useful investigation tool in the management of GIST as they are usually strongly FDG avid. It can help stage the patient and monitor response to treatment with imatinib.

Biopsy

Histologic examination is essential for diagnosis and treatment planning and should be assessed by a specialist pathologist. When the histologic diagnosis of sarcoma is uncertain, expert review of the biopsy can help determine if a mass is traumatic, inflammatory, carcinomatous or lymphomatous. There are several methods of biopsy available.

Fine Needle Aspiration Cytology

Fine needle aspiration cytology (FNAC) involves a small needle being passed multiple times through the abnormality. The sample is then fixed and stained to a slide. It is accurate at determining if a lesion is malignant; however, due to the limited sample size, it is difficult to assess tissue architecture and it is often insufficient for immunohistochemistry. FNAC can be useful in GIST and leiomyosarcoma, particularly in visceral sarcomas which are often diagnosed via the endoscopic route but not for other STS subtypes.

Core Needle Biopsy

Core needle biopsy (CNB) is the preferred method for biopsy and it can be performed in an outpatient setting for superficial lesions or with USS or CT guidance for deeper lesions. Generally uses a 16-G core needle to take a 1.5-cm sample of tissue and is performed under local anaesthesia. Unlike FNA, a large enough sample is taken to allow ancillary diagnostic tests. The risk of seeding is negligible in percutaneous biopsy. One study showed the rate was 0.8% with CNB versus 32% in open biopsy.[7] CT and USS scans can be used to help obtain CNB in deeper or anatomically sensitive areas. A CNB should be ideally performed by locating the incision site in a site that may be incorporated into any planned incision for sarcoma.

Open Biopsy

Open biopsy is incisional, where a portion of the lesion is removed and sent for histology, or excisional, where the whole lesion is removed. Incisional biopsies are generally discouraged. Open biopsies should be a last resort, performed by a specialist surgeon who would review the case and, if required, would perform the procedure in a fashion to minimize disease spread. Incisional biopsy has been replaced by CNB and as such should be discouraged. Excisional biopsy implies a planned marginal resection of the lesion with the assumption that it is benign. Incisional biopsies should be planned so the entire tract can be removed en-bloc at the time of the definitive surgery. All tissue exposed during the incisional biopsy must be excised in the definitive procedure, including nerves and blood vessels if exposed. A poorly planned incision can compromise later surgery. Incisional biopsy results in approximately threefold higher risk of recurrence and more extensive surgery.

Pathology

Firstly, the gross (macroscopic) appearance of the specimen is examined along with the clinicoradiological appearance. The specimen is then examined under a microscope to assess its microscopic appearance. The aim of pathological investigation is to determine the cell lineage, the degree of differentiation and, if a sarcoma is suspected, the grade of the tumour and the margin of clearance. Differentiation measures the amount a tumour resembles the original cell linage. In some cases of STT, the histological line of the tumour may be obvious such as smooth muscle, skeletal muscle, vascular and neural. Sometimes, however, the line of differentiation of a tumour may be less obvious and the histomorphological pattern is used to aid diagnosis. These include adipocytic (fat cell), spindle cell (narrow elongated cells), myxoid (clear mucoid substance), round cell (small round undifferentiated cells), epithelioid (morphologically resembles epithelial cells) and pleomorphic (suggests variation in shape and size of cells; see Fig. 33.8). Because the differential diagnosis for these histological patterns is still long, further tests can narrow the choice. This is where ancillary tests such as immunohistochemistry (IHC) and cytogenetics play an important role.

Immunohistochemistry

IHC is the process where antibodies bind to specific antigens in cells. This is designed to cause a colour reaction which can be visualized under microscopy. Table 33.4 demonstrates some selected common cell-type markers commonly used in IHC. Cytokeratins are found in epithelial cells, neurofilaments in neural cells, desmin in muscle cells and vimentin in mesenchymal cells. Neoplasms arising from these cell types still express characteristics from their cell of origin. Carcinomas express cytokeratin, sarcomas often express vimentin, neural tumours express neurofilaments and myogenic tumours express desmin. Unfortunately, many of these markers are not class specific. Cytogenetics involves studying chromosomes by testing samples of tissue specifically looking for broken, missing or extra chromosomes. These markers are often more specific to certain neoplasms and can narrow down the differential diagnosis further. Examples of these are listed in Table 33.5.

The diagnosis of STT is complex as it represents a heterogenous group of neoplasms with overlapping features. A combination of clinicoradiological information, histomorphological pattern, IHC and molecular techniques are often all required to make the final pathological diagnosis.

Grading

The grade of a tumour describes how normal or abnormal a tumour's cells appear. Histologic grade aids the clinician by giving the team an idea of how quickly the cancer is growing and how likely it is to spread. This is key to staging many sarcomas and in planning treatment. Assessing grade

TABLE 33.4 Common Cell-Typic Markers in Immunohistochemistry

	Keratin	Desmin	SMA	CD31	CD34	FLI-1	S-100	HMB-45	Other Diagnostic Markers
Epithelioid sarcoma	+	–	–	–	+	–	–	–	INI1-
Epithelioid hemangioendothelioma	±	–	–	+	+	+	–	–	ERG
Epithelioid sarcoma-like hemangioendothelioma	+	–	–	+	+	+	–	–	ERG
Epithelioid angiosarcoma	±	–	–	+	+	+	–	–	ERG
Benign epithelioid peripheral nerve sheath tumour	±	–	–	–	–	–	+	–	SOX10
Epithelioid malignant peripheral nerve sheath tumour	–	–	–	–	–	–	+	–	INI1- (epithelioid)
Epithelioid leiomyosarcoma	±	+	+	–	–	–	–	–	h-caldesmon
Sclerosing epithelioid fibrosarcoma	±	–	–	–	–	–	±	–	
Extrarenal rhabdoid tumour	+	–	–	–	–	–	–	–	INI1-
Myoepithelioma/ parachordoma	+	–	±	–	–	–	+	–	
Alveolar soft part sarcoma	–	±	±	–	–	–	±	+	TFE3
Clear cell sarcoma	–	–	–	–	–	–	+	+	
Carcinoma	+	–	–	–	–	–	–	–	
Melanoma	–	–	–	–	–	–	+	+	

TABLE 33.5 Genetic and IHC Markers Associated with Some STT

Neoplasm	Positive Markers	Newer Genetic Markers
Atypical lipomatous tumour	S100	MDM2 / CDK4
Spindle cell lipoma	CD34	–
Dedifferentiated liposarcoma	–	MDM2 / CDK4
Nodular fasciitis	α-SMA/Vimentin/Calponin/CD10/DGP9.5	MYH9-USP6
DFSP	CD34	COLIA1-PDGFB
DFSP with fibrosarcomatous transformation	CD34 negative	COLIA1-PDGFB
Solitary fibrous tumour	CD34/EMA/SMA/CD99	STAT6
Malignant peripheral nerve sheath tumour	S100/SOX-10	p75NTR
Synovial sarcoma	EMA/CD99/Bcl-2/CD34 negative	TLE1, SS18
Clear cell sarcoma	SOX-10	EWSR1-ATF1
Myxofibrosarcoma	–	–

DFSP, Dermatofibrosarcoma protuberans; *IHC*, immunohistochemistry; *STT,* soft tissue tumour.

involves studying the specimen under a microscope. The most common grading system used in STT is known as the French Federation of Comprehensive Cancer Centres (FNCLCC) system and incorporates the degree of differentiation, mitotic rate and extent of necrosis (Box 33.3). Differentiation is how closely cancer cells resemble normal cell structure and function, the mitotic rate suggests how quickly the cancer is dividing and necrosis is the amount of dead tissue in the sample. More aggressive tumours, which are faster growing, outgrowing their blood supply (causing necrosis) and have limited differentiation, are termed high grade. Those which are slower growing and resemble normal tissue cells more closely are low grade.

Staging

Ideally a surgical staging system should incorporate the most significant prognostic factors, divide these risks into progressive stages with specific implications for surgery and provide guidelines for the use of adjuvant treatments. This has proved difficult in sarcoma surgery and therefore multiple systems exist. The most common staging system used is the American Joint Committee on Cancer (AJCC) staging system, which uses tumour size (T), evidence of nodal metastasis (N) and distant metastasis (M) and grade (G) (Box 33.4). The staging system varies for extremity/trunk, retroperitoneal and visceral sarcomas.

These systems are, however, flawed as they fail to incorporate many important factors into the staging system, such as histological subtype. This was particularly evident for RPS as most are large at presentation (>10 cm). Nodal metastases are rare and therefore metastatic spread and grade are the only useful predictive factors. This led to the development of a validated nomogram by Gronchi et al.[8] which included age, tumour grade, size, histological subtype, multifocality and extent of surgical resection. This nomogram predicted disease-free survival and seven-year overall survival in primary RPS.

Treatment

Soft tissue masses are common; however, due to the rarity of STS, ideally treatment should be carried out in a centre which specializes in the treatment of sarcomas. The treatment is multimodal and requires specialists in surgical oncology, plastic surgery, medical and radiation oncology. The treatment aims in limb sarcoma surgery are to remove the tumour with adequate surgical margins and at the same time preserve limb function.

In retroperitoneal sarcoma, the aim is to achieve a resection with microscopically negative margins (R0) or microscopically positive margins (R1) en-bloc, meaning removing all involved organs within the limits of anatomical constraints. Complete resection provides the only chance of cure. Local recurrence is the major oncological concern for RPS as local recurrence and not distant metastasis is the leading causes of death. In other forms of sarcoma, metastasis is the leading cause of death.

• BOX 33.3   FNCLCC Grading System

Tumour differentiation

Score 1	Sarcomas closely resembling normal adult mesenchymal tissue (e.g. well differentiated liposarcoma and leiomyosarcoma)
Score 2	Sarcomas for which histological typing is certain (e.g. myxoid liposarcoma & conventional leiomyosarcoma)
Score 3	Embryonal and undifferential sarcomas, pleomorphic sarcomas, synovial sarcomas, osteosarcomas, PNET)

Mitotic count

Score 1	0–9 mitoses per 10 HFP
Score 2	10–19 mitoses per 10 HFP
Score 3	≤20 mitoses per 10 HFP

Tumour necrosis: determined on histologic sections

Score 0:	No tumour necrosis
Score 1:	Less than or equal to 50% tumour necrosis
Score 2:	More than 50% tumour necrosis

Histological grade

Grade 1	Total score 2,3
Grade 2	Total score 4,5
Grade 3	Total score 6,7,8

FNCLCC, French Federation of Comprehensive Cancer Centres; *HPF*, high power field; *PNET*, primitive neuroectodermal tumour.

Surgery

In sarcoma surgery, appropriate diagnostic work-up of patients enables the correct surgery to be employed. Inadvertent excision due to inadequate work up or unexpected sarcoma is still a frequent problem in sarcoma surgery. This leads to increased local recurrence, further surgery and worse overall survival for patients. Most soft tissue sarcomas have a pushing border which forms a pseudocapsule at the periphery. This capsule is the reactive zone between normal tissue and the tumour. Microsatellites of tumour may be present in the pseudocapsule. Resections performed along this plane have high rates of local recurrence. Obtaining an accurate diagnosis and understanding the differing pathological courses of STT allows various surgical approaches including those discussed in the following sections.

Marginal Resection

The tumour is removed with a very narrow cuff of normal tissue. This is generally reserved for benign lesions, lesions with a low risk of local recurrence or where a wider margin is not possible or would cause unacceptable morbidity. This is the preferred method of treatment for atypical lipomatous tumours.

T category	T criteria	Staging	
TX	Cannot be assessed	Stage IA	T1; N0; M0; G1,GX
T0	No evidence of tumour	Stage IB	T2-4; N0; M0; G1,GX
T1	<5 cm	Stage II	T1; N0; M0; G2–3
T2	5–10 cm	Stage IIIA	T2; N0; M0; G2–3
T3	10–15 cm	Stage IIIB	T3–4; N0; M0; G2–3
T4	>15 cm	Stage IV	T1–4; N1[a]; M0; G any or T1–4; N0; M1; G any
N category	N criteria		
N0	No lymph nodes		
N1	Regional lymph nodes		
M category	M criteria		
M0	No distant metastasis		
M1	Distant metastasis		
Grade	G criteria		
GX	Cannot be assessed		
G1	Low grade		
G2	High grade		
G3	High grade		

[a]American Joint Committee on Cancer (AJCC) staging: N1 classifies a stage IV grading using the French Federation of Comprehensive Cancer Centres (FNLCC) grading system.
With permission from Wittekind CW, Brierley JD, Gospodarowicz MK. TNM Classification of Malignant Tumours, 8th ed. Wiley Books, Chichester, UK, pp. 125–126.

Wide Local Resection

The tumour is removed en-bloc with a margin of normal tissue. In the limb or trunk, this usually includes skin, fascia, muscle and fat. If adjacent to bone, the periosteum can be removed as long as the bone deep to this is free of tumour. Advised margins vary; however, most surgeons would accept a 1-cm margin or a natural tissue barrier such as fascia or peritoneum. If nerves or blood vessels are directly involved, they can be sacrificed or reconstructed if required, or, if preoperative radiotherapy is given, a planned positive microscopic margin may be accepted at these critical sites. Wide local resection is the initial treatment choice for multiple sarcomas including dermatofibrosarcoma protuberans. With large wounds it may be necessary to reconstruct the defect with the assistance of plastic surgeons to perform local or free flap coverage of the defect. This is even more important if postoperative radiotherapy is to be considered as wounds closed under tension or with skin grafts will often breakdown in this setting.

Compartmental Resection

For higher risk or locally advanced lesions, the tumour is removed along with all the muscles, nerves and blood supply of the compartment containing the tumour, which greatly reduces the risk of local recurrence and is potentially curative. The aim of this surgery is to remove the tumour, but preserve a functional limb. The need for compartment resection has become less with the advent of radiotherapy.

Amputation

Once the primary therapy for extremity sarcoma, amputation is now rarely used. Amputation does not lower the risk of metastatic spread compared to limb-sparing surgery.[9] If a functional limb cannot be preserved, better functional outcomes may be obtained with modern prostheses. Amputations chosen judiciously can provide excellent disease control and survival. Indications can include salvage surgery after initial limb-sparing surgery (delayed amputation), multiple compartment involvement, neurovascular compromise, joint involvement, multifocal tumours and large tumour size. Amputation is still used in approximately 6% of high-grade extremity sarcomas.

Isolated Limb Perfusion

This type of surgery is reserved for locally advanced sarcomas which are irresectable or would require amputation to treat. It involves heating the limb (hyperthermia) and perfusing the limb with chemotherapy agents, often melphalan and tumour necrosis factor alpha (TNF-α). This treatment may act as a palliative measure or sometimes downsizes the tumour, thereby allowing less aggressive surgery. Suggested management strategies for extremity STS are shown in Table 33.6.

Retroperitoneal Sarcomas

Local recurrence is high in RPS, between 30 and 50% in some studies.[10] The aim of treatment is to achieve macroscopically negative margins if possible (R0 resection) and to minimize microscopically positive margins (R1 resection); however, this is difficult to achieve due to anatomical restraints. En-bloc resection (removing surrounding organs) has been shown to reduce local recurrence rates and therefore improve overall survival. This can often mean performing an additional colectomy, nephrectomy, splenectomy, pancreatectomy or diaphragmatic resection and sometimes hepatectomy with appropriate reconstructions (Fig. 33.17). Surgical inoperability is often determined by vascular involvement such as the superior mesenteric artery or post-hepatic IVC. The four main types of retroperitoneal sarcoma are: liposarcoma (well and dedifferentiated), leiomyosarcoma and solitary fibrous tumour. Histological type should play a role in surgical decision making.

TABLE 33.6   Management Strategies for Extremity STS

Extremity/Superficial Trunk Sarcoma	Recommended	Optional
G1, superficial	Wide excision	
G1, deep, <5 cm	Wide excision	
G1, deep, >5 cm	Wide excision + adj RT	
G2–3, superficial	Wide excision	Radiotherapy (RT)
G2–3, deep, <5 cm	Wide excision	Wide excision + RT
		Compartmental resection
G2–3, deep, >5 cm	Wide excision + RT	Adjuvant chemotherapy
	Compartmental resection	Isolated limb perfusion
		Amputation
Local recurrence, G1	Wide excision + RT	Wide excision only
Local recurrence, G2–3	Wide excision + adj RT (if possible)	Adjuvant chemotherapy
	Compartmental resection	Isolated limb perfusion
		Amputation

Adapted from European Society for Medical Oncology (ESMO) guidance.

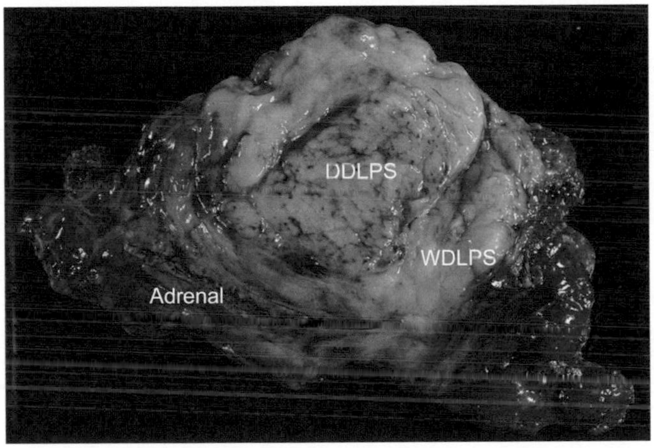

• **Fig. 33.17** Dedifferentiated Retroperitoneal Liposarcoma with Central High-Grade Tumour Adrenal gland incorporated in bottom right of picture. *DDLPS,* Dedifferentiated liposarcoma; *WDLPS,* well differentiated liposarcoma. (Courtesy Silvia Bagué, MD.)

Visceral Sarcomas

The most common visceral sarcomas are GISTs and leiomyosarcomas. GISTs can occur anywhere along the gastrointestinal tract, most commonly the stomach (55%), small bowel (30%), duodenum (5%) and colon or rectum (5%). Many of the principles which apply to RPS apply to visceral sarcomas. Understanding how sarcomas metastasize plays a key role in the differences between surgical treatments of visceral sarcoma and adenocarcinomas. Adenocarcinoma tends to spread via the lymph nodes and therefore wide resection of these lymphatic structures are required for staging and cure. On the other hand, sarcomas rarely spread in this manner and if lymph node metastases are present, resection rarely results in long-term survival. Lymph node metastasis implies an aggressive disease process. Therefore, the aims of treatment are to achieve negative surgical margins and avoid peritoneal seeding, caused by rupturing the tumour resulting in peritoneal sarcomatosis. Laparoscopic resection may be performed for tumours less than 5 cm or as long as the principles of complete excision without tumour rupture.

Radiotherapy

Modern radiotherapy (RT) has allowed limb preserving surgical approaches to become the primary mode of surgery in sarcoma patients. Wide local excision with RT is the treatment of choice in many cases where radical compartment resections or amputations would have been necessary to obtain local control in the past. Wide local resections with RT have similar local control and overall survival outcomes compared to compartmental resections and amputations. Preoperative and postoperative RT are equally effective in control and survival in STS (Fig. 33.18) therefore, preoperative radiotherapy is often the preferred approach, as it reduces the overall dose of radiotherapy, reduces the size of the radiotherapy field, may allow for a planned positive margin on critical structures, and may afford better functional outcomes in the longterm. The caveat, is that there is a higher rate of perioperative infection in comparison with postoperative radiotherapy. It is considered standard treatment for all intermediate or high-grade STS of the extremities. Some larger deeper low-grade tumours are also considered for RT on a case-by-case basis. Radiotherapy has not been definitively proven to affect disease-free survival with RPS or uterine leiomyosarcomas. GIST is a radiosensitive tumour and RT can be used in certain cases; however,

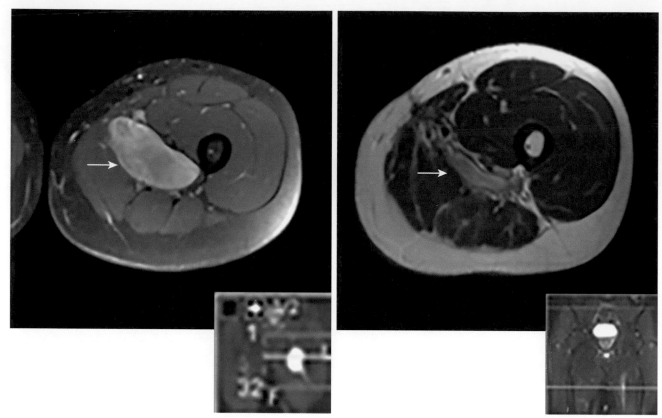

• **Fig. 33.18** Pre- and Postradiotherapy Response for Myxoid Liposarcoma of the Lower Limb

due to bowel sensitivity to radiation and other adjuvant treatments such as imatinib, it is rarely used. For some tumours that are particularly radiosensitive, i.e. myxoid liposarcoma, a small preoperative RT dose may be given to downsize the tumour and postoperatively if margins are positive.

Adjuvant Radiotherapy

Adjuvant radiotherapy is radiotherapy given after surgical resection. RT should be considered for marginal and R1 resections where further resection is inappropriate. In the retroperitoneum, tumours are often too large and surrounding structures are too near to allow routine recommendation of RT and can result in worse outcomes. Advantages of postoperative RT include fewer wound complications compared to neo-adjuvant treatment (17%) and tumour pathology is easily available. Disadvantages include higher radiation doses with larger fields as the whole operative wound and drain site needs to be covered in the radiation field and a greater risk of long-term fibrosis and oedema, with worse functionality. There is often greater delay in receiving RT due to wound complications pre-treatment.

Neo-Adjuvant Radiotherapy

Neo-adjuvant radiotherapy is given before surgery. The advantages of preoperative RT include a short interval between RT and surgery, ease of targeting the lesion and a smaller field and lower overall dose compared to postoperative radiotherapy. Preoperative radiotherapy may downsize the tumour in specific subtypes such as myxoid liposarcoma, allowing smaller surgical resections as well as inactivating the tumour reducing the

risk of intra-operative spillage of tumour. The disadvantages include a greater wound morbidity which can be as high as 40% in some studies with 20% of patient needing further surgery. Pathological evaluation of the tumour may also be more difficult due to cell death. Preoperative RT in RPS is generally well tolerated and may reduce local recurrence in some cases (e.g. liposarcoma) but overall survival is unchanged. The recently published STRASS trial[11] looking at preoperative RT and surgery versus surgery for RPS concluded preoperative RT should not be considered the standard of care in RPS as it did not improve overall survival over surgery alone.

Chemotherapy

Tumour biology and therefore the effectiveness of chemotherapy varies greatly with histological subtype (Table 33.7). The role of chemotherapy has been unequivocally accepted into the treatment of certain types of sarcomata, such as Ewing's sarcoma.

Due to the relatively poor outcomes of patients with high-grade extremity sarcomas larger than 5 cm (50% mortality at 5 years), multiple studies have examined the role of adjuvant and neo-adjuvant chemotherapy in this group with mixed results. Research has been hampered by small cohorts of patients, due to the rarity of disease, with mixed histological subtypes and differing treatment regimes, making meta-analysis less precise. The results were mixed but an updated meta-analysis showed a 6% increase in overall survival at 5 years, which was significant.[12] Doxorubicin combined with ifosfamide is the favoured regime in adjuvant

TABLE 33.7	Relative Chemosensitivity			
	Chemosensitive	Moderately Chemosensitivity	Low Chemosensitivity	Chemoresistant
	Ewing's sarcoma	Pleomorphic sarcoma	Malignant peripheral nerve sheath tumour	Alveolar soft part sarcoma
	Embryonal / alveolar rhabdomyosarcoma	Angiosarcoma	Myxofibrosarcoma	Extraskeletal myxoid chondrosarcoma
	Synovial sarcoma	Pleomorphic rhabdomyosarcoma	Dedifferentiated liposarcoma	Clear cell sarcoma
	Desmoplastic small round cell tumour	Epithelioid sarcoma	Adult fibrosarcoma	Gastrointestinal stromal tumour
	Myxoid liposarcoma	Leiomyosarcoma	Haemangiopericytoma	
			Endometrial stromal sarcoma	

treatment for STS. The role of adjuvant and neo-adjuvant chemotherapy is unclear, with arguably no clear benefit in most cases, over local therapy. Overall, the beneficial effects are small and must be weighed against adverse effects such as neutropenia with sepsis, long-term risks of cardiomyopathy and infertility. Evidence suggests that synovial sarcoma and myxoid/round cell liposarcoma (MRCL) are more chemosensitive with prolonged overall survival from 12 to 18 months in MRCL patients and 12 to 15 months in synovial sarcoma patients with metastatic disease.

For RPS there is no evidence that adjuvant chemotherapy improves survival. Neo-adjuvant chemotherapy may be beneficial to downsize the tumours, particularly for more chemosensitive subtypes. The STRASS II trial is examining the utility of this approach in high grade RPS.

The primary treatment for GIST, the most common mesenchymal visceral sarcoma, is resection. However, even after curative resections, 40% of patients go on to develop disseminated disease and require effective systemic treatments. The pathogenesis of GIST is associated with the activation of oncoproteins KIT and PDGFRA (platelet-derived growth factor receptor-α). Conventional chemotherapy is ineffective in GIST; however, imatinib, a tyrosine kinase inhibitor of KIT, is highly effective (Fig. 33.19). This targeted oncological therapy has proven to be very effective and has vastly improved overall survival to 91% at 5 years with recurrence-free survival of 71% when given in the adjuvant setting. Imatinib treatment has been used both for neo-adjuvant treatment for cytoreduction prior to surgery to reduce the need for multivisceral resections and ongoing adjuvant treatment for lesions at greater risk of recurrence, i.e. large tumours (>5 cm), R1 resections or tumour rupture, small or large bowel lesions and a mitotic index of greater than 5/50 high powered fields.

Treatment of Systemic Disease

The treatment intent for systemic disease is palliative. The median survival after diagnosis is 12 months. Palliative treatment options are complex with many clinical trials currently underway.

Palliative Systemic Anti-Cancer Therapy

Published response rates to chemotherapy vary enormously; however, good functional status, young age and absence of liver metastases predict a good response. The first-line therapy in Europe is doxorubicin given 3-weekly for six cycles, maximum, due to the risk of cardiotoxicity. Second-line treatment is ifosfamide when doxorubicin is contraindicated. Angiosarcoma is highly susceptible to taxanes such as paclitaxel and docetaxel and other options include doxorubicin and ifosfamide. Imatinib is the first-line therapy for metastatic GISTs and is a small molecule tyrosine kinase inhibitor. Second-line agents include TKIs sunitimib and regorafenib. Imatinib can be used with dermatofibrosarcoma protuberans if surgery is contraindicated or in the rare event of metastatic disease.

Palliative Radiotherapy

Palliative RT is often used for symptomatic control. Bone metastases may cause pain, and visceral or other STS may bleed and benefit from radiotherapy. Late morbidity is less of a concern in this group, therefore high fractions can be given. Unresectable tumours either due to anatomy or the patient's fitness, may be given definitive radiotherapy treatment in order to slow disease progression.

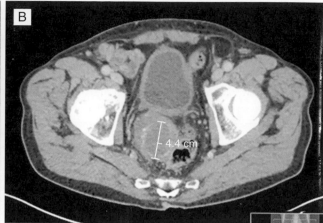

• **Fig. 33.19** Pelvic GIST Response to Imatinib After 10 Months (A) Prior to treatment. (B) 10 months after treatment.

Palliative Abdominal Surgery

For recurrent RPS if isolated and potentially resectable, the aim should be curative surgery. Well differentiated liposarcomas carry a more favourable prognosis. One study found the local recurrence rates were 71% at 5 years for recurrent RPS compared to 36% for primary RPS with similar rates of distant metastases (11% at 5 years).[13] Disease-free survival was 27% at 10 years for primary resections and 4.6% for recurrent resections. Surgery should be decided on a case-by-case basis and depends on the duration to disease recurrence. Patients with well differentiated liposarcoma may have indolent disease and can be watched to determine appropriate timing of surgery. Planned R2 resections with macroscopically positive margins can be considered for symptomatic reasons, but the morbidity of the procedure must be weighed against expected survival.

Surgery for Distant Metastases

This is controversial due to a lack of randomized data to support the practice. Treatment does not aim to be curative but can be performed for symptomatic reasons or in an effort to prolong disease-free survival. Surgery can be considered for lung metastases, but depends on the disease-free period prior to recurrence, the total number of lesions (i.e. oligometastatic disease) and tumour growth. Surgery has been shown to improve overall survival compared to historical controls in very selective patients (30–50% 5-year overall survival but with recurrence rates upto 83%.[14] Recurrence though is still high and decisions should be made on a case-by-case basis. Isolated hepatic metastases may also be amenable to hepatectomy but evidence is limited to small studies. One study with 38 patients found 5-year survival to be 42%.[15]

GIST

GIST outcomes have been greatly improved with the introduction of tyrosine kinase inhibitors. Of patients presenting with advanced disease, 81% benefit from imatinib therapy,

with median survival times of 55 months compared to 18 months prior to this.[16] Irresectable tumours can be down staged with neo-adjuvant treatment to allow definitive surgery and then continued as adjuvant treatment to reduce the risk of recurrence. Systemic disease can also be treated with long-term imatinib.

Prognosis

The overall 5-year survival in England for STS is 53%.[17] Data from the National Cancer Institute (NCI) demonstrates that as a sarcoma spreads, survival time is diminished and once metastasis occurs, the tumour is generally incurable. Five-year survival is 83% for localized disease, 54% for regional disease and 16% for distant disease.[18] Site of a sarcoma can also affect outcomes. Retroperitoneal lesions and intra-abdominal lesions have a higher risk of recurrence compared to extremity lesions, partly due to anatomical constraints when performing primary resections. Retroperitoneal survival was worse compared to extremity sarcoma at 45% 5-year survival; however, with modern surgical techniques, including en-bloc resections of involved organs, survival has increased to 70% at 5 years in some studies for primary RPS.[19]

References

1. Hartley AL, et al. Patterns of cancer in the families of children with soft tissue sarcoma. *Cancer*. 1993;72:923–930.
2. McIntyre JF, et al. Germline mutations of the p53 tumor suppressor gene in children with osteosarcoma. *J Clin Oncol*. 1994;12:925–930.
3. Farid M, Ngeow J. Sarcomas associated with genetic cancer predisposition syndromes: a review. *Oncol*. 2016;21(8):1002–1013.
4. López-Lázaro M. The stem cell division theory of cancer. *Crit Rev Oncol Hematol*. 2018;123:95–113.
5. Knudson A. Alfred knudson and his two-hit hypothesis. (Interview by Ezzie Hutchinson). *Lancet Oncol*. 2001;2(10):642–645.
6. Choi H, et al. CT evaluation of the response of gastrointestinal stromal tumors after imatinib mesylate treatment: a quantitative

analysis correlated with FDG PET findings. *Am J Roentgenol.* 2004;183:1619–1628.

7. Strauss DC, Qureshi YA, Hayes AJ, Thway K, Fisher C, Thomas JM. The role of core needle biopsy in the diagnosis of suspected soft tissue tumours. *J Surg Oncol.* 2010;102(5):523–529.

8. Gronchi A, et al. Outcome prediction in primary resected retroperitoneal soft tissue sarcoma: histology-specific overall survival and disease-free survival nomograms built on major sarcoma center data sets. *J Clin Oncol.* 2013;31:1649–1655.

9. Alamanda VK, Crosby SN, Archer KR, Song Y, Schwartz HS, Holt GE. Amputation for extremity soft tissue sarcoma does not increase overall survival: a retrospective cohort study. *Eur J Surg Oncol.* 2012;38(12):1178–1183.

10. Trans-Atlantic RPS Working Group. Management of recurrent retroperitoneal sarcoma (rps) in the adult: a consensus approach from the Trans-Atlantic RPS Working Group. *Ann Surg Oncol.* 2016;23(11):3531–3540.

11. Bonvalot S, et al. Preoperative radiotherapy plus surgery versus surgery alone for patients with primary retroperitoneal sarcoma (EORTC-62092: strass): a multicentre, open-label, randomised, phase 3 trial. *Lancet Oncol.* 2020;21(10):1366–1377.

12. Sarcoma Meta-analysis Collaboration (SMAC). Adjuvant chemotherapy for localised resectable soft tissue sarcoma in adults. *Cochrane Database Syst Rev.* 2000;(4):CD001419.

13. Neuhaus SJ, Barry P, Clark MA, Hayes AJ, Fisher C, Thomas JM. Surgical management of primary and recurrent retroperitoneal liposarcoma. *Br J Surg.* 2005;92(2):246–252.

14. Digesu CS, Wiesel O, Vaporciyan AA, Colson YL. Management of sarcoma metastases to the lung. *Surg Oncol Clin N Am.* 2016;25(4):721–733.

15. Grimme FAB, et al. On behalf of the Dutch liver surgery working group. Liver resection for hepatic metastases from soft tissue sarcoma: a nationwide study. *Dig Surg.* 2019;36(6):479–486.

16. Kelly CM, Gutierrez Sainz L, Chi P. The management of metastatic GIST: current standard and investigational therapeutics. *J Hematol Oncol.* 2021 5;14(1):2.

17. Cancer Research UK, https://www.cancerresearchuk.org/health-professional/cancer-statistics/statistics-by-cancer-type/soft-tissue-sarcoma/survival.

18. American Cancer Society, https://www.cancer.org/.

19. Ferrario T, Karakousis CP. Retroperitoneal sarcomas: grade and survival, *Arch Surg.* 2003;138(3):248–251.

Further Reading

Almond LM, et al. Neoadjuvant and adjuvant strategies in retroperitoneal sarcoma. *Eur J Surg Oncol.* 2018;44:571–579.

Bashir U, et al. Soft-tissue masses in the abdominal wall. *Clin Radiol.* 2014;69:422–431.

Bleloch JS, et al. Managing sarcoma: where have we come from and where are we going? *Ther Adv Med Oncol.* 2017;9(10):637–659.

Brennan MF, Antonescu CR, Maki RG. *Management of Soft Tissue Sarcoma.* New York: Springer Science + Business Media; 2013.

Bridge JA. The role of cytogenetics and molecular diagnostics in the diagnosis of soft-tissue tumours. *Mod Pathol.* 2014;27:S80–S97.

Casali PG, et al. Soft tissue and visceral sarcomas: ESMO-EURACAN clinical practice guidelines for diagnosis, treatment and follow-up. *Annual Oncol.* 2018;(suppl 0):1–17.

Fairweather M, Gonzalez RJ, Strauss D, Raut CP. Current principles of surgery for retroperitoneal sarcomas. *J Surg Oncol.* 2018;117(1):33–41.

Farid M, Ngeow J. Sarcomas associated with genetic cancer predisposition syndromes: a review. *The Oncologist.* 2016;21:1002–1013.

Fletcher CDM, Bridge JA, Hogendoorn PCW, Mertens F. *WHO Classification of Tumours of Soft Tissue and Bone (World Health Organization Classification of Tumours),* 4th ed. Vol. 5. Lyon, France: IARC Publications; 2013.

Gladdy RA, Gupta A, Catton CN. Retroperitoneal sarcoma fact, opinion, and controversy. *Surg Oncol Clin N Am.* 2016:697–711.

International Agency for Research on Cancer. World Health Organization: WHO Classification of Soft Tissue Tumors.

Jagannathan JP, Tirumani SH, Ramaiya NH. Imaging in soft tissue sarcomas: current updates. *Surg Oncol Clin N Am.* 2016;25:645–675.

Jakob J, et al. Regional chemotherapy by isolated limb perfusion prior to surgery compared with surgery and post-operative radiotherapy for primary, locally advanced extremity sarcoma: a comparison of matched cohorts. *Clin Sarcoma Res.* 2018:8.

Kong SH, Yang HK. Surgical Treatment of gastric gastrointestinal stromal tumour. *J Gastric Cancer.* 2013;13:3–18.

Larrier NA, Czito BG, Kirsch DG. Radiation therapy for soft tissue sarcoma. *Surg Oncol Clin N Am.* 2016;25:841–860.

Pencavel T, et al. Excision and radiotherapy for large extremity sarcomas results in excellent local control and limb salvage rates. *Eur J Cancer Conference.* 2011; Conference Publication 47(suppl 1):S668.

Tan BT, Park CY, Ailles LE, Weissman IL. The cancer stem cell hypothesis: a work in progress. *Lab Invest.* 2006;86:1203–1207.

34

Bariatric and Metabolic Surgery

CHAPTER OUTLINE

Introduction

Obesity is an accumulation of excess body fat; it is a serious but a preventable and reversible chronic condition. Any person with a body mass index (BMI) equal to or more than 30 kg/m^2 is classified as obese and those between 25–29.9 kg/m^2 are considered overweight (Box 34.1). The causation is often multifactorial, with both genetic and environmental factors playing a part. The underlying pathophysiology involves an imbalance between calorie consumption and expenditure, with the excess calories being stored as fat in the human body.

Obesity subsequently increases the risk of developing the obesity-related comorbidities listed in Box 34.2. As a result, if left untreated, life expectancy is significantly shortened.

Epidemiology

On a global scale, this condition has reached an epidemic level and is not just confined to high-income countries. The World Health Organization recognizes that obesity is one of the greatest public health challenges of the 21st century. In 2016, there were 650 million obese adults worldwide, which equates to approximately 13% of the population. This number is expected to continue to rise at an alarming rate to the extent that obesity is now associated with more deaths than underweight across the globe. In the UK, over half the population are considered to be overweight or obese.

Therapeutic Options of Obesity

As with most conditions, therapeutic options can be divided into conservative, medical and surgical.

Weight management in the UK is also divided into tiers.

Tiers 1 and 2 cover health promotional and lifestyle interventions at a primary care level. Tier 3 extends to hospital-based specialist weight management programs. This includes diet, behavioural modifications and exercise. Several pharmacological options are also available, but none have been proven to be highly successful. Furthermore, it is now well-established that even if patients achieve successful weight loss, most often suffer from weight regain several years later.

Tier 4 service is surgery for obesity or its associated co-morbidities; this is known as bariatric or metabolic surgery. Initially intended only for weight loss, we are now seeing significant beneficial effects also to obesity related co-morbidities such as type 2 diabetes and hypertension. What is even more exhilarating is that some of these effects take place before weight loss has occurred and are sometimes weight independent. The precise underlying mechanisms are yet to be fully understood.

Effective weight loss not only improves a patient's medical co-morbidities, reduces cancer risk and improves life expectancy but it is evident than improvements are also seen in overall quality of life and social and psychological well-being.

• BOX 34.1 Classification of Obesity (World Health Organization)

Classification	BMI (Kg/m^2)
Normal	18.5–24.9
Overweight	24.9–29.9
Obese	30.0–34.9
Morbidly Obese	35.0–39.9
Super Morbidly Obese	≥40.0

• BOX 34.2 Obesity Related Co-Morbidities

- 'Metabolic syndrome': type 2 diabetes, hypertension and obesity
- Hypercholesterolemia or dyslipidaemia
- Asthma
- Coronary heart disease
- Stroke
- Gastro-oesophageal reflux disease (GORD)
- Increased cancer risk
- Osteoarthritis
- Obstructive sleep apnoea (OSA)
- Polycystic ovarian syndrome
- Obesity related infertility
- Depression
- Liver and kidney disease

Indications for Surgery

In the UK, the current NICE criteria for surgery under the national health system are as follows:

- BMI >40 kg/m^2
- BMI between 35–40 kg/m^2 with obesity related co-morbidities such as type 2 diabetes
- The patient has tried all appropriate non-surgical measures to achieve or maintain adequate weight loss
- The patient has been or will receive tier 3 intensive obesity management services
- Fitness for general anaesthesia
- Willingness to engage in long-term follow-up
- No contraindications for bariatric surgery

There are lower thresholds in two cohorts of patients:

- Consider surgery for patients with severe type 2 diabetes who have a BMI of 30 or above
- In patients with Asian family origins, the BMI threshold can be reduced by a further 2.5 kg/m^2

Selection for Surgery

Patient selection for surgery is extremely important. Those who seek a 'quick fix' with surgery often do not achieve satisfactory results as surgery is only a part of the weight loss pathway. Good patient engagement is essential. Significant behavioural modifications, eating habits and exercise are also required to achieve a good end result.

Following on a referral from the general practitioner to a bariatric centre, the patient should be independently assessed

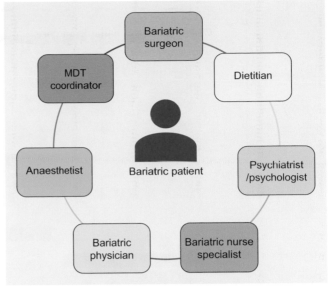

• Fig. 34.1 The Patient-Centred Bariatric MDT Approach

by members of the multidisciplinary team (MDT) before a decision for surgery is made. Members of this team include the surgeon, anaesthetist, dietitian, bariatric nurse specialist, bariatric physician and bariatric psychiatrist or psychologist (Fig. 34.1). A consensus should be reached by the MDT and with the patient before surgery is to proceed. This process is important for patient safety, particularly in complex cases.

Surgical Procedures

Common Surgical Procedures

Bariatric procedures were historically divided into two categories of 'restrictive' or 'malabsorptive'. Restrictive indicated procedures where food intake was physically constrained and malabsorptive indicating a reduction in nutrient absorption due to intestinal diversion. We now know that the beneficial effects of surgery are in fact multi-factorial and involve a wide range of mechanisms which we will discuss further in the chapter.

The significant majority of these procedures are performed laparoscopically. This particular cohort of patients benefit massively from the minimally invasive nature of surgery. This includes, and is not limited to, reduced rates of infection, pain and hernia risk. Early discharge and a return to ambulatory state reduces the risk of hospital acquired pneumonia (Fig. 34.2).

Intra-Gastric Balloon: This procedure can be performed under conscious sedation or under general anaesthesia. A balloon approximately 500–700 mL in size is placed in the stomach fundus endoscopically and filled with saline. An intra-gastric balloon is often used as a temporary measure for weight loss or as a first-stage procedure pre-surgery for the super morbidly obese patient. The balloon is removed endoscopically after 6 months.

Laparoscopic Adjustable Gastric Band (LAGB) (Fig. 34.3): The LAGB is laparoscopically placed just below the

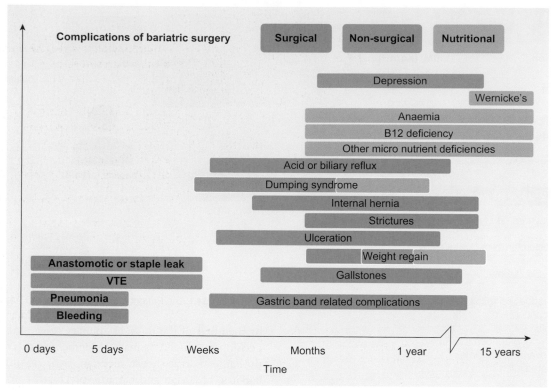

• **Fig. 34.2** Timeline of Complications

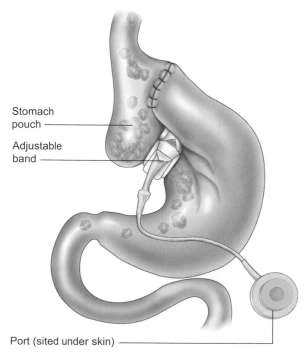

• **Fig. 34.3** Adjustable Gastric Band

gastro-oesophageal junction. The band is connected to a subcutaneous port via tubing. The port is secured to the patient's fascia on the abdomen. Through this, the gastric band can be adjusted by injecting or removing fluid into the system using a non-coring Huber needle. The therapeutic effects are achieved by limiting the amount of food a patient

can tolerate; eating slower leads to behavioural change. It also promotes early satiety.

There is a high variability in therapeutic success with LAGB as, in addition to the procedure, patients are required to make significant changes to their eating and behavioural habits. There is also a life-time risk of complications leading to the need for band removal.

Laparoscopic Sleeve Gastrectomy (LSG) (Fig. 34.4)**:** In this procedure, a large portion of the stomach is essentially 'resected' along the greater curve. This usually leaves a new tube-like stomach with a volume of approximately 80 mL. This is formed using a series of laparoscopic stapler firings. The staple line extends from approximately 3–5 cm proximal from the pylorus to just lateral of the gastro-oesophageal junction. The sleeve gastrectomy has gained significant popularity in Europe, North America and especially the Middle East. This has become the predominant procedure worldwide. It has shown both good weight loss and positive metabolic outcomes in several large published studies.

Laparoscopic Roux-En-Y Gastric Bypass (LRYGB) (Fig. 34.5): Until recently, the LRYGB was the most common bariatric procedure performed worldwide. The operation involves creating an egg-sized gastric pouch and anastomosing this with the distal jejunum. Food enters the pouch and 'bypasses' the excluded stomach remnant, duodenum and proximal jejunum. This new channel is known as the Roux limb. The divided proximal jejunum is anastomosed in the Y shape fashion downstream to allow passage of the biliary and pancreatic digestive excretions. This limb is known as the biliary pancreatic (BP) limb. Distal to the

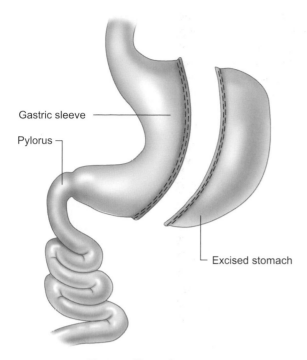

• **Fig. 34.4** Sleeve Gastrectomy

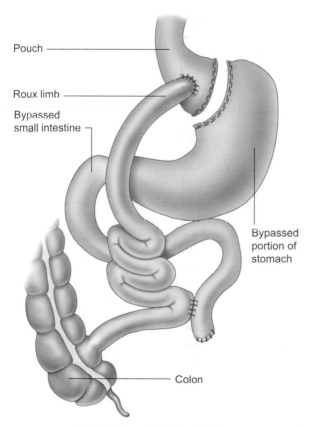

• **Fig. 34.5** Roux-En-Y Gastric Bypass

anastomosis, the passage is known as the common channel. This procedure leads to a permanent change to the patient's digestive system and has also been shown to produce significant weight loss and produce a positive impact on metabolic outcomes.

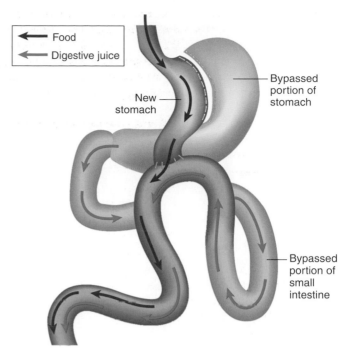

• **Fig. 34.6** Mini Gastric Bypass. (Modified from Deitel M, Rutledge R, International Journal of Surgery 71:119-123, 2019, Fig. 1, ©Elsevier.)

Mini Gastric or One Anastomosis Gastric Bypass (MGB/OAGB) (Fig. 34.6): This procedure takes the principals of an RYGB but requires only one anastomosis. Of all the 'newer' procedures, this by far has shown the most promise for weight loss and resolution of co-morbidities. It is gaining popularity throughout the globe yearly. A gastric pouch is created in a similar fashion to RYGB, but the size of the pouch is slightly longer and in a tubular shape. Afterwards, a loop of small bowel is brought up distally and the bypass is completed via a loop anastomosis. One major side-effect of this procedure is severe biliary reflux which is hard to treat.

Single Anastomosis Duodeno-Ileal Bypass with Sleeve Gastrectomy (SADI-S): This procedure takes the principals of the BPS-DS, SG and MGB put together. A sleeve gastrectomy is performed and following on, the duodenum is divided and re-anastomosed with a distal loop of small bowel. This bypasses a significant portion of the bowel but allows the biliary-pancreatic content to mix. The procedure is still classified as experimental but shows early promise.

Other Surgical Procedures

As with all surgical specialties, there are always newer and more innovative procedures that are being performed. Some are experimental or gaining more popularity but have not reached a stage of being standardized yet. There are also those that have been superseded by newer procedures.

Historical Procedures

Vertical Banded Gastroplasty (VBG): This procedure is now no longer commonly performed. A small stomach pouch is created using a combination of bands and staples.

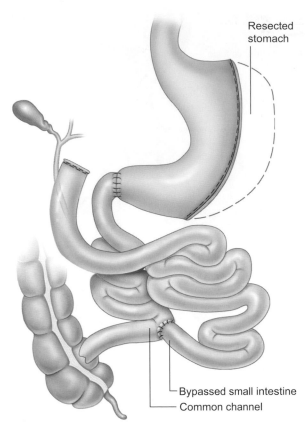

• **Fig. 34.7** Biliopancreatic Diversion with Duodenal Switch

At the base of the pouch, a 1cm opening is left allowing food to enter the rest of the stomach. The adjustable gastric band has far more advantages compared to this procedure, is it safer and also adjustable, making it a much more attractive alternative.

Biliopancreatic diversion with duodenal switch (BPD-DS): This is a more extensive procedure and has not picked up popularity in the UK. The stomach is tubulized like a sleeve gastrectomy and subsequently the duodenum is divided just past the gastric outlet. This is anastomosed to a segment of small bowel so that approximately three-quarters of the total bowel length is 'bypassed'. The limb that has been bypassed is then re-connected at the last part of the small bowel to allow bilious and pancreatic digestive enzymes to mix with the food stream (Fig. 34.7). This procedure has a higher rate of morbidity and mortality compared to other bariatric procedures. Long-term severe nutritional deficiencies can also occur.

Endoscopic Procedures

There are also other devices which are being trialled aimed at reproducing the effects of bariatric/metabolic surgery but without surgery. One example of such devices is the Endobarrier. This is an endoscopically inserted plastic sleeve which covers the inner lining of the first 60 cm of the small bowel. The device acts as a barrier to absorption, aimed at achieving a similar effect to having a gastric bypass. This device is not permanent and is endoscopically removed after a period of use. The full results from clinical trials evaluating the therapeutic effect of this class of device are expected later in 2022.

Another procedure of interest is endoscopic gastric plication. In this procedure, an endoscopic suture placating device is used to plicate the stomach endo-luminally. This results in a reduction of gastric volume and may have effects on satiety. The medium to long term effects of this procedure are still relatively unknown.

Future Procedures

Some patients may not be fit for surgery and this had led to some other innovative procedures being trialled. Embolization of the left gastric artery, in theory, reduces blood flow to the gastric fundus. Some studies have shown that patients who undergo this procedure also have subsequently reduced levels of circulating ghrelin. This may lead to benefits in weight loss and a change in gut hormone homeostasis.

Duodenal resurfacing is another procedure that has been trialled. In this procedure, patients undergo endoscopic hydrothermal ablation of their duodenal mucosa. The segments can vary in length and the aim is to achieve the same effect as bypassing the duodenum without any surgery or foreign device. This procedure has yet to undergo any randomized controlled trial.

Robotic-Assisted Surgery

All the procedures mentioned above can also be achieved using robotic surgery. Although to date there has not been any evidence to suggest robotic is superior to conventional laparoscopic techniques, it is certainly a feasible method used around the globe, including in the UK and North America.

Effects of Surgery

Following on from surgery, there is a complex system-wide cascade of effects that take place. An acronym of BRAVE describes some of the effects of bariatric surgery. This stands for Bile flow alteration, Reduction of gastric size, Anatomical gut rearrangement with altered flow of nutrients, Vagal manipulation and Enteric gut hormone modulation. A separate acronym of SLIMMER describes the role of bile acids in modulating Satiety, Lipid and cholesterol metabolism, Incretins and glucose homeostasis, energy Metabolism, gut Microbiota and Endoplasmic Reticulum stress.

Weight loss occurs due to the restrictive and/or malabsorptive nature of the procedures, leading to a reduced calorie intake. This, however, takes time to occur and, at the same time, a change in diet, exercise and behaviours is required to achieve significant and sustained weight loss.

Biliary diversion leads to a malabsorptive effect. On top of this, there has been significant interest in the effects of bile diversion and glucose haemostasis. Changes also occur to the gut microbiome and subsequent signalling molecules metabolized and activated by the altered gut microbiome include short chain fatty acids and bile acids, which may also contribute to the beneficial effects of surgery.

Hormonal changes also occur after surgery; for example the 'hunger hormone' ghrelin is shown to have reduced plasma concentrations after surgery. This hormone plays a role in the body's energy haemostasis and has an effect on the hunger centres. Glucagon and glucagon-like peptide 1 (GLP-1) have also been shown to change in serum concentrations post-surgery. These have an effect on inhibiting appetite. Changes in gut hormone profiles are key to the weight-independent and weight-dependent effects of bariatric surgery.

Bariatric surgery has also been shown to have a positive effect on all the obesity related co-morbidities, including type 2 diabetes, hypertension, ischaemic heart disease, and also modifies patient's cancer risk. Some of these effects are weight-dependent but, what is more intriguing, is that some of these effects are weight-independent. The precise underlying mechanisms are yet to be fully understood.

In particular, the therapeutic effects of bariatric surgery on type 2 diabetes cure is astounding. Patients requiring insulin often find themselves leaving hospital several days postoperatively not requiring insulin or a significantly reduced dose to achieve glycaemic control. Weight loss at this point has yet to begin and a whole host of factors contribute to this effect. Several large-scale clinical trials comparing bariatric surgery to medical treatment found surgery to be up to five times superior in sustained diabetic resolution. This is now recognized by multiple medical diabetic associations worldwide. In the UK, surgery has been listed within its guidelines for treatment of severe diabetes. The effects are so dramatic that surgery is considered in those severe diabetics who are below the surgical threshold BMI of 35.

Risk Stratification

There are several scores that can be used to help stratify risk in this cohort of patients. The STOP BANG (Snoring, Tiredness, Observed apnoea, Pressure, BMI, Age, Neck, Gender) score originates from a group in Canada and is a quick scoring questionnaire that determines risk of obstructive sleep apnoea. The American College of Surgeons National Surgical Quality Improvement Program (ACS NSQIP) risk calculator is another example that could be used to quantify a patients' risk of developing postoperative complications. The use of scores can assist the surgeon in counselling patients regarding operative risk prior to surgery and is an important part of the informed consent process.

Postoperative Complications

As with all surgical procedures, there are associated risks to bariatric surgery. With advances in laparoscopic surgery, bariatric surgery is extremely safe. Within the UK, the complication and mortality rate is approximately 2% and 0.05%, respectively. This compares well with other leading European and North American countries.

General postoperative complications are no different in those who are obese. Often their pre-existing co-morbidities may be exacerbated by general anaesthesia and surgery. Patients presenting with complaints postoperatively should be thoroughly investigated. Box 34.3 lists a selection of tests which should be considered, depending on the presenting complaint.

Obesity associated hypoventilation leads to an increased risk of basal atelectasis and hospital-acquired pneumonias. Early mobilization, good pain relief, CPAP and the use of an incentive spirometer is used to reduce this risk. Venous thromboembolic events occur higher in those patients with a higher BMI. Appropriate weight-adjusted pharmacological and mechanical prophylaxis should be used.

Patients who undergo bariatric surgery are at higher risk of gallstone formation due to rapid weight loss. Ursodeoxycholic acid is used by many centres as a prophylactic agent. Obstructive biliary symptoms can be difficult to treat in patients who have undergone a Roux-en-Y gastric bypass as the biliary tree is not immediately accessible via the oral route due to the altered anatomy. Alternate strategies include trans-gastric endoscopic retrograde cholangiopancreatography (ERCP) or laparoscopic bile duct exploration. There has been no benefit shown in performing simultaneous or prophylactic cholecystectomy at the index procedure in asymptomatic patients and thus it is not routinely performed in most centres.

Nutritional deficiencies can also occur in any patient who has undergone a bariatric procedure. This can occur with any micro-nutrient and life-time monitoring and replacement is essential. There is also a higher risk of patients developing depression. This can be particularly exacerbated in those who previously used eating as a stress coping mechanism. This illustrates why pre- and postoperative psychological follow-up is important.

Weight Regain

Weight regain can occur with any of the described procedures. Weight regain needs to be thoroughly investigated and there can be many reasons, including surgical, lifestyle and psychological causes.

The patient should be assessed anatomically for any potential surgical complications, such as band slippage in those who underwent LAGB. Pouch or stoma dilatation can occur with other procedures and, in rare cases, entero-gastric or gastro-gastric fistulae may be found. At times, surgical revision of the same procedure or conversion to another may be required. A summary of conversion procedures can be seen in Table 34.1.

Assessment should also include non-surgical factors. A dietitian review is required to ensure the patient is eating the right types of food; snacks and sweets which are low-volume and highly calorific can contribute to such issues. Eating habits and behaviours should also be assessed. Finally, undiagnosed or untreated eating and psychiatric disorders may also be the cause of weight regain and thus psychological or

TABLE 34.1 **Summary of Bariatric Surgery.**

Operation	Advantages	Disadvantages	Can be Converted Into
Intra-Gastric Balloon	• Day case procedure • Useful first stage • Minimal risks • Does not require general anaesthetic • Reversible	• Temporary measure and weight regain after removal • Can migrate distally to cause gastric outlet obstruction • Nausea and vomiting • Worsening reflux	• Any procedure
Adjustable Gastric Band (AGB)	• Adjustable • Removable • Relatively low-risk procedure • No permanent anatomical alteration • Reversible	• Foreign body – Band slippage and erosion • Risk of port site infection • Nausea and vomiting • Worsening reflux • High rate of band removal • Less weight loss compared to other procedures • Requires strict follow-up and diet modifications	• SG/MGB/RYGB/ SAID-S
Sleeve Gastrectomy (SG)	• Rapid and significant weight loss • Positive metabolic outcomes comparable to RYGB • Shorter operation • Can be used as a first stage procedure	• Non-reversible • No foreign body or re-routing of anatomy • Worsening reflux • Barrett's oesophagus • Surgical risk – staple line bleed and leak • Nutritional deficiencies	• SAID-S/MGB/ RYGB/DS
Roux-En-Y Gastric Bypass (RYGB)	• Current 'gold standard' procedure • Established significant effect on weight loss and obesity related co-morbidities • Reversible	• Highest morbidity • Surgical risk of bleeding, anastomotic leak and stenosis • Risk of internal hernia • Biliary or gastric remnant disease difficult to treat • Nutritional deficiencies • Dumping syndrome	• Banded bypass • Minimizer ring • Distalization
Mini Gastric Bypass/One Anastomosis Gastric Bypass (MGB/OAGB)	• Significant weight loss shown in early studies • At least equal to RYGB in co-morbidity resolution • Only one anastomosis • Reversible	• New procedure – long-term effects yet to be fully established • Significant biliary reflux	• RYGB • Distalization
Biliopancreatic Diversion with Duodenal Switch (BPD/DS)	• Allows 'normal' meal volumes • Effective against diabetes	• Highest risk of complications • Significant long-term nutritional deficiencies • Surgical risk – bleed, leak, stenosis	• Common channel lengthening
Vertical Banded Gastroplasty (VBG)	• No dumping syndrome	• Not adjustable • Complex reversal • No longer performed and superseded by other procedures	• RYGB
Single Anastomosis duodeno-ileal bypass with sleeve gastrectomy (SAID-S)	• Aims to combine the advantages of DS, SG and RYGB	• Can worsen reflux • Significant nutritional deficiencies • Surgical risk – bleed, leak, stenosis • New procedure – still classified as experimental with long-term effects unknown	• MGB/RYGB

psychiatric reassessment should also form part of the investigative chain.

It is prudent that any eventual findings should be discussed in an MDT setting at a specialist centre prior to any invention to try help achieve the best outcomes for the patient involved.

Procedure-Specific Complications

Adjustable Gastric Band: A slipped or eroded gastric band are the two most common long-term complications related to this procedure. Slippage can occur both acutely and chronically. The stomach herniates via the proximal end of the band, which leads to symptoms of dysphagia, vomiting and reflux. Associated abdominal pain is rare but gastric ischaemia due to herniation should be considered if a patient presents with such symptoms. Urgent band decompression via the subcutaneous port and gastric decompression via a nasal gastric tube is vital. Subsequent laparoscopic band removal is the required treatment.

Erosion of the band into the stomach can also occur. The most common presentation related to this is a port site infection. Those who present with such should be investigated with an upper GI endoscopy. Symptoms can include abdominal pain, weight regain and even obstruction. Removal of the band can be performed trans-orally if a significant portion of the band has become intra gastric. Otherwise, laparoscopic removal with suture repair of the stomach is required. Other complications include tube fracture, tube leak, port slippage or port leakage, all of which potentially require surgical correction.

Sleeve Gastrectomy: A significant portion of patients suffer from a high degree of nausea in the immediate postoperative period. Other major complications in this period are rare but bleeding and leakage can occur from the gastric staple line. Staple line leaks which present early is often associated with a technical failure or several days or weeks later, which is more in keeping with ischaemia or thermal injury during dissection. Leaks, especially from the proximal staple line, are very difficult to treat. Endoscopic stenting or further surgical salvage procedures may be required.

Staple line bleed patients should be managed as per any postoperative bleed. Re-intervention can be conservative, endoscopic or a return to the operating theatre.

Later complications include gastro-oesophageal reflux progressing to Barrett's oesophagus, gastric tube stricture and stenosis. Any reflux or dysphagia should be investigated with an upper GI endoscopy and contrast swallow. The presence of a hiatus hernia is important to establish and treatment for reflux should be with proton pump inhibitors. Failing that, a conversion to RYGB is sometimes required. Patients who undergo this procedure are also more prone to vitamin B_{12} deficiency and pernicious anaemia.

Roux-en-Y Gastric Bypass: With this procedure, there are general anastomosis-related complications but also procedure-specific complications due to the anatomical rearrangement. The most serious complication is an anastomotic leak. The most common site for this to occur is the gastro-jejunal anastomosis. Patients can present with abdominal pain or sepsis but sometimes with more subtle features such as a paralytic ileus or failure to progress. Bleeding can again also occur early or late. Treatment will depend on the identified source of bleeding and the physiological state of the patient. Not all cases require re-operation.

Ulceration can occur, particularly at the gastro-jejunal anastomosis, especially in patients who continue to smoke postoperatively. Bleeding can occur and symptoms include post-prandial pain, haematemesis, melena or fresh per rectal bleeding. Recurrent ulceration can also lead to strictures.

Specific to the RYGB, internal hernias are a rare but potentially serious and difficult to diagnose complication. Due to the anatomical rearrangement, there are two mesenteric defects which bowel can herniate through. The first is Peterson's defect where the roux limb or the mesentery overlies the transverse mesocolon. The second is the defect within the small bowel mesentery at the jejunal-jejunal anastomosis. Most surgeons close these defects but despite this, rapid weight loss can cause the defect to re-open. Herniation causes obstruction but often signs are subtler such as positional abdominal pain. Bowel ischaemia related to this can be catastrophic. There should be a high index of suspicion in patients who re-present with unexplained abdominal pain and/or obstruction. Cross-sectional imaging should be arranged urgently with low threshold to return to theatre for diagnostic laparoscopy.

Dumping syndrome occurs when highly calorific and osmotic content enters the distal jejunum rapidly. This can lead to symptoms of nausea, vomiting, dizziness, sweating and abdominal cramping due to rapid fluid and electrolyte shifts.

Mini Gastric Bypass: Complications related to RYGB can be related to this cohort as well. On top of this, other complications can include diarrhoea, biliary reflux and an increased risk of gastro-jejunal ulceration. These patients also have a higher risk of developing anaemia.

Social and Lifestyle Considerations

There are several common social and lifestyle considerations that bariatric patients need to be counselled about. It is strongly recommended that patients cease to smoke prior to surgery as smoking increases the risk of developing postoperative complications. Smokers are also at an increased risk of developing marginal ulcers and subsequent anastomotic strictures. For alcohol drinkers, in particular any patient who has undergone a bypass procedure, they must be counselled that, postoperatively, alcohol absorption rates increase; thus, a small volume of alcohol will rapidly lead to levels that are illegal for driving.

Patients who are also substance abusers or have polypharmacy need to be thoroughly assessed by the MDT team prior to any decision for surgery.

Sexual function and fertility initially decrease postoperatively before increasing over time. It is recommended that women of child-bearing age use appropriate contraception for at least the first 18 months postoperatively due to the effects of surgery on the patient's body and nutritional state.

Revision Surgery

Any procedure performed on a patient who has had previous surgery can be classified as revisional surgery. In the case of this cohort of patients, this is not just limited to bariatric procedures. In some cases, patients may have undergone other operations such as anti-reflux procedures.

The indications for revisional surgery can be due to one or multiple factors. These include complications relating to the index procedure, failure to lose weight or weight regain or failure of resolution or improvement of a co-morbidity. In very rare cases, reversal operations are done for excessive weight loss or malnutrition. Some examples include revision or removal of a slipped gastric band, or conversion from a sleeve gastrectomy to a Roux-en-Y gastric bypass for severe gastro-oesophageal reflux. In most cases, the main indication is the treatment of side-effects. Inadequate weight loss or weight regain can also be a reason for further surgery but this itself is controversial as there are currently no defined international guidelines related to revisional surgery.

There is no consensus on what is the best revisional procedure nor the precise definition of weight regain or inadequate resolution of obesity related co-morbidities. In countries where funding is based on a public system, eligibility can be debatable, as is the increasing numbers of health tourists seeking financially cheaper operations abroad and returning with complications.

Surgical risks in revisional surgery are certainly higher. The operations are more complex and take longer due to scaring and adhesions. Risk of complications such as leaks, bleeding and even postoperative VTE events are higher. However, if further weight loss is to be achieved along with further co-morbidity resolution, revisional surgery should be considered. Overall mortality is no different from a primary procedure. The final column in Table 34.1 describes which procedures can be converted into which subsequently.

Summary

Bariatric/metabolic surgery is a growing field with significant therapeutic potential. Initially designed for weight loss, we are now seeing benefits extending far beyond weight. However, services should only be provided in centres of expertise as caring for such a cohort of patients is not straightforward. Patients often come with a significant number of obesity-related co-morbidities and their management requires an all-round approach. Recognition of postoperative complications is important and failure to rescue can result in catastrophe. Any decision for surgery should be made collectively with the MDT and the counselled patient. The overall outcome not only relies on a successful operation but also with patient engagement and motivation. From a medical point of view, evidence continues to grow with regards to the highly successful therapeutic effects of surgery on obesity and its related co-morbidities.

Further Reading

Chang SH, et al. The effectiveness and risks of bariatric surgery: an updated systematic review and meta-analysis, 2003–2012. *JAMA Surg.* 2014;149(3):275–287.

Colquitt JL, et al. Surgery for weight loss in adults. *Cochrane Database Syst Rev.* 2014;(8):CD003641.

Mingrone G, et al. Bariatric-metabolic surgery versus conventional medical treatment in obese patients with type 2 diabetes: 5-year follow-up of an open-label, single centre, randomized controlled trial. *Lancet.* 2015;386(9997):964–973.

Schauer PR, et al. Bariatric surgery versus intensive medical therapy for diabetes – 5-year outcomes. *N Engl J Med*. 2017;376(7):641–651.

Sjostrom L, et al. Effects of bariatric surgery on mortality in Swedish obese subjects. *N Engl J Med.* 2007;357(8):741–752.

35

Trauma and Orthopaedic Surgery

CHAPTER OUTLINE

Orthopaedics is concerned with the surgical treatment of bone and joint conditions. The word is derived from the Greek for 'straight child', and the symbol that has been adopted by most orthopaedic associations is the twisted sapling (symbolizing the bent child) lashed to a straight supporting stick.

Orthopaedic terms. A number of terms with particular definitions are used in orthopaedic practice, and these are summarized in Box 35.1.

Special Features of Orthopaedic History and Examination

History

Pain

This is usually the presenting symptom. Onset and duration are important. Was it sudden or was it gradual over a few months? Is the pain constant or exacerbated by standing or mobilizing? The site of pain can aid detection of the cause. However, it is important to recognize that pain can be referred from one area to another. It is common for hip pain to refer to the knee region, and vice versa. Children may find it difficult to express the location and to realize that the adjacent joint may be the source of pain. Hence it is important, following history taking, to examine possible surrounding sites. There are some characteristic patterns. Hip pain is classically felt in the groin. Radicular pain from a spinal nerve root impingement can cause arm or leg pain. Such situations can cause paraesthesia which is described as 'pins and needles'. Joint pain may be relieved by rest, load reduction with a walking stick or analgesics.

Pain from meniscal tears in the knee can be exacerbated by twisting movements and can be associated with locking.

Night pain is important as it can signify the severity of joint arthritis and be an indicator of the need for joint replacement. It is also an important sign for a neoplasm, including classically benign osteoid osteoma. Early morning pain with stiffness is common with arthritic joints.

Weakness

This can be secondary to pain, neurological or soft tissue injury such as to muscles or tendon tears, as in rotator cuff injuries of the shoulder. Weakness due to neurologic damage will usually be associated with sensory disturbances unless it is a pure motor nerve damage (e.g. posterior interosseous nerve damage). Even the so-called pure motor nerves carry proprioceptive sensations to the joints they cross.

• BOX 35.1 Orthopaedic Terms

Proximal[a] Closer to the trunk
Distal[a] Further away from the trunk
Varus[b] Deformity or angulation towards the midline
Valgus[b] Deformity or angulation away from the midline
Genu Knee
Recurvatum Abnormal hyperextension of the knee joint
Cubitus Elbow
Coxa Hip
Pes Foot
Cavus[c] Abnormally arched
Planus[c] Flat
Alta[d] High
Baja[d] (pronounced Ba-ha) Low
Scoliosis[e] Abnormal lateral curvature
Lordosis[e] Posterior curvature – normal in cervical and lumbar regions
Kyphosis[e] Anterior curvature – normal in thoracic region
Crepitus Grating or grinding sound or sensation from an abnormal joint (usually degenerative) when moved
Ankylosis Joint fusion secondary to a pathological process (usually inflammatory) – usually fibrous
Arthrodesis Joint fusion brought about by operation – always bony
Osteoporosis Normal bone mineral content but reduction in bone mass or matrix
Osteosclerosis Increased bone mineral content
Osteomalacia Reduced bone mineral content
Polydactyly Duplication of digits
Macrodactyly Enlarged digits
Syndactyly Fused digits
Camptodactyly Deformed digits

[a]The position of body part in relation to another.
[b]The description is applied to the distal part.
[c]Terms applied to the foot.
[d]Terms describing the position of the patella.
[e]Terms used to describe the shape of the spine; may be combined.

Stiffness and Loss of Function

Stiffness and pain are hallmarks of arthritis but are also a feature of contractures around any joint (a typical example is hamstring contracture in cerebral palsy).

Joint Instability

This occurs with altered joint stabilizers as seen with cruciate ligament injuries of the knee, labral tears of the shoulder or fractures. Instability can result in deformity such as in ulna deviation of the metacarpophalangeal joints in rheumatoid arthritis.

Trauma

Is there a history of injury? Mechanism of injury is important as it gives a clue to the degree of potential damage and the type of fracture. Spiral fractures are associated with twisting forces, whilst transverse fractures are common in direct blows. Understanding the direction of fracture displacement can allow one to reverse the mechanism to reduce the fracture. This is utilized in Colles' distal radius fracture reduction.

Secondary osteoarthritis may follow:
- direct disruption of a joint
- malunion which places undue loads on a joint

Need to Use an 'Aid'

The need for a walking stick or special cutlery may give an indication of the severity of the problem or of the use of past conservative management by the patient or doctors.

Occupation

Certain occupations which involve continued or repetitive movements can cause tenosynovitis (tendon inflammation), for example in typists, chicken pluckers or keyboard operators. Osteoarthritis of the spine is seen in miners and farm workers. Osteonecrosis of the femoral heads occurs in deep sea divers and is termed 'caisson's disease'.

Dominant Hand

The dominant hand may be affected more commonly, as in carpal tunnel syndrome.

Past Medical History

This includes:
- Similar problem on the contralateral side
- Recent infections – urethritis, gastroenteritis or a streptococcal sore throat, all of which predispose to reactive arthritis
- Pregnancy – which often precipitates low back pain or carpal tunnel syndrome
- Diabetes – which is often associated with frozen shoulder

Family History

Dupuytren's contracture, gout, rheumatoid arthritis and bone dysplasias may all run in families.

Medication

Current and past medication should be identified. The use of steroids predisposes to osteonecrosis of the femoral head.

Patients on steroids often have problems with wound healing. Dupuytren's contracture is observed in association with phenytoin.

Examination
General Assessment

Two classes of information result:
- specific indications of the cause of the problem
- suitability and fitness for surgery to correct the condition

Joints

The examination of any joint has four components:
- look
- feel
- measure (not always applicable)
- move and special tests pertinent to the joint examined
  Look at:
- Gait – assessment is made when the patient walks into the clinic or takes a few steps on the ward; normal gait has

TABLE 35.1	Phases of Normal Gait.
Heel strike	The heel makes contact with the ground
Stance	Weight is being transferred from the heel to the toes
Toe-off	A final push is given to the foot as it leaves the ground
Swing-through	The leg is brought forward with the knee lightly flexed to allow the foot to clear the ground

• BOX 35.2 Abnormal Gaits

Antalgic Painful and with a short stance phase; seen in any condition of the lower leg where the pain is exacerbated by weight-bearing, e.g. osteoarthritis of the hip

Stiff leg A fused hip or knee joint causes abnormal swing-through when the pelvis has to be rotated to bring the leg through

Trendelenburg With proximal muscle weakness, the pelvis on the opposite side sags during the stance phase – seen in developmental dysplasia of the hip, poliomyelitis and in osteoarthritis of the hip

Short leg During the stance phase, the short leg results in the pelvis and shoulder on the affected side sagging down

Shuffling Seen in Parkinson's disease, it has a short swing-through and no real heel strike or toe-off

Stamping The swing-through phase is abnormal with a broad base and high stepping – often caused by peripheral neuropathy with tabes dorsalis

Ataxic Broad-based with unsteadiness on turning – cerebellar disease, multiple sclerosis or head injury

Foot drop During swing-through, the foot scuffs on the ground – an L5 root lesion, common peroneal nerve palsy or old poliomyelitis

Scissor Occurs in children with cerebral palsy with adductor spasm, so the swing-through of one leg is blocked by the other

four phases (Table 35.1) which flow smoothly one into the other but there are many abnormalities (Box 35.2)
- Skin – for scars and colour
- Shape of the joint in general, the presence of swelling and lumps, and the position of the limb
- Muscle-wasting – can be secondary to disuse from pain, contracture or deformity
Feel for:
- temperature
- swelling – is it fluctuant and therefore fluid, or soft tissue or bone?
- abnormal movement
- crepitus

Measure the length of the limb to determine inequality between the two sides. True length is measured using a fixed bony prominence, whereas apparent discrepancy utilizes a fixed point and is different due to position of deformity.

Is it possible to determine if the whole limb or only a part of it is short? Muscle wasting can be documented by measuring and comparing girths.

Move: Joint movement may be painful, and care should be taken not to cause pain. First, the patient is asked to move the joint in question actively. This gives the examiner an indication of the degree of pain and disability within an affected joint. Next the limb is passively moved. Often there is no significant difference between the active and passive ranges. Local weakness due to muscular or neurological dysfunction may result in limited active movement but a full range of passive movement.

However, a tendon injury can cause a difference. In the shoulder, rotator cuff tears may limit active abduction, but passive abduction is often unaffected.

The range of movement can be recorded using a goniometer and serial documentation in the notes will allow comparison of progress with treatments (Table 35.2).

Investigation

Imaging

Plain X-ray is one of the simplest forms of imaging yet it can provide a wealth of information and is hence often the first choice. Although bone pathology can be identified, the surrounding soft tissues can be visualized. Fractures are often associated with soft tissue swelling and, occasionally, an X-ray may be the first investigation to highlight a soft tissue mass such as a sarcoma. Healed fractures, arthritis in joint, calcification on cartilage (chondrocalcinosis) (Fig. 35.1) and typical infection changes such as osteomyelitis and TB can be detected.

Arthrography. Injection of a radio-opaque contrast medium into a joint delineates its anatomical boundaries and shows abnormal communications such as those that occur in rotator cuff tears of the shoulder. Intra-articular structures may become apparent, e.g. loose bodies or the menisci in the knee. Arthrography can be used to supplement CT and MRI. Labral tears in the hip and shoulder can be identified and this can direct surgical treatments.

Computed tomography (CT) is used for imaging bony pathology, fractures, bone tumours and specific locations such as the pelvis, foot and ankle and spine. It is sensitive in detecting bone graft fusion and fracture healing and hence it is useful in determining safe timing for loading postoperatively. The extent of bone defects can be determined to help with augment use in joint replacement surgery.

Magnetic resonance imaging (MRI). This is now the standard investigation for many musculoskeletal problems. This technique (see Ch. 15) provides excellent images in both coronal and sagittal planes, and with appropriate computer software, three-dimensional reconstruction is possible. MRI now provides unparalleled detail (Fig. 35.2) and can be combined with contrast to enhance diagnosis. MRI scans are useful in the staging of bone tumours: intraosseous as well as extracompartmental spread can be identified and local bone and soft tissue extension can be defined to ensure surgery achieves adequate resection margins.

TABLE 35.2	Radiological Appearances in Arthritis.	
Feature	Osteoarthritis	Rheumatoid arthritis
Loss of joint space	Yes	Yes
Sclerosis	Yes	No
Osteophytes	Yes	No
Subchondral cysts	Yes	No
Erosions	No	Yes
Osteoporosis	No	Yes

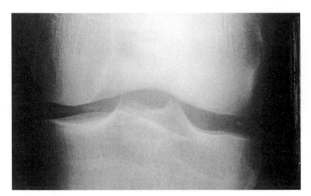

• **Fig. 35.1** Radiological calcification in a meniscus in the knee joint.

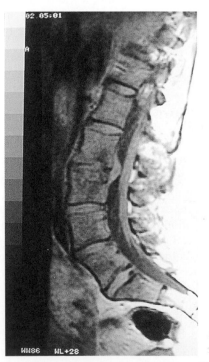

• **Fig. 35.2** MRI of a disc abscess in the spine at L2/3

Isotope scanning is frequently used in orthopaedics. Technetium-99m diphosphonate is concentrated in areas of increased osteoblastic activity usually associated with increased blood supply. These areas occur in such conditions as arthritis, fractures and bone tumour metastases. Scans also reveal zones of relative underactivity when the blood supply is reduced, such as in osteonecrosis. Radiolabelled white blood cells are used to localize infection within a painful joint replacement or a nidus of osteomyelitis (see later).

Ultrasound is useful in soft tissue conditions and can aid detection of tendinopathies, tendon and muscle tears, bursitis, oedema, joint effusions, neoplasms and congenital hip dislocations in children.

It can be combined with needle biopsy and fluid aspiration, for example in suspected septic arthritis of a joint. Early use and microbiology assessments on aspirations can be vital to prevent cartilage and joint destruction and the development of sepsis.

Blood Investigations

ESR and C-reactive protein (CRP) are non-specific markers of inflammation which can be used to follow the course of an orthopaedic disease and its treatment. They are raised in conditions such as osteomyelitis, active rheumatoid arthritis, malignant disease and infected joint replacement.

Rheumatoid factor is an IgM autoantibody present in the serum of patients with a number of conditions, including rheumatoid arthritis (80%), Sjögren's syndrome (90%) and systemic lupus erythematosus (50%). Cyclic citrullinated peptide antibody (CCP test) is a newer test for rheumatoid arthritis, being useful particularly in early disease and rheumatoid factor negative patients.

Uric acid. Raised serum levels predispose to gout but are not always raised in acute attacks.

Antistreptolysin (ASO) titres are increased in recent streptococcal infection, which may be helpful in confirming an occult infection in a joint replacement.

Protein electrophoresis for a specific monoclonal antibody is diagnostic of myeloma.

Alkaline phosphatase is raised in Paget's disease, secondary malignancy in bone and osteomalacia.

Synovial Fluid Examination

Joint aspiration is generally an outpatient procedure which must be performed with aseptic technique. In a situation where there is a joint replacement, it is even more important to reduce the risk of introducing infection around an implant and procedures are generally undertaken in the sterile operating theatre.

Findings may include:

- the presence of crystals in both gout and pseudogout (seen using a polarizing light microscope)
- organisms and a very high white cell count (50×10^9/L) in septic arthritis and lower levels in any inflammatory arthritis ($1-3 \times 10^9$/L)

Arthroscopy

The interior of the knee joint was first examined in 1918, using a cystoscope. The techniques were refined over subsequent years until 1957 when the first purpose-built instrument was introduced. An arthroscope is a rigid instrument with an outer sheath and an inner lens system. Almost any joint can be arthroscoped, although some require specialized instrumentation. The commonest ones are the knee (most frequent), shoulder, elbow, wrist, hip and ankle. Arthroscopy of the phalangeal joints has been described, as well as that of the facet joints of the lumbar spine. The technique consists of the introduction of the sheath into the joint by a small puncture wound (portal) followed by distension with saline. The lens system can be slid down within the sheath and the joint inspected. Procedures can be performed with instruments introduced through other portals. A large variety are available. They range from simple hooked probes to scissors, grasping forceps, knives, specialized meniscal sutures and powered tools to shave or cut. Lasers can also be used to trim intra-articular structures such as meniscal tags or to shrink the capsule in unstable shoulder or ankle joints.

Arthritis

Osteoarthritis

Epidemiology and Aetiology

Osteoarthritis (OA) is the most frequent type of arthritis and is more common in women than in men. The incidence increases with age, and by 80 years, 80–90% of hips show radiographic evidence of osteoarthritis. The condition is usually primary but can be secondary to other conditions (Box 35.3). Primary OA is of unknown cause, although repeated minor trauma and a genetic predisposition are probable factors. It affects the main weight-bearing joints – the spine, hips and knees – although it rarely occurs in the ankle. The distal interphalangeal joints of the hand and, in the thumb, the carpometacarpal joints can also be sites of the disorder. Secondary osteoarthritis can affect any joint.

Clinical Features

History

Joint pain and stiffness are usual and tend to be progressive over time but they may be variable from day to day. Pain initially occurs on weight-bearing, then at rest and subsequently wakes the patient at night. As well as pain during movement, joint crepitus may be felt and heard by the patient. Deformity of the affected joint from local swelling and destruction may be noted and, on weight-bearing, these may increase.

Physical Findings
- *Look* for:
  - local swelling
  - deformity – weight-bearing may make this worse
  - scars or sinuses that suggest a secondary cause

• BOX 35.3   Causes of Osteoarthritis

Primary (or idiopathic)
- Unknown

Secondary
- Abnormal joint contour
- Trauma (dislocation in particular)
- Developmental dysplasia of the hip
- Slipped upper-femoral epiphysis
- Osteonecrosis
- Kienbock's disease of the lunate
- Panner's disease of the capitellum
- Scheuermann's disease of the vertebral end plates
- Perthes' disease of the hip
- Osgood–Schlatter's disease of the tibial tuberosity
- Sever's disease of the calcaneum
- Kohler's disease of the navicular
- Freiberg's disease of the metatarsal heads
- Drugs
  - Systemic steroids and cytotoxics
  - Intra-articular steroids
- Local radiotherapy
- Sickle cell disease
- Alcoholism
- Neoplasia – leukaemia and lymphoma
- Occupational – caisson's disease
- Cartilage destruction
  - Infection
  - Recurrent haemarthrosis – haemophilia
  - Gout and pseudogout
  - Rheumatoid arthritis

Metabolic and endocrine disorders
- Alkaptonuria
- Wilson's disease
- Acromegaly

Neuropathic disorders
- Diabetes mellitus
- Tabes dorsalis

- *Feel* to detect if:
  - the swelling is bone, soft tissue or fluid
  - crepitus is present
- *Move* the joint to test:
  - active and then passive range of movement
  - stability of ligaments

Investigation

Few investigations are required. Plain X-rays are needed to assess the extent of the disease, but the radiological appearances (Table 35.3) may not correlate well with clinical symptoms.

Rheumatoid Arthritis

Epidemiology and Aetiology

This is a systemic inflammatory disease which affects 3% of the female and 1% of the male UK population. Small joints in the hands and wrists, elbows, shoulders, cervical spine

TABLE 35.3	Normal Degrees of Large Joint Movement.					
Joint	Flexion	Extension	Abduction	Adduction	External rotation	Internal rotation
Shoulder	180	50	180	30	80	100
Elbow	150	5	–	–	–	–
Wrist	Dorsi-90	Palmar 90	Ulnar 30	Radial 15	Supination 90	Pronation 90
Hip	150	0	45	30	80	45
Knee	140	10				
Ankle	Dorsi-15	Plantar 70	Eversion 10	Inversion 25		

and feet are particularly involved, but any joints may be affected except the lumbar spine and the distal interphalangeal joints. The cause remains unknown, although various organisms and an exaggerated immune response to them have frequently been invoked.

Clinical Features

History
There is usually a long history of systemic illness with multiple joint involvement and extra-articular problems including weight loss, low-grade fever, subcutaneous nodules, arteritis and tendon sheath involvement. Joint symptoms are pain, morning stiffness and progressive deformity with loss of function.

Physical Findings
- *Look*:
  - at the hands, which have the characteristic deformity of ulnar deviation of the fingers and subluxation at the metacarpophalangeal joints
  - for rheumatoid nodules on the subcutaneous border of the ulna
- *Feel* for:
  - subcutaneous nodules
  - local warmth in the affected joint
  - soft-tissue swelling around joints and tendon sheaths
  - joint crepitus
- *Move* to detect:
  - active rather than the passive range of movement
  - abnormal joint mobility secondary to subluxation

Investigation
The diagnosis of rheumatoid arthritis has usually been made by the time the patient is seen in the orthopaedic clinic.

Imaging
Plain X-ray may help to confirm the diagnosis (see Table 35.2). However, there may be radiological features of superimposed (secondary) osteoarthritis. MRI scanning is best for investigation of early disease.

Blood Examination
Anaemia is common and is either a leucoerythroblastic type or reflects iron deficiency (secondary to chronic gastrointestinal bleeding after NSAID ingestion). ESR is usually raised. Rheumatoid factor is detectable in 80% of cases. CCP test is usually positive (see earlier).

Management
Rheumatoid arthritis is predominantly managed by medical means. Patients are referred to the orthopaedic clinic or to one conducted jointly with rheumatologists when surgical correction of deformity and restoration of function has been considered beneficial.

Other Arthritides

Systemic Lupus Erythematosus (SLE)
This systemic inflammatory condition mainly affects young women. Ninety percent of patients develop joint symptoms that include polyarthritis of the hands.

Polymyalgia Rheumatica
This affects the elderly and is more common in women. It presents with aching and morning stiffness in the shoulders and pelvis. Locally, there is muscle tenderness and a reduced range of active movement but normal passive movement. There may be associated temporal arteritis. The ESR is markedly raised (>100). Management is with steroid therapy.

Gout
Arthropathy with urate crystal deposition affects mostly men at the metacarpophalangeal joint of the big toe, although the knee is also a common additional site. Acute attacks may occur spontaneously or be precipitated by local trauma. Gout may also be secondary to myeloproliferative disorders with increased purine production or renal disease with reduced urate excretion. Urate crystals may also be deposited as tophi in soft tissues: the Achilles tendon, around joints, in bursae and on the pinna of the ear. The diagnosis is made by demonstrating the presence of

TABLE 35.4	Surgical Options for an Arthritic Joint.	
Procedure	**Effects**	**Example**
Arthrodesis	Stiff but pain-free joint	Fusion of the lumbar spine, ankle or wrist
Excision	Removal of one aspect of the joint may relieve pain; shortening of the limb beyond the resection	Keller's operation on the big toe for hallux valgus
Osteotomy	Alteration of the line of load transmission to an unaffected part of the joint – now an infrequently performed procedure	High tibial osteotomy for unicompartmental osteoarthritis of the knee
Prosthetic replacement	Excision of diseased joint surfaces and replacement of surfaces with metal and high-density polyethylene	Hip, knee and shoulder and other joints

urate crystals within the joint or soft tissues. Management includes treatment of the acute attack with NSAIDs and long-term prophylaxis with allopurinol to reduce uric acid production after the acute attack has settled.

Management of Arthritis

Arthritis is rarely reversible, and treatment is directed at symptomatic relief and the preservation or restoration of function.

Non-Operative

Conservative Management
Conservative measures are tried initially in patients with osteoarthritis. Pain relief with simple analgesics, NSAIDs or cyclo-oxygenase 2 (COX-2) selective inhibitors will be helpful. For patients with early rheumatoid arthritis, treatment with disease modifying anti-rheumatic drugs (DMARDs) provides good results. The medical treatment of rheumatoid and other forms of arthritis is beyond the scope of this chapter.

Intra-Articular Steroid Injection
The role of this is controversial and it is not used in young people. An intra-articular injection often provides pain relief because the inflammatory reaction within the joint is reduced, but repeated steroid injections may increase joint degeneration by the inhibition of the normal processes of repair. In general, two or three injections should be the maximum at any one point.

Weight Reduction
Weight loss is encouraged. Not only is the load transmitted through the damaged joint reduced but also obesity is associated with an increase in the complications of operation should this ultimately be required.

Aids to Daily Living (ADLs)
These should be considered; they include walking sticks and crutches. The rheumatoid patient with limited hand function may require special large-handled cutlery and easy-open containers for medication.

Operative
When conservative measures have failed, surgical options need to be considered.

Arthroscopy
A joint that is swollen and inflamed may benefit from an arthroscopic washout which removes inflammatory mediators, fragments of cartilage and loose bodies and to evaluate articular and meniscal damage and direct debridement. There is no evidence of benefit for simple washout procedures.

Synovectomy
The role of synovectomy has reduced as more effective medical treatments for rheumatoid arthritis have become available. Surgical excision of the synovium or tendon sheath in rheumatoid arthritis can occasionally be beneficial. In the past it was performed as an open procedure with consequent considerable joint morbidity, but this has been replaced by arthroscopic synovectomy with special powered instruments.

Joint Surgery
Long-term or permanent relief of the symptoms of arthritis requires surgery on the bones of the affected joint. A variety of options are available (Table 35.4) and the choice depends on a number of factors, including:
- age
- patient expectation
- occupation
- the joint affected

In the younger patient with osteoarthritis, prosthetic replacement (Table 35.5) is avoided, if possible, because of the limited lifespan of the prosthesis. The results of further replacements after initial failure (revision surgery) are not as good as those of the primary procedure, and with each subsequent attempt, the surgery becomes more challenging. Almost any joint in the arm or leg can be replaced. Usually, the replacement consists of a metal component bearing on a high-density polyethylene surface. The prosthesis may be cemented into place with methyl-methacrylate bone cement or be uncemented, with the surface textured to encourage bone ingrowth. New surfaces include the use of hydroxy-apatite (HA), which is the basic mineral of bone. With

TABLE 35.5	Types of Joint Replacement.			
Type	**Nature**	**Comments**	**Examples**
Constrained	Simple hinge	Loosening because of inevitable rotational movement	Elbow, wrist
Semi-constrained	Simple hinge, but some rotation possible	Still subject to loosening	Elbow, wrist
Unconstrained	Two independent parts so that stability depends on sound anchorage in bone and the soft tissues	Most common type in use; highly satisfactory	Hip, knee, ankle, shoulder, elbow

In the knee, the replacement can be unicompartmental if one side only is affected; more usually, all three compartments are replaced

HA chemically bonded to the surface of the prosthesis, the patient's bone can directly bind the implant. The first successful replacement was the hip joint developed by Charnley in the 1960s, although previous attempts had been made to replace the hip as far back as the 1930s. The modern hip joint can be expected to last for 15–20 years but this depends upon:

- surgical experience and implant alignment
- state of the recipient bone
- prosthesis design
- stresses placed upon the implant
- the materials used at the bearing surfaces – recent research has supported hard-on-soft articulations with metal on polyethylene/ceramic on polyethylene or hard-on-hard ceramic-on-ceramic articulations.
- infection related loosening

Approximately 101 000 hip replacements and 108 000 knee replacements were implanted in 2016–2017 in England, Wales and Northern Ireland.[1]

Complications of joint replacement surgery include:

- General complications of any major operation
- Specific complications of the procedure, including intra-operative fractures, postoperative dislocations and fractures, infection of the implant and loosening

Loosening may be secondary to infection or an aseptic mechanical process. If the prosthesis is mechanically loose, it can be removed and replaced, but when infection is present, the safest option is to remove all the foreign material, identify the infective agent and treat this vigorously. At a second procedure, it may then be possible to insert another prosthesis.

Joint replacement surgery in rheumatoid arthritis carries particular risks. The immune response is altered, and infection rates are higher. At operation, the bones are often osteoporotic with an increased risk of intra-operative fractures. When multiple joints are involved, the surgeon may be embarking on an extended programme of replacement.

Infections

Acute Osteomyelitis

Before the introduction of antibiotics, acute osteomyelitis was a common infection with a 50% mortality. In the Western world, the condition has now become much less common – although the reason for this is not entirely clear – and fatalities are rare.

Aetiology

Haematogenous

Organisms transported by the bloodstream from a distant site lodge in the capillaries of bone (usually, but not always, the metaphysis of a long bone) and set up a focus. Their origin is usually not clear but occasionally there may be a distant infected focus, such as a boil. Localization of the infection may be determined by a minor injury to the bone, although this is not well established in pathological terms.

Individuals of any age may be infected but the condition is more common in children.

Exogenous

Direct inoculation of bone from the outside takes place as a result of a surgical procedure or after an open fracture.

Pathological Features

Organisms

In haematogenous osteomyelitis, the agent is most commonly *Staphylococcus aureus* (85%), now often penicillin resistant.

Streptococcus pyogenes and *Pseudomonas aeruginosa* are other pus-producing organisms sometimes involved. Occasionally, *Salmonella typhimurium* is found either with or without an intestinal infection and is more common in patients with sickle cell disease. *Escherichia coli* may infect the bones of neonates.

Infection from without can be with any organism and is often mixed.

Pathological Course

In haematogenous osteomyelitis, a short period of intense inflammation is speedily followed by pus formation within the medulla. Because bone is not expandable, pressure rises rapidly with two effects:

- pus is forced through the Haversian canals to reach the periosteum, so forming a subperiosteal abscess
- blood vessels in the Haversian canals thrombose, and the bone dies; stripping of periosteum contributes to this infarction

Eventually, if treatment does not take place, pus breaks through the periosteum, tracks up to the skin surface and discharges to produce an infected sinus. There is dead bone in its depths which gradually separates to form a sequestrum.

Exogenous infection does not usually pursue such an acute course, and damage to bone is less. However, it is often persistent and chronic.

Clinical Features

History
There is often a history of minor trauma. The patient, usually a child, is unwell with a high pyrexia and – if old enough to voice this – a complaint of severe localized bone pain. The affected limb is held still (pseudoparalysis).

Physical Findings
- *Look*:
  - redness and oedema may be seen over the affected metaphysis
  - the limb is held still
- *Feel*:
  - warmth at the affected site
  - focal bony tenderness – an important sign
  - fluctuant swelling overlying the bone
- *Move*:
  - pain on movement

Investigation

Imaging
Plain X-ray is initially normal. Changes occur after 10–14 days, when the periosteum is lifted and there is local rarefaction. Later, dead bone and sequestra show up as sclerosis.

Ultrasound may identify a subperiosteal abscess.

Radioisotope bone scan shows increased activity after a few days but well before anything is seen on X-ray.

MRI is extremely sensitive in identifying intraosseous oedema and pus.

Blood Examination
White cell count, ESR and CRP are raised.

Blood culture (before the administration of antibiotics) is positive in half of those with haematogenous osteomyelitis.

Management

Non-Operative
High-dose intravenous antibiotics are begun immediately after a blood culture has been taken. The affected limb is elevated and splinted because this helps to relieve pain.

Antibiotic therapy is continued until the ESR has returned to normal, which may take 6 weeks or longer.

Surgical
If the patient fails to respond by speedy return of temperature to normal and relief of pain, or if there is a fluctuant abscess on presentation, then the site is explored. The periosteum is incised and the underlying bone drilled to drain and decompress the medullary cavity.

Complications
Complications are:
- acute septic arthritis secondary to direct spread from adjacent bone
- pathological fracture through bone that is rarefied because of infection
- growth impairment from epiphyseal involvement
- chronicity because of dead bone
- chronic osteomyelitis

Chronic Osteomyelitis

This condition occurs because of inadequate treatment of acute osteomyelitis, or it may complicate the management of an open fracture or the surgical treatment of a closed one.

It is now rare in the UK.

Clinical Features

History
There has usually been an episode of acute haematogenous osteomyelitis, often followed by a discharging sinus. Evidence of infection is dormant for months or years with an occasional flare-up in which there is local pain and swelling with discharge of pus.

Physical Findings
There are often scars from old sinuses, one or more of which may still be open with a purulent discharge.

Investigation

Imaging
Plain X-ray shows grossly abnormal bone with areas of rarefaction and sclerosis. A sequestrum appears as a separate piece of dense bone lying within a cavity.

Isotope bone scan may show increased activity although, if there is a sequestrum, reduced uptake is present in relation to it.

CT may give useful information on the exact size and position of a sequestrum.

Examination of the Blood
This is usually unhelpful, but the ESR may be raised. Blood culture is negative except during a flare-up.

Management

Non-Operative
Antibiotics are insufficient by themselves as they are unable to penetrate the dense soft-tissue fibrosis and the relatively ischaemic bone. The occasional flare-up can be managed with dry dressings until the sinus stops discharging.

Surgical
The aim of surgery is to remove all dead bone and infected material. A chain of antibiotic impregnated beads can then be implanted in the cavity to give a very high but localized concentration of antibiotic.

Complications

Complications are:
- pathological fracture
- amyloidosis
- squamous cell carcinoma in the sinus tract

Septic Arthritis

Any joint may be affected but the common site is the knee and hip.

Aetiology

Causes are:
- Haematogenous spread from a distant focus of infection
- Secondary to acute osteomyelitis
- Direct inoculation after trauma or surgery – the incidence after arthroscopy is less than 0.2%

Pathological Features

Organisms
- *S. aureus*
- *S. pyogenes*
- *Neisseria gonorrhoeae*

Course

The hyaline cartilage is destroyed by a combination of ischaemia and toxic enzymes released by white blood cells and bacteria. As with osteomyelitis, unchecked development of pus eventually ruptures the joint capsule, and discharge occurs through the skin. Such a damaged joint heals with either a fibrous or a bony ankylosis.

Clinical Features

History

The patient complains of increasingly severe pain in the joint and is unwell with a high swinging pyrexia.

Physical Findings
- *Look* for:
  - a red and swollen joint
  - immobility because of pain
  - rarely, evidence of a local wound
- *Feel* for:
  - local warmth
  - local tenderness
- *Move*:
  - marked pain on movement

Investigation

Imaging

Plain X-ray is normal in the early stages. After 2–3 weeks, there is local rarefaction of the adjacent bone and loss of joint space. Still later, the necrosis of cartilage reduces the joint space still further. Finally, bony ankylosis can be seen.

Blood Examination

The white cell count, ESR and CRP are raised and blood culture may be positive.

Joint Aspiration

This should always be done (before commencing antibiotics) and is both diagnostic and therapeutic. The aspirate is sent for culture. At the same time, the toxic content of the effusion can be reduced by washing out the joint cavity.

The reduction of intra-articular pressure provides relief from pain.

Management

Medical

High-dose intravenous antibiotics are begun (flucloxacillin up to 8 g 6-hourly or clindamycin up to 1.2 g 6-hourly if allergic to penicillin), adjusted on the results of culture and continued until the ESR has returned to normal, which may take 6 weeks. The joint is rested.

Surgical

Pus within a joint must be washed out as a matter of some urgency. This may be performed via an arthrotomy; however, some joints such as the knee, ankle, shoulder and elbow can easily be washed out through the arthroscope. This is simply because of the larger bore of the instrument, a more efficient form of aspiration.

Complications

Complications are:
- dislocation – in particular, the hip in children
- joint stiffness
- secondary osteoarthritis

Bone Tumours

These are either primary or secondary. Primary tumours may be either benign or malignant, but some are in an intermediate group which, although showing locally invasive features, do not metastasize. A detailed classification is given in Table 35.6.

Clinical Features

History

When the tumour is secondary, there may be symptoms from the primary malignancy, although sometimes the first presentation is with bone pain or a pathological fracture. Pain is common and is localized at the site of the tumour. It is usually constant with no relieving factors and often worse at night.

A lump may be noticed.

Physical Findings

A thorough general examination is required. Most bone tumours are secondary deposits, and so the common sites of a possible primary (breast, lung, prostate, thyroid and kidney) must be examined (Table 35.7):
- *Look* for a lump.
- *Feel* for:
  - a lump
  - local bony tenderness
  - crepitus under the fingers when there is a history of possible pathological fracture

TABLE 35.6	Bone Tumours.			
Cell of origin	**Benign**	**Intermediate**	**Malignant**
Osteoblast	Osteoid osteoma	Osteoblastoma	Osteosarcoma
Osteoclast		Giant-cell tumour (osteoclastoma)	
Chondroblast	Chondroma Osteochondroma		Chondrosarcoma
Fibroblast	Non-ossifying fibroma (unicameral bone cyst)		Fibrosarcoma
Vascular	Haemangioma	Aneurysmal bone cyst	Haemangiosarcoma
Marrow		Plasmacytoma	Ewing's sarcoma Lymphoma Myeloma Leukaemia

TABLE 35.7	Common Sites of Primary in Secondary Bone Tumour.
Site	**Incidence (%)**
Breast	35
Prostate	30
Bronchus	10
Kidney	5
Thyroid	2

- *Move* – Restricted movement due to pain or possible abnormal movement in the presence of a pathological fracture.

Investigation

Imaging

Plain X ray is always needed. Benign tumours have a sharp, well-defined margin and the cortex is intact. By contrast, malignant growths are expansive with indistinct margins and destruction of the cortex. In osteosarcoma, new bone formation is seen – so-called 'sun-ray spicules'. *Isotope scan* differentiates secondary deposits – which produce multiple areas of increased activity – from a primary tumour in which there is usually a solitary active area. *MRI* is also useful for the assessment of local spread within the bone and adjacent soft tissues.

CT is required to assess the local spread of malignant tumours and so to aid in the planning of surgery. The lungs are scanned for evidence of metastases. *Biopsy* is essential for a histological diagnosis for all suspicious lesions.

Benign Tumours

These occur in young adults. They may be found in any bone; however, chondromas favour metacarpals, metatarsals and the phalanges.

Clinical Features

History

Benign tumours are often without symptoms unless a pathological fracture occurs. Constant local pain, often worse at night, may be the presenting feature. In osteoid osteoma, relief is obtained from aspirin but not opioid analgesics. Local pressure symptoms are typical of osteochondromas.

Physical Findings

- *Look* for any evidence of a fracture – chiefly deformity.
- *Feel* for:
  - a hard lump
  - localized bony tenderness
  - crepitus
- *Check* for pain restricting movement and test for unusual movement – indicative of a pathological fracture.

Management

If there are symptoms, curettage and bone grafting may be required. A pathological fracture through the tumour can lead to spontaneous cure.

Locally Aggressive Tumours

These tumours are not truly malignant, and metastatic spread is very rare. There is, however, local destruction, and there may be local recurrence after surgery.

Aneurysmal Bone Cysts

These are blood-filled cavities that usually occur in the spine and at the ends of long bones. On plain X-ray, the cyst is seen as an expansive lesion with thinning of the cortex. The management is curettage and bone grafting, which is usually curative. Radiotherapy may be required for recurrent lesions.

Embolization may represent optimal treatment for inaccessible lesions.

Giant-Cell Tumour (Osteoclastoma)

This occurs at the end of long bones in adults between the ages of 20 and 40 – the knee is a common site. There is local pain and possibly a pathological fracture. The X-ray appearance is that of a multiloculated lesion; the tumour extends up to the joint surface. Metastases are rare but can occur, especially after local recurrence.

Curettage with bone grafting is often followed by recurrence.

The cavity should be filled with bone cement which sets by an exothermic reaction that is cytotoxic to residual tumour cells. Local recurrence necessitates wide excision and then either bone grafting or a prosthesis.

Malignant Tumours

These are rare – only 125 new osteosarcomas and 60 new chondrosarcomas a year in the UK. They spread via the bloodstream to the lungs and other sites.

Osteosarcoma

This tumour occurs mainly in the young between the ages of 10 and 30 years. There is a second peak in the elderly in association with Paget's disease of bone.

The tumour occurs in the metaphyseal region of long bones, the knee being the most common site. Its management used to be by amputation, but now, with more effective chemotherapeutic agents and consequently a better prognosis, surgical resection is less radical. Excision of the affected bone and replacement with a custom-made or modular prosthesis now form the standard approach. Radiotherapy is usually reserved for inaccessible sites or for recurrence. With radical surgery and chemotherapy, there is a 90% survival at 1 year and over 50% at 3 years. Survival for more than 3 years means a probable cure.

Chondrosarcoma

This occurs in an older age group than that of osteosarcoma: between 30 and 70 years. Tumours commonly involve the flat bones: scapula, ribs and pelvis. They vary widely in their degree of differentiation, from high-grade anaplastic to low grade with only slow growth. Their management is by wide local excision with bone grafting or reconstruction with a custom-made prosthesis. Radiotherapy is ineffective. The 5-year survival ranges from 20% to 80%, depending on size, location and histological grade.

Fibrosarcoma

This is a rare growth in the age range of 40–60 years and occurs at any site. Management is surgical, with wide excision or amputation. The outlook is poor, with a 5-year survival rate of about 30%.

Ewing's Sarcoma

This is a highly malignant tumour that affects children and adolescents of 5–20 years. Males are slightly more frequently affected. The common site is the diaphyseal region of long bones. The clinical features, in addition to local pain and a lump, may include general ill health and fever. The lump maybe red and warm. Ewing's sarcoma is often initially misdiagnosed as acute osteomyelitis. On the plain X-ray, a characteristic 'onion peel' appearance is typically seen due to periosteal reaction. Management is by chemotherapy followed by surgical excision and radiotherapy. The outlook has been poor. However, with radical and aggressive treatment, survival rates are now approaching 50% or more at 5 years.

Plasmacytoma

This condition is rare and consists of a mass of plasma cells in bone or soft tissue which may prove to be a focal manifestation of multiple myeloma. Isolated lesions may be excised followed by a course of radiotherapy.

Secondary Tumours

Secondary bone tumours are common: about 30% of patients who die of a malignancy have bone secondaries. Common sources of the primary growth are given in Table 35.7. The patients are often over 60, because of the nature of the primary. Any bone may be affected, but the skull, vertebrae, ribs and pelvis are common sites. On plain X-ray, most secondary tumours are osteolytic but bone deposits from carcinoma of the prostate and about 10% of breast cancers are osteosclerotic. Treatment which is appropriate for the primary – such as hormone manipulation in breast and prostate cancer and chemotherapy – may alleviate the symptoms of secondary deposits. The pain may respond to anti-inflammatory drugs and local radiotherapy. Pathological fractures do not unite spontaneously. Internal fixation for medically fit patients can improve quality of life, mobility, aid nursing care and reduce analgesia requirements, although life expectancy remains unchanged. Prophylactic internal fixation should be considered when there is:

- rapid increase in local pain
- destruction of 50% or more of shaft diameter in a long bone
- a femoral lesion greater than 3 cm in diameter.
- a destructive lesion in the subtrochanteric region of the femur

SHOULDER

The shoulder is the most mobile of all joints and, with the elbow, has the prime function of manoeuvring the hand to the best position required for function, particularly to the mouth.

General Clinical Features

History

Pain is felt over the deltoid insertion in impingement syndromes (see later); at the front in arthritis; and at the top in acromioclavicular disorders. Radiation down the arm is common.

Pain from sites such as the heart, lung, diaphragm or cervical spine can be referred to the shoulder region and so it is important to take a full history and examination to determine if other pathologies co-exist.

Stiffness is a common symptom in shoulder disease, and loss of function such as inability to brush the hair or to dress oneself can be disabling.

Trauma frequently figures in the history and may cause fractures, dislocations or soft-tissue injury to the joint capsule, particularly the rotator cuff.

Mechanical derangement may be a presenting symptom, as in recurrent dislocation.

Physical Findings

- *Look* for:
  - muscle wasting of the deltoid, biceps, supraspinatus and infraspinatus
  - scars – indications of previous injury or surgery
  - the contour of the shoulder – in dislocation, the normal rounded appearance is lost and the shoulder looks squared off because of the prominence of the acromion
  - winging of the scapula because of weakness of the serratus anterior muscle
- *Feel* for the belly of biceps during resisted elbow flexion – rupture of the long head of biceps tendon results in an abnormal contour of the muscle.
- *Move:*
  - through the active and passive ranges (see Table 35.2)
  - note any painful arcs of movement during elevation of the arm – pain during mid-elevation is caused by subacromial impingement, but pain at full elevation is from an acromioclavicular disorder

Investigation
Imaging

Plain X-ray is required, both an anteroposterior and an axillary view. This can show degenerative arthritis, loose bodies and abnormal calcification – usually in tendons. In recurrent dislocation, a defect (Hill–Sachs lesion) may be seen on the posterosuperior humeral head and is caused by repeated impingement of the rim of the glenoid on the humerus.

Ultrasound scanning is commonly used as the first investigation after plain X-rays.

Arthrograms were commonly performed and are still used where MRI is unavailable. Rotator cuff tears are demonstrated by leakage of contrast medium into the subacromial bursa. Alternatively the rotator cuff can be assessed by ultrasound scan.

CT and MRI are of increasing value. A tear may be visualized, loose bodies seen and bicipital tendonitis can be diagnosed.

Arthroscopy

The procedure is both a diagnostic tool and of therapeutic value. It is possible to repair tears in the labrum of the glenoid, to stabilize the shoulder in recurrent dislocation, to

decompress the subacromial space, to repair rotator cuff, or SLAP (superior labrum from anterior to posterior at the point where the biceps tendon inserts on the labrum) lesions, synovectomy or release contractures and remove loose bodies.

Acromioclavicular Disorders

Acromioclavicular Osteoarthritis
Aetiology

This condition is often secondary to trauma.

Clinical Features
History

Pain is the usual feature often felt on the top of the shoulder in relation to the joint and aggravated by lifting the arm above the head or across the body.

Physical Findings
- *Look* for:
  - prominence of the acromioclavicular joint
  - muscle wasting, in particular in the supraspinatus
- *Feel* for:
  - localized tenderness at the joint
  - crepitus on movement
- *Test movement* – Pain is found when passive movement above shoulder level is attempted.

Management

Surgical excision of the outer end of the clavicle provides relief.

Rheumatoid Arthritis

The shoulder and acromioclavicular joint are often affected by rheumatoid arthritis. In addition to pain, there is often prominent swelling.

Management
Non-Operative

Medical management of the disease is important and provides pain relief.

Surgical

Excision of the outer end of the clavicle is performed.

Subacromial Disorders

The subacromial bursa, the rotator cuff and the tendon of biceps lie between the acromion and the head of the humerus. Any one of these structures may become trapped between the two bones and cause pain.

Impingement

This often affects the rotator cuff tendons of subscapularis and supraspinatus.

Clinical Features

A painful arc occurs on abduction of the humerus. On examination, the arc is confirmed and can be precisely defined. There is tenderness in the anterior cuff and signs of impingement are present. The most commonly used is the Hawkins sign where a forceful internal rotation on a forward flexed shoulder at 90 degrees produces subacromial pain.

Management

Non-Operative

Analgesics such as NSAIDs may help the local swelling to settle. Local steroid injection into the subacromial space is also helpful.

Surgical

If symptoms fail to improve with conservative measures, then surgery is advisable. The subacromial space is decompressed by excising the undersurface of the acromion as a wedge.

Rotator Cuff Tears

There are two causes:

- acute injury as a result of trauma and seen with dislocations of the shoulder in the elderly
- more commonly, chronic lesions from degeneration within the cuff

Pathological Features

There is a spectrum of disorders that are interconnected and which range from superficial abrasions of the rotator cuff from impingement through incomplete (partial-thickness) tears to complete full-thickness ones. However, there is not inevitable progression from one to another. Other factors such as ischaemic degeneration within the cuff coupled with trauma may determine the extent of tear.

Clinical Features

History

There may be a history of significant shoulder injury, but more usually there is chronic shoulder pain felt over the deltoid muscle, especially at one point of abduction. Adduction may also be difficult.

Physical Findings

- *Look* for muscle wasting – especially in the supraspinatus.
- *Feel* for localized tenderness along the lateral border of the acromion.
- *Test for shoulder movement* – Active movement, particularly abduction, is reduced but there is a full range of passive movement.

Management

Non-Operative

Partial tears of the cuff heal and the symptoms settle after resting the shoulder. Once acute symptoms have settled, a graduated programme of rehabilitation is begun. Tears in the elderly can be managed conservatively; surgical repair in this age group can be pursued if other treatments such as physiotherapy have failed. Severe stiffness after surgery is a complication.

Surgical

When symptoms fail to settle, then it is likely that the tear is complete. In the young, it should be repaired. The rotator cuff is exposed and repaired with interrupted sutures, which is now achieved by arthroscopic surgery, reducing morbidity. Very large tears may require grafts to close the defect. Autografts, allograft and synthetic grafts can be used.

Acute Calcific Tendonitis

Deposition of calcium hydroxyapatite within the tendon of supraspinatus may occur for unknown reasons. There is a local inflammatory reaction.

Clinical Features

History

The inflammation that takes place causes pain that is dull initially but, over a few hours, becomes increasingly severe. There is considerable muscle spasm, and a septic arthritis may be suspected, but the joint itself is not inflamed.

Physical Findings

- *Look* for:
  - a pale, sweaty patient in severe pain
  - the arm held still by the side
- *Feel* for diffuse tenderness of the whole shoulder region.
- *Test* for movement, which will be resisted because of pain.

Management

Non-Operative

Rest, anti-inflammatory drugs and local anaesthetic injections may help.

Surgical

Incising the tendon releases the calcific deposit. It squeezes out under pressure like toothpaste from a tube, and pain relief is immediate.

Adhesive Capsulitis (Frozen Shoulder)

This condition is characterized by increasing pain and relative immobility of the joint. It fundamentally is a contracture of the shoulder capsule. The aetiology is unknown, but there may be a history of minor trauma, and the disorder may also complicate other illnesses such as a myocardial infarct or pneumonia. Recent research has highlighted an association between adhesive capsulitis, insulin-dependent diabetes and Dupuytren's contracture.

Clinical Features

Pain and stiffness are the only complaints. Joint movement is limited, especially external rotation. Attempts to increase the range of passive movement cause pain. Over a period of about a year, the symptoms may gradually improve, and within 2 years the shoulder may have returned to normal but sometimes the stiffness can be protracted.

Management
Non-Operative
The mainstay of treatment is that resolution eventually takes place. Cautious physiotherapy is helpful, and steroid injections into the shoulder joint may also help during the painful phase.

Surgical
When recovery is slow and stiffness persists, a manipulation under anaesthesia is often beneficial.

Glenohumeral Disorders

Osteoarthritis

This condition is uncommon and usually secondary to trauma. Pain is felt at the front of the joint and may radiate through to the posterior aspect. Conservative measures such as anti-inflammatory agents and steroid injections into the joint help in the early stages. Persistent disability requires:

- arthroscopy – the joint is washed out and any loose bodies are removed, which gives some relief for most patients
- arthroplasty – replacement with a prosthesis; many designs are available but most consist of a metal humeral head and a high-density polyethylene glenoid
- arthrodesis – fusion of the shoulder is rarely done except as a salvage procedure after failed joint replacement

Rheumatoid Arthritis

The shoulder is commonly affected by this disease. Management is usually non-operative by treating the underlying condition and using intra-articular steroid injections. Surgical options are the same as for osteoarthritis.

Avascular Necrosis of the Humeral Head

This is much less common than the same condition in the femoral head. The causes and mechanisms are the same. Management is by treating any underlying cause and by the use of anti-inflammatory agents and physiotherapy. Surgical core decompression is indicated in early disease to arrest progress. In the late stages, when there has been collapse of the humeral head and secondary osteoarthritis has developed, an arthroplasty may be required.

Elbow

The elbow joint is a hinge that works in consort with the shoulder in positioning the hand.

General Clinical Features
History
- **Stiffness** is noticed early by patients because of difficulty in getting the hand to the mouth.
- **Pain** is common and often aggravated by movement.
- **Locking** is an occasional feature, particularly in degenerative disease.
- **Past trauma** to the joint is not uncommon.

Physical Findings
- *Look* at:
  - the shape of the joint – compare with the other side
  - contour for swellings – a bursa, rheumatoid nodule or effusion
  - carrying angle of the arm in extension – normal is 8–10 degrees of valgus.
- *Feel* for:
  - crepitus
  - bony landmarks – two epicondyles and the olecranon: do they form an equilateral triangle with the elbow flexed (Fig. 35.3)?
  - effusion – best felt between the lateral epicondyle and the olecranon; the normal hollow is filled out by a soft swelling
  - radial head during pronation and supination – does it dislocate as the forearm moves?
- *Test* for:
  - ulnar nerve function in the hand
  - movements – ask the patient to demonstrate the active range of movement; measure the passive range of movement (see Table 35.2)

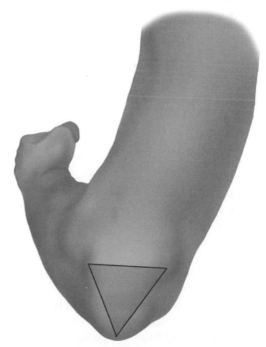

• **Fig. 35.3** Equilateral triangle formed at the elbow by two epicondyles and the olecranon

Investigation
Imaging

Plain X-ray is valuable and can show old injuries, the presence of arthritis, loose bodies and subluxation of the radial head. MRI can provide further information regarding the articular surfaces, loose bodies and surrounding soft tissues, including inflammation of the common flexor and extensor tendon origins and nerve entrapment.

Nerve Function

If an ulnar nerve lesion is suspected, electromyography is required.

Osteoarthritis
Clinical Features

The condition is almost always secondary to trauma. Pain and stiffness are the common symptoms. Locking can sometimes occur.

Management
Non-Operative

The usual initial – and often the only – treatment required consists of analgesia, local strapping and physiotherapy.

Surgical

The indications for surgery are:
- Symptomatic loose bodies that can be removed arthroscopically
- Ulnar neuritis – usually the consequence of a valgus deformity; this is treated by transposition of the nerve in front of the medial epicondyle. Fusion is indicated when there is failure of conservative treatment, with severe pain. The joint is fixed in a position of function that allows the hand to reach the mouth – about 100 degrees of flexion. Total elbow replacement is possible, but the long-term results are less satisfactory in the joint with degenerative disease as compared with rheumatoid arthritis.

Rheumatoid Arthritis

The elbow is often involved in rheumatoid arthritis, and clinical features are of pain, swelling and stiffness.

Management
Non-Operative

Most patients can be managed by control of the systemic disease and local measures including splints.

Operative

If conservative measures are not sufficient, then there are a number of surgical options.
- **Synovectomy** can produce good relief of pain and is usually performed using arthroscopy.
- **Excision of the radial head** can reduce symptoms if this structure is particularly involved.
- **Fusion and replacement** can both be considered.

Hand and Wrist

Loss of hand function is very disabling in that nearly all daily activities require the hands to a greater or lesser extent. The wrist, in conjunction with the elbow and shoulder, positions the hand in space whilst the fingers and thumb hold and manipulate.

General Clinical Features
History

Pain is often felt in the wrist but less commonly in the hand. Pain which originates in the hand may be felt across the wrist joint or be localized to a styloid process. In the fingers, it is usually related to pathological change in a joint. Pain at night which affects the hand and is associated with numbness is characteristic of compression of nerves in the carpal tunnel.

Stiffness in the wrist may not cause significant problems, but in the fingers it is an early complaint because it is so disabling.

Swelling in the hand or fingers is noticed early. Rings may become tight and so draw attention to the fingers.

Paraesthesia is usually in the distribution of a peripheral nerve.

Weakness is a common symptom in median or ulnar nerve lesions. Patients often complain of difficulty in fine finger movements such as in knitting or writing.

Physical Findings
- *Look* for:
  - the position of the hand at rest – are the fingers in fixed flexion because of fascial contractures in the palm (e.g. Dupuytren's contracture)?
  - finger deviation with ulnar drift as seen in the rheumatoid hand
  - muscle function in the hand – the thenar eminence may be atrophied in median nerve compression, and the hypothenar eminence and interossei in ulnar nerve compression
  - the pattern of any swelling at the joints of the fingers; Heberden's nodes are seen at the distal interphalangeal joints in osteoarthritis
- *Feel*:
  - the palmar aponeurosis – thickened areas may indicate aponeurotic fibrosis
  - the skin – warmth and dryness are present if there is a peripheral nerve lesion
- *Test*:
  - sensation to light touch and pinprick and establish the distribution of any loss found
  - for crepitus at the wrist on movement
  - ulnar and median nerves for Tinel's sign; this is often positive in fascial compression at the wrist or other causes of nerve excitability
  - active and passive ranges of movement (see Table 35.2)

Investigation
Imaging

Plain X-ray is often needed and can confirm if a lump arises from bone. Arthritic change and its underlying cause can be demonstrated (see Table 35.3). Old trauma may be evident. Unusual conditions such as Kienbock's disease (osteochondrosis of the lunate – often post-traumatic) or Madelung's deformity (subluxation of the distal radioulnar joint, see later) can be confirmed.

Electromyography (EMG)

If a peripheral nerve lesion is suspected, EMG is essential. It confirms the diagnosis and site of the lesion and may help to avoid unnecessary surgery.

Arthritis at the Wrist

At the wrist, osteoarthritis is often secondary to trauma. Rheumatoid arthritis also affects the wrist.

Clinical Features

The symptoms are pain, stiffness and swelling. The swelling is often accompanied by deformity from a previous fracture. Crepitus may be felt.

Management

Non-Operative

Measures such as a removable wrist splint can relieve symptoms, as do mild analgesics.

Surgical

The indications for surgery are pain and incapacity which have failed to respond to non-operative measures, such as in the young adult with post-traumatic arthritis. Of the options available (see Table 35.4), fusion is the procedure of choice. The joint is removed and a bone graft inserted. A plate is normally required for stabilization until the bone unites. Wrist joint replacement is technically feasible but remains controversial.

Arthritis of the Hand

The distribution in the hand follows a pattern characteristic of the cause.

Clinical Features

Stiffness and deformity of the fingers are common symptoms. In rheumatoid arthritis, the hand deforms in a characteristic way. Progressive destruction of the metacarpophalangeal joints causes the fingers to drift to the ulnar side, and later there is subluxation at these joints. In addition, inflammatory tenosynovitis may lead to tendon rupture with one or more dropped (semi-immobile and flexed) fingers.

Management

Because arthritis, in particular rheumatoid, is a continuing process, management varies with the stage of the disease. A series of procedures may be required as deformities develop and progress.

Non-Operative

Physiotherapy to conserve and improve hand function is essential. The occupational therapist can provide crucial aids to assist in the activities of daily living: modified cutlery with curved or flattened handles, special fasteners for clothes, and other devices may all preserve independence. Hand splints are often used. They rarely prevent deformity but do allow rheumatoid joints to be rested during an acute exacerbation of the disease.

Surgical

Various operative procedures are appropriate at different stages of the disease, but the potential problems of undertaking surgery should always be carefully discussed. Many badly deformed hands are still able to function usefully. Ruptured tendons should be repaired and, in rheumatoid arthritis, early synovectomy may delay destruction. In later stages, or in osteoarthritis, damaged joints may be replaced by Silastic implants. These correct deformities and relieve pain but rarely increase grip strength and some residual stiffness persists.

Dupuytren's Contracture

This is a condition of the hand in which there is thickening and contraction of the palmar aponeurosis, which may be due to a local change in collagen metabolism.

Aetiology and Pathological Features

The precise cause is not known, but there are nevertheless a number of well-recognized associated factors, including:

- a family history
- male sex
- regular high consumption of alcohol
- insulin-dependent diabetes mellitus
- adhesive capsulitis
- phenytoin therapy
- trauma

Contracture is bilateral in 45%; similar lesions in the plantar aponeurosis (Ledderhose disease) occur in 5%; and the penile fascia (Peyronie's disease) is affected in 3%.

Clinical Features

The condition usually develops at the base of the ring and little fingers. As the lesion progresses, the fingers gradually develop fixed flexion deformities, and the thumb web may also be involved.

Management

Non-Operative

Although many measures have been tried, none is effective. The condition may be self-limiting but is usually progressive.

Surgical

Five operations may be considered, and these are outlined in Table 35.8. The choice depends on the extent of the disease,

TABLE 35.8 **Operations for Dupuytren's contracture of the palmar fascia**

Procedure	Technique	Outcome
Percutaneous fasciotomy	Simple division of fibrous bands through percutaneous stab wounds	Recurrence rates high and damage may occur to nerves and blood vessels
Selective fasciectomy	Thickened areas are excised	Most common operation; successful in limited disease
Complete fasciectomy	Whole aponeurosis excised even if not obviously involved	Potentially curative but high incidence of skin necrosis
Complete fasciectomy and skin graft	Aponeurosis excised together with the skin of the palm followed by split-skin grafting	Curative but requires high skills
Amputation	Removal of a single digit (usually little finger), severely contracted into the palm and interfering with hand function	Can be procedure of choice in special circumstances

the degree of disability and whether or not previous operations have been done.

Nerve Entrapment Syndromes

These commonly affect the hand. Usually it is compression of the median nerve that gives rise to symptoms, but ulnar nerve entrapment at the elbow or occasionally the wrist can also occur.

Aetiology

Median nerve compression in the carpal tunnel is associated with direct compression or reduced space, although an identifiable cause cannot always be identified.

The carpal tunnel consists of a space bordered radially by the scaphoid and trapezium and ulnarly by the pisiform and hamate carpal bones and by the flexor retinaculum at its roof.

The transverse carpal ligament crosses this area and may be found to be tight at surgery. Compression at the wrist is considered a low lesion, whereas high lesions occur at the elbow and forearm.

Causes of carpal tunnel syndrome (CTS) include:

- wrist fracture – early from local haematoma and oedema or late because of a malunion and bony encroachment
- ganglion within the carpal tunnel
- tenosynovitis from rheumatoid arthritis or repetitive strain injury
- changes in the interstitial space – obesity, diabetes mellitus, hypothyroidism, pregnancy, acromegaly and amyloidosis

Ulnar nerve compression is usually at the elbow adjacent to the medial epicondyle of the humerus. There may not be an obvious cause, but a distal humeral fracture which causes a valgus deformity of the elbow may attenuate the nerve. Compression at the wrist in the ulna canal (Guyon's canal) formed between the pisiform medially and the hook of the hamate laterally is far less common.

Clinical Features

History

In **median nerve compression** – the characteristic CTS – there is often pain in the distribution of the median nerve, and this is frequently worse at night where patients wake up with tingling of the radial three and half fingers. Loss of grip and clumsiness in handling objects or 'dropping things' are other complaints.

In **ulnar nerve compression** at the elbow there may be a past history of trauma in the region of the elbow joint. Weakness and clumsiness of the hand are the chief complaints in association with shooting pain down the ulna border of the forearm.

Physical Findings

Median nerve: Wasting of the thenar eminence is seen. There is loss of sensation in the median nerve territory of lateral three and a half fingers. A positive Durkan's test is the most specific test and involves applying direct pressure over the carpal tunnel for 30 seconds with reproduction of symptoms.

Ulnar nerve: If the compression is at the elbow, evidence of elbow deformity may be apparent with an abnormal carrying angle. An elbow lesion also causes weakness of the ulnar half of flexor digitorum profundus, but flexor carpi ulnaris is weak only when the lesion is above the elbow. Wasting of the hypothenar and interosseous muscles is present (most noticeable in the first web space). The hand may appear flattened with the ring and metacarpophalangeal joints hyperextended because of lumbrical paralysis. Attempts to grip a sheet of paper between the thumb and index finger cause the trick movement of flexion of the interphalangeal joint of the thumb to compensate for the weak interossei (Froment's sign; Fig. 35.4).

Management

Non-Operative

Underlying causes of CTS at the wrist are treated. In pregnancy, the symptoms often resolve rapidly after delivery. Injections of steroid into the carpal tunnel may help in mild

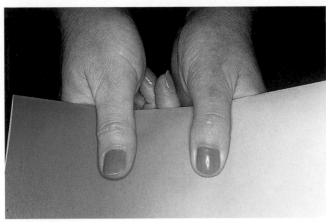

• **Fig. 35.4** Froment's sign, positive in the patient's left thumb.

cases but should not be repeated more than twice or irreversible fibrosis may take place around the median nerve. Night splints may help. Non-operative treatment of ulnar nerve compression usually fails.

Surgical

Median nerve: Decompression of the median nerve by dividing the transverse carpal ligament is a highly effective and simple procedure that can be carried out under local or general anaesthesia. Relief of symptoms is often immediate but recovery of thenar muscle wasting is not guaranteed.

Ulnar nerve: For lesions with their cause at the elbow, the nerve is released in situ (releasing the nerve as it pierces the flexor carpi ulnaris distally and proximally at the medial intermuscular septum). The nerve can be transposed to lie in front of the medial epicondyle after dividing the medial intermuscular septum which, if left intact, can irritate the nerve and cause ongoing problems. At the wrist, the volar carpal ligament is released, which forms the roof of Guyon's canal to decompress the ulna nerve. Recovery is often slower compared with the median nerve but symptoms do generally improve.

Ganglion

Ganglions are tense cysts containing viscous, jelly-like material. They frequently occur on the dorsum of the wrist and originate from joints or tendon sheaths. They are commonly found around the wrist and ankle but also occur in the hand and in the foot.

Aetiology and Pathological Features

Many explanations have been advanced but none has been conclusively established. It is possible that they are derived from small extra-articular fragments of synovium and, at times, a communication with the underlying joint or tendon sheath can be demonstrated and this would certainly explain both their inspissated contents and their tendency

to recur if incompletely removed. They are mucoid rich with no true epithelial lining.

Clinical Features

Symptoms are usually cosmetic unless previous inadequate surgical excision has caused secondary problems. Signs are of a tense, fluctuant usually globular swelling deep to skin and incompletely mobile on the deep aspect because of attachment to a neighbouring joint or tendon sheath.

Management

Non-Operative

An asymptomatic lesion which does not cause cosmetic embarrassment is best left alone. Traditional treatment has also included subcutaneous rupture – the family bible was often used. Modern therapy consists of aspiration followed by steroid injection, but this has recurrence rates of approximately 50%.

Surgical

Excision of the ganglion is effective provided the technique is meticulous and undertaken in a bloodless field and the underlying stalk/portion of adjacent capsule is also removed. In a distal interphalangeal joint ganglion (mucous cyst), the underlying osteophyte must be removed.

Trigger Finger

The cause is unknown, but is more commonly seen in diabetics. There is localized inflammation and thickening of the flexor tendon sheath, thereby restricting smooth passage of the flexor tendon, under the entrance to the synovial sheath at the base of the finger (A1 pulley).

Clinical Features

The patient complains of clicking and catching of the affected finger or 'locking' of the finger in a flexed position that requires manual straightening associated with a sharp snap.

Management

Surgical treatment is the mainstay. The A1 pulley is incised to allow the tendon to move freely.

de Quervain's Syndrome

Tenosynovitis of the tendon sheaths of the first dorsal compartment (extensor pollicis brevis and abductor pollicis longus) may be the result of local trauma, but usually no cause is found. It is most frequent in middle-aged women.

Clinical Features

The symptoms are radial-sided wrist pain and weakness of the thumb. The sheath is palpably thickened and tender. Adducting the thumb and moving the hand/wrist ulnarward (Finkelstein's test) is painful.

Management

Non-Operative

Injection of steroid into the tendon sheath is often effective, but it is important that only the sheath (and not the tendon) is injected otherwise the tendon is prone to rupture.

Surgical

The tendon sheath is released, so allowing free movement of the tendons. The procedure is curative and used when non-operative treatment fails or the condition is chronic.

Kienbock's Disease

This condition is avascular necrosis of the lunate. In most instances the cause is unknown, but it may occasionally follow dislocation of the bone. The patient – a young adult – complains of local dorsal wrist pain and stiffness. There may be no clinical findings except slight tenderness over the dorsum of the wrist with restricted wrist movement.

Investigation and Management

Plain X-ray show sclerosis of the lunate. As the condition progresses, there is fragmentation, and secondary osteoarthritis develops in the wrist joint. In the early stages a splint may help. Attempts have been made to revascularize the bone with part of the pronator quadratus muscle, but these have met with limited success. Other surgical options include:

- Removal of the bone and insertion of a Silastic prosthesis
- Shortening of the radius to decompress the lunate
- Fusion if osteoarthritis is present

Madelung's Deformity

This is a growth disorder of the distal radial epiphysis. It becomes apparent after the age of 10 years and is more common in girls. The patient complains of a prominent lump alongside the ulnar styloid with stiffness at the wrist. Examination of the mother's wrist often reveals the same deformity. There is some limitation of the range of movement.

Investigation and Management

Plain X-ray shows the distal radius to be shortened slightly and curved, with the lunate tending to subluxation between the radius and ulna. The ulna is of normal length and therefore appears more prominent. Operations should be avoided if possible. Excision of a segment of distal ulna leaves a weak wrist. In gross deformity, elongation of the abnormal radius may improve the appearance and function of the wrist but is technically challenging.

Hip

General Clinical Features and Examination

History

Pain originating from the hip tends to be felt in the groin or thigh. It may be referred to the knee, particularly in children. Pain is worse at the end of the day and on weight-bearing. Nocturnal pain may cause much loss of sleep.

Past trauma: In chronic disorders there may be a past history of trauma, e.g. fracture of the pelvis and dislocation or a fracture-dislocation of the femoral head.

Limp and gait: Limp may be noticed by others or by the patient, and there may be increasing difficulty in walking. Causes may be:

- pain as the patient tries to protect the joint
- shortening of the leg secondary to proximal migration of the femoral head
- muscle weakness.

For abnormal gaits associated with hip disorders, see Box 35.2.

Physical Findings

- *Look* at:
  - the skin for scars
  - the position of the hip – in established osteoarthritis the hip is in fixed flexion, external rotation and adduction
  - gait; this can be protective (antalgic), Trendelenburg (abnormal abductor mechanism which included the hip joint fulcrum), short- or stiff-legged
- *Feel:*
  - for crepitus on hip movement
  - measure leg length – from the anterior superior iliac spine to the medial malleolus
- *Move:*
  - Establish active range of movement.
  - Measure the passive range of movement. The normal range is shown in Table 35.2. It is important to ensure that movement is taking place at the hip alone and not the pelvis as well. Fully flex the other hip to abolish the normal lumbar lordosis to demonstrate a fixed flexion deformity as the affected leg rises up off the examination couch. On flexion, a hand under the lumbar spine can feel when the pelvis starts to tilt (Thomas hip flexion test). During abduction and adduction, a forearm resting on both anterior superior iliac spines (ASIS) across the front of the pelvis prevents pelvic tilt.

Investigation

Imaging

- **Plain X-ray** is usually sufficient to confirm a clinical diagnosis.
- **Isotope scan.** In osteoblastic lesions, there is increased uptake; avascular necrosis appears as a relatively dense area.
- **CT and MRI** can help to determine the site or extent of bony and other damage in more detail.

Blood Examination

In osteoarthritis, the ESR is normal and rheumatoid factor is absent. The reverse is usually true in rheumatoid arthritis.

Osteoarthritis

This condition is extremely common. The treatment aims to relieve pain and restore mobility, and management has been revolutionized by the development of prosthetic hip joints.

Epidemiology and Aetiology

Numerous factors contribute to the development of osteoarthritis. By far the most common is wear and tear on the joint in a population with an increased life expectancy – by the age of 80 years, 80–90% of hips show radiographic changes of osteoarthritis. Women are more commonly affected than men (3 : 1). The condition can be unilateral or bilateral. More than 10% of unilateral instances become bilateral over 5–8 years.

Management

Decisions on management depend on:
- degree of disability and its interaction with lifestyle
- general physical condition
- age – although, with modern techniques of surgery and anaesthesia, chronological age is rarely a contraindication
- the wishes of the patient

Non-Operative

Those with only minor symptoms can be managed by losing weight, physiotherapy, a walking stick and NSAIDs. Loss of 1 kg of body weight reduces the forces acting across the hip by roughly 3 kg.

Surgical

Surgery for osteoarthritis of the hip is now essentially joint replacement, although in the past there were other options (see Table 35.4). An osteotomy can provide short-term relief of pain, but a subsequent joint replacement may be difficult because of the altered anatomy. Excision arthroplasty is reserved for infected hip replacements. The modern total hip replacement was introduced in 1961 by Sir Jon Charnley and can be expected to last for approximately 15 years. However, longevity is multifactorial and affected by factors such as implant alignment, amount of loading, bearing surface wear and infection. Outcomes of individual implants are indicated in Joint Registries.[1]

The chief causes of failure are:
- aseptic loosening (without infection) with resultant pain and instability.

- infection – infection rates should ideally be less than 1%. Established prosthetic infection necessitates removal of the prosthesis, usually as part of a two-stage procedure, with reinsertion of a hip replacement once the infection has been eradicated. Loosening without infection is treated by a single stage revision procedure. A variety of surgical approaches to the hip are used, as shown in Table 35.9. Typical pre- and postoperative management is given in Clinical Box 35.1.

Rheumatoid Arthritis (RA)

This is a systemic condition which is initially managed medically. The hip and knee are involved but, in particular, it affects the upper limbs and the feet. There are a number of problems encountered with hip joint replacement in the patient with RA. When, as is often the case, multiple joints are involved, rehabilitation may be difficult. Bone quality is poor, thereby necessitating a cemented hip replacement.

CLINICAL BOX 35.1

Preoperative
- Obtain adequate and up-to-date radiological images
- Exclude intercurrent infection
  - Midstream urine sample
  - Skin infection and venous ulcers
- MRSA swabs to groin and axilla to determine carrier status
- Anaesthetic assessment
- Group and save

Postoperative
- Abduction wedge for 24 hours, to minimize risks of dislocation
- Early mobilization
- Low molecular weight heparin, dabigatran etexilate, fondaparinux sodium or rivaroxaban continued for 4–5 weeks to reduce risks of venous thrombosis (unfractionated heparin in patients with renal failure).
- Crutches or sticks to reduce risk of falling
- Inpatient stay for 3–5 days
- Standard hip precautions:
  - Raised toilet seat for 6 weeks
  - Avoid low chairs for 6 weeks
  - Do not bend down and twist

TABLE 35.9 Surgical Approaches to the Hip Joint.

Approach	Advantages	Disadvantages
Anterior/anterolateral	Reduced risk of dislocation Sciatic nerve not at risk	Increased muscle dissection Femoral nerve at risk Possible increased risk of infection
Posterior	Faster and easier approach Muscle-splitting approach, so preserving muscle power Femoral nerve not at risk Improved access to femoral canal and acetabulum, especially in revision hip surgery	Increased risk of dislocation Sciatic nerve at risk

Infection rates in RA are higher than in OA patients. Nevertheless, hip replacements in RA have a definite place for improving pain and restoring mobility provided that the hip joint is the principal site of the problem.

Osteonecrosis of the Femoral Head

In this condition, the femoral head becomes ischaemic and infarcts secondary to a disruption in the blood supply. As a result, there is structural weakness and collapse of the bone.

Aetiology

The underlying process is not fully understood. The following have been postulated:
- arterial insufficiency following a fracture or dislocation
- venous occlusion – a feature of Perthes' disease
- raised intraosseous pressure – possibly the cause in sickle cell disease, alcoholism, systemic steroids and decompression from high atmospheric pressure with the formation of gas bubbles (the bends in deep-sea-divers)

Management

Non-Operative

Treatment of any correctable underlying cause is instituted. Anti-inflammatory drugs are symptomatically helpful.

Surgical

Surgery is often required to provide pain relief:
- Core decompression – Drilling a core of bone out of the femoral head and neck is thought to be effective by reducing the intraosseous pressure and improving venous drainage. This is less helpful in later stages III or IV where structural collapse has occurred.
- Arthroplasty is reserved for the late stages post femoral head collapse and secondary osteoarthritis.

Tuberculosis

Aetiology and Pathological Manifestations

The disease is now less common, although the incidence has recently increased in the poor and in groups with immunosuppression from such causes as AIDS. The route of infection is haematogenous and the pathological features are the same as for tuberculosis in other organs – tissue destruction, abscess formation and fibrosis. Untreated, the joint progresses to fibrous ankylosis.

Clinical Features

As well as systemic symptoms of malaise and fever, local ones include a mild ache and limp. Initially, there is little to be found – only the features of an irritable hip. Later, there is marked muscle wasting, joint stiffness, pain and shortening. This chronic picture is in contrast to the acute, severe pattern of septic arthritis.

Investigation and Management

X-ray changes are of osteoporosis and, later, joint destruction. As in septic arthritis, pus is drained, samples are taken and the organism is cultured to establish sensitivity to chemotherapy and appropriate anti-tuberculosis therapy commenced. With these measures, damage can be limited. A hip that heals with ankylosis may require a shoe raise when walking is resumed. A painful joint may need to be arthrodesed. Arthroplasty is considered with caution because of risks of reactivation of the infection.

Knee

General Clinical Features

History

Age: Young adults commonly suffer injury in sport; their first presentation is often to general practitioners and casualty departments. In older individuals, the joint is more frequently affected by osteoarthritis, although injury may be a precipitating factor. In an acute event, the patient may be able to pinpoint the exact moment of injury.

Pain: Generalized or localized pain is a frequent symptom. The location is important because it provides clue to the diagnosis. Generalized pain over the whole knee is a feature of arthritis and acute injury. In meniscal tears, pain is localized to the joint line, including posteriorly in the popliteal fossa. Collateral ligament sprains cause pain above or below the joint line. Anterior pain is a symptom of disorders of the patella such as chondromalacia. Such anterior pain is frequently worse when the knee is loaded in flexion – characteristically when going up or down stairs. Deficiency of the anterior cruciate ligament is often associated with a sensation of giving way and associated diffuse pain.

Mechanism of injury: Commonly, there is a twisting injury, often with an associated tearing or popping sensation from the joint which is accompanied by pain. The patient may well fall to the ground and, if playing sport, has to stop.

Swelling may be immediate (within an hour) and implies an acute haemarthrosis (the usual causes are given in Table 35.10). Swelling delay for several hours suggests a meniscal injury. Arthritic knees are chronically swollen from either an effusion or thickened synovium.

Locking and giving way occur when the knee is unstable, or if a loose body or tear in the meniscus is present. Locking prevents the knee achieving full extension – in the acute presentation, this is commonly known as 'locked knee' and commonly due to a bucket handle tear of the meniscus.

The arthritic knee may also give way because of instability and may lock because of loose bodies trapped in the joint.

Physical Findings

- *Look* for:
  - swelling in the joint – by assessing contour and fluid in the medial and lateral aspects of the knee
  - wasting of the quadriceps

TABLE 35.10	Causes of Acute Haemarthrosis of the Knee.	
Lesion[a]		**Percentage**
Anterior cruciate ligament rupture		39
Peripheral meniscal tear		26
Collateral ligament injury		13
Capsular tear		9
Osteochondral fracture		7
Posterior cruciate ligament rupture		6

[a]Seventy percent have more than one lesion, 29% have only one lesion, and in 1%, no cause is found

- position at rest – is the joint in fixed flexion or is there a varus or valgus deformity?
- scars – previous arthroscopy portals can be missed unless examination is meticulous
- abnormal skin colour
- *Feel* for:
  - swelling – if present, is it bony or a boggy synovial thickening or fluid?
  - the presence of an effusion (see below)
  - altered temperature
  - the joint line – medially, laterally and in the popliteal fossa. Local joint line tenderness suggests a meniscal pathology
  - tenderness over the femoral condyles when the knee is flexed; may occur in arthritis
  - the patella – is it very mobile; when pushed laterally, does the patient flinch or grimace (called a positive apprehension test, as seen in patients with recurrent dislocations); is there tenderness on the retropatellar surface?
  - loose bodies maybe palpable
  - crepitus when the joint is moved

Effusion is diagnosed by two methods. The first, cross-fluctuation, is the more sensitive of the two. The second, the patellar tap test, confirms a large effusion but may not be elicited with a small collection.

Cross-fluctuation. The suprapatellar pouch is emptied by placing one hand proximal to the patella, so pushing any fluid down into the main cavity of the joint. The hand stays in position and the medial and lateral sides are examined. In the normal knee, a soft hollow is seen, but this is absent with a large effusion. With a stroking motion of the other hand to the medial and lateral sides, fluid can be pushed across the joint. In the presence of an effusion, a soft swelling appears on the opposite side of the knee to the hand.

Patellar tap. The suprapatellar pouch is emptied as before and kept empty by leaving the hand above the patella. The other hand gently presses the patella down onto the underlying femoral condyles. There is a distinct feeling of the patella sinking down and coming to a sudden stop when it hits the condyles with a 'tap'.

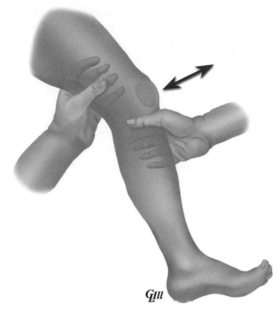

• **Fig. 35.5** Lachman's test for integrity of the anterior cruciate.

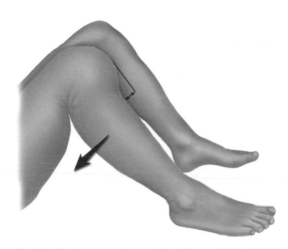

• **Fig. 35.6** Posterior sag in a lesion of the posterior cruciate.

Collateral ligament stability is assessed with the knee in 20 degrees of flexion. A varus strain is applied to test the lateral collateral ligament; a valgus strain for assessing integrity of the medial collateral ligament.

Cruciate ligaments The integrity of the anterior cruciate is assessed by performing the Lachmans test (Fig. 35.5) or anterior draw test and the posterior cruciate by looking for a 'posterior sag' (Fig. 35.6).

Quadriceps wasting. The circumference of the leg is measured on both sides at a fixed distance (usually 10 cm) above the upper border of the patella.

Movement. The patient is asked to walk. On bearing weight, does the knee go into a valgus or varus deformity? There may be an antalgic, short leg or stiff leg gait (see Box 35.2). The range of active movement is then assessed and compared with the passive range. Is it possible to get the knee to full extension, or is there a block? Finally, in a normal knee, the patella tracks evenly on the trochlear surface of the femur. Maltracking occurs when the patella is seen to subluxate or dislocate laterally as the knee moves.

Investigation
Imaging

Plain X-ray reveal any arthritis. Loose bodies may be seen, often in the intercondylar notch. On the lateral film, the length of the patella should be about equal to the distance from the inferior pole of the patella to the tibial tuberosity. If it is less than this, then the patella is riding high (patella alta) which predisposes to dislocation. *Skyline views* show the patellofemoral joint and are taken with the knee flexed. The patella should be horizontal and centrally positioned within its trochlear groove. *Tunnel views* are taken with the knee flexed to 45 degrees and provide a view of the intercondylar notch. They are useful if loose bodies are suspected. If an avulsion of the anterior cruciate is possible, then a small flake of bone torn off the tibial plateau may be seen. *Weight-bearing films* accentuate any loss of joint space and also show up varus/valgus deformities.

Arthrography can show meniscal and capsular tears. With the advent of MRI and diagnostic arthroscopy, its use is declining.

CT is not often used in the knee but can show arthritis, loose bodies and patella malalignment.

MRI can demonstrate meniscal and cruciate injuries. It is non-invasive and in most centres has replaced arthrography.

Radioisotope scan shows increased activity in degenerative conditions which may be localized to one compartment, but are rarely used nowadays.

Meniscal Injuries

A meniscus trapped between the joint surfaces may tear. There are five main types of tear (Fig. 35.7). The distribution is:

- medial meniscus 70%
- lateral meniscus 25%
- both 5%

The more frequent involvement of the medial meniscus is because it is firmly adherent to the medial capsule and therefore less mobile than the lateral one.

Clinical Features
History

There has usually been a painful twisting injury, often during sport. There may be an associated 'pop', 'crack' or tearing sensation within the joint and swelling quickly appears. Subsequently, there is persistent swelling and a feeling of something catching. Occasionally, the knee locks as the torn meniscus becomes lodged within the joint (locked knee).

Physical Findings

- *Look* for:
  - effusion
  - wasted quadriceps by comparison with the other side
- *Feel* for:
  - effusion
  - tenderness at the joint line
- *Test movement* for:
  - springy feel in a locked knee
  - McMurray's test – with the knee at 90 degrees of flexion, the tibia is rotated on the femur to try to trap the meniscal tear between the femoral condyle and tibial

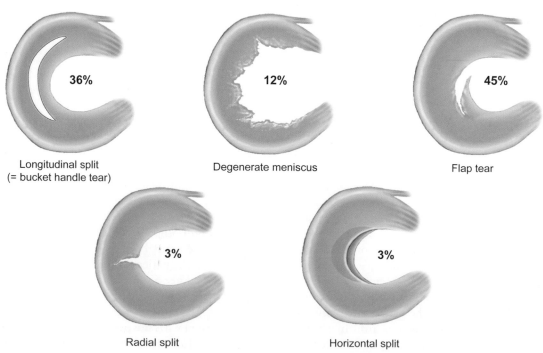

Longitudinal split
(= bucket handle tear)   36%

Degenerate meniscus   12%

Flap tear   45%

Radial split   3%

Horizontal split   3%

• **Fig. 35.7** Types of meniscal tear in the knee.

plateau; internal rotation of the tibia catches a lateral meniscus and external rotation the medial; in either event, pain is felt at the joint line

Management

Non-Operative

When there is doubt about the diagnosis, then it is reasonable to treat the symptoms with a review in 2–3 weeks, with appropriate MRI cross-sectional imaging. In those with improvement, a graduated programme of knee rehabilitation is continued. When symptoms and signs persist, surgery should be considered.

Surgical

When the clinical features are typical, then the management is surgical. Arthroscopy (see later) is both diagnostic and therapeutic – the tear can be seen and then either excised or repaired depending on the type of tear. Acute repairable tears of the meniscus are present in the red-red peripheral zone (the only region of meniscus that has a viable blood supply). After surgery, it is vital that formal rehabilitation is undertaken to improve the chances of a full recovery. This starts immediately with quadriceps exercises and, once the arthroscopic portals have healed, swimming, cycling and resistance training can begin. Only when all these activities are managed with ease is a return to impact loading exercises such as jogging, low-impact aerobics and, finally, high-impact sporting activities are allowed.

Anterior Cruciate Ligament (ACL) Injuries

Mechanism and Pathological Features

These injuries are sustained after a twisting and valgus strain is applied to the knee. Typically, they are seen in the footballer who twists on the knee during a tackle against an opposing player. In women, the most common cause of ACL rupture is skiing. The medial collateral ligament and medial meniscus are often damaged at the same time. Hyperextension on its own can also produce an isolated ACL rupture. Occasionally, any of these mechanisms may avulse a fragment of bone at the insertion of the ACL onto the tibial plateau, something more common in adolescents.

Clinical Features

Physical examination demonstrates only about 70% of ruptures of the ACL. The diagnosis is confirmed by MRI.

Management

Non-Operative

The knee with a ruptured ACL can often be managed without the need for surgery. Intensive rehabilitation is used to strengthen the hamstring and quadriceps muscles and improve proprioception at the knee. Swimming, cycling and weight training followed by gentle jogging can then be attempted. Change in lifestyle with withdrawal from some sports or other activities may be necessary. A brace can help to stabilize the knee during the rehabilitation phase, of which a large variety are available but all rely on firm strapping above and below the knee, with metal or carbon fibre supports for tennis or skiing.

Surgical

With effective non-operative management, surgery may often be avoided. If it is, an urgent operation has no advantage over delayed reconstruction. The only unequivocal indication for early repair is when a fragment of bone has been avulsed from the tibial plateau, in which case the fragment should be reattached with a screw. Delayed reconstruction may be required if the torn ACL continues to cause instability (giving way). Various methods to stabilize the knee have been used in the past, including an extra-articular reconstruction or use of synthetic intra-articular grafts; however, the current favoured surgical technique is an intra-articular reconstruction using either the patellar tendon or autologous hamstring tendons harvested from the patient's own knee.

Posterior Cruciate Ligament (PCL) Injuries

Rupture of the posterior cruciate ligament is much less common than that of the ACL and is often not recognized. The tibia is forced posteriorly on the femoral condyles – as in a head-on car crash when the lower leg hits the dashboard.

Clinical Features

The functional instability after PCL rupture may be minimal, with the symptoms of pain, stiffness and an effusion only developing after degenerative changes in the knee have occurred. In an acute injury, there is a tense haemarthrosis with perhaps soft-tissue abrasions on the front of the tibia.

Investigation and Management

Plain X-ray shows an effusion and sometimes a piece of bone that has been avulsed off the back of the tibia (PCL insertion). A change in lifestyle, including types of sporting activity, may allow the patient to lead a near-normal life. An avulsed fragment should be exposed through the popliteal fossa and reattached. In a rupture with chronic problems, the indications for surgical treatment are the same as for reconstruction of the ACL, and the methods are also similar.

Recurrent Dislocation of the Patella

The patella is a mobile sesamoid within the quadriceps tendon and is in a vulnerable position in front of the knee. True dislocation must be differentiated from maltracking in which there is painful subluxation.

Clinical Features

History

Full dislocation. The patella always dislocates laterally, and there is usually a history of direct trauma to the medial side, often during sport. The patient sees and feels the bone displaced, and the knee is locked in 30–40 degrees of flexion. Anterior pain and rapid swelling develop.

Subluxation. The patella is felt to 'pop' out of place, often during a turning movement. Pain is momentary and sharp over the front of the knee, which may feel unstable or give way. Minor swelling is noted over 24 hours.

Physical Findings in Acute Dislocation

- *Look* for:
  - the patella on the lateral side of the knee
  - knee locked in flexion
  - presence of an effusion
- *Feel* for:
  - lateral based position of the patella
  - tenderness on the medial side of the patella after reduction over the MPFL (medial patella femoral ligament)
  - effusion
- *Test* for reducibility by applying firm pressure on the lateral side and simultaneously extending the knee; the bone may reduce with a 'snap'.

Investigation

Plain X-ray shows the displacement. After reduction, patella alta (see below) may be seen. Skyline views are essential and may reveal an osteochondral fracture that occurs as the patella dislocates over the lateral femoral condyle, something that must not be missed as it will require fixation. In subluxation, X-rays may be normal or show patella alta (high riding patella).

Arthritis

Arthritis of the knee is very common, and the usual form is osteoarthritis. Rheumatoid arthritis also occurs but less frequently. As in the hip, the management of this painful, disabling condition has been transformed by the development of prosthetic replacement, as well as modern day disease-modifying drugs.

Clinical Features

History

Pain is the main complaint. Initially this is felt only after activity but later also at rest. Accompanying stiffness and swelling is initially intermittent but eventually becomes permanent. It is also common for the joint to lock because of loose bodies and painfully give way.

Physical Findings

- *Look* for:
  - varus or valgus deformity with the patient standing
  - swelling
- *Feel* for:
  - an effusion
  - tenderness over the joint line and the femoral condyles
  - crepitus

- *Test* for:
  - movement – fixed flexion deformity is common
  - collateral ligament laxity, especially in the presence of varus or valgus deformity

Management

Non-Operative

Weight loss, analgesics, physiotherapy, a walking stick and foam heel wedges all help in those with mild symptoms.

Surgical

There are several surgical options. The choice depends on:

- wishes of the patient
- age
- degree of disability

Arthroscopy is a useful first step and allows the surgeon to assess the extent of the cartilage degeneration/destruction. Debris in the joint can be washed out, and any chondral flaps or loose bodies can be removed and degenerative meniscal tears trimmed, all of which may provide short- to medium-term symptom relief. In rheumatoid arthritis, an arthroscopic synovectomy is symptomatically useful in that synovial hypertrophy contributes to the inflammatory process.

Osteotomy. Often the medial compartment of the knee is the main compartment affected by the arthritis and the lateral side is relatively spared. An osteotomy can be performed to realign the knee, and weight-bearing axis transferred to the relatively healthy side. This procedure is of use in the younger patient and may provide 8–10 years of pain relief. Once the lateral side starts to wear, a knee replacement can be performed.

Total knee replacement. Knee replacements with a hinge were inserted in the early 1950s, and later in that decade, metal discs were interposed but with poor results. However, it was not until the early 1970s, with the development of dedicated instrumentation and unconstrained (no hinge) prostheses, that the results improved. 'Unconstrained' means that stability relies on the surrounding tissue tension to hold the two parts in correct alignment. A large variety of knee replacements are now available. These fall into three main groups as shown in Table 35.5.

The majority of primary knee replacements are unconstrained and either retain the PCL (Cruciate Retaining) or sacrifice it (Posterior Stabilized). It is imperative that the soft tissues are balanced to ensure stability. Bone cuts can be based on anatomical structures (measured resection) or by soft tissue tension (gap balancing) by employing a calibrated measuring device (e.g. Gobot, Stryker UK). Outcomes of individual implants are indicated in Joint Registries.[1]

Arthrodesis. This operation has largely been superseded by joint replacement. It can be a salvage procedure after joint replacement has failed. The knee is fused in a functional position of about 5–10 degrees of flexion, which allows the limb to be swung through during the relevant phase of the gait cycle.

ANKLE AND FOOT

Ankle

General Clinical Features

History

Pain from the ankle joint is often felt as a band across the front. When there is a problem involving the malleolus, the symptoms may be to one side or the other. Pain from the subtalar joint tends to be felt below the ankle and may radiate forwards into the foot.

Instability is a sensation of unusual movement, usually from side to side, and is common because of the frequent exposure of the ankle to twisting strains.

Swelling around the ankle may be the consequence of local disease such as arthritis or of more general problems—cardiac or renal. In chronic instability, it is often localized at one or other malleolus.

Trauma is often an important factor. In addition to predisposing to chronic instability, it can also cause secondary osteoarthritis – the result of damage to the articular cartilage at the time of injury and subsequent joint surface irregularity or from avascular necrosis following a talus fracture.

Physical Findings
- *Look* for:
  - swelling
  - scars
  - Inspect the gait (see Box 35.2). It may be antalgic (pain avoidance) or there may be foot drop, which causes the toes to contact the ground when normally the heel should strike first; this is a high stepping gait seen after injury to the sciatic nerve at the buttock, or the common peroneal nerve at the knee.
- *Feel* for:
  - localized tenderness in the malleoli
  - crepitus (perform this gently) in the area
  - swelling – boggy synovial thickening, pitting oedema or an effusion within the joint
  - local warmth
- *Move* the ankle for:
  - active and passive range – the ankle joint is capable of both plantarflexion and dorsiflexion from a neutral position; inversion and eversion occur at the subtalar joint; this test is done by holding the lower leg with one hand and grasping the heel with the other so that the subtalar joint can then be moved separately.
  - excessive movement – laxity of the collateral ligaments is detected on inversion and eversion; drawing the foot forwards and backwards on the lower leg may reveal subluxation.

Investigation

Imaging
- **Plain X-rays** may show arthritis or evidence of old trauma. When the history is one of instability, there may be localized arthritic changes at the malleolus with perhaps a loose body at the tip of the malleolus from an old avulsion fracture. Avascular necrosis of the talus results in sclerosis and collapse of the bone. If the history and examination suggest that the site of the problem is in the subtalar joint, it may be necessary to request plain films of this joint.
- **Stress X-ray** are performed by applying a valgus or varus strain to the joint while X-rays are taken – when this is painful, general anaesthesia may be required. If there is significant instability, the talus may be shown to tilt within the mortise of the ankle joint.
- **Isotope bone scan** may show an increase in activity in the ankle or subtalar joint or at a malleolus. In avascular necrosis of the talus, there is an area of reduced uptake.
- **CT or MRI** confirm the presence of arthritis and are also helpful when avascular necrosis is suspected, as its extent can be clearly seen. MRI highlights any ligament or reticular cartilage pathology.

Chronic Instability

This condition is better prevented than cured. The cause is an inversion or eversion injury that tears the collateral ligament under stress.

Clinical Features

There is usually a history of the relevant injury. There is tenderness over the ligament just distal to the malleolus. Evidence of bruising is only present in the early stages.

Investigation and Management

Stress X-rays will demonstrate talar tilt, although this investigation may be difficult in the acute phase because of pain. In a patient with an acute injury in whom a diagnosis of a collateral ligament tear has been made, the traditional treatment has been 3 weeks in a below-knee plaster cast to allow the ligament to heal. More recently, early intensive physiotherapy with proprioceptive training on a 'wobble board' (a board balanced on a ball) has been advocated, and the results are better than cast immobilization. In spite of adequate treatment, chronic instability may become established and this is treated:
- *Non-operatively* – This may be sufficient if the patient alters lifestyle, changes to a different sport or wears boots that support the ankle.
- *Surgically* – A number of operations have been described; as well as reconstituting the affected ligament with synthetic grafts, further support is provided by using a local structure such as the tendon of peroneus brevis. The joint capsule may be shrunk with a thermal technique.

Arthritis

As a weight-bearing joint, the ankle is prone to osteoarthritis but much less commonly than the hip or the knee. The reason is unclear but may be in part because the ankle is essentially a hinge joint, whereas at the hip and knee, there is also rotation and therefore extra shear forces on the cartilage. Nevertheless, post-traumatic secondary osteoarthritis of the ankle is common in young adults involved in athletics. Involvement by rheumatoid arthritis is to a similar extent as the hip and knee.

Management
Non-Operative
This is the most common method: a walking stick; firm boots that go above the ankle, thereby limiting movement at the joint; and anti-inflammatory drugs are used.

Surgical
Operation is less satisfactory in the ankle than in the hip or knee; the options are fusion, providing a stiff painless joint, or arthroplasty. Prosthetic replacements are available but the long-term results are not as good as in the hip or knee and ankle fusions generally do better, especially in the younger, more active population.

Foot

Painful feet are very common. The hazard of attempts at surgical management of an individual lesion is that it may merely transfer the problem from one part of the foot to another and so never achieve a cure.

Clinical Features
History
Pain is the usual presenting symptom, most commonly localized to one area, but it may radiate, be worse on weight-bearing and be relieved by rest. There is often difficulty in finding shoes that can be worn without pain.

Physical Findings
The appearance of the foot can be the presenting feature.
- *Look* for:
  - shape, including any callosities over bony prominences
  - the shoes and in what areas they show signs of wear – an indication of how load is being transferred
  - evidence of vascular insufficiency – the presence of peripheral vascular disease may contraindicate surgery on the foot
- *Feel* for:
  - local tenderness
  - pulses in the foot (dorsalis pedis and posterior tibial)
- *Move:*
  - the midtarsal joint by holding the heel with one hand and the forefoot with the other
  - the toes – are any deformities correctable?

Investigation
Imaging
Plain X-ray of the foot may be required so as to plan an operation. The presence of radiological evidence of arthritis may influence what procedure, if any, is performed. Films taken during weight-bearing provide more useful information.

Other Investigations
Pedobarography produces a pressure profile of the foot. However, the device is not widely available. It can confirm the areas of high pressure and can be used to assess the effect of surgical procedures. MRI imaging would be the other investigation that is useful. A very painful, red and swollen first metatarsophalangeal joint should raise the suspicion of gout.

Hallux Valgus

This is a progressive valgus deformity of the big toe. Once the toe starts to angulate, progression is inevitable because the pull of the tendons increases the deformity.

Aetiology
A number of factors can be identified in the development of hallux valgus:
- family history
- sex – more common in females
- age – tends to occur in the middle-aged; with the passage of time the foot tends to splay, so making any deforming forces worse
- metatarsus primus varus – if the first metatarsal is in varus, there is a greater tendency for the big toe to go into valgus because of the pull of the extensor tendon
- shoes – modern shoes tend to be very tight at the toes, so forcing the big toe into valgus; hallux valgus rarely occurs in those who do not wear shoes or who wear slippers

Clinical Features
History
There is cosmetic deformity and discomfort over the prominent bunion at the metatarsophalangeal joint. Inflammation occurs as this rubs on the shoes. Crossing of the first toe under or over the second and third increases discomfort.

Physical Findings
- Look for the deformity and the bunion.
- Feel for localized tenderness.
- Test for movement, which is often reduced, and check to see if the valgus deformity is reducible.

Management
Non-Operative
In the elderly with poor peripheral blood flow, conservative management is best. Using shoes with a wide toe box or surgical shoes can be made to fit the foot, as opposed to the normal practice of squashing the deformed toe and foot

into the shoe. Regular chiropody is important to care for the skin and nails.

Surgical

Over 40 operations have been described for hallux valgus. A simple bunionectomy is usually not enough because the deformity will recur. In the younger age group, surgery in the form of an osteotomy of the first metatarsal is performed (Chevron or Scarf), directed at correcting the underlying deformity – the varus displacement of the first metatarsal. Various operations have been described to correct the deformity. When there is osteoarthritis at the joint, surgery is either a fusion or joint replacement (with a Silastic or ceramic implant) or an excisional arthroplasty (Keller's), which is seldom performed these days. These relieve the pain and correct the deformity, but the joint is often stiffer than normal and, after a Keller's procedure, the big toe is considerably shorter.

Hallux Rigidus

This condition of a stiff, painful big toe is caused by degenerative arthritis at the first metatarsophalangeal joint. During walking, the big toe is unable to extend as the foot rolls forwards to toe-off (see Table 35.1) resulting in significant pain.

Management

Non-Operative

A rocker-bottom sole on the shoe allows the foot to roll forward more easily during walking. This is often cosmetically unacceptable but useful in those not keen on surgery.

Surgical

A dorsal cheilectomy is performed. This operation involves excision of the dorsal osteophytes and so allows a greater range of extension. Arthrodesis of the metatarsophalangeal joint provides pain relief although the big toe will rest in a somewhat extended position. Other methods such as excisional arthroplasty may be useful in the frail or elderly population.

Metatarsalgia Foot

In this condition, the distal foot (forefoot) is painful. The source of the pain is high pressure on the metatarsal heads as the patient walks. It is often associated with claw toes (see later), and as a result, instead of the toes sharing in weight-bearing, all the weight is taken on the metatarsal heads. It can also occur when the foot has a high longitudinal arch (pes cavus) for either unknown reasons or in neuromuscular conditions such as cerebral palsy, spina bifida or Friedreich's ataxia. Morton's metatarsalgia (neuroma) is a specific condition in which there is an interdigital neuroma between the metatarsal heads. This is then irritated by the adjacent bones, so resulting in pain and sensory disturbance between the corresponding toes.

Management

Non-Operative

A padded metatarsal bar fitted into the shoes to offload the metatarsal heads helps to spread the load across the foot. Surgical shoes may also be required to accommodate the foot more comfortably.

Surgical

An oblique osteotomy of the metatarsal necks (Weil's osteotomy) allows the heads of the metatarsals to ride up. It is important to perform the osteotomy on the second, third and fourth metatarsals because operating on one alone is not sufficient. In Morton's metatarsalgia, the affected space is explored and the neuroma excised. After operation, sensation is absent in the cleft/between the toes.

Claw Toes

Toes hyperextended at the metatarsophalangeal joints and flexed at the interphalangeal joints is termed clawing and so they do not touch the ground. As a result, they rub on the shoes and callosities develop over the dorsal proximal interphalangeal joints. There is also a tendency to develop associated metatarsalgia. The cause is usually unknown, but claw toes are seen in neuromuscular disorders such as spina bifida.

Management

Non-Operative

Local measures such as felt pads and attention to footwear may be sufficient.

Surgical

Fusion of the proximal interphalangeal joint allows the toe to straighten. This is usually done by excising the joint and then using a small wire, inserted through the end of toe to hold it straight for 6 weeks until the bone ends unite. A single, grossly deformed toe should be amputated.

Plantar Fasciitis

This is a painful condition of the heel caused by a localized area of inflammation of the plantar fascia at its origin from the os calcis. It is sometimes precipitated by local trauma or excessive weight-bearing.

Clinical Features

A relevant history of focal trauma may be obtained. Otherwise, the only complaint is of well-localized pain in the heel on weight-bearing. There is tenderness over the most prominent point of the calcaneus in the sole of the foot.

Investigation and Management

Plain X-ray may show a spur on the plantar aspect of the os calcis. Non-operative management with use of a cushioned heel wedge, night splints or local steroid injection is usually successful. Surgery to release the plantar fascia is occasionally required.

Achilles Tendonitis

This is a similar condition to plantar fasciitis in which there is an area of local inflammation at the insertion of the Achilles tendon. It may be precipitated by local trauma or a new pair of shoes that rub on the heel. Treatment consists of a heel wedge to reduce the tension in the tendon and a local steroid injection into the tendon sheath. Surgery is occasionally required to incise the inflamed tendon sheath or any bony spurs that may be responsible.

Freiberg's Disease

This condition is of an unknown cause in which there is fragmentation and collapse of the second metatarsal head. It occurs in young adults, and there may be a history of local trauma. The enlarged metatarsal head produces local pressure symptoms and metatarsalgia. Treatment is conservative with felt pads to relieve pressure. Surgery is occasionally done to reduce the size of the metatarsal head.

Gout

This is a medical condition which does not usually concern the orthopaedic surgeon, but patients may present initially to the A & E department or the orthopaedic clinic. The metatarsophalangeal joint is red, hot, swollen and extremely painful, mimicking a septic arthritis. There may be a precipitating history of minor trauma to the big toe, dietary excess, recent surgery or the use of drugs such as a thiazide diuretic. In the acute stage, the treatment is with NSAIDs. Prophylaxis with allopurinol may prevent recurrent attacks and should be undertaken if these are frequent, under the care of a rheumatologist.

PAEDIATRIC ORTHOPAEDICS

Hip

Problems with the hip in the paediatric age group are common. Patients present with pain, which may be felt in the knee alone, limp or leg length discrepancy; any child with knee pain must have his or her hip examined. Whereas trauma and infection can occur at any age, other conditions tend to occur within particular age brackets (Table 35.11).

Developmental Dysplasia of the Hip

The hip is unstable at birth either because of ligamentous laxity or because of dislocation out of an undeveloped (dysplastic) acetabular socket.

Epidemiology

The incidence is 15/1000 at birth but falls to 1.5/1000 at 6 weeks. The left side is affected in 60%, the right in 20% and the condition is bilateral in 20%.

TABLE 35.11   **Age ranges for paediatric hip conditions**

Age	Condition
0–5 years	Congenital dislocation of the hip
5–10 years	Perthe's disease
10–15 years	Slipped upper-femoral epiphysis

Aetiology

Genetic

There may be a family history:
- affected sibling – 6% chance
- affected mother – 12% chance
- affected sibling and mother – 35% chance

Sex

It is more common in girls than in boys, in a ratio of 9:1. This is probably because the female fetus is more sensitive to the maternal hormone relaxin secreted during pregnancy.

Perinatal

Associated factors are:
- first born
- an extended breech presentation
- coexistent talipes (see later)
- any other congenital anomaly
- oligohydramnios

Postnatal

Wrapping the infant in extension and adduction can cause a hip dislocation.

Clinical Features

History

Often the condition is diagnosed at birth, as part of the routine postnatal check where clicky hips are noted. Occasionally, the parents may notice asymmetry of the skin creases. In older children, there is a history of abnormal gait (see Box 35.2).

Physical Findings
- *Look:*
  - at the skin creases – there may be asymmetry of the gluteal creases but not if the condition is bilateral
  - for limited abduction in flexion
  - at the gait of an older child – it is a characteristic Trendelenburg gait
- *Feel and move* – The head may dislocate and relocate when Ortolani's or Barlow's tests are performed (Box 35.4); they must be done gently and not repeated, because avascular necrosis of the femoral head may result.

Barlow's test

With the hips adducted and flexed to 90 degrees, gentle pressure is applied along the femoral shaft to dislocate the head posteriorly.

Ortolani's test

The femoral head is dislocated as for Barlow's test. The hips are then abducted and the head is felt to relocate with a 'clunk'

Investigation

Plain X-ray. Up to 15 signs can be identified on a plain X-ray of the pelvis. The common ones are shown in Fig. 35.8. The ossification centre of the femoral head does not appear until the age of 5 months. For the acetabulum to develop normally, the femoral head must be within it. If not, it remains shallow with a large acetabular angle.

Ultrasound. In experienced hands, as well as being diagnostic, it is a useful screening technique. Under the age of 5 months, it is the investigation of choice to diagnose a dislocated hip.

Arthrography is required only for planning surgical correction in the older child.

Management

The final result depends to a great extent on the age at which the diagnosis is made and treatment begun. If this is at birth, the developed hip is normal. The aim of treatment is to achieve a complete and stable reduction. Patients who are missed at birth may present late – up to the age of 3 or 4 years – and in these circumstances, the outlook for good function is poor and treatment difficult.

Birth to 6 Months

A splint is used to hold the hip joint in approximately 60 degrees of abduction and 90 degrees of flexion. A variety is available, but the most common type used is the Pavlik harness. The splint is worn all the time until the acetabulum is seen to be developing normally.

Six Months to Walking

At this age, the hip is dislocated. Gentle traction is applied over a few weeks with progressive abduction (an adductor tenotomy may be required). The hip is then assessed under a general anaesthetic. If it is stable, a plaster of Paris hip spica is applied. If unstable or still dislocated, then an arthrogram is done which may show an inverted, thickened and folded acetabular labrum (limbus). This requires surgical removal to permit reduction.

The Older Child

An open operation is required to remove the limbus (contracted acetabular labrum and capsule) which is in the way of reduction of the femoral head into its socket. At a later stage, femoral osteotomy may also be required. Over 7 years of age, there is a case for non-operative management and, when secondary osteoarthritis develops in adult life, a total hip replacement.

Perthes' Disease

There is, in this condition, a variable degree of osteonecrosis of the femoral head.

Aetiology and Pathological Features

The cause is essentially unknown. An effusion forms, perhaps as a result of minor trauma or a viral infection. Pressure within the joint rises and impairs venous return from the femoral head, which then undergoes avascular necrosis. The incidence is 1:9000, and the condition occurs four times more frequently in boys than in girls. It is bilateral in 10%. The degree of collapse of the femoral head and the subsequent secondary arthritis is such that, by the age of 45, nearly half require a hip replacement, and by 65, secondary osteoarthritis is evident in 86%.

Clinical Features

The age of onset is between 5 and 10 years with a limp and a complaint of a dull ache. There are few signs, but abduction in flexion is reduced.

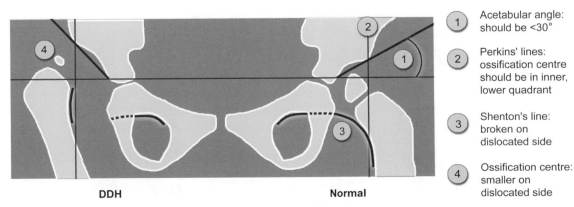

DDH   Normal

1. Acetabular angle: should be <30°
2. Perkins' lines: ossification centre should be in inner, lower quadrant
3. Shenton's line: broken on dislocated side
4. Ossification centre: smaller on dislocated side

• **Fig. 35.8** Common radiological features of the dislocated hip. *DDH*, developmental dysplasia of the hip.

Investigation

Imaging

Plain X-ray. An effusion may be seen. As the condition progresses, the femoral head becomes increasingly sclerotic and fragmented. Collapse of the head is associated with lateral subluxation.

Bone scan is rarely required but, if undertaken, shows an area of reduced uptake that corresponds to the femoral head.

Blood Examination

Standard tests are normal.

Management

Non-Operative

Weight-bearing should be avoided while there is pain. The child should rest the hip whilst it is painful. A conservative approach can be employed if the progression of the disease is slow with limited involvement of the femoral head.

Surgical

If the femoral head is subluxed laterally on X-ray, surgery is aimed at containing it within the acetabulum. This can be achieved by wide abduction of the hip in a hip spica, or a femoral osteotomy to bring the head back into the acetabulum.

Slipped Upper-Femoral Epiphysis

The upper-femoral epiphysis can sometimes slip on the adjacent cartilaginous growth plate (physis). The epiphysis then slides off posteriorly.

Epidemiology

The incidence varies with race. In Caucasians it is 2 in 100 000, but in Afro-Caribbeans it is 7 in 100 000. Boys are affected twice as often as girls. The age of onset is between 10 and 15 years and is younger in girls (12 years) than in boys (14 years). The condition is slightly more common on the left side and is bilateral at presentation in 10%. If one side slips, there is a 25% chance that the other side will follow.

Aetiology

Trauma

There may be an acute slip after injury to the hip.

Hormonal

A relative deficiency of sex hormones, which play a part in the ossification of cartilage, is thought to be a factor in the development of a chronic slip. As growth progresses, the cartilaginous plate is then unable to resist the increasing load placed upon it.

Clinical Features

History

In 70%, the history is of chronic pain and a limp. In 30%, there is an acute slip with a correspondingly short history.

Physical Findings

- Look:
  - the child is often overweight and sexually underdeveloped
  - the hip is held in extension, external rotation and adduction.
- Measure – the leg is short by 1–2 cm
- Move:
  - abduction in flexion is reduced – there may be fixed external rotation
  - possibly a Trendelenburg gait (see Box 35.2)

Investigation

On an anteroposterior X-ray, the presence of a mild slip may be missed: look at Trethowan's sign which utilized Klein's line (Fig. 35.9). On a lateral film, however, the slip is easily seen. The amount is usually expressed as the percentage of the head uncovered on the lateral film.

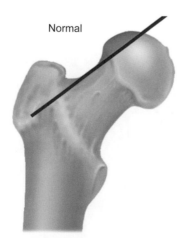
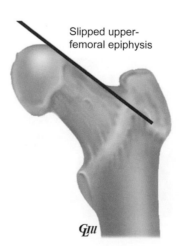

• **Fig. 35.9** Trethowan's sign: Klein's line in slipped femoral epiphysis compared with normal.

Management

There is no place for conservative management. When there is a mild slip of up to 30%, the epiphysis should be pinned where it is without attempting reduction, because forcible manipulation may precipitate avascular necrosis. Greater than 30% displacement is managed by either of the following:

- Open reduction and pinning – There is a 14% risk of avascular necrosis of the femoral head.
- Pinning without reduction and later femoral osteotomy to bring the epiphysis back into the correct position – Late secondary osteoarthritis frequently occurs when there has been a slip of 50% or more.

It is generally accepted that, if there is unreliable parental care or follow-up, consideration should be given to pinning the contralateral hip prophylactically.

Talipes

This term is applied to a congenital deformity of the foot. A more detailed classification follows below.

Epidemiology and Aetiology

The incidence is 2 in 1000 live births in the UK. It is twice as common in boys as in girls and is bilateral in one-third. In most instances, the condition is present at birth, and it used to be thought that the intrauterine position might be causative. However, deformities from this cause rapidly recover after birth. Other causes are neuromuscular, e.g. spina bifida, polio and arthrogryposis – the last is a joint malformation of unknown but possible neurogenic cause.

Types

The disorder is classified by the direction in which the heel points and the deviation of the forefoot. A foot that points down is said to be in equinus and one that points up calcaneus. The forefoot may be in either varus or valgus.

The types in order of frequency are then:

- equinovarus – most common
- calcaneovalgus – second most common; may be associated with congenital dislocation of the hip
- equinovalgus – rare
- calcaneovarus – rare

Clinical Features

The deformity is usually noticed at routine postnatal examination or by the parents within a few days or weeks of birth. Physical findings are of uncorrectable deformity in one of the directions described above.

Management

Non-Operative

The initial treatment is to gently stretch and manipulate the foot into the correct position. A number of methods have been described to do this. The Ponseti[2] technique of serial casting is started in the first week after birth and can result in a very good outcome in experienced hands. The technique is time-consuming and requires close attention to detail. With this technique, an Achilles tenotomy may be required after 4 to 6 weeks of casting and this can be performed in the clinic. After the deformity has been corrected, the baby will need to continue to wear special shoes (Dennis Brown boots) for 3 to 4 years.

Surgical

If non-operative methods are unsuccessful or if there is a relapse in the older child, then surgery will need to be considered. The tight soft tissue posteriorly and medially will need to be released and, in the older child, bony surgery may also be required.

Minor Leg Deformities

Knock-knees, bow-legs and an in-toeing gait are all common and a source of much parental anxiety.

Knock-Knee and Bow-Leg

In babies and toddlers, there is physiological bowing that corrects at 2–3 years of age. Later, at 4 or 5, there may be knock-knee of unknown cause. All but 2% of these correct spontaneously. In a few children, there is an underlying cause. Rickets is rare in the UK (but not unknown in some dark-skinned ethnic groups accustomed to more sunlight than they get in Britain). However, worldwide it is a common cause. Osteochondrosis deformans is a rare epiphyseal dysplasia which is associated with knock-knee.

In-Toeing

This is the consequence of torsional deformity of either the tibia or the femur. Children then have a tendency to trip over their own feet. Treatment is not required until at least 6 or 7 years because almost all will correct spontaneously. If correction is required, then the affected long bone is derotated by an osteotomy.

References

1. National Joint Registry for England, Wales, Northern Ireland and the Isle of Man. 18th Annual Report 2021. Surgical Data to 31 December 2020. ISSN 2054-183X (Online).

2. Ponseti IV. 2008. *Congenital Clubfoot. Fundamentals of treatment.* 2nd ed. New York: Oxford University Press. ISBN-13 978-0192627650.

36

Trauma Surgery/Principles of Trauma Care

CHAPTER OUTLINE

Introduction

The description of the tri-modal distribution of death by Trunkey in 1983 classically divides injuries into three modalities of mortality. Acute primary mortality is due to injuries that are incompatible with life and patients normally die within seconds. Typical injuries include severe head injuries, mediastinal and cardiac disruption, high cervical vertebral (C3 and above) and airway obstruction.

The secondary mortality occurs within minutes to hours and is potentially preventable by early and appropriate medical intervention. Examples include intracranial haemorrhage, pneumothorax, cardiac tamponade, haemothorax, intra-abdominal haemorrhage, pelvic fracture or long bone fracture.

The third mortality occurs within days or weeks following the injury. The triggering of multiorgan failure and subsequent death is usually on a continuum and starts with potentially reversible physiological dysfunction, usually caused by sepsis or cardiorespiratory failure.

Head and spinal-cord injuries form a great proportion of the causes of disability in high-income countries, whereas there is an immense burden of disability in developing countries due to extremity injury alone, suggesting that relatively simple intervention such as improved orthopaedic

care and rehabilitation could provide significant benefit and relief to these communities.

Injuries are due to either blunt or penetrating trauma. The ATMIST mnemonic provides a way of succinctly giving the paramedic the information necessary to give to the emergency department staff on initial handover. ATMIST corresponds to the age of the patient, time of injury, mechanism of injury, where the injury is, signs and symptoms pertaining to the injury and the treatment given. The mechanism of injury relates to the energy dissipated. For example, a driver slamming into a tree at 70 miles an hour can be expected to have a head and cervical spine injury from hitting the windscreen, a potential aortic transection from the sudden acceleration/deceleration injury where the relatively mobile mediastinum moves forward on the relatively fixed thoracic aorta, a pneumothorax or haemothorax from fractured ribs, lung and cardiac contusion injury from the steering wheel, a pancreatic injury from the safety belt, a lower lumbar or pelvic fracture, a hip dislocation, femoral shaft fracture, patella dislocation and ankle injuries from the sudden deceleration injury and potentially also arterial and venous injuries from the bony injuries.

Compare that to a single stab wound in the chest for example. The injury is low energy but the effects could be devastating depending on the trajectory of the knife. This can range from a small puncture wound in the lung causing a simple pneumothorax treated with a chest drain to a penetrating injury to the heart and its outflow vessels causing a cardiac tamponade and, if not treated immediately, rapid death.

The time of the injury is of course paramount in survival. Most major trauma units rely on a time of less than 45 minutes from injury to transfer to a major trauma centre as it is known that a time delay increases mortality. Depending on the resources available, it is sometimes better to scoop and run to bring the patient to the hospital rather than to spend time performing on the road or site of injury treatment.

Assessment by the prehospital paramedic using the pneumonic CABCDE (derived from ATLS) is mandatory for the initial triage of the patient. It is repeated when the patient is handed over to the accident and emergency staff. 'C' stands for catastrophic haemorrhage, whereby bleeding in a limb is controlled using a tourniquet or direct pressure. 'A' stands for airway and those who are in unconscious or in shock benefit from immediate endotracheal intubation. Some may require a surgical airway in cases of significant bleeding and facial trauma with oedema or laryngeal fracture. Breathing can be assessed by respiratory rate, chest movement and tracheal deviation. Have no hesitation in placing bilateral chest drains if necessary. Assessment of the circulation 'C' follows the standard palpation techniques for radial pulse (90 mmHg), carotid pulse (80 mmHg), femoral pulse (70 mmHg), with an assessment of the peripheries for capillary return. Look at the neck veins: they may be distended and point to the diagnosis of tension pneumothorax, cardiac tamponade and cardiac contusion. However, these signs may be absent in someone with significant haemorrhage. 'D' for disability, equating to neurological status, eye response, best verbal response and motor response. The Glasgow coma scale is the gold standard and significantly provides a better level of conscious understanding rather than the AVPU (alert, verbal, pain and unresponsive) method. 'E', for the environment can be done during the secondary survey where clothes are removed for a top to toe and front to back examination, including log roll and assessment of the anal sphincter tone. This is especially important in penetrating injuries, but care must be taken that the patient does not become hypothermic. Core temperatures fall very rapidly in patients who have had significant haemorrhage with the added issues of delay in extraction. On arrival to the emergency department, warming blankets should be available and fluids given at body temperature or higher (Table 36.1).

Apart from examination, investigative adjuncts are also necessary: chest X-ray, pelvic X-ray and focused abdominal sonography in trauma (FAST) scan will identify blood in the inaccessible areas such as the chest, including cardiac tamponade, abdomen and pelvis. The X-rays will define any bony injury. Bloods, including full

TABLE 36.1	Indications for Damage Control Surgery.
Conditions	High energy blunt trauma
Complexes	Multiple torso penetration
	Haemodynamic instability
	Presenting coagulopathy and/or hypothermia
	Major abdominal vascular injury with multiple visceral injuries
	Multifocal or multi-cavity exsanguinations with concomitant visceral injuries
	Multi-regional injury with competing priorities
Critical factors	Severe metabolic acidosis (pH <7.3)
	Hypothermia (temperature <35C)
	Resuscitation and operative time >90mins
	Coagulopathy as evidenced by development of non-mechanical bleeding massive transfusion requirements (>10 packed red cells units)

blood count, urea and electrolytes, glucose (especially in children), and group and save and cross-matching should be sent off immediately. Passage of a nasogastric tube and also a urinary catheter is helpful, but in the confines of the injury present. A patient with a pelvic fracture should have the passage of the urinary catheter attempted just once, in pelvic haematoma blood at the meatus and a high riding prostate are contraindications to the attempt.

Emergency Department Surgery

ATLS protocols should be adhered to and a careful monitoring of the blood pressure with response to fluids should be under the watchful eye of the surgeon and the trauma team leader. A blood pressure of 90 systolic must be maintained, which will provide adequate perfusion of the major organs. Initial crystalloid infusion while waiting for a response in the blood pressure falls into three groups. A responder to fluid implies that the bleeding has stopped, a transient responder suggests ongoing bleeding and a non-responder suggests catastrophic bleeding which may require immediate surgery in the emergency department. Non-responders with falling blood pressure due to massive haemorrhage or cardiac tamponade require emergency department thoracotomy via a left antero-lateral incision.

Damage Control

The term damage control was first coined by the Navy as early as the 1600s. It meant saving the ship at any cost if it was damaged. That is controlling the flooding and the fire as quickly as possible before the ship sank and rescuing an engine so that the ship could return to port and undergo repairs. The same concept is used in damage control for the patient. That is saving the patient at any cost. Controlling the flooding which is the bleeding, the fire which is the sepsis, and the engine which is maintaining oxygen to the organs i.e. the heart and blood vessels which, if they are damaged, require shunts. The whole purpose of resuscitation is to normalize the oxygen delivery to vital organs and allow cells to respire aerobically.

Haemorrhage remains the leading cause of death in both civilian and military trauma. Significant blood loss leads to tissue hypoperfusion, thus causing diminished oxygen delivery to the cells which very rapidly switch to anaerobic respiration and produce lactic acid. Anaerobic respiration produces only two ATPs as opposed to 38 ATPs in aerobic respiration and therefore the temperature of the patient begins to fall. This is added to the fact that the patient may well be in a cool environment. The lactic acid reduces the pH of the blood and the hypothermia compounds the abnormal homeostatic environment. Enzyme kinetics begin to slow down and the coagulation efficacy is significantly reduced. An early form of coagulopathy was found mainly in patients with hypoperfusion, 'acute traumatic coagulopathy', a complex multifactorial endogenous process occurring in up to one-third of patients which independently predicts death. This acute traumatic coagulopathy is characterized by regulation of endothelial thrombomodulin which, forming complexes with thrombin, promotes anticoagulation as well as endothelium dysfunction-induced hyper-fibrinolysis.

This form of coagulopathy is present in the most severely injured patients and is usually associated with poor outcomes. The more coagulopathic the patient is on arrival, the greater mortality. Based on the above, haemostatic resuscitation could be considered as the utilization of blood and blood products in the early treatment phases of traumatic coagulopathy. Adequate detection and treatment of post-traumatic coagulopathy mandates early and repeated monitoring of prothrombin time (PT), activated partial thromboplastin time (aPTT), fibrinogen levels and platelet count. Moreover, utilization of recently introduced viscoelastic testing such as thromboelastography is useful for better characterization of an existing coagulopathy and management of haemostatic therapy. An ideal test (rapid, highly sensitive, etc.) does not yet exist. For this reason, in the very early acute phase of trauma management, decision to initiate clotting factor replacement is based mainly on clinical considerations.

If rapid treatment is not instigated, the patient will enter the so-called trauma triad of death of acidosis, hypothermia and coagulopathy (Fig. 36.1). Hypothermia will increase fibrinolysis, affect platelet function by decreasing platelet aggregation and alter platelet surface molecule expression, increasing platelet sequestration in the liver and spleen. Acidosis has an effect of reducing cardiac activity and reducing enzymatic conversion of coagulation factors, particularly thrombin generation and, by alteration of platelet activity through decreasing platelet count, modification of

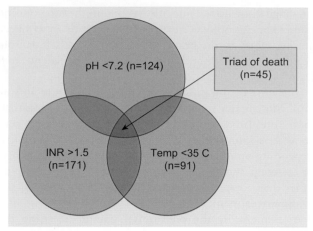

• **Fig. 36.1** 'Triad of death.' (From Mitra B, et al., Recombinant factor VIIa in trauma patients with the 'triad of death', Injury. 2012; 43(9): 1410, Fig. 1)

calcium-iron binding site morphology. The whole mantra of damage control is to check and reverse this process in the shortest possible time on the operating table, as patients tend to lose 1°C per hour, which compounds the hypothermia.

In 1993, Rotondo first applied the concept of damage control in surgery.[1] His indications still hold true and provide a useful guide.

However, in 1993 when the concept was first muted, resuscitation used high-volume crystalloids *followed* by packed red cells. Although it was shown that there was a significant initial reduction in mortality in those patients undergoing damage control surgery as opposed to definitive surgery, there was significant complications due to the third space extravasation of isotonic fluid as well as significant dilution of clotting products. Abdominal tamponade became a real problem with retroperitoneal and intestinal oedema causing abdominal pressure symptoms, including kidney failure. In addition, uncontrolled crystalloid infusion in trauma causes acute lung injury, worsening coagulopathy and reduced end-organ perfusion.

Much research was performed by the British military in both the Iraq and Afghanistan wars into the resuscitation aspect of damage control. Changing the fluid from crystalloid to replacing blood with blood was the key. Damage control resuscitation (DCR) is now in line with damage control surgery and the two have become synonymous with the aim of improving the physiology of the patient by replacing blood and blood products at the outset. Military and austere environment surgery rely on giving fresh whole blood but most civilian trauma systems are reliant on packed red blood cells, fresh frozen plasma, platelets and cryoprecipitate given in a ratio of 1:1:1. This approximates whole blood equivalents and can be converted to specific directed therapy guided by thromboelastography. DCR also requires hypotensive resuscitation, such that, initially, the blood pressure can be kept to organ perfusion levels, such as 90 mmHg, so as not to 'pop the clot', limiting the amount of crystalloids, if any, that are given, and all fluids are given at body temperature or higher. Adjuncts, such as tranexamic acid, a synthetic derivative of the amino acid lysine, act as an anti-fibrinolytic by inhibiting the activation of plasminogen to plasmin and have been shown, in the CRASH-2 trial,[2] to significantly reduce the risk of death in up to one-third of patients if given within the first 3 hours of injury.

Viscoelastic coagulation, otherwise known as rotational thromboelastometry, is a very useful bedside test to evaluate the clotting haemodynamics during damage control resuscitation. It evaluates the time to clotting by using a small amount of blood placed in a beaker which is agitated. Using the on-screen results, it is possible to evaluate platelet function and also the degree of activation of fibrin and thrombin. Based on these results, it would be possible to titrate the amount of clotting factors necessary.

Once haemostasis is achieved, the goal is to reverse the end-organ ischaemia and the acidosis. Vasopressors are avoided in haemorrhagic shock to minimize further peripheral acidosis and facilitate faster base deficit clearance. Base deficit provides an indirect indicator of hypoperfusion and forecasts transfusion requirements. This also correlates with mortality and, therefore, makes for an effective resuscitation marker. Active methods to prevent and reverse hypothermia are used, including warming intravenous fluids and intraoperative fluids for washout, increasing the temperature of the operating theatre and forced air patient warming.

Effective DCR starts at the point of injury and often the receiving hospital is given advance warning of the necessity to give blood immediately by the paramedic crew. The word 'code red' implies significant haemorrhage and the necessity for damage control. The surgeon must be prepared to act immediately to stem the bleeding. This may necessitate an emergency department thoracotomy to cross clamp the aorta to stem the haemorrhage below the diaphragm and also assess the heart.

Although not a new concept, aortic occlusive balloons were first used in the 1950s in the Korean War and were used sparingly over the following four decades. Since the 2000s, resuscitative endovascular balloon occlusion of the aorta (REBOA), has seen an upsurge in interest, especially in pre-hospital use in London by the Helicopter Emergency Medical Service (HEMS) team from the Royal London Hospital. As 35% of all haemorrhagic deaths occur prehospital, it may prove to be an exciting significant advance in the armamentarium of the trauma team. In hospital, it may be suitable for those patients in the systolic bracket of between 60 and 80 mmHg with an infra-diaphragmatic bleed and certainly, from initial reports, it has proved very beneficial in those patients who have bleeding from pelvic injuries. Essentially, the device is passed through the common femoral artery using a sheath and a balloon directed using anatomical landmarks and external measuring tape. The balloon is blown up to occlude the blood flow in the aorta.

There are three separate areas where the balloon can be inflated. Zone 1 is in the descending thoracic aorta to above the diaphragm; zone 2, below the diaphragm to below the renal arteries; and zone 3 from the infrarenal abdominal aorta to the bifurcation. It is a temporizing modality used to increase perfusion pressures of the heart and brain but will need to be removed and the downstream bleeding fixed either surgically or radiologically. In general terms, the balloon occlusion should be the shortest time possible. For Zone 1, under 30 minutes is optimal and over 60 minutes is very dangerous due to the ischaemic insult and consequently perfusion injury. For Zone 2, due to the high-risk of ischaemia to the major abdominal organs and intestines, only a few minutes is desirable and in zone 3, up to 2 to 3 hours may be tolerated. There have been significant complications reported, including limb loss and small bowel infarction. At the present time there are ongoing randomized, controlled trials to assess both its clinical relevance and risks.

Although the majority of trauma does occur in the adult population under the age of 45 and it is appropriate to apply all the strategies of damage control, two groups of vulnerable populations need to be considered. Children under the age of 8 years have very different fluid requirements each year of their life and it is very easy to overload the heart and lungs; particular attention should be paid to fluid requirements using standard paediatric protocols. As the population gets older, decreased physiological reserve and co-morbidities such as heart failure and chronic obstructive airways disease causing pulmonary hypertension, as well as the plethora of drugs including anticoagulants which are taken, mean that caution needs to be taken when submitting patients in this group to massive transfusion protocols.

Definitive anatomical surgery takes place when the physiology of the patient (i.e. pH, base deficit, core temperature and coagulation) has been normalized. This usually takes place within 24 to 48 hours but, most importantly, the surgeon and the team need to be vigilant with constant careful examination of the patient, especially if arterial and venous shunts are in place as these can often thrombose when the clotting becomes normalized.

VASCULAR TRAUMA

For patients presenting with active haemorrhage, diagnosis is straightforward and no additional evaluation is required. As a general principle, the presence of a hard sign of vascular injury (Box 36.1) warrants immediate operation for exploration and earliest possible control of vascular haemorrhage. Patients who present with soft signs suggestive of occult vascular injury, however, benefit from additional diagnostic imaging. A variety of imaging options are available, each with important capabilities and limitations to consider.

Doppler Waveform Analysis

The handheld Doppler is an easy tool to provide quick diagnosis. The Doppler probe placed on a normal blood vessel, for example the radial artery, angled towards its flow will reveal a tri-phasic wave form. The initial systolic forward flow hits an organ of high resistance producing a reversed waveform, followed by the diastolic relaxation of the elasticity within the artery providing next forward

Hard signs

- Absent pulsatile bleeding
- Absent pulses distal to the injury site
- Expanding or pulsatile haematoma
- Bruit or thrill at the site of injury
- Unexplained shock

Soft signs

- Diminished pulses distal to the injury site
- Stable, small haematoma
- Injury in proximity major vessels
- Peripheral nerve deficit
- History of haemorrhage at the scene
- Suspicious pattern of fracture or dislocation

flow. If there is a significant injury, then the flow may be almost absent, giving a monophasic signal or no signal at all. If the flow is tri-phasic, then one can assume no injury; anything less than that, assume a more proximal injury.

Duplex Ultrasonography

Duplex ultrasonography is Doppler combined with ultrasound and is probably more useful as a follow-up of injuries as the presence of associated haematoma, soft tissue injury and bony injuries makes the reliability of spectral waveform analysis and colour-flow examination much more difficult.

Computed Tomography Angiography

CT has become the primary imaging modality in patients who suffer significant trauma. With the advent of the multidetector CT (MDCT) technology, high resolution images with shorter acquisition times are now routine and the quality of multi-planar and 3D re-formations has revolutionized the evaluation of trauma victims. These technological advances, in particular the shorter image acquisition times, enable complex, multi-phasic imaging studies of the entire body specifically aimed at determining the integrity of the vasculature.

In patients who sustain poly trauma, the main purpose of thoracic CT is evaluation of the thoracic aorta and brachiocephalic arteries. Acute traumatic injuries of thoracic aorta are highly lethal. It is estimated that 85% to 90% of patients who suffer acute aortic trauma expire prior to reaching hospital and 50–70 percent of the survivors die within a week without proper treatment. A significant force is needed to tear the aorta and is usually the result of high-speed trauma such as motor vehicle collisions with sudden deceleration injury. The most likely location for aortic injuries is at the proximal descending aorta at the level of the ligamentum arteriosum just below the take-off of the subclavian artery where the relatively mobile aortic arch connects to the fixed ascending aorta and where more than 90% of injuries occur.

The aortic transection haematoma contains about 150–200 mL of blood and looks like an aubergine due to the blood being just held by the adventitia. It is not the cause of haemodynamic instability and that is what needs to be addressed first. Endovascular stenting has become the first-line treatment.

Surgical Treatment

Although definitive surgical treatment of vascular trauma remains the ultimate objective of care for patients requiring surgery, there are important caveats to consider. Vascular repairs can prove technically demanding and time-consuming and is not the primary option in the patient who is physiologically unwell. Similarly, damage control approaches may be more beneficial to the patient with multiple injuries. For example, a shunt can be used to restore temporary perfusion to a distal limb so that a craniotomy can be conducted to prevent herniation in the setting of a severe traumatic brain injury. The options for vascular damage control are ligation and temporary vascular shunting.

Ligation

As a general rule, all major named arteries should be repaired or reconstructed if at all possible. In the setting of damage control, however, ligation may be considered for specific vessels. Specific anatomic redundancies of the vascular system and collateral pathways for distal perfusion can be accepted in the patient whose physiology is abnormal or the circumstances require this. Applicable situations of this type include ligation of the radial artery in the upper extremity that has a dominant ulnar perfusion to the palmar arch or ligation of the two out of three crural vessels in a patient without peripheral arterial disease.

The collateral circulation around the shoulder often is good enough for ligation of the subclavian artery if necessity demands it. Ligation carries with it the risk of distal ischaemia and, certainly for vessels such as the popliteal artery, which is an end artery, the chance of ischaemia is greater than 90%. Ligation of the internal carotid artery carries a stroke rate of around 40% in those without an intact circle of Willis. Although ligation in these more extreme situations has been espoused as an effective method of salvaging life, one has to remember that, in the trauma situation, the blood pressure is often low and there may not be enough collateralization to afford a good perfusion and reconstruction of the subclavian artery may be necessary in the form of a carotico-subclavian bypass.

Temporary Vascular Shunts

Endoluminal temporary shunt should be used in damage control situations that involve injuries to large or medium sized arteries. Commercially available shunts such as the Javid and Pruitt shunts used in elective vascular surgery are ideally suited for this purpose. However, any sterile tube can suffice, e.g. nasogastric tubes, intravenous giving set tubes, paediatric endotracheal tubes and umbilical feeding tubes. Careful insertion of the shunt is required to prevent intimal damage and distal dissection. Prior to insertion, the injured vessel should be cleanly cut and all thrombus removed proximally and distally using Fogarty embolectomy catheters and copious amounts of heparinized saline (5000 units of heparin in 500 mL of saline) used to flush the proximal and distal vessels. The shunts should always be tied down using two number one silk ligatures on both ends of the shunt and vessel. Following removal of the shunt and definitive surgery, this part of the artery and vein, if shunted, will need to be removed in case of intimal damage.

Definitive Repair

Definitive vascular repair may take place following stabilization of the patient following damage control or as initial treatment in patients who are stable enough to tolerate the time required for repair at the first operation. The technologies at our disposal, such as rotational thromboelastometry (ROTEM), and massive transfusion protocols affords a variety of potential definitive solutions to most vascular injury problems. The choice of repair must be made with careful consideration of the potential role of each approach.

Primary Repair

Primary repair of both venous and arterial injuries can be considered for clean lacerations of vessels. However, the gap between the proximal and distal ends after debridement must be able to come together in a tension free fashion. Traditional dogma suggested that 2 cm was the maximal gap that can be bridged to achieve this goal. In practice, however, if the length of the mobilization of the proximal in distal arteries, including division of side branches, proves problematical, the safer principle is to always place an interposition graft to reduce any tension in the anastomosis which, in the event of any infection, will inevitably end up with secondary haemorrhage.

Conduit

Interposition repair using autogenous reversed vein grafts remains the standard of vascular injury repair for appropriately-sized vessels. The technique involves harvesting the long saphenous vein from the groin, which is better than at the ankle because it is thicker and less prone to aneurysmal blowout. The vein graft is reversed and distended with heparinized saline and all side branches which are still leaking are sutured with 7/0 prolene. The best technique for suturing if a mismatch occurs is the fish mouth technique using interrupted 5/0 or 6/0 prolene. Prosthetic grafts are an effective and durable alternative when used in surgical fields that are not compromised by gross contamination. Expanded polytetrafluoroethylene (PTFE) is preferable to Dacron in this situation due to its higher resistance to infection.

Intraoperative Anticoagulation

Although the use of systemic heparinization is ubiquitous in elective vascular surgery, its role in traumatic vascular surgery remains debateable. In the damage control situation, one can assume that the patient is already coagulopathic and therefore it is not necessary to give heparin. In addition, the patient may already be unstable haemodynamically with the presence of traumatic brain injury and/or bleeding from major organs or the pelvis.

Intra- and Postoperative Evaluation

After any intervention or repair, restoration of perfusion is confirmed. The handheld Doppler probe is a necessary intraoperative device which, when held over the proximal artery and vein graft and distal artery, should provide evidence of biphasic flow on all sides of the vessel. It is also possible to pick up an increase in frequency suggestive of a stenosis. Intraoperative duplex is another tried and tested modality. More invasive techniques, such as intraoperative angiogram using direct placement of a needle or catheter in the proximal vessel with a contrast agent diluted with 50% saline and using a C-arm or a one-shot angiogram, is also necessary to confirm patency of repair and detect a missed additional injury.

Specific Injuries

Head and Neck/Cerebral Vascular Injuries

The neck is classically divided into three distinct anatomical zones.

Zone 1 extends from the clavicle to the cricoid cartilage. Surgical access to this zone may require thoracotomy or sternotomy. Major arteries and veins, trachea and nerves, oesophagus, lower thyroid and parathyroid glands and thymus are located in this area.

Zone 2 is from the cricoid cartilage to the angle of the mandible. This contains the internal and external carotid arteries, jugular veins, pharynx, larynx, oesophagus, recurrent laryngeal nerves, spinal cord, trachea, thyroid and parathyroid glands. Injuries in zone 2 are most accessible for direct surgical exposure.

Zone 3 is from the angle of the mandible to the base of the skull. This contains the extracranial carotid and vertebral arteries, jugular veins, cranial nerves IX–XII and sympathetic nerve trunk. Surgical exposures of injuries in zone 3 are challenging which makes these lesions best treated with an endovascular approach.

Exposure in zone 2 requires a long incision from the mastoid process down to the sternal notch. The carotid sheath is then exposed by moving the sternomastoid muscle back and dividing the facial vein, which is the gateway to the carotid arterial complex. Often, there is significant haematoma which distorts the anatomy and increases the risk of cranial nerve damage. Proximal and distal control is then obtained and the injury carefully evaluated. All non-viable tissue should be debrided and a decision made regarding the need for an interposition graft. In the author's opinion, the long saphenous vein conduit has an increased likelihood to thrombose in the carotid arterial complex and for that reason the author would always use a PTFE interposition graft. If possible, a shunt should be used to reduce the risk of cerebral ischaemia during reconstruction.

Internal Jugular Vein

Unilateral internal jugular vein injuries are best managed with simple lateral sutures if possible. If not, then ligation is the preferred option. In the rare occasion of bilateral internal jugular vein injuries, at least one of the veins must be repaired because bilateral ligation invariably results in cerebral venous congestion and increases mortality.

Thoracic-Penetrating Neck Injuries

Zone 1 neck injuries require proximal control and this can really only be managed with an incision into the chest. The approach is usually a median sternotomy but a clamshell manoeuvre will give just as much exposure. This will also allow access to injuries to the aortic arch. The median sternotomy incision can also be extended into the neck for additional exposure of the thoracic outlet. The gateway to the aortic arch is to divide the brachiocephalic vein. Restoration of flow requires proximal and distal control, patching and grafting. Most gunshot wounds in this area are unsurvivable.

Blunt Descending Thoracic Injury

The treatment for acute aortic transection involves endovascular stenting. If cover of the subclavian artery orifice (in very rare instances) produces significant ischaemia, then subclavian revascularization can be performed using a carotid-subclavian bypass. Consider also a spinal drain in cases requiring a long stent in case of spinal ischaemia.

Abdominal Vascular Surgery

In contrast to those with peripheral arterial injuries which can be compressed, the abdomen is non-compressible and cannot be controlled by external pressure. Abdominal vascular injuries are usually associated with additional intra-abdominal injuries such as small and large bowel defects with gross contamination.

The retroperitoneum is systemically compartmentalized into four anatomic zones: a single central zone 1, paired lateral zones 2s, and a distal zone 3. Zone 1 is the central area of the retroperitoneum and extends from the aortic hiatus to the sacral promontory and contains the aorta with its major branches and the inferior vena cava. Zone 2 is located laterally and includes the kidneys and the hilar renal vessels. Zone 3 is located in the space of the pelvic retroperitoneum and contains the iliac arteries and veins.

Zone 1 Exploration

It is necessary to explore all haematomas in zone 1 to rule out the possibility of a major vascular injury regardless of the injury mechanism. The haematoma is central. Depending on the mechanism of injury and confidence of the site of the injury, which has either been diagnosed on CT scan or by the trajectory of the wounding implement, the surgeon can decide to enter the haematoma to gain proximal control in the chest. The problem is knowing which central vascular structure has been damaged. The safest method is to perform a left anterolateral thoracotomy and control the arterial inflow to the abdomen by cross-clamping the aorta above the diaphragm. Once an arterial clamp is placed on the aorta, a laparotomy can be performed. If there is damage to the aorta at the hiatus then a thoraco-abdominal incision can be made through the eighth or ninth interspace by dividing costal cartilage.

To gain access to the suprarenal aorta and visceral branches once cross-clamping is established, the left visceral medial rotation can be performed. The white line of Toldt on the left is divided and the left colon mobilized from the anterior abdominal wall. The dissection plane at the retroperitoneum is carried out anteriorly to Gerota's fascia, leaving the left kidney in place. The dissection is extended in a cephalad direction. The splenophrenic ligament is divided and an en bloc medial rotation of the spleen, pancreas, colon and small bowel is performed. Exposure of the coeliac axis, superior mesenteric artery (SMA) and left renal artery is achieved. If an injury to the posterior aspect of the aorta it suspected, the same manoeuvre is performed but instead of the plane of dissection staying anterior to the left kidney, it extends posterior to the left kidney which is included in the en bloc medial distal rotation.

Visceral Arteries

The coeliac artery emerges anteriorly from the aorta and trifurcates into the left gastric, common hepatic and splenic arteries. In addition to the medial vessel rotation described previously, the coeliac trunk and its branches can also be approached through the lesser sac. This exposure, however, requires division of the median arcuate ligament and the coeliac ganglion, which is difficult in the trauma setting. A rich network of collaterals make ligation of the coeliac trunk the treatment of choice when injuries are encountered in this situation. Ligation of the coeliac branches, including the common hepatic artery, can also be performed with negligible risk of visceral ischaemia. Injuries to the proper hepatic artery which are distal to the gastroduodenal artery should be repaired.

Superior Mesenteric Artery, Superior Mesenteric Vein and Portal Vein

A left visceral medial rotation provides adequate exposure to the retro-pancreatic segment, the SMA. The SMA segment distal to the inferior pancreatic border is best exposed to the root of the mesentery by retracting the transverse colon cephalad, dividing the ligament of Treitz and mobilizing the duodenum to the right. Injuries to the SMA require repair or reconstruction. Ligation is not an option as this will lead to small bowel infarction. Autogenous conduits are preferable for SMA reconstructions but prosthetic grafts can be used if enteric contamination is not present. The reconstruction is usually via a lazy S from the iliac artery to the posterior aspect of the SMA.

Injuries to the superior mesenteric vein and portal vein are highly lethal. Ligation is probably not an option as venous infarction is very high. Direct damage to the portal vein requires interposition grafting using the internal jugular vein as lateral suture will probably cause severe stenosis and subsequent venous and portal hypertension.

Inferior Vena Cava

Injuries to the IVC are usually associated with significant blood loss and are highly lethal. Sometimes it is difficult to know in a retroperitoneal zone 1 area whether it is the aorta or the IVC which is damaged. Sometimes it is both. The exposure is achieved using the Cattell-Braasch manoeuvre extended with kocherization of the of the duodenum and full mobilization of the duodenopancreatic complex. This exposes the entire extent of the IVC from the common iliac veins confluence to where the cava becomes retrohepatic. Because of the easily torn lumbar veins, control is best achieved using direct sponge stick control. Immediate control is also important to avoid air embolism. Primary repair without significant stenosis can be achieved in the majority of cases. If greater than 50% stenosis is expected with primary repair, then a vein patch or, if damage control necessitates, ligation can be performed. The subsequent venous hypertension in the leg compartment may necessitate bilateral thigh and leg fasciotomy.

Zone 2 Exploration

Proximal renal artery exposure is achieved by division of the ligament of Treitz and mobilization of the duodenum to the right. The left renal vein is identified and usually needs to be mobilized to allow exposure of the aortic segment where the renal arteries originate. The management of renovascular injuries is determined by the duration of warm ischaemia, haemodynamic status of the patient and condition of the contralateral kidney. Active bleeding from a renal hilum is best managed by a nephrectomy in a haemodynamically unstable patient, but renovascular reconstruction should be considered for a haemodynamically stable patient with less than 6 hours of warm renal ischaemia.

Zone 3 Exploration

Expanding haematomas from penetrating trauma in zone 3 should be explored to rule out injuries to the iliac vessels. Proximal control prior to haematoma exploration is obtained at the distal aorta. Distal control it is usually easy at the external iliac artery. Autogenous vein bypass can be used or patching techniques or a prosthetic graft. In the confines, though, of enteric soiling, copious washout is necessary with possibility of cover with an omental patch.

However, right common iliac vein injuries may require division of the right common iliac artery to get access. If possible, lateral repair would be more suitable than ligation but, in the damage control situation, ligation can be life-saving.

In blunt injuries, non-expanding haematomas should not be explored. In patients with significant bony pelvic injuries with an expanding haematoma, this is more likely to be due to an arterial cause principally due to superior gluteal or pudendal artery shearing. With significant haemodynamic instability, the haematoma should be opened (the haematoma does most of the dissection) and the extra peritoneal space on both sides of the rectum should be packed as tight as possible with packs from the sacroiliac joint to the pubic ramus on both sides. Packing should be performed using unrolled large packs with a long forceps. Tight packing is necessary if one is to reduce the amount of arterial flow. Once haemodynamic stability has been assured, then the patient can be transferred to the interventional radiology suite for formal embolization.

Peripheral Vascular Injuries

Typical vascular patterns in blunt trauma due to fractures are common in the peripheries. A clavicular fracture can cause subclavian artery injury. Axillary artery thrombosis due to intimal damage caused by stretching is a risk factor in shoulder dislocation. Supracondylar fracture of the elbow commonly causes brachial occlusion especially in children. The forearm vessels are most commonly injured in penetrating injuries. In the lower extremity, the popliteal artery is the most commonly injured vessel after blunt mechanisms such as knee dislocation, whereas a superficial femoral artery is the most common penetrating location of vascular injury.

Proximal and distal vascular control should be, in theory, outside the zone of injury. For example, a brachial artery injury should have proximal axillary artery control using an infraclavicular incision. The technique is to spread the pectoralis major muscle followed by division of the pectoralis minor muscle to gain access to the axillary artery. The haematoma can then be opened without significant arterial bleeding from the injury. Once vascular control has been obtained, the decision to use damage control principles as discussed previously, should be evaluated.

A low threshold should exist for performing prophylactic fasciotomy. In the upper limb, one incision is made on the palmer aspect including the carpal tunnel and one on the dorsal aspect.

Fasciotomy of the lower limb is a two-incision, four-compartment fasciotomy. The incision is made one fingerbreadth below the tibial spine on the lateral aspect and one fingerbreadth below the inferior part of the tibia in the medial aspect. In that way, one still preserves the perforators to the skin to allow for rotational flaps. After making a long incision on the lateral aspect of the leg, the fascia over tibialis anterior is then divided in the whole length of the wound. The inferior border of the tibialis anterior is then retracted such that the fascia can be divided to enter the lateral peroneal compartment. The medial/posterior aspect of the leg has two compartments, a superficial and a deep. There are three muscles in the superficial compartment (gastrocnemius, soleus and plantaris) and there are four muscles in the deep compartment (popliteus, flexor digitorum longus, flexor hallucis longus and tibialis posterior). The first medial incision is made over the superficial muscles, the soleus is then taken off its origin from the tibia, and the fascia can be found overlying the posterior tibial artery. This artery confirms entrance into the deep fascial compartment.

Accessing the Upper Limb Vessels

The subclavian artery is divided into three parts by the scalenus anterior muscle. The first part is from the origin to the border with the scalenus anterior, the second part is behind the scalenus anterior and the third part is from the scalenus anterior to the outer border of the first rib. A supra-clavicular incision is made, platysma divided and the scalenus fat pad mobilized laterally to expose the scalenus anterior muscle with the phrenic nerve (the only nerve in the body which goes from lateral to medial). The muscle is divided, taking great care to avoid the phrenic nerve, and the subclavian artery can be slinged. Great care should be taken in doing this because the subclavian artery is probably the most fragile artery in the body and pulling can easily disrupt the intima.

Dissection of the axillary artery has already been discussed above. The axillary artery becomes the brachial artery at the lower border of teres major. It can easily be accessed in the group between biceps and triceps. The median nerve tends to run with the brachial artery and its venae comitantes and is a useful adjunct in finding the vessel. At the elbow, the biceps aponeurosis must be divided to gain access. The radial and ulnar arteries can be followed from the brachial at the elbow. If both arteries are damaged, then it is better to repair the ulnar artery as it is commonly the dominant source of palmar arch arterial supply.

Lower Limb

Significant injuries to the common femoral vessels mandate proximal control performed via an extraperitoneal suprainguinal incision with division of the external oblique aponeurosis followed by division of the internal and transversus muscles. The peritoneum is preserved and mobilized medially. The anatomical landmark is the psoas muscle with the external iliac artery lying medial to the muscle. Careful blunt dissection allows for slinging of the artery and clamping.

The common femoral artery lies at the mid inguinal point, between the anterior superior iliac spine and the pubic symphysis. The inguinal ligament can be divided if additional proximal exposure is required. The common femoral, superficial femoral and popliteal are all relatively medium-size vessels which lend themselves to intra-arterial shunting in damage control. Definitive repair is performed using the long saphenous vein, preferably from the other leg.

Popliteal Artery

Blunt popliteal arteries are commonly associated with tibial plateau fractures and posterior knee dislocation. Missed injuries and injuries not promptly repaired have high rates of amputation. Medial exposure of the retrogeniculate popliteal artery is accomplished with separate incisions above and below the knee. Further exposure is performed by dividing the three tendons of the hamstring muscles, semitendinosus, semimembranosus and sartorius. Selective short segment popliteal injuries in the retrogeniculate location may be repaired through a posterior approach. The majority of popliteal artery injuries can be repaired with either an end-to-end anastomosis or saphenous vein interposition. Associated venous injuries should be repaired if possible and, of course, fasciotomy must be performed in all traumatic vascular damage in the lower limb.

Paediatric Vascular Injuries

In young children, supracondylar humeral fractures are associated with high-risk brachial artery injury. If the radial pulse is not restored after reduction of these fractures, brachial artery exploration should be performed. The vessels of young children are prone to vasospasm during the manipulation required for repair. Topical or intra-arterial nitroglycerin or papaverine may prove helpful in treatment of this arterial vasospasm. For extremity arterial injuries, a limb with normal neurological function and distal Doppler signals can be managed non-operatively. Long-term follow-up is required, however, due to the risk of stunted limb growth with age. When required, paediatric arterial repairs should be performed with interrupted 8/0 sutures.

HEAD AND NECK SURGERY

Severe maxillofacial and neck trauma exposes patients to life-threatening complications such as airway compromise, haemorrhagic shock and management of vision threatening injuries. Penetrating maxillofacial and neck injuries result in a complex of lacerations, open fractures, profuse bleeding, tissue avulsions, eye injuries and burns. The critical immediate life-threatening injury following maxillofacial injury results from airway compromise due to oropharyngeal bleeding, swelling and loss of mandibular structural integrity.

The airway is maintained and secured by tracheal intubation or via surgical airways such as cricothyroidotomy or tracheostomy. Once the airway is secured, direct pressure and aggressive packing of open bleeding wounds will control all but the most catastrophic haemorrhages. External fixation of unstable anterior mandibular fractures using available means such as pin fixators or wiring may assist in preventing airway compromise as well as reducing profuse bleeding, pain and morbidity often associated with such injuries. More significant bleeding can be controlled by angiographic embolization or selective ligation of the external carotid artery, whilst simultaneously protecting the brain, cervical spine and eyes from further injury. Early fixation of the flail mandible is also mandatory because it may destabilize tongue musculature insertions, thus compromising the airway, and also cause bleeding, significant pain and morbidity. Head and neck injuries should be copiously irrigated, wound contaminants removed, clearly nonviable tissue fragments should debrided and the wounds covered to prevent further contamination. Suturing of soft tissue lacerations covering underlying bone fractures should be deferred so that such fractures should not be overlooked during subsequent examination of the patient.

Airway Control and Breathing Support in Maxillofacial Trauma

Initial casualty assessment determines whether the airway is patent and protected, and if breathing is present and adequate. Normal speech may suggest that the airway is patent, at least for the time being, whilst wheezy breathing usually indicates partial airway obstruction by the tongue and hoarseness or stridor usually suggest a laryngeal cause. The oral cavity must be thoroughly cleared, visualized and inspected under proper lighting, taking care not to extend or to rotate the neck. Blood, loose and fractured teeth, foreign bodies, dirt and mucus are meticulously removed. The midface and mandible are inspected for structural integrity and the anterior neck inspected for penetrating wounds. Crepitus upon palpation of the neck may suggest airway injury or communicating pneumomediastinum. Diminished breath sounds on auscultation may result from atelectasis, pneumothorax, haemothorax or pleural effusion. Wheezing and dyspnoea may imply lower airway obstruction, agitation may represent hypoxia at tissue level and cyanosis indicates arterial blood hypoxaemia.

Despite active bleeding and gaping facial wounds, the fastest and most straightforward technique to establish a definitive airway is often direct laryngoscopy and endotracheal intubation using a rapid sequence technique. If this fails, a cricothyroidotomy is an expedient technique to establish a definitive airway. If right-handed, hold the tracheal cartilage in the left hand and palpate with the right hand the space between the cartilage and the cricoid cartilage, make a vertical incision and plunge the blade of the scalpel into the membrane. Once achieving an airway, rotate the scalpel and put the handle into the space created and put a size 4–6 endotracheal tube into the trachea. In an emergency situation, a surgical cricothyroidotomy is preferred to tracheostomy because it is more rapidly executed, the distance from the skin is shorter (10 mm versus 20–30 mm) and the risk of violating the vascular thyroid isthmus resulting in haemorrhage is lower.

Head and Neck Trauma Surgery

From the faciomaxillary perspective, emergency care in facial trauma effectively means airway management, control of profuse bleeding and the management of vision threatening injuries (VTI). Most maxillofacial trauma is in the context of other major life-threatening injuries, especially in blunt trauma, and life-saving surgery may be required

before tackling other injuries. Most facial injuries can be placed into one of four groups:

1. Immediate life- or sight-saving treatment as required, e.g. surgical airway, controlling profuse haemorrhage and sight-preserving surgery such as lateral canthotomy for retrobulbar haemorrhage.
2. Treatment is required within a few hours. This applies to clinically urgent injuries such as heavily contaminated wounds and some contaminated open fractures (especially skull fractures with exposed dura). The patient is otherwise clinically stable.
3. Treatment can wait 24 hours if necessary (some fractures and clean lacerations).
4. Treatment can wait for over 24 hours if necessary (most fractures).

When assessing injuries above the collarbones, consider them under four main anatomic subheadings:

a. the brain
b. the neck
c. the eyes
d. the face

In all trauma patients, the first priority is to assess the airway. In facial trauma, reduction in conscious level may be due to alcohol consumption, brain injury or hypoxaemia due to hypovolaemia, and early intubation may be required. Retropharyngeal haematoma secondary to cervical spine injury can also occasionally result in airway obstruction, as well as from food debris, dentures, teeth, blood and secretions or displaced/swollen tissues. The most common obstructed materials in facial injuries are blood and vomit. Accumulation of blood in the stomach can give rise to unexpected vomiting. Trauma to the front of the neck (bicycle injuries, car crashes, falls, sports injuries, clothesline injuries and hanging) can also result in direct injuries the upper airway and, occasionally, expanding haematoma. In most awake patients, blood and secretions are normally swallowed; however, in midface or mandibular fractures, swallowing may be painful and ineffective. Be aware also that the mandibular support of the tongue may be compromised in jaw fractures and can easily obstruct the airway, in addition to soft tissue swelling and retropropulsion of mid-face fractures.

Although facial injuries are not a common cause of hypovolaemia, clinically significant haemorrhage has been reported to occur in approximately 10% of pan-facial fractures. Unfortunately, bleeding may not always be immediately apparent. It can also be difficult to control due to the extensive collateral blood supply to the face. External blood loss from the scalp, face and neck are usually more obvious and can be profuse. In children, this can quickly result in hypovolaemia. In the pan-facial fracture, bleeding comes from multiple sites along the fractures and torn soft tissues rather than a named vessel. This makes control difficult. Significant concealed bleeding may occur in the supine patient, and it should therefore be considered in cases of persisting shock. These patients are also likely to develop significant soft tissue swelling and the airway may need to be secured early. Once intubated, blood loss becomes more apparent as blood is no longer swallowed or overspilled from the mouth and nose.

Damage control maxillofacial surgery should be performed at this stage with significant blood loss. External bleeding should initially be controlled by direct pressure, clips or sutures. With displacement midface fractures, early manual reduction not only improves the airway but helps to control blood loss and can be performed following intubation. Oral bleeding can be controlled with sutures or local gauze packs. Epistaxis, either in isolation or associated with midface fractures, may be controlled using a specifically-designed balloon or, if not available, two urinary catheters can be used, each passed via the nostril into the pharynx under direct vision and inflated with saline and then gently withdrawn until the balloon wedges in the postnasal space. The nasal cavity can then be packed. Packs are normally removed after 24 to 48 hours.

If haemorrhage persists despite these interventions, it is important to consider coagulation abnormalities. These may either be pre-existing (e.g. haemophilia, chronic liver disease, warfarin therapy) or acquired (dilutional coagulopathy). Facial fractures may be temporarily stabilized in various ways. These include wires, splints, intermaxillary fixation (IMF) or plating techniques. The aim of all these treatments is to rapidly reduce and stabilize fractures. Separation of fractures and movement between them is not only painful but can result in significant bleeding and swelling. External fixation is also very effective in providing rapid stabilization. It can also be used long-term with significant soft tissue damage. If bleeding continues despite all these measures, further interventions include ligation of the external carotid and ethmoidal arteries via the neck and medial wall of the orbit.

Vision Threatening Injuries

In the alert patient, it only takes a few seconds to assess for vision in each eye (during the assessment of the GCS), check pupil size and reaction and, if the eye is proptosed, carefully palpate the globe through closed eyelids. Ocular injuries range from simple corneal abrasions to devastating injuries resulting in total and irreversible loss of sight. Because of the close proximity of the structures within the anterior and middle cranial fossa to the orbit (separated by some of the thinnest bones in the body), penetrating intracranial injury must always be considered in penetrating orbital injuries.

Vision threatening injuries (VTIs) commonly present with severe visual impairment or blindness immediately after injury.

Loss of sight maybe due to the following mechanisms:
1. Direct injury to the globe
2. Direct injury to the optic nerve e.g. bony impingement
3. Indirect injury to the optic nerve (decelerating injury resulting in shearing and stretching forces)
4. Reduction in tissue perfusion (anterior ischaemic optic neuropathy, retrobulbar haemorrhage, nutrient vessel disruption)
5. Loss of eyelid integrity

Visual acuity testing and colour perception are the reliable tests in the conscious patient. In the unconscious patient, pupil size and funduscopy for the detection of intraocular haemorrhage and the red reflex suggest abnormal or normal signs. Critically raised retrobulbar pressures need to be recognized and treated promptly. Irreversible optic and retinal ischaemia can occur within 60 minutes and permanent vision loss within 2 hours.

The orbit is mostly a rigid box apart from anteriorly and any increase in volume from bleeding or swelling will quickly increase interstitial pressure. This decreases the perfusion pressure, resulting in ischaemia and infarction eventually. Traditionally, the tense, proptosed non-seeing eye with a non-reacting dilated pupil following facial trauma is considered to be a surgical emergency that requires immediate decompression by performing a lateral canthotomy. This is performed using local anaesthesia and the lateral canthal raphe is divided. This allows the globe to move forward, partially relieving the pressure and effectively increasing the retrobulbar volume.

The formal evacuation of the haematomas is carried out under general anaesthesia. The orbital and intraconal spaces are opened allowing blood and oedema to escape. Occasionally, proptosis can be seen on CT, the classic balloon-on-a-string sign. Management of globe injuries depends on whether the injury is open or closed. Analgesia and antiemetics should be administered and tetanus status checked. Hard plastic shields should be taped over the orbit to protect open globes. Primary surgical repair of an open globe should be performed under general anaesthetic as soon as possible but within 24 hours after the trauma. Inability to effectively close the eyelids rapidly results in drying of the cornea, ulceration and, potentially, loss of sight. Until the defect is repaired, eyelid remnants should be pulled over to provide corneal cover, if necessary using a traction suture, liberal application of chloramphenicol should be administered and the whole area covered with sterile wet gauze swab. Full-thickness skin grafts are often used in the reconstruction of the eyelid.

Management of Facial Fractures

Mandibular Fractures

The hallmark of a mandibular fracture is a change in the patient's occlusion.

If a mandibular fracture can be reduced manually, a bridal or tie wire should be passed around the teeth on either side and tightened. This provides temporary support, preventing painful movement. In a sense, this can be regarded as the maxillofacial equivalent of an orthopaedic back slab.

Intermaxillary fixation (IMF), also known as maxillo-mandibular fixation, is commonly used in the management of mandibular fractures. This is based on the assumption that if the upper and lower teeth are repositioned back into the patient's preinjury occlusion, the bones will be anatomically reduced. Although open reduction and internal fixation (ORIF) is now preferred in many centres, in those countries that do not have the resources for expensive plating systems, IMF is still commonly and successfully used. The principle of IMF is straightforward. Arch bars, books or eyelets are applied to the upper and lower dentition using circumflex dental wires or adhesives. These are then used to hold the teeth into occlusion. If dentition is a problem, then IMF screws can be placed into the dentoalveolar bone between the roots of the teeth and wires or bands can be placed between the screws. Most maxillofacial units tend to surgically expose, anatomically reduce, and then repair fractures (ORIF). Compared to orthopaedic surgery, salivary growth factors and the excellent blood supply to the face provide favourable conditions for healing. Fractures can therefore be more extensively exposed, with less risk of infection or avascular necrosis.

The main role of external fixation in maxillofacial trauma as to provide rapid first-aid stabilization (damage control) in the multi-injured patient. With gunshot wounds or other types of contamination, this method also provides good long-term temporary fixation until the contaminated wounds have healed. In order to attain effective stability, two pins are placed on either side of the fracture. Many types of devices exist, some specifically designed for the mandible, others fabricated from general external fixation kits. If a kit is unavailable, acrylic connecting bars can easily be fabricated with the aid of an endotracheal tube for chest drain filled with acrylic resin.

Midface Fractures

The term midface is often used to refer collectively to those structures situated between the skull base and the occlusal plane. Many of these bones are extremely thin. The two maxillary bones are joined in the midline to form the bulk of the middle third of the face. They support the teeth in the roof of the oral cavity. They also form the floor and part of the lateral wall of the nasal cavity, contain the maxillary sinus and contribute to the medial part of the infra-orbital rim and orbital floor.

Fractures of the mid-face can be classified under the LeFort classification. They can be divided into three types:

* Type I: this is often due to a direct horizontal impact to the upper jaw and causes a transverse fracture through the maxillary sinuses, lower nasal septum and pterygoid plates
* Type 2: it is usually due to a direct impact of the central midface causing an oblique fracture crossing the zygomaticomaxillary suture, inferior orbital rim and nasal bridge
* Type 3: this causes craniofacial dissociation and is a fracture above the zygomatic arch through the lateral and medial orbital walls and nasofrontal suture

In theory, the level of the LeFort fracture can be determined by a detailed clinical examination. Abnormal mobility of the midface can be detected by grasping the front teeth and holding the nasal bone and gently rocking the

maxilla. If the teeth and palate move but the nasal bones are stable, then this is a LeFort 1 fracture. If the teeth, palate and nasal bones move but the lateral orbital rims are stable, then this is a LeFort II fracture. If the whole of the midface feels unstable, it is probably a LeFort III.

Although plain films provide some useful information, patients with suspected midface fractures should ideally undergo CT scanning of the face.

Treatment

The goal of faciomaxillary fracture treatment is to concentrate on reduction and fixation of the main struts of the facial skeleton such as the zygomaticomaxillary strut, the maxilla-alveolar strut, infra-orbital nasal rim and fronto-cranial skull base. If these structures are not adequately re-positioned and stabilized, then varying degrees of disfiguration and functional disability will occur.

However, in patients in whom the maxilla is not displaced and stable, non-operative management may be appropriate. In cases of maxillary impaction, it is wise to dis-impact the structure before soft tissues begin to fibrose and contract, ideally within 48 hours. Digital manipulation using a gentle rocking motion is enough to free the maxilla and re-establish the occlusion. It is important to watch out for any CSF leakage, excessive bleeding or proptosis as these may indicate serious complications. Instruments are applied into the nose and mouth designed specifically to be placed on the hard palate from above and below to pull the maxilla into position. Operative fixation of these fractures, aided by careful planning with open reduction and mini plating, is the treatment of choice, based on detailed CT scans.

External fixation may be indicated for blast injuries, rapid mobilization or in severe comminution. In such cases, the occlusion is used to align the fractures, which are then immobilized by fixing them to the cranium or frontal bone. External fixation is generally carried out using supraorbital pins or a halo frame connected to the maxilla with a bar. Other methods to fix the maxilla include using wires placed around the zygoma onto an arch bar placed on the teeth of the mandible. Mandibular fractures in this context can either be wired by IMF or externally fixated depending on the resources available.

Head Trauma

Primary brain injury is injury to the actual fabric of the brain. It is often untreatable and generally determines outcome. Secondary brain injury is the response of the body to the primary brain injury which, if not treated, will inevitably lead to clinical deterioration. Secondary brain injury involves managing raised intracranial pressure and is extremely time-sensitive. For example, in a patient with a subdural haematoma, the primary injury is to the hemisphere of the brain and, as a result, the hemisphere bleeds and swells, causing the secondary injury, which then causes a rise in intracranial pressure.

The cranium is a rigid box which contains the brain and three fluids, cerebral spinal fluid (CSF), venous blood and arterial blood. The intracranial volume is around 1500 mL: the brain and arterial blood take up around 1300 mL, the rest is CSF and venous blood. The pressure within the cranium, the intracranial pressure (ICP), is usually less than 10 mmHg and any increase in the volume will cause the ICP to rise, which is governed by the Monro-Kellie doctrine. In the context of trauma, the brain volume and the arterial volume generally remain stable, but there can be variations in the amount of CSF and venous blood. An expanding mass within the skull such as a haematoma initially displaces CSF and venous blood to compensate for the volume change. This is the lucid interval following a head injury. As the mass gets bigger, the compensatory mechanisms are exhausted when all the CSF has been expelled down into the lumbar region and venous blood into the venous circulation, and the ICP suddenly increases and, if not treated early, the patient will become unconscious and die due to the coning effect of the brain.

There are many different types of brain coning. The most common is the movement of the cingulate gyrus under the falx cerebri, seen on a CT scan as midline shift. The next is the movement of the uncus of the temporal lobe under the tentorium cerebri putting pressure on the third cranial nerve causing a blown pupil on the same side as the lesion. One which is more dramatic and can cause rapid death is the whole of the pons and midbrain being pushed down toward the tentorium incisura causing rapid respiratory failure and death.

As in all forms of trauma, the injury can be divided into blunt and penetrating. Blunt trauma characteristically causes subdural haematoma, extradural haematoma and brain contusions.

Subdural Haematoma

Acute subdural haematoma, a traumatic venous bleed due to stretching and tearing of the veins on the brain surface, occurs in the space under the dura on the outside of the brain substance and distributes itself alongside the whole side of the brain as there are no divisions. On CT, it is characteristically concave. The degree of primary injury to the brain in an acute subdural is what makes the difference in the outcome. The necessity to treat the secondary brain injury is of paramount importance by performing a craniotomy and removing the source of the raised intracranial pressure but, if the primary brain injury is significant, the outcome following an acute subdural haematoma may not be optimal.

Extradural Haematoma

This occurs secondary to a skull fracture mainly in the temporal region, which causes a tearing of the middle meningeal artery. The dura has two layers, a superficial layer which serves as the skull's inner periosteum, called the endocranium, and a deeper layer, called the meningeal layer. In an extradural haematoma, the arterial blood collects between the bone and the endocranium. Because the endocranium of the skull goes up into the sutures, an extradural haematoma does not cross any of the sutures lines and is often quite contained and does not cover the side of the brain as does a subdural. It is characteristically lens shaped. It takes quite a high pressure to strip the dura off the inside of the skull. This again will cause midline shift. So, in this case, there is no primary brain injury; what causes the bleeding is a skull fracture. As the extradural haematoma expands, it compresses the brain and, unless something is done, the patient will rapidly lose consciousness and potentially die, but if it removed quickly enough, then the patient will make an excellent recovery as there is no underlying brain injury. Extradural haematomas are time-sensitive emergencies and are potentially fatal. They often occur in young people and, if treated promptly, the patient can have an excellent outcome.

Cerebral Contusions

Mainly a primary brain injury, often due to a patient hitting the back of the head and causing a contrecoup injury with the brain being thrown forward inside the cranial vault and the base of the frontal lobes hitting the base of the frontal fossa floor. At the same time, the olfactory nerve is torn and, if patients survive, they often complain of anosmia. Primary brain injury can be seen as a diffuse brain oedema with intra-cerebral haematoma.

The secondary injury which is treated is brain oedema which causes raised ICP. Often, pressure monitoring equipment can be used to measure the ICP and guide the clinicians in management. Several non-surgical techniques are used to reduce ICP, e.g. raising the head of the bed, keeping the patient fully sedated, hyperosmolar diuretics such as mannitol to reduce brain swelling, careful management of the pCO_2, increasing the cerebral perfusion pressure by increasing the mean arterial pressure, cooling the patient or inducing coma using thiopentone.

Surgery

Targeted burr holes for relief of the intracranial haematoma diagnosed on CT can be performed using powered tools such as the perforator drill bit, which works with electric or pneumatic energy to perforate the skull. The hole is then enlarged using a burr, which stops at the dura. Manual burr holes can be performed using the Hudson brace, which relies on the operator drilling a hole using the perforator until the dura can just be seen underneath its tip and then a burr is applied to widen the hole. It is important to stand correctly, with one foot forward and the other one back, and apply just the correct amount of pressure to the drill.

In the case of an extradural haematoma, the burr hole made over the fracture line is usually 1 cm above the tip of the ear and 1 cm forward of the site where one would be greeted with arterial blood. This can then be converted into conventional craniotomy using multiple burr holes to raise a craniotomy flap and then treat the bleeding middle meningeal artery with either cautery or suture. The burr holes can be joined up using a Gigli saw or an electrically operated craniotome.

Similar techniques are used for subdural haematomas, raising an inverted question mark incision and subsequent craniotomy. The dura is then opened either using a semicircle incision or cruciate incision and the clot washed out and any bleeding vessels, which may be arterial or venous, on the brain surface are coagulated. In case of brain swelling, the craniotomy may be placed in an abdominal wall pocket for future placement.

In austere environments, without using a CT scan, exploratory burr holes are made over the side of the fracture or where the signs of raised intracranial pressure are made, such as a blown pupil. Penetrating injuries such as those with bomb blasts and fragmentation wounds are treated first of all by a proper wound toilet, with removal of all the scalp hair and exploration of the scalp wounds. Motor signs such as localizing to pain, which involves movement of the hand above the chin line on supra orbital pressure, will give an indication on whether surgery may be necessary. In this environment, any motor signs lower than this render surgery futile. If surgery is appropriate, several burr holes are placed next to the entrance the fragmentation wound and a craniotomy raised, the dura is then opened to allow any blood under pressure to be extruded. Wound debridement is then performed removing all dead and infected looking material, followed by copious saline. The dura does not need to be repaired and the craniotomy flap can be sutured back into place.

EXTREMITY AND SOFT TISSUE TRAUMA

The goal and the management of extremity and soft tissue trauma is to prevent secondary or tertiary deaths and subsequently minimize morbidity related to musculoskeletal injury. Typically, secondary mortality can be minimized by stabilization of fractures of the pelvis and long bones. Stabilization of such injuries not only helps with the reduction of blood loss but also decreases the pain stimuli, reducing the analgesia and anaesthetic requirements, which helps with normalizing physiology. Furthermore, stabilization of the long bones can also minimize the risk of pulmonary complications due to fat emboli and pulmonary embolism.

Open fractures involve a direct communication of the injured bone with the environment and are often the reflection of high-energy injury. Not only does the potential for contamination worsen the injury burden but the high-energy indicates severe damage to local soft tissues, both leading to wound complications and increased potential for infection. Open fractures are classified by the Gustilo Anderson classification into three types:

- Type I is a wound which is less than 1 cm with minimal soft tissue injury.

- Type II is a wound greater than 1 cm in length with moderate soft tissue injury
- Type IIIA is extensive soft tissue injury with degloving or periosteal stripping but where soft tissue closure is possible
- Type IIIB is extensive soft tissue injury with periosteal stripping which requires a flap coverage
- Type IIIC is associated with an arterial injury requiring repair

The most important predictor of infection following open fracture seems to be the timeliness of antibiotic administration, with antibiotics given more than 60 minutes after the injury being an independent risk factor for infection. Typically, a first-generation cephalosporin is recommended with additional broader coverage only in certain scenarios. Surgical debridement and irrigation should be performed within 24 hours, and ideally sooner, depending on the level of contamination. The type of fixation, which can be either temporary or definitive, depends on the level of soft tissue injury and contamination and also the degree to which resuscitation is necessary. Wound coverage should be ideally performed within 5 to 7 days.

In the presence of haemodynamic instability even in the context of a closed femoral fracture, blood loss can be as much as 2.2 L. In such situations, it is advocated that skeletal immobilization of long bone fractures be performed during the primary survey. The femur can be immobilized by external fixation or skeletal traction until early operative skeletal stabilization can be performed.

Because of the energy needed to create a pelvic ring injury, there is often concomitant significant haemodynamic instability and possibly head injury, thoraco-abdominal injuries and long bone fractures. Pelvic fractures resulting in blood loss and hypovolaemia have a mortality rate up to 20%. With increasing fracture severity and more posterior pelvic disruption, the pelvic venous plexus and the internal iliac vessels are at an increased risk of injury and subsequent uncontrolled haemorrhage. Stabilization of the pelvic ring is necessary to close the injury using pelvic binder initially followed by external fixation.

Acute compartment syndrome (ACS) is defined as pressure within a closed space with the potential to cause irreversible damage to the contents of the closed space. There is progressive myoneural ischaemia due to the accumulation of fluid within a confined myofascial space or prolonged elevated pressure due to an external source such as a crush injury. ACS is considered a surgical emergency because irreversible muscle necrosis can begin within six hours of injury. The six Ps normally describe this: Pressure with a turgid compartment with shiny skin, Pain out of proportion with movement and late findings such as Paraesthesia, Paralysis, Pallor and Poikilothermia. Once ACS is diagnosed, emergent fasciotomies are performed to relieve the pressure and prevent further myoneural ischaemia. These have been described earlier.

A vascular injury should be suspected if the injured extremity shows signs of pallor, reduced temperature, prolonged capillary refill and reduced pulses. Gross limb length and alignment should be obtained and the limb re-examined. The ankle brachial pressure index should be obtained if a vascular injury is suspected, with a value of 0.9 or lower having a high positive predictive value for an associated vascular injury. Re-establishment of the blood supply to the limb is an emergency because muscle necrosis begins to occur within 6 hours of injury. The damage control method involves inserting a shunt into the blood vessel to establish arterial flow and then performing skeletal stabilization and, following this, a definitive repair if the physiology is normalized.

The close proximity and tethering of neurovascular structures to joints places them at significant risk of injury in joint dislocation. Localized soft tissue swelling, distal extremity oedema, abnormal neurology or signs of vascular compromise are all markers for a high index of suspicion of a major joint dislocation. Expedient joint relocation and stabilization in a splint or traction may be necessary. Unlike most dislocations, a hip dislocation is considered as an orthopaedic emergency and should be reduced immediately on recognition because of an increased time reduction associated with the subsequent development of avascular necrosis.

In the polytrauma patient, there is much discussion about the appropriate timing to stabilize fractures. Ideally, the correct surgery is performed for each patient, personally tailored to their physiologic status. In the orthopaedic arena, there are two ongoing arguments with protagonists for both early total care (ETC) and for damage control orthopaedics (DCO).

Patients with unstable fractures of the femur, pelvis, acetabulum and spine are often forced into a recumbent position, which predisposes to pulmonary complications and prolonged systemic inflammation. Early stabilization of these fractures can lead to improved pain relief and mobility. Several studies have clearly demonstrated the benefits of ETC. Harvin[3] published a decade of experience comparing femur fractures definitively stabilized with intra-medullary nails before and after 24 hours. It was found that early fracture fixation was independently associated with a reduction in pulmonary complications by nearly 60%, a reduction in ventilator days and hospital length of stay. As evidence suggests, early definitive treatment may be safely used for patients with multiple injuries. However, ETC is not ideal for all patients as there is a subset of patients who will benefit more from DCO.

Damage Control Orthopaedics

Not all patients benefit from early definitive stabilization. In certain patients, particularly those with abdominal, pulmonary or head injuries, a less aggressive approach to fracture fixation is needed. Trauma causes sustained response of the immune system and the early hyper-inflammatory response is often followed by a hypo-inflammatory stage. In the polytrauma patient, extended surgery, which can lead to increased blood loss, hypovolaemia and surgical trauma, can

result in an excessive inflammatory reaction, which has been termed the 'second hit'. In these patients, extensive surgical procedures can overwhelm the immune system, which can trigger a pulmonary complication such as ARDS or multiple organ failure.

Although modern skeletal stabilization techniques, such as internal fixation, have become the primary method of treatment, there is the occasional patient who requires extensive resuscitation where this would be inappropriate. DCO involves stabilizing the fracture, using external fixation of long bones, and unstable pelvic ring injuries. This avoids open, lengthy and often bloody surgical procedures, the second hit is theoretically avoided and definitive reconstruction can occur at a later point, after the patient's physiological parameters have improved. The benefits of this strategy on the immune system have been demonstrated by Pape[4] who showed that, in those patients with ETC (intramedullary nail), there was a sustained increase in serum inflammatory markers, which was not seen in the DCO group following both the initial external fixation and subsequent conversion to definitive fixation with an intramedullary nail.

It has also been shown that the risk of multiorgan failure is higher with ETC than with DCO, emphasizing the impact that the second hit can have and the importance of planning the definitive fixation based on physiological improvement. Indeed, as in all damage control surgical and resuscitation scenarios, treating the physiology rather than the anatomy is mandatory, performing quick, safe, orthopaedic stabilization using external fixation and soft tissue debridement of all devitalized tissue, skin, fascia and bone. If the patient needs to go back to theatre several times for sequential debridement, then that is an indication for DCO. It is so important to make sure that the wound is clean before definitive treatment such as an intramedullary nail or plate.

Coverage of the bone, especially the tibia, is necessary when it is clean and free from infection. The lower leg is characteristically divided into three zones, the proximal third, middle third and distal third. Exposed tibia in the proximal third can be covered by a medial gastrocnemius flap and a split skin graft, the middle third by a soleal flap and, in the lower third, by a cross leg flap or sural flap. Both of these flaps are fasciocutaneous flaps which rely on blood supply from perforators from the posterior tibial artery and sural artery.

PRINCIPLES OF TRAUMA CARE TO THE SOLID ORGANS OF THE THORAX AND ABDOMEN

Thorax

It only takes around 50 mL of blood to cause the effects of cardiac tamponade, low blood pressure, distended neck veins and muffled heart sounds – the so-called Beck's triad.

Treatment requires a left anterolateral thoracotomy in the 5th intercostal space. The incision is made from the sternum to the operating table and follows the line of the rib. The intercostal muscle is incised on the superior border of the rib below so as not to damage the intercostal vessels and nerve.

The pericardium is opened longitudinally above the phrenic nerve as it passes to innovate the diaphragm on the pericardium. This releases pressure on the heart from the blood in the pericardial space. An assessment is then made on whether the heart is beating, whether it contains a good amount of blood or is partially empty.

There is not much room following this incision apart from relieving the tamponade and performing internal cardiac massage, using four fingers from both hands to massage the heart if required. To improve exposure of the heart, the incision traverses the sternum, which is divided using a strong pair of scissors or a Lebsche sternal knife. The heart can be exposed by this extended left anterolateral thoracotomy or, if required, by extending the incision to perform a right anterolateral thoracotomy – the so-called clamshell procedure. Two finochietto retractors are placed to elevate the rib cage. It may be necessary to divide some of the sternopericardial ligaments that are attached to the back of the sternum to expose the heart fully. The pericardium is then fully opened to the arch of the aorta where it becomes joined to the adventitia of the aorta.

In the majority of cases, it is the right ventricle which has been lacerated. The tamponade effect of pressure on the heart is usually pressure on the atria reducing preload. If the heart is beating, then light finger pressure over the lacerated right ventricle will allow the operating surgeon to place a pledgeted, 4/0 prolene, double-ended, round-bodied needle through-and-through the heart to close the defect. It is very important that the suture is pledgeted with either PTFE felt or pericardium as the suture can easily tear the heart and make the defect larger. If the injury is close to a coronary vessel, the stitch is placed further away from the laceration so as to elevate the coronary vessel and not cause occlusion and subsequent infarction of the heart muscle.

The muscle of the right ventricle is thin and can easily be damaged by pressure of a digit such as the thumb and so distributed, four-finger pressure when performing internal cardiac massage is highly recommended. If the heart is empty, then it may be necessary to increase afterload by applying a clamp on the distal thoracic aorta. In this case, the pleura over the aorta needs to be divided for a distance of 2 to 3 cm to allow the adventitia to be exposed, and careful digital manipulation of the aorta at this area will help in application of a clamp as intercostal vessels are easily damaged. It is very important to constantly assess the heart as it is possible to cause crashing heart failure following overdistention, especially in children. If the ventricles fibrillate, then internal cardiac paddles can be used with an initial energy of 20 J. If the operation is successful, then the pericardium does not need to be reconstituted. There have been anecdotal reports of the atria herniating into the small gap of pericardium causing sudden death.

Lungs

Bleeding through-and-through injuries of the lung can undergo tractotomy. A GIA stapler can be placed across the entry and exit point to open up the track. Bleeding vessels can then be sutured using 3/0 or 4/0 prolene or the stapler refired. If a stapler is not available, then the track can be opened up using two soft bowel clamps and oversewn.

Occasionally, a haemothorax is due to a bleeding intercostal artery following a rib fracture. This can easily be sutured from within using a figure-of-eight suture going around the superior and inferior aspects of the rib including the artery.

Massive bleeding from the hilum and significant air, which can cause systemic air embolism, can be temporarily arrested by performing a lung twist. In this manoeuvre, the inferior pulmonary ligament is divided and the lung twisted 180 degrees on its axis. Once the acute situation is over, the hilum can be clamped using a vascular clamp and the bleeding point in the vascular pedicle sutured.

In those circumstances where there is massive damage to a lobe, a formal lobectomy can be performed but more likely, in the trauma situation, a non-anatomic lung resection just concentrating on the damaged lung is more appropriate. In those cases that require a pneumonectomy due to such disruption, be aware that the pulmonary vascular resistance may suddenly increase causing the patient to suddenly go into crashing right heart failure, especially if the patient has other morbidities.

Abdomen

The computed tomography scan and the technical expertise of the interventional radiologist has changed the management of blunt injuries to the abdomen. Patients who are responders to fluid challenge and continue to remain in a haemodynamically relatively normal state can be managed with a non-operative approach. Indeed, 75% of all organ injuries can be managed non-operatively. A blush of contrast on CT angiography may indicate active arterial bleeding, which may proceed to embolization. Haemodynamically stable patients, even those with stage IV or V injuries, can be managed with embolization and most careful monitoring.

Severe abdominal pain or tenderness, peritonitis, evisceration or haemodynamic instability not responding to fluids warrant an exploratory trauma laparotomy. A long xiphisternum to pubis incision is made and the abdomen opened rapidly. The operating team prior to the incision will have at least two large suckers and at least 12 abdominal packs at the ready. The first manoeuvre of the surgeon is to pull out all the small bowel and drape the bowel and mesentery over the side of the right abdominal wall. This tamponades any significant bleeding within the mesentery and small bowel and allows the left upper quadrant, left paracolic gutter and left lower quadrant and left pelvis to be packed. The small bowel is then transferred and draped over the left abdominal wall and the right upper quadrant above and below the liver is packed, then the right paracolic gutter, the right lower quadrant and the right pelvis, and then the central pelvic area. The small bowel and mesentery are then looked at and, if not bleeding, placed centrally and pack placed over that. This is general packing; targeted packing assumes that the area of injury is known and packing is concentrated in that area.

Liver

Its large size and position under the right costal margin make the liver the most frequently injured abdominal organ. Significant liver injuries due to blunt trauma cause a shattering of the liver substance. There can be massive rents within the liver substance down to the porta hepatis. There have been many attempts to grade liver injuries from grade 1 to grade 5. This is usually a radiological or pathological grading system. For the operating surgeon, it does not really matter which grade the liver injury falls within, the most important aspect is to stop the bleeding. On opening the abdomen via long xiphoid to pubic incision, the abdomen is packed and then the packs are removed sequentially to assess the damage. In the case of the liver, the falciform ligament is divided to get access to right and left lobes. The first action of the surgeon and the assistant is to compress the liver to try and stem the haemorrhage using the assistant's and surgeon's hands. The second action is to assess the damage of the liver. Significant haemorrhage from the liver substance may require careful packing using abdominal packs. At least eight packs need to be available to effectively sandwich the liver between the superior and inferior and lateral border. If bleeding is successfully controlled, then the abdomen is closed and the patient brought back to the operating theatre 48 hours later for removal of packs with copious amounts of saline The surgeon needs to be aware that it is possible to compress the IVC and then reduce preload to the heart and that packing needs to be carefully conducted.

Through-and-through liver injuries due to gunshot wounds or stabbing can be managed by placing a balloon within the track to tamponade the walls of the bleeding liver. This can be performed with a Sengstaken tube or using a balloon created from a finger of a size-eight glove and tied over a Foley catheter. This can be left in for a period of 72 hours and slowly deflated and removed. The catheter can be brought out of the abdominal wall and the abdomen closed. The deflated balloon and catheter are taken out in the operating theatre in case of secondary bleeding.

Bleeding that persists despite packing may be arterial in origin. In this case, a Pringle manoeuvre can be performed. The operating finger is placed into the foramen of Winslow and above the finger will be the portal vein and hepatic artery. These can be then gently compressed using a Rumel tourniquet or a soft clamp. The warm ischaemia time of the liver is only about 20 minutes and therefore it is mandatory to note times. Clamping and un-clamping the inflow will be necessary to perfuse the liver and, during the clamp time, active surgical work must be performed on the bleeding parts of the liver to find the bleeding artery, which can be packed with an omental plug or other topical agents such as an absorbable gelatin sponge. Alternatively, in the appropriate setting, the patient may undergo arterial embolization. Significant bleeding that persists after a Pringle manoeuvre can also indicate bleeding from the hepatic veins.

Lacerations of the liver can be sutured using pledgeted liver sutures and occasionally supplemented using the omentum acting as an omental pack placed into the liver substance to tamponade the liver capsule. Finger fracture technique also allows the surgeon to reach a vessel for ligation, but care should be taken and each individual artery, vein or bile tributary should be ligated and cut.

Bleeding from posterior area parts of the liver will have a high mortality and, if possible, this area should be packed. If it is uncontrollable, then a thoraco-abdominal incision and division of the diaphragm, following right triangular ligament division, will give good access to the posterior IVC. Suturing of the torn hepatic veins can then be attended to, but be aware that this can be torrential and careful placement of pledgeted prolene sutures is mandatory.

Spleen

Although in the past the traditional management of splenic injury was invariably splenectomy, over the past 20 years the importance of splenic preservation has been emphasized for preventing overwhelming post-splenectomy infection. Non-operative management may be indicated in patients with haemodynamic stability and is often used in association with angio-embolization. There is a risk of rebleed and delayed spleen rupture with higher grade injuries. However, in the case of haemodynamic instability whereby the patient may be already coagulopathic, then a total splenectomy would be more appropriate. In those patients who have an isolated injury to the lower third of the spleen and if the patient is haemodynamically stable with a normal coagulation profile, then suturing the lower pole using Teflon-pledgeted sutures would be acceptable. Other techniques such as linear stapling and division of the spleen or placing the damaged spleen in a Vicryl mesh bag should only be performed if splenic haemostasis is assured.

The spleen is mobilized by dividing the lienorenal ligament, splenophrenic ligaments and the splenocolic ligament and is moved to the midline for assessment. For total splenectomy, the short gastric vessels are divided superiorly and, inferiorly, the gastroepiploic vessels. A double suture is placed on the splenic artery and splenic vein which can be taken either separately or together, keeping close to the spleen in order to avoid damage to the tail of the pancreas.

Post-emergency splenectomy vaccines for prevention of infections from pneumococcus, *Haemophilus influenzae* and meningococcus must be given within 14 days. If fever occurs at any stage, then appropriate antibiotics are given.

Duodenal Injuries

Duodenal injuries are rarely isolated, although blunt injures are associated with seat belt injuries causing compression of the duodenum on the first and second lumbar vertebrae which is part of the injury fracture, the so-called 'chance fracture'. Non-operative treatment can be appropriate if a haematoma of the duodenum can be assured. More commonly, penetration due to knives, bullets and fragments will cause injuries requiring a full laparotomy. The duodenum is mobilized as part of the laparotomy using a Kocher's manoeuvre to mobilize the whole of the second and third parts, including the pancreatic head. Injuries to the duodenum can be classified into five categories; however, it is the assessment of the duodenum by careful inspection by the operating surgeon that will dictate management. Small injuries less than 1 cm can be primary sutured using a non-absorbable suture such as 3/0 PDS. Larger defects can be sutured primarily by extending the wound and closing the defect transversely with a single- or double-layer closure; however, great care must be taken not to narrow the lumen. The author always buttresses the anastomosis with omentum where possible. Technically difficult injuries involve the area around the ampulla and head of the duodenum. Destruction of the ampulla can warrant a trauma Whipple's procedure. If this is beyond the expertise in the austere environment, then large suction drains can be placed but this invariably ends in high mortality. Very large injuries involving greater than 75% of the wall above the ampulla will necessitate a pyloric exclusion and gastroenterostomy or below the ampulla may require Roux-en-Y anastomosis. The author has performed all these operations and careful meticulous observation of good blood supply and tension free anastomoses will produce a good outcome.

Pancreatic Injuries

Significant injuries to the main body of the pancreas occur with crush injuries against the lumbar spine. Penetrating injuries invariably involve the stomach. Exposure of the pancreas is performed after opening the lesser sac by dividing the gastrocolic ligament. Damage to the anterior wall is readily seen with bruising and breach of the pancreatic substance. Exposure of the posterior head and neck is with a Kocher's manoeuvre and exposure of the tail by mobilization of the spleen. Damage which requires treatment involves the main pancreatic duct, a small structure not often seen but is most likely damaged when a transection or near transection occurs. Injuries to the duct beyond the body and neck require a distal pancreatectomy. In the trauma situation, the spleen should be removed as well. The pancreas can either be oversewn or stapled.

Injuries in the head of the pancreas involving the duct should be treated with large drains expectantly. The pancreas should be rested and allowed to heal and nutrition given parenterally for at least 6 weeks.

Hollow Organ Injuries

As in all blunt or penetrating injuries, the physiology of the patient is paramount in making the correct judgement call for damage control or definitive surgery. Stomach injuries can be directly sutured in two layers. The blood supply of the stomach is so rich that partial wedge resection of the damaged area can be undertaken. Significant damage to the stomach may require a gastrectomy and gastroenterostomy.

Injuries to the small bowel require resection with an anastomosis using a single layer serosal suture with 3/0 PDS. Mesenteric vessel injuries have already been covered in the vascular section.

Damage to the large bowel will inevitably require resection and, if the physiology of the patient is normal, the decision needs to be made on the amount of soiling present in the abdomen. Penetrating injuries with little soiling can be primarily sutured but if a significant amount of soiling is apparent, then the safest procedure is to exteriorize the colon as a double-barrelled colostomy or Hartman's procedure. Blunt injuries causing bruising are best treated with resection. Injuries to the rectum are treated using a faecal diversion colostomy.

Urogenital Trauma

The kidneys lie in zone 2 of the retroperitoneum. Exploration is only required for expanding haematomas or penetrating injury. Indeed, there are some schools who would not explore a kidney even for a penetrating wound in the absence of significant haematoma. In those cases of massive vascular disruption at the hilum, access can be gained via the line of Toldt and mobilizing either the right or left hemi-colon to the major midline vessels and kidneys. It is always better to try to preserve the kidney if at all possible and an on-table IVP in those cases of severe disruption will indicate the presence of the other kidney. In those patients who are haemodynamically stable with grade 5 injuries, there have been many reports of selective angiography, stent placement and embolization with preservation of the injured kidney. In blast injuries of the retroperitoneum involving the kidney, mobilization of the omentum to wrap the kidney after debridement of the renal parenchyma has been shown to prevent delayed complications such as urinoma or abscess in the de-vascularized area. A urinoma spontaneously resolves in the majority of cases but occasionally requires drainage.

Injuries to the ureters are extremely rare and most are due to penetrating or iatrogenic trauma. Diagnosis is made with IVP, CT or injection of methylene blue into the renal pelvis. Partial tears can be closed primarily with a ureteric stent. End-to-end spatulated anastomosis with an omental wrap and ureteric stent is used for transections. Upper- and mid-ureteric injury can be repaired primarily. In mid-ureteral trauma, an omental wrap is recommended because of the poor blood supply and the distal ureter can be re-implanted into the bladder using a Boari flap or psoas hitch procedure.

Intra-peritoneal bladder repairs are generally straightforward, using a two-layer absorbable suture. Extraperitoneal injuries are usually managed with a large Foley catheter for 2 weeks.

Injuries to the urethra are usually due to pelvic trauma. A single pass of the Foley catheter is warranted in the case of a suspicion of urethral injury with blood at the meatus; otherwise a retrograde urethrogram is the best radiographic study to diagnose urethral trauma. In cases of complete urethral transection, suprapubic catheterization provides urinary diversion until early urethral alignment is attempted using proximal and distal endoscopic techniques.

ADVANCED TRAUMA/MILITARY SURGERY

This is usually the trauma related to ballistics.

Ballistics and physics go hand-in-hand and reflect energy transfer from one source to another, such as the transfer of energy from a bullet or a bomb to a person or structure with devastating effects on physical integrity. This energy, kinetic energy (KE), is given by the equation:

$$KE = \frac{1}{2}MV^2$$

where M equals the mass of the missile and V its velocity.

Doubling the mass doubles the kinetic energy, but doubling the velocity will quadruple the kinetic energy.

If one considers a gunshot wound with an entry and exit, then, assuming that the mass stays the same:

$$KE = \frac{1}{2}M\left(V^2entry - V^2exit\right)$$

If there is no exit, then all the energy will be dumped into the patient:

$$KE = \frac{1}{2}M\left(V^2entry + exit\right)$$

How much energy is dumped by a bullet depends on the retardation (drag) force of the organ which is penetrated and depends on the penetration of the bullet, the velocity, the area of the bullet presented and the density of the target organ. Low-density structures such as lung and muscle will present little retardation force compared to high-density such as the liver and very high-density such as bone.

A bullet damages living tissue via two mechanisms depending on the energy transferred. In the first mechanism, a track is made following crushing of tissue and in the second mechanism, a temporary cavity is produced. A low-energy bullet may simply produce a permanent track and no temporary cavity, whereas a high-energy bullet will cause devastating internal injuries with a combination of the track and dissipation of energy to the surrounding structures.

In high-energy gunshot wounds from an assault rifle, the temporary cavity will, for a microsecond, be sub-atmospheric and will suck in bacteria and debris into the wound. That is the main reason for the increased contamination and debridement that is necessary in high-energy wounds compared to those of lower energy, say a pistol wound.

Apart from the increase in contamination, the expanding walls of the temporary cavity are capable of doing severe damage. There is compression, stretching and shearing of the displaced tissue. Injuries to blood vessels, nerves or organs not struck by the bullet, and a distance from the path, can occur, as can fractures of bones.

The size of both the temporary and permanent cavities is determined not only by the amount of kinetic energy deposited in the tissue but also by the density and elastic cohesiveness of the tissue. Because liver and muscle have similar densities (1.01–1.02 and 1.02–1.04, respectively), both tissues absorb the same amount of kinetic energy per centimetre of tissue traversed by the bullet. Muscle, however, has an elastic, cohesive structure; the liver has a weak, less cohesive structure. Thus, both the temporary and the permanent cavities produced in the liver are larger than those in the muscle. In muscle, except for where the bullet passed, the tissue displaced by the temporary cavity returns to its original position. Only a small rim of cellular destruction surrounds the permanent track requiring limited debridement. In liver struck by high energy bullets, the undulation of the temporary cavity loosens the hepatocytes from the cellular supporting tissue and produces a permanent cavity approximately the size of the temporary cavity. Lung, with a very low-density (specific gravity of 0.4–0.5) and a high degree of elasticity, is relatively resistant to the effects of temporary cavity formation and has only a very small temporary cavity formed with very little tissue destruction.

There is a critical amount of kinetic energy loss above which tissue destruction becomes radically more severe. This level is different for each organ or tissue. When a bullet exceeds the kinetic energy threshold, it produces a temporary cavity which the organ or tissue can no longer contain and exceeds the elastic limit of the organ and, when the elastic limit is exceeded, the organ bursts. Wounds of the head are especially destructive because of the formation of a temporary cavity within the cranial cavity. The brain is enclosed by the skull, a closed, rigid structure that can relieve pressure only by bursting. Thus, high-energy missile wounds to the head tend to produce bursting injuries. That these bursting injuries are the result of temporary cavity formation can be demonstrated by shooting through empty skulls. A high energy bullet fired through an empty skull produces a small entrance and exit with no fractures. The same missile fired through a skull containing brain causes extensive fracturing and bursting injuries.

Often, the full metal jacket casing of the bullet when it hits a hard object such as the bone will break up and the lead contents will act as secondary projectiles causing increased damage.

Management of Gunshot Wounds

Because of the low energy from a handgun, to cause a significant injury the bullet must traverse a major blood vessel or nerve. High energy rifle bullets fall into two general categories, hunting bullets and military bullets. Hunting bullets are designed to expand on contact and dissipate their energy rapidly over a short distance. Military bullets are non-deforming and wounding is due to the combination of the crushed and shredded tissue generated by the bullet perforating tissue and the effects of the temporary cavity on tissue adjacent to the bullet (shearing, compression and stretching). Temporarily cavitation does not always cause a large zone of tissue damage and skeletal muscle is relatively tolerant. For this reason, it may be unwise to try to excise all the tissue which may have been affected by the cavitation.

A bullet is not sterilized by firing and may carry bacteria into the wound. In addition, high-energy gunshot wounds draw bacteria in to the temporary cavity due to the low pressure. The bacterial flora of a gunshot wound changes with time. In the first few days, it is mainly commensals but after that Gram-positive and Gram-negative bacteria, including clostridia, may take hold if proper debridement is not performed.

Wound Management

Although it is of interest to assess for an entry and exit wound, it is often not possible. In the limbs especially, it is important to assess for neurological, vascular and bony damage. If there is an entrance and exit wound and no major soft tissue damage, then it is probably not necessary to explore the wound and lay it open. Often all that is necessary is to apply a fluffy gauze to the entrance and exit areas to allow drainage.

If the wound is large with a lot of soft tissue damage and possible bony involvement, then debridement is necessary. All bone not attached to periosteum will die and be a focus of infection and therefore should be removed. Damaged subcutaneous fat and shredded fascia should be removed with a sharp knife or scissors. The deep fascia is incised for the length of the incision or beyond it to relieve pressure within the wound and associated compartments and copious amounts of saline are used for irrigation. Any evidence of raised or increasing pressure in compartments is treated by complete fasciotomy.

Muscle is assessed for colour, consistency, contractility and capillary bleeding. The muscle is cut back until one can be sure of viability. The wounds are all left open and either fluffed up gauze or negative pressure dressings are applied. The principal of staged treatment using delayed primary closure to close wounds with no excessive loss of skin is widely accepted. Wounds may be re-inspected in the operating theatre after 48 hours, but closures should be planned 4 or 5 days after injury. If unable to close the wound primarily, then a split skin graft is applied. A few areas of skin that have sufficient vascularity such as the face, neck, scalp and genitalia may be sutured to allow primary closure but only after careful wound excision.

It is advisable to splint the injured limb for support and stabilization using a back slab or plaster cast to protect the soft tissues even when there is no fracture. If there is a fracture, then this should be stabilized first with a back slab and then assessment of the soft tissue and fracture. In the majority of unclean cases, a combination of external fixation and soft tissue management will suffice. There is a case for internal fixation provided one can be sure that there is no contamination.

Surgeons faced with gunshot wounds need to make carefully reasoned clinical decisions based on the understanding of the mechanisms involved. It is often difficult to know whether the injury was due to a high-energy or low-energy bullet but the old adage 'the surgeon should not treat the weapon' holds. Decisions need to be made on the extent of the soft tissue damage and the fracture involved. The aim is the preservation of healthy soft tissue with minimal non-viable tissue and contamination. This will allow fracture healing with any of a variety of different methods of stabilization appropriate to the fracture pattern. For massive wounds, a viable soft tissue environment must be established before addressing the bony problem. Treatment must be based on careful assessment of the wound and available expertise and facilities. There is no dogmatic treatment of choice for gunshot wounds.

Blast Injuries

Explosions result from the almost instantaneous conversion of a solid or liquid into gas after detonation of an explosive material. Gas rapidly expands outwards from the point of detonation and displaces the surrounding medium, usually air or water. This expansion of gas causes an immediate rise in pressure creating a blast wave that subsequently dissipates over distance and time.

The blast wave consists of two parts, a shock wave of high pressure, followed closely by a blast of wind or air in motion which can be several hundred km/h depending on the size of the explosion. These blast winds can immediately propel objects or people, causing injury. The blast wave which is produced following the explosion decays immediately after the peak is reached, followed by an immediate decay to a negative pressure phase. The positive phase of the blast wave is usually characterized by the overpressure and is defined as the time between the shock arrival and the beginning of the negative phase of the overpressure. High-order explosives such as TNT and Semtex produce a supersonic overpressure wave, whilst low-order explosives such as gunpowder, which burns rapidly, do not produce an overpressure wave. The blast wave lasts for a few milliseconds.

Several factors affect the magnitude of the blast wave, e.g. water, which is non-compressible, causes a greater potential for injury than that of air. Secondly, the energy of the blast decreases inversely proportional to the cubed root of the distance. This means that at 10 feet from the explosion, the blast wave is eight times more powerful than at 20 feet. The third factor is the effect of amplification of the pressure wave due to confined areas such as a bus or a restaurant. This confinement raises the peak overpressure and duration of the positive pressure phase.

Types of Explosives

Explosives are classified into low-order or higher-order explosives. Low-order explosives such as gunpowder burn rapidly (deflagrate) with a velocity of less than 1000 m/s and produce large volumes of gas that only explode if confined (e.g. a pipe bomb). High-order explosives such as TNT, dynamite and Semtex do not burn, but instead detonate when a shock wave passes through the material, generating a substantial blast overpressure, even if unconfined. Dynamite was used in the 2004 train bombing in Madrid, Spain and Semtex in the 1988 downing of Pan Am flight 103 over Lockerbie. Dense inert metal explosives (DIME) are composed of a high-order explosive and small particles of chemically inert materials such as tungsten. These explosives are designed to produce a small but very effective explosive radius, lethal at close range. Improvised explosive devices are broadly any makeshift incendiary device constructed to explode using triggers such as mobile telephones, motion and pressure detectors.

The Effect of Blast Injuries

Blast injuries are usually divided into four categories. However, in the majority of bomb blast injuries, there is usually significant overlap of all categories even in the same patient.

Primary Blast Injuries

These are caused by barotrauma, either over pressurization or under pressurization relative to atmospheric pressure. There are three explosive forces that cause injury: spallation, implosion and inertia. These forces usually affect the air tissue interface. Spallation takes place when a pressure wave passes from a dense medium to a less dense medium. For example, an explosion detonated underwater will cause the dense water to spall into the less dense air, causing fragmentation represented by an upward splash. This can be represented in the lung, whereby a blast wave travelling through relatively incompressible blood disrupts the endothelium of the capillary wall as the wave enters the alveolus. An implosion occurs when blood and air mix in the alveolus causing air emboli and bleeding, leading to adult respiratory distress syndrome and acute lung injury.

The tympanic membrane is the structure most frequently damaged. An increase in pressure of as little as 5 psi above atmospheric pressure (1 atm is equivalent to 14.7 psi or 760 mmHg) can rupture the human eardrum which manifests as deafness, tinnitus and vertigo. If the dynamic pressure is high enough, the bones of the middle ear can be dislocated and traumatic disruption of the oval or round window will both cause permanent hearing loss. In the Madrid bombing, rupture of the tympanic membrane occurred in 99 of 243 victims.

The lung is the second most susceptible organ to undergo primary blast injury. Pressure differentials across the alveolar/capillary interface cause disruption, haemorrhage, pulmonary contusion (appearing as a butterfly pattern and chest radiographs), pneumothorax, haemothorax, pneumomediastinum and subcutaneous emphysema. Pulmonary injuries are life-threatening and the immediate onset of pulmonary oedema with frothing at the mouth carries very grave prognosis. Systemic acute air embolism from pulmonary disruption is believed to affect the blood vessels of the brain or spinal canal and must be differentiated from the direct effects of head trauma and concussion.

Forty percent of those who die do so because of pulmonary complications and of those, 50% present immediately and the next 50% over the next 12 to 24 hours.

Secondary Blast Injuries

These are caused by debris which cause a combination of penetrating and blunt trauma. Penetrating injuries include primary fragments from the weapon (shrapnel) and secondary fragments (those that result from the explosion) and are the leading cause of death and injury apart from major building collapse. The crush syndrome in victims of structural collapse is a metabolic derangement resulting from damage to muscle tissues and the subsequent release of myoglobin, urates, potassium and phosphates causing death from asphyxiation, compartment syndromes and renal failure.

The compartment syndrome results from the compression of damaged, oedematous muscle within its inelastic sheath. Such confined swelling promotes local ischaemia, which then continues a vicious cycle of swelling, increased compartment pressures, decreased tissue perfusion and further ischaemia. Fasciotomy or compartment decompression should be performed as soon as possible.

One to seven percent of people injured by explosions have traumatic amputations. These injuries result from high blast overpressure forces causing bony fractures while concomitant strong blast winds rupture soft tissue structure leading to partial or complete extremity amputation. Those that suffer from traumatic amputations also have a very high mortality rate from other primary blast injuries.

The distance over which fragments travel and can cause injury is much greater than the distance over which the blast overpressure travels. Thus, fragments can cause secondary blast injury hundreds to thousands of metres from the explosion's epicentre, whereas primary blast injury usually happens within tens of metres. Hence, secondary blast injuries are more common than primary blast injuries.

Tertiary Blast Injuries

These are caused when a person is physically displaced by the force of the peak overpressure and blast wind and sustains blunt trauma such as closed head injuries, blunt abdominal trauma, tissue contusions and fractures.

Quaternary Blast Injuries

These include burns (chemical or thermal), toxic inhalation, exposure to radiation, asphyxiation (including carbon monoxide and cyanide after incomplete combustion of materials) and inhalation of dust containing coal or asbestos. Dust inhalation was the commonest form of death in Syria following barrel bombs. Burns are present in up to 30% of those injured by blast and are associated with increased mortality as inhalation increases the pulmonary damage. They are also complicated by crush injuries, making debridement difficult compounded with high infection rates. Aggressive crystalloid resuscitation is crucial in thermal burns, although abdominal compartment syndrome and extremity myonecrosis occurs with over-excessive resuscitation.

General Treatment

Initial stabilization of victims, like any other trauma victims, includes assessment and management of airway, breathing and circulation. Maintenance of a radial pulse pressure of around 90 mmHg provides circulation to the major organs and cerebral mentation. When treating patients with crush injury, therapy with fluids must maintain renal perfusion whilst avoiding fluid overload. Once immediate life support measures have been instituted, it is very important to check for eardrum perforation. If tympanic membranes are intact, then the likelihood of severe primary blast injury can be reasonably excluded in the absence of other symptoms such as dyspnoea, respiratory distress and abdominal pain. Patients with rupture of the tympanic membrane should undergo chest X-ray and be observed for at least eight hours or as clinically indicated. As previously stated, blast injuries are notorious for their delayed onset. These patients should have their oxygen saturation monitored by pulse oximetry. Decreased oxygen saturation probably signals early blast lung.

Ten percent also suffer from ocular trauma with conditions varying from ruptured globes, hyphemas and conjunctival haemorrhage. Additionally, cardiac confusion, myocardial wall haemorrhage and atrial rupture have been described in the cardiovascular system.

A primary and secondary survey is tantamount to careful treatment regimens. Knowledge of the cause and effect of the blast injury should be paramount in making the right decisions for treatment.

Mine Injuries

There are at present a total of around 85 million landmines around the world. They languish in 65 countries and it is estimated that there are around 250 million mines stockpiled for use. The cost of producing a landmine is around $3. The Halo Trust, which specializes in clearing mines, puts a figure of $1000 for the safe removal of a single mine. Eighty percent of victims are civilians who have less than 10% access to healthcare. The medical bill on average from point of wounding to rehabilitation with a prosthetic limb is on average $10 000. Landmines continue to claim more than 26 000 new victims annually. Around the world one person steps on a landmine every 22 minutes. A landmine can be triggered by a number of things including pressure, movement, sound, magnetism and vibration.

The effect of stepping on a mine produces a blast wave and fragmentation injury. The mine is usually under the ground and therefore the fragmentation comprises both shrapnel from the mine and mud and dirt from the ground.

The muscle forms an umbrella around the tibia. The foot is blown off and the effect of the blast wind strips the muscle from the tibia. Fragmentation is in effect the dirt and mud blown into the muscles of the remaining leg. To be able to treat the injury described takes a lot of time and manpower. Initially, a social scrub is used using copious amounts of Betadine/soap and water. This scrubs off all the mud and dirt. Following that, the muscle is debrided with a sharp scalpel and scissors until actively bleeding and contracting muscle is seen. The wounds are then dressed and packed with fluffy gauze and the patient returned to the operating theatre 2 to 3 days later where further debridement is performed or the dressings changed and the bone of the lower leg removed in preparation for a below knee amputation around the fifth or sixth day.

Reference

1. Rotondo MF, Schwab CW, McGonigal MD, et al. 'Damage control': an approach for improved survival in exsanguinating penetrating abdominal injury. *J Trauma*. 1993;35(3):375–382; discussion 382–383.
2. Roberts I, Shakur H, Coats T, et al. The CRASH-2 trial: a randomised controlled trial and economic evaluation of the effects of tranexamic acid on death, vascular occlusive events and transfusion requirement in bleeding trauma patients. *Health Technol Assess*. 2013;17(10):1–79. https://doi.org/10.3310/hta17100.
3. Harvin JA, Harvin WH, Camp E, et al. Early FEMA fixation is associated with a reduction in pulmonary complications and hospital charges: a decade of experience as 1376 diaphyseal femur fractures. *J Trauma Acute Care Surg*. 2012;73(6):1442–1448.
4. Pape HC, Grimme K, van Griensven M, EPOFF Study Group, et al. Impact of intramedullary instrumentation versus damage control for femoral fractures on immunoinflammatory parameters: prospective randomised analysis by the EPOFF Study Group. *J Trauma*. 2003;55(1):7–13.

Surgical Specialties

37

Leadership and the Surgical Team and Management

CHAPTER OUTLINE

Strong Surgical Leadership for Future

With over 230 million major surgical procedures performed worldwide every year, surgery constitutes a large number of healthcare interactions.[1] Indeed, there remain a substantial number of deaths due to preventable surgical activities, which is estimated to contribute to half a million mortalities per year across the world.[2] We must aim to deliver high-quality care in times of economic austerity. Healthcare faces many challenges worldwide due to economic and social pressures with ageing populations, increasingly complex treatment options and a focus on not just cure but delivering excellent quality of life and living better for longer. Furthermore, these challenges are in the context of reduced training time and increased necessary clinical governance.

For surgeons, such challenges are particularly demanding to deliver with increasing sub-specialization and the widespread understanding that 'postcode' lotteries are not acceptable and all patients should be offered the best quality care.

Surgery, in particular, is a high-risk environment with a greater number of adverse events. Clear and effective surgical leadership is required to drive healthcare towards being a high-safety, high-performance environment. Steps have been made in this direction through regulation, the introduction of surgical checklists, where appropriate centralization of surgical care and the focus on safety and quality in healthcare. Such a transition to a 'safe' industry will require strong leadership in surgery. Furthermore, this will need to be driven within individual specialities to work in collaboration with healthcare providers, government, policy makers, industry and the public. Strong leadership will be needed to engender a culture of positive safety attitudes, safety management and high reliability.[3]

This chapter outlines key definitions of what constitutes effective leadership. We seek to explore the differences and overlaps in the leadership and management paradigms and outline the development of leadership theory and leadership styles. Leadership is an art to be nurtured and developed. We will, therefore, describe ways in which leadership skills can be developed throughout surgical training and honed during clinical practice as part of continuous professional development.

The Definition of Leadership

There are innumerable definitions of leadership available. In essence, leadership is a means of influencing others to achieve a shared goal. Chatman and Kennedy's definition is particularly descriptive, suggesting that leadership is 'a process of motivating people to work together collaboratively to accomplish great things', with these 'great things' being defined in the minds of the leader and their followers.[4] Hence, leadership can be explained as having influence, and exerting that influence towards a clear vision. Furthermore, effective leadership also involves sharing that vision with others so that it becomes a collective vision that everyone in an organization can work towards. It involves providing the resources to deliver the goals, and bringing together and balancing all stakeholders to realise that vision.[5]

• BOX 37.1 **Key Goals of Leadership Within an Organization**

Recognition that the work of leadership involves an inward journey of self-discovery and self-development
Clarity of organization values
Clear communication of purpose and vision
Creation of a culture of quality and accountability throughout the whole organization
Development of individuals within an organization and build the future leaders

Reprinted from Souba W. Building Our Future: a Plea for Leadership. *World J Surg.* 2004;28:445-450.[7]

Leadership and Management

Effective leadership and management are key skills for high-performing organizations. There are meaningful differences between management and leadership to consider.

Management is focused on planning, controlling and putting appropriate structures in place. It can be thought of as the day-to-day running of an organization.

Leadership is about ensuring the future of an organization through predicting, facilitating and adapting to change and adopting a visionary stance. Radical change often requires stronger leadership.[6]

'Vision without a strategy is a day-dream; strategy without vision is a nightmare.'

JAPANESE PROVERB

Hence, we can theorize that the key to leadership is having a clear strategy and vision.

The above often-quoted Japanese proverb emphasizes the need for both these elements together in effective leadership.

Box 37.1 describes the key goals of leadership within an organisation.

The Evolution of Leadership Theory

The study of leadership theory began in earnest in the last century and has undergone a gradual evolution to the current theories on leadership. Though there have been many coexisting theories of what makes effective leadership, the main development of leadership theories can be summarized as follows.[8]

Eras in Leadership Theory

The first significant leadership theory to gain traction was the *Great Man* period, which evolved into the *trait* period. These theories were characterized by emphasizing the personality traits of an individual. Such theories suggested that adopting behaviours and traits of renowned leaders would enhance an individual's leadership qualities. The Achilles heel of these personality-driven theories was the recognition that many notable leaders had significantly varied personalities and approaches. Such variation means that a single individual characteristic cannot be translated directly into effective leadership.

These personality theories of leadership then evolved into the *influence* era. These theories focused on the relationships needed to underpin effective leadership and the need for such leaders to influence others to be successful. The drawback of these theories was that they concentrated very much on a top down approach to leadership and did not recognize the need to empower followers within an organization.

The *behaviour* era moved away from the concepts of the personality and influence of an individual to focusing on the actions of that individual. This theory recognized key behaviours in an individual that were effective. Such behaviours include taking action, accomplishing goals and consideration for individuals within the wider organization.

The *situation* era of leadership theory developed the behaviour theory further to recognize that leadership is not just about the individual but also about the environment in which that individual operates. There are many factors beyond the control of individuals that influence events within an organization. Indeed, even the individual assuming leadership can be fluid depending on the particular situation.

The *contingency* era of leadership theory recognized the merits of all the preceding paradigms and suggested that leadership was multifaceted, including an individual's behaviours and personality, their ability to influence and the wider context in which they are acting.

During the evolution of leadership theory, Kurt Lewin, well renowned as the father of psychology, developed his own theory of leadership in 1939. This incorporated three leadership styles commonly described today – the autocratic, the democratic and the laissez-faire leadership styles.

The Autocratic Leadership Style

The autocratic leaders are also known as dictatorial leaders. All decisions are made by the leader, who tells staff or team members what to do. The team members have little opportunity to make suggestions or question instructions. Of course, this is efficient, as decisions are made quickly without group discussion and are implemented by the team without question[9]; thus, there is good control and discipline and group members are aware of their own role. However, diminished freedom is known to decrease creative decision making, and can cause rivalry amongst group members, as well as nurture resentment towards the leader. Modern generations including Generation 'X' team members have been proven to respond poorly to such an autocratic leadership style.[10]

Such a leadership style does have a role within organizations. Autocratic leadership is best used when there is little time for group decision making, such as in a crisis situation. We often see this autocratic style of leadership in the emergency setting to provide specific direction. It is important to remember that overuse, or inappropriate use, of this leadership style can lead to poor morale and misunderstandings.[11] When the critical emergency period has passed, other leadership styles are more effective.

The Democratic Leadership Style

The democratic leader is known as the participative leadership style. Team members are actively involved in the decision-making process. The leader facilitates and encourages these discussions but ultimately makes the final decision. Under a democratic leader, team members tend to have high job satisfaction rates, productivity and creativity. On the other hand, speed and efficacy can be sacrificed to group discussion.[10]

The Laissez-Faire Leadership Style

Laissez-faire, or 'let it be' style is the hands-off approach to leadership. There is complete freedom for the team members to make decisions without any leader participation. The leaders will provide advice and resources if needed, but otherwise do not get involved. The group has complete freedom and independence. However, this can cause unproductivity if left to a group of inexperienced or unmotivated people. The laissez-faire style of leadership should only be used when leading a team of highly-skilled and driven people who are trustworthy and experienced.[12]

In 1978, James MacGregor Burns, an American historian and political scientist, introduced his theory of transactional and transformational leadership styles which have largely superseded Kurt Lewin's descriptions of leadership.

The Transactional Leadership Style

This type of leadership style is characterized by the concept exchange of work for reward. It involves the leader setting tasks and objectives. They have to motivate the team with rewards and incentives. Some obvious examples of incentives are linking monetary rewards with increased productivity, or tax incentives for votes in an election. Thus, there are clear objectives and hence decreased workplace anxiety. Such leadership recognizes good performance and accomplishments. However, this leadership style does not create long-term relationships between the leaders and the team.[13] It can mean a failure to take responsibility and make key decisions. There are three key aspects to transactional leadership: contingent reward, management by exception-active and management by exception-passive. Contingent reward is the process whereby the leader sets up task-reward transactions and makes clear the rules around such transactions. Management by exception-active is the proactive monitoring and taking corrective action to ensure that tasks are achieved. This aspect seeks to manage situations early before problems arise. Management by exception-passive is a less proactive style where action is taken after a problem arises.[14]

TABLE 37.1 Transformational and Transactional Leadership

Transformational	Transactional
Charisma	Contingent reward
Inspirational motivation	Management by exception—active
Intellectual stimulation	Management by exception—passive
Individualized consideration	

Adapted from Judge TA, Piccolo RF. Transformational and transactional leadership: a meta-analytic test of their relative validity. *J Appl Psychol.* 2004;89:755-768.[14]

The Transformational Leadership Style

The transformational leader is also known as the charismatic leader. These leaders inspire loyalty and enthusiasm to help team members to see the importance and overall organizational benefit of the task.[11] This means that team members develop an emotional involvement with the goal and are motivated in their work. Such leaders place great emphasis on caring for each employee individually. The transformational leadership style has been studied in both the United States and Canadian Military. This behaviour is increasingly seen among those of senior ranks in the military, and has been proven to be linked with increased motivation and commitment.[15,16]

The two styles have been compared by Hu and colleagues. Transactional (task-focused) leaders achieve minimum standards. Transformational (team-oriented) leaders inspire performance beyond expectations.[17] Transformational leadership improves team behaviours in the operating theatre and increases information-sharing and supportive behaviours within their teams.[17] Table 37.1 describes the main elements of each leadership theory.

Effective Leadership in Surgery

There are certain key tenets that are particularly applicable to surgical leadership. This focuses on emotional intelligence, which is characterized by humanized relationships and mentorship.[6,18] It is a non-cognitive skill that requires self-awareness, self-management, social awareness and relationship management.[6] As surgeons, these skills are required to establish collaboration and cooperation within the team, and hence develop and share a vision for the values and goals of the team. Table 37.2 describes key skills associated with successful surgical leadership.

Leadership and Safety

We have learnt from industrial investigations into major incidents such as the Piper Alpha oil incident and the Chernobyl

TABLE 37.2	Key Areas for Effective Surgical Leaders	
Personal skills	**Skills in relations with others**	
Acute diagnostician with knowledge, expertise and technical competence	Communication	
Professionalism and integrity	Team-work	
Selflessness	Effective teaching	
Business acumen	Motivate others	
Innovative		
Effective decision making		
Resilience		
Flexibility		
Self-awareness		

Adapted from Chatman and Kennedy,[4] Lobas,[19] Patel[20] and Souba.[21]

• BOX 37.2 Pathways for Developing Effective Leadership Skills

Mentorship (at an individual level and through dedicated mentor partnership programs)
Coaching
Development of networks of individuals within and between organizations
Leadership courses
Organizational leadership development programs
Formal qualifications and degrees in leadership and management such as Masters in Business Administration (MBAs)

From Patel et al[20] and Maykel.[25]

disaster that safety issues and poor safety cultures are as a result of significant leadership failings. More recently in healthcare, the Bristol inquiry and the Francis report into the Mid-Staffordshire NHS Trust have highlighted the results of poor leadership and management. These investigations and reports have emphasized the need for system-based approaches to safety without reliance on single individuals on the frontline. A senior led commitment to safety within an organization is essential to drive a culture of safety and high performance.[22]

Flin and Yule summarize the leadership behaviours necessary for engendering a safety culture according to organizational seniority of a leader. Such leadership serves to create a culture where safety is the norm. Supervisors should monitor and reinforce safe behaviours, participate and be supportive of safety initiatives and encourage the participation of others. Middle managers have a role in emphasizing the paramount importance of safety over other corporate objectives, as well as translating the overall organizational vision for supervisors and individual staff. Senior managers need to ensure that regulatory frameworks are adhered to and provide the financial and time investment in a broad-ranging programme of safety. In addition, senior managers need to lead by example and exhibit a clear and explicit commitment to safety. Such commitments should include encouraging the participation of others as well as committing to and championing safety initiatives.[22] In the healthcare industry, the hierarchy of healthcare is ill-defined with both senior organizational managers and healthcare professionals serving as key opinion makers. The leadership roles of individuals in healthcare can be, at times, fluid. An individual's position in the leadership hierarchy can change depending on the situation. All individuals, therefore, have a responsibility towards creating a culture of safety within the healthcare organization.

Training in Leadership

Leadership skills, like any other aspect of surgical training, can be taught. The 'Good Surgical Practice' guidance from the Royal College of Surgeons of England emphasizes the need for individual surgeons to possess and develop effective leadership skills.[23] Indeed, it has been shown that one's leadership style can change and adapt. Rooke and Torbert performed an interesting study which demonstrated how an individual's leadership style evolved over time and how it can be adapted to suit a role or seniority within an organization.[24]

There are many different avenues available for surgical trainees to develop their leadership skills.

Box 37.2 outlines the various different pathways available for leadership training with surgery.

Mentoring and Coaching

Mentorship and coaching are often thought to be interchangeable; however, there are key differences in the two training mediums. Mentorship is a longer term relationship between individuals where the mentor facilitates the mentee to make developments in knowledge, work and thinking.[20,26] Until recently, this was an informal process within organizations but, more recently, healthcare training organizations such as the Academy for Medical Sciences have formalized these arrangements. Such mentorship arrangements should be as objective and confidential as possible.

Coaching, on the other hand, is a more specific dedicated program to improve a defined area over a defined period of time.[20] Such coaching tends to be carried out by independent specialized coaches.

In healthcare systems, leadership training should encompass how to lead change, drive innovation, create a vision and strategy and build teams. Certain aspects of healthcare administration are particularly important for surgical leaders. These include finance, marketing, operations, legislation and healthcare policy.[27,28]

It should be noted that leadership training does require continuous appraisal and feedback to allow development. Such feedback can form part of an individual's regular appraisal. Furthermore, independent means of assessing leadership skills in healthcare have been developed,[29,30] which allow for a more objective tool to measure an individual's leadership development over time.

Conclusion

Effective surgical leadership is essential to drive up quality in surgical care and promote innovations in surgery. Leadership skills can be taught. Steps should be taken to train the surgical leaders of the future. The supreme test of our leadership skills is the ability of the team to function in our absence. We should all be seeking to help others succeed and make ourselves redundant.

References

1. Weiser TG, Regenbogen SE, Thompson KD, et al. An estimation of the global volume of surgery: a modelling strategy based on available data. *Lancet*. 2008;372:139–144.
2. Weiser TG, Gawande A. Excess surgical mortality: strategies for improving quality of care. In: Debas HT, Donkor P, Gawande A, Jamison DT, Kruk ME, Mock CN, eds. *Essential Surgery: Disease Control Priorities*. 3rd ed. Vol. 1. Washington (DC); 2015.
3. Hudson P. Applying the lessons of high risk industries to health care. *Qual Suf Health Care*. 2003;12(suppl 1):i7–i12.
4. Chatman J, Kennedy J. Psychological perspectives on leadership. In: Nohria N, Khurana R, eds. *Handbook of Leadership Theory and Practice : an HBS Centennial Colloquium on Advancing Leadership*. Boston, Mass: Harvard Business Press; 2010.
5. What is leadership? WebFinance Inc; 2018. Available from: http://www.businessdictionary.com/definition/leadership.html.
6. Buchler P, Martin D, Knaebel HP, Buchler MW. Leadership characteristics and business management in modern academic surgery. *Langenbecks Arch Surg*. 2006;391:149–156.
7. Souba W. Building our future: a plea for leadership. *World J Surg*. 2004;28:445–450.
8. King AS. Evolution of leadership theory. *Vikalpa*. 1990;15:43–54.
9. Amanchukwu RN, Stanley GJ, Ololube NP. A review of leadership theories, principles and styles and their relevance to educational management. *Management*. 2015;5:6–14.
10. Khan MS, Khan I, Qureshi QA. The styles of leadership: a critical review. *Public Policy Admin Res*. 2015;5:87–92.
11. Brophy J. *Leadership Essentials for Emergency Medical Services*. Jones and Bartlett Publishers; 2010:13–21.
12. Khan ZA, Nawaz A, Khan I. Leadership theories and styles: a literature review. *J Res Develop Manag*. 2016;16
13. McCleskey JA. Situational, transformational, and transactional leadership and leadership development. *J Business Stud Quart*. 2014;5:117–130.
14. Judge TA, Piccolo RF. Transformational and transactional leadership: a meta-analytic test of their relative validity. *J Appl Psychol*. 2004;89:755–768.
15. Kane TD, Tremble Jr TR. Transformational leadership effects at different levels of the army. *Military Psychol*. 2000;12(2):137–160.
16. Ivey GW. Transformational and active transactional leadership in the Canadian military. *Leadership Org Develop J*. 2010;31:246–262.
17. Hu YY, Parker SH, Lipsitz SR, et al. Surgeons' leadership styles and team behavior in the operating room. *J Am Coll Surg*. 2016;222:41–51.
18. Rosengart TK, Kent KC, Bland KI, et al. Key tenets of effective surgery leadership: perspectives from the society of surgical chairs mentorship sessions. *JAMA Surg*. 2016;151:768–770.
19. Lobas JG. Leadership in academic medicine: capabilities and conditions for organizational success. *Am J Med*. 2006;119:617–621.
20. Patel V, Warren O, Humphris P, Ahmed K. What does leadership in surgery entail? *ANZ J Surg*. 2010;80:876–883.
21. Souba WW. The new leader: new demands in a changing, turbulent environment. *J Am Coll Surg*. 2003;197:79–87.
22. Flin R, Yule S. Leadership for safety: industrial experience. *Qual Saf Health Care*. 2004;13(suppl 2):ii45–ii51.
23. Good Surgical Practice, Standards and Research. The Royal College of Surgeons of England. Available from: https://www.rcseng.ac.uk/standards-and-research/gsp/.
24. Rooke D, Torbert WR. Seven transformations of leadership. *Harvard Business Review*. 2005;83:66–76.
25. Maykel JA. Leadership in surgery. *Clin Colon Rectal Surg*. 2013;26:254–258.
26. Clutterbuck D. *Everyone Needs a Mentor*. 2nd ed. London: Institute of Personnel Management; 1991.
27. Mulholland MW. Leadership in surgery. In: Kibbe M, Chen H, eds. *Leadership in Surgery*. Springer International Publishing; 2015.
28. Kao L, Chen H. *Success in Academic Surgery*. Springer International Publishing; 2016.
29. Horwitz IB, Horwitz SK, Daram P, Brandt ML, Brunicardi FC, Awad SS. Transformational, transactional, and passive-avoidant leadership characteristics of a surgical resident cohort: analysis using the multifactor leadership questionnaire and implications for improving surgical education curriculums. *J Surg Res*. 2008;148:49–59.
30. *The Leadership Framework and 360 Feedback*. NHS Leadership Academy; Available from: https://www.leadershipacademy.nhs.uk/.

38

Evidence Based Medicine

CHAPTER OUTLINE

History and Development

Perhaps the most commonly cited definition of evidence based medicine (EBM) is from the seminal paper by Sir David Sackett, widely thought of as the pioneer of EBM, in which he stated that EBM is the 'conscientious, explicit and judicious use of current best evidence in making decision about the care of individual patients'.[1] In its broadest definition, EBM is the application of scientific methodology to optimize medical decision making in the care of individuals or to shape national healthcare policy. Early in its development, EBM was utilized as a methodology for the teaching of medical personnel in order to improve their decision-making skills; however, since then, EBM has been applied to all aspects of medicine, including policy formulation, guidelines and regulations.

Whilst some level of scientific methodology has been applied to everyday medical practice since the Age of Enlightenment of the 17–18th centuries, it was really only in the late 19th and early 20th century that it became increasingly apparent that current medical practice was more often than not presumptive rather than based on any real scientific evidence. Decision making for the same pathologies/patient groups was often extremely varied, treatments often relied on what was taught by elders and peers rather than backed by hard scientific evidence. A growing movement of pioneers such as Ernest Codman, Archie Cochrane, Alvan Feinstein, John Wennberg and David Sackett, amongst others, questioned previously assumed 'robust' medical practices leading to the age of randomized control trials (RCTs), meta-analyses and large cohort/population studies with clear end points. By the 1980s and 1990s, the practice of EBM and with it RCTs, observational studies, systematic reviews and meta-analyses, guidelines and laboratory studies had grown exponentially internationally.

Organizations across a variety of medical specialties began developing guidelines which, in turn, helped shape political healthcare policy as well as individual practice. Transnational collaborations, trials and studies developed rapidly. The Cochrane Collaborative is one of many examples of such international cooperation leading to improved evidence synthesis in healthcare. Presently, there are increasingly sophisticated studies, research collaboratives, networks and organizations aimed at improving healthcare through sound scientific methodology as highlighted by the meteoric rise in the number of medical journals as well as the volumes of papers published each week.[2,3]

Evidence Based Medicine: Principles of Evidence

Levels of Evidence

One of the key pillars of the practice of EBM is the quality of the scientific evidence that it generates and how much weight should that evidence carry given its level of quality in any given clinical scenario. In order to solve the issues regarding evidence quality, scientific studies are scrutinized for their quality by attributing them to a 'Level'. Since the inception of this hierarchy, there have been sub-groups, variations and even slight disagreements with regards as to what attributes a study must have in order for it to occupy a particular level in the hierarchy. The levels of evidence are presented in Table 38.1. Level 1 is the highest level of evidence and comprises of RCTs and, ideally, even systematic reviews and meta-analysis of homogenous RCTs, that is RCTs similar in design and outcome measures. Level 2 evidence largely consists of good quality large cohort studies with adequate follow-up periods and a low drop-out rate

	TABLE 38.1	Levels of Evidence.

Level	Characteristics
1a	Systematic review and meta-analysis of homogenous RCTs
1b	One well designed and executed RCT with narrow confidence interval
2a	Systematic review and meta-analysis of homogenous cohort studies
2b	One good quality cohort study with adequate follow-up
3a	Systematic review and meta-analysis of case-control studies
3b	Individual case-control study
4	Case series
5	Expert opinion

of participants. Level 3 evidence comprises of case-control studies, whilst level 4 and 5 are usually attributed to case series and expert/panel opinions.

Effect Size and Uncertainty

Often in medical research, a group or certain groups of patients are compared with one another in terms of the outcome (for example, male to female, old to young, those with the disease to those without, etc.). In order to have a meaningful, quantifiable comparison, an effect size is used. An effect size is a way of objectively quantifying the difference between two (or more) groups. There are a variety of effective sizes as highlighted in the three most commonly used, which are odds ratio (OR), hazard ratio (HR) and relative risk/risk ratio (RR).

The OR is the chance (odds) of an event/outcome occurring in one group compared with another. In survival and other time-dependent analyses, a HR is used instead. The HR is the ratio of risk comparing one group to another. The relative risk (also known as the risk ratio) is the probability of an event occurring. Both the OR and RR are similar in that they measure the association between a predictor and an outcome. However, where they differ is in exactly what this measurement is. In the case of OR, it is a comparison of two odds, whereas in RR, it is a comparison of two probabilities, bearing in mind that probability and odds are slightly different. A probability is the fraction/percentage of time you would expect to witness an event, whereas the odds are the probability that the event will occur over the probability that the event will not.

In the case of all these three effect sizes, the OR, HR or RR is essentially a best 'estimate', i.e. it is our best prediction as to what the difference between the two (or more) groups will be. However, we cannot be 100% certain, therefore

there is always a degree of uncertainty. We use the 95% confidence interval (CI) to be sure that 95% of the time, the effect size will lie in this range. In other words, the 95% CI demonstrates that if the experiment was repeated 100 times, in 95 out of those 100, the effect size will lie between the values. For example, the odds that Group B suffer a stroke compared with Group A is OR 1.5 (95% CI 1.4–1.6, $P<.05$). Essentially this means that our best estimate is that Group B is 1.5 times more likely to suffer a stroke compared with Group A. However, we are confident that, should we repeat this experiment 100 times, 95 out of these 100 will produce a result in which Group B is between 1.4 and 1.6 times more likely than Group A to suffer a stroke. In this instance, the P value is less than .05, therefore we can be confident that this has not occurred by chance.

Sample Size

It would be impossible for us to observe the entire population of humans or conduct experiments on all tissue samples or give a drug to everyone, so a sample of the population is chosen instead. Therefore, in a given study, the sample size is the number of observations we accept to be representative of the overall population. How large the sample size should be is mainly determined by how accurate we would like to be versus how feasible the study is to perform. To be 100% accurate, the only sure way is to include the entire population. This, however, is often not feasible or ethical. Therefore, a certain margin of error must be accepted. To calculate sample size, we need three variables:

1. **Precision (Margin of Error):** The margin of error is how close we want the mean from our sample to be from the true sample of the population. The more accurate we want the results to be (i.e. the smaller the margin of error), the more observations we will need. We may choose to accept a 5% or 10% margin of error, meaning that any result we produce will be 'give or take' 5% or 10% either way from the real result had we included the entire population in our study and not just a sample.

2. **Confidence Level:** This pertains to how confident we want to be that the mean we calculated will fall within our confidence interval. We often accept a 95% confidence interval, but we could accept (within reason) any degree of error, including 1% error (99% confidence interval) or 10% (90% confidence interval). Our confidence level corresponds to the *Z-Score* and, depending on how confident we want to be, there is a given mathematical constant. If we want to be 99% confident, the constant is 2.576, 95% confident the constant is 1.96 and for 90% it is 1.645. Irrespective of any of the other variables or the situation, the constant is always as above.

3. **Variation (Standard Deviation):** We would also need to take into account that there will be a certain degree of variation in responses/outcomes from the mean; this is the *Standard Deviation*. However, since we do not know what degree of variation there would be in the population, we would have to make an educated guess, usually

either based on findings of previous research in the field by ourselves or others. If other studies in the same field of interest have reported the standard deviation in the population they studied, we can simply use their findings. In the absence of any previous study, we would have to come up with a figure of variation that would be reasonable.

Once we have these three, we can calculate our sample size, i.e. how many patients, observations or laboratory samples we will require for our study by the following formula:

$$\text{Sample Size}(n) = \frac{\text{Z - Score}^2 \times \text{Standard Deviation}^2}{\text{Margin of Error}^2}$$

For example, if, in our study, we want to be 95% confident and we have a standard deviation of 0.6 and we accept that our results will be within 5% of the real results (margin of error), the number of patients, samples or observations we would need would be:

$$\text{Sample Size}(n) = \frac{1.96^2 \times 0.6^2}{0.05^2}$$

$$\text{Sample Size}(n) = \frac{3.841 \times 0.36}{0.0025}$$

$$n = 553.1$$

Therefore, based on the parameters we have entered, we would need 553 patients, observations or samples for us to be 95% confident that our results would fall within 5% (give or take) of the result we would obtain had we enrolled or sampled the entire population. We can safely assume that these 553 are likely to be representative of the entire population.

Weighting Data

Whilst we often treat all the data we collect or obtain as the same, in certain circumstances we may need to give more **weight** to a certain group of survey respondents, laboratory samples or studies. For example, if we were to collectively compile and analyse data from three studies to answer a specific scientific question and one study had 1000 participants, whilst the other two had less than 200 participants, should all studies be treated equal or should we give more weight to the results of the study with 1000 patients? In surveys, some groups of patients may be under represented i.e. lower response to the survey amongst elderly patients, therefore we may wish to give responses from this group a greater weight (maybe count each of their responses as two responses instead of one) when it comes to the overall analyses.

There are many ways to weight data; however, the simplest is to multiply the number of respondents by >1.0 if we want them to have a greater weight or by <1.0 if we want to them to have a lesser weight.

Quality of Evidence

Evidence quality remains an ongoing issue in healthcare research. Up until recently, research quality was largely subjective, relying on the opinions of peers for validation. Over the years, concerted efforts have materialized in an attempt to develop scoring and quality assessment tools/checklists. Various validated checklists exist for different types of studies. The Jadad Oxford Quality Scale for trials, Newcastle Ottawa Scale (NOS) for observational studies, and National Institute for Health and Care Excellence (NICE) and the Cochrane GRADE (Grading of Recommendations, Assessment, Development and Evaluations) scale for study assessment, amongst others, are widely used in an attempt to objectively assess the quality of studies. In more recent years, there have even been checklists developed to assess the quality of guidelines (the Appraisal of Guidelines for Research and Evaluation – AGREE).

Limitations to Evidence Based Medicine

Despite its enormous potential and the large improvements that have been made in the delivery of healthcare, drug and surgical therapy, EBM does have certain limitations. The conducting of high-level, good-quality research is often expensive and time-consuming and the practicality of applying best practice into everyday practice is sometimes difficult. Evidence based medicine has also resulted in a large amount of research that will ultimately contribute very little or, in some cases, not at all to patient care and the delivery of healthcare, making it a wasteful practice. The vast number of studies published every week is also causing difficulties amongst clinicians in keeping up to date and knowing what the best practice is. Sometimes, EBM cannot even establish best practice as the experiment the issue requires is costly, unethical or otherwise impossible to do. Clinicians also require new skills and training to adequately analyse and use the best evidence.

Searching for Evidence

Identifying the Evidence

All modern clinicians should be able to identify and choose the best current available evidence. They must be able to formulate a question that has clinical relevance, perform a focused literature search, critically appraise the evidence, integrate the information and act in accordance to the best available evidence.[4]

PICO Model

Defining a clinical question in terms of the specific patient problem aids the clinician in finding clinically relevant evidence in the literature. The PICO Model is a good format to employ in defining the question one needs answering.

P: Patient, Population or Problem: This is the group of interest that you need evidence for.

I: Intervention, Prognostic Factor, or Exposure: Which main intervention, prognostic factor, or exposure am I considering?

C: Comparison or Intervention (if appropriate): What is the main alternative to compare with the intervention?

O: Outcome one would like to measure or achieve: What are the effects and end points of intervention?

The PICO format is best suited to answer foreground questions i.e. specific knowledge questions that affect clinical decisions and include a broad range of biological, psychological and sociological issues. Foreground questions generally require a search of the primary medical literature. In contrast, background questions concern general knowledge and can best be answered by using a textbook or consulting a clinical database.

Sources of Evidence

Clinical questions should be answered on the best available knowledge, but there is a wide range of relevant information sources in the form of databases, clinical search engines, professional organizations, patient support groups, networks, libraries, etc., all containing fluctuating levels of evidence. These resources can provide access to evidence, such as systematic reviews and RCTs from journal articles, books, conference proceedings, reports, etc. Many sources will be reliable, but others may contain poorer quality evidence.

To avoid selection bias and have a balanced information, one should use a reputable source of summarized evidence, for example, the following, which are all freely available:

- **National Institute for Health and Care Excellence (NICE) Evidence Search**: publishes evidence updates containing the best available evidence on the major health conditions, based on systematic and comprehensive searching of the research evidence.
- **Turning Research into Practice (TRIP) Database**: provides access to evidence synopses, guidelines, Cochrane systematic reviews, health technology assessment reports, RCTs and case reports.
- **Cochrane Library**: contains high-quality systematic reviews.

Clinical databases, such as **Medline, Embase, Google Scholar and CINAHL**, are only available via subscription, although Medline content is freely available via **PubMed** (http://www.pubmed.gov). However, the content on these databases will not have been appraised or standardized by any assessing body. It is therefore the responsibility of the reader/researcher to critically appraise the content and determine the quality of the evidence obtained during the search process.

Tools for Evidence Synthesis

Evidence Synthesis

The exponential rise of published evidence on a yearly basis has generated the need for a systematic method that can best summarize evidence towards its application to patient care. The information overload that we are facing in today's biomedical world and its scattered nature makes the work of the modern enthusiastic clinician very difficult if he or she chooses to apply current evidence to their practise. The presence of conflicting results amongst the individual studies that may have been derived either by chance or by the presence of systemic error also adds to the problem. The narrative review was the suggested solution to this problem; however, the use of miscellaneous review methodologies, lack of disclosure and transparency in techniques and the inability to statistically combine the results of individual studies rendered the narrative review ineffective.

Similarly, relying on single RCTs may be unreliable due to their inherent limitations. RCTs often require numbers of trial participants to ensure adequate statistical power and need longer follow-up periods to compensate for the low incidence or prevalence of certain diseases as well as the multivariate nature of the 'real world'. Also, the number of surgical RCTs is relatively small and cohort series are still the predominant publication type, with the heterogeneous differences in study quality, insufficient sample size and unclear methodologies. The above issues demonstrate that a more objective method of summarizing research evidence was needed and this has led to the development of a formalized set of processes and methodology in the form of systematic review and meta-analysis.

Synthesizing Data

Often in EBM, we come across a collection of previous studies conducted in our field of interest and we may want to collate the results of these studies to arrive at a single answer, such as does treatment X work better than treatment Y for condition Z? We could just read all the studies conducted on this very question and attempt to arrive at an answer by getting a 'feel' of what each study reports. However, we are at risk of a variety of biases, we may not have all the studies, we may be subconsciously prejudiced in favour of one treatment or another just because we are more familiar with it or it is cheaper, etc., and how would we deal with differences in the number of patients/observations/samples in each study? Would all studies be of equal value and contribute the same to the final judgement? In order to obtain more subjective scientific data, we can combine the data in either *pooled analysis* or *meta-analysis*, both of which are examples of data synthesis, that is, the creation of new data from existing published data. A pooled analysis is the addition of all patients in all studies in each treatment group to determine what proportion of patients benefited from treatment X compared with Y for the condition Z. A meta-analysis only entails data collated together from comparative studies (i.e. all studies must contain outcomes for both groups); however, it remains a more robust analysis of studies, generating an OR, HR or RR for the groups.

What is a Systematic Review?

A systematic review is a scientific evaluation of several studies that have been conducted on a specific clinical question.

By pooling together the results of several studies, the evidence drawn from systematic reviews can be very powerful and influential indeed.

Every systematic review is composed of a discrete number of steps which includes:
- Definition and refinement of a clinical problem.
- Formation of an explicit and objective protocol on how the systematic review is to be conducted. This protocol should include methodology, search strategies, inclusion and exclusion criteria, other validity criteria for included studies and instruments to be used for extracting data such as data extraction sheets, checklists, etc.
- Comprehensive search in order to identify relevant studies. The search for published or unpublished studies should be thorough and exhaustive.
- Application of exclusion and inclusion criteria on the selected studies. Most protocols should also state how any disagreements are to be dealt with so as all studies considered are subject to the same degree of scrutiny, reducing the chance of selection bias.
- Critical appraisal of each individual study using explicit appraisal criteria.
- Data extraction by the use of the instruments stipulated in the protocol so as to reduce the observer bias.
- The methodology of a systematic review should also include a meta-analysis calculation if appropriate

In systematic review, two types of synthesis can be performed: a qualitative synthesis where selected studies are summarized and quantitative synthesis where the results of the studies are statistically combined.

What is a Meta-Analysis?

A meta-analysis is a statistical summation of the results from the studies that have been conducted to answer a specific clinical question. Meta-analysis pools the results from several studies to produce an overall estimate of the effect-size. A meta-analysis can help in synthesizing the results of individual studies when they show no effect due to small sample size or varying directions of effect. The statistical summation can combine findings from similar studies to help increase the power to detect statistical differences.

Analysis of the Evidence

Any variability seen to occur from study to study can be due to chance, systematic differences or both. A collection of studies that have similar and consistent results where any observed differences are simply due to random variation are said to have homogenous results. Real differences can exist between the selected studies even after allowing for random variation. Such a scenario with significant differences between study variability are said to have heterogeneous results. There are different ways to assess for heterogeneity with, e.g. the Cochrane's Q test that follows a chi-square or the analysis of variance (ANOVA). The meta-analytic approach used when heterogeneity has been ruled out is

called 'fixed–effect model' i.e. this way of performing meta-analysis assumes that there is no heterogeneity between the studies. When it occurs, heterogeneity should raise doubts about the respective methodologies of the selected studies and should prompt investigation of the reasons for the discrepancy. The meta-analytic approach used when heterogeneity exists is called a 'random–effects model' as this type of analysis makes less assumptions about how homogenous the studies are.

Reporting of the Evidence

According to the consensus statement that was published in 2000 in Journal of the American Medical Association (JAMA) entitled *Meta-analysis of observational studies in epidemiology – a proposal for reporting*[5] reporting of the results should include:
- Graphic summarizing of individual study estimates and overall affect
- Table giving descriptive information for the selected studies
- Results of sensitivity testing
- Indication of statistical uncertainty of the findings

A forest plot is the graphical display of the results from each trial together with their 95% CI. Each study is represented by a black square and a horizontal line which correspond to the effect size and its 95% CI. The size or area of each black square reflects the weighting ascribed to each study. The midline of a forest plot corresponds to no effect of a treatment such as OR or RR of 1. The solid diamond represents the overall affect size of the selected studies.

The robustness of the findings of the meta-analysis needs to be assessed by performing a sensitivity analysis:
- Both fixed and random effects should be used
- Methodological quality of the studies needs to be assessed using an arbitrary scoring scale and the meta-analysis can be repeated for high- and low-quality studies
- Identification of publication bias

Funnel plots work on the assumption that, if all studies conducted about a similar subject were represented graphically by plotting effect size against respective sample size, a funnel-shaped distribution would be formed. The funnel shape results from the fact that large studies generally have more precise results, which hardly vary about a mean estimate, whereas small studies generally have widely varying results about the mean estimate. Publication bias can be detected by constructing a funnel plot of the selected studies and, if a study lies outside the lines of the funnel plot, this is a sign of potential bias.

Sub-group analysis can be used to explain the heterogeneity by determining which component of the study might be contributing to treatment effect. Meta-regression is also another option if the researcher wants to better understand the causes of heterogeneity between study groups. Multiple continuous or categorical variables could be investigated simultaneously to identify their association with the effect size.[6]

Comparative Effectiveness

Meta-Analysis of Individual Patient Data

Detailed datasets of individual trials are studied, the data are standardized and merged together and overall summary results are calculated. This method provides the ability to assess the implementation of trial methodology, the adequacy of randomization, the demographics of each group and the missing data. On the other hand, the implementation and conduction of this type of meta-analysis could be very costly and time-consuming.

Meta-Analysis of Observational and Epidemiological Studies

RCT results are the most objective form of evidence; however, there are instances where RCTs are unfeasible and only observational studies are available, especially in studies which might involve small disease prevalence and incidence, moderate effect sizes and long follow-up periods. The meta-analysis of observational studies would help in combining results allowing for increased power but the major forms of bias in these studies such as confounding bias, selection/recall bias and study methodology heterogeneity will still need to be accounted for.

Meta-Analysis of Survival Data

In studies reporting survival, the primary outcome is an event occurrence (death, recurrence of disease, etc.) after study initiation and the events are summarized in a Kaplan-Meier curve with an accompanying summary statistic such as HR/log HR. A meta-analysis of such survivorship data involves the summary of their effect sizes. There is a variety of methods and different types of summary measures available to achieve this estimation, including mathematical conversions of numerical data or via direct calculation off of a survival curve.

Cumulative Meta-Analysis

Cumulative meta-analysis allows you to perform or update an already existing analysis every time that a study fulfilling the selection criteria is published. This can be achieved either prospectively or retrospectively. Using a prospective method, there is continual update of the overall effect size as more studies are published and this in turn creates spontaneous reflection on clinical practice. Alternatively, this update of the cumulative meta-analysis can be performed retrospectively, i.e. after a specified time period has lapsed (12, 24, 36 months, etc.). In this manner, time lag bias and effect on temporal changes on current practice and population can also be observed.

Mixed Treatment Comparison Meta-Analysis

Mixed treatment comparison (MTCs), otherwise known as network meta-analyses, allow the comparison of several treatment regimens, or even combinations of them, on an outcome(s). This allows the clinician to incorporate all of the available evidence as opposed to the best available evidence and rank the benefits and harms of each treatment modality so that the most superior one can be suggested for clinical use.

Umbrella Review

With the increase in the number of systematic reviews available, umbrella reviews have been developed in which systematic reviews are themselves subjected to the review process. An umbrella review allows the findings of reviews relevant to a specific question to be compared and contrasted. An umbrella review's most characteristic feature is that this type of evidence synthesis only considers for inclusion the highest level of evidence, namely other systematic reviews and meta-analyses. Umbrella reviews are conducted to provide an overall examination of the body of information that is available for a given topic, and to compare and contrast the results of published systematic reviews. The wide picture obtainable from the conduct of an umbrella review is ideal in highlighting whether the evidence base around a topic is consistent or contradictory, and to explore the reasons for possible discrepancies in the evidence.

Implementing Evidence Based Medicine

Despite a growing trend in the up-take of adopting EBM in everyday practice, its actual implementation remains variable amongst clinicians, different hospitals and different healthcare systems. Implementing EBM can be challenging, time-consuming and expensive; this is despite a generally positive view of EBM amongst clinicians.

Issues to Consider

Perhaps the greatest difficulty in implementing EBM is that, for it to effective, it needs to be implemented diffusely (i.e. across multiple departments/units), it requires championing (i.e. staff dedicated to implementing change), needs auditing to ensure adopted practice is having a positive impact on outcomes and requires planning.[7] Broadly, there are seven key areas to focus on in implementing EBM:

1. **Applicability:** Before implementing any guideline or policy, it is always wise to discuss whether this guideline/policy is appropriate/applicable or suitable for one's particular department in its full state or whether it needs customization. Not all the points within a guideline/policy may be applicable and therefore a workshop/group meeting of all stakeholders in the project (including patient advocacy groups where possible) may be a good start.
2. **Trials and Customizing:** Healthcare departments and institutions are different, as are the populations they serve. Therefore a 'one size fits all' approach is unlikely to be successful and experimentation with different ways

of implementing a certain policy or guideline is essential for success. Often many different pilot trials/experiments may need to be conducted in how to implement an EBM policy before the desired outcome is achieved.

3. **Monitoring and Audit:** This aspect of implementation is often ignored. A guideline/policy is adopted often with little objective monitoring or data collecting. Over time, a policy that was initially meant to be a flexible tool for delivering better care mutates into a rigid set of 'rules' blindly followed (or sometimes ignored altogether) without any checks as to what effect the policy has had on patient care. Objective collection of data, continual monitoring and changes to any newly implemented evidence-based policy/guideline is vital.

4. **Dialogue and Human Factors:** Communication between healthcare workers as well as with patient groups, hospital management, information technology teams and policy makers will greatly increase chances of success in implementing a sustainable evidence-based practice. The opinion of front-line staff is usually invaluable as they are more likely to identify potential risks or areas for improvement. Unfortunately, in policy implementation, the opinion of this key group is often ignored.

5. **Leadership and Champions:** A group of dedicated individuals are required to 'champion' the cause of the newly adopted guideline or policy. Ultimately, any new policy that is not fully supported by the department/institution and practising members is unlikely to be successful. Consensus agreement and discussion with all stakeholders is important to ensure the evidence-based practice survives.

6. **Cost:** The adoption of any new practice will incur some costs in the short run (even if it potentially cuts cost in the long-term). In an ideal world, cost would not be an issue and the best evidence-based practice would be adopted irrespective of cost. However, in reality there will always need to be a compromise between the ideal treatment/care and the cost to ensure that a cost-effective, sustainable policy is implemented. Many healthcare care policies rooted in evidence do not survive because of their unmanageable and unrealistic costing.

7. **Size and Scope:** Healthcare institutions often undertake grandiose plans to implement EBM. However, small and well-targeted measures are more likely to be successful. The scope of the new policy should be clear and reproducible.

How to Implement an EBM Project

Implementation of EBM is a cyclical process in which an important issue/problem is identified, knowledge on how to approach the problem is acquired from the existing literature (or sometimes from trials that others have successfully conducted), the policy is appraised by the stakeholders, the policy is applied and then finally evaluated/audited. Data from the evaluation/audit is then fed back into the process to further improve the implemented policy (Fig. 38.1).

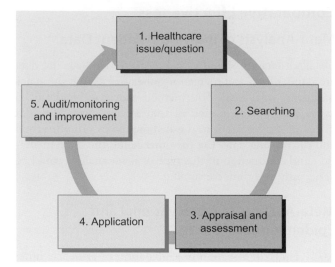

• **Fig. 38.1** The Key Steps in Implementing Evidence-Based Practice

1. **Healthcare Issue/Question:** Typically, this is identified by a member of the 'front-line' healthcare team, although non-clinical staff often raise issues as well. In this step, the identified issue is discussed with the relevant stakeholders (sometimes in a team in a large organized workshop). The team should be as multi-disciplinary as possible with inclusion from patient groups if appropriate.

2. **Searching:** Literature searches, contact with other hospitals or departments are made in order to determine what evidence there is to resolve this issue. Experience from other hospitals (perhaps even hospitals in other countries) can be invaluable and prevent repetition of effort or use of implementation techniques/ways that do not work. A group of selected motivated personnel with specific roles are chosen to find the answers to the questions formulated by the meeting/workshop in step 1. There must be an appropriate length of time dedicated to this to prevent delay in the project.

3. **Appraisal and Assessment:** Once the evidence (the answer to the question) has been obtained, it needs to be critically appraised to determine how appropriate the solutions are and how applicable they are to the particular department/hospital. During this stage, the stakeholders scrutinize the scientific evidence to determine what is likely to succeed, be cost-effective and possible. This stage also requires discussion/meeting/workshop with the stakeholders (ideally the same personnel that were involved in stage 1). The end result of these consultations should be a definitive plan of action with timelines as to how (and over what timeframe) the project will be implemented, how it will be monitored/audited, what additional human and material resources will be required. etc.

4. **Application:** In stage 3, a clear and precise plan with protocol should have been created. A team with designated roles, duties and responsibilities should also be selected to oversee the implementation of the policy/guideline. Initially, it may be sensible to carry out a pilot or trial

run to identify potential 'teething problems' and arrange solutions to minimize these issues. Once this has been achieved, the policy can be implemented on an agreed date with front-line staff.

5. **Audit, Monitoring and Improvement:** Continual monitoring of the established policy is required to ensure further improvement. Prospective data collection and audit are important to objectively assess how well the implemented policy is working. This data is then analysed, presented at clinical governance meetings and further healthcare issues/questions are raised, thus taking the process back to stage 1.

Evidence Based Medicine and Quality of Care

The very aim of EBM from its early beginnings has been to improve the quality of the care delivered to patients, not just by assessing the efficacy of the treatment offered but also grounding the very decision of the clinician in science. To this end, EBM has always had an unbreakable link with direct patient care, largely due to the fact that EBM can be applied to every stage of the patient journey, from diagnosis through treatment and onto prognosis. Over the last few decades, huge leaps in quality of care have been achieved, largely thanks to the application of scientific methods obtained through practicing EBM. Randomized control trials, for example, have played a decisive role in determining the superiority (or at least non-inferiority) of treatments across a variety of subspecialties. However, adopting an EBM approach does not automatically translate into a greater quality of care.

Technology, Innovation and Diffusion of Ideas

In the last 60 years, there has been an explosion of human innovation and technology with many ideas/products rapidly taken up across the world. The smartphone and the tablet computer are perhaps the latest amongst a long line of examples. In healthcare, it is no different. The advent of fibre optics and improving high-definition (now 4K) cameras and screens has made access to the smallest part of the human body not only possible but routine. Endoscopy of the gastrointestinal tract, upper respiratory, thoracic and abdominal cavities is not only feasible but routine and, in many cases, the preferred modality. All of this has occurred within 25 years. Laparoscopic, thoracoscopic, arthroscopic and robotic surgery, amongst countless other medical equipment for monitoring and altering human physiology, is now widespread for a variety of conditions even in the developing world.

Part of this drive for innovation and uptake of technology has been at least in part due to EBM. The practice of EBM has helped develop critical thinking and new, ingenious solutions have been developed to deal with real life, everyday problems. These ideas have then been subjected to rigorous development, trial and then diffusion across healthcare systems. Industry has undoubtedly played a central role. However, it is not just hardware that has benefitted. With increasing miniaturization of computer technology and processors, smart phones and tablet computers have become valuable tools for medical education, training and medical reference applications. What used to require a trip to the library and hours of laborious searching only to find EBM information/data that was years out of date can now be obtained instantaneously at a touch of a screen. Dissemination of these ideas and technologies (which are becoming increasingly cheaper) has resulted in a truly international practice of EBM across the world. Ideas and innovations born in one location can be rapidly taken up across the other side of the world.

Artificial Intelligence and The Future

If current predictions are to be believed, artificial intelligence (AI) will change human society and innovation to an almost unfathomable level in the next 30–40 years. Much of the decision-making process will be taken over by objective AI, with access to the findings of the latest meta-analyses and trials. Already, we routinely use computer algorithms and online calculators to predict survival, peri-operative mortality and life expectancy across a variety of specialities. The next logical step will be AIs capable of a high degree of machine learning that can utilize ever increasing data points about a patient's physical characteristics, morbidity, disease pathology and even genomics to determine what treatment modality is most likely to be successful. Some fear that this may result in a slavish adherence to computer decisions, removing the human and emotional factor that is important in our everyday clinical practice but ultimately how we choose to employ such technology is up to us and the future is far from a foregone conclusion.

References

1. Sackett DL, Rosenberg WM, Gray JA, Haynes RB, Richardson WS. Evidence based medicine: what it is and what it isn't. *BMJ*. 1996;312(7023): 71–72.
2. Moher D, Schulz KF, Altman DG. The CONSORT statement: revised recommendations for improving the quality of reports of parallel-group randomised trials. *Lancet*. 2001;357(9263): 1191–1194.
3. Sackett DL, Wennberg JE. Choosing the best research design for each question. *BMJ*. 1997;315(7123): 1636.
4. Mulrow CD. Rationale for systematic reviews. *BMJ*. 1994;309 (6954): 597–599.
5. Stroup DF, Berlin JA, Morton SC, et al. Meta-analysis of observational studies in epidemiology: a proposal for reporting. Meta-analysis of Observational Studies in Epidemiology (MOOSE) group. *J Am Med Assoc*. 2000;283(15): 2008–2012.
6. Moher D, Tetzlaff J, Tricco AC, Sampson M, Altman DG. Epidemiology and reporting characteristics of systematic reviews. *PLoS Med*. 2007;4(3): e78.
7. Dixon E, Hameed M, Sutherland F, Cook DJ, Doig C. Evaluating meta-analyses in the general surgical literature: a critical appraisal. *Ann Surg*. 2005;241(3): 450–459.

39

Surgical Ethics

CHAPTER OUTLINE

Introduction

Surgeons in training emerge into ethical and legal landscapes radically different to their predecessors. Paternalism is less welcome and deference to professional authority has declined. Legal judgements and even criminal convictions have reshaped behaviours and practice, while public faith has been dented by publicized failings and scandals.[1] Most patients still place immense trust in the person who operates on them, but surgeons are increasingly expected to explain and justify decisions and actions. Many complaints relate to inadequate communication and consent, and thus, in addition to being a competent operator, surgeons must act as advisors and counsellors to patients, as well as leaders, trainers and role models. They must be fully aware of all the legal and ethical issues that apply to their work. In this chapter, we explore areas of medical ethics which have the greatest bearing on surgical practice, highlighting common examples where ethical dilemmas may arise. Where appropriate, case law and legislation is presented, but variation across nations means that this is for illustration only.

Evolution of Surgery and Ethics

Surgery evolved in medieval Europe thanks largely to *Barber Surgeons* within military organizations, operating in the precursors of field hospitals. Mortality (frequently secondary to haemorrhage and infection) was high.[2,3] Anatomical study advanced surgical techniques during the *Renaissance* and, in the mid-19th century, the germ theory of sepsis, effective hand-washing and general anaesthesia allowed the modern speciality of surgery to develop.[4-6] Society very rarely questioned surgeons' judgement even when mortality rates were high. At the same time, the 'ethic of surgery' was often defined by the virtues of resilience in the face of hard work and sleep deprivation; personal certainty in decision making and courage when faced with extreme risks and poor outcomes. New techniques, modern anaesthesia and perioperative care have enabled huge advances.[7,8] They provide operative and postoperative conditions for complex operations, reducing the 'brutality and violence' of surgery and offering prospects of survival for even the frailest of patients (Box 39.1). However, potential benefits of modern surgery can be accompanied by much greater ethical dilemmas.

Medical Ethics and Law

Ethics is the branch of philosophy dealing with the moral content of our conduct. It aims to establish what is right and wrong, although a number of theories compete to do this. Religious texts originally provided moral codes, and professions such as medicine have also developed their own e.g. the Hippocratic Oath. The morality of actions can also be judged against outcomes *(consequentialism)* or against a deeper set of duties.[9] Virtue ethics is another theory, which holds that the right ethical behaviours should conform to what the virtuous person would do. Most well-known, however, is the four principals account of medical ethics,[10] which is presented in Box 39.2 with examples relevant to surgical practice. Current social norms and ethical accounts appear to place the greatest value on respect for autonomy over other duties. However, autonomy is an elusive philosophical concept[11] and the extent that most patients wish to be fully autonomous remains vigorously debated.[12]

Ethical dilemmas imply that a choice needs to be made and that one or more ethical principles are in conflict. Ethical theories do not offer complete answers but they provide templates for debate, where facts and values can be established leading to rational and defensible decisions. Box 39.3 offers suggested components for the process of ethical reasoning.

Law is a set of codified rules of conduct, with a moral foundation. It is specific to given jurisdictions, but countries frequently follow precedent examples from others. Various sources of law may apply to surgical practice.

- Common (or case) law – whereby the law relating to specific situations e.g. consent is refined by successive court judgments over the years. In the UK, the UK Supreme Court is now the highest court authority.

• BOX 39.1   What Is Surgery?

Surgery is a profession defined by its authority to cure by means of bodily invasion. The brutality and risks of opening a living person's body have long been apparent, the benefits only slowly and haltingly worked out. Nonetheless, over the past two centuries, surgery has become radically more effective, and its violence substantially reduced – changes that have proved central to the development of mankind's abilities to heal the sick.

Gawande, A., 2012. Two hundred years of surgery. NEJM. 266, 1716–1723

• BOX 39.2   The Four Principles of Medical Ethics with Examples for Surgical Practice

Respect for autonomy

- Providing information and support to allow patients to make informed decisions
- Honesty regarding complications and errors
- Confidentiality of medical information
- Consideration and respect for patients' dignity

Beneficence (doing good)

- Practising to the highest standards, striving to improve knowledge and skills
- Leading perioperative teams to maximize patient outcomes
- Making decisions in the best interests of incompetent patients/protecting vulnerable patients
- Supporting teaching and research to improve care

Non-maleficence (avoiding harms)

- Contributing to a professional culture that promotes safety
- Operating within one's expertise e.g. recognizing fatigue
- Being prepared to report hazards or inappropriate/dangerous practices
- Conducting training and research in a way that minimizes patient harm

Justice

- Treating patients equally
- Using scarce resources wisely and allocating them fairly
- Preventing financial considerations from influencing clinical decisions
- Refusing to participate in state activities that contravene medical codes

---

- Statutory legislation – e.g. acts passed by parliament e.g. the Mental Capacity Act 2005, or the Health and Social Care Act 2008 which now contains the duty of candour
- Human Rights law (see Box 39.9)
- European Law – whilst the UK still adheres to this legislation
- Quasi law – in the UK, the General Medical Council (GMC) is legally empowered to regulate doctors' practice and conduct, and GMC guidance is binding.

• BOX 39.3   Steps in Ethical Reasoning

A number of models of ethical reasoning exist, but some common steps can be identified in the context of making ethical decisions in surgery.[13]

1. Establish all the clinical facts relating to this patient as far as possible, i.e. the exact problem, the nature of non-surgical and surgical options, and the likely outcomes, burdens and risks associated with each.
2. Establish who this decision affects – above all, it will be the patient, but also their family and close associates, and also other colleagues who may have views or an interest.
3. Confirm that all key parties share the same objective clinical facts, and be sure that all clinicians understand the patient's values and preferences in the fullest context of their life e.g. attitude to medical treatment, occupation, family life and future plans etc.
4. Establish how law and other professional guidance apply to this situation – e.g. which actions are not permissible, what is obliged or recommended
5. Explore the ethical principles that apply and identify where these are in potential conflict.
6. Evaluate each clinical option to examine how it fits best with the requirements above. Discuss fully with the patient if possible, and place their wishes at the very centre of the debate. Include also all those who they wish to be involved and also other colleagues. Document the steps taken to justify the decision and why other options were rejected.

Based on data from Wall, A., Angelos, P., Brown, D., Kodner, I. J., Keune, J. D. Ethics in surgery. *Curr Probl Surg*, 2013;50: 99–134.

Civil law aims to resolve a dispute between two parties, e.g. a patient suing their surgeon for negligence. The criminal law operates when actions are felt sufficiently serious to warrant prosecution by the state, e.g. gross negligence or manslaughter.

Decision Making

This is often the hardest part of surgical management. Beyond the technical considerations of operating,[13] most decisions have ethical and legal components. It is vital to consider the broader goals of medicine such as restoring quality of life and alleviating suffering, as well as the technical feasibility of an operation. With competent patients, decision making should be shared and the process of informed consent forms the framework for doing this. However, making autonomous decisions in the context of being unwell or in fear can be very difficult. Patients may know much about their own conditions but often lack knowledge and experience to make confident surgical decisions, resulting in significant asymmetry of knowledge and power. Surgeons will also have to seek consent from parents before they operate on children and make decisions on behalf of adults who lack the capacity to decide by themselves. Difficult, challenging judgements also have to be made at the end of life, e.g. knowing when not to operate and helping patients to achieve a dignified death.

Consent

Competent patients have sovereignty over their own bodies, and the duty of doctors to seek consent is grounded in the principal of respect for autonomy. This was first expressed conclusively in law as:

> *Every human being of adult years and sound mind has a right to determine what is done with his (or her) own body and a surgeon who performs an operation without consent commits an assault...*[14]

> **J. CARDOZO**

Seeking consent for invasive procedures has evolved significantly since 1914. Law and professional guidelines increasingly reflect patients' rights to make fully informed decisions via shared decision making. At the same time, levels of litigation are increasing, and deficiency in consent has increasingly become a route for recovering damages from surgical complications (Box 39.4).

Key Points for Optimal Process of Consent

A new diagnosis can leave patients in emotional shock, and unable to decide 'rationally.' Most patients need time to understand their diagnoses and available treatments. Consent should usually, therefore, be a process and not a single event, beginning well before the day of surgery. Indeed, consent taken on the day of surgery can be regarded as placing pressure on a patient to proceed and may be invalid.

Consent should usually be taken by a surgeon competent to perform the operation, or someone specifically trained to take consent for the proposed procedure, such as a *termination of pregnancy* counsellor. Trainee surgeons must learn to seek consent but should be competent when doing so for a given operation. They must have the guidance and authorization of their senior. All patients should meet with an experienced surgeon at some point in their care in order to answer specific queries and discuss the pros and cons of treatment options, for example surgery versus chemotherapy/radiotherapy in cancer treatment. A clear explanation of the condition and range of treatments available is essential. Surgeons are not obliged to offer procedures that they feel are unlikely to benefit patients or have unacceptable risks (although referral to a second opinion can be wise at times).

Providing Adequate Information

Surgeons face major challenges in judging what information to share. Some operations are urgent necessities, e.g. laparotomy for life-threatening haemorrhage, whilst others are finely-balanced decisions, e.g. prostate cancer surgery vs radiotherapy. Patients also range from those who wish to

---

• **BOX 39.4** **The Principal Roles of Consent, and the Key Elements of Valid Consent**

Roles played by the consent process

1. Good clinical practice necessitates seeking patients' agreement prior to surgery. Active dialogue promotes trust and hopefully selects operations that are best for individuals. Informed and engaged patients are likely to have better outcomes.
2. Seeking consent fulfils an ethical duty to respect patients' autonomy; something represented in multiple ethical theories
3. Valid consent provides surgeons with legal protection against charges of assault (unlawful touching) and claims of negligence, e.g. failure to warn of complications. Law varies across jurisdictions but the principal that competent patients must give informed agreement before surgery is consistently upheld.

Three key elements of valid consent

1. Patients must be competent to make decisions. In England and Wales, this is defined as capacity, as set out in the Mental Capacity Act 2005 (see Box 39.6).
2. Patients should be acting freely. The role of the surgeon is to provide recommendations, but this should not extend to pressure or coercion (regardless of good intentions). Patients have the right to decline surgery (even if the decision appears to be unwise) and should be supported and protected to make such choices uninfluenced by any external pressures.
3. Patients must be adequately informed in order to make an autonomous decision for themselves. This can provoke uncertainty as to what should be discussed and disclosed, and we discuss this at greater length in the main text.

---

know (and challenge) every detail to those who simply want to place their trust in someone and receive good advice.

Previously, the required level of information disclosure was judged by the professional standard, i.e. what would a responsible body of surgeons think appropriate to warn patients of (the *Bolam Principal.*) Since then, law has evolved in favour of patients' rights to make fully informed decisions. In the UK, the recent landmark *Montgomery Judgment* (2015) stated that doctors should take 'reasonable care to ensure patients are aware of *any* material risks involved in any recommended treatment and of *any* reasonable alternative or variant treatment' [author's italics][15]. The implication is that patients must be informed of all relevant information that may be significant and that could affect their decisions. This is echoed in many other professional guidelines, i.e. that patients should 'know the risks'.

There is, however, minimal legal guidance as to which actual risks must be disclosed and conversely, most patients do not know what questions to ask. The Montgomery judgment cautions against 'bombarding patients with information,' although the increased volume of information now presented to patients may amount to this. Most patients are principally seeking good advice and honesty. Establishing trust and good communication is therefore the foundation for effective consent.[16] It should also be remembered that information is not provided solely to prevent litigation in the event of complications. Patients wish to be informed so that they can plan for the future, involve families and close friends, and generally feel engaged with care.[17]

Information can only be withheld in exceptional circumstances if it would cause real physical or psychological harm, but not to avoid distress or through concerns that the patient might decide against surgery. Patients do also have rights to decline to hear every single risk, although this should be carefully documented, with advice that there are some risks that they may, in hindsight, wish that they had been aware of. There is also a basic minimum of information, namely the nature, purpose and likely outcome of an operation, together with the alternatives, that would be essential to constitute valid consent.

Surgeons should establish through dialogue what particular information is relevant to an individual patient faced with a particular decision. Guidance from professional bodies can be useful but should not replace experienced counselling. Box 39.5 contains broad categories of information that most patients should know before making decisions about surgery. For patients undergoing major surgery and/or those with significant co-morbidities, the early input of anaesthetists is important in helping to assess perioperative risk and discuss these matters with patients.

The ultimate goal is to educate and empower patients to understand and engage in decisions. They should be provided with all relevant available information in an intelligible format before they commit themselves to a given option. Despite improved national datasets for outcomes, establishing the risks that apply to individuals remains difficult. Online risk tools can help refine estimates of risk for mortality, morbidity and specific complications, but remain population based.[18] Shared decision making can be further enhanced using procedure-specific consent forms or 'decision records' that patients can take home.[19] Interactive decision aids and other online resources can also help improve understanding of clinical conditions and treatment options.[20]

Finally, consent must also survive hindsight, particularly if complications have arisen. Patients must still feel that their consent was taken adequately and without pressure. Numerous studies reveal that patients recall and understand little of their consent process and this is a significant concern.[21] Clear communications and good records that are shared with patients will be essential in minimizing the impact of potential disputes and also helping patients remember why they agreed to surgery. Written consent is not usually required by law, but is fundamental good practice for any procedure with risks or requiring anaesthesia.

Caring for Adults Who Lack Capacity

Many adults are unable to make their own decisions about surgery or may appear to be making very unwise choices. Surgeons have a duty to respect the autonomous decisions of competent patients but must work without prejudice

> ### • BOX 39.5 Information to be Provided During the Consent Process
>
> - An explanation of the patient's current problem
> - All other options available for this patient, including having no treatment
> - The prospects for benefit for each option, but also the possibility of failure
> - The nature, purpose and likely outcome of the proposed operation
> - Whether general anaesthesia, sedation or local anaesthesia will be required
> - Common side-effects and information about recovery, hospital stay and convalescence
> - Complications, particularly those causing pain, loss of function and change of appearance
> - Adverse outcomes, particularly those that might affect independence, employment and personal life, e.g. fertility
> - Serious complications, particularly where these might cause prolonged recovery, poor functional outcome or death
> - Specific risks that might be significant to an individual patient (e.g. loss of dexterity in a skilled worker or vocal cord injury in a singer, etc.)
> - Who will be performing the procedure, and who will also be present
>
> NOTE: all risk information should, as far as possible, be applicable to the individual patient having their operation in a given institution.

to make the best decisions for patients lacking capacity. This section explores principles contained in the Mental Capacity Act 2005 (MCA), but readers must always be aware of the exact legislation that applies in their country of practice.

Making decisions on behalf of others can be intensely difficult. There may be a distinct difference between what appears best for a patient as they are now, compared with what that person may have previously wished for themselves. Living wills and advance decisions introduce the problem of precedent autonomy, i.e. can a past version of a person dictate what happens to their future self with complete authority?[22] Relatives or advisors cannot claim to know another person's mind fully, and thus decision making by a proxy is equally problematic.[23] However decisions do have to be made, and these will need to be justified ethically and remain within the law.

In England and Wales, the legal criteria for testing capacity are set out in the Mental Capacity Act 2005 (MCA), accompanied by a check list of factors to consider when making a best interests decision (Box 39.6). Other countries have legislation to cover decision making on behalf of adults without capacity. Capacity is a legal criterion referring to the ability to make a specific decision. It forms a spectrum

> **• BOX 39.6** | **Mental Capacity Act (2005) England and Wales**
>
> Patients must be able to do the following to demonstrate the capacity to make a given decision.
> - Understand relevant information about the decision to be made
> - Retain that information in their mind (for long enough to make a decision)
> - Use or weigh that information as part of the decision making
> - Communicate their decision (by talking, using sign language or any other means)
>
> All 'practicable steps' must be taken to promote a patient's capacity e.g.:
> - Use of appropriate language or sign language or other educational aids
> - Reversing any temporary causes of incapacity e.g. acute confusion or drug effects
> - Choosing the optimum environment and time of day
> - Providing support, e.g. family, close friends or official advocates
>
> Does the patient have a disturbance of mind or brain causing their loss of capacity?
> - If the patient does not have any known cause, consider the possibility of coercion or undue external influence.
>
> If a patient lacks capacity to make this decision, the following issues must be considered:
> - Can the decision be deferred if the person is likely to regain capacity in the future?
> - Does the patient have any documented advance care plan, or advance decisions to refuse treatment?
> - Is another individual such as a *Lasting Power of Attorney* (for welfare) holder or Court Appointed Deputy authorized to make this decision?
> - Can anyone (family, close friends, other professionals) offer information about the patient's values and beliefs?
> - For patients lacking family and friends, an independent mental capacity advocate (IMCA) should be appointed where serious medical treatments are being considered
>
> The act does not define 'best interests' but provides a checklist of factors to be reviewed:
> - All circumstances relating to the person and the decision must be considered
> - Encourage, enhance the person's ability to participate in the decision
> - Consider person's past and present wishes and feelings and any statements written when they had capacity, as well as their beliefs, values and other factors
> - Consult with carers, anyone named by the person, any attorney under Lasting Power of Attorney, Court Appointed Deputy and previous representatives.
> - If the decision concerns life-sustaining treatment – no assumption about quality of life should be made, and the decision must not be motivated by any desire to bring about the person's death.
>
> Much more guidance and information is provided in the MCA Code of Practice. In addition, NICE guidance on implementing the Act has been published. See www.nice.org.uk Decision-making and mental capacity NICE guideline [NG108]Published: 03 October 2018

in that some patients lack capacity to make any decision, whereas others may reach this threshold with support. However, for all patients, capacity should be judged against the specific decision that needs to be made. Lack of capacity should not be presumed from the patient's appearance, age or behaviour, and nor should it be ascribed to decisions that appear unwise or that could lead to bad outcomes. Capacity is related to the intellectual difficulty of the decision rather than the gravity of the consequences, although it is understandable to want greater reassurance that a patient is competent to make a life-changing decision. All reasonable efforts must be made to support a patient's decision making and these should be documented.

If a patient lacks capacity, the surgeons will need to make a best interests decision. This should not simply be a 'good surgical decision' but should be made in the fullest sense of the patient's interests including their past wishes and values, and present psychological and social welfare. It is also important to seek the views those who know the patient well. Their role is not to decide or impose their views, but to present what they think this patient would want in the circumstances. Adults who hold valid powers of attorney can make the decisions on patients' behalves; however, they cannot demand procedures which are thought to be futile, and they must also act responsibly.

Consent for Children

Most countries allow consent to be given by a parent or authorized caregiver but, increasingly, the views of children must be included as they develop through childhood. At 14 years of age, many children have decision-making skills that match adults. Courts have upheld their decisions where they have sufficient maturity and understanding to make a given decision. However, they may be more easily overwhelmed by sickness or anxiety in hospitals and need support to reach decisions. Box 39.7 summarizes the current law in England and Wales. Readers should always be fully aware of laws and professional guidance in their own country. Children need kindness and respect to help engagement, and sufficient honesty to preserve trust for future encounters. Overriding the refusal of a child may be necessary on occasions, but will also carry risks for the current procedure and their future

• BOX 39.7 Legal Aspects of Consent for Children in England and Wales

What does English law state in regard to consent by children and young people?

- Under 16 years, children cannot normally give valid consent*, and parents (or those with parental responsibility**) must give consent on their behalf. Parents can authorize others to take on some aspects of parental responsibility. Other persons, e.g. teachers or grandparents, may do what is 'reasonable to promote the welfare of a child', e.g. take them to A&E, but cannot give valid consent.
- Young persons aged 16–18 years may give consent if they wish***, but parents may also consent on their behalf if their child is unwilling or unable.
- Parents should act in the best interests of their children. Clinicians may apply for a court order if parental wishes appear to be against a child's best interests.
- Once young persons reach 18 years of age, they must give consent for themselves, and parents cannot consent on their behalf.
- Urgent treatment may be given without consent to prevent harm or deterioration from occurring.
- United Nations Convention on the Rights of the Child (UNCRC) 1989 (adopted by the UK in 1991) states in Article 12 that: *When adults are making decisions that affect children, children have the right to say what they think should happen and have their opinions taken into account.*

*The legal concept of *Gillick* competence allows children less than 16 years with sufficient maturity and understanding to consent to some treatment without parental knowledge.
**Parental responsibility is a legal term giving a parent rights and responsibilities over their child. Married mothers and fathers have parental responsibility, as do unmarried fathers of children born after 1/12/2003, providing they are named on the birth certificate. Unmarried fathers of children born before this date must acquire legal responsibility via a Parental Responsibility Agreement or court order. Parents do not lose responsibility if they divorce, but they do if they give up their child for adoption.
***The capacity of a young person of 16 years or greater to give consent is judged by the criteria set out in the Mental Capacity Act 2005.

health and development. Additionally, all doctors should know how to act on concerns about a vulnerable child or signs of abuse or neglect.

Consent for Organ Donation and Receipt

Demand for transplanted organs greatly outstrips supply, and thus the enrolment of consenting donors must be maximized, and their organs allocated in an ethical manner. Most countries have an 'opt in' system, i.e. potential donors must have indicated their previous willingness by carrying a donor card or leaving some form of instructions. Family and next of kin will routinely be consulted and their refusal may override the previous wishes of the donor. In future, 'opt out' systems may become more widespread, i.e. willingness to donate is assumed by default unless there is evidence to the contrary. Living donors can donate to family or close

relatives, but at present, few countries sanction open markets in organs, due to concerns of coercion or exploitation.

Organs from the deceased donor are harvested after brain death has been certified, or in some cases after circulatory arrest has occurred. Diagnosis of brain death and organ retrieval practice varies between countries. Allocation of available organs must conform to a principal of justice and will typically be based on length of wait and/or clinical urgency for the recipient. Some have argued that priority for the more 'deserving' patient should also be considered, e.g. should a patient whose liver failure arises from self-harm such as alcohol or paracetamol abuse have a lesser right to receive an organ? However, allocating merit to patients is highly problematic, as alcoholism can equally be viewed as a disease rather than a moral failing. Utilitarian arguments might suggest that patients who are most likely to benefit from their transplanted organ should have priority, but this should also be cleared of any unjust judgments about entitlement or moral worth of recipients.[22] This topic will be covered in greater detail in Chapter 12.

Organ donation in the United Kingdom is regulated by the Human Tissue Act (2004) except for Scotland where the Human Tissue (Scotland) Act 2006 applies.

Patients Refusing Treatment

It is well-established in English law and other jurisdictions that competent patients are entitled to refuse any treatment, providing it is a voluntary decision and they are fully aware of the possible consequences. If the test for capacity is satisfied, surgeons are not entitled to coerce or make undue efforts to encourage patients to agree to surgery. This may feel ethically difficult on occasions, e.g. if a young adult makes a decision which they might later bitterly regret (if they are still alive). This conflicts with a clear duty to prevent harm and promote recovery and presents a concern that a patient is being abandoned to an ill thought-out decision. There is criticism that respect for autonomy has emerged as the pre-eminent principal in ethical accounts and court room judgements.[25] Ethical approaches would be to explore the underlying reasons for refusal from the patient's perspective and engage in dialogue at least. If, after engagement in balanced (and documented) dialogue, the patient with capacity continues to refuse treatment, then a best practice approach has at least occurred.

Patients can also refuse treatment via advance decisions. Surgeons must ensure these are valid and applicable to the circumstances, and if so, they must be followed. Competent patients, however, can reverse previous advance decisions. Under the MCA, attorneys can decide against surgery, but they cannot refuse life-saving procedures unless separately authorized to do so by a valid advance decision.

Problems can arise when patients' stipulations make a procedure increasingly risky or difficult to complete. For example, a patient might consent to laparotomy for bowel surgery but refuse a stoma under any circumstances. Surgeons are not obliged to offer operations where the risks greatly outweigh benefits and the rights for patients to refuse treatment do not automatically extend to the component parts of the procedure.

One quite common scenario arises with members of the Jehovah's Witness community who routinely refuse transfusion of blood or blood products. Most Jehovah's Witness patients have stable and sincerely held views and will present these as advance decisions to refuse treatment (ADRTs) which cannot be lawfully overridden. Difficult dilemmas can arise with young persons and others whose refusal might not feel fully committed or individually made. Dialogue should aim to establish their true wishes and also their acceptance of techniques such as cell salvage or pre-donation of blood. Second opinions should be offered where surgeons feel unable to offer an operation. For unconscious patients and children of Jehovah's Witnesses, emergency court orders may be needed.

Futility and End-of-Life Care

Adults are increasingly dying in hospital after prolonged periods of deterioration associated with *eleventh hour* interventions (including surgery) that may have no long-term benefit. Life-saving treatments can become tortuous and degrading interventions. To develop best practice, surgeons must be able to define *Serious Medical Treatments* (Box 39.8) and understand physiological and holistic aspects of futility. This will improve abilities to directly discuss matters with patients who have capacity and, when capacity is lost in the absence of ADRTs or Lasting Power of Attorneys (LPAs), to develop ethical and legal templates for best interests decisions.

Medical Futility

The concept of futility has quantitative and qualitative components reflecting scientific and holistic aspects of care. Quantitative futility is recognized as something that cannot accomplish intended physiological goals.[26] It can be easy for doctors to conceptualize as it involves assessing the severity of acute conditions and the related impact of co-morbidities, often via outcome prediction scores. However, the population-based nature of such scores means they do not apply to individuals and cannot become uniform guides. Clinicians' experience with similar cases should also be considered, but again case histories do not refer to individuals whose care is being discussed. Therefore, when considering each case on its merits, further thought should be given to *normative futility* reflecting holistic care.

This requires information about patients' beliefs and values to gauge what is meaningful to them. In ideal circumstances, this will have been discussed with competent patients; however, during acute illness, patients may lose capacity and there may be an absence of ADRTs or LPAs. Comparatively few patients have considered making such preparations for serious illness or terminal disease. In these circumstances, best interests are discussed and determined. Effective, empathic communications are vital to minimize conflict.

• BOX 39.8   **Serious Medical Treatments**

Serious medical treatments are treatments that have a fine balance between benefit and risk. Institution, withdrawal or withholding has *serious consequences,* e.g. likely death, serious pain and distress, serious impact on future life choices (orchidectomy, oophorectomy.) This term has had a specific meaning under the MCA Code of Practice, although this is under review.

Debate considers the relative value and potential conflicts of *beneficence, non-maleficence, autonomy* and *distributive justice* (see Box 39.2). The desire to perform altruistic acts *(beneficence)* motivates healthcare professionals but, for dying patients, surgery may become harmful if precipitating a degrading death. Here, doctors should consider philosophical as well as physiological aspects of life. Patients may have autonomous desires to live but situations can develop whereby prolonging treatments infringes their right of having a good, natural death and thus a complete life.[27] When cultural or religious contexts are applied, a good natural death can be perceived as enabling a step towards a further stage of existence. In summary, good end-of-life care can avoid tortuous treatments and provide the circumstances for the final part of a fulfilling autonomous life. In countries that are aligned to the European Convention on Human Rights, dilemmas can be discussed in the context of Articles 2, 3 and 8 which express fundamental human rights (Box 39.9).

Prognostic uncertainty exists in many scenarios and therapeutic trials may need to be considered with well-defined goals in specific time frames, e.g. responses to changing antibiotics over 48–72 hours. If conflicting views become embedded and an impasse arises, formal channels for debate and decision making should be opened. The scope of this chapter is too limited to provide in-depth analyses of such matters; however, they include processes of second or third opinions, clinical ethics committees and recourse to the courts.

Provision of End-of-Life Care

Recognition of dying precipitates a duty to provide effective end-of-life care. The specifics of this are dealt with in Chapter 11 but it includes the *desire to have minimal pain and suffering, achieve a sense of control, have burdens relieved, to ensure that there is no inappropriate prolongation of dying* and *to strengthen relationships with loved ones.* Doctors must be capable of organizing care reflecting such needs, balancing individuals' needs to 'put their affairs in order' against unnecessarily prolonging pain and suffering.

In a medical context, this includes administering analgesia and withholding or withdrawing life-sustaining treatments to allow a natural death. Actions and omissions should be considered in the context of relative harms and benefits, which is rarely an all-or-nothing process. The three most prominent discussions frequently relate to opiate analgesia, do not attempt cardiopulmonary resuscitation (DNACPR) and withholding/withdrawing nutrition and hydration.

Administering Opiate Analgesia to the Dying Patient

This can raise fear of intentionally precipitating death. Reality is usually different; firstly, there is a therapeutic window between analgesic and lethal effects of opiates; secondly, staff will be judged on their intent via the *Doctrine of Double Effect* or DDE (Box 39.10). This distinguishes between *foreseeing* and *intending*, i.e. administering opiate analgesia may result in a so-called 'bad' result (death) but if intentions were to provide pain control to a dying patient the 'good' result is beneficial. The DDE also applies to other acts or omissions, e.g. withdrawing or withholding cardiovascular support.

It has been argued that the DDE provides a 'moral loophole' to avoid assault charges, manslaughter or murder and with respect to 'intent' such *purity of thought* does not exist. Evidence and experiences, however, demonstrate under-used analgesia near the end of life. The DDE therefore has the potential to justify improved analgesia, even if this may shorten life.

DNACPR

CPR was devised as a resuscitation tool for previously well patients suffering a sudden collapse, often due to acute out-of-hospital cardiac events. It has a role in other forms of cardiac arrest but its quantitative success rate (return of spontaneous circulation or ROSC) has to be balanced against the qualitative outcome of survival, including hypoxic brain injury. Cardiac arrests with poor outcomes are frequently associated with hours or days of deterioration, debilitating chronic illness and metastatic disease. There is thus a requirement in certain patient groups to consider *Do Not Attempt CardioPulmonary Resuscitation* (Box 39.11).

Chest compressions and defibrillation can cause direct physical harm to dying patients (musculoskeletal injury and burns). Significant consideration should therefore be given to discussions with patients and their relatives making it clear that they relate specifically to CPR and do not equate to the withdrawal of care, which can include supplementary oxygen, intravenous fluids and antibiotics. It should also be made clear that DNACPR is a means of minimizing unnecessary harm and not a process of neglect.

Additionally, DNACPR orders are not necessarily permanent. They can be put in place during a period of severe illness where cardiac arrest would be non-survivable, but if patients subsequently improve, the decision can be reviewed and if necessary revoked. Likewise, patients with long-standing DNACPR orders can be advised to consider temporary suspension if they were to undergo elective surgery.[28] The unique circumstances of an operating theatre may allow rapidly reversible causes of cardiac arrest to be managed immediately, and the physiological instability that can occur under anaesthesia is quite distinct from the natural process of dying.

Within the UK, there is now clear legal guidance for healthcare organizations when considering DNACPR discussions. They have to be patient-centred with policies that are 'clear and accessible' and compatible with a recent Court of Appeal judgement brought by a family against an NHS Trust for not providing consultation with their mother (Box 39.12).

• BOX 39.12 Key Findings for NHS Organizations and DNACPR Discussions

1. Patients (except in exceptional circumstances) should always be consulted in relation to advance DNACPR decisions and that Article 8 of the European Convention on Human Rights (right to respect for private and family life) is engaged by the decision to impose DNACPR

2. There has to be a convincing reason not to engage the patient in DNACPR discussions even if such a treatment is deemed futile, i.e. they have lost capacity or discussions would cause direct physical or psychological harm. Distress alone is not sufficient reason

3. DNACPR decisions must be made in accordance with a 'clear and accessible' policy. Local policies should be available and clearly directed and disseminated to patients.

Court of Appeal 2014. Tracey v Cambridge University NHS Foundation Trust

---

Withholding or Withdrawing Hydration and Nutrition

There is significant symbolism attached to food and drink as basic expressions of humanity and social interaction. Furthermore, the interplay of fasting and feasting has multiple religious associations. Withholding or withdrawing nutrition has also led to court cases and appeals about 'starving to death'. A decision to withhold or withdraw hydration can therefore invoke strong feelings within individuals, but such matters need to be dealt with case by case.

Hydration and nutrition can provide significant comfort care in many patients; however, this must be balanced against the possibility of causing harm, e.g. biochemical disturbances associated with dehydration and starvation (particularly uraemia) can enhance analgesia and sedation via *starvation euphoria*. Additionally, oral feeding may cause gagging and choking as might the insertion of enteral feeding tubes, with the added indirect discomfort of gastric distension when feed is administered. The risk of vomiting, regurgitation and possible aspiration may also be increased. Methods of hydration can also be harmful, i.e. relieving the discomfort of thirst has to be balanced against the discomfort of tissue swelling and breathing difficulties from fluid overload and pain from cannulae insertion. Clinically-assisted nutrition and hydration (CANH) is the current terminology that applies to this therapy in the UK. As a medical treatment, it does not have to be offered or can be withdrawn if it is not providing benefit or is not in patients' best interests. Decisions to continue or withdraw such treatments continue to be difficult and can require a court decision.

Euthanasia and Physician Assisted Suicide (PAS)

Euthanasia is defined as 'intentional killing of an individual (by intervention or omission) for their alleged benefit.' If there is no intention to kill, euthanasia has not occurred. PAS is where a doctor 'knowingly and intentionally' provides persons with the knowledge and/or means to commit suicide. This includes counselling about lethal drug doses and prescribing and supplying such drugs.

PAS is currently legal in four European countries (Switzerland, The Netherlands, Belgium and Luxembourg) and five states within the USA (Oregon, Montana, Vermont, Washington and California). There have been strong moral arguments presented to support such interventions for competent patients within the UK who are dying. Despite debate however, both remain illegal due to concerns about adequate safeguards for vulnerable and at-risk patients.

Other Professional Duties

The modern role of the surgeon requires being a clinician, scholar and leader, as well as an expert technical operator. The skills and traits required have been listed by the Royal College of Surgeons.[29] Surgeons also have a wider range of ethical duties extending beyond their interactions with individual patients. These include obligations to other colleagues and shared resources, as well as a duty to promote safer healthcare and conduct training and research ethically. These are increasingly part of postgraduate curricula requirements, and in the UK have been formalized into the Generic Professional Capabilities framework by the GMC. Box 39.13 lists the nine domains, and these can be explored in full online. Below we highlight a few particular areas of ethical relevance for the practicing surgeon.

Innovation and Research

Scientific and medical research is founded on the process of randomized controlled trials (RCTs) whereby an idea or innovation is compared to a control or current practice according to a strict protocol. Surgery, however, has largely progressed from primitive procedures to highly elaborate operations by the efforts of individual innovators. Improvements in surgical technique have also been accrued incrementally over time, often driven by the unanticipated demands of particular cases. As a consequence, RCTs (which represent the minority of published research in surgical journals) are difficult to conduct due to challenges of blinding and ethical difficulty of performing sham surgery as a control. Furthermore, the success of surgical procedures also depends on individuals' operating skills and relative experience. Surgeons have a responsibility to refine and continue to improve surgical techniques and adopt new proven procedures but in doing so, patients must be made aware of when novel procedures are being offered. Patients will increasingly request evidence that the procedure they are being recommended to have offers the best outcome for

Domain 1: Professional values and behaviours
Domain 2: Professional skills
    Practical skills
    Communication and interpersonal skills
    Dealing with complexity and uncertainty
    Clinical skills
Domain 3: Professional knowledge
    Professional requirements
    National legislative requirements
    The health service and healthcare system in the four
        countries
Domain 4: Capabilities in health promotion and illness
    prevention
Domain 5: Capabilities in leadership and team working
Domain 6: Capabilities in patient safety and quality
    improvement
    Patient safety
    Quality improvement
Domain 7: Capabilities in safeguarding vulnerable groups
Domain 8: Capabilities in education and training
Domain 9: Capabilities in research and scholarship

them, and it is vital to have data on the risks and benefit to patients. Surgical innovation should occur with the open collaboration of peers and approval from regulatory bodies. Whilst this may slow the pace of innovation at times, the strength of larger data registries and incident reporting promotes safety and openness. Proper ethical oversight and peer approval will also protect surgeons from accusations of lone, idiosyncratic practice. The IDEAL collaboration[30] is an example of such collaborative endeavour to guide and facilitate surgical research and innovation.[31]

Teaching, Training and Education

Patients benefit from all the experience that a surgeon has accrued from previous cases and arguably they have some shared obligation (though a principal of justice) to participate in teaching and training. However, patients still have the expectation and right to be managed by a competent surgeon. Acquiring this experience is likely to become more difficult. Traditionally, teaching hospitals offered free care to patients in return for the acceptance that they would participate in medical training. Surgeons in training would often work with limited supervision acquiring a large case experience before becoming consultants. The challenge for the future is to conduct surgical training without significant risk to patients, but produce accredited surgeons capable of operating independently. Increasingly, today's surgical trainees must achieve the same standards within greatly reduced training hours and with much higher levels of supervision than previously provided. Above all, patients should be entitled to know who will be operating on them, and what their

level of experience is. This was a feature of a recent medico-legal case, where notification of a last-minute change of surgeon was judged to have invalidated the patient's consent. Procedures performed for training purposes only, e.g. additional examinations under anaesthesia, should also be carried out with the patients' explicit consent.

Simulation, part task trainers and virtual reality technology all offer great future prospects to augment training, but cannot wholly replace the experience of performing a real operation. Accredited trainers must have the judgment and temperament to allow trainees to take over operations as their skill and confidence grows. Transitional handover partnerships should become more widespread when taking up first consultant posts, and in future the role of mentors will hopefully become the norm.[32]

Probity and Other Professional Duties

Financial pressures (particularly in independent practice) often present the greatest challenges to personal probity. An old adage warns that 'a bag of gold lies between the surgeon and a private patient'. Given such statements, it is important to ensure that financial incentives do not influence decision making and recommendations for care. With the increasing influence of commercial pressures within public medicine and potential fragmentation of publicly funded health systems, surgeons will need to navigate between inducements to use certain equipment and the prioritization of patients for factors other than clinical need. Financial conflicts of interests should be disclosed. Clinical decisions and outcomes should be shared openly within an MDT setting.

Candour, Truth Telling and Confidentiality

Hippocrates counselled his students to divulge as little information as possible to patients for fear that bad news might harm them. Today, however, patients increasingly expect to be told of their diagnosis, all available treatment options and their future prognosis. Information can be withheld under 'therapeutic privilege' but this should be exercised rarely and only justified if certain information could cause true psychological or physical harm.

Family members withholding information from elderly relatives or young adults can also create difficult situations. Whilst understandable and possibly conforming to traditions within certain cultures, continuing to treat patients when they are ignorant of vital facts leaves them unable to make valued, informed decisions and prepare for the future. Patients live within the context of their family and culture but they are also situated within a society and legal codes relating to respect for autonomy. Furthermore, such an approach is contrary to professional guidance. With most facts likely to emerge over time, there is the risk of trust being diminished either between the patient and both their doctor and family. In England and Wales, the *Montgomery Judgment* (2015) emphasizes that patients should know all information that may affect their decisions. In essence, this extends to all advice and counselling given beyond the formal context of consent.

The duty of candour specifically requires doctors to explain and apologize to patients when things have gone wrong and harm has occurred. In the UK, this includes a written apology with an explanation when harm has been at least moderate or severe. It should be combined with local critical incident reporting to prevent future recurrence if possible. Guidance is available from the Royal College of Surgeons of England.[33]

Other difficulties can arise when surgeons become aware of previous errors or poor practice that has occurred to patients in other institutions. This can range from an unorthodox treatment to criminally negligent errors. Patients may be oblivious to these but are nevertheless entitled to know what has happened. Here guidance for surgeons is less clear cut; however, it would be wise to establish all facts with the referring team first. Direct questions from patients should thereafter be answered honestly and fully, being clear where the issue is a simple difference of opinion, or whether negligent harm has occurred. An ethical duty to the patient should be stronger than any sense of professional loyalty. Candour at this point will prevent the future loss of trust as information emerges over time, and promotes the continued clinical relationship.

Confidentiality of patient data remains a core duty of doctors and in the UK is explicitly set out in GMC guidance. There are specific circumstances where breaching confidentiality may be required by a court, or in the event of a notifiable disease. Disclosure of information about a patient who is unconscious or refuses to give consent may also be justified if it is strongly in the public interest, e.g. to prevent serious harm to others. In the UK, the police force should usually be notified if a person presents with a gunshot wound, or a non-accidental knife injury; however, the patient's identity should not be disclosed without their consent. Similarly, medical insurers and government agencies do not have automatic rights to know individual patients' records without their consent.

Modern IT and social-media present great risks for breaches of confidentiality, and legislation such as the Data Protection Act sets the standard in the UK for how medical records should be maintained, stored and shared. Any text or image shared via email text message or social media has unlimited potential to be disseminated over the internet, and this should be avoided. Images of patients for educational, training and research purposes must be taken with their explicit consent, even if the material appears anonymous. Past images in collections may be retained for their educational value, but publishing any images should be done in accordance with GMC or applicable national guidance.

Participating in Safer Surgery

Ethical duties extend beyond those directly affecting the patient undergoing surgery, i.e. surgeons have a duty to promote safer practice for all patients by reducing the risks of error and patient harm. This includes participating in team briefs, safety checks and actively identifying latent risks in the perioperative environment. Surgeons must increasingly be willing to reflect on personal performance and ensure that their skills and knowledge are up to date. Fatigue and sleep deprivation are major contributing factors to error and, despite the culture of continuing to work even when tired, it is imperative to acknowledge the effects of these factors on performance and act upon them when they arise. Errors represent critical moments at which to review practice. Sadly, the process of reflection and learning may be inhibited by the continued trend to punish individuals even where systems' failures may be just as much to blame.[34]

In addition to reflecting on their own practice, there is an imperative to assist others to reflect and develop their own work. Judging the practice of peers can be difficult as professional solidarity and a sense of 'there but for the grace of God go I' can inhibit effective critique. Nevertheless, surgeons must be increasingly prepared to identify shortcomings and errors in order to protect patients. Many serious cases of surgical mismanagement (sometimes criminal) have occurred where surgeons have been allowed to continue their practice unchallenged. Increasingly, there is closer scrutiny and even sanctions against those who should have been aware of misconduct but failed to act to protect patients.

Within the UK a number of these scandals have often occurred in the independent sector, where clinical networks, peer review and audit may previously have been less robust. General recommendations are that all surgeons should work in MDTs with a willingness to audit their own results and have their practice scrutinized and at times challenged. The honest input from colleagues may be the best strategy to preserve good standards, and prevent ethical misjudgements. Engaging in a robust process of annual appraisal covering all areas of practice can assist surgeons in engaging in these processes.

The Surgeon as Role Model

A final duty of surgeons is to act as ethical role models to those with whom they work, in particular surgeons in training, who will naturally absorb standards of behaviour and conduct from their seniors. In difficult circumstances, it may help to consider what an idealized role model surgeon would do. This follows from virtue ethics, a theory which holds that the right course of action is that which the virtuous person would follow. Cardinal surgical virtues have included prudence, justice, bravery and temperance, but more could be suggested, e.g. humility. Aspiring to such levels of virtuous behaviour should accompany the quest for technical expertise and clinical judgment; the goal of *Surgical Mastery* suggested by Rothenberger:[14]

> *Master surgeons have an intuitive grasp of clinical situations and recognize potential difficulties before they become a major problem. They prioritize and focus on real problems. They possess insight and find creative ways to manage unusual and complex situations. They are realistic, self-critical, and humble. They understand their limitations and are willing to seek help without hesitation. They adjust their plans to fit the specifics of a situation. They worry about their decisions but are emotionally stable.*

Summary

Mastering of operative skills remains at the core of surgical training, but in 21st century surgical practice, surgeons must be fully aware of the ethical and legal frameworks within which they work and also strive to be ethical role models themselves.

Further Reading

Buchanan AE, Brock DW. *Deciding for Others: The Ethics of Surrogate Decision Making*. Cambridge: Cambridge University Press; 1990.

Gawande A. *Complications: A Surgeon's Notes on an Imperfect Science*. New York: Metropolitan Books; 2002.

Hope RA, Savulescu J, Hendrick J. *Medical Ethics and Law: The Core Curriculum*. Edinburgh: Churchill Livingstone Elsevier; 2008.

Jones JW, Mccullough LB, Richman BW. *The Ethics of Surgical Practice: Cases, Dilemmas, and Resolutions*. Oxford; New York: Oxford University Press; 2008.

Laurie GT, Harmon S, Porter G. In: *Mason & McCall Smith's Law & Medical Ethics*. 10th ed. Oxford: Oxford University Press; 2016.

Sade RM. *The Ethics of Surgery: Conflicts and Controversies*. Oxford: Oxford University Press; 2015.

References

1. *GMC Statement on the Sentencing of Ian Patterson*. May 2017. https://www.gmc-uk.org/news/news-archive/ian-paterson-sentencing.

2. Robinson JO. The Barber-surgeons of London. *Arch Surgery*. 1984;119:1171–1175.

3. McVaugh M. When universities first encountered surgery. *J Hist Med Allied Sci*. 2017;72:6–20.

4. Toledo-Pereyra LH. Joseph Lister's surgical revolution. *J Invest Surg*. 2010;23:241–243.

5. Manor J, Blum N, Lurie Y. "No good deed Goes Unpunished." Ignaz Semmelweiz and the story of Puerperal Fever. *Infect Control Hosp Epidemiol*. 2016;37:881–887.

6. The Royal College of Anaesthetists. https://www.rcoa.ac.uk/about-college/heritage/history-anaesthesia.

7. Gawande A. Two hundred years of surgery. *N Engl J Med*. 2012;366:1716–1723.

8. Older P, Levett DZ. Cardiopulmonary exercise testing and surgery. *Ann Am Thorac Soc*. 2017. https://doi.org/10.1513/AnnalsATS.201610-780FR.

9. Heubel F, Biller-Andoron N. The contribution of Kantian moral theory to contemporary medical ethics: a critical analysis. *Med Health Care Philos*. 2005;8:5–18.

10. Beauchamp T, Childress J. In: *Principles of Biomedical Ethics*. 4th ed. Oxford: Oxford University Press; 1994.

11. Frankfurt H. *Necessity, Volition, and Love*. Cambridge: Cambridge University Press; 1998.

12. Schneider CE. *The Practice of Autonomy. Patients, Doctors and Medical Decisions*. Oxford University Press; 1998.

13. Wall A, Angelos P, Brown D, et al. Ethics in surgery. *Curr Probl Surg*. 2013;50:99–134.

14. Rothenberger DA. "If you can keep your head.": clinical decision making in the age of evidence-based medicine. *Dis Colon Rectum*. 2004;47:407–412.

15. Cardozo J. *In Mary E. Schloendorff V. The Society of New York Hospital*, 105 N.E. 92; 1914.

16. O'Neill O. *Autonomy and Trust in Bioethics: The Gifford Lectures*. University of Edinburgh, 2001. Cambridge: Cambridge University Press; 2002.

17. Manson NC. Why do patients want information if not to take part in decision making? *J Med Ethics*. 2010;36:834–837.

18. Moonesinghe SR, Mythen MG, Das P, et al. Risk stratification tools for predicting morbidity and mortality in adult patients undergoing major surgery: qualitative systematic review. *Anesthesiology*. 2013;119:959–981.

19. Choudry MI, Latif A, Hamilton L, Leigh B. Documenting the process of patient decision making: a review of the development of the law on consent. *Future Hospital Journal*. 2016;3:109–113.

20. Stacey D, Legare F, Lewis K, et al. Decision aids for people facing health treatment or screening decisions. *Cochrane Database Syst Rev*. 2017;4:CD001431.

21. Falagas ME, Korbila IP, Giannopoulou KP, et al. Informed consent: how much and what do patients understand? *Am J Surg*. 2009;198:420–435.

22. Sheather JC. Should we respect precedent autonomy in life-sustaining treatment decisions? *J Med Ethics*. 2013;39:547–550.

23. Wrigley A. Proxy consent: moral authority misconceived. *J Med Ethics*. 2007;33:527–531.

24. Simpson PJ. What are the issues in organ donation in 2012? *Br J Anaesth*. 2012;108(suppl 1):i3–i6.

25. Foster C. *Choosing Life, Choosing Death: The Tyranny of Autonomy in Medical Ethics and Law*. Oxford: Hart; 2009.

26. Kon AA, Shepard EK, Sederstrom NO, et al. Defining futile and potentially inappropriate interventions: a policy statement from the Society of Critical Care Medicine Ethics Committee. *Crit Care Med*. 2016;44:1769–1774.

27. Parkins P. How to have a better death. *The Economist*. London; 2017.

28. Association of Anaesthetists of Great Britain and Ireland. *Do Not Attempt Resuscitation (DNAR) Decisions in the Perioperative Period*; 2009. London.

29. Surgical Training Curriculum. Royal College of Surgeons of England. https://www.rcseng.ac.uk/careers-in-surgery/trainees/st3-and-beyond/surgical-training-curriculum/.

30. The IDEAL Collaboration. Idea, Development, Exploration, Assessment, Long-term Follow-up, Improving the Quality of Research in Surgery. www.ideal-collaboration.net.

31. Hirst A, Agha RA, Rosin D, Mcculloch P. How can we improve surgical research and innovation?: the IDEAL framework for action. *Int J Surg*. 2013;11:1038–1042.

32. Gawande A. *Personal Best*. New York: The New Yorker.; 2011.

33. Royal College of Surgeons of England. *Duty of Candour: Guidance for Surgeons and Employers*; 2015.

34. Cohen D. Back to blame: the Bawa-Garba case and the patient safety agenda. *BMJ*. 2017;359:j5534.

40

Global Surgery

CHAPTER OUTLINE

Introduction

The Global Burden of Surgical Conditions

There are 5 billion people around the world who lack access to safe and affordable surgical and anaesthesia care, and surgical conditions account for 11–32% of the total global health burden. In 2010, there were 16.9 million excess deaths attributable to untreated surgical conditions, which is more than HIV, malaria and TB combined. There is disproportionate access to care in low-resource areas, and surgeries performed in countries where the poorest 33.7% of the global population live account for only 6.3% of the total operations done around the world. Examples of common conditions managed by both operative and non-operative surgical care include injuries, maternal disorders, malignancy and congenital anomalies. Over the years, there has been a steady increase in the number of deaths due to injuries, now leading to more than 5 million deaths annually. Maternal disorders account for a large proportion of mortality each year, and 99% of the 250 000 maternal deaths occur in low- and middle-income countries (LMICs). Since the Millennium Development Goals, maternal mortality has decreased by 50%. Malignancies were the cause of 8.2 million deaths in 2012, and predictions show that this figure will increase by 70% in the coming 20 years. This is partly because of an ageing population, as well as the behavioural changes associated with rapid urbanization. Congenital anomalies cause around a quarter of a million of newborn deaths annually and can result in life-long disability contributing to the loss of millions of disability-adjusted-life years, which could be averted with provision of basic surgical care.

In 2015, the World Health Assembly resolution 68.15 called for inclusion of emergency and essential surgical and anaesthesia care as a component of universal health coverage. This coincided with the Lancet Commission on Global Surgery which recommends ways on how to achieve universal access to safe, affordable surgical and anaesthesia care when needed. As a response, the G4 Alliance was founded with a mission to provide a collective voice for increased access to safe, essential and timely surgical, obstetric, trauma and anaesthesia care for patients around the globe. More than 85 organizations have come together to make the strong argument that providing basic surgical care is necessary, feasible and cost-effective with the appropriate collaboration and mobilization of international and national funds. Currently, many initiatives are established that elevate efforts and resources to improve access. For example, several LMICs are developing and implementing National Surgical and Anaesthesia plans, which aim to improve access and affordability of essential surgical care for underserved populations.

Perspective for Surgical Visitors from Developed Countries

A considerable challenge for the surgical visitor is the relevance of experience gained in highly-technical surgical settings to resource-poor environments. Twenty-first-century developed surgery is highly technical and managed within narrow sub-specialties. In contrast, surgery in poor rural communities is usually delivered by the diverse skills of a generalist working with little technical support. Visiting surgeons frequently have to cover a wide range of surgical specialties, especially in isolated rural areas.

The ideal model for support from visiting teams is to develop long-term partnerships, built on mutual respect, two-way learning from poor to rich and vice versa, with capacity-building a prime goal.

Many experienced surgical teams working in LMICs attest to the overwhelming importance of training and capacity-building in developing surgical resources for sustainable development in the longer term. Currently, there are four main types of surgical platforms, consisting of disaster and crisis relief platforms, short-term surgical missions, specialty hospitals and capacity-building and academic partnerships. The four types have different goals and educational focus with their respective advantages and disadvantages.

Although an ideal platform for support from visiting teams does not exist due to the diversity of need, the most valuable partnerships between high-income countries (HICs) and LMICs are multi-professional. Long-term relationships flourish in contrast to short, one-off, visits and longer-term exchanges of professionals are extremely beneficial. When short-term visits are undertaken, visitors must be prepared to empathize with local challenges faced by national colleagues working in LMICs, respect cultural differences, make an effort with the language and readily accept that they will probably receive more than they can give both professionally and personally. Not surprisingly, many surgeons from developed countries will attest to the impact of a surgical elective – undertaken whilst a medical student – on their career choice. Further into their career, surgeons may have opportunities to return to a developing country for varied periods of time, as part of a global health training program or fellowship. In the past, the focus of these trips has been surgical service provision. However, in recent years, the focus has shifted towards partnerships in teaching and training, and collaboration between surgeons, surgical departments and institutions is now encouraged. Furthermore, online resources or courses and Master's degrees are available as an alternative approach to global health education.

It is beyond the remit of this chapter to discuss the specific management of all diseases that present to the surgeon.

In fact, many of the diseases encountered are found in HICs and have been discussed in previous chapters. The focus of this chapter will be on:

- General environmental challenges faced in LMICs
- Surgical disease and challenges faced in LMICs
- Surgical presentations rarely seen in HICs.

Environmental Challenges

Currently, there are 5 billion people worldwide who do not have access to basic, life-saving surgical care. Limited infrastructure and inadequate resources are a major contributing factor in the limitations of providing surgical care. Box 40.1 summarizes the many challenges faced by the healthcare workers and patients in LMICs.

Approachability, Poverty and Low Literacy Rates

Two indicators for health include the life expectancy at birth and the infant mortality rate (IMR). These indicators are influenced by the gross domestic product (GDP) and the percentage of GDP spent on health. Fig. 40.1 shows the correlation between GDP per capita and infant mortality

---

> **• BOX 40.1 Challenges to Patients and Healthcare Workers in LMICs**
>
> - Approachability, poverty and low literacy rates
> - Lack of clean water and basic sanitation
> - Availability: poor infrastructure, civil unrest, military conflict, distance from health centres and lack of patient transport
> - Acceptability: cultural, social and personal belief and values
> - Appropriateness: poor health facilities and limited trained human resources
> - Infectious diseases, malnutrition and the immunocompromised patient
> - Problems in perioperative management

---

rates. In LMICs, the percentage of GDP spent on education mirrors that spent on health, and consequently adult literacy rates are low. This adversely impacts awareness of public health priorities and overall societal health.

Many people have no health insurance due to poverty; therefore, few are protected from catastrophic expenditure from out-of-pocket (OOP) payments for health services. It is estimated that 25% of the people worldwide who receive a surgical procedure will face catastrophic healthcare expenditure. The World Bank and WHO have targeted 100% financial protection by 2030.

Lack of Clean Water and Basic Sanitation

Inadequate water, sanitation and hygiene contributed to 842 000 deaths in 2012 in LMICs, mostly due to diarrhoeal illnesses. Availability of water is essential for providing safe surgical care, and clean water is necessary for washing instruments, surgical scrubbing and wound irrigation. Yet less than two-thirds of hospitals that provide surgical care in 19 LMICs have a reliable water source.

Availability: Poor Infrastructure, Civil Unrest, Military Conflict, Distance from Health Centres and Lack of Patient Transport

Patients living in rural areas have limited access to healthcare facilities and often have to travel great distances to urban areas where these resources are located. Travel to the healthcare facilities takes patients away from work and family, and the travel itself may be difficult due lack of infrastructure and poor roads, compounded by weather conditions. In addition, areas affected by civil unrest and military conflict may have disruption of healthcare provisions, destruction of infrastructure and additional surgical burden due to the traumatic injury.

Appropriateness: Inadequate Health Facilities and Limited Trained Human Resources

Lack of trained surgery, obstetrics and anaesthesia providers is one of the most significant causes of the unmet need for

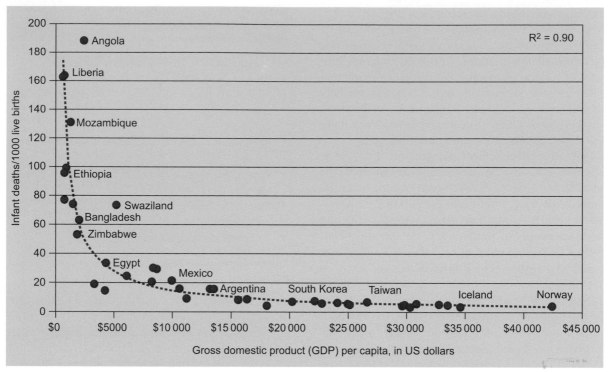

• **Fig. 40.1** Infant Mortality Rate and GDP per Capita (CIA Worldfactbook 2006)

surgical care in LMICs. Reasons for this disparity include lack of education and training opportunities and migration to higher income countries. Up to 28% of all physicians in HICs are international medical graduates, and of those, up to 70% come from lower-income countries, thus exacerbating the problem of lack of workforce. It is estimated that an additional 2.2 million surgeons, obstetricians and anaesthetists are needed to reach an acceptable workforce density worldwide. A first realistic target is to reach 20 per 100 000, requiring training of 1.27 million specialist providers, and several initiatives have been established that aim to train surgeons (e.g. Ghana College of Physicians, or COSECSA which collaborates with the Royal College of Surgeons in Ireland to train surgeons in east, central and southern Africa).

Lack of a trained workforce is compounded by inadequate health facilities with basic equipment, unreliable source of electricity, water and medication. Surgical instruments are often old or of poor quality, demanding greater expertise from the surgeon. Suture material may also be poor quality or in low supply. As a result, surgeons may have to compromise either with the type of needle or suture material and have to frequently modify their technique.

One way to address the shortage in the surgical workforce is the approach of surgical task sharing. This concept involves the delegation of tasks from highly qualified workers (i.e. specialists care providers) to clinicians with fewer qualifications, e.g. physician assistants, medical officers or midwives. The redistribution of task maximizes the potential of the human resources that are available. When associate clinicians receive adequate training, supervision and assistance, they can perform essential surgical procedures with good outcomes. Additional non-clinical staff such

as administrators, pharmacists, maintenance and accountancy, are also needed to successfully manage a hospital system.

Acceptability: Cultural Social and Personal Beliefs and Values

Cultural beliefs and religious practices vary across regions and can contribute to an increased mortality and morbidity by delaying presentation of patients to hospital. Surgeons often encounter patients at a late stage of their pathology due to initial treatment from traditional healers, making delayed medical management more difficult. Traditional herbal medicines can also delay recovery from surgical disease, for example by inducing a postoperative ileus.

Female genital mutilation/cutting (FMGC) is an ongoing practice and can be found in parts of Africa, the Middle East and Asia. Although there is an overall decline in the rate of FMGC, a large number of girls and women (estimated 200 million) have already been subjected to this mutilation. The sequelae of FMGC are both mental and physical, and include increased risk of post-partum haemorrhage, obstetric tears, obstetric fistulas and perinatal risks. Ending FMGC is part of the United Nations Sustainable Development Goals (SDG5), which also strives to achieve gender equality and empower women and girls.

Infectious Disease, Malnutrition and Immunocompromised Patients

Patients presenting to the surgical team are often malnourished and may suffer from an infectious disease such as HIV, tuberculosis and malaria. These pose a special challenge to the recovery and management of these patients.

HIV: It was estimated that at the end of 2016, 36.7 million people were living with HIV and 1 million died due to HIV-related illnesses. Nearly two-thirds of patients with HIV lived in sub-Saharan Africa, which remains the most severely affected area despite global efforts to increase testing, antiretroviral therapy and reduce mother-to-child transmission.

Challenges HIV poses to the surgical community include:
- Immunocompromised patients
- Surgical presentations related to HIV
- Risk to staff from needlestick injury and mucous membrane contact
- Lack of antiretroviral prophylaxis after exposure

Malaria: This is a life-threatening disease caused by *Plasmodium* parasite, the deadliest one being *falciparum* malaria. It is endemic in areas like sub-Saharan Africa and South East Asia. Severe falciparum malaria can affect multiple organs causing convulsions, circulatory collapse, renal impairment and pulmonary oedema. In addition to these, treatment with quinine can affect the perioperative care of a patient because it can cause hypoglycaemia, cardiac arrhythmias and prolonged neuromuscular blockade.

Tuberculosis is caused by *Mycobacterium tuberculosis*. It killed 1.7 million people in 2016 and more than 95% of these deaths occurred in low- and middle-income countries. Most of the cases occurred in India, but Indonesia, China, the Philippines, Pakistan, Nigeria and South Africa have higher prevalence than the rest of the world. TB can affect the general health and multiple organ systems of a patient, which can in turn affect their response to a general anaesthetic. Multidrug-resistant TB is a public health crisis and ending TB by 2030 is one of the health targets of the Sustainable Development Goals.

Malnutrition is defined as the 'deficiency, excess or imbalance in the intake of energy and/or nutrients'. Approximately 45% of deaths in children younger than 5 years old are linked to undernutrition. Surgical patients who are malnourished are more likely to have prolonged hospital stay, experience postoperative complications and adverse effects on their immune function. Perioperative nutrition (enteral and parenteral) is normally managed by specialist nutrition teams in HICs. It is therefore even more of a challenge in the setting of LMICs, given the lack of nurses, equipment and nutritional supplements.

SURGICAL CONDITIONS

General Surgery

The Disease Control Priorities (DCP) 3 group has proposed a list of 44 essential surgical conditions and procedures. These address a large health burden and are cost-effective and can be implemented in resource limited settings. Describing the presentation of general surgical conditions and their management has already been done in this book and is beyond the scope of this chapter.

We will instead describe common general surgical conditions prevalent in LMICs.

Trauma and Injuries Surgery

Surgeons in LMICs are burdened with severe pathology due to injuries and violence. Recent years figures show a steady increase in injuries and violence as a cause of death globally compared to other causes of death, now leading to more 5.8 million deaths annually and accounting for 10% of the world's deaths. This is partly explained by the increase of motorized traffic without sufficient road safety measurements in LMICs. Besides the fatal injuries, many more people suffer from injuries leading to disability, with 16% of the disabilities globally being caused by injuries. Ninety-three percent of the world's deaths on the roads occur in LMICs. The United Nations General Assembly aims to halve the number of deaths and injuries from road traffic accidents by 2030.

Primary Trauma Care

As in HICs, all surgical clinicians working in first-level hospitals or higher levels of care should be trained in the primary management of severely injured patients. Primary trauma care (PTC) is available for LMICs, an advanced trauma life support training module which is appropriate for resource-limited settings. It is a 2-day course, followed by a 1-day instructors' course. Doctors and nurses are trained to treat injuries quickly and systematically, learn to prioritize patients and use equipment that is available. It is also promoted to adapt PTC principles in their respective hospitals.

Clinicians working in a first-level hospital will frequently be involved in the following procedures: chest drain, trauma laparotomy, fracture reduction, open fracture treatment (irrigation, debridement and external fixator, traction), escharotomy, fasciotomy, trauma-related amputations, skin grafting and burr holes.

The Acute Abdomen

Initial management of patients with acute abdominal pain follows the same principles as in HICs. Resuscitation, correction of electrolyte disturbances, antibiotic treatment for the sepsis and analgesia are paramount.

Definitive diagnosis is difficult, so the decision to proceed to surgery is really challenging in this setting. A laparotomy is indicated when a diagnosis has been made, i.e. perforated peptic ulcer, or when a diagnosis is uncertain but the patient does not improve despite resuscitation.

Peritonitis has a high incidence rate in LMICs. Conditions with a high incidence are: gastric perforation, typhoid fever perforation (largely affecting the ileum), visceral injuries, appendicitis (perforated and bacterial peritonitis due to late presentation) and TB peritonitis.

Abscesses

Drainage of abscesses is the commonest procedure for the general surgeon. This is due to inadequate hygiene, immunosuppression and malnutrition. The abscesses are often large in size and chronic in nature.

Bowel Obstruction

Bowel obstruction causes and presentation has already been described in Chapter 13 but we will discuss specific causes of intestinal obstruction which is commonly seen in LMICs.

Volvulus

Volvulus is an obstruction caused by 'twisting' of the stomach, small or large bowels around its mesentery and is a common cause of bowel obstruction in LMICs.

Sigmoid Volvulus

Aetiology and Epidemiology. The high-fibre diet consumed in these areas is considered to be a predisposing factor. Increased bowel motility is also thought to be a contributing factor, as incidence of volvulus tends to be higher during harvest seasons when farmers tend to eat one large meal a day, with dehydration due to poor oral fluid intake exacerbated by physical exercise. Patients also tend to be younger and it is commoner in males. It is associated with high mortality especially if the bowel becomes gangrenous.

Clinical Features. The condition may present acutely, but in many instances, a history of subacute episodes can be elicited.

The clinical features of large-bowel volvulus generally commence with constipation (for flatus), followed by increasing abdominal distension. The abdomen can distend to huge proportions, but often little pain is experienced and tenderness is minimal. This disparity between the patients' apparent comfort and the abdominal signs is often striking. When available, abdominal radiography will classically display the 'coffee-bean' appearance of a sigmoid volvulus, although this is only evident in 65% of cases.

Management. Management of sigmoid volvulus depends largely on the type of volvulus that presents. In most instances, the volvulus is subacute and there is no impairment of intestinal blood supply. The aim should be to treat this group conservatively if possible. In acute cases, however, the mesenteric blood supply to the large bowel is impaired and septic shock can occur rapidly. These cases will require aggressive resuscitation as well as prompt intervention.

In the first instance, if there are no signs of compromise to the blood supply and if the facilities are available, decompression can be attempted with a sigmoidoscope and flatus tube. This technique is successful in 75% of cases. When successful, a flatus tube can be placed into the sigmoid colon to aid decompression and prevent recurrence. When successful decompression has been achieved, an elective sigmoid colectomy should be considered, as the incidence of recurrence is high. It is important to note that most patients present with an acute obstruction and quite late, therefore more likely to suffer from complications like perforation.

If, however, in the acute setting, the sigmoid decompression fails or there are signs of strangulation and gangrene, a laparotomy will be required. At operation, if the affected large bowel is viable, it requires untwisting with insertion of a rectal tube and/or suturing the colon to the abdominal wall to prevent further attacks. If there are signs of gangrene or strangulation, however, resection will be required with a primary anastomosis if the sigmoid appears viable or Hartmann's procedure or defunctioning with a double-barrelled stoma in case of gangrene. Much consideration is required prior to creating a stoma. Poverty and lack of specialist nursing staff and materials (e.g. colostomy bags), makes stoma management difficult.

Caecal Volvulus

Caecal volvulus is rare in high-income countries. In some instances, the caecum, ascending colon and ileum are all free to rotate and undergo volvulus. The clinical presentation of this condition is much the same as that of an acute sigmoid volvulus. Plain abdominal radiographs may demonstrate a large gas shadow placed centrally with a suspicious absence of gas in the right lower quadrant.

Management. Caecal volvulus in the absence of access to colonoscopy will almost always require a laparotomy. If the caecal volvulus can be untwisted and appears viable at operation, a caecopexy procedure may be performed to anchor the caecum to the anterior abdominal wall. Alternatively, a caecostomy with a Foley catheter passed through the anterior abdominal wall is fashioned. If, however, the bowel is not viable, a right hemicolectomy will be required.

Small-Bowel Volvulus

Aetiology. Volvulus of the small gut is rarely encountered in the high-income countries. When it does occur, it is usually seen in infants as a result of intestinal malrotation or another congenital anomaly. In adults, this condition is extremely rare and usually results from a 'twist' that has occurred around a fixed postsurgical adhesion. In contrast, however, small-bowel volvulus is seen frequently in LMICs in all age groups, with the highest incidence in young males. The aetiology commonly arises from a congenital band which tethers the bowel from the posterior abdominal wall to a point a few centimetres proximal to the ileocaecal valve. In other cases, post-surgical adhesions are to blame. Intestinal ascariasis, which is very prevalent in LMICs, can also cause a small bowel volvulus.

Clinical Features and Management

The characteristic clinical features of small-bowel volvulus include the sudden onset of colicky abdominal pain, distension and vomiting. The impact of rapid cessation of blood flow to the bowel is profound. Over a short period of time, haemodynamic instability supervenes, secondary to hypovolaemia and sepsis. For this reason, these patients require aggressive resuscitation with intravenous fluid and antibiotics.

In theory, treatment is easy if the condition is detected early. In these cases, 'untwisting' of the affected gut can be performed at laparotomy if irreversible bowel wall strangulation has not already occurred. In many cases small-bowel resection will be necessary, however. At the time of surgery, care must be taken not to rupture the affected bowel loop. Under these circumstances, overall mortality rises to approximately 30%.

Adhesional Obstruction

Postoperative adhesions can cause intestinal obstruction many years following previous abdominal surgery. Management of obstruction that occurs secondary to adhesions virtually always affects the small bowel. Treatment for this form of obstruction is usually non-operative. Replacement of fluid and electrolyte losses as well as nasogastric decompression ('drip and suck') is the main treatment. Operative intervention is indicated if there are signs of peritonism or sepsis which could indicate bowel infarction or perforation.

Intussusception

Epidemiology and Aetiology

Intussusception is rarely seen in adults in high-income countries. In the developing world, however, it is encountered more frequently, although the condition still predominates in infants and young children. Telescoping of the ileum into the caecum (ileocaecal intussusception) is the type most commonly seen. In addition, adult caeco-colic, colo-colic and ileo-ileal intussusceptions are seen in parts of Nigeria and East Africa. Sometimes intussusception occurs secondary to a polyp or tumour acting as a lead-point but in many cases, no specific cause is identifiable.

Clinical Features

The combination of colicky abdominal pain, bloody diarrhoea and an abdominal mass should alert the surgeon to the possibility of intussusception. On digital rectal examination, bloody mucous is often found. Often, in case of late presentation, a period of bloody diarrhoea is followed by obstipation.

Management

In children, an intussusception will sometimes resolve spontaneously. This is not the case in adults. In HICs, it is sometimes possible to achieve reduction of an intussusception hydrostatically using contrast media. This is rarely possible in developing countries and should not be attempted without adequate access to surgical services. When an operation is required, an attempt at manual reduction of the intussusception should be afforded. This is successful in approximately 80% of cases. When reduction is not possible, or the intussuscepted segment has strangulated or the cause is due to a tumour, resection of the affected bowel segment will be necessary.

Obstruction Due to *Ascaris* Worms

Aetiology

Ingested *Ascaris* ova grow into worms within the gut lumen. *Ascaris* infestation is generally an indication of poor sanitation and consequently is seen frequently where poverty prevails. Only rarely is intestinal contamination so heavy that bowel obstruction occurs. Indeed, obstruction often follows an attempt at decontamination, as paralysis of the worms may result in a bolus and predispose towards complete blockage.

Clinical Features

A diagnosis of ascaris bowel obstruction may be considered when a child presents with a history of having passed worms rectally or having vomited them. In some cases, an irregular mobile abdominal mass can be palpated.

Management

When ascaris obstruction has been diagnosed, and there are no features of peritoneal irritation, conservative management should be started with intravenous fluids and nasogastric tube insertion. Anthelminthic medication, e.g. mebendazole, should not be attempted until the obstruction has resolved, as there is a risk of aggravating the condition. In most instances, non-operative treatment is successful and surgery is not required.

When surgery is required for uncomplicated obstruction, every attempt should be made to avoid enterotomy, and instead attempts should be made to milk the worms into the caecum from where they can be passed safely. If there is evidence of a gangrenous bowel, then bowel resection is advocated.

In case of invasion of the gallbladder, then cholecystectomy with common duct exploration and T-tube insertion until the patient is treated is necessary. This, of course, depends on the equipment availability and local expertise.

Hernia

Although this topic is extensively covered in Chapter 30, its clinical presentation in LMICs is very different from HICs, as they tend to present late with associated complications. This makes elective repair a much less common occurrence compared to HICs. Around 60% of hernias are repaired as an emergency and 24% require a bowel resection. Reasons for late presentation vary but include lack of patient awareness, limited access to surgeons and anaesthetists and patient reluctance to leave their families and work to travel and see specialists.

In elective cases, mesh repair is the method of choice in HICs. However, it is currently not affordable in LMICs and so hernias are repaired with either the Bassini McVay or Shouldice procedure, which have a recurrence rate of up to 30%. A randomized controlled trial by Lofgren in 2017, showed that if the hernia repair is performed under local anaesthesia with low-cost mesh (i.e. sterilized mosquito net), its overall cost is lower compared to non-mesh repair, in a research setting. The Desarda technique for hernia operation, which does not require a mesh, has shown similar recurrence rates to the Lichtenstein repair and may be an important alternative repair method for LMICs.

Plastic Surgery

Plastic surgery, or the surgery of reconstruction, is frequently neglected in the provision of comprehensive surgical care in developing countries. This is unfortunate, since at least 20% of the surgical case load of a hospital in rural

Africa is likely to require plastic surgical methods as part or all of the management (Box 40.2). Plastic surgery frequently requires no more than basic surgical resources, with little of the specialized equipment that can be associated with other surgical disciplines.

Its primary role is in restoring tissues to their normal form and function, thereby enabling the patient to feel more confident and function socially.

Plastic surgery methodology includes careful discipline for tissue handling, the use of grafts of all tissue types (which are transferred without their blood supply) and a wide repertoire of flaps (which are transferred with a nutrient blood supply). Basic principles are a thorough understanding of the anatomy, dealing adequately with the underlying pathology before reconstruction (which may follow immediately or be delayed) and not expecting grafted material to 'take' on sites which have exposed, dried bone or are otherwise denuded of nutrient supply for wound healing. Tissues which are raised for transfer must be mobilized with a clear understanding of the anatomy and tissue capabilities, and put into the new position without tension, underlying blood or exudates, and with careful handling to avoid early damage or loss.

Burns

Burn injuries are one of the commonest conditions in hospitals in LMICs and common causes include: falls into open fires used for cooking, petrol, electric shock and house fires. Annually, 11 million people require medical attention for burn injuries and over 200 000 patients die due to burns. Globally, burn injuries are in the top 15 causes of burden of disease. Of all burn injuries, 95% occur in resource-limited settings, and sub-Saharan Africa is particularly afflicted. This is compounded by conflict-related burns and acid burns following domestic violence. Burn care is acknowledged as essential surgical conditions, as surgical care is essential in the treatment of severe burn injuries in minimizing morbidity, mortality and preventing complications.

Despite this, research on surgical burn care in resource-limited settings is sparse.

One of the most difficult issues for low resource settings is the choice between early or delayed excision and grafting. The International Society for Burn Injury (ISBI) guideline defines early excision as the removal of necrotic tissue before 10 days after burn injury and delayed excision between 10 days and 3 weeks after burn injury.

Immediate Care

Many burns cases in rural areas present late. In urban areas, however, they may arrive early, and require first aid. Initial assessment should include the following:

- ABCDE primary survey should be done

  A: Airway: assess, open and clean airway (jaw thrust). Assess risk of inhalation burn. (Singed nasal hairs, soot visible in back of throat, dyspnoea)

  B: Breathing: Assess respiratory rate, chest expansion, recessions, accessory muscles, stridor and saturation. Provide O_2, perform escharotomy in circumferential burns of the chest

  C: Circulation: Assess pulse, BP, bleeding, capillary refill, warm hands, circumferential burn with compromised circulation. Give two large-bore i.v. lines. Escharotomy in circumferential burns of extremities

  D: Disability GCS, pupillary reaction. Admission to ICU if impaired consciousness (consider CO intoxication)

  E: clothing, body temperature

- **Evaluation:** What is the approximate body surface area of the burn?

  - 'rule of nines' in adults (see Ch. 31); palm = 1%; children, the head and trunk have a higher proportion of surface area, therefore use Lund & Browder chart.

- **Evaluation:** What is the depth of the burn?

  - full thickness/deep burns: blotch red to white, dry, hard, capillary refill impaired, dull sensation
  - superficial burns: pink/red, can blister, moist, normal capillary refill and painful

- Fluid management: in burns >20% TBSA, give fluids. In the first 24 hours provide resuscitation fluids, using the Parkland Formula and add maintenance fluid.

Burn Management

Ideally, when resources are available for excision and skin grafting, early excision of full-thickness burns should be considered, before they become infected and can be grafted 'cleanly'. Moreover, early excision reduces the deteriorating systemic reaction to large necrotic areas and early grafting and closure of the wound limits contracture formation, reduces mortality and shortens length of stay.

However, one of the most difficult issues for resource-limited settings is the choice between early (before 10 days) or delayed excision and grafting (between 10 days and 3 weeks). Early grafting requires many resources, equipment, dressings, means of resuscitation and trained clinicians, of which all are frequently unavailable. A recent study determined burn management capacity in 458 hospitals in 14 low-and middle-income countries around the world.[3] Capacity was defined by using seven criteria, showing limitations in the presence of surgeons (0.71 surgeons available per hospital), presence of anaesthesiologists (0.18 per hospital), the capability of hospitals to provide skin grafting (35.6% provided skin grafts) or basic resuscitation (82.3% provided resuscitation). Therefore, delayed excision and grafting can be the only option in resource-limited settings, although rates of infection are higher and hospital stays longer.

Hand burns are usually best managed in plastic bags with some antiseptic fluid, in order to maintain mobility. Eyelid burns must be managed urgently to prevent exposure of the corneas.

Many hospitals in the developing world do not operate early on severe burns because of the lack of facilities to undertake safe surgical excision with the inevitable fluid loss. This is unfortunate, since many of the later consequences of burn contracture and infection could be avoided if this were possible.

If burns are to be dressed, areas which might be expected to heal spontaneously should be dressed early with non-stick dressings and left intact for 4–5-day periods to prevent secondary contamination.

Deeper burns are ideally dressed daily with silver sulfadiazine (Flamazine) or a hypertonic agent such as pure honey. There is no role for topical antibiotics.

Facial burns can be covered with simple liquid paraffin for comfort and washed regularly. Regular washing with clean water is a cheap, comfortable and often life-saving action which reduces the overall bacterial concentration in the wound colonization, thereby reducing the incidence of invasive cellulitis (which is the first cause of septicaemia in burns). There is no evidence that washing with normal saline or antiseptics is superior to water washing.

In larger burns, a staged excisions and grafting approach can be followed. Areas of up to 15% of body surface area burn can be excised and split skin grafted at one session, depending upon surgical equipment, anaesthetic and postoperative support. With modern equipment (electrical dermatomes and mesh machines), the donor sites can be kept small while larger areas can be grafted. Modern mesh machines can increase the surface of the donor skin with a ratio of 1:9. Areas which often require more than a split skin graft include eyelids, exposed skull, tendons and nerves, and the neck. These may be best treated with flap cover or full-thickness grafting (challenging technique for large areas).

Longer-Term Management and Contracture Prevention

The paramount importance of splintage and mobilization to prevent contractures following burn injury cannot be over-emphasized. Six rules can help to prevent contractures:
1. Positioning (wrist extended, metacarpophalangeal joints flexed, phalangeal extended)
2. Splinting of limbs which are not used (backslab POP)
3. Physiotherapy
4. Daily cleaning on the ward
5. Debriding of eschar in theatre
6. Covering underlying skin graft early (flaps or skin grafts)

Simple plastic rings fashioned from strips of suction tubing connected together and placed around the neck can prevent severe neck flexion contracture developing. Hands which are not being used must be splinted, usually with wrist extended, metacarpophalangeal joints flexed and fingers straight.

The social needs of badly burnt patients must also be addressed. Significant scarring and loss of function may often be unavoidable, and it is vital to begin to help the victim and their family early on in coming to terms with this, as well as planning for future occupation and social reintegration.

Burn Contracture

Burn contractures present one of the most common and enduring images of disabling injury in the developing world (Fig. 40.2). The loss of function of limbs, and hands in particular, is all the more devastating to lives where physical function is an essential component in personal or family

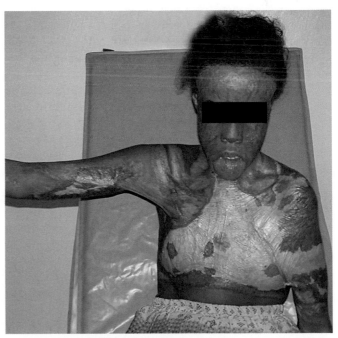

• **Fig. 40.2** Burn Contracture

survival. These disabilities also influence future marriage prospects and social integration.

Contracture release requires careful planning, and a certain amount of overall skin loss can be compensated by flap transfers, which relates to using tissue from one healthy area to repair another, as done in V-Y flaps and rotation flaps. Important techniques for flap transfer are the V-Y plasty, Z-plasty and jumping man flap. In Z-plasty, transposition of two triangular flaps is followed after a Z-shaped incision, and aims to elongate the scar of burn contracture. The V-Y plasty, is performed via a V-shaped cut, which is then sealed in a Y-shape. The jumping man flap is a hybrid of two techniques; first a Y-V advancement is performed, then two Z-plasties.

However, many contractures do not have enough adjacent healthy tissue and require the defect to be covered with additional skin. Skin grafting consists of two main techniques, which differ in the portion of skin used; full-thickness grafts (FTG) contain the full dermis, whilst split-thickness grafts (SSG) only consist of parts of the dermis. Thinner grafts are more likely to take and vascularize, but thicker grafts are usually the main option for important functional or cosmetic regions such as the digits and the face. Grafts may be harvested from the patient (autograft), someone who is genetically identical to the patient (isograft), an individual who is of the same species as the patient (allograft) or from another species (xenograft). The latter three are only used as temporary grafts. In patients with high TBSA% (total burn surface area), skin grafts need to be modified or enlarged to be applied, which happens through 'meshing'. After graft transfer surgery, dressings and splints may be attached to keep grafts in place.

Paediatric Surgery

It is important to acknowledge the role of paediatric surgical care in the context of global surgery. In LMICs, children make up a significantly larger proportion of the population than in HICs, and account for an estimated 40% of the global burden of disease in these areas.[1] It is estimated that 85% of children will have a surgically treatable condition by age 15.[2] In many areas, there is a shortage of paediatric surgical specialists and many paediatric conditions are cared for by adult surgeons. This section attempts to highlight common conditions for which all surgeons should have a basic understanding of their appropriate management in a child.

Injury and Burns

Injuries account for more deaths in children under 5 years old than HIV, tuberculosis and malaria combined.[4] In children, special attention must be paid to the physiologic differences in stress response and physiologic reserve, and apparently stable children with severe injury should be resuscitated and monitored closely. The detailed management of burns is discussed in depth previously in this chapter.

Gastrointestinal Emergencies

Gastrointestinal emergencies are a common presentation for children in all areas of the world, and should be managed expediently with adequate resuscitation and appropriate surgical intervention. Commonly seen conditions in LMICs include intestinal obstruction, intussusception, perforation and pyloric stenosis. The management of many of these conditions is discussed previously in this chapter.

Pyloric stenosis is a disease of the infant in which hypertrophy of the pylorus muscle causes gastric outlet obstruction, leading to projectile emesis, dehydration, metabolic alkalosis and electrolyte disturbances. Infants most commonly present between 2 and 8 weeks of age and diagnosis can be made on physical examination with palpation of an 'olive-shaped' mass in the upper abdomen. Infants with pyloric stenosis should first be managed with volume resuscitation and correction of electrolyte disturbances, particularly hypokalaemia. Once resuscitation is adequate, open or laparoscopic pyloromyotomy should be performed.

Abdominal Wall Defects

Gastroschisis and exomphalos are major congenital wall defects that pose a significant challenge to surgeons in LMICs. Exomphalos is a midline defect where the herniated bowel and viscera are encased by the amniotic membrane, and is often associated with other congenital anomalies. Gastroschisis has no covering membrane over the herniated bowel and occurs lateral to the umbilical cord. As with other paediatric conditions, nasogastric decompression and adequate resuscitation of the newborn is the first priority, followed by protection of the herniated bowel. In areas with limited resources, there is often a lack of access to necessary medication and supplies such as abdominal silos and parenteral nutrition. For exomphalos, when immediate primary closure is not feasible, the hernia sac should be painted with antiseptic and supportive care initiated with bowel rest and parenteral nutrition where available. Management of gastroschisis includes placement of a Silastic silo or other external management system for careful reduction of the herniated viscera, followed by delayed abdominal closure. Unfortunately, due to a lack of specialized facilities, trained personnel and limited resources, the mortality rate for these conditions can reach as high as 98% in some developing areas.[5]

Anorectal Malformations/Hirschsprung's Disease

Anorectal malformations (ARM) and Hirschsprung's disease (HD) are two congenital conditions where management in LMICs is often different than HICs due to delayed presentation and lack of specialized resources. A much lower proportion of these cases present as neonates, and often children have significant fluid and electrolyte derangements. All management of these conditions should start with adequate resuscitation prior to any surgical intervention.

Complex ARMs, particularly high and intermediate types, require highly specialized, interdisciplinary care and should be managed at a centre with experience with these conditions. Stable infants with low anomalies may undergo a definitive pull-through and avoid the morbidity of diverting colostomy. For HD, diagnosis should be confirmed with barium enema and full-thickness rectal biopsy, available in many LMICs.[6] For children who present in the neonatal period and are well resuscitated, a single-stage transanal pull-through may be performed by trained surgeons and anaesthesia providers. Otherwise, children can be managed with a traditional three-stage procedure.

Hydatid Cyst

Whilst rarely seen in HICs, hydatid liver cysts are a common condition in children worldwide. The disease is caused by the *Echinococcus* tapeworm, and is a faecal-oral disease primarily transmitted though sheep and dogs. Children may present with abdominal pain, fever and jaundice, or may be asymptomatic. Diagnosis can be made with ultrasound imaging demonstrating round, thin-walled cystic lesions that may be solitary or polycystic, or may also contain floating daughter cysts within a primary lesion. When an echinococcal cyst is suspected, biopsy is contraindicated as systemic dissemination of the organism will lead to anaphylaxis. Treatment includes perioperative albendazole followed by surgical resection of the lesion. Intraoperatively, the abdomen should be carefully prepped to avoid spillage of cystic contents in the abdomen, and the cyst is injected with hypertonic saline prior to excision.

Club Foot

Club foot is a congenital anomaly where the foot is rotated inward; it can be idiopathic or associated with other genetic conditions. When identified early during infancy, non-operative treatment is often successful and many children will grow to live normal lives. The Ponseti method, which consists of serial stretching and casting followed by Achilles tenotomy, has shown to be successful in 68–98% of cases treated early.[7] However, if not corrected, this condition can lead to life-long debility, stigmatization and loss of economic productivity.

Ophthalmology

There is an estimated 314 million people who have a visual impairment worldwide, of which 45 million are blind. Ninety percent of them live in LMICs especially Asia and sub-Saharan Africa. Disease burden from visual loss can markedly reduce quality of life as it prevents patients from performing their routine activities (i.e. walking, driving)

and also causes additional morbidity (e.g. increased risk of fall and fragility fractures).

Cataract Disease

In 2004, the WHO reported that cataract was responsible for blindness in 17.7 million people, which makes it the leading cause of blindness globally. The only treatment for cataracts is surgical and it has several advantages over other ophthalmic treatments as it is a one-time surgical intervention and achieves near-normal visual acuity postoperatively. This makes it the most cost-effective surgical intervention, although postoperative outcomes vary in different settings.

In sub-Saharan Africa, there are three ophthalmologists per 1 million population, compared to 79 ophthalmologists per 1 million population in HICs. Apart from the surgical expertise, a good infrastructure is also required in order to provide good service.

Although cataract surgeries have improved with the collaboration between governmental and non-governmental organization (NGOs) funding, the rate of affected individuals continues to increase at a rate which is faster than the rate of growth of the surgical services and so effective strategies with long-term follow up and better education of patients are required.

Dental

The WHO defines oral health as: 'a state of being free from chronic mouth and facial pain, oral and throat cancer, oral sores, birth defects such as cleft lip and palate, periodontal (gum) disease, tooth decay and tooth loss, and other diseases and disorders that affect the oral cavity'.[8]

Periodontitis and caries affect 50% of the world. These diseases are largely preventable bacterial infections and yet are increasing in prevalence. Noma is a gangrenous infection of the mouth, which is associated with high morbidity and mortality. Predisposing factors include malnutrition and immunodeficiency disease, e.g. AIDS.

Oral health services in LMICs are mostly limited to pain relief or emergency care. In Africa, there is one dentist for 150 000 patients, making it difficult to give priority to preventative or restorative dental care.

The WHO Oral Health Program promotes the establishment of oral health services that match the needs of each country. A basic package of oral care has been developed to meet the Primary Health Care principles; it includes three key components: affordable fluoride toothpaste, oral urgent treatment and atraumatic restorative treatment.

In 2016, the WHO launched a manual proposing effective and sustainable oral health solutions for Africa, which includes a set of 10 protocols specifically addressing primary healthcare staff to help with diagnosis and management of specific oral diseases.

References

1. Ozgediz D, Poenaru D. The burden of pediatric surgical conditions in low- and middle-income countries: a call to action. *J Pediatr Surg*. 2012;47(12):2305–2311.
2. Bickler SW, Rode H. Surgical services for children in developing countries. *Bull World Health Organ*. 2002;80(10):829–835.
3. Gupta S, Wong EG, Mahmood U, Charles AG, Nwomeh BC, Kushner AL. Burn management capacity in low and middle-income countries: a systematic review of 458 hospitals across 14 countries. *Int J Surg*. 2014;12(10):1070–1073.
4. WHO Mathers C, Boerma T, Ma Fat D. *The Global Burden of Disease: 2004 Update*. Geneva: World Health Organization; 2008.
5. Wesonga AS, Fitzgerald TN, Kabuye R, et al. Gastroschisis in Uganda: opportunities for improved survival. *J Pediatr Surg*. 2016;51(11):1772–1777.
6. Chirdan LB, Ngiloi PJ, Elhalaby EA. Neonatal surgery in Africa. *Semin Pediatr Surg*. 2012;21(2):151–159.
7. Smythe T, Mudariki D, Kuper H, Lavy C, Foster A. Assessment of success of the Ponseti method of clubfoot management in sub-Saharan Africa: a systematic review. *BMC Musculoskelet Disord*. 2017:453.
8. WHO. *Promoting Oral Health in Africa: Prevention and Control of Oral Diseases and Noma as Part of Essential Noncommunicable Disease Interventions*. Geneva: World Health Organization; 2016.

Index

Page numbers followed by "f" indicate figures, "t" indicate tables, and "b" indicate boxes.